HLA

Genetic diversity of HLA Functional and Medical Implication

Dominique Charron
EDITOR

EDK
MEDICAL AND SCIENTIFIC INTERNATIONAL PUBLISHER

EDK
Medical and Scientific International Publisher
10, rue Champfleury, 92310 Sèvres, France
Tel. : (33) 1 45 07 27 49 - Fax : (33) 1 45 07 85 29
E-mail: martinek@francenet.fr
ISBN: 2-84254-003-4

Proceedings of the Twelfth International Histocompatibility Workshop and Conference

Volume I : Workshop
Volume II : Conference

Edited by
Dominique Charron

INTERNATIONAL HISTOCOMPATIBILITY COUNCIL

Corresponding address: Pr. Dominique Charron
Institut Biomédical des Cordeliers, 15, rue de l'École de Médecine,
75006 Paris - France - Tel.: (33) 1.40.46.81.76 - Fax: (33) 1.43.29.96.44
E-mail: charron@ccr.jussieu.fr
charron@histo.chu.stlouis.fr

12th INTERNATIONAL HISTOCOMPATIBILITY WORKSHOP AND CONFERENCE

COUNCIL

Chairman

D. Charron, Paris (F)

European Committee

E. Albert, München (D)
J. Bodmer, London (UK)
A. Cambon-Thomsen, Toulouse (F)
L. Degos, Paris (F)
R. Fauchet, Rennes (F) Executive Organiser
J. Hors, Paris (F)
A. Piazza, Torino (I)
I. Schreuder, Leiden (NL)

Presidents

T. Sasazuki, Fukuoka (J)
K. Tsuji, Isehara (J)

Past-Presidents

D. B. Amos, Durham (USA)
J.J. van Rood, Leiden (NL)
R. Ceppellini, Milano (I)
J. Dausset, Paris (F)
F. Kissmeyer-Nielsen, Aarhus (DK)
W. Bodmer, London (UK)
P.J. Terasaki, Los Angeles (USA)
E. Albert, München (D)
W. Mayr, Wien (A)
B. Dupont, New York (USA)

Honorary Councillors

M. Aizawa, Sapporo (J)
R. Payne, Palo Alto (USA)

International Councillors

E. Albert, München (D)
D. B. Amos, Durham (USA)
F. Bach, New York (USA)
J. Batchelor, London (UK)
J. Bodmer, London (UK)
W. Bodmer, London (UK)
C.B. Carpenter, Boston (USA)
D. Charron, Paris (F)
R.L. Dawkins, Perth (AUS)
L. Degos, Paris (F)
B. Dupont, New York (USA)
C. Engelfriet, Amsterdam (NL)
G.B. Ferrara, Genova (I)
J.A. Hansen, Seattle (USA)
P. Ivanyi, Amsterdam (NL)
T. Juji, Tokyo (J)
Z. Layrisse, Caracas (VEN)
W. Mayr, Wien (A)
P. Morris, Oxford (UK)
P. Parham, Stanford (USA)
A. Piazza, Torino (I)
P. Rubinstein, New York (USA)
T. Sasazuki, Fukuoka (J)
I. Schreuder, Leiden (NL)
A. Svejgaard, Copenhagen (DK)
P.I. Terasaki, Los Angeles (USA)
E. Thorsby, Oslo (N)
R. Tosi, Roma (I)
K. Tsuji, Isehara (J)
J.J. van Rood, Leiden (NL)
R.L. Walford, Los Angeles (USA)
E.J. Yunis, Boston (USA)

ORGANISING COMMITTEES

EUROPEAN COMMITTEE - 12th IHWC Saint-Malo and Paris

D. Charron, *Chairman*
R. Fauchet, *Executive Organiser*
E. Albert
J. Bodmer
A. Cambon-Thomsen
L. Degos
J. Hors
A. Piazza
I. Schreuder

ORGANISING COMMITTEE - Workshop in Saint-Malo

Chair: R. Fauchet
Co-Chair: D. Charron

Secretariat: M. Sorel
M. Brandel
N. Meynard

E. Albert
J. D. Bignon
J. Bodmer
A. Cambon-Thomsen
J. Clayton
G. Dejour
B. Drenou
M. Gueguen-Delamaire
M. Jeannet
T. Lahaye
C. Lonjou
S. Marsh
M. Onno
A. Piazza
A.M. Prieur
I. Schreuder
G. Semana

ORGANISING COMMITTEE - Conference in Paris

Chair: D. Charron
Co-Chair: R. Fauchet

Secretary: M. Brandel

J.C. Bensa
J. Bodmer
M. Busson
S. Caillat-Zucman
L. Degos
J.F. Eliaou
E. Gluckman
J. Hors
V. Lepage
P. Loiseau
C. Raffoux
C. Stavropoulos
H. Teisserenc
M.M. Tongio
A. Toubert

Scientific Honorary Committee

M. Aizawa, Sapporo (J)
E. Albert, München (D)
B. Amos, Durham (USA)
J.F. Bach, Paris (F)
M. Boiron, Paris (F)
W. Bodmer, London (UK)
J. Dausset, Paris (F)
R. Dawkins, Perth (AUS)
L. Douay, Paris (F)
B. Dupont, New York (USA)
J. Goldman, London (UK)
T. Kishimoto, Osaka (J)
H. Kreis, Paris (F)
N. Le Douarin, Paris (F)
B. Mach, Genève (CH)
W. Mayr, Wien (A)
H.O. McDevitt, Stanford (USA)
P. Morris, London (UK)
R. Payne, Palo Alto (USA)
T. Sasazuki, Fukuoka (J)
J. Strominger, Cambridge (UK)
A. Svejgaard, Copenhagen (DK)
P. Terasaki, Los Angeles (USA)
K. Tsuji, Isehara (J)
J.J. van Rood, Leiden (NL)

EFI Executive Committee

H. Betuel
J. Bodmer
F. Claas
G.B. Ferrara
F. Garrido
G. Mueller Eckhardt
G. Petranyi
P. Richiardi
I. Schreuder
M. Thomsen
M.M. Tongio
R. Tosi
J. Trowsdale

Société Francophone d'Histocompatibilité et d'Immunogénétique (SFHI)

Committee

M. Abbal (Toulouse)
D. Alcalay (Poitiers)
F. Amesland (Paris)
R. Bardi (Tunis)
P. Bierling (Créteil)
M. Bois (Poitiers)
M.D. Boulanger (Tours)
B. Cavelier (Rouen)
A. Cesbron (Nantes)
J. Cohen (Reims)
C. Coussedière (Clermont-Ferrand)
M. Drouet (Limoges)
F. Dufossé (Lille)
E. Dupont (Bruxelles)
F. El Chenawi (Mansoura)
H. Farahmand (Villejuif)
D. Fizet (Bordeaux)
C. Freidel (Lyon)
L. Gebuhrer (Lyon)
A.M. Griveau (Caen)
F. Guignier (Dijon)
G. Hauptmann (Strasbourg)
C. Kaplan (Paris)
J.C. Lepetit (St-Étienne)
A. Moine (Grenoble)
P. Mercier (Marseille)
P. Merel (Bordeaux)
J.Y. Muller (Nantes)
P. Perrier (Vandœuvre-les-Nancy)
I. Theodorou (Paris)
P. Tiberghien (Besançon)
J.M. Tiercy (Genève)
A. Wackenheim Urlacher (Strasbourg)

ACKNOWLEDGEMENTS

The Organising Committee of the ***Conference*** *wishes to extend its thanks and appreciation to the following institutions and companies for their support*

INSTITUTIONS

Major partners: Agence Française du Sang
European Community- Biomed
Ligue Nationale Française contre le Cancer
HLA et Médecine

Partners: European Science Foundation
Établissement Français des Greffes
Fondation Saint-Louis
Comité de Paris de la LNFCC
Faculté de Médecine Saint-Louis Lariboisière
Institut Biomédical des Cordeliers
Institut Universitaire d'Hématologie
Association France Transplant
Imperial Cancer Research Fund
Comités Départementaux de la LNFCC
(Ardèche, Ardennes, Drôme, Hauts de Seine, Oise et Vendée)
Société Francophone d'Histocompatibilité et d'Immunogénétique
CREG

COMPANIES

Major Sponsor: Perkin Elmer

Sponsors: Pharmacia Biotech
Innogenetics & Murex

Contributors: ALK
Chugai Pharmaceutical
One Lambda
Produits Roche/Roche Diagnostic
Sandoz

We also acknowledge the support of:
France Biochem
Genset
Biotest AG

Special thanks to Mairie de Paris, Air France

We would like to specially acknowledge the contribution and the dedication of Convergence *in organizing the 12th IHWC in Saint-Malo and in Paris.*
Special Thanks to François Contenay, Emmanuelle Viau, Olivier Ravasse and Jean-Baptiste Mündler.
The contribution of Muriel Brandel, Mireille Sorel and Nadia Meynard is greatly appreciated.
We are indebted to Martine Krief and her team at EDK for their help and understanding in the publishing process of the 12th IHWC Proceedings.

Volume II
Conference

Proceedings of the Twelfth International Histocompatibility Conference

FOREWORD

PLENARY LECTURES

1. HLA genes and molecules

2. HLA diversity

3. Expression and function of HLA genes

4. HLA in medicine

SUMMARY

SYMPOSIUM COMMUNICATIONS

1. HLA DIVERSITY

• HLA diversity of alleles and haplotypes

• New HLA region genes and markers. TNF and Complement

• HLA-G. Reproductive immunology

2. HLA TYPING AND SEQUENCING

• Technical advances in HLA typing

- **Sequencing Based HLA Typing**

3. FUNCTION OF HLA

- **Assembly and traffic of MHC molecules. Antigen processing and presentation**

• **HLA and peptides in Physiology and Diseases**

• Signal transduction. NK receptors and function

4. TRANSPLANTATION BIOLOGY AND MEDICINE

• Allorecognition. Tolerance and immunosuppression in transplantation

• Modulation of HLA. Soluble HLA

• Immunologic monitoring of transplantation. HLA matching

• HLA and Rheumatism

• HLA and Diseases

• HLA and Cancer

FOREWORD

The twelfth International Histocompatibility Workshop and Conference (12th IHWC), the last of the XXth century were held in Saint-Malo and Paris respectively in June 1996. Ultimate successor of a series of memorable workshops, it perpetuated the spirit of the International Histocompatibility community. It is now apparent that, 30 years after the concept of HLA workshops was initiated by the pionneers to catalyse and to federate international studies on the newly described and enigmatic HLA system, no other field in biological and medical sciences has been equally committed and successful in developing such large scale international studies and no other field has benefited so much from this unique form of cooperation. From the first workshop at Duke University in 1964 to the previous 11th Workshop in Yokohama and to the most recent in Saint-Malo, the IHWCs have been an ever growing forum for scientific exchange at the forefront of science and medicine.

The aim of each workshop has been to compare results generated in different laboratories, to combine findings and to distribute summaries worldwide which benefit the Histocompatibility and more generally the medical and scientific communities. The everyday life of HLA laboratories in every part of the world has now been for several decades influenced by the IHWs, from the pre-workshops excitement to the post workshops "depression" (rapidly overcome by the planning of the next HLA workshop). The language itself reflects this professional obsession. For scientists and technologists, the term "Workshop" has become a designation for sera, cell lines, antibodies and cells panels and Nomenclature.

Sharing is indeed the word which best defines the HLA workshops. That is the sharing of reagents, data and protocols in order to generate a wealth of new information that no single laboratory or group of laboratories could have generated alone but also sharing solidarity and concern for the patients who are the ultimate beneficiaries of this unique organisation. It is only by comparison with other fields that one realises how "advanced", truly international and united the HLA community is in terms of organisation and thoroughness thanks to the IHWCs. It is no surprise that IHWCs have became a model for other areas of biological and medical research. International workshops on lymphocyte differenciation antigens (CD) and part of the Human Genome studies are now successfully organised according to the previous experience of the IHWCs. The absence of written rules of the International Histocompatibility Council also facilitates the adjustments which have become necessary and has allowed the development of more HLA Immunogenetics related research. The organisation of the HLA community, a cooperation which federates over 200 laboratories worldwide may be initially viewed as futuristic by people who are unaware of what has been achieved in the previous workshops. The proceedings of each workshop are the definitive documents which aknowledge this unique activity.

The 12th IHWC was held in Europe for the 7th time and was the 2nd IHWC in France, following the one in Evian in 1977 which was chaired by Jean Dausset. The decision to launch the 12th IHWC was made in Yokohama in November 1991 by the International Histocompatibility Council (IHC) with the agreement that it should take place in Europe but also that it should be organised for the first time by Europe as a whole and not by a single or two nations. A European search committee was rapidly formed to suggest and select candidates to organise the 12th IHWC. After a friendly discussion a proposal was outlined which was accepted by the European search committee and the IHC. The 12th IHWC European committee was constituted of colleagues known in the HLA community for their personal enthusiasm and commitment to hard work. Renée Fauchet, Julia Bodmer, Anne Cambon, Ieke Schreuder, Ekkehart Albert, Alberto Piazza, Jacque Hors, Laurent Degos and I. My election as chairman was an honour although I immediately felt that the next 4 years of my life would be obsessed and overwhelmed by this task.

The study of the "Genetic diversity of the HLA region and its functional and medical implications" was the objective of the 12th IHWC. The first decision (in fact an obligation) was to propose to build up the structure of the Workshop on the commitment of individuals each of which would be asked to take responsibility for part of the organisation. "A Workshop to do together what each of us likes to do best" was our idealistic concept. Every chairperson or technical coordinator must now feel that we put heavy pressure on them to make this ideal become reality. Their commitment has been essential to the success of the 12th IHWC. The volume I of these proceedings is the written record of their contribution.

Since its discovery, the HLA complex has been one of the most rewarding fields of investigation in biological sciences and medicine. Our limited knowledge of the highly complex HLA system has developed to allow us to understand the roles this system in the control of the immune response and therefore its impact in transplantation medicine, auto-immunity, infectious diseases allergy and cancer. For the first time, in addition to genetics and anthropology, the 12th IHWC chose to promote a clear and strong emphasis on the medical implications of the HLA system. This was possible because of the recent technological developments which permit reliable and reproducible genetic typing of the HLA diversity. It is impressive to notice how fast the HLA field benefited from and contributed to the development of novel technology of genetic typing from the first application of the PCR 10 years ago to the present sequencing based typing.

The 12th IHWC illustrates how greatly our knowledge of the HLA system has benefited over the years from the combined contributions of Technology, Science and Medicine.

While the workshop volume (I) provides the detailed reports of the experimental work carried out throughout the last 4 years by the participating Laboratories, the conference volume (II) presents contemporary knowledge of the HLA system with regard to different basic science aspects such as Genetics, Anthropology and Immunology as well as the medical implications of the HLA system emcompassing an ever increasing number of disciplines from Immunology to Oncology, Hematology to Infectious Diseases and Transplantation Medicine. The 12th IHWC proceedings constitute an international landmark documenting the state of the art for the HLA community at this end of the century.

Paris. Europe

Dominique Charron, MD Ph/D
Chairman
Twelfth International
Histocompatibility Workshop
and Conference

WELCOME INTRODUCTION

As chairman of the 12th International Histocompatibility Workshop and Conference and on behalf of the European organizing committee I am pleased and honored to welcome all of you here in Paris for the Conference. Over 600 of you representing 65 nations have just comeback from a week in Saint-Malo.

In spite of the sunny weather and of the numerous sites of interest to visit you spent all your time in the Palais du grand Large working very hard in many different ways.

We all knew that we had to report here in Paris to over 1400 participants. "The HLA community at Large" the work which has been done during the past 3 years in 400 laboratories worldwide.

This will happen this morning.

Emphasis will be given on the two central themes of the workshop "Diversity and medicine".

The genetic diversity with regard to the description new alleles and of many more new haplotypes, at the population level a large amount of anthropological data and the medical implications of this diversity were extensively studied.

This Workshop examined for the first time not only disease associations but also the physiology as well as the physiopathology of HLA associated diseases providing concepts and tools for prevention, prediction and treatment.

THE HLA system is moving fast from histocompatibility *stricto sensu* to modern Immunogenetics with equal emphasis on both. Immunology and Genetics.

HLA has therefore become a central player in biological science and medicine.

This is exemplified by the diversity of the topics which will be presented and discussed in the plenary sessions and in the symposia of this conference.

Many of these topics clearly indicate the way ahead.

- Antigen presentation and peptides, natural killer cell receptors and ligands and their implication in infectious diseases, auto immunity as well as allergy, cancer and transplantation.
- From serology to sequencing, from manual calculation to sophisticated computing from hand writing to internet the HLA community has always been at the forefront of our society in biology and medicine and also in ethics and communication.

It is symbolic that this International Conference, the last of the Century, is held in the city of Claude Bernard and in the city of Jean Dausset.

Paris has become this week the city of HLA.

The organisation of this conference has only been possible through the help of many sponsors and contributing Institutions and Companies.

More than sponsors they have been partners of the 12th IHWC.

I now declare the 12th International Histocompatibility Conference open.

Dominique Charron
Paris, June 10th 1996

Plenary lectures

Contents

Plenary lectures

1 • HLA genes and molecules

The 12th International MHC map

J. Trowsdale[1], R.D. Campbell[2]

1 Human Immunogenetics Laboratory, Imperial Cancer Research Fund, PO Box 123, 44 Lincoln's Inn Fields, Holborn, London WC2A 3PX, UK
2 MRC Immunochemistry Unit, Department of Biochemistry, South Parks Road, Oxford, UK

More than 200 genes have been located in the human MHC, many of which have immunological functions in antigen processing and presentation *(Figure 1)*. The MHC is divided into class I, class II and class III regions. The class I region (distal) contains genes encoding the classic transplantation antigens, HLA-A, B and C. The class II region is at the opposite (centromeric) end of the complex. The class III region, lying between the other two clusters, is densely packed with genes encoding a variety of functions, including some components of the complement system. A list of genes in the human MHC is provided in *Table I*. Information on the loci and their functions are provided in *Figure 1*. Further details may be found in [1-4].

Table I. Human MHC genes, their common alternative names and their protein products

Class II region	
Gene	**Protein, function or prominent feature**
HSET(mouse Tctex)	Kinesin-related
KE1.5	GDS-related protein (guanine nucleotide dissociation stimulator of G proteins such as Ras, Rho, Rac and Rab)
HKE2(mouse KE-2)	-
RPS18(KE3; D6S219)	Protein S18 component of the ribosome
RING1(D6S111E)	Prototype RING finger
RING2(D6S111E HKE6)	Steroid and prostaglandin dehydrogenase-related protein
KE4(RING5)	membrane protein with his-and gly-rich domains
RXRB	retinoid X receptor β transcription factor for HLA class I genes
COL11A2	Collagen type 11A2
HLA-DPB2 Ψ	DPB pseudogene
HLA-DPA2 Ψ	DPA pseudogene
HLA-DPB1	DPβ chain DPB expressed gene
HLA-DPA1	DPα chain DPA expressed gene antigen presentation
HLA-DNA (DZα/DOα)	DNα chain Equivalent to mouse Oa gene. Class IIA-related gene with accessory function
RING3(D6S113E) (Y5/Y4)	Similar to *Drosophila female sterile homeotic (fsh)* mitogen-activated nuclear kinase
DMA(RING6)	Class II-related. Non-polymorphic. Expressed intra-cellularly. Function in loading peptides onto conventional class II molecules in MIIC vesicles
DMB(RING7)	Class II related. Non-polymorphic. Expressed intra-cellularly. Function in loading peptides onto conventional class II molecules
Z1	HLA-class I fragment Ψ
PPP1R2P (IPP2)	phosphatase inhibitor Ψ
LMP2(RING12)	Proteasome ß component
TAP1(D6S114E) (RING4/Y3/PSF1)	TAP1 Heterodimer with TAP2 IFN γ inducible. Modifies proteasome activity
RING9(D6S215)Ψ	Expresssed mRNA. Not known to make a protein
LMP7(D6S216E) (RING10/Y2)	Proteasome ß component (see LMP2)
TAP2(D6S217E) (RING11/Y1/PSF2)	1/2 of peptide TAP2 transporter with TAP1. See TAP1
HLA-DOB	Class II related sequence. Product probably pairs with HLA-DNA. Equivalent to mouse Ob
HLA-DQB2 Ψ	DQB pseudogene
HLA-DQA2 Ψ	DQB pseudogene
HLA-DQB3(D6S205) (DVß) Ψ	DQB pseudogene fragment

Table I. Continued

HLA-DQB1	DQβ protein Expressed polymorphic DQβ gene Antigen presentation
HLA-DQA1	DQα protein Expressed polymorphic DQA gene Antigen presentation
HLA-DRB1-9	DRβ Expressed polymorphic DRB genes and pseudogenes Antigen presentation Numbers of DRB genes differ in different haplotypes
HLA-DRA	DRα Expressed non-polymorphic DRα product pairs with DRβ Antigen presentation

Class III region

Gene	Protein, function or prominent feature
NOTCH3 (INT3)	Cellular interactions? Counterpart of mouse int3-site of MMTV integration
G18	-
PBX2	Homeobox gene related to PBX1
RAGE	RAGE Receptor for advanced glycosylation end products of proteins (AGEs)
G16	-
G15	2.1 kbp mRNA single copy
G14	-
G13	Transcription factor of CREB family
TN-X(XB)	TN-X
XB-S	XB-S Truncated TN-X (C-terminal 673 amino acids)
YB	-
CYP21B(P450c21B)	21-OH Mineralocorticoid and glucocorticoid biosynthesis
ZB	-
C4B	C4 Complement classical pathway thioester containing protein
XA	TN-X(Ψ) Pseudogene
YA	-
CYP21Ps(P450c21A)	21-0H(Ψ) Pseudogene
ZA	-
C4A	C4 Complement classical pathway thioester containing protein
G11	G11 Protein kinase?
G11a	SK12W Helicase
RD	RD
Bf(Factor B)	Factor B Complement alternative pathway serine protease
C2	C2 Complement classical pathway serine protease
G10	-
G9a	G9a Regulation of transcription?
G9	G9 Sialidase enzyme, acidic pH optimum
G8	G8
HSP70-2	HSP70 (HSP72) Heat-inducible hsp70. Chaperone in recovery of cells from stress
HSP70-1	HSP70 (HSP72) Heat-inducible hsp70. Chaperone in recovery of cells from stress
HSP70-HOM	HSP70-HOM Constitutive hsp70
G7b	-
G7a	Valyl tRNA synthetase
G7c	-
G7d	-
G7	-
G6	-
G6a	-
BAT5(D6S82E)	-
G5b	-
CKIIß(G5a)	Casein kinase IIß Cell growth?
G5	-
G4	-
G3a	-
G3(BAT3)	BAT3
G2(BAT2)	BAT2 Proline-rich. Contains novel repeat elements. 228 kD-protein
G1	G1 Encodes 10 kD protein with 2 potential 'EF-hand' type calcium-binding domains in N-terminal half. Restricted to T-cells, monocytes and macrophages
K18L	Cytokeratin (Ψ)
B144(Lst-1)	Lst-1
1C7	-
LTB	LTß Cytokine. Anchors LTα to cell membrane

Table I. Continued

TNF	Cytokine. Antitumor activity. Roles in inflammation/ immuno-modulation
LTA	LTα. Cytokine. Role in lymphoid organ development and germinal centre formation
NB6	-
IkBL	Ikβl Inhibitor of Rel family of transcrip-tion factor(s)?
BAT1	BAT1 RNA helicase?
MICB (PERB11.2)	MICB
PERB6	TNF-receptor-associated-protein-like?
PERB10	-
MICA (PERB11.1)	MICA
NOB1	
PERB3	MHC class I-like pseudogene or gene fragment?
NOB2	-
P5-6 (PERB7; NOB6)	-
DHFRPs (NOB8)	-
17	MHC class I gene fragment
NOB3	-
PERB1	Tyrosine kinase receptor?
PERB10	-
PPIPs	Cyclophillin (peptidyl-propyl iso-merase) (Ψ) Pseudogene

Class I region

Gene	Protein, function or prominent feature
B	HLA-B expressed polymorphic class I gene
RPL3-Hom (NOB7)	-
C	HLA-C expressed polymorphic class I gene
NOB5	-
NOB4	
POU5F1 (OTF-3; OCT-3/4)	Octamer transcription factor 3-Transcription factor containing a POU domain
TCF19(SC1)	5C1
S	high S, G, P protein expressed in keratinocytes
TUBB	Tubulin ß
X	-
P5-1	Multicopy MHC gene family. 25KD protein
CAT53	'Gly-rich' sequence
CAT54 (4419)	Probable ATP-dep. transporter
CAT55	-
CAT56	'Pro-rich' like Wiskottt-Aldrich gene
CAT57	'Gln-rich' sequence
CAT59	-
HSR-1(GNL-1?)	putative GTP-binding protein
E (HLA-E) (6.2)	HLA-E class I gene. Low level expression
CAT60	proline-rich motifs
MICC (PERB11.3)	Class I related MIC family. Truncated gene fragment
CAT62	
TC4	GTP-binding nuclear protein
CAT63	-
CAT64	-
CAT65	TIMP-3
30	MHC class I gene fragment
CAT66	-
CAT67	-
92	MHC class IΨ
VI	-
I	-
B30.2(Cat 72)	C-terminus butyrophilin
CAT70	-
ZNF173(CAT69, 71/ AFP, VLG51)	Acid finger protein Contains two domains rich in Cys and His similar to those characteristic of metal-dependent DNA binding proteins
HTCTEX-5	Human equivalent of mouse Tctex-5 gene
ZNF 178	C-terminus butyrophilin
hSUP45.1 (clone 58, HCGVII)	Related to yeast SUP45 gene - translation factor
VIII.1	-
VEF	-
J(HLA-J), D6S203, HLA-59, cda12	MHC class I Ψ
IV-2	Multicopy MHC gene family
P5-2	Multicopy MHC gene family
CAT73A/B	
3.8-1.2	Multicopy MHC gene family
IX-1	-
HUMCAT75X	-
II-1	-
80	MHC class I truncated gene
IV-3	Multicopy MHC gene family
P5-3	Multicopy MHC gene family
HUMMHCFANC	-
A (HLA-A)	HLA-A MHC class I gene - antigen presentation.
IV-4	Multicopy MHC gene family
MICD (PERB11.4)	MHC class I-related. Truncated gene fragment

Table I. Continued

21	MHC class I gene fragment
70	MHC class I Ψ
IV-5	Multicopy MHC gene family
P5-4	Multicopy MHC gene family
3.8-1.3	Multicopy MHC gene family
ZNFA3	C4-type zinc finger
PERB2	BAT1-related gene
B30.7 (CAT 78,80)	TFIIS zinc ribbon domain
11.2	-
16	MHC class I gene fragment
P5.7	Multicopy MHC gene family
CAT81	-
H (HLA-H)	-
IV-6	Multicopy MHC gene family
VLG20	-
VIII.2	-
P5.C	-
10.0-1	-
CAT79	-
3.8-1.4 (PERB6-like)	Multicopy MHC gene family
HUMMHCFANE (FAT1, FAT2, FAT4)	-
HUMMHI (FAT3)	-
G (HLA-G)	Class I gene
IV-7	Multicopy MHC gene family
P5-5	Multicopy MHC gene family
FAT5	-
II-3	-
90	MHC class I gene fragment
IV-8	Multicopy MHC gene family
FAT6/15	class I-related
75	MHC class I truncated gene
IV-9	Multicopy MHC gene family
FAT 7	-
P5-6	Multicopy MHC gene family
3.8-1.5	Multicopy MHC gene family
FAT8	60s ribosomal protein L23A
IX-2	-
MICE	Class I-related MIC family truncated gene fragment
F (HLA-F)(5.4)	HLA-F class I protein
IV-10	Multicopy MHC gene family
CAT82	-
CAT83	beta glucuronidase
FAT9	-
MOG	myelin oligodendrocyte glycoprotein
FAT10	ubiquitin-like family of proteins
HUMORLMHC (FAT11, OL42)	Family of olfactory receptor genes, at least one of which is expressed as a mRNA. Some polymorphism
MHCOR2	olfactory receptor family
MAD2	-
MAD1	-

Markers which are not precisely mapped	
FB146-1	Size-related (Sez-6)
WI-9441	-
B12-7	zinc finger protein
B10-7	-
B38-3	ORFI 3' to speb, *E. coli*
B38-7	-
HUMORFKG1A	-
CAT 75h	human TRAM protein
960-205	-
1-8U	interferon-inducible protein Gene family
903-182	-
903-7	-
903-11	-
903-12	-
903-14	-
903-49	-
903-102	-
903-128	-
903-137	-
903-179	-
903-180	-
903-213	-

Ψ, Pseudogene

References

1. Campbell RD, Trowsdale J. *Map of the human MHC. Immunol Today* 1997, in press.
2. Gruen JR, Nalabolu SR, Chu TW, Bowlus C, Fan WF, Goei VL, Wei H, Sivakamasundari R, Liu Y-C, Xu HX, Parimoo S, Nallur G, Ajioka R, Shukla H, Bray-Ward P, Pan J, Weissman SM. A transcription map of the major histocompatibility complex (MHC) class I region. *Genomics* 1996;36: 70-85.
3. Feder JN, Gnirke A, Thomas W, Tsuchihashi Z, Ruddy DA, Basava A, Dormishian F, Domingo RJ, Ellis MC, Fullan A, Hinton LM, Jones NL, Kimmel BE, Kronmal GS, Lauer P, Lee VK, Loeb DB, Mapa FA, McClelland E, Meyer NC, Mintier GA, Moeleer N, Moore T, Morikang E, Prass CE, Quintana L, Starnes SM, Schatzman RC, Brunke KJ, Drayna DT, Risch NJ, Bacon BR, Wolff RK. A novel MHC class I-like gene is mutated in patients with heriditary haemochromatosis. *Nature Genet* 1996; 13: 399-403.
4. Albertella MR, Jones H, Thomson W, Olavesen MG, Campbell RD. Localisation of eight additional genes in the human major histocompatibility complex, including the gene encoding the casein kinase II beta subunit. *Genomics* 1996; 36: 240-51.

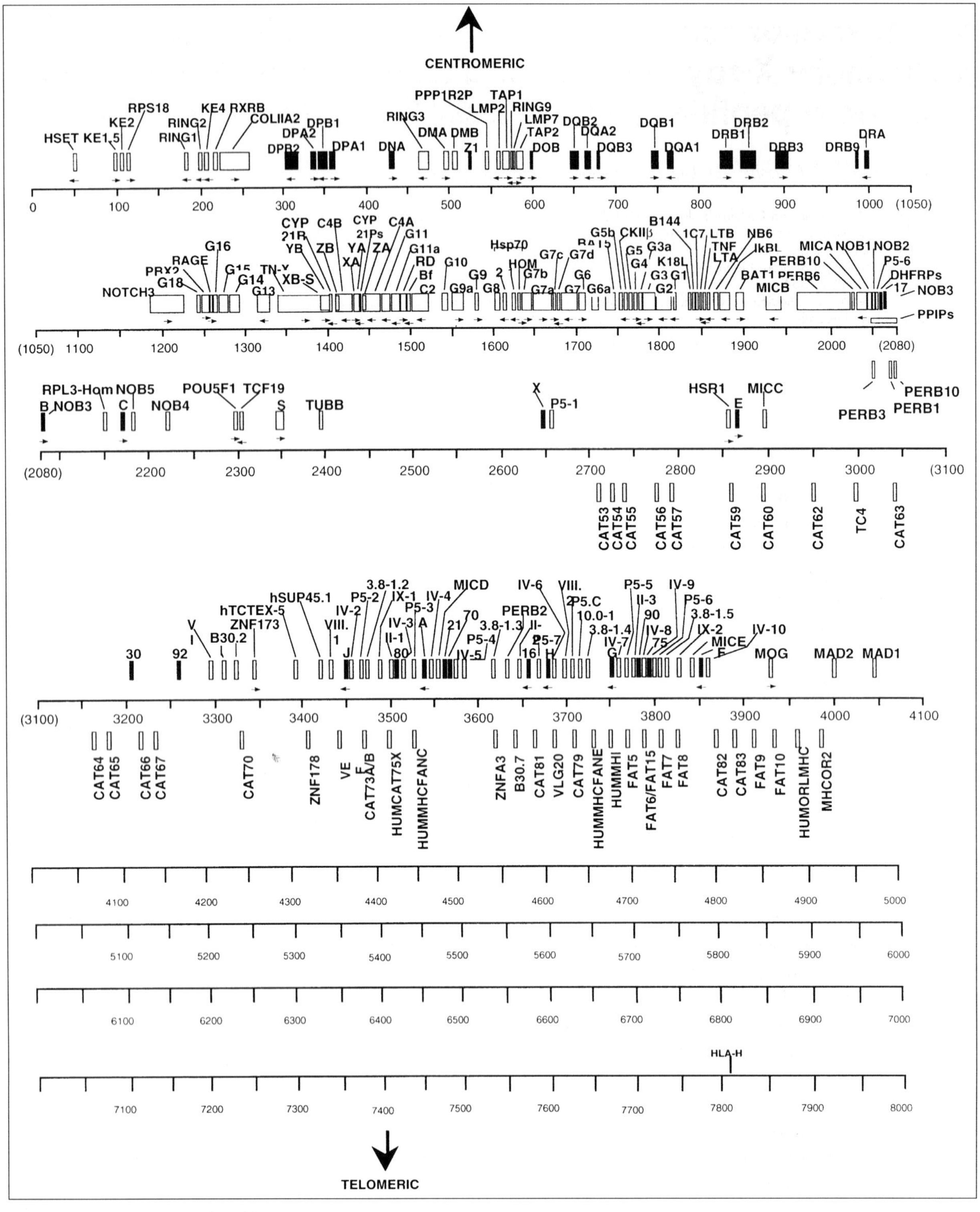

Figure 1. The human MHC (1997).

A trimolecular complex: production, crystallization and preliminary X-ray analysis of a human alpha/beta T cell receptor, a peptide, and the class I MHC molecule HLA-A2

D.N. Garboczi[1], P. Ghosh[1]*, U. Utz[3], W.E. Biddison[4], D.C. Wiley[1,2,5]*

1. Department of Molecular and Cellular Biology, Harvard University, 7 Divinity Avenue, Cambridge, MA 02138, USA
2. Howard Hughes Medical Institute, Harvard University, 7 Divinity Avenue, Cambridge, MA 02138, USA
3. Laboratoire d'Immunologie, Institut de Recherches Cliniques de Montréal, 110 Avenue des Pins Ouest, Montréal, H2W 1R7 Canada
4. Molecular Immunology Section, Neuroimmunology Branch, National Institute of Neurological Disorders and Stroke, National Institutes of Health, Bethesda, MD 20892, USA
5. Laboratory of Molecular Medicine, Howard Hughes Medical Institute, The Children's Hospital, Boston, MA 02115, USA

*Authors contributed equally

In the cellular immune response, antigen-specific T cell recognition results from the binding of a TCR to the complex of an antigenic peptide bound to a MHC glycoprotein located on the surface of an antigen-presenting cell [1]. Specific binding by the TCR triggers signals within the T cell that are central to the development of the T cell repertoire, the regulation of the immune response, and the activation of cytolytic T cells (CTL). Human cells infected by viruses display on their cell surfaces peptides from viral proteins bound to MHC molecules. CTL expressing a TCR specific for a viral peptide/class I MHC complex are activated to cause lysis of infected cells and/or release of cytokines following specific recognition of the complex.

For biochemical and structural studies, we chose to study a human alpha/beta TCR specific for the Tax peptide from HTLV-1 in complex with HLA-A2. HTLV-1 is associated with adult T cell leukemia and a slowly progressive neurological disease, HTLV-1-associated myelopathy/tropical spastic paraparesis (HAM/TSP). In patients with HAM/TSP, the frequency of virus-specific CD8+ precursor CTL is at least 40-fold higher than in asymptomatic, but virus-infected individuals. In HLA-A2+ patients, the great majority of CD8+ HTLV-1-specific CTL recognize a peptide (LLFGYPVYV) from residues 11-19 of the Tax protein [6]. One such CTL clone, identified as A6, exhibits specific lysis of HLA-A2+ target cells that have been exposed to the Tax 11-19 peptide [7].

We have expressed the extracellular domains of the A6 TCR alpha and beta subunits separately as inclusion bodies in *E. coli*. The refolded TCR heterodimer binds to the complex of the Tax peptide with HLA-A2 with a specificity that appears to be identical to that of the A6 T cell clone from which it was isolated [2]. The ternary complex, forms crystals which diffract X-rays and will enable the determination of the structure of this antigen-specific cell-cell interaction complex.

Expression of alpha and beta TCR polypeptides

For expression of the A6 alpha and beta polypeptides, translation stop codons were placed just before the predicted transmembrane residues or at the C-terminal-most cysteine of each chain, producing a long and short version of each subunit, respectively. The longer form of each subunit includes the C-terminal-most cysteine residue which takes part in the interchain disulfide bond. Both forms of each subunit were expressed in large quantities as inclusion bodies. Lysing the bacteria with lysozyme and detergents, washing the inclusion bodies with detergent-containing buffer, and dissolving the insoluble protein in 8M urea, yielded highly purified proteins, typically yielding 40 mg of protein per liter of bacterial culture.

Without further purification, the alpha and beta chains could be refolded to form either covalently- or non-covalently-associated heterodimers. To form covalently-associated dimers, the longer versions of the alpha and beta subunits were refolded separately by dialysis under dilute conditions. The specific formation of interchain disulfide bonded alpha/beta heterodimers rather than homodimers was accomplished by treating the refolded beta chains with the sulfhydryl reagent 5,5'-dithiobis(2-nitrobenzoic acid) (DTNB) forming a labile TNB-cysteine disulfide with the C-terminal-most cysteine of beta. Upon mixing the DTNB-treated beta with the refolded alpha, the TNB-cysteine disulfide bond of beta is attacked by the free cysteine of the alpha chain, displacing TNB to form a disulfide bond between alpha and beta. The disulfide between the chains was demonstrated by SDS-PAGE analysis under reducing and non-reducing conditions (not shown). Although the covalent heterodimer produced in this way bound specifically to HLA-A2 (see below), it did not crystallize.

To form non-covalently-associated heterodimers, a mixture of the denatured shorter versions of the alpha and beta chains were refolded by rapid dilution. The second free cysteine in the constant domain of beta was replaced by an alanine residue to help prevent the mispairing of cysteines during folding. Typically, refolding was carried out on about 100 mg of each subunit and approximately 20% of the diluted alpha and beta protein refolded and dimerized. The non-covalently-associated TCR appeared on non-reducing SDS-PAGE to be much more homogeneous than the covalently-associated TCR preparations (data not shown). The refolded non-covalently associated TCR is stable and is soluble at 100 mg/ml. The refolded non-covalently linked alpha/beta heterodimer elutes during purification by gel filtration chromatography at a volume expected for a 40 kD protein; the calculated molecular weight of the heterodimer is 50.2 kD. An initial screen of crystallization conditions with a mixture of this TCR protein and the HLA-A2/Tax complex yielded crystals.

Refolded alpha/beta TCR bind specifically to peptide/HLA-A2 complexes

The specific interaction of soluble alpha/beta TCR with the soluble HLA-A2/Tax peptide complex [8] was demonstrated using native (non-denaturing) PAGE without heating or reducing the samples. A typical experiment of this type is shown in *Figure 1.* A mixture of either the covalently-associated (not shown) or the non-covalently-associated TCR and the HLA-A2/Tax peptide complex exhibited a prominent shifted band (lanes 3, 5, 7, and 9) that migrated at a position distinct from either TCR alone (lanes 2, 4, 6, and 8) or HLA-A2/Tax alone (lanes 1 and 10). No shifted band appeared when the TCR was mixed with HLA-A2 complexed with single-residue mutants of the Tax peptide (see below). Neither the alpha subunit alone nor the beta subunit alone showed any binding to HLA-A2/Tax in the native gel shift assay (data not shown). The non-covalently associated TCR exhibits two bands (for example, lane 6), both of which shift mobility in the presence of HLA-A2/Tax.

The soluble alpha/beta TCR also bound to HLA-A2 complexed with a Tax peptide modified at position 1 of the peptide from leucine to cysteine (L1C) and with HLA-A2 complexed with a Tax peptide modified at position 5 of the peptide from tyrosine to alanine (Y5A). Tax peptides modified at position 4 (G4V), 6 (P6Q), or 8 (Y8A), all of which bind to and promote the refolding of HLA-A2, did not mediate binding of soluble HLA-A2 to soluble TCR under the conditions used in the gel-shift assay. The L1C and Y5A peptides are recognized by the A6 T cell in cell-killing assays, while G4V, P6Q, and Y8A are not recognized. The Y5A peptide seems to be a partial agonist peptide since it induces different cell-killing/cytokine production in T cell assays as compared to the wild-type Tax peptide (data not shown).

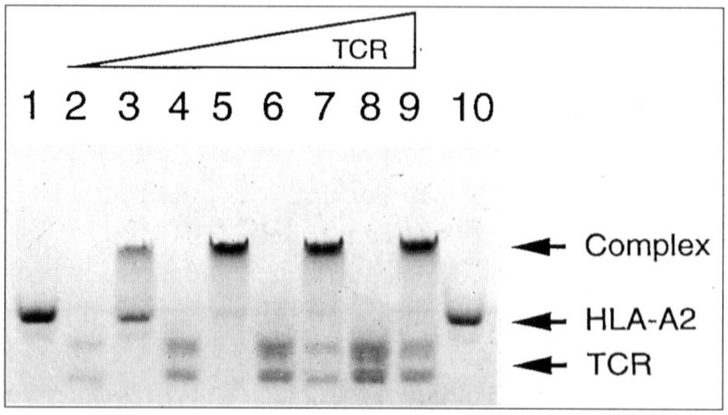

Figure 1. Native gel-shift assay with the non-covalently-associated TCR and the HLA-A2/Tax peptide complex.
Lanes 2, 3, TCR (6 μg)
Lanes 4, 5, TCR (12 μg)
Lanes 6, 7, TCR (18 μg)
Lanes 8, 9, TCR (24 μg)
Lanes 1, 3, 5, 7, 9, 10, HLA-A2/Tax (6 μg).
TCR loaded alone in lanes 2, 4, 6, and 8. HLA-A2/Tax peptide loaded alone in lanes 1 and 10.

The native gel-shift assay was essential as the functional test that guided the development of the procedure for refolding recombinant alpha/beta TCR. It is a rapid assay that checks the quality of a refolding experiment without column chromatography or other more time-consuming techniques. Native-PAGE can separate proteins based on slight differences in overall charge and size. For example, we have observed differences in the mobility on native gels of HLA-A2 complexed with various peptides that have single amino acid residue changes that do not involve charged side chains (data not shown).

Crystallization of the alpha/beta TCR/HLA-A2 complex

The disulfide-linked TCR heterodimer complexed with HLA-A2/Tax did not crystallize, probably due to the heterogeneity of the disulfide-linked TCR. Although the part of the covalently-associated TCR preparation that bound HLA-A2/Tax and shifted its mobility was relatively homogeneous, even the covalently-associated TCR/Tax/HLA-A2 complex isolated from preparative native gels did not crystallize. One source of heterogeneity is the formation of non-native disulfide bonds. The refolded alpha subunit often yielded three bands on non-reducing SDS-PAGE, an indication of mispairing of cysteines (data not shown).

Non-covalently associated TCR in complex with HLA-A2 showed no such heterogeneity and readily crystallized. TCR (36 mg/ml) and Tax peptide/HLA-A2 complex (12 mg/ml) were mixed at a 1:1 molar ratio and crystallized by vapor diffusion in hanging-drops consisting of 1 µl of protein solution and 1 µl of each solution from a screen of crystallization conditions. Crystals appeared at the buffer conditions of 10% polyethylene glycol 8000, 100 mM MgAcetate, 50 mM NaCacodylate pH 6.5. Crushing crystals for microseeding was very useful in that seeding new hanging drops with 10-fold dilutions of a crushed-crystal suspension readily produced large (700 x 400 x 200 mm) crystals. SDS-PAGE revealed that the alpha and beta chains of the TCR and the two chains of HLA-A2 were present in the crystals (data not shown).

The ease of purification and of crystallization proved to be important for the success of the project. At two points during the project, we were granted synchrotron time with insufficient advance notice to allow time to prepare all the crystals. Some of the cysteine mutant proteins used for mercury derivatives were refolded, but were not purified by gel filtration or crystallized in time for the trip to the synchrotron. At the synchrotron, we discovered that most of the misfolded protein and impurities could be precipitated with 50 mM MgAcetate and 25 mM NaCacodylate, pH 6.5. The supernatant could then be used to grow microseeded crystals, without further purification. Crystals large enough for data collection were grown in 12-24 h at the synchrotron, soaked in 1 mM ethylmercury phosphate, and immediately exposed to the x-ray beam for data collection.

X-ray analysis

Crystals diffracted X-rays from a laboratory X-ray generator to about 3.5 Å resolution at room temperature but stopped diffracting after overnight exposure to x-rays. Crystals could be flash frozen to -160°C in a stream of cold nitrogen gas after being soaked in the crystal growth solution with 20% glycerol added as cryoprotectant. Diffraction was observed to about 3.3 Å from frozen crystals. Using the synchrotron X-ray source at CHESS (Cornell High Energy Synchrotron Source), diffraction data to beyond 2.8 Å resolution could be collected from crystals at -160°C. Analysis of the diffraction intensities of a partial dataset collected on a laboratory X-ray source (90% complete to 3.5 Å, 46% complete from 3.5 to 3.3 Å) indicated the space group to be C2 with unit cell dimensions: a= 228.2 Å, b= 49.6 Å, c= 94.7 Å, beta= 91.3°. The size and symmetry of the unit cell are consistent with the presence of one TCR/Tax peptide/HLA-A2 complex per asymmetric unit assuming 56% solvent content.

Molecular replacement calculations with the HLA-A2/Tax model [5] clearly revealed the location of HLA-A2 in the unit cell, as the top solutions in both the rotation and translation functions were well above and separate from the next most significant solutions. Viewing the positioned HLA-A2 and its symmetry mates revealed planes of HLA-A2 molecules arranged within the crystal. Within each plane the molecules are oriented in an alternating fashion, with the bound peptides of adjacent molecules exposed to opposite sides of each plane. The planes do not touch each other making it clear then that the TCR will fill the spaces between the planes.

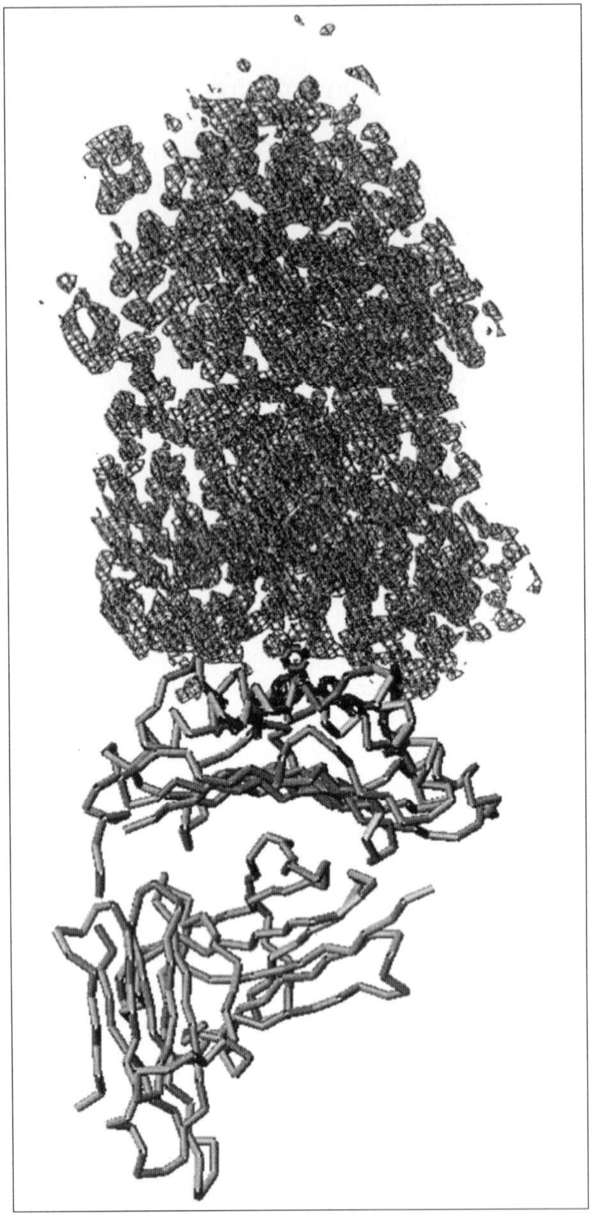

Figure 2. A 2Fo-Fc map revealing electron density over the peptide-binding site of HLA-A2. The HLA-A2 model was positioned within the unit cell with the AMORE program of the CCP4 (Collaborative Computing Project 4) package. The positioned model of HLA-A2 was used to generate calculated structure factors which were combined with experimentally-measured structure factor amplitudes to calculate this 2Fo-Fc map. The density is displayed in the graphics program O at a greater than one sigma contour level, covering the models of the TCR beta subunit [3] and the TCR Valpha domain [4] positioned by molecular replacement.

A 2Fo-Fc electron density map using calculated structure factors from the positioned HLA-A2 model was generated *(Figure 2)*. Examination of this map showed density located directly over the peptide-binding site of HLA-A2. This new electron density appeared to show direct interactions with the bound peptide of HLA-A2. After density modification using the program DM (CCP4), a few strands of beta sheet of the Vbeta region could be identified, but overall the map was not of a sufficient quality for protein model-building. Experiments to identify heavy atom derivatives to allow improved phasing by multiple isomorphous replacement were begun.

Conclusions

Soluble alpha/beta TCR has been assembled by refolding the extracellular domains of the alpha and beta chains expressed as insoluble inclusion bodies in *E. coli.* Inclusion body yields of 40 mg per liter of bacteria and a 20% refolding efficiency allow routine purification of 40 mg of pure alpha/beta TCR. The soluble alpha/beta TCR binds specifically to the complex of HLA-A2 with the Tax peptide of HTLV1 as shown in gel-shift assays. Assembly of the complex of TCR/peptide/HLA-A2 does not require any of the carbohydrate of either glycoprotein, nor does it require the presence of the interchain disulfide bond of the alpha/beta TCR. The refolding methods developed during this work may be useful in the refolding of other TCRs, as the sequences of alpha/beta TCRs are similar and the TCRs are expected to have essentially the same structure. A second, class II-restricted human TCR in this laboratory has been produced in bacteria and refolded using these methods. This alpha/beta TCR was shown to bind both a specific class II/peptide complex and a superantigen using gel-shift assays (J. Park, D.N.G., A. Seth, D.C.W., unpublished results). For structural studies low affinities between some pairings of the alpha and beta chains may be overcome by using the high concentrations of the polypeptides now available from bacterial expression.

A study of the crystals of the alpha/beta TCR/peptide/HLA-A2 complex reported here should reveal the atomic details of the antigen-specific cell-cell recognition that is central to the activation of T cells

Acknowledgments

D. N. G. was supported by a postdoctoral fellowship (DAMD 17-94-J-4060) from the Department of the Army; no official endorsement by the government should be inferred. P. G. was supported by the Irvington Institute for Medical Research. This research was supported by the National Institutes of Health (HD-17461) and the HHMI. D. C. W. is an investigator of the Howard Hughes Medical Institute.

References

1. Hedrick SM, Eidelman FJ. T lymphocyte antigen receptors. In : Paul WE, ed. *Fundamental immunology,* 3rd ed. New York : Raven Press Ltd : 1993 : 383-420.
2. Garboczi, DN, Utz, U, Ghosh P, Seth, A, Kim, J, VanTienhoven, EAE, Biddison, WE, Wiley, DC. Assembly, specific binding, and crystallization of a human alpha/beta T cell receptor with an antigenic tax peptide from HTLV-1 and the class I MHC molecule HLA-A2. *J Immunol* 1997 (in press).
3. Bentley GA, Boulot G, Karjalainen K, Mariuzza RA. Crystal structure of the beta chain of a T cell antigen receptor. *Science* 1995 ; 267 : 1984-7.
4. Fields BA, Ober B, Malchiodi EL, Lebedeva MI, Braden BC, Ysern X, Kim JK, Shao X, Ward ES, Mariuzza RA. Crystal structure of the Valpha domain of a T cell antigen receptor. *Science* 1995 ; 270 : 1821-4.
5. Madden DR, Garboczi DN, Wiley DC. The antigenic identity of peptide/MHC complexes: a comparison of the conformations of five viral peptides presented by HLA-A2. *Cell* 1993 ; 75 : 1-20.
6. Elovaara I, Koenig S, Brewah AY, Woods RM, Lehky T, Jacobson S. High human T-cell lymphotropic virus type 1 (HTLV-1)-specific precursor cytotoxic T lymphocyte frequencies in patients with HTLV-1-associated neurological disease. *J Exp Med* 1993 ; 177 : 1567-73.
7. Utz U, Banks D, Jacobson S, Biddison WE. Analysis of the T-cell receptor repertoire of human T-cell leukemia virus type 1 (HTLV-1) Tax-specific CD8+ cytotoxic T lymphocytes from patients with HTLV-1-associated disease: evidence for oligoclonal expansion. *J Virol* 1996 ; 70 : 843-51.
8. Garboczi DN, Hung DT, Wiley DC. HLA-A2-peptide complexes: refolding and crystallization of molecules expressed in *Escherichia coli* and complexed with single antigenic peptides. *Proc Natl Acad Sci USA* 1992 ; 89 : 3429-33.

The molecular basis of MHC class II deficiency and regulation of MHC class II genes

W. Reith, B. Mach

L. Jeantet Laboratory of Molecular Genetics, Department of Genetics and Microbiology, University of Geneva Medical School, 1, rue Michel-Servet, CH-1211 Geneva 4, Switzerland

Major histocompatibility complex class II (MHC-II) antigens are cell surface molecules playing a pivotal role in the immune response. They initiate immune responses by presenting exogenous peptides to the receptor of CD4$^+$ T helper lymphocytes, they shape the T cell repertoire by directing positive and negative selection events in the thymus and they participate in the activation of the antigen presenting cells on which they are expressed. Considering these three key functions, it is not surprising that expression of MHC-II molecules is tightly regulated and largely restricted to professional antigen presenting cells, thymic epithelial cells and cells exposed to a variety of stimuli including immune regulators such as interferon-γ (IFN-γ). Precise regulation of this expression profile is crucial for the immune system. For instance, ectopic or abnormal levels of MHC-II expression have been implicated in the pathogenesis of autoimmune diseases, while the lack of MHC-II expression results in a severe immunodeficiency syndrome called MHC-II deficiency.

Expression of MHC-II genes is controlled primarily at the level of their transcription by a short promoter proximal enhancer region consisting of four highly conserved cis-acting DNA sequences referred to as the S, X, X2 and Y 'boxes'. A major breakthrough in the elucidation of the molecular mechanisms controlling MHC-II gene transcription *via* these *cis*-acting sequences has come from the study of patients suffering from MHC-II deficiency. MHC-II deficiency is a genetically heterogeneous disease resulting from defects in *trans*-acting regulatory factors required for transcriptional activation of MHC-II promoters. Patients have been classified into four different genetic complementation groups (A, B, C and D) reflecting the existence of four distinct regulatory factors. The genes that are affected in three of the groups (A, C and D) have now been isolated, and this has led to the identification of two key regulatory proteins, the class II transactivator CIITA and regulatory factor X (RFX). Both CIITA and RFX are absolutely essential and highly specific for transcriptional activation of MHC-II genes.

RFX is a ubiquitously expressed multimeric protein complex that binds to the X box *cis*-acting sequence present in all MHC-II promoters. RFX is essential for the occupation of MHC-II promoters *in vivo* because it is a key participant in co-operative protein-protein interactions that are required for stable and specific recruitment of other DNA binding proteins to the adjacent X2 and Y box sequences. Binding of RFX is deficient in complementation groups B, C and D, and cells from these patients thus exhibit unoccupied MHC-II promoters and a lack of constitutive and inducible MHC-II gene transcription. The genes encoding two different subunits of the RFX complex, RFX5 and RFXAP, have now been isolated and shown to be defective in complementation groups C and D, respectively.

The gene encoding CIITA is defective in patients in complementation group A, and both constitutive and IFN-γ induced MHC-II expression is consequently abolished. In contrast to RFX, CIITA is a non-DNA binding transactivator of MHC-II genes. It is a differentially expressed protein that functions as a master controller determining the level, cell type specificity and inducibility of MHC-II expression. Constitutive expression of CIITA is restricted to cell types that express MHC-II genes constitutively. In MHC-II negative cell types, the CIITA gene is silent. However, exposure of these cells to inducers such as IFN-γ leads to the activation of CIITA expression, which in its turn mediates the induction of MHC-II gene transcription. Expression of the CIITA gene is controlled by at least three independent promoters differing in their tissue specificity and inducibility by IFN-γ. It is thus the differential usage of the different CIITA promoters that ultimately determines the cell type specificity and inducibility of MHC-II expression.

Regulation of MHC-II expression

Given the vital functions of MHC-II molecules, the molecular mechanisms regulating their expression obviously represent an important parameter in the normal physiological control of the immune response. For instance, the level of MHC expression on professional APCs can determine their competence for antigen presentation, and can thus influence the efficiency of T cell activation and the immune response that is elicited. In addition, defects in the regulation of MHC-II expression can have profound immunopathological consequences. Ectopic or pathological upregulation of MHC-II expression has been suggested to contribute to the aberrant T cell activation observed in certain autoimmune diseases. Autoimmune diseases in which abnormal MHC-II expression has for example been implicated include rheumatoid arthritis, autoimmune nephritis, insulin-dependent diabetes mellitus, inflammatory bowel disease and multiple sclerosis. Conversely, a lack of MHC-II expression is known to result in the severe immunodeficiency syndrome called MHC-II deficiency, also referred to as the bare lymphocyte syndrome (BLS) [1-3]. The elucidation of the mechanisms that control the regulation of MHC-II gene expression thus represents a major challenge in both molecular immunology and immunopathology.

In contrast to the relatively ubiquitous expression of MHC-I, the pattern of MHC-II expression is complex and very tightly regulated. Under most normal conditions, the different MHC-II A and B genes are all regulated in a co-ordinated fashion. As expected from their role in antigen presentation by MHC-II molecules, the Ii and HLA-DM (H-2M) genes are in general also co-regulated with MHC-II genes. Two distinct modes of expression are generally recognised. Certain specialised cells express MHC-II genes constitutively, while in many MHC-II negative cell types, expression can be induced by a variety of stimuli, particularly by interferon-γ (IFN-γ) (for reviews see [2,4]). This situation is complicated further by the fact that both constitutive and IFN-γ induced expression can be modulated positively or negatively, in a cell type dependent manner, by quite a large number of secondary stimuli (for reviews see [2,4]).

Both constitutive and IFN-γ inducible expression of MHC-II genes are controlled primarily at the level of transcription by a highly conserved promoter proximal region.

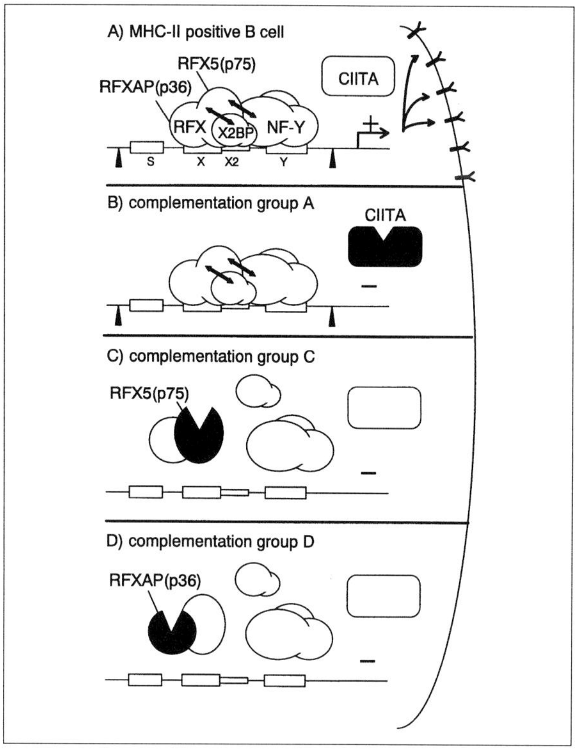

Figure 1. Molecular defects in MHC-II deficiency. MHC-II promoter occupancy and transcription status of MHC-II genes in normal MHC-II positive B cells and in B cells from complementation groups A, C and D. The open boxes represent the S, X, X2 and Y regulatory DNA sequences present in the promoter proximal regions of all MHC-II genes. The protein complexes RFX, X2BP and NF-Y bind respectively, to the X, X2 and Y boxes. Proteins binding to the S box remain poorly characterised. CIITA (rounded rectangle) is shown hovering over the promoter because its mode of action remains elusive. Co-operative protein-protein interactions between RFX, X2BP and NF-Y are indicated schematically by double-headed arrows. Solid arrow heads indicate the presence of DNAse I hypersensitive sites. CIITA is mutated in complementation group A. Mutations in CIITA do not modify promoter occupation *in vivo* or the presence of DNAse I hypersensitive sites. In complementation groups C and D, the 75 kD (RFX5) and 36 kD (RFXAP) subunits of RFX are mutated, respectively. A deficiency in RFX leads to a bare promoter *in vivo*, and the absence of DNAse I hypersensitive sites.

The promoter proximal regions of all MHC-II genes contain four essential cis-acting sequence motifs referred to as the MHC-II S, X, X2 and Y boxes (*Figure 1*) [2,4]. The same sequence elements are also present in the promoter proximal regions of the non-classical HLA-DM

Table I. MHC-II deficiency patients and regulatory mutants in complementation groups A to D

	MHC-II deficiency complementation groups			
	A	B	C	D
Prototypical patient	BLS-2	BLS-1	SJO	DA, ABI, ZM
Number of unrelated families	5	15	3	6[(1)]
Prototypical *in vitro* mutant	RJ2.2.5	none	none	6.1.6
Number of *in vitro* mutants	3	none	none	1
main ethnic origin	Hispanic	North African	North American European	Turkish North African

[(1)] numbers are based on somatic cell fusion experiments and/or on mutation analysis of the affected genes (see text).

genes and of the Ii chain gene. The S, X, X2 and Y elements are highly conserved with respect to their sequence, relative position, orientation and spacing, and they function together as a single unit [2,4]. Much of what we have learned about the trans-acting regulatory factors controlling the activity of MHC-II promoters has come from the elucidation of the molecular basis of MHC-II deficiency, a disease resulting from regulatory defects in MHC-II gene expression.

MHC-II deficiency, a disease of MHC-II gene regulation

The availability of a genetic approach for the identification and isolation of regulatory factors controlling expression of MHC-II genes has represented an enormous advantage. This approach relies on the existence of regulatory mutants that are deficient in trans-acting factors required for expression of MHC-II genes. The majority of these regulatory mutants are cell lines derived from patients suffering from MHC-II deficiency, a severe hereditary immunodeficiency syndrome resulting from the lack of MHC-II expression. The disease has represented an ideal model system for the dissection of the molecular mechanisms controlling transcriptional activation of MHC-II genes. It has indeed permitted the identification and isolation of the relevant regulatory factors on the basis of a powerful functional criterion, namely the ability to complement the genetic defect and restore expression of the endogenous MHC-II genes.

Direct measurements of the transcriptional activity of MHC-II genes in cells from the patients has demonstrated that the lack of MHC-II expression is due to a deficiency in transcription of the MHC-II genes [5]. This suggested that the disease was due to defects in regulatory factors controlling transcriptional activation of MHC-II genes. Direct evidence for this interpretation was provided by four independent observations. First, family studies demonstrated that the genetic lesions responsible for the disease do not co-segregate with the MHC [6]. Second, reporter genes fused to the DNA sequences controlling transcription of MHC-II genes (*see below*) remain silent upon transfection into cells from the patients. Third, in *in vitro* transcription experiments, nuclear extracts from the patient's cells are unable to activate transcription from MHC-II promoters [7]. Finally, expression of the endogenous MHC-II genes of the patient's cells can be reactivated in somatic cell fusion experiments.

It is now clear that defects in several distinct MHC-II regulatory factors can give rise to MHC-II deficiency. This genetic heterogeneity was first demonstrated by means of somatic cell fusion experiments performed with a panel of cell lines derived from different patients. In addition, several experimentally generated cell lines exhibiting an MHC-II negative phenotype indistinguishable from the patient's cell lines were also included. Patients from 29 unrelated families and four experimentally generated mutants have now been included in this analysis. The results of these experiments indicate that the patients and experimentally derived cell lines can be assigned to at least four different complementation groups (*Table I*, A to D), believed to reflect the existence of mutations in four distinct MHC-II regulatory genes. The majority of the patients (18 patients from 15 different families) fall into complementation group B. Group A contains patients from five different families, as well as three experimentally derived mutants of which the most well known is RJ2.2.5. Group C contains patients from three families. Group D was first defined by cell fusion experiments with the experimentally generated cell line 6.1.6. Subsequent cell fusion experiments and isolation of the gene affected in 6.1.6 (*see below*) has now permitted the classification of patients from 6 unrelated families in this group ([8]; J. Villard, W. Reith, B. Lisowska-Grospierre, A, Fischer, P. van den Elsen and B. Mach, manuscript submitted).

The spectrum of clinical manifestations and immunopathologies associated with the disease encompass all four complementation groups. No distinctive phenotype restricted to one of these complementation groups has been identified. Despite the genetic heterogeneity in the cause of MHC-II deficiency, the syndrome is therefore clinically homogeneous. There is on the other hand an interesting correlation between the complementation groups and the ethnic origin of the patients (*Table I*). The majority of patients in group B are of North African origin. Four out of five families in group A are Hispanic. The majority of patients in group D are either of Turkish or North African descent. Finally, all patients in group C are Caucasians of North American or European origin.

Molecular basis of MHC-II deficiency

A combination of biochemical and genetic approaches has now elucidated the molecular defects responsible for MHC-II deficiency patients in complementation groups A, C and D [8-10]. The isolation, characterisation and function of the genes affected in these three groups (CIITA, RFX5 and RFXAP) are discussed in detail below. *Figure 1* summarises schematically what the affected genes have taught us about the regulation of MHC-II genes and the molecular basis of MHC-II deficiency.

Binding of RFX discriminates between two molecular defects

RFX (regulatory factor X) is a protein complex that was first identified in nuclear extracts from MHC-II positive B cell lines on the basis of its ability to bind *in vitro* to the X box of MHC-II promoters [5]. It has been purified to near homogeneity by affinity chromatography, and shown to be a heteromeric protein consisting of at least two subunits of 75 kD and 36 kD (*Figure 1*) [7]. The binding activity of this RFX complex has been analysed extensively by *in vitro* binding studies using nuclear extracts prepared from MHC-II deficiency cell lines and from the experimentally generated regulatory mutants [5, 7, 11]. Based on the presence or absence of RFX binding activity, two types of mutant cells were recognised (*Figure 1*); RFX binding activity is normal in cell lines classified in complementation group A, but is deficient in cell lines assigned to complementation groups B, C and D (reviewed in [1,2]). The lack of RFX binding activity in cells from complementation groups B-D is specific since other known MHC-II promoter binding proteins are detected normally in these cells [5,11]. Moreover, the absence of RFX is functionally relevant because MHC-II promoter activity can be restored to normal levels in *in vitro* transcription experiments when transcriptionally silent extracts from cells in groups B and C are supplemented with purified RFX [7].
Examination of DNAse I hypersensitive sites and *in vivo* footprint experiments have revealed that the lack of RFX binding activity observed *in vitro* correlates with a bare promoter *in vivo* (*Figure 1*) (reviewed in [1,2]). In RFX positive cells (normal MHC-II positive B cells as well as B cells from complementation group A), MHC class II promoters exhibit characteristic DNAse I hypersensitive sites and are occupied by DNA-binding proteins *in vivo* (*Figure 1*). In RFX deficient B cells, on the other hand (complementation groups B-D), the DNAse I hypersensitive sites are missing and all of the MHC-II promoter elements, including the X, X2 and Y boxes, are unoccupied (*Figure 1*).

CIITA, the gene affected in complementation group A

A genetic approach based on cDNA expression cloning was developed to identify the genes affected in MHC-II deficiency [9]. This approach is based on functional complementation of the genetic defects. Briefly, cell lines established from the patients, or experimentally generated cell lines, were transfected with cDNA expression libraries and cells carrying cDNA clones capable of restoring MHC-II expression were selected for. This approach was first successful in RJ2.2.5, a cell line from complementation group A. Complementation of RJ2.2.5 led to isolation of the MHC-II transactivator CIITA, a novel 1130 amino acid protein exhibiting no homology to any other known proteins [9]. Transfection with the CIITA cDNA restores expression of all MHC-II isotypes (DR, DQ, DP) to wild type levels in all cell lines from complementation group A [9]. It also restores normal expression of the Ii, DMA and DMB genes in these cells.
Mutations in the CIITA gene have been documented in two patients, BLS-2 and BCH, and the experimentally generated mutant RJ2.2.5 from complementation group A [9]. In BLS-2, a homozygous splice donor site mutation leads to exon skipping and hence to an in-frame 23 amino acid deletion near the C-terminal end of CIITA. In BCH, one allele contains a point mutation generating a premature stop codon, while the second allele contains a splice donor site mutation that leads to skipping of a 27 amino acid exon and thus to an in-frame deletion

27 amino acid exon and thus to an in-frame deletion near the C-terminus. In RJ2.2.5, both alleles are disrupted by genomic deletions; one allele contains a deletion within the CIITA gene, while the second allele is deleted entirely. Transfection experiments have confirmed that all mutations abolish the ability of CIITA to activate transcription of MHC-II genes.

The human CIITA gene is localised on chromosome 16 (16p13), and the corresponding mouse gene is situated in a syntenic region of mouse chromosome 16 (M. Haas, V. Steimle, L. Otten, J. Lieman, D.C. Ward, B. Mach, unpublished data). This localisation is in accordance with the findings that regulatory genes present on human and mouse chromosomes 16 are required for expression of MHC-II genes.

RFX5, the gene affected in complementation group C

The same complementation approach used to isolate CIITA was used to elucidate the molecular defect leading to a lack of RFX binding activity in patients from complementation group C (*Figure 1*). Complementation of a cell line derived from patient SJO led to the isolation of a cDNA encoding the 75 kD subunit of RFX [10]. The gene isolated was called RFX5 because it encodes the fifth member of a growing family of DNA-binding proteins sharing a novel and highly characteristic DNA-binding domain [10,12]. This DNA-binding motif has been strongly conserved in evolution, and has been identified in a variety of different proteins having diverse regulatory functions in organisms ranging from yeast to man [12]. Transfection of the RFX5 cDNA restores RFX binding activity and thus reactivates expression of all MHC-II isotypes (DR, DQ, DP) in cell lines from patients in complementation group C [10]. It also restores expression of the Ii, DMA and DMB genes in these cells.

Mutations disrupting the RFX5 gene have been identified in all patients in complementation group C [10]. All of the mutations result in a severely truncated RFX5 protein. In Ro, there is a homozygous point mutation generating a premature stop codon downstream of the DNA-binding domain. In SJO, one allele contains a point mutation disrupting a splice acceptor site, such that a cryptic splice acceptor site situated 5 nucleotides downstream is used instead. This leads to a 5 nucleotide deletion in the mRNA and thus to a frame shift that is followed 18 nucleotides downstream by an out of frame stop codon. No transcripts derived from the second allele of SJO have been detected. In the siblings TF and EVF a homozygous splice donor site point mutation leads to the use of a cryptic splice donor site situated 10 nucleotides upstream. This results in a 10 nucleotide deletion in the mRNA and thus to a frame shift followed 18 nucleotides downstream by an out of frame stop codon.

The human RFX5 gene is situated in a subcentromeric region of the long arm of chromosome 1, and the corresponding mouse gene maps to a syntenic region of chromosome 3 (W. Reith, L. Stubs, B. Mach, unpublished data). This localisation is in accordance with independent evidence that a regulatory gene situated on human chromosome 1 is required for expression of MHC-II genes.

RFXAP, the gene affected in complementation group D

Until recently the experimentally generated cell line 6.1.6 was the only representative of complementation group D. The molecular defect responsible for the lack of RFX binding activity in the 6.1.6 cell line has recently been elucidated [8]. The affected gene was isolated and shown to encode a novel protein corresponding to the 36 kD subunit of the RFX complex (*Figure 1*). This protein was called RFX associated protein (RFXAP) because it is clearly a subunit of the RFX complex, and interacts with the RFX5 subunit, but does not contain the DNA binding domain motif characteristic of the RFX family of DNA binding proteins. Transfection of the RFXAP cDNA restores RFX binding activity and thus reactivates expression of all the endogenous MHC-II genes (α and β chain genes of HLA-DR, -DP and -DQ) in the 6.1.6 cell line. Each allele of the RFXAP gene in the 6.1.6 cell line contains a frame shift mutation resulting from the insertion of a single G nucleotide (*Figure 2*).

Isolation of the RFXAP gene has permitted the identification of several MHC-II deficiency patients belonging to complementation group D. Transfection of the RFXAP cDNA was found to complement cell lines derived from three patients that had not been classified into the existing complementation groups by somatic cell fusion experiments ([8], J. Villard, B. Lisowska-Grospierre, A. Fischer, P. van den Elsen, W. Reith and B. Mach, manuscript submitted). These patients are DA, ABI and ZM (unpublished patient). Patients DA and

ZM have the same mutation: they contain a homozygous frame shift mutation resulting from the deletion of a single G nucleotide in the RFXAP gene (*Figure 2*) ([8]; J. Villard, B. Lisowska-Grospierre, A. Fischer, P. van den Elsen, W. Reith and B. Mach, manuscript submitted). Although patients DA and ZM have the identical mutation, they come from different families and share no known common ancestry. In ABI, the RFXAP gene contains a homozygous point mutation generating a premature stop codon (*Figure 2*) (J. Villard, B. Lisowska-Grospierre, A. Fischer, P. van den Elsen, W. Reith and B. Mach, manuscript submitted). Patients from three additional families have been placed in group D by means of cell fusion experiments with ABI (B. Lisowska-Grospierre, personal communication).

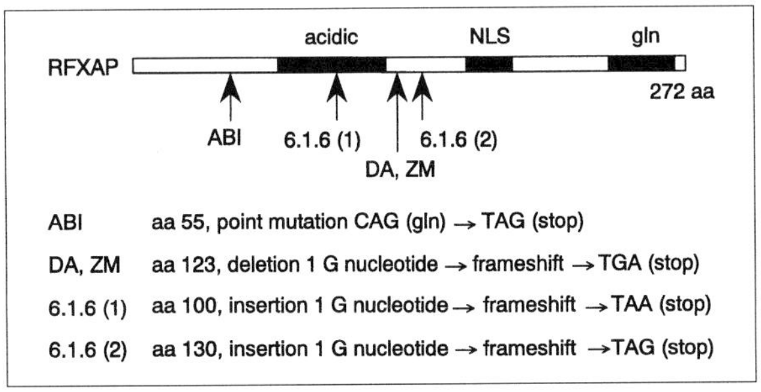

Figure 2. Structure and mutations of the RFXAP gene. The upper line represents a schematic map of the wild type 272 aa RFXAP protein, and indicates the positions of a putative bipartite nuclear localisation signal (NLS), and regions resembling transcription activation domains, namely a segment that is rich in acidic aa and a segment that is rich in glutamine (gln). Mutations in the RFXAP gene have been characterised in the *in vitro* generated mutant 6.1.6, and in three patients (ABI, DA, ZM) from complementation group C. All of the mutations result in the synthesis of severely truncated RFXAP proteins. In 6.1.6, each allele contains a frameshift mutation resulting from the insertion of a single G residue, at aa 100 and 130 respectively. The frame shifts lead to the use of out of frame stop codons further downstream (TAG and TAA). In patients DA and ZM, there is a homozygous frameshift mutation resulting from the deletion of a single G nucleotide at aa 123. The frame shift leads to the use of an out of frame TGA stop codon further downstream. In patient ABI there is a homozygous point mutation (CAG to TAG) generating a premature stop codon at aa 55.

The molecular defect in complementation group B

The gene affected in patients from complementation group B has not yet been identified. However, this gene must be essential for either the integrity or the binding activity of RFX, because cell lines in group B are characterised, like those in groups C and D, by a deficiency in binding of the RFX complex, the absence of DNAse I hypersensitive sites, and a bare promoter phenotype. Two possibilities come to mind; RFX may contain other subunits in addition to the two that have already been isolated (RFX5 and RFXAP), or binding activity of RFX may require activation by post-translational modifications such as phosphorylation. We currently favour the first possibility, because a third 41 kD polypeptide indeed co-purifies with RFX5 and RFXAP when RFX is immunoprecipitated from nuclear extracts with either RFX5 or RFXAP specific antibodies (W. Reith, K. Masternak and B. Mach, unpublished data).

Function and mode of action of CIITA

MHC-II genes, and the Ii, DMA and DMB genes required for antigen presentation by MHC-II molecules, are currently the only known target genes of CIITA. It is unlikely that CIITA plays an essential role in other systems, because all of the clinical manifestations exhibited by patients in which CIITA is mutated can be attributed to the deficiency in MHC-II expression.

CIITA functions as a "master regulator" controlling the cell-type specificity, inducibility and level of MHC-II expression. The CIITA gene is expressed in a cell type specific manner that correlates closely with MHC-II expression ([9,13], L. Otten, V. Steimle, B. Mach, unpublished results). In addition, the following characteristic features of MHC-II expression have been attributed directly to the expression status of CIITA.

a. Constitutive expression of MHC-II genes in B cells is determined by constitutive expression of CIITA [9].

b. CIITA expression is essential for the activation of MHC-II gene transcription in response to IFN-γ, and induction of MHC-II expression by IFN-γ is in fact mediated by induction of CIITA expression (*Figure 3*) [13].

c. Differentiation of B cells into mature plasma cells is accompanied by the loss of MHC-II expression, a process believed to be mediated by a dominant repression mechanism. This loss of MHC-II expression has been shown to result from silencing of the CIITA gene.

d. It has long been a puzzle that MHC-II gene expression is induced in human T cells following their activation but not in activated mouse T cells. This has recently been shown to be due to a species specific difference in CIITA expression; CIITA is expressed in activated human T cells but not in activated mouse T cells.

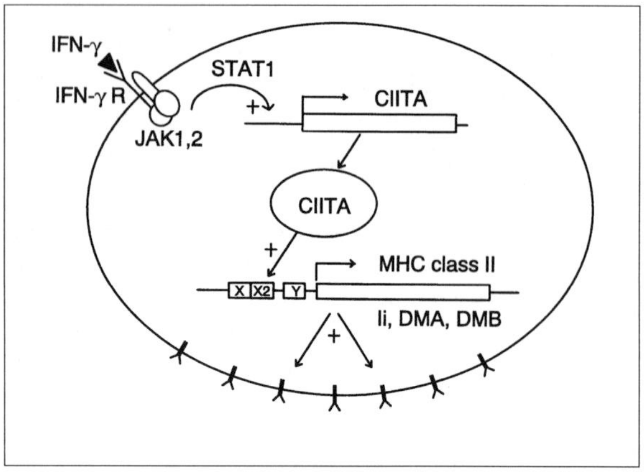

Figure 3. Schematic representation of the role of CIITA in the induction of MHC-II expression by IFN-γ. Activation of the interferon γ receptor (IFN-γR) generates intracellular signals that induce transcription of the CIITA gene. These intracellular signals are known to include activation of the receptor associated Jak1 and Jak2 kinases (Jak: Janus kinase), followed by recruitment of STAT1 to the receptor/kinase complex, and then phosphorylation, dimerization and nuclear import of the STAT1 (STAT: signal transducer and activator of transcription). STAT1 probably contributes directly to the activation of CIITA expression by binding to and activating promoter IV of the CIITA gene (see *Figure 4*). Induced CIITA expression then activates transcription of the MHC-II, Ii and DM genes.

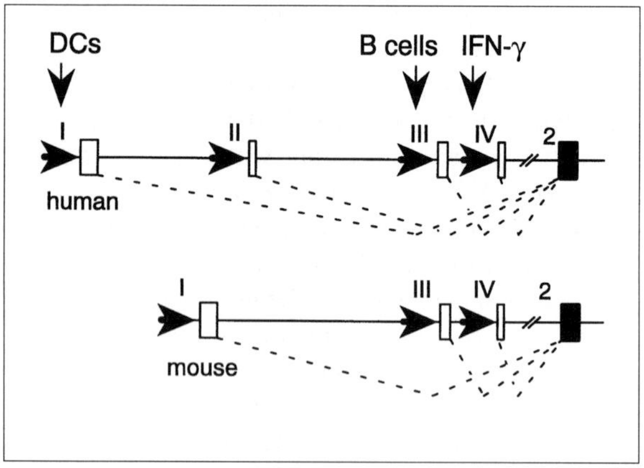

Figure 4. Expression of the CIITA gene is controlled by alternative promoters. Four independent promoters (I, II, III, IV) drive expression of the human CIITA gene. In mice, only three promoters have been identified (I, III, IV). Each promoter precedes an alternative first exon (open boxes) that is spliced (dotted lines) to the common second exon (solid box). In both man and mice, promoter I is used specifically in dendritic cells (DCs), promoter III is used mainly in B cells, and promoter IV is responsible for the induction by IFN-γ. The specificity of promoter II in the human gene has not been established. Figure is adapted from reference [14].

e. The level of MHC-II expression is modulated by the level of CIITA. Analysis of a large number of human and mouse cell lines and tissues has demonstrated that there is a tight quantitative correlation between the level of MHC-II expression and that of CIITA expression (L. Otten, A. Mottet, V. Steimle, B. Mach, in preparation). In addition, experimental modulation of CIITA expression using a tetracycline inducible system has shown that the level of CIITA expression directly determines the level of MHC-II expression (L. Otten, A. Mottet, V. Steimle, B. Mach, in preparation).

Interestingly, expression of both the human and mouse CIITA gene is directed by at least three independent promoters (promoters I, III and IV) preceding three alternative 5' exons (*Figure 4*) [14]. A fourth promoter (promoter II) has been identified in the human gene but not in the mouse gene (*Figure 4*) [14]. These promoters differ in their cell-type specificity and response to IFN-γ. It is thus the differential activity of the different CIITA promoters that ultimately determines the cell-type specificity and inducibility of MHC-II gene expression. Promoter I is used specifically in dendritic cells. Promoter III primarily controls constitutive expression in B cells. Promoter IV is largely responsible for IFN-γ induced expression. The specificity of promoter II is not known [14].

Although the crucial biological function of CIITA in the activation of MHC-II expression is now firmly established, its mode of action remains unsolved. It activates MHC-II gene transcription *via* the promoter proximal region containing the S, X, X2 and Y regulatory sequences [13], but does not appear to achieve this directly by binding to DNA [9]. No known DNA-binding domain is apparent in CIITA, and no DNA-binding activity has been demonstrated. On the other hand, it does contain acidic and proline/serine/threonine rich regions reminiscent of the transcription activation domains commonly found in transcription factors [9]. Evidence that the acidic region is indeed an activation domain relies on the findings that it is essential for the activity of CIITA, can be replaced by activation domains from heterologous transcription factors, and can indeed function as an activation domain when fused to a heterologous DNA-binding protein (V. Steimle, B. Mach, unpublished data). This has led to the hypothesis that CIITA may be a non-DNA-binding co-activator that is recruited to MHC-II promoters indirectly *via* protein-protein interactions with DNA-binding proteins such as RFX, X2BP and NF-Y, and activates transcription *via* its acidic region. However, protein-protein interactions between CIITA and proteins that bind to MHC-II promoters remain to be demonstrated.

Whatever its mode of action will turn out to be, there appears to be a requirement for binding of ATP or GTP. CIITA contains an ATP/GTP binding motif that is essential for its ability to activate transcription of MHC-II genes, and can indeed bind ATP and GTP (V. Steimle, B. Mach, unpublished results). The function of this ATP/GTP binding activity remains unknown.

References

1. Reith W, Steimle V, Mach B. Molecular defects in the bare lymphocyte syndrome and the regulation of MHC class II genes. *Immunol Today* 1995; 16:539-46.
2. Mach B, Steimle V, Martinez-Soria E, Reith W. Regulation of MHC class II genes: lessons from a disease. *Annu Rev Immunol* 1996; 14:301-31.
3. Reith W, Steimle V, Lisowska-Grospierre B, Fischer A, Mach B. Molecular basis of major histocompatibility class II deficiency. In: Ochs H, Puck J, Smith E eds. *Primary immunodeficiency diseases, a molecular and genetic approach.* New York: Oxford University Press, 1997 (in press).
4. Glimcher LH, Kara CJ. Sequences and factors: a guide to MHC class-II transcription. *Annu Rev Immunol* 1992; 10:13-49.
5. Reith W, Satola S, Herrero Sanchez C, Amaldi I, Lisowska-Grospierre B, Griscelli C, Hadam MR, Mach B. Congenital immunodeficiency with a regulatory defect in MHC class II gene expression lacks a specific HLA-DR promoter binding protein, RF-X. *Cell* 1988; 53:897-906.
6. De Preval C, Lisowska-Grospierre B, Loche M, Griscelli C, Mach B. A *trans*-acting class II regulatory gene unlinked to the MHC controls expression of HLA class II genes. *Nature* 1985; 318:291-3.
7. Durand B, Kobr M, Reith W, Mach B. Functional complementation of MHC class II regulatory mutants by the purified X box binding protein RFX. *Mol Cell Biol* 1994; 14:6839-47.
8. Durand B, Sperisen P, Emery P, Barras E, Zufferey M, Mach B, Reith W. RFXAP, a novel subunit of the RFX DNA binding complex is mutated in MHC class II deficiency. *EMBO J* 1997; 16: 1045-55.
9. Steimle V, Otten LA, Zufferey M, Mach B. Complementation cloning of an MHC class II transactivator mutated in hereditary MHC class II deficiency (or bare lymphocyte syndrome). *Cell* 1993; 75:135-46.
10. Steimle V, Durand B, Barras E, Zufferey M, Hadam MR, Mach B, Reith W. A novel DNA binding regulatory factor is mutated in primary MHC class II deficiency (bare lymphocyte syndrome). *Genes Dev* 1995; 9:1021-32.
11. Herrero Sanchez C, Reith W, Silacci P, Mach B. The DNA-binding defect observed in major histocompatibility complex class II regulatory mutants concerns only one member of a family of complexes binding to the X boxes of class II promoters. *Mol Cell Biol* 1992; 12:4076-83.
12. Emery P, Durand B, Mach B, Reith W. RFX proteins, a novel family of DNA binding proteins conserved in the eukaryotic kingdom. *Nucleic Acids Res* 1996; 24:803-7.
13. Steimle V, Siegrist CA, Mottet A, Lisowska-Grospierre B, Mach B. Regulation of MHC class II expression by Interferon-gamma mediated by the transactivator gene CIITA. *Science* 1994; 265:106-9.
14. Muhlethaler-Mottet A, Otten L, Steimle V, Mach B. Expression of MHC class II molecules in different cellular and functional compartments is controlled by differential usage of multiple promoters of the transactivator CIITA. *EMBO J* 1997 (in press).

Plenary lectures

2 • HLA diversity

Definition and importance of HLA class I null alleles: a new role for serological HLA class I typing

P. Parham

Department of Structural Biology, Fairchild Building, Stanford University, Stanford, CA 94305-5400, USA

At the eleventh International Histocompatibility Workshop and Conference I reported on molecular analyses of HLA class I of Amerindian populations and the insights they had provided as to the mechanism and manner by which new class I alleles are formed. In the research leading to the twelfth workshop, analysis of HLA class I in many Amerindian groups has been performed, confirming and extending the earlier results of Belich *et al.* [1] and Watkins *et al.* [2]. New HLA class I alleles are usually formed by conversion or recombination between pairs of existing alleles or genes and only rarely by point substitution. New HLA-B alleles are formed at a higher rate than HLA-A or -C, with HLA-A evolving new alleles somewhat more rapidly than HLA-C. The indigenous populations of Latin American countries have evolved many more HLA class I alleles than their counterparts in northern America, a difference that is primarily due to the HLA-B locus. In the populations of southern America, older HLA-B alleles have been, to a considerable extent, replaced by newer recombinant alleles, revealing the general trend for allele turnover and demonstrating that 10,000-35,000 years (the time that human populations have lived in America) can be sufficient to replace a founding set of HLA-B alleles by a derived set of recombinants. These observations and their possible interpretations have been recently reviewed in Parham and Ohta [3]. Here I describe a complementary study of the evolutionary mechanisms that inactivate functioning HLA class I alleles and their implications for typing and matching for transplantation. These studies were performed in collaboration with the groups of Derek Middleton, Jim McCluskey, XiaGong Gao and their colleagues, and are described in detail by Magor *et al.* [4].

Structures of three inactivated alleles of HLA-A*2402

Since the eleventh workshop a number of groups have identified HLA class I alleles that do not express normal levels of class I antigen at the cell surface [5-8]. Such "null" alleles have been identified in three ways: family study showing the segregation of a serologically blank allele; comparison of DNA and serological typing revealing individuals who are positive for an allele but lack the antigen; and the discovery of individuals who lack expression of any HLA-A antigens and are therefore homozygous for a null allele. The null alleles so far characterized are all of the HLA-A locus: subtypes of A1, A2, A3 and A24. We have now determined the structure and defect of three null variants of HLA-A*2402, the common allele encoding the HLA-A24 antigen.

The HLA-A*2409N allele

Using serological methods Middleton's group discovered an A*24null that segregates within a family. The null allele has the property of conferring apparent homozygosity to any expressed allele with which it is paired, thereby producing a pattern of homozygosity within a family that cannot be explained by Mendelian segregation of the typed antigens. When the family was submitted to HLA class I DNA typing the null allele typed as an A*2402 allele, with no differences from the common A*2402 allele being detected.

To determine the cause of the null phenotype we had initially hoped to adapt procedures that had been successfully used in analyses of expressed HLA-A, B and C alleles. We reasoned, incorrectly as it turned out, that the chance of the defect in the A*24null allele interfering with both protein and mRNA expression was slight and that an mRNA-based cloning approach to structure determination should work [9]. To this end a B cell line (SUS-NF) was made from a family member expressing the A*24null allele. Messenger RNA was isolated from the cell line and used as starting material for the isolation and sequencing of HLA-A clones [9-10]. Partial sequence determination of more than 50 HLA-A cDNA clones revealed no single clone resembling A*2402: every clone isolated corresponded to A*0205, the allele responsible for the HLA-A2 antigen of SUS-ND. Either the mRNA levels of the A*24null allele were highly reduced, or the null allele contained changes in the sequences of the priming sites used for polymerase chain reaction (PCR) amplification. To address these questions a pair of oligonucleotide primers derived from HLA-A coding region sequences was used to amplify SUS-NF cDNA, in place of the primers from the 5' and 3' untranslated regions used in our routine cDNA cloning method [10]. Again, only cDNA clones corresponding to A*0205 were obtained, suggesting mRNA levels for the A*24null allele are very low. Genomic DNA from SUS-NF cells was then used as the template for PCR amplification of a fragment of the HLA-A gene encompassing parts of exons 3 and 4. After cloning the amplification product, random clones were selected for sequence analysis. This strategy produced equal numbers of genomic clones corresponding to A*0205 and the null A*24 allele. Moreover within the regions of exon 2 and 3 sequenced, the null allele was identical to A*2402. Similar analysis of a cell expressing "wild-type" A*2402 in conjunction with A*0202 gave similar numbers of A*2402 and A*0202 clones, irrespective of whether the analysis was performed at the cDNA or genomic DNA level. In conclusion, the presence of a null allele related to A*2402 in the SUS-ND genome was confirmed and the cause of defective expression was shown to reduce the level of mRNA expression as well as that of antigenic protein.

From this preliminary analysis it was apparent that the strategy necessary for identifying the cause for non-expression of the null A*24 allele, was characterization of the structure and function of full-length genomic clones. Given that potential sites for inactivation exist at sites throughout the gene it was essential that the entire gene be sequenced and that *a priori* assumptions not be made as to the likely site of inactivation or the number of changes contributing to the phenotype. No matter where the defect resides, an essential part of the analysis had to be comparison of the sequence of the null allele with that of a functional "wild-type" A*2402 allele. One of the very first HLA class I sequences obtained was that of an A*24 allele and N'guyen et al had indeed completely sequenced a genomic clone [11]. This sequence, originally designated as A*2401, proved to have a number of errors in the coding region and the A*2401 designation was later dropped. With this background it was highly likely that additional sequence errors were present in the noncoding regions of the A*2401 sequence, and given this possibility a meaningful analysis of the A*24 allele from SUS-NF necessitated independent sequencing of a wild-type A*2402 genomic clone. Previously we had sequenced A*2402 cDNA from SHJO and this cell line was therefore selected for the isolation of HLA-A genomic clones [12]. The second HLA-A allele of SHJO is A*2301, an allele we had previously shown to be closely related to A*2402 [12]. We decided to perform parallel analysis of the A*2301 gene, reasoning that pairwise comparison of A*2402 to a closely related functional allele (A*2301) and to the related non-functional null allele could provide additional insight regarding the evolution of HLA class I alleles.

Genomic DNA preparations from SUS-NF and SHJO were digested with the restriction enzyme *Eco* RI and fractionated on agarose gels. The 6.7kb fragments corresponding to HLA class I genes were used to make genomic libraries from which clones corresponding to the A*24null and A*0205 alleles of SUS-NF and the A*2402 and A*2301 alleles of SHJO were isolated. The complete nucleotide sequences of each clone in both orientations were determined [4]. As anticipated the previously determined A24 genomic sequence of N'guyen *et al.* [11] differed at many positions from that of the A*2402 sequence obtained from SHJO [12]. In contrast the introns and non-coding regions of the A*2402 and A*2301 alleles from SHJO had identical sequences, the only differences between the two alleles being the five exonic substitutions previously described [12].

The homogeneity in the non-coding sequences of the A*2301 and A*2402 genes suggested that the functional differences between A*2402 and the A*24null allele of SUS-NF would not be obscured by an accumulation of other neutral changes. This proved to be the case: the A*24null allele of SUS-NF differs from A*2402 by a single nucleotide change in exon 4 that causes translation termination at residue 225 of the mature class I heavy chain. (This substitution was just outside the segment of exon 4 that had been characterized in the earlier PCR characterization of the two HLA-A alleles of SUS-ND.) According to the agreed procedures the null A*24 allele of SUS-NF has been named A*2409N [13].

The predicted consequence of a stop codon in exon 4 is that the heavy chain protein made from the A*2409N allele would consist of a leader peptide, α1 and α2 domains, and a piece of the α3 domain. The expectations of such a heavy chain protein are that it would not associate with β2 microglobulin or be membrane-bound, but be secreted from the cell by the constitutive pathway of exocytosis. Not obvious from the position of the stop codon was why mRNA levels were undetectable in SUS-NF cells, although that observation was consistent with our inability to immunoprecipitate any protein product from the A*2409N allele, either from cell lysates or the culture medium. To determine if the single substitution in exon 4 was responsible for loss of mRNA expression as well as cell surface A24 antigen, the A*2402 and A*2409N genomic clones were transfected into the class I deficient cell line LCL.721.221 [4]. The transfected cells were assayed for cell surface expression of HLA class I using the monomorphic anti-class I monoclonal antibody W6/32 and for polyadenylated A*24 message using a reverse transcriptase PCR assay. The results of this experiment showed that the A*2402 transfectant had high levels of mRNA and of protein at the cell surface, whereas neither mRNA nor protein were detectable for the A*2409N transfectant. In conclusion the single nucleotide substitution that distinguishes A*2409N from A*2402 and introduces a nonsense codon in exon 4, reduces mRNA levels to the point of their being undetectable. In reality it is the reduction of mRNA in the cytoplasm that is the direct cause of the null phenotype rather than the truncated nature of the encoded protein. We were initially surprised that a single nucleotide substitution had such a profound effect upon the levels of mRNA. However, a search of the literature revealed that the introduction of nonsense codons within genes often has this type of effect and that its magnitude increases with proximity of the nonsense codon to the 5' end of the reading frame. In immunoglobulin genes the effect is particularly strong and the same would seem true for HLA class I [4].

The A*2411N allele

When the A*2409N allele was first examined by DNA typing it was indistinguishable from the functional A*2402 allele. Once the difference between the two alleles had been determined it became trivial to design oligonucleotides for either SSO typing or SSP typing that would distinguish the two alleles. From further screening of the population of Northern Ireland, Middleton and coworkers had identified additional persons who typed genotypically for A*24, but were serologically negative. These ten donors were then assayed for the substitution in codon 249 found in A*2409N: eight of the ten typed identically to A*2409N, whereas the other two still typed identically to A*2402. The latter individuals were presumed to carry A*24null alleles that are inactivated differently to A*2409N and further investigation was directed toward their characterization. A transformed B cell line was made from one of the two individuals (BM2406) and a genomic clone for the A*24null allele isolated and sequenced. The BM2406 cell line was indeed found to possess a novel A*24null allele, which was similar to A*2409N, in that it differs from A*2402 by a single nucleotide change in exon 4. The change, however, is an insertion of a nucleotide in codon 183, the first codon of exon 4, which by changing the frame of translation induces chain termination at codon 196. This second inactivated A*24 allele, now designated A*2411N [13], is again similar to A*2409N in producing undetectable levels of mRNA as was shown by studying a transfectant of LCL.721 expressing A*2411N [4].

Our next goal was to determine whether the A*24null allele from the second individual (BM2307) who typed negatively for A*2409N, was A*2411N. The nucleotide insertion in exon 4 of A*2411N adds an additional cytosine to a run of seven cytosines, a change that could be difficult to type using SSO or SSP. As an alternative approach to typing BM2307 we PCR amplified the region containing the run of cytosines from BM2307 genomic DNA and determined its sequence. The sequence contained the additional cytosine, consistent with BM2307 expressing the A*2411N allele [4].

The A*2402^{low} allele (A*2402102L)

A different type of A*24null allele was discovered by McCluskey, Gao and Lienert in Adelaide, South Australia. This allele was found segregating in the family of a patient with leukemia who needed a bone marrow transplant. A transformed cell line (6319) was made from the peripheral blood B cells of one family member who expressed the A*24null allele and, after a preliminary analysis to identify the likely defect, a 6.7kb *Eco* RI genomic clone encoding the allele was isolated and fully sequenced [4]. Like A*2409N and A*2411N the third A*24null differs from A*2402 by a single nucleotide change, but the change is different: a point substitution at the 3' end of intron 2, near exon 3 and seven nucleotides upstream of the intron 2 acceptor splice site. Transfection of the gene into LCL.721.221 cells produced cells expressing small amounts of W6/32-reactive protein and of messenger RNA [4]. We estimate that A*24 expression is on the order of 1% of the normal A*2402 level. Thus this A*24null allele, provisionally called A*2402low, is qualitatively different from A*2409N and A*2411N in that it encodes the same protein as A*2402 and makes a small amount of it. To reflect this difference the A*2402low allele has been designated as A*2402102L, to reflect low expression, and the common A*2402 allele renamed A*2402101. The A*24 mRNA made by the A*2402low transfectant consists of two species present in roughly equal amounts: a normal A*2402 message and an alternatively spliced species that lacks exon 3. Consistent with this pattern of alternate splicing was the finding that cDNA cloning from the 6319 cell line only gave A*24 messages that lacked exon 3. This analysis shows that point substitution in intron 2 has the combined effect of greatly reducing the level of mRNA while changing the pattern of splicing [4]. The A*24null allele described by Marie-Marthe Tongio and colleagues appears identical to A*24low (A*2402102) [14].

Mechanisms of HLA-A*2402 inactivation

HLA-A*2402 is found throughout the world and in eastern Asian and Amerindian populations reaches frequencies as high as 64% [15]. Each of the three A*24null alleles differs from A*2402 by a single nucleotide change: A*2409N and A*2402low by point substitution and A*2411N by a nucleotide insertion *(Figure 1).* Each of the A*24null alleles has independently evolved from functional A*2402 alleles by a

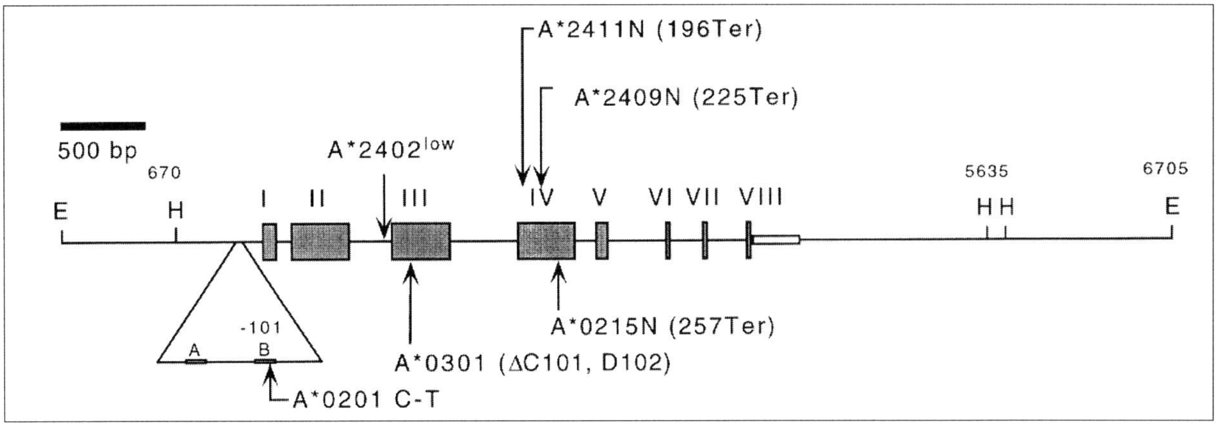

Figure 1. Location within the gene of inactivating mutations in HLA-A null alleles. A schematic map of the locus is shown with blocks and Roman numerals designating the the exons. Inactivating mutations in the A*2409N, A*2411N and A*2402low alleles are indicated above the map, while those characterized by other investigators are shown below. The location of the nonsense codons (Ter) and deleted (D) codons are indicated following the allele designation. *Eco* R1 and *Hind* III sites are indicated by E and H respectively. Only for the three A*24null alleles have complete sequences been determined and the identified substitutions proven to be responsible for the phenotype. For the HLA-A null alleles substitutions additional to those shown may exist and contribute to the null phenotype. Reference to the other HLA-A null alleles are: A*0201 [6], A*0301 [8] and A*0215N [7].

single mutational event. Such events have had the effect of inactivating the expression and function of A*2402. The nucleotide substitution distinguishing A*2409N is unique amongst the known HLA class I genes, indicating this allele was formed by point substitution. In contrast the nucleotide substitution distinguishing A*2402low from A*2402 is also present in the pseudogenes HLA-K and HLA-L. Thus A*2402low could have evolved from A*2402, either by point substitution or by intergenic conversion with HLA-K or HLA-L. On balance we favour the latter hypothesis because conversions rather than point substitutions are the predominant events that evolve new HLA class I alleles from the old [3]. The nucleotide insertion that distinguishes A*2411N is also present in a pseudogene, HLA-J. Again there are two possibilities for the evolution of this allele from A*2402: de novo insertion due to slippage of DNA polymerase during replication, or intergenic conversion with HLA-J. As we have no knowledge of the frequency of de novo insertion events in HLA class I genes it is difficult to hazard which of these two mechanisms is more likely.

Significance of HLA class I null alleles for transplantation

Although the inactivated A*24null alleles only differ from the common, functional A*2402 allele by single nucleotide changes the potential effect of these changes on function and histocompatibility are immense. This can be seen by considering imaginary transplant situations in which the donor and the recipient are completely HLA matched except one expresses A*2402 and the other a null allele, for example A*2409N.

If an A*2402 kidney or heart were transplanted into an A*2409N recipient, the recipient's immune system would recognize A*2402 as a completely histoincompatible class I antigen against which potent alloreactive antibody and cytotoxic T cell responses could be made. The reciprocal situation, transplantation of an A*2409N organ to an A*2402 donor would not stimulate the recipient's immune system in a comparable fashion. Donor lymphocytes carried in the graft have the potential to be activated by the A*2402 antigen of the recipient while natural killer (NK) cells of the recipient, which are reactive to loss of self class I, could attack cells of the graft.

In bone marrow transplantation the situation is reversed. The combination in which the graft has A*2409N and the recipient expresses A*2402 is that creating the greatest histoincompatibility. Here the B cells and T cells of the graft could mount a strong alloreactive response against the A*2402 of the recipient leading to graft-versus-host disease. In the reciprocal situation, where A*2402 bone marrow is transplanted into an A*2409N recipient, the B and T cells of the graft will see the recipient as self. The recipient's response to the graft will generally be of secondary consequence unless the pretreatment has failed to eliminate haematopoietic elements. In the latter circumstances the recipient's immune system could reject the graft by raising antibodies and cytotoxic T cells against A*2402. As the recipient lacks the A*2402 antigen of the graft, NK cells from the graft might attack cells of the recipient. This could be advantageous in eliminating residual elements of the recipient's haematopoietic system including leukemia cells, but could also endanger other tissues.

In the context of this discussion the functionality of A*2402low is unknown and of interest. Expression of A*2402 at only 1% of the normal level must greatly reduce antigen presentation to T cells and the inhibitory regulation of NK cells. On the other hand there is precedent for alloreactive cytotoxic T cells being able to kill target cells expressing comparably reduced levels of HLA-B*3503 [16]. Whether such levels can stimulate an alloreactive response or select a CD8+T cell repertoire is another question, but one central to the impact of A*2402low in the transplant setting.

Serological typing is needed to search for HLA null class I alleles

Although the difference between null and normal subtypes of an allele has the potential to produce major histoincompatibility in certain transplant situations, the overall relevance of HLA class I null alleles will depend upon their frequency within the populations of patients seeking transplants and of donors providing tissue. Given that HLA class I DNA typing is still in its infancy, the number of HLA class I null alleles that has emerged so far is impressive *(Figure 1).* Moreover, a number of them have been discovered in the families of patients seeking treatment. From study of the population of

Northern Ireland there is every indication that A*24null alleles are at a frequency (0.14% in a screen of 5000 individuals) that suggests their detection should be incorporated into high resolution HLA typing in that locale (personal communication). Similarly, other HLA class I null alleles may be preferentially found in particular populations.

Comparison of serological and DNA typing is the best approach for the identification of HLA class I null alleles, and the need to define the null alleles provides a compelling reason for maintaining serological typing while the DNA-based methods are implemented and refined. Once gene cloning and sequencing have identified the nucleotide changes that distinguish a null allele from its expressed progenitor it will then usually be possible to incorporate the unequivocal identification of the null allele into schemes for DNA typing. This approach should prove effective in the definition of HLA-A and B null alleles. Less clear is how null alleles of the HLA-C locus, for which serological typing is inadequate and levels of expression are already low, are to be defined. From the present set of data it appears as though HLA-A null alleles are more common, but that might merely reflect the more advanced state of development of DNA typing for HLA-A and the less complicated serology for that locus.

As a final point, I wish to emphasize the effects that the inactivating nucleotide changes have on messenger RNA levels. In general mRNA levels of null alleles are dramatically lower than for other alleles and often are at levels which are difficult to detect. Thus DNA systems of typing based on mRNA are less compatible with the typing of HLA class I null alleles than are those based upon genomic DNA.

Acknowledgements

Research in the author's laboratory was supported by NIH grant AI-24258. The author acknowledges the essential contributions of K.E. Magor, E. Taylor, S. Shen, E. Martinez-Naves, R.S. Wells, J.E. Gumperz, E. Adams, A.-M. Little, F. Williams, D. Middleton, X. Gao, J. McCluskey and K. Lienert to the research described here.

References

1. Belich MP, Madrigal JA, Hildebrand WH, Zemmour J, Williams RC, Luz R, Petzl-Erler ML, Parham P. Unusual HLA-B alleles in two tribes of Brazilian Indians. *Nature* 1992 ; 357 : 326-9.
2. Watkins DI, McAdam SN, Liu X, Strang CR, Milford EL, Levine CG, Garbe TL, Dogon AL, Lord CI, Ghim SH, Troup GM, Hughes AL, Letvin NL. New recombinant HLA-B alleles in a tribe of South American Amerindians indicate rapid evolution of MHC class I loci. *Nature* 1992 ; 357 : 329-33.
3. Parham P, Ohta T. Population biology of antigen presentation by MHC class I molecules. *Science* 1996 ; 272 : 67-73.
4. Magor KE, Taylor E, Shen S, Martinez-Naves E, Wells RS, Gumperz JE, Adams E, Little AM, Williams F, Middleton D, Gao X, McCluskey, Parham P, Lienert K. Natural inactivation of a common HLA allele (A*2402) has occurred on at least three separate occasions. *J Immunol* 1997, in press.
5. Lardy NM, Bakas RM, Van der Horst AR, Van Twuyver E, Bontrop R, de Waal LP. *Cis*-acting regulatory elements abrogate allele-specific HLA class I gene expression in healthy individuals. *J Immunol* 1992 ; 148 : 2572-7.
6. Balas A, Garcia-Sanchez F, Gomez-Reino F, Viccario JL. HLA class I allele (HLA-A2) expression defect associated with a mutation in its enhancer B inverted cat box in two families. *Hum Immunol* 1994 ; 41 : 69-73.
7. Ishikawa Y, Tokunaga K, Tanaka H, Nishimura M, Muraoka M, Fujii Y, Akaza T, Tadokoro K, Juji T. HLA-A null allele with a stop codon, HLA-A*0215N, identified in a homozygous state in a healthy adult. *Immunogenetics* 1995 ; 43 : 1-5.
8. Lienert K, Russ G, Lester S, Bennett G, Gao X, McCluskey J. Stable inheritance of an HLA-A "blank" phenotype associated with a structural mutation in the HLA-A*0301 gene. *Tissue Antigens* 1996; 48: 187-91.
9. Ennis PD, Zemmour J, Salter RD, Parham P. Rapid cloning of HLA-A,B cDNA by using the polymera-

se chain reaction: frequency and nature of errors produced in amplification. *Proc Natl Acad Sci USA* 1990 ; 87 : 2833-7.

10. Domena JD, Little A-M, Madrigal JA, Hildebrand WH, Johnston-Dow L, du Toit E, Bias WB, Parham P. Structural heterogeneity in HLA-B70, a high-frequency antigen of black populations. *Tissue Antigens* 1993 ; 42 : 509-17.
11. N'Guyen C, Sodoyer R, Trucy J, Strachan T, Jordan BR. The *HLA-AW24* gene: sequence, surroundings and comparison with the *HLA-A2* and *HLA-A3* genes. *Immunogenetics* 1985 ; 21 : 479-89.
12. Little AM, Madrigal JA, Parham P. Molecular definition of an elusive third HLA-A9 molecule HLA-A9.3. *Immunogenetics* 1992 ; 35 : 41-5.
13. Marsh SGE. Nomenclature for factors of the HLA system, update April 1996. *Tissue Antigens* 1996 ; 48 : 69-70.
14. Laforet M, Parissiadis A, Froelich N, Tongio MM. Lack of HLA-A1 and A24 antigenic expression in normal individuals carrying HLA-A*01 and A*24 alleles. *Hum Immunol* 1996 ; 47 : 16.
15. Imanishi T, Akaza T, Kimura A, Tokunaga K, Gojobori T. W15.1: allele and haplotype frequencies for HLA and complement loci in various ethnic groups. In: Tsuji K, Aizawa M, Sasazuki T, eds. *HLA 1991, Proceedings of the Eleventh International Histocompatibility Workshop and Conference*, vol. 1. Oxford, New York, Tokyo : Oxford University Press , 1992 : 1065-220.
16. Zemmour J, Little AM, Schendel DJ, Parham P. The HLA-A,B "negative" mutant cell line C1R expresses a novel HLA-B35 allele, which also has a point mutation in the translation initiation codon. *J Immunol* 1992 ; 148 : 1941-8.

Allele specific peptide motifs of HLA molecules

H.G. Rammensee

Eberhard-Karls-Universität Tübingen, Interfakultäres Institut für Zellbiologie, Abteilung Immunologie, Auf der Morgenstelle 15, 72076 Tübingen, Germany

HLA class I and class II molecules are peptide receptors whose function is to sample peptides intracellularly and to present them on the cell surface for inspection by T cells. Peptide loading of class I molecules occurs mainly in the endoplasmatic reticulum(ER); the peptides are produced by cytolytic proteases and are transported into the ER by TAP molecules, or are produced, respectively trimmed, in the ER. In addition, class I molecules can be loaded in endocytic or phagocytic vesicles independent of cytosolic proteases and TAP. Class II molecules are loaded in endosomal compartments under contribution of a population of local enzymes like cathepsine D.

The structure of both HLA classes are remarkably similar [1]. Both have a peptide accommodating groove capable of interacting with a peptide stretch of 9 amino acids. For class I molecules, peptide ligands are 9mers or slightly longer. One or both of the termini is tightly hold by the edge of the groove. The side chains of 2 of the amino acids, one at position 2, 3, or 5 and the other at the C-terminus are anchored specifically by complementary pockets in the groove. In addition, some of the other residues, most notably P1, interact with complementary sites of the groove in a more degenerate way. The remaining residues point out of the groove and are available for interaction with the CDR3 region of the T cell receptor.

The termini of peptides presented by class II molecules are not fixed in the groove's ends and protrude at either side. Thus, class II ligands are longer than the groove; their length ranges anywhere from 12 to 25 amino acids. The nine amino acid stretch accomodate by the groove is designated by relative position numbers, P1 through P9, whereby P1 is defined as the residue anchored in the first pocket (located around amino acid 86 of the ß chain in HLA-DR molecules). Additional anchors are frequently at P4, P6, and P9.

Motifs

The characteristics shared by most of the peptides presented by a particular HLA molecule (allelic product) are summarized as a motif. Such motifs reflect the structure and the spacing of the respective pockets in the HLA groove, as well as additional interactions between peptide and groove. Motifs are useful for analysis of the relation between HLA sequence and structure, and, for practical purposes, for determining T cell epitopes.

HLA class I

A basic class I motif is defined by peptide length, usually 9 amino acids, and by the position and specificities of anchors. For a complete motif, preferences or abhorrences at non-anchor positions are included. Motifs are determined by sequence analysis of natural HLA ligands, preferentially by combining the results of pool sequencing of peptide mixtures, alignment of individually sequenced ligands, and peptide binding assays [2,3]. The numbers of HLA alleles are in excess of 50 for HLA-A, 100 for HLA-B, and 30 for HLA-C (*see elsewhere in this volume*). Each of the respective gene products carries its own individual peptide motif. The basic motifs of 46 HLA molecules are compiled in *Table I.* Identical or similar specificities of anchors are usually correlated with similar composition of the respective pockets in the HLA groove. For example, A*6801 and A*6901 share P2 specificity and show very similar amino acid residues in the B-pocket area positions 7,9,45,63,66,67,70,and 99. On the other hand, A*6901 and A*0201 share P9 specificity and also striking similarities in the amino acids contributing to the P9-binding pocket (77, 80, 81, 116, 123, 143, 147) [4].

The basic motifs in *Table I* give the impression that some HLA molecules are almost identical in their pep-

Table I. HLA class I motifs

	Position										
	1	2	3	4	5	6	7	8	9	10	11
A*0101		TS	**DE**	P			L		**Y**		
A*0201		**LM**				V			**VL**		
A*0202		**LA**							**LV**		
A*0205		**VQLI**				ILV			**V**		
A*0214		**VQL**				ILVF			**L**		
A*0301		**LVM**							**KYF**		
A*1101		**VI**	ML				LI		**KR**	**KR**	**KR**
A*2401		**Y**			IV	F			**LIF**		
A*3101	KR	LVYF	FLYW			LFVI			**R**		
A*3302	DE	AILF							**R**		
A*6801	DE	**VT**							**RK**		
A*6901	E	**VTA**	IFLM			IFL			**VL**		
B*0702	A	**P**	R						**LF**		
B*0801			**KR**		**KR**				LFM		
B*1402		**RK**	**LYF**		**RH**	**IL**			**L**		
B*1501		**QL**			IV				**FY**		
B*2702	K	**R**							**FYILW**		
B*2705	R	**R**							**LFRK**		
B*3501		**P**							**YFMLI**		
B*3503		**P**							**MLF**		
B*3701		**DE**			VI			**FML**	**IL**		
B*3801		H	DE						**FL**		
B*39011		**RH**				IVL			LVIM		
B*3902		**KQ**			ILFV				LFM		
B40		**E**	FIV						LWMA		
B*4006	GR	**E**	FILVY			I			**V**		
B*40012		**E**					IV		**L**		
B*4402		**E**							**FY**	FY	
B*4403		**E**							**YF**	YF	
B*5101	D	**APG**							**FI**		
B*5102		**PAG**	Y						**IV**		
B*5103		**APG**	Y						**VIF**		
B*5201		Q	FYW		LIV			IVMF	**IVMF**		
B*5301		**P**							**LIVMY**		
B*5401		**P**	FMR						A		
B*5501	A	**P**	RMY	T	V	FG		M	A		
B*5502	A	**P**	RMY	H				M	A		
B*5601	A	**P**	YNR						**AL**		
B*5801	KRI	**AST**		PEK	VILMF				**FW**		
B*6701	A	**P**	FM	G					**L**		
B*7801		**PAG**				ILFV		A			
C*w0301			VIYL	P		FY			**LFMI**		
C*w0401		**YPF**				VIL			**LFM**		
C*w0602					ILFM	VIL			LIVY		
C*w0702		YP			VYIL	VILM			**YFL**		
G		**IL**	P						**L**		

Compiled from [3,4,8-12]. Letters refer to the single letter amino acid code. Bold, anchors; Regular type, preferred residues.

Table II. HLA class II motifs

	Relative Position									
	1	2	3	4	5	6	7	8	9	10
DRB1*0101	**YVLF** **IA**M W			**LAIV** MNQ		**AGST** P			LAIV NFY	
DRB1*0301	**LIFM** **V**			**D**		KREQ N			YLF	
DRB1*0401	**FYW**I LVM			FWIL VAD E ***no*** ***RK***		NSTQ HR	polar chgd. aliph.		polar aliph. K	
DRB1*0402	**VILM**			YFWI LMR N ***no DE***		**NQST** **K**	RKH NQP		polar aliph. H	
DRB1*0404	**VILM**			FYWI LVM ADE ***no RK***		NTSQ R	polar chrgd. aliph.		polar aliph. K	
DRB1*0405	**FY**W VILM			VILM DE		NSTQ KD	polar chrgd. aliph.		**DEQ**	
DRB1*1101	WYF			MLV		RKH			AGSP	
DRB1*1201	**IL**FY V		**LMN** **VA**			VYFI NA			**YFMI** **V**	
DRB1*1501	LVI			FYI			ILVM F			
DRB5*0101	**FY**L M			QVIM					**RK**	
DQA1*0501/DQB1*0301	**FYIM** LV				**VL**IM Y		YFM LVI			
DPA1*0201/DPB1*0401	**FLY** MIVA						**FLY** MVIA			**VYI**A L
DPA1*0102/DPB1*0201	**FLM** **VWY**				**FLM** **Y**			**IAM** **V**		

from [3,7].

tide specificity. However, even very closely related HLA molecules sharing the same basic peptide motifs differ in their fine specificity (especially at the non-anchor positions). Thus, even closely related HLA molecules will present different if overlapping population of peptides, and for T cell epitope predictions, detailed motifs should be used, as compiled, *e.g.*, in [3].

HLA class II

A class II motif describes the sum of characteristics common to the nine amino acid stretches acommodated in the HLA groove of most of the peptide ligands associated with a particular class II molecule. Typically, this stretch starts at absolute position 3, 4, or 5 of class II ligands, with a considerable number of exceptions, however. Motifs are determined in principally the same way as for class I; due to the variable length of ligands, however, interpretation of pool sequencing results as well as alignment of individual ligands is more difficult [5,6].

Anchors of class II motifs are frequently more degenerate than those of class I molecules, allowing a number of different amino acids with similar characteristics (*e.g.*, all aromatic or most of the aliphatic amino acids). A few anchors, like P4 of DRB1*0301 (strictly aspartate) or P9 of DRB1*0405 (strictly D, E, or Q), are, in contrast, very specific. An important feature of class II motifs are residues not allowed at otherwise degenerate anchors. The positively charged amino acids arginine and lysine, for example, are not allowed at P4 of DRB1*0401 and 0404, whereas the acidic amino acids aspartate and glutamate are not liked by P4 of DRB1*0402. Again, anchor specificity is well reflected by pocket structure. For example, the specificity of the P1 anchor is strongly influenced by the nature of the residue at position ß86 of the DRB1 chain. Whenever this dimorphic position is occupied with a glycin, the resulting P1 pocket acommodates bulky aromatic side chains (*e.g.*, DRB1*0101, 0401, 0405); if ß86 is a valine, the P1 pocket is more limited to the smaller side chains of aliphatic amino acids (*e.g.*, DRB1*0402, 0404).

Since most autoimmune diseases are associated with particular HLA class II molecules, comparison of the peptide motifs of the disease associated alleles with that of closely related alleles not associated with the disease should be informative with respect to the disease inducing self or foreign peptides [7] *(Table II).*

References

1. Stern LJ, Wiley DC. Antigenic peptide binding by class I and class II histocompatibility proteins. *Structure* 1994;2:245-51.
2. Falk K, Rötzschke O, Stevanovič S, Jung G, Rammensee H-G. Allele-specific motifs revealed by sequencing of self-peptides eluted from MHC molecules. *Nature* 1991;351:290-6.
3. Rammensee HG, Friede T, Stevanovič S. MHC ligands and peptide motifs. First listing. *Immunogenetics* 1995;41:178-228.
4. Barouch D, Friede T, Stevanovič S, *et al.* HLA-A2 subtypes are functionally distinct in peptide binding and presentation. *J Exp Med* 1995;182:1847-56.
5. Falk K, Rötzschke O, Stevanovič S, Jung G, Rammensee HG. Pool sequencing of natural HLA-DR, DQ, and DP ligands reveals detailed peptide motifs, constraints of processing, and general rules. *Immunogenetics* 1994;39:230-42.
6. Hammer J, Valsasnini P, Tolba K, *et al.* Promiscuous and allele-specific anchors in HLA-DR-binding peptides. *Cell* 1993;74:197-203.
7. Friede T, Gnau V, Jung G, Keilholz W, Stevanovič S, Rammensee HG. Natural ligand motifs of closely related HLA-DR4 molecules predict features of rheumatoid arthritis associated peptides. *BBA* 1996; 1316: 85-101.
8. Barber LD, Gillececastro B, Percival L, Li XB, Clayberger C, Parham P. Overlap in the repertoires of peptides bound *in vivo* by a group of related class I HLA-B allotypes. *Curr Biol* 1995;5:179-90.
9. DiBrino M, Parker KC, Margulies DH, *et al.* The HLA-B14 peptide binding site can accommodate peptides with different combinations of anchor residues. *J Biol Chem* 1994;269:32426-34.
10. Diehl M, Münz C, Keilholz W, *et al.* Nonclassical HLA-G molecules are classical peptide presenters. *Curr Biol* 1996;6:305-14.
11. Lee N, Malacko AR, Ishitani A, *et al.* The membrane-bound and soluble forms of HLA-G bind identical sets of endogenous peptides but differ with respect to TAP association. *Immunity* 1995;3:591-600.
12. Steinle A, Falk K, Rötzschke O, *et al.* Motif of HLA-B*3503 peptide ligands. *Immunogenetics* 1996;43:105-7.

Nature of the minor histocompatibility antigens

E. Goulmy

Department of Immunohaematology and Blood Bank, University Hospital, Bulding 1, E3-Q, PO Box 9600, 2300 RC Leiden, The Netherlands

Human bone marrow transplants performed as therapeutical treatment of severe aplastic anaemia, leukaemia and immune deficiency disease became available in the seventies. For the present, the long-term results of allogeneic bone marrow transplantation (BMT) have greatly improved due to the use of HLA-matched siblings as marrow donors, advanced pretransplant chemoradiotherapy, the use of potent immunosuppressive drugs as Graft-versus-Host-Disease (GvHD) prophylaxis, better antibiotics and isolation procedures. Nonetheless, the results of clinical BMT reveal that the selection of MHC identical donors/recipients is not a guarantee of avoidance of GvHD or disease free survival even when donor and recipient are closely related. Allogeneic BMT especially in adults results, depending on the amount of T cell depletion of the graft, in uptil 80% of the cases in GvHD. In the HLA genotypically identical situation it amounts to 15-35% whereas in the phenotypical HLA matched recipient/donor combinations, the occurrence of GvHD is significantly higher *i.e.* 50-80% [1]. It is believed that disparities for minor histocompatibility antigens (mHag) between donor and recipient constitute a potential risk for GvHD or graft failure, which necessitate life long pharmacologic immunosuppression of organ and bone marrow transplant recipients. mHag can evoke strong MHC restricted cytotoxic (CTL) and proliferative T (Th) cell responses which can be measured *in vitro* [2]. Our laboratory has a series of well defined CTL and Th cell clones which are specific for sexlinked and non-sexlinked mHag, all of them are recognized in a classical MHC restricted fashion.

Functional studies

We studied the male specific mHag H-Y and five non-sexlinked mHag (designated HA-1 to HA-5) at three levels *i.e.* immunogenetics, immunogenicity and tissue distribution (as reviewed in [2]).

Immunogenetics

Immunogenetic studies revealed that some mHag appeared frequent (69-95%), others occurred with lesser frequencies (7-16%) in the healthy population. An analysis of the genetic traits demonstrated a Mendelian mode of inheritance independent of HLA.

Immunogenicity

Three sets of data are indicative for a hierarchy in immunogenicity among mHag. Firstly, CTL clones reactive to the same mHag HA-1 were obtained from peripheral blood lymphocytes of 3 out of 5 individuals each transplanted across a multiple and probably distinct mH barrier. Secondly, recent results indicate that the latter HA-1 specific CTL clones derived from different individuals, all seemed to use an identical TCR Vβ, showed remarkable similarities within the N-D-N regions, but used distinct Vα and γ segments. Thirdly, in a retrospective study, comprising 148 bone marrow donor/recipient pairs, investigating the influence of mHag HA-1 to HA-5 mismatching on the development of GvHD, we observed a significant correlation (P = 0.02) between mHag HA-1 mismatch and GvHD [3].

Tissue distribution

Tissue distribution studies revealed differential expression: some mHag (*i.e.* H-Y, HA-3 and HA-4) are expressed on haematopoietic as well as on non-haematopoietic cells, while the expression of other mHag (HA-1 and HA-2) is limited to cells of the haematopoietic lineage only. Moreover, all mHag are present on clonogenic leukemic precursor cells [4] as well as on circulating leukemic cells of lymphocytic and myeloid origin [5].

We may conclude from the results of the clinical related studies that mHag are involved in both Graft-versus-Host and Graft-versus-Leukemia activities.

Molecular nature of minor histocompatibility antigens

Using immuno and biochemical isolation and purification procedures combined with sensitization of target cells for T cell recognition, mHag peptide containing fractions responsible for target cell sensitization were identified. Subsequent mass spectometric analysis determined the amino acid (AA) sequence of to our knowledge the first mHag, *i.e.* HA-2, identified. Synthetic peptides generated accordingly sensitized an HA-2 negative target cell to lysis by the mHag HA-2 specific CTL and herewith confirmed the correct mHag HA-2 AA sequence. This peptide most probably originates from a member of the non-filament-forming class I myosin family [6].
Another mHag we recently identified is the male specific antigen H-Y [7], an antigen searched for since 1955. The first report on H-Y as a transplantation antigen is an untitled communication by Eichwald and Silmser. These authors observed that within two inbred strains of mice, most of the male-to-female skin grafts were rejected, whereas transplants made in other sex combinations nearly always succeeded [8]. In the human situation the first report on involvement of H-Y in transplantation appeared in 1976 [9]. It concerned a clinical observation of a bone marrow graft rejection of a male HLA identical sibling donor by his HLA identical sister. *In vitro* analysis of the posttransplant peripheral blood lymphocytes (PBLs) of this female patient (HLA phenotype: HLA-A2, -A2, -B44, -B60, -Cw3, -Cw5, -DR4, -DRw6) showed unambiguously strong CTL responses specific for male HLA-A2 positive target cells. Besides, this study also evidenced the first demonstration in man of the classical phenomenon of MHC restricted recognition of foreign antigen [9].
Sensitization to the H-Y antigen extends to organ transplantation, bloodtransfusion and possibly also pregnancy wherein MHC restricted T cell responses to the mHag H-Y in association with different MHC molecules are observed (reviewed in [2]).
The same isolation and identification techniques as applied for the characterization of mHag HA-2 (*described above*) was used to identify the human mHag H-Y. The H-Y antigen presented by HLA-B7 appears an 11-residue peptide derived from SMCY, an evolutionarily conserved protein encoded by the Y chromosome [7, 10]. The human Y gene coding for the mHag H-Y is possibly functioning as a gene controlling spermatogenesis. We are currently characterizing the mHag HA-1 as well as H-Y T cell epitopes eluted from other HLA molecules.
Summarizing, mHag are peptides from polymorphic self proteins. They are derived from evolutionarily conserved genes with important biological function.

Clinical applications

As more mHags become biochemically identified, molecular typing can now be used for diagnostic in bone marrow donor selection. Dissection of the major from the minor minors and their biochemical identification may aid in immunomodulatory approaches. Designing mHag peptide analogues which function as MHC or T cell receptor antagonists might interfere with the harmful anti-host T cell reactivities post HLA identical BMT. The potential application of mHag with broad tissue distribution like H-Y and HA-3 may aid in induction of tolerance in mHag negative bone marrow donors to prevent GvHD and in mHag negative bone marrow recipients to prevent rejection. The mHag H-Y peptide information may also be used in the generation of genetic probes to be used for prenatal diagnosis in sex-linked congenital abnormalities and investigating minimal residual disease and chimerism. Most promising is immunotherapy using CTLs specific for mHag peptide for the treatment of refractory, residual or relapsed leukemia. The mHag with restricted tissue distribution (*e.g.* HA-1 and HA-2) are candidates for adoptive immunotherapy of leukemia. Upon transfusion, the mHag peptide specific CTLs will kill the haematopoietic cells including the leukemia cells and will spare non-haematopoietic cells.

References

1. Beatty PG, Hervé P. Immunogenetic factors relevant to acute GvHD. In: Burakoff SJ, Deeg DHJ, Ferrara S, Atkinson K eds. *Graft-versus-host-disease, immunology, pathophysiology and treatment.* New York: Dekker, 1989: 415-23.
2. Goulmy E. Human minor histocompatibility antigens. *Curr Op Immunol* 1996; 8: 75-81.
3. Goulmy E, Schipper R, Pool J, Blokland E, Falkenburg JHF, Vossen J, Gratwohl A, Vogelsang

GB, van Houwelingen HC, van Rood JJ. Mismatches of minor histocompatibility antigens between HLA-identical donor and recipient and the development of graft-versus-host disease after bone marrow transplantation. *N Engl J Med* 1996; 334: 281-5.

4. Falkenburg F, Goselink H, van der Harst D, Van Luxemburg-Heijs SAP, Kooij-Winkelaar YMC, Faber LM, De Kroon J, Brand A, Fibbe WE, Willemze R, Goulmy E. Growth inhibition of clonogenic leukemic precursor cells by histocompatibility antigen-specific cytotoxic T lymphocytes. *J Exp Med* 1991; 174: 27-33.
5. Van der Harst D, Goulmy E, Falkenburg JHF, Kooij-Winkelaar YMC, Van Luxemburg SAP, Goselink HM, Brand A. Recognition of minor Histocompatibility antigens on lymphocytic and myeloid leukemic cells by cytotoxic T cell clones. *Blood* 1994; 83: 1060-66.
6. Den Haan JMM, Sherman NE, Blokland E, Huczko E, Koning F, Drijfhout JW, Skipper J, Shabanowitz J, Hunt DF, Engelhard VH, Goulmy E. Identification of graft versus host disease-associated human minor histocompatibility antigen. *Science* 1995; 268: 1476-80.
7. Wang W, Meadows LR, Den Haan JMM, Sherman NE, Chen Y, Blokland E, Shabanowitz J, Agulnik AI, Hendrickson RC, Bishop CE, Hunt DF, Goulmy E, Engelhard VH. Human H-Y: a male-specific histocompatibility antigen derived from the SMCY protein. *Science* 1995; 269: 1588-90.
8. Eichwald EJ, Slimser CR. *Transplant Bull* 1955; 2: 148-9.
9. Goulmy E, Termijtelen A, Bradley BA, Van Rood JJ. Alloimmunity to human H-Y. *Lancet* 1976; 2: 1206.
10. Den Haan JMM, Bontrop RE, Pool J, Sherman N, Blokland E, Engelhard VH, Hunt DF, Goulmy E. Conservation of minor histocompatibility antigens between human and non-human primates. *Eur J Immunol* 1996; 26: 2680-5.

NK cell receptors for polymorphic MHC class I molecules

L.L. Lanier

DNAX Research Institute of Molecular and Cellular Biology, 901 California Avenue, Palo Alto, California 94304, USA

T cells and Natural Killer (NK) cells are types of lymphocyte that arise from a common progenitor cell originating in the bone marrow [1]. Rearrangement of the T cell antigen receptor (TcR) genes and T cell maturation occurs in the thymus. By contrast, NK cells do not rearrange TcR genes and do not require a functional thymus for differentiation and maturation. While differing in expression of the TcR complex, NK cells and T cells share many common properties, reflecting their common origin. Both cell types mediate cytotoxicity by using a lytic process that involves the perforin or fas pathways. Upon activation, NK and T cells secrete many of the same cytokines, including interferon-γ, GM-CSF, IL-5, and TNF-α. Protective immunity against certain viruses, intracellular bacteria, and parasites is mediated by the cooperative efforts of NK and T cells, with the NK cells serving as a first line of defense during the early phases of the response.

While antigen receptors for B and T cells have been identified, no unique "NK receptor" has been found. However, NK cells express most of the "costimulatory" receptors and adhesion molecules that are present on T cells and it is possible that NK cells use these receptors to initiate cytotoxicity and cytokine secretion. Early during an infection, neutrophils and macrophages secrete a variety of pro-inflammatory cytokines and chemokines, as well as IL-12 and IL-15. These many serve to recruit and activate NK cells. In addition, cells at sites of inflammation often up-regulate cell surface molecules (e.g. the ICAMs, VCAM-1, CD58, etc.) that are ligands for the costimulatory receptors present on NK cells. These "non-specific" receptor-ligand interactions may be sufficient to deliver the "positive signals" that initiate NK cell effector function. The obvious disadvantage of this type of recognition system is that it would fail to discriminate between infected or abnormal cells and normal, bystander tissues that also up-regulate their adhesion molecules due to cytokine exposure.

A solution to this paradox was provided by Kärre and colleagues [2] who observed that NK cells preferentially killed certain tumors that had lost expression of H-2 class I molecules. While down-regulation of H-2 would circumvent recognition by CD8+ cytotoxic T lymphocytes (CTL), this apparently elicited a response by NK cells. Presumably, the NK cells initially bind and form conjugates with the tumor cells using undefined adhesion/costimulatory molecules. However, a central and unique aspect of NK cell recognition is their ability to determine whether or not the antigen presenting cell (APC) expresses normal amounts of major histocompatibility complex (MHC) class I on the cell surface. NK cells may kill APC lacking class I, but are inactivated and therefore do not lyse APC expressing class I molecules. Therefore, the function of NK cells is determined by a "positive signal" from the APC (possibly provided by costimulatory molecules or cytokines) and the lack of a "negative signal" generated by interactions between class I molecules on the APC and inhibitory MHC class I receptors on the NK cells. This model of opposing positive and negative signals to determine a functional outcome may represent a general theme in the immune system, as supported by recent studies demonstrating the agonist - antagonist relationship between CD28 and CTLA4 in T cell responses [3].

NK cell receptors for polymorphic MHC class I molecules

In rodents, the Ly49 receptors present on NK cells bind polymorphic H-2K, D, and L ligands and inhibit NK cell-mediated cytotoxicity [4]. At least 8 Ly49 genes are present on mouse chromosome 6 and these encode type II membrane proteins that form disulfide-linked homodimers [4]. The Ly49A, Ly49C, and Ly49G2 receptors are expressed on overlapping subsets of NK cells and function to prevent lysis of target cells expressing H-2 alleles that function as ligands for these receptors. Ly49 receptors have been implicated in the elimination of transplanted tumors lacking H-2 and in the rejection of allogeneic bone marrow grafts. The phenomenon of hybrid resistance, whereby parental bone marrow is rejected in F1 recipients, is mediated by NK cells and determined by Ly49 and H-2 interactions [5].

While human homologs of the rodent Ly49 genes have not been identified, another family of receptors, the Killer Cell Inhibitory Receptors (KIR), bind HLA class I ligands and inhibit human NK cell function [6]. Unlike Ly49, KIR are type I membrane glycoproteins of the immunoglobulin (Ig) superfamily that are expressed as monomers on subsets of NK cells and T cells. KIR are encoded by a family of related genes present on the telomeric end of chromosome 19. Two subgroups of KIR genes can be distinguished based on the presence of two or three Ig domains in their extracellular region [7-9]. These receptors bind HLA class I molecules and inhibit NK cell and T cell cytolytic function and cytokine production [10], presumably by their ability to recruit a phosphatase, SHP-1 [11, 12]. As yet, rodent homologs of the KIR genes have not been found and Southern blot analysis of genomic DNA isolated from several species indicated the existence of KIR homologs in primates, but not other mammals or birds.

Ly49 and KIR recognition of MHC class I

While structurally distinct, the KIR and Ly49 receptors interact with common regions of the human and mouse class I molecules, respectively. Binding of Ly49A to H-2Dd is blocked by antibodies directed against the $\alpha1/\alpha2$ domain of class I, but not antibodies against the $\alpha3$ region [4]. Similarly, interactions between KIR and their HLA-B and HLA-C ligands involve sites localized in the $\alpha1$ domain of the human class I heavy chain. A polymorphism at residues 77 and 80 in the HLA-C alleles is recognized by KIR molecules that are identified by their reactivity with the monoclonal antibodies GL183 and EB6 [13]. Similarly, KIR reactive with the monoclonal antibody DX9 serve as receptors for HLA-B alleles expressing the Bw4 serological epitope, also present in the $\alpha1$ domain of the class I heavy chain [14, 15]. KIR reacting with the Bw6 polymorphism have not been detected, raising the question of why the Bw4 structure is uniquely identified by these receptors.

MHC class I molecules expressed on the cell surface are typically composed of the class I heavy chain bound to peptide and $\beta2$-microglobulin. Interactions between Ly49A and H-2 apparently are not influenced by the nature of the peptide [16]. In contrast, Malnati and colleagues [17] have shown that recognition of HLA-B27 by human NK cells is influenced by the bound peptide. However, the biological relevance of peptide diversity is as yet uncertain because these NK cells were unable to discriminate "self" from "foreign" peptides bound to the MHC molecules. Further studies will be needed to determine whether these findings with HLA-B27 also apply to recognition of other HLA-B and HLA-C molecules and if KIR can discriminate between individual peptides when they are presented in complex mixtures (*i.e.* mimicking their presentation in a normal cell). Given the relatively limited diversity of KIR and Ly49 receptors, it seems unlikely that peptide discrimination will play a major role in the function of these molecules unless certain pathogens can dramatically alter the composition of the MHC bound peptides after infection of the host.

Concluding remarks

The concept that recognition of MHC class I by receptors expressed on T cells and NK cells can inhibit an immune response is an important advancement in our understanding of the immune system. This implies that MHC molecules are necessary not only for presentation of foreign peptides to activate T cells, but also to engage receptors on T cells and NK cells that may limit the extent of the response and possibly prevent autoimmune destruction of normal tissues. Although conceptually appealing, further work is necessary to test this hypothesis in the context of bona fide immune responses *in vivo*. Moreover, there are many unanswered questions about these novel receptors for MHC class I. How does an individual acquire KIR or Ly49 receptors reactive with self MHC ligands during development? What controls transcription of these genes, providing for expression of these receptors on some, but not all, NK and T cells? Can Ly49 and KIR inhibit certain signaling pathways and not others? Have rodents and humans evolved distinct receptors or do both KIR and Ly49 exist in these species? Undoubtedly, these problems will direct the nature of experimentation in the near future. Hopefully, insights from these studies will impact future directions in clinical transplantation and suggest new strategies for the treatment of autoimmunity.

Acknowledgments
DNAX Research Institute is supported by Schering Plough Corporation.

References

1. Spits H, Lanier LL, Phillips JH. Development of human T and natural killer cells. *Blood* 1995; 85: 2654-70.
2. Karre K, Ljunggren HG, Piontek G, Kiessling R. Selective rejection of H-2-deficient lymphoma variants suggests alternative immune defense strategy. *Nature* 1986; 319: 675-8.
3. Walunas TL, Lenschow DJ, Bakker CY, Linsley PS, Freeman GJ, Green JM, Thompson CB, Bluestone JA. CTLA-4 can function as a negative regulator of T cell activation. *Immunity* 1994; 1: 405-13.
4. Karlhofer FM, Ribuado RK, Yokoyama WM. MHC class I alloantigen specificity of Ly-49+ IL-2- activated natural killer cells. *Nature* 1992; 358: 66-70.
5. Yu YYL, George T, Dorfman JR, Roland J, Kumar V, Bennett M. The role of Ly49A and 5E6 (Ly49C) molecules in hybrid resistance mediated by murine natural killer cells against normal T cell blasts. *Immunity* 1996; 4: 67-76.
6. Lanier LL, Phillips JH. Inhibitory MHC class I receptors on NK cells and T cells. *Immunol Today* 1996; 17: 86-91.
7. Colonna M, Samaridis J. Cloning of Ig-superfamily members associated with HLA-C and HLA-B recognition by human NK cells. *Science* 1995; 268: 405-8.
8. D'Andrea A, Chang C, Franz-Bacon K, McClanahan T, Phillips JH, Lanier LL. Molecular cloning of NKB1: A natural killer cell receptor for HLA-B allotypes. *J Immunol* 1995; 155: 2306-10.
9. Wagtmann N, Biassoni R, Cantoni C, Verdiani S, Malnati MS, Vitale M, Bottino C, Moretta L, Moretta A, Long EO. Molecular clones of the p58 natural killer cell receptor reveal Ig-related molecules with diversity in both the extra- and intracellular domains. *Immunity* 1995; 2: 439-49.
10. D'Andrea A, Chang C, Phillips JH, Lanier LL. Regulation of T cell lymphokine production by killer cell inhibitory receptor recognition of self HLA class I alleles. *J Exp Med* 1996; 184: 789-94.
11. Burshtyn DN, Scharenberg AM, Wagtmann N, Rajagopalan S, Berrada K, Yi T, Kinet JP, Long EO. Recruitment of tyrosine phosphatase HCP by the killer cell inhibitory receptor. *Immunity* 1996; 4: 77-85.
12. Fry A, Lanier LL, Weiss A. Phosphotyrosines in the KIR motif of NKB1 are required for negative signaling and for association with PTP1C. *J Exp Med* 1996; 184: 295-300.
13. Moretta A, Vitale M, Bottino C, Orengo AM, Morelli L, Augugliaro R, Barbaresi M, Ciccone E, Moretta L. p58 molecules as putative receptors for major histocompatibility complex (MHC) class I molecules in human natural killer (NK) cells. Anti-p58 antibodies reconstitute lysis of MHC class I-protected cells in NK clones displaying different specificities. *J Exp Med* 1993; 178: 597-604.

14. Gumperz JE, Litwin V, Phillips JH, Lanier LL, Parham P. The Bw4 public epitope of HLA-B molecules confers reactivity with NK cell clones that express NKB1, a putative HLA receptor. *J Exp Med* 1995; 181: 1133-44.
15. Litwin V, Gumperz J, Parham P, Phillips JH, Lanier LL. NKB1: an NK cell receptor involved in the recognition of polymorphic HLA-B molecules. *J Exp Med* 1994; 180: 537-43.
16. Correa I, Raulet DH. Binding of diverse peptides to MHC class I molecules inhibits target cell lysis by activated natural killer cells. *Immunity* 1995; 2: 61-71.
17. Malnati MS, Peruzzi M, Parker KC, Biddison WE, Ciccone E, Moretta A, Long EO. Peptide specificity in the recognition of MHC class I by natural killer cell clones. *Science* 1995; 267: 1016-8.

Plenary lectures

3 • Expression and function of HLA genes

Incomplete tolerance to nuclear self-antigens: a model for HLA-restricted induction and diversification of autoantibodies in systemic autoimmunity

J. McCluskey, P. Reynolds[1], M. Rischmueller[1], C. Keech[1], S. Lester, T.P. Gordon[1]

Transplant Services, Red Cross Blood Transfusion Service, 301 Pirie Street, Adelaide, South Australia, 5000 Australia
1 Department of Clinical Immunology, Flinders Medical Centre, Bedford Park, South Australia, 5042 Australia

Susceptibility to many autoimmune disorders is associated with particular alleles of genes encoded in the major histocompatibility complex [1]. For example HLA class II alleles are associated with organ-specific diseases like insulin dependent diabetes mellitus (IDDM-associated with DQ2) and multiple sclerosis (DR2) as well as systemic autoimmune conditions such as systemic lupus erythematosus (SLE-associated with DR3) and primary Sjögren's syndrome (DR3-DQ2/DR2-DQ1). These observations have long suggested a role for products of the MHC in regulating autoimmune responses in addition to their known role in controlling immunity to microbial pathogens [1]. However the precise mechanism by which polymorphic MHC products influence disease susceptibility remains unsolved. One theory suggests that class II alleles strongly associated with an autoimmune disease might selectively present self-antigens to autoreactive T cells. This is a popular explanation for why HLA DQ2 is associated with IDDM which is characterised by specific destruction of β-islet cells. However, a plethora of candidate autoantigens have been implicated in islet cell autoimmunity and selective presentation of all these antigens to autoimmune T cells by a single HLA product seems highly improbable. This objection might be less significant if the autoimmune response in IDDM was nearly always initiated towards the same autoantigen in islet cells with subsequent spreading of the immune response to involve other islet antigens. In this way selective presentation of the initiating autoantigen to T cells might represent a major susceptibility point in the pathway to autoimmunity. Experimental support for this notion is evident in the sequential development of autoantibodies and T cell responses to islet cell autoantigens in the NOD model of IDDM [2].

The mechanism of determinant spreading in autoimmune responses is not clear, nor is it proven that the pattern of spreading is always the same in different MHC-identical individuals. Nonetheless determinant spreading is now well recognised in tissue specific autoimmunity such as IDDM [1, 2], experimental allergic encephalomyelitis (EAE) [3] and autoimmune gastritis associated with pernicious anemia [4]. In these disorders the target antigens are sequestered in localised tissues such as the islets of Langerhans, myelinated nerve fibres or the gastric parietal cells of the stomach. This anatomical isolation of specialised antigens is associated with a lack of central or thymic T cell tolerance involving intrathymic antigen presentation during development of the T cell repertoire. Thus, spreading of the autoimmune response in organ-specific autoimmunity is probably facilitated by the absence of central tolerance to tissue specific antigens.

More difficult to understand is the determinant spreading observed in models of systemic autoimmunity where multiple autoantibodies are often directed towards ubiquitously distributed intracellular host antigens. These autoantibodies are relatively disease-specific and often recognise multiple components of discrete subcellular particles. For instance autoantibodies recognising nucleosomes, dsDNA and small nuclear ribonucleoproteins (snRNPs) are characteristic of systemic lupus erythematosus whereas antibodies recognising components of the Ro (SS-A)/La (SS-B) RNP are most commonly associated with primary

Sjögren's syndrome. Clustering of autoantibody responses probably reflects the physical association of the various target structures within distinct subcellular particles and may occur through determinant spreading of an autoimmune response initially directed to only a single component of the particle. This notion is supported by experiments in normal animals showing spreading of autoimmunity towards the different components of the cellular RNPs [5] including the Ro/La RNP [6-8] after initiation of immunity to a single component of the RNP complex. Autoantibodies appear to develop in a T helper-dependent manner in both experimentally induced autoimmunity [5-8] and in clinical autoimmune diseases. The apparent failure of immune tolerance to nuclear self-antigens in systemic autoimmunity is at odds with the widespread availablility of these antigens to the developing and adult immune system. To address some of these issues we have studied experimental and clinical autoimmunity to the La (SS-B)/Ro (SS-A) ribonucleoprotein complex (RNP). The results of our experiments are discussed below.

Clustering of anti-La/Ro autoantibodies in primary Sjögren's syndrome probably results from the physical association of La and Ro proteins within the RNP particle

Approximately 90% of patients with primary Sjögren's syndrome (a systemic autoimmune condition) have high titer circulating autoantibodies towards components of the La (SS-B)/Ro (SS-A) ribonucleoprotein complex. The autoantibody response is usually highly polyclonal and specifically involves all components of the complex including the Ro60kDa antigen (Ro60), the Ro52kDa antigen (Ro52), La (48kDa) and snRNAs. However, some patients develop anti-Ro without anti-La even though anti-Ro52 is almost always associated with anti-Ro60. The mechanism by which autoantibodies towards Ro60, Ro52 and La autoantigens are strongly linked is believed to reflect the fact that these proteins are physically linked intracellularly in a RNP particle. A prediction of this concept is that the La/Ro RNP might behave like a single antigenic complex so that induction of T helper immunity to any component of the complex would result in molecular spreading of the autoantibody response to involve all other components.

To evaluate whether the induction of experimental immunity to any component of the La/Ro RNP would result in spreading to involve other components we immunised normal inbred mice with either recombinant Ro52, Ro60 or La protein and examined the respective immune sera for evidence of spreading of the immune response. Antibodies raised against any one protein component of the Ro/La RNP cluster resulted in a delayed, lower titer response to each of the other components, see *Figure 1*. Some variation in spreading was observed between strains of mice suggesting the likelihood of background genetic factors controlling the immune repertoire. This feature of the autoantibody spreading resembles the clinical variation in anti-La/Ro autoantibody patterns seen in patients with primary Sjögren's syndrome and in SLE. Diversification of the autoimmune response occurred rapidly in mice immunised with Ro60, La or Ro52 autoantigens. For instance immunisation with Ro52 protein resulted in the production

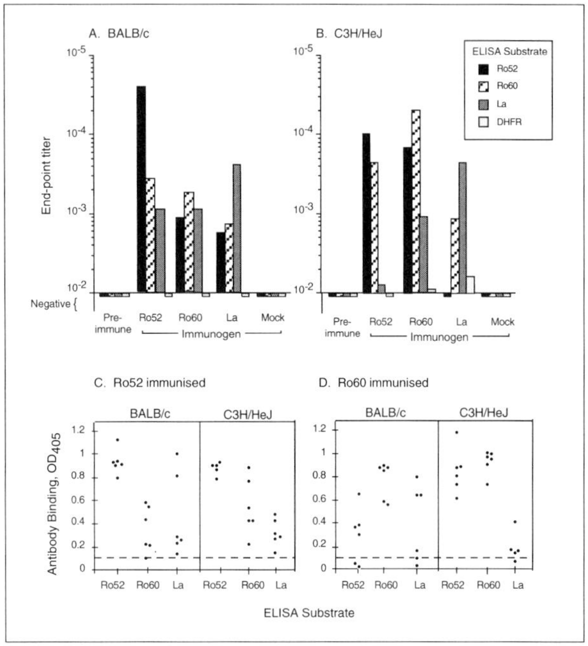

Figure 1. Experimental autoimmunity to Ro autoantigen induces autoantibodies to La antigen and *vice versa*. Groups of (A) BALB/c and (B) C3H/HeJ mice were immunised with recombinant 6xHis-mouse Ro52 (Ro52), 6xHis-human Ro60 (Ro60), 6xHis-human La (La) antigens or mock immunised with saline in Freund's complete adjuvant (Mock). Pre-immune sera (Pre-immune) and immune sera from day 42 post-immunisation were titered for reactivity with recombinant 6xHis-mouse Ro52 (Ro52), 6xHis-human Ro60 (Ro60), 6xHis-mouse La (La) and 6xHis-DHFR (DHFR) by ELISA. End-point titers were determined as the dilution of sera resulting in an OD_{405} of 0.2. Serial dilutions began at 1:125. (C) and (D) show OD_{405} values from individual mouse serum samples. Adapted with permission from reference [7].

of high titer antibody to Ro52 detectable within 7-14 days (not shown). This was followed a further 7-14 days later by a lower titer autoantibody production to Ro60. In BALB/c mice, but not C3H/HeJ mice, spreading of autoimmunity towards the La autoantigen also occurred 7-14 days after the first appearance of anti-Ro-52 antibodies. Immunisation with Ro60 led to the production of antibody to the Ro60 protein followed by lower titer autoantibody production to Ro52 and La with similar delayed kinetics. Similarly, spreading of the immune response was observed following immunisation with La, resulting in the production of anti-Ro60 antibodies and in BALB/c mice the production of anti-Ro52 antibody. Thus, the time course of antibody production was generally consistent with an initial response directed towards the primary immunogen followed within 1-3 weeks by an independent autoimmune response to the other components of the Ro/La RNP. These observations implied that immune tolerance to nuclear self antigens may be absent or incomplete and suggested that a degree of immune ignorance may be physiologically normal despite the ubiquitous expression of these autoantigens.

Ignorance of self-antigens like the La/Ro RNP is understandable in the B cell compartment because of the low level of circulating La/Ro RNPs present under physiological conditions. B cell silencing requires threshold concentrations of circulating antigen in order to aggregate sufficient surface Ig receptors to induce tolerance in developing B cells. In contrast to B cell ignorance of La/Ro RNPs, the T cell compartment is likely to be at least partly tolerised because the ubiquitous nature of the La/Ro RNP might be predicted to engender proper antigen presentation. Nonetheless, self-reactive T cells are critical for the development of autoantibodies. Therefore we hypothesised that incomplete self-tolerance in the T compartment may permit the initiation of T helper immunity which could then augment B cell proliferation and differentiation leading to autoantibody production. Incomplete self tolerance to sequestered self-antigen is described in some models of tissue specific autoimmunity where non-tolerogenic cryptic peptides are believed to play an important role in driving autoreactive T cells and antibody diversification [1-4]. Since the induction of diversified anti-La/Ro RNP immunity is presumed to be a T-dependent process, non-tolerogenic T cell determinants almost certainly exist in La/Ro RNPs despite their ubiquitous distribution and presence throughout lymphocyte development.

T helper reactivity to nuclear self-antigens in normal mice

As discussed above the precise extent to which the helper T cell compartment is tolerised to nuclear/cytoplasmic antigens is not known and the general nature of the self-determinants recognised by T helper cells in systemic autoimmunity is unclear. One of the problems of defining tolerance to self antigens is that any non-responsiveness following autoimmunisation could be explained in many ways other than self-tolerance. For a complete assessment of the extent of self-tolerance it is necessary to examine the host immune response in the presence and absence of expression of the self antigen. Generally speaking this is only experimentally possible in genetically engineered or natural knock out mice. In the experiments reported here we have immunised mice with a surrogate self-antigen, viz. the human La antigen (hLa) which is 77% identical to mouse La (mLa) [9]. We hypothesised that any tolerogenic mLa determinants might be highly immunogenic as their xenogeneic hLa homologue because of species polymorphisms. At the same time we argued that the sequence identity between hLa and mLa would result in a number of tolerogenic and non-tolerogenic T helper determinants being identical in these two proteins.

To test this hypothesis we mapped the mouse T cell response to hLa antigen. Lymph node T cells were isolated 9 days after immunisation of healthy mice with recombinant hLa (6xHis-hLa) and tested for reactivity with a panel of 155 overlapping peptides spanning the complete hLa molecule. Peptides were pooled as pairs of 15mers overlapping by 2 or 3 residues with the next peptide. A summary of these experiments is shown in *Table I.* One determinant, hLa288-302 (core amino acids 289-299), was stimulatory in every experiment and always induced maximal proliferation of responding T cells (stimulation index usually ≥ 10). The core amino acid sequence of this dominant epitope revealed it was a xenogeneic determinant differing from the homologous mLa determinant by a single residue (hLa295Q→mLa294L) from the mouse homolog (mLa288-298) (*Table I*). At least 6 other xenogeneic hLa determinants were identified as defined by clustering of the relevant T cell response to involve two or more pairs of overlapping peptides with a SI ≥ 2 in one or more experiment [8]. However a feature of the responses to these additional xenogeneic determinants was the generally low level of T cell stimulation (SI = 2-6) and the failure to stimulate T cells in every experiment, consistent with the determinants being either subdominant or facultatively cryptic.

In addition to these xenoresponses, significant T cell reactivity was identified towards several hLa peptide determinants containing identical amino acid sequences to the homologous peptide regions of mLa. Two of these 'autoepitopes' corresponded to peptides in common with hLa and mLa at amino acid residues 13-30 (reactivity in 75% experiments) and 25-44 (reactivity in 37% experiments). These auto determinants behaved like cryptic or subdominant epitopes in that they produced only low levels of T cell proliferation and in some experiments were non-stimulatory. Taken together these findings confirmed the suspicion that hLa and mLa protein contained shared, notionally autologous T cell epitopes, in addition to xenogeneic hLa determinants recognised by the murine immune system.

Table I. Selected mouse T cell determinants within human La

(a) Comparison of hLa peptide sequence and homologous mLa sequence	(b) Nature of determinant	Predicted amino acid residues	(c) Positive experiments
h LEAKIC**HQIEYYFGD**FNL m ------------------	AUTO	13-30	6/8
h FGDFNL**PRDKFLKEQIKL**DE m --------------------	AUTO	25-44	3/8
h D**ANNGNLQLRNK**EVT m N------**L**----K--	XENO	288-302	8/8

(a) The predicted minimum peptide epitopes are shown in bold type. A single amino acid deletion in the mLa sequence corresponding to hLa residue 217 and a 16 residue insertion in mLa after position 332 alters the numbering between equivalent mLa and hLa peptides following these positions.

(b) Auto = determinant of hLa where the same sequence is present in mLa; xeno = determinant sequences which differ between hLa and mLa. The hLa288-302 peptide was defined as immunodominant based upon the magnitude (SI generally $\geqslant 6$) and frequency of its reactivity. Although hLa13-30 was reactive in 75% experiments the magnitude of these responses was consistently marginal (SI~2) and so this determinant was defined as subdominant.

(c) Positive proliferative T cell responses are defined as an SI $\geqslant 2$ present in two or more adjacent pairs of peptides and occurring in one or more experiment. Adapted with permission from reference [8].

T cell tolerance to the dominant $mLa_{287\text{-}301}$ determinant in normal mice

The immunodominance of the homologous $hLa_{288\text{-}302}$ determinant suggested that the $mLa_{287\text{-}301}$ region might be highly tolerogenic in normal mice. To test whether this was the case groups of normal H-2^a mice (I-A^k) were immunised with either $hLa_{288\text{-}302}$ or $mLa_{287\text{-}301}$ in complete Freund's adjuvant and draining lymph node T cells were tested for proliferative reactivity 9 days later. In addition a group of mice were boosted with peptides in incomplete Freund's adjuvant and sera were tested for anti-La antibody approximately 4 weeks later.

T cells from mice primed with the $hLa_{288\text{-}302}$ determinant responded vigorously to this peptide (50%max response at ~20 nM; *Figure 2A*) and the response was recalled on the intact hLa antigen *(Figure 2B)*. In contrast T cells from mice primed with $mLa_{287\text{-}301}$ proliferated poorly to the mLa287-301 peptide even at high concentrations (50%max response~1 mM; *Figure 2A)* and failed to respond at all to the intact mLa antigen *(Figure 2B)*.

The lack of T cell reactivity to $mLa_{287\text{-}301}$ was not due to a failure to bind I-A^k since this peptide bound I-A^k as efficiently hLa288-302 in peptide binding studies [8]. The $mLa_{287\text{-}301}$ peptide was also found to act as a specific antagonist for recognition of the $hLa_{288\text{-}302}$ peptide and this property allowed us to demonstrate comparable antigen processing and presentation of the two determinants by splenic and L cell APC [8]. However, it was possible that the $mLa_{287\text{-}301}$ peptide might induce autoreactive T helper cells which proliferated poorly despite providing helper support for specific autoantibody responses. Therefore we tested the sera of animals immunised with $mLa_{287\text{-}301}$ peptide for the development of anti-La antibodies. Neither the $mLa_{287\text{-}301}$ nor the $hLa_{288\text{-}302}$ peptides provoked an autoantibody response under conditions where immunisation with intact 6xHis-mLa induced a significant anti-La response *(Figure 2C)*. Presumably the lack of autoantibody production despite efficient T immunity to $hLa_{288\text{-}302}$ reflects the absence of B epitopes in this peptide and the failure of reactive T helper cells to recognise the mouse homologue of this determinant. Therefore we assumed that the T cell repertoire in normal mice was specifically tolerant of the $mLa_{287\text{-}301}$ determinant, presumably because of its efficient presentation to the T cell compartment relative to other determinants. Accordingly, we considered that the induction of autoimmunity to mouse La protein was

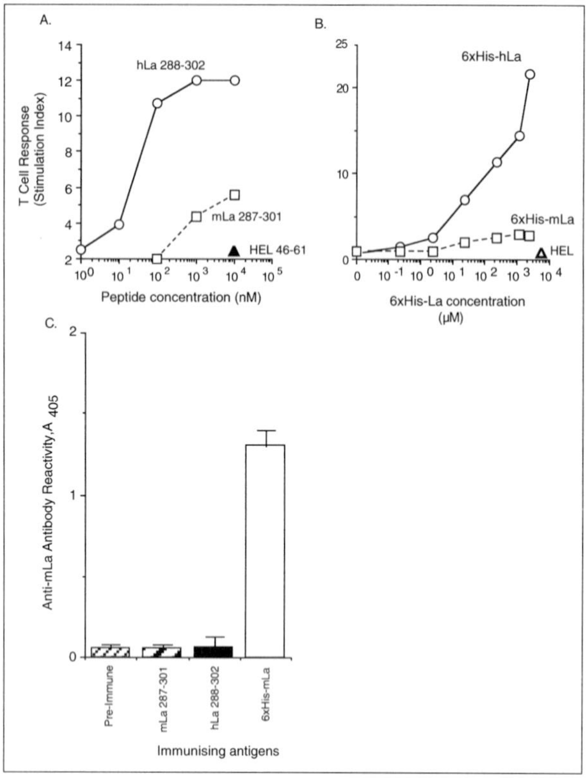

Figure 2. Immune tolerance to the mLa287-301 determinant in normal mice. A/J mice (12 per group) were immunised subcutaneously in the hind foot pad and at the base of tail with 20 μM of hLa288-302 (○—○) or mLa287-301 peptide (□----□) in CFA. The proliferation of T-enriched LN cells from hLa- or mLa-primed A/J mice was assayed 9 days later by co-culture with irradiated syngeneic spleen cells (2000 rads) in the presence of graded amounts of the immunising peptide shown in (A); hLa288-302 peptide (○) or mLa287-301 peptide (□), or intact recombinant antigen containing the immunising peptide shown in (B); 6xHis-hLa antigen (○) or 6xHis-mLa antigen (□). There was no T cell reactivity to HEL46-61 peptide (▲) or HEL protein (Δ) (SI=1). The stimulation index shown represents the mean value of triplicate assays. The whole experiment was carried out twice. In (C) groups of 6-8 A/J mice were immunised with 20 μM of either mLa287-301 peptide (▨), hLa288-302 peptide (■) or 100 μg of 6xHis-mLa protein antigen (□) and then boosted twice at 10 day intervals with 10 μM of the corresponding peptide or 50 μg of protein antigen in IFA. 3-4 days after the last boost individual sera tested individually at 1/100 for anti-mLa antibody reactivity by ELISA using 6xHis-mLa coated microtitre plates. The reactivity of pre-immune serum also is shown. Adapted with permission from reference [8].

likely to depend upon helper T cell responses recognising non-tolerogenic subdominant mLa determinants such as mLa_{13-30} and mLa_{25-44}.

Induction of T cell immunity and a diversified anti-La/Ro RNP autoantibody response by a non-tolerogenic subdominant determinant of mLa

To test whether the subdominant La determinants mLa_{13-30} and mLa_{25-44} could initiate anti-La autoantibodies we immunised groups of normal mice with one or other of these peptides in Freund's adjuvant and boosted the response 2-3 times over a 4-5 week period. Sera were then tested by western blots for the presence of autoantibodies recognising recombinant La [either fused to glutathione S transferase (GST) or a 6xhistidine tag (6xHis)] and control proteins. In A/J mice immunised with mLa_{25-44} the autoantibody response was restricted to the La A subfragment (aa 1-107) containing the mLa_{25-44} peptide and did not involve other regions of La including the hLaA3 subfragment (aa 46-107) immediately adjacent to the mLa_{25-44} peptide *(Figure 3)*. Pooled sera from mice immunised and boosted with mLa_{13-30} also specifically reacted with recombinant and mammalian sources of intact La antigen in immunoblots *(Figure 3)*. However, mLa_{13-30}-immune sera reacted with multiple regions of the mLa polypeptide as shown by immunoblots of La subfragments spanning four non-overlapping regions of the mLa molecule, LaA (aa 1-107), LaC (aa 111-243), LaF (aa 244-345) and LaL2/3 (aa 346-416), *(Figure 3)*. In addition mLa_{13-30}-immune sera reacted with the $hLaA_3$ subfragment (aa 46-107). In some lanes (*eg.* Bac. hLa) immune mouse sera reacted with multiple bands representing proteolytic degradation products of the recombinant antigens. Absorption of pooled immune sera with one subfragment of La (*eg.* the La C) specifically removed immunoblot reactivity to that fragment without affecting binding to the other subfragments (data not shown). By contrast, absorption with recombinant GST protein had no significant effect on the reactivity of the pooled serum with La subfragments (data not shown), confirming that reactivity with different regions of the La polypeptide was not due to cross-reactive antibodies. In addition immunoblot reactivity of the immune sera was not observed with the control proteins 6xHis-DHFR, 6xHis-HEL or with other nuclear proteins such as Sm polypeptides known to be present in the rabbit thymus extract *(Figure 3)*.

To determine whether intermolecular spreading of autoimmunity also occured after immunisation with

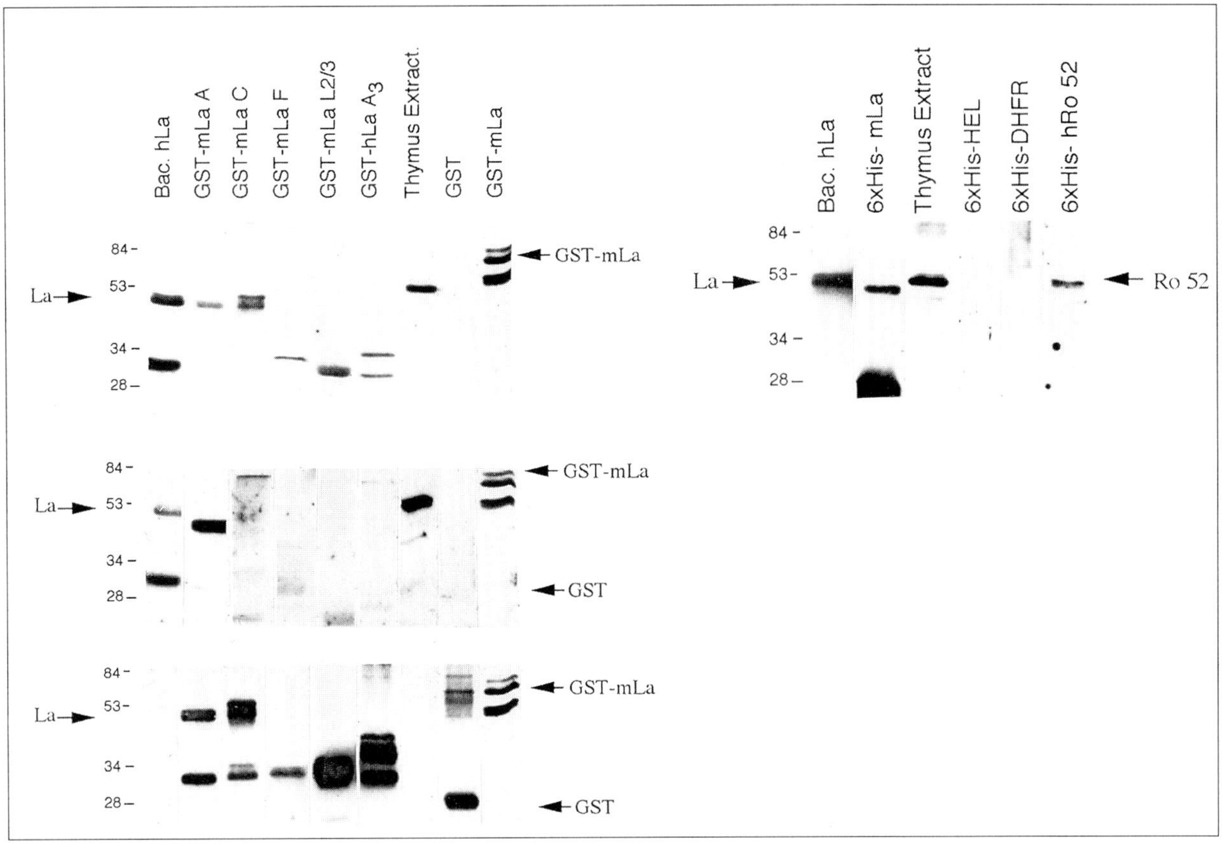

Figure 3. Intra- and intermolecular diversification of anti-La autoimmunity following immunisation with the subdominant mLa13-30 peptide. Pooled sera (diluted 1/500) from A/J mice immunised and boosted twice with either mLa13-30 (left, upper panel) or mLa25-44 peptides (left, middle panel) were used to immunoblot baculovirus 6xHis-hLa (Bac. hLa), the GST-mLa subfragments; GST-LaA (aa 1-107 predicted mol wt ~41kDa), GST-LaC (aa 111-242 predicted mol wt ~43kDa), GST-LaF (aa 243-345 predicted mol wt ~33kDa), GST-LaL2/3 (aa 346-416 predicted mol wt ~31-33kDa), GST-hLaA3 (aa 46-107 predicted mol wt ~30-33kD), rabbit thymus extract (containing several nuclear and cytoplasmic antigens, i.e. Sm antigens and La) (Pel-Freez Biologicals, Arkansas, USA), GST protein (predicted mol wt ~26kDa), and recombinant GST-mLa (predicted mol wt ~74kDa) separated on a 12.5% SDS-PAGE prior to electrotransfer. The same proteins were immunoblotted with a rabbit anti-GST antiserum at 1:3000 (left, lower panel). Right panel, pooled immune serum (diluted 1/250) from A/J mice immunised with mLa13-30 peptide was also reacted with baculovirus 6xHis-hLa (Bac. hLa), 6xHis-mLa, rabbit thymus extract, 6xHis-HEL, 6xHis-DHFR and 6xHis-hRo52 (Amrad, Melbourne, Australia) separated by SDS-PAGE and electrotransferred to nitrocellulose membrane. Bound antibodies were detected by ECL (Amersham, Buckinghamshire, England) using goat anti-mIgG (Sigma, USA) as second antibody. Bands corresponding to lower molecular weight degradation production are seen in some lanes. Adapted with permission from reference [8].

mLa_{13-30}, pooled immune serum was examined for immunoblot reactivity with the Ro autoantigens *(Figure 3)*. Pooled sera from mice immunised with the La_{13-30} peptide reacted specifically with recombinant Ro 52 *(Figure 3)* however, reactivity with recombinant Ro60 was equivocal and not observed in all experiments (data not shown). The titre of anti-Ro52 antibodies was significantly lower than that of the anti-La response (1/500 for anti-Ro52 and 1/3000 for anti-La antibodies). Nonetheless, this reactivity was specific since binding to control recombinant HEL and DHFR proteins (6xHis-DHFR and 6xHis-HEL) was not observed under the same conditions *(Figure 3)*. We conclude that immunisation with the subdominant mLa_{13-30} peptide is sufficient to induce intramolecular spreading of autoimmunity to La autoantigen as well as a low level of intermolecular antibody spreading of the autoimmune response.

Possible pathways for autoimmunisation in systemic autoimmunity

The tolerogenicity of mLa*287-301* indicates that endogenous La polypeptides are indeed processed and presented to host T cells, presumably by catabolism of La/Ro RNP particles. This putative turnover and antigen presentation of endogenous RNPs clearly does not lead to autoimmunity under normal conditions. However once autoreactive T cells have been primed towards poorly tolerogenic determinants within the La/Ro RNP, antigen presentation following the natural uptake of these RNPs appears to be potentially autoimmunogenic. In our experimental model the poorly tolerogenic determinants appear to be subdominant or possibly behave as facultatively cryptic regions of the La molecule which are only presented under special circumstances. Even so, humoral immunity to mLa is easily triggered experimentally and is associated with T cell responses to subdominant determinants. Although our assays have measured proliferative T cell responses, these responses are associated with functional T helper cells revealed by the isotype switching of autoantibody responses.

The diversification of the autoimmune response towards endogenous La/Ro described here occurred without the need for any challenge with exogenous intact La/Ro RNPs suggesting that the autoimmunisation driving the spreading of the response was due to endogenous turnover of intracellular RNPs. Notably then, the autoreactive T cell response induced by the $mLa_{13\text{-}30}$ subdominant peptide was recalled on intact La antigen [8] even though T cell responses to this and other subdominant mLa peptides were not evident in every experiment involving immunisation with intact La protein.

We propose that under normal conditions subdominant self-determinants are continuously being presented to T cells by APC, including self-reactive B cells, but this presentation is qualitatively and quantitatively insufficient to prime naive self-reactive T cells. In particular, the necessary costimulatory signals are likely to be absent under conditions of constitutive antigen presentation and the density of subdominant determinants presented on the surface of the APC probably falls below the threshold for activation of naive T cells. It seems likely that experimentally induced autoimmunity to the La/Ro RNP occurs because immunisation overcomes the priming threshold by using larger amounts of antigen than is normally encountered *in vivo* and by using adjuvants to activate APC and induce the qualitative costimulatory APC functions necessary for T cell priming. In other words, experimental induction of autoimmunity exposes the extent of immune self-ignorance.

We speculate that the initial diversification of the autoimmune response in primary Sjögren's syndrome is driven by selective constitutive uptake of endogenous "native" La/Ro RNP complexes by self-reactive B cells of diverse specificity. Our view is that uptake of La/Ro RNPs by these B cells leads to La/Ro processing and presentation of subdominant determinants to autoreactive T cells. T cells specific for only one subdominant determinant might provide helper signals to diverse autoreactive B cells with differing specificities within the RNP complex. It is also possible that once the autoimmune response is initiated, natural presentation of multiple subdominant (or cryptic) determinants will lead to spreading of the T cell response. Spreading of T cell autoimmunity may depend upon priming by specific autoreactive B cells but could also involve enhanced antigen presentation through FcR uptake of autoantibody-autoantigen complexes. Either way HLA-restricted presentation of new autoepitopes would be necessary for efficient spreading of autoimmunity. In this way the HLA class II phenotype of an individual may influence the pattern of autoimmune determinant spreading by controlling the presentation of distinct molecular determinants within different components of complex autoantigens.

A study of the anti-La/Ro RNP autoantibody response in primary Sjögren's syndrome

The notion that systemic autoimmunity involving ubiquitous self antigens is initiated by T cell responses to one or two subdominant self peptides has several implications for understanding clinical autoimmunity. For instance selective antigen presentation might explain HLA class II allele associations with the development of certain anti-nuclear autoantibodies. Similarly, if determinant spreading occurs in both the T and B compartments then HLA class II alleles may also influence the patterns of diversification of immune responses. To examine these possibilities further we have studied the distribution of HLA class II alleles in a population of patients with primary Sjögren's syndrome as described below.

Patients fulfilling at least 4 of the 6 European consensus criteria for the diagnosis of primary Sjögren's syndrome were examined for clinical features such as salivary gland enlargement, Raynaud's phenomenon, arthralgia and joint stiffness. Control sera were collected from 25 healthy donors and HLA typing was performed on 164 healthy South Australian blood donors. High resolution DRB1, DRB3, DRB5, DQA1 and DQB1 typings were performed by PCR-SSO using 11th and 12th International Histocompatibility Workshop protocols and an enhanced chemiluminescent (ECL) system.

Precipitating autoantibodies were detected by counter immune electrophoresis using rabbit thymus extract and extracts of K562 (a human myeloid cell line) as sources of autoantigen [10]. ELISA estimations of autoantibody levels were carried out using recombinant soluble human Ro and La [6-10] produced in bacteria as in-frame six-histidine fusion proteins in the pQE vector (Qiagen, Chatsworth, CA) and purified by nickel ion affinity chromatography [6-8].

A spectrum of diversification of the autoimmune response to the La/Ro RNP occurs in patients with primary Sjögren's syndrome

The 80 patients with primary Sjögren's syndrome were stratified into 4 categories based on the extent of diversification of their autoimmune response to the La/Ro RNP: (1) seronegative for anti-Ro and anti-La antibodies (11 patients); (2) anti-Ro antibodies only (10 patients); (3) anti-Ro and non-precipitating anti-La antibodies (15 patients); and (4) anti-Ro and precipitating anti-La antibodies (44 patients). Previously we have shown that the specificity of anti-La antibodies in patients with anti-Ro and nonprecipitating anti-La is highly restricted [10]. Therefore these subsets define points within a spectrum of diversification and amplification of the autoimmune response to the La/Ro RNP. All sera containing anti-Ro precipitins on counter immune electrophoresis were also positive by indirect immunofluorescence on Ro60-transfected HEp-2 cells, consistent with a B cell response to conformational epitopes on Ro60 [11]. Autoantibodies were not detected in sera from the 25 normal controls or in previously examined blood bank donors [11].

Diversification of La/Ro autoimmunity is influenced by distinct HLA class II alleles

Since the function of HLA class II molecules is to present antigen to CD4-positive T cells, including T helper cells, we next determined whether the expression of distinct HLA class II haplotypes influenced diversification and amplification of the autoantibody response in patients with primary Sjögren's syndrome. *Table II* shows the phenotypic frequency of HLA class II alleles in patients stratified according to the spectrum of autoantibody diversity. Notably 12/15 (80%) of the anti-Ro, precipitin-negative anti-La group expressed HLA DR2, and 40/44 (91%) of the anti-Ro, precipitin-positive anti-La group expressed HLA DR3. The DR2-DQA1*0102-DQB1*0602 (DR2-DQ1) haplotype was strongly associated with autoantibodies to Ro alone (DR2, relative risk, RR=7.5, $P<0.01$) or to Ro in conjunction with non-precipitating anti-La antibodies (DR2, RR=16.6, $P<0.001$). In contrast, the DR3-DQA1*0501-DQB1*02 (DR3-DQ2) haplotype was predominantly associated with precipitating anti-La antibodies (DR3, RR 47.1, $P<0.001$), and to a lesser extent with anti-Ro in the absence of anti-La precipitins (DR3, RR 4.7-5.8, $p<0.05$). Only 5 of the 80 patients lacked both DR2 and DR3 - one seronegative, one precipitin-negative anti-La with anti-Ro, and three patients with precipitin-positive anti-La and anti-Ro. Each of these patients expressed DR5 (three DR11 and two DR12 subtypes), which was found overall to be strongly associated with anti-Ro in association with both non-precipitating (RR 12.0, $P<0.001$) and precipitating (RR 7.1, $P<0.01$) anti-La antibodies.

A role for DQA1*0501 in controlling anti-La/Ro autoimmune diversification

All of the DR5-positive/DR2-negative/DR3-negative patients expressed DQA1*0501, which is known to be in linkage disequilibrium with both DR3 and DR5. This finding suggested that DQA1*0501 may be an important determinant in T cell recognition of the La/Ro RNP. In support of this notion the frequency of DQA1*0501 increased in patient subgroups with increasing diversification of the autoantibody response to the La/Ro RNP *(Table II)*. To identify the individual contributions of DQA1*0501 and the DQB1*02 allele (in strong linkage disequilibrium with DQA1*0501) we examined the effect of coexpression of these two alleles upon diversification of autoantibody responses to Ro and La. We observed that when

Table II. HLA class II influence on the pattern of anti-La/Ro autoantibody response in primary Sjögren's syndrome*

HLA allele	Controls	Sjögren's syndrome subsets based on CIE and La ELISA							
		Seronegative		Anti-Ro only		Anti-Ro, ppt-ve anti-La		Anti-Ro, ppt+ve anti-La	
	(n=164)	(n=11)		(n=10)		(n=15)		(n=44)	
	%	%	¶RR	%	RR	%	RR	%	RR
DR2	29	46	NS	70	7.5†	80	16.6§	39	NS
DR3	27	46	NS	60	5.8‡	40	4.7‡	91	47.1§
DR5	12	27	NS	10	NS	40	12.0§	16	7.1†
DQA1*0501	43	60	NS	67	4.6†	73	5.9†	93	21.4§
DQA1*0102	33	50	NS	78	6.5†	80	11.6§	48	2.9†
DQB1*02	44	55	NS	60	NS	47	NS	91	13.8§
DQB1*0602	27	27	NS	70	7.5†	73	8.2 §	41	2.3‡

* Phenotype frequencies are shown (%);¶ HLA associations were analysed by odds (or cross-product) ratios which are approximations to the relative risk (RR) in the case of retrospective data. Simple, single associations were tested by the 2x2 table odds ratio (with 0.5 added to each cell count when there were zero counts in any cell). Significance was assessed by χ^2 values. Possible multiple phenotypic HLA associations were analysed by base-line logistic regression with each group of patients compared in turn to the controls with variables included for each allele. Regression was performed in a forward step-wise manner to select the most parsimonious model. The (antilog) of the regression coefficients are the odds ratios. The probability of the regression coefficients were taken as the significance (probability) values of the odds ratios. ppt-ve = precipitin-negative; ppt+ve = precipitin-positive. NS = not significant; DR2 = DRB1*1501, DRB1*1502, DRB1*1601; DR3 = DRB1*0301; DR5 = DRB1*1101, DRB1*1102, DRB1*1103, DRB1*1104, DRB1*1201. † = 0.001<p<0.01; ‡ = 0.01<p<0.05; § = p<0.001. Adapted from Rischmueller *et al.* [13].

DQA1*0501 and DQB1*02 were coexpressed anti-La antibodies were more likely to be diversified (*ie.* precipitating; RR 8.7, p<0.01) but when DQA1*0501 was expressed in the absence of DQB1*02 the imune response was less diversified with only non-precipitating anti-La antibodies (RR 5.6, p<0.05; *Table III*). One interpretation of the data is that La peptide determinants may be efficiently presented to T cells by DQ molecules composed of the DQA1*0501 and DQB1*02 chains, and less efficiently presented by DQ molecules bearing DQA1*0501 α-chains in conjunction with other DQβ chains (see *Figure 4).*

A model for MHC class II control of autoantibody diversification in primary Sjögren's syndrome

This study reveals a spectrum of autoantibody diversification in the immune response to the La/Ro RNP in patients with primary Sjögren's syndrome. Autoantibody responses can vary from undetectable to high titer responses involving anti-Ro and anti-La precipitins. In our experience patients with intermediate levels of autoantibody diversification remain stable in their expression of anti-Ro without anti-La or anti-Ro with low titer non-precipitating anti-La antibodies. This is consistent with our hypothesis that diversification of La/Ro autoimmunity observed in primary Sjögren's syndrome is likely to be genetically determined. More specifically, we predict that separate HLA class II associations might reflect T cell recognition of unique peptides derived from either or both of the La/Ro proteins. The model shown in *Figure 4* suggests how DQA1*0501 may act differentially in regulating the anti-La/Ro response, however this observation alone cannot explain the influence of HLA phenotype on diversification of the autoantibody response in primary Sjögren's syndrome. Comparison of HLA class II phenotypes between the patient subgroups and the normal control population *(Table II)* clearly demonstrated that HLA alleles present on the HLA DR2-DQA1*0102-DQB1*060 (DR2-DQ1)

Table III. Coexpression of DQA1*0501 with DQB1*02 is associated with precipitating anti-La antibodies, whereas DQA1*0501 in the absence of DQB1*02 is a risk factor for nonprecipitating anti-La

	Anti-Ro, ppt-ve anti-La (n=15)	**Anti-Ro, ppt+ve anti-La (n=44)**
HLA DQ phenotype	**❒Relative risk**	
DQA1*0501/DQB1*02	NS	8.7‡
DQA1*0501/DQB1*X	5.6†	NS

❒ = Relative risk estimates calculated as odd ratios, see also *Table II* footnote; ppt-ve = precipitin-negative; ppt+ve = precipitin-positive. NS = not significant; † = 0.001<p<0.05; ‡ = 0.01<P<0.05. X = other DQB1 alleles. Adapted from Rischmueller *et al.* [13].

haplotype were strongly associated with autoantibodies to Ro polypeptides with or without a restricted anti-La antibody response (nonprecipitating). On the other hand the tendency to develop a more amplified polyclonal autoimmune phenotype characterised by precipitating anti-La antibodies was markedly increased in patients carrying alleles frequently encoded on the DR3-DQA1*0501-DQB1*02 (DR3-DQ2) haplotype.

A simple model to explain our findings is proposed in *Figure 5*. The model proposes the normal existence of circulating, surface Ig-positive B cells with autospecificity for both La and Ro polypeptides. Following uptake and processing of La/Ro RNPs through capture by the Ro-specific B cell receptor, anti-Ro antibody responses in autoimmune patients are driven by cognate interactions between Ro-specific B cells and helper T cells. Initiation of anti-Ro autoimmunity can occur when autoreactive B cells present HLA DR2- or DQ1-restricted Ro peptides to Ro-specific T helper cells *(Figure 5A*, upper panel). We propose that the DR2-DQ1 haplotype is deficient at activating La-specific T cells. However in patients with DR2-DQ1, La-specific B cells can also take up La/Ro RNP *via* their surface Ig, and may then present HLA DR2- or DQ1-restricted Ro peptides to Ro-specific T helper cells, thereby gaining intermolecular help for anti-La antibody production (*Figure 5A*, lower panel). This intermolecular help is limited as reflected by the production of only nonprecipitating anti-La antibodies, because only a subset of La molecules are associated with Ro RNP and thus restricted numbers of La-specific B cells are able to simultaneously capture La/Ro RNPs by surface Ig. These La-specific B cells might compete poorly with Ro-specific B cells for T cell help, resulting in the production of low titer, low affinity, pauciclonal anti-La antibodies lacking the ability to form latticed precipitates.

In contrast, we propose that patients with the DR3-DQ2 haplotype can present peptides derived from both Ro and La antigens to specific helper T cells. Thus, high titer, high affinity precipitating anti-La antibody responses are driven by La-specific T helper cells following presentation of HLA DR3-DQ2-restricted La peptides by polyclonal La-specific B cells (*Figure 5B*, upper panel). In addition a strong anti-Ro response is driven by polyclonal B cell presentation of Ro peptides to Ro-specific T cells also restricted by the HLA DR3-DQ2 haplotype (*Figure 5B*, lower panel). It follows from this model that both anti-Ro and anti-La antibody responses may also be driven by intermolecular T helper cells recognising HLA DR3-DQ2-restricted La/Ro peptides, further amplifying autoimmune responses. The influence of HLA DQA1*0501-DQB1*02 may modulate the propensity for antibody diversification associated with the DR3-DQ2 haplotype, as suggested in *Figure 4*.

The models proposed here are clearly speculative and not all studies have observed the same distribution of HLA class phenotypes in Sjögren's syndrome [12]. Our study has focussed on primary Sjögren's syndrome in a racially homogeneous population of caucasians. We have also distinguished different degrees of autoantibody diversification in the patient cohort. Nonetheless, alternative explanations for our results are obviously possible. For instance the data are entirely consistent with effects of non-structural HLA class II or other MHC genes in linkage disequilibrium with specific class II alleles. Such

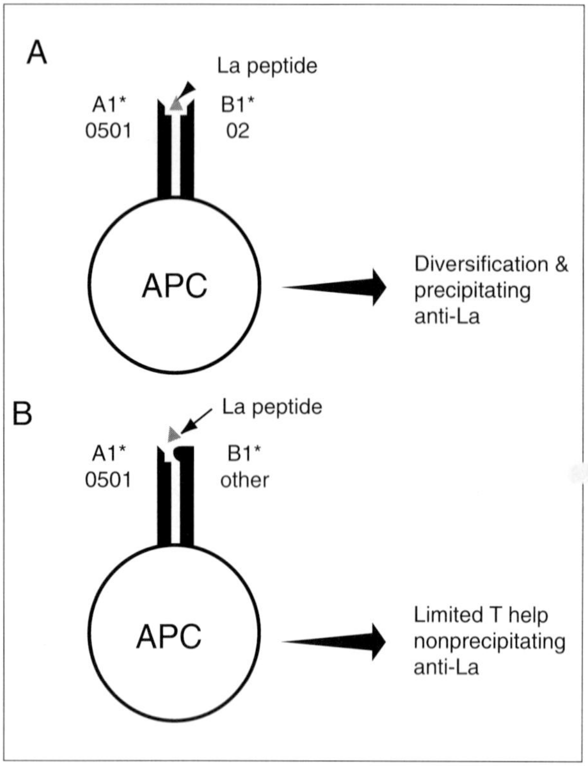

Figure 4. Model to explain the influence of HLA DQA1*0501 in anti-La/Ro autoantibody diversification. The model proposes that high affinity precipitating anti-La antibody responses are partly driven by La-specific T helper cells recognising an HLA DQA1*0501-DQB1*02-restricted La peptide presented by polyclonal La-specific B cells. This model suggests that the DQA1*0501 α-chains play an important role in the selective binding of a La peptide especially in the context of the DQB1*02 β -chain but also to a lesser extent in the context of other DQ β-chains.

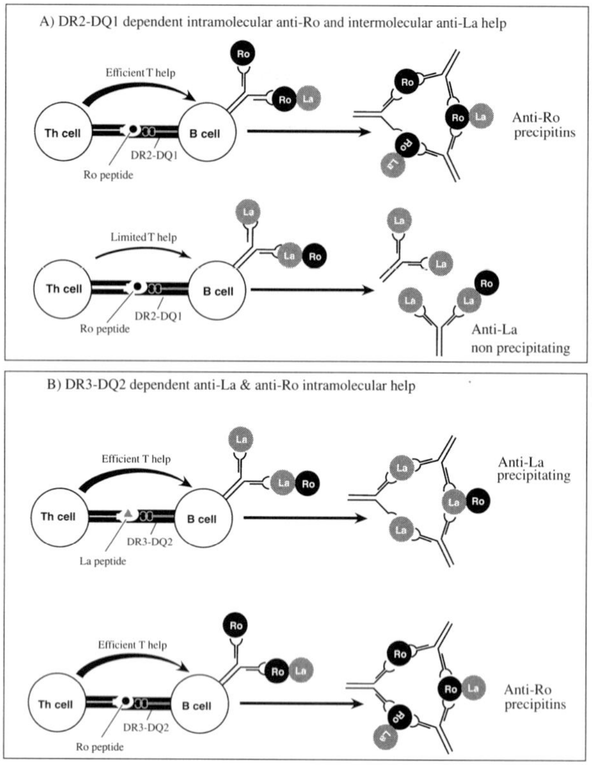

Figure 5. Model showing HLA-restricted control of anti-La/Ro autoantibody diversification. (A), the model proposes that anti-La/Ro autoimmunity can be initiated when anti-Ro T cells are activated and provide helper signals for Ro-specific B cells presenting HLA DR2- or DQ1-restricted processed Ro peptides (upper panel). Ro-specific B cells selectively bind La/Ro RNPs through their membrane Ig which then undergoes receptor-mediated endocytosis leading to antigen processing and presentation of captured proteins. La-specific B cells also take up La/Ro RNP *via* their mIg receptor and also present HLA DR2- or DQ1-restricted Ro peptides to Ro-specific T helper cells, thereby gaining intermolecular help for anti-La antibody production (lower panel). The latter intermolecular help is limited because there is a pool of free La which restricts the number of anti-La B cells able to take up La and Ro together. This results in the production of low titer, low affinity, pauciclonal anti-La antibodies lacking the ability to form latticed precipitates. (B), Anti-Ro autoimmunity can also be initiated by T helper cells recognising Ro peptides presented by DR3 or DQ2 (lower panel), however these HLA molecules can also present La peptides (upper panel). Thus, high affinity precipitating anti-La antibody responses are driven by La-specific T helper cells following presentation of HLA DR3-DQ2-restricted processed La peptides by a broad range of La-specific B cells. It follows from this model that both the anti-Ro and anti-La antibody responses may receive intermolecular T helper signals. This may explain why anti-La autoantibodies rarely occur in the absence of anti-Ro antibodies. Adapted from Rischmueller *et al.* [13].

influences could either act alone or concurrently with HLA-encoded risk. Candidate genetic factors might include polymorphisms at gene promoters, genes associated with antigen presentation, TNF genes or as yet uncharacterised genes within the MHC. Nonetheless our findings in an animal model of autoimmunity towards the the La/Ro RNP show that defined peptide determinants within nuclear self antigens can induce complex patterns of autoimmunity to ribonucleoprotein complexes. This observation suggests how HLA control of an initial autoimmune response involving just one or two non-tolerogenic (perhaps subdominant) peptides within a self antigen might control subsequent diversification and amplification of autoimmunity.

Acknowledgments
We thank the NHMRC, AFA and ARC for grant support; and the Arthritis Foundation of South Australia Lupus/Scleroderma group for informing primary Sjögren's syndrome patients about this work. Additional thanks to Mr Greg Bennett for his assistance in coordination of the HLA typing.

References

1. Sinha AA, Lopez T, McDevitt HO. Autoimmune diseases: the failure of self tolerance. *Science* 1990; 248: 1380-8.
2. Kaufman DM, Clare-Salzler M, Tian J, Forsthuber T, Ting GSP, Robinson P, Atkinson MA, Sercarz EE, Tobin AJ, Lehmann PV. Spontaneous loss of T-cell tolerance to glutamic acid decarboxylase in murine insulin-dependent diabetes. *Nature* 1993; 366: 69-72.
3. Tuohy VK, Fritz RB, Ben-Nun A. Self-determinants in autoimmune demyelinating disease: changes in T-cell response specificity. *Curr Opin Immunol* 1994; 6: 887.
4. Alderuccio F, Toh BH, Tan P, Gleeson P, Van Driel I. An autoimmune disease with multiple molecular targets abrogated by the transgenic expression of a single autoantigen in the thymus. *J Exp Med* 1993; 178: 419.
5. Van Venrooij WJ, Pruijn GJM. Ribonucleoprotein complexes as autoantigens. *Curr Opin Immunol* 1995; 7: 819-24.
6. Topfer F, Gordon T, McCluskey J. Intra- and intermolecular spreading of autoimmunity involving the nuclear self-antigens La (SS-B) and Ro (SS-A). *Proc Natl Acad Sci USA* 1995; 92:875-9.
7. Keech CL, Gordon TP, McCluskey J. The immune response to 52 kDa Ro and 60 kDa Ro are linked in experimental autoimmunity. *J Immunol* 1996; 157: 3684-99.
8. Reynolds P, Gordon TP, Purcell AW, Jackson DC, McCluskey J. Hierarchical self -tolerance to T cell determinants within the ubiquitous nuclear self antigen La (SS-B) permits induction of systemic autoimmunity in normal mice. *J Exp Med* 1997 (in press).
9. Topfer F, Gordon T, McCluskey J. Characterization of the mouse autoantigen La (SS-B). *J Immunol* 1993; 150: 3091-100.
10. Gordon T, Mavrangelos C, McCluskey J. Restricted epitope recognition by precipitin-negative anti-La/SS-B-positive sera. *Arthritis Rheum* 1992; 35: 663-6.
11. Keech, C, McCluskey J, Gordon T.P. Transfection and overexpression of the human 60kDa Ro/SS-A autoantigen in Hep-2 cells. *Clin Immunol Immunopathol* 1994; 73:146-51.
12. Arnet FC. Immunogenetics: a tool to analyse autoimmunity. In: Latchman DS ed. *From genetics to gene therapy. autoimmune diseases: focus on Sjögren's syndrome.* London: Bios Scientific Publishers, 1994.
13. Rischmueller, Lester S, Chen Z, Champion G, Van Den Berg R, Beer R, Contes T, McCluskey J, Gordon TP. HLA class II phenotype controls diversification of the autoantibody response in primary Sjögren's syndrome. 1996 (submitted).

A role for HLA class II molecules in B lymphocyte activation and/or apoptosis

N. Mooney [1], J.P. Truman [1], F. Garban [1], C. Choqueux [1], J. Lord [2], D. Charron [1]

1 INSERM U396, Institut Biomédical des Cordeliers, 15, rue de l'École de Médecine, 75006 Paris, France
2 University of Birmingham Medical School, Birmingham, UK

Histocompatibility workshops have been designed in order to explore the extreme polymorphism of the products of the Major histocompatibility complex (MHC) gene locus. The MHC class I and class II molecules are characterized by their extreme polymorphism coupled with monomorphic regions. The benefits of polymorphism are clear in the light of the stringent specificity of the immune response We propose that the monomorphic regions may have a role in HLA class II molecule mediated signal transduction.

HLA class II molecules serve as receptors for both their physiological ligand, the TCR-CD4 complex and for the pathological ligands, the bacterial superantigens (SA) [1]. Bacterial exoproteins are derived from a variety of species including *Staphylococcus aureus, Streptococcus pneumoniae* and *Mycoplasma arthritidis*. SA act by forming a bridge between the MHC class II molecule on the antigen presenting cell (APC) and the T-cell receptor in a Vβ restricted fashion. The specific binding of SA underlines the importance of MHC class II expressing cells in SA mediated diseases.

Signal transduction via HLA class II molecules was initially indicated by Palacios *et al.* who used anti-HLA class II antibodies to replace T-helper cells for B cell activation. A number of reports followed indicating either inhibition or potentiation of B lymphocyte proliferation. In hindsight, these differences could perhaps be explained by differences in the physiological origin of the B lymphocytes, their state of activation and/or the degree of cross-linking of the MHC class II molecules. The generation of second messengers was first examined in the mouse. Activation of murine B lymphocytes *via* MHC class II molecules led to the activation of protein kinase A and the production of cyclic adenosine monophosphate (cAMP). A nuclear translocation of the serine/threonine kinase Protein Kinase C (PKC) was then demonstrated [2]. Studies in the human demonstrated the activation of phospholipase C and the rapid generation of an intracellular calcium flux (Ca^{++}_i) [3]. PKC translocation was then examined in the human and activation was detected by measuring both the enzymatic activity and by detecting translocation by immunoblotting [4]. It was particularly interesting to note that increased mRNA levels of PKC were also detected after signalling *via* HLA class II and that the increase was detected even after a relatively short period of stimulation. Further study of mRNA levels after stimulation of the EBV transformed B cell line Raji *via* either HLA class II or polyclonal activators suggested that the principal PKC isoforms affected were alpha, beta and delta [5]. This was the first indication of which PKC isoforms were involved in HLA class II mediated signaling. We have recently used anti-PKC isoform specific monoclonal antibodies in order to answer three questions: the identity of the PKC isoforms involved in primary B lymphocytes, the localization of the PKC isoforms pre and post-HLA signalling and finally the differences in PKC protein levels after HLA class II signalling. Firstly, we have confirmed that it is the isoforms α,β and δ which are affected in one way or another after HLA class II mediated signalling. Secondly, the relocalization of PKC α, β and δ involves translocation to either/both the plasma membrane and the nuclear membrane. Finally, increased protein levels of PKC were observed even after only twenty minutes of stimulation. It is crucial to note that B lymphocyte stimulation with bacterial superantigens or monoclonal anti-HLA-DR mAbs affected the same PKC isoforms therby confirming the importance of this signalling pathway in HLA class II mediated signal transduction. The observation of PKC activation in both activated and in resting B lymphocytes provides further confirmation.

On the contrary to PKC activation, generation of cAMP has only been observed in murine cells after stimulation via MHC class II. Although human B lymphocytes from different physiological origins have been examined, the absence of cAMP generation has been a consistent feature. This is in marked contrast to tyrosine kinase activation which has been observed after HLA class II signalling on B lymphocytes from either adult or foetal origin. Tyrosine kinase activation and an Ca^{++}_i was only observed in pre-activated murine B lymphocytes [6]. Human foetal B lymphocytes are essentially located in the Go/G1 stage of the cell cycle and migrate as dense cells on Percoll density gradients further suggesting that they are resting rather than activated. Tyrosine kinase activation is conserved in these cells although an Ca^{++}_i is not observed. Tyrosine kinase activation is necessary for downstream signalling events including activation of phospholipase C and generation of the intracellular calcium flux in adult B lymphocytes. Furthermore, HLA class II mediated aggregation requires tyrosine kinase and PKC activation. Overall these data suggest that tyrosine kinase activation is a fundamental step in HLA class II mediated signalling.

The intracellular calcium flux is an early event following signalling *via* HLA class II molecules. The precise targets for this increase in intracellular calcium are unknown and recent data suggest that it is not an obligatory second messenger for cellular proliferation [7].

Foetal B lymphocytes express HLA class II molecules (albeit to a lower extent than adult B lymphocytes) and the integrity of the HLA class II signalling pathway on these cells is indicated by their ability to activate both tyrosine kinases and protein kinase C. Interestingly, the isoforms of the protein kinase C family that are stimulated via HLA class II in foetal versus adult B lymphocytes are the same, that is α,β and δ.

In marked contrast to HLA class II signalling in adult B lymphocytes, we have failed to observe an intracellular calcium flux after HLA class II signalling in B lymphocytes of foetal (isolated from umbilical cord blood) origin. This pathway was nonetheless intact in neonatal B lymphocytes since it was possible to generate an Ca^{++}_i *via* sIg in these cells. These data suggest that the observed PKC activation *via* HLA class II in foetal B lymphocytes is not therefore dependent on the simultaneous generation of an Ca^{++}_i and that the tyrosine kinase activation is independent of the intracellular calcium generation. Finally, since foetal B lymphocytes proliferated in response to HLA class II mediated signalling, these data suggest that the HLA class II mediated intracellular calcium flux is not essential for HLA class II mediated B lymphocyte proliferation.

Programmed cell death via MHC class II antigens has also been described in the mouse, although in marked contrast to the human only resting murine B lymphocytes were affected [8]. This demonstrates yet another difference between signal transduction *via* MHC class II versus HLA class II. Initially, we observed HLA class II mediated apoptosis in an EBV transformed B cell line and in activated *(in vivo or in vitro)* primary B lymphocytes. Studies using previously reported inhibitors of apoptosis revealed that cytoskeletal integrity and activation of a serine threonine phosphatase were required. Since these second messengers had not previously been implicated in HLA class II mediated signalling, we have tried to distinguish the signalling pathway involved in HLA class II mediated apoptosis from that leading to proliferation. Pretreatment with an inhibitor of either protein synthesis or mRNA significantly decreased the number of cells proliferating in response to HLA class II signalling. Therefore having effectively blocked proliferation, this allowed us to study signals leading to apoptosis. Essentially, the PKC family of iso-enzymes and both intra-and extracellular calcium were crucial. Two different inhibitors of protein kinase C were used which are believed to be specific for PKC at the concentrations shown. The extracellular calcium chelator inhibited apoptosis to a greater degree than the intracellular chelator although it is difficult to be conclusive since intra and extra-cellular calcium concentrations are intimately linked and since the specificity of the chelators is not absolute.

Our previous data suggesting a role for a serine/threonine phosphatase was confirmed as was the necessity for cytoskeletal integrity since cytochalasin B was a major inhibitor. Resting B lymphocytes are most sensitive to HLA class II mediated proliferative signals and are practically insensitive to apoptotic signals. We therefore used resting B cells to examine the second messengers involved in proliferation. On the contrary to apoptosis, a role for tyrosine kinases was clearly indicated as were the PKC iso-enzymes inhibited by GF109203X. Extracellular calcium was again implicated to an equivalent degree as that observed for induction of apoptosis, this is probably a consequence of the ubiquitous nature of calcium dependent signals. It appears that HLA class II mediated proliferation is indifferent to cytoskeletal integrity since cytochalasin B did not at all affect cell proliferation. It is interesting to note that foetal B lymphocytes did not undergo apoptosis as a consequence of HLA class II mediated signalling *(Figure 1a* and *1b)*. However, addition of a non-toxic concentration of the calcium ionophore ionomycin at the same time as a signal HLA class II DR resulted in apoptosis *(Figure 1d)*. It therefore appears that the relatively low basal level of calcium limits HLA class II DR mediated apoptosis in foetal B lymphocytes.

The Fas, Apo-1 or CD95 molecule is a member of the TNF receptor superfamily (which includes CD27, CD30, CD40,

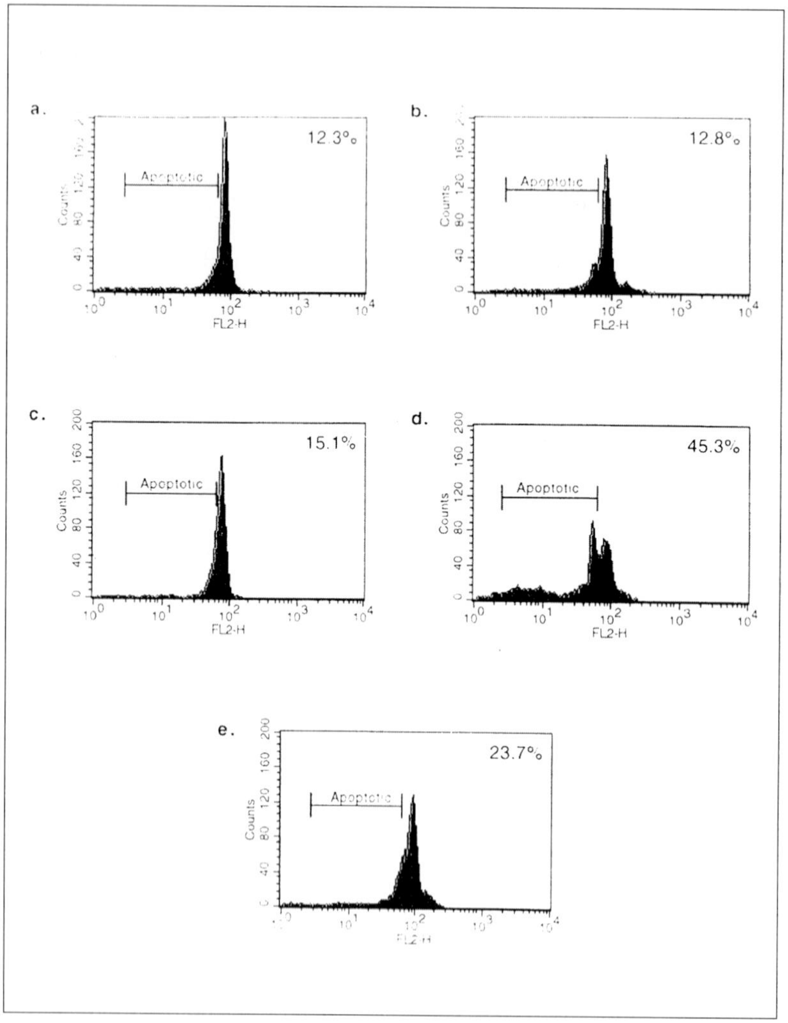

Figure 1. HLA class II mediated apoptosis of foetal B lymphocytes depends on addition of extracellular calcium.

Apoptosis was detected by quantifying the number of hypodiploid nucleii after lysis of the cells. Propodium iodide labelling of nucleii reveals their distribution throughout the cell cycle. 10,000 events were read using the red sensitive detector of a FACScan and the debris was removed by raising the forward scatter threshold.

a. Cell cycle analysis of non-stimulated cord blood B lymphocytes
b. 63Cell cycle analysis of cord blood B lymphocytes after stimulation *via* HLA class II for 24 hours.
c. Cell cycle analysis of cord blood B lymphocytes after addition of ionomycin (0.6uM) during 24 hours.
d. Cell cycle analysis of cord blood B lymphocytes after stmulation *via* HLA class II for 24 hours in the presence of ionomycin (0.6uM). Note the large increase of hypodiploid or apoptotic nucleii.
e. Cell cycle analysis of cord blood B lymphocytes after stmulation *via* HLA class II for 24 hours in the presence of ionomycin (0.6uM) and the calcium chelator E.D.T.A. Calcium chelation strongly inhibited the apoptosis observed with ionomycin and HLA-DR signalling.

OX40 and 4-1BB). This molecule was initially described as a death inducing molecule and the importance of the molecule was pinpointed since a mutation in the Fas gene was found in *lpr* and a mutation of the FasL gene in *gld* mice. Both *lpr* and *gld* inbred mice have a large expansion of the TCR α/β CD4+/CD8- as well as hypergammaglobulinemia and accumulation of autoantibodies. Recent studies have indicated that with regard to homeostasis of lymphocyte subpopulations, the Fas/FasL interaction is particularly involved in peripheral rather than in thymic selection. A role for Fas in activation induced cell death of T lymphocytes *via* CD3 was described. Since our observation of apoptosis of B lymphocytes *via* HLA class II was limited to activated cells we were interested in the possible contribution of this molecule to HLA class II mediated B lymphocyte apoptosis. The molecule Fas was detected on activated B lymphocytes and on EBV transformed B cell lines and did lead to oligosomal fragmentation of the DNA. A suggestion of the role of Fas/FasL in HLA class II mediated apoptosis was obtained when a B cell line from a patient with a mutation in the *Fas* gene [9,10] did not die in response to HLA class II mediated signalling. This mutation is due to a large deletion in the intracellular region of the Fas molecule. Since it was possible to induce

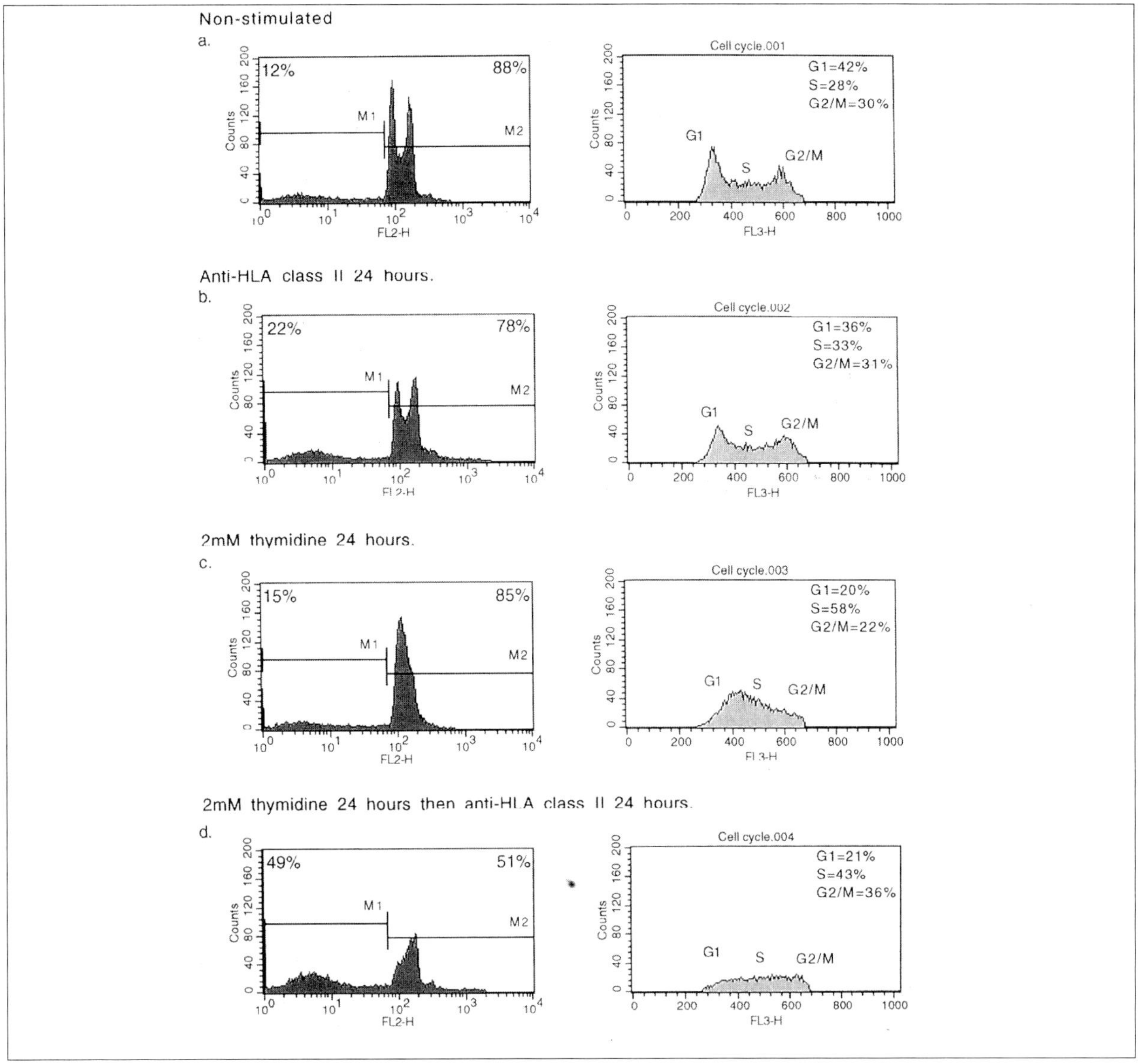

Figure 2. HLA class II signalling induces a G_1-S phase block in the B cell line Raji
a. Cell cycle analysis of isolated nucleii from non-stimulated Raji B cells.
b. Cell cycle analysis of Raji B cells which had been stimulated via HLA-class II DR for 48 hours. Note the decreased number of pre-S phase nucleii indicating progression from Go/G1 to S phase. Since the number of nucelii does not increase in or beyond the S phase this indicates that cell death is ocurring at this point.
c. An S-phase block was imposed by adding thymidine (2mM) for 24 hours.
d. HLA class II mediated apoptosis of Raji is increased by imposing an S phase block before beginning signalling *via* HLA class II DR.

HLA class II mediated apoptosis of highly purified B lymphocyte populations and since the Fas molecule could behave as an effector molecule on these cells we examined the ability of HLA class II molecules to signal for expression of the Fas ligand. Suicide, or a *cis* interaction of Fas-Fas L on the same cell has been documented in T lymphocyte activation induced cell death although a role for fraticide or a *trans* interaction of Fas-Fas L has not been excluded. An anti-FasL antibody (kindly provided by J. Tschopp) was used to detect induction of FasL in B lymphocytes activated *via* HLA class II. The induction of expression of FasL was confirmed by immunoprecipitation of the FasL from metabolically labelled cells. An increase of the mRNA was observed using a semi-quantitative RT-PCR assay. Finally, HLA class II mediated apoptosis was almost completly inhibited in the presence of either an anti-Fas or an anti-FasL Ab while isotype matched control antibodies did not have any effect. These data lead us to suggest that a HLA class II restricted antigen specific signal can lead to apoptosis mediated by a non-antigen specific system. Further these data support the idea of cytotoxic B lymphocytes. The FasL belongs to the TNF family and also exists in a bioactive soluble form after cleavage by a metalloprotease. We have detected the soluble form of the Fas ligand in supernatants of cells stimulated *via* HLA class II and we suggest that the soluble effector molecule may also have a role in HLA class II mediated apoptosis.

Disruption of the cell cycle has been implicated in a variety of apoptotic systems. We therefore examined whether or not HLA class II signals actually influence the cell cycle. For this purpose we have employed the Raji EBV transformed B cell lymphoma and the HTLV transformed T cell line HUT78. HLA class II signalling led to a block in the S phase and subsequent death from this phase in the cell cycle (*Figures 2a* and *2b*). We interpret these data with caution since an S phase block is more difficult to detect in primary B cells. Nonetheless HLA class II signalling does cause apoptosis of cells in the G_1 to S transition and imposition of an S phase block using thymidine (*Figures 2c* and *2d*) does actually increase the degree of apoptosis observed. The relationship between the S phase block and apoptosis is currently under examination.

The role of HLA class II antigen density in signal transduction has not been established although it is clear that the intensity of signalling is not directly proportional to the level of HLA class II molecule expression. We have approached this question by examining HLA class II signalling in foetal B lymphocytes. Despite the much lower expression of HLA class II on these cells, signalling was both conserved and altered since PKC was activated although an intracellular calcium flux was not observed. With regard to the influence of peptide binding to HLA class II molecules, signal transduction occurs on foetal B lymphocytes although a significant proportion of these molecules are 'empty'. We cannot conclude anything about the optimal HLA class II structure with regard to signalling for the moment since signalling function may be like antigen presentation and require few molecules to generate a successful response.

In summary, HLA class II molecule signalling influences the antigen presenting cell and in the case of human B lymphocytes, this may result in proliferation or in apoptosis. HLA class II signalling appears to be conserved throughout B lymphocyte ontogeny and it is the activation state of the APC which determines the response to HLA class II mediated signals.

References

1. Fraser JD. High affinity binding of staphlococcal enterotoxins A and B to HLA-DR. *Nature* 1989; 339: 221-3.
2. Cambier JC, Newell MK, Justement LB, Mc Guire JC, Leach KL, Chen ZZ. Ia binding ligands and cAMP stimulate nuclear translocation of PKC in B lymphocytes. *Nature* 1987; 327: 629-32.
3. Mooney NA, Grillot-Courvalin C, Hivroz C, Ju L, Charron D. Early biochemical events after MHC class II mediated signaling on human B lymphocytes. *J Immunol* 1990; 145: 2070-6.
4. Brick-Ghannan C, Huang FL, Temine N, Charron D. Protein kinase C (PKC) activation *via* human leucocyte antigen class II molecules. *J Biol Chem* 1991; 266: 24169-75.
5. Brick-Ghannan C, Ericson ML, Schelle I, Charron D. Differential regulation of mRNAs encoding protein kinase C isoenzymes in activated human B cells. *Hum Immunol* 1994; 41: 216-24.
6. André P, Cambier JC, Wade TK, Raetz T, William Wade. Distinct structural compartmentalization of the signal transducing functions of major histocompatibility complex class II (Ia) molecules. *J Exp Med* 1994; 179: 763-8.
7. Truman JP, Choqueux C, Charron D, Mooney N. HLA class II molecule signal transduction leads to either apoptosis or activation *via* two different pathways. *Cell Immunol* 1996; 172: 149-57.
8. Newell NK, Vanderwall J, Scott Beard KS, Freed J. Ligation of major histocompatility complex class II molecules mediates apoptotic cell death in resting B lymphocytes. *Proc Natl Acad Sci USA* 1990; 87: 10459-63.
9. Rieux-Leucat F, Le Deist F, Hivroz C, Roberts I, Debatin KM, Fischer A, De Villaraty JP. Mutations in Fas associated with human lymphoproliferative syndrome and autoimmunity. *Science* 1995; 268: 1347-50.
10. Truman JP, Choqueux C, Le Deist F, Charron D, Mooney N. HLA class II mediated death is induced *via* Fas/Fas ligand interactions in human splenic B lymphocytes. *Blood* 1997; 89: 1996-2007.

Positive and negative CD4$^+$ thymocyte selection by a single MHC class II/peptide ligand *in vivo*

T. Sasazuki, Y. Fukui

Department of Genetics, Medical Institute of Bioregulation, Kyushu University, 3-1-1 Maidashi, Higashi-Ku, Fukuoka 812-82, Japan

While the diversity of αβ T cell receptors (TCRs) theoretically reaches to 10^{15} by random rearrangement of five gene segments (Vα, Jα, Vβ, Dβ, Jβ) and random nucleotide addition, mature T cells express highly selected TCRs in that they exhibit tolerance to self-antigenic peptides and restriction to self-major histocompatibility complex (MHC) molecules. This mainly results from two reciprocal selection processes, positive and negative selection, acting during T-cell development in the thymus. Several evidence has been accumulated to indicate that self-peptides bound to self-MHC molecules mediate both positive and negative selection.

One explanation for the conceptual paradox between positive and negative selection has led to a differential avidity model that the fate of T cells is determined by the cell-surface density of MHC/peptide complexes as well as the intrinsic affinity of TCRs for the ligands. Supporting this model, *in vitro* experiments using fetal thymic organ culture have clearly shown that the cell-surface density of a single MHC class I/peptide complex affects the fate of CD8$^+$ T cells expressing the transgenic TCR [1, 2]. However, the effect of TCR-ligand density on thymic selection remains unclear under physiological T-cell differentiation where T cells express a diverse set of TCRs with various specificities and various affinities or kinetics for a given ligand differently expressed on distinct thymic stroma cells. Especially, very little is known about thymic selection of CD4$^+$ T cells, because of the lack of the appropriate experimental system to follow the fate of CD4$^+$ T cells directed by a given ligand.

The peptide derived from MHC class II Eα chain (Eα52-68) binds to MHC class II I-A^b molecules. To follow the fate of CD4$^+$ T cells directed by a given MHC class II/peptide complex, we have developed three lines of transgenic mouse expressing I-A^b/Eα52-68 complex as a single species, B2H $A^{0/0}Ii^{0/0}$, H3 $A^{0/0}Ii^{0/0}$, and B2L $A^{0/0}Ii^{0/0}$, by introducing the chimeric gene to encode I-Aβ^b chain covalently bound to Eα52-68 into mice carrying H-2^b haplotype but lacking both wild-type I-Aβ^b and invariant chains [3]. The evidence that I-A^b molecule covalently bound to Eα52-68 is expressed as a single MHC class II/peptide complex in these transgenic mouse lines comes from the following two results. First, pre-incubation of spleen cells or short-term cultured thymic epithelial cell line with YAe specific for this complex completely inhibited the staining with Y3P which recognizes I-A^b molecules irrespective of the binding peptides. Second, spleen cells from transgenic mouse lines were unable to present the other I-A^b-binding peptide, even though high concentration of the peptide was used. All these results are consistent with the recent report by Ignatowicz [4] on a line of transgenic mice expressing the same MHC class II/peptide complex as a single species. Since spleen cells from transgenic mouse lines stimulated a hybridoma specific for I-A^b/Eα52-68 complex in the absence of the exogenous Eα52-68, it is also clear that I-A^b molecules covalently bound to Eα52-68 are expressed in these mice as appropriate form to be recognized by a given TCR.

The mean intensity for YAe in B cell population of B2H $A^{0/0}Ii^{0/0}$ was 24.2 times higher than that of C57BL/6 (B6 [H-2^b]) which lack the expression of I-A^b/Eα52-68 complex, whereas that of H3 $A^{0/0}Ii^{0/0}$ and B2L $A^{0/0}Ii^{0/0}$ showed only 3.6 and 1.8 times higher level, respectively (*Table I*). Immunohistochemical analysis using YAe revealed that I-A^b/Eα52-68 complexes were expressed in thymic cortex and medulla in both B2H $A^{0/0}Ii^{0/0}$ and B2L $A^{0/0}Ii^{0/0}$. The expression of I-A^b/Eα52-68 complexes, however, was scarcely detected in thymic cortex in H3 $A^{0/0}Ii^{0/0}$, although weak positive staining was observed in thymic medulla in this line (*Table I*). Since staining was done simultaneously under the same condition, it was concluded that the expression level of I-A^b/Eα52-68 complexes in B2H $A^{0/0}Ii^{0/0}$ was considerably higher than that in B2L $A^{0/0}Ii^{0/0}$ and H3 $A^{0/0}Ii^{0/0}$ in the thymus and periphery.

Having established transgenic mouse lines expressing a single MHC class II/peptide complex at different levels in the thymus, we compared CD4$^+$ T-cell differentiation in the thymus among these lines. Since a considerable number of CD4$^+$CD8$^-$NK1.1$^+$ T cells (8 - 25 % of CD4$^+$CD8$^-$ T cells depending on the analyzed lines) selected by non-classical MHC class I molecules such as CD1 were found, we analyzed the expression of CD4 and CD8 on thymocytes which did not express NK1.1. Immature CD4$^+$CD8$^+$ T cells differentiated into mature CD4$^+$CD8$^-$ T cells *via* CD4$^+$CD8^{int} stage in B2L A$^{0/0}$Ii$^{0/0}$ and H3 A$^{0/0}$Ii$^{0/0}$. Surprisingly, however, no definite CD4$^+$CD8$^-$ T cells were observed in B2H A$^{0/0}$Ii$^{0/0}$ with the highest expression level of I-A^b/Eα52-68 complex in the thymus among three lines of transgenic mouse (*Table I*). It is unlikely that the failure of CD4$^+$ T-cell differentiation in B2H A$^{0/0}$Ii$^{0/0}$ resulted from some T-cell defects causing differentiation arrest, because a considerable number of CD4$^+$CD8$^-$NK1.1$^-$ T cells were observed in B2H A$^{0/0}$Ii$^{+/+}$ in which part of Eα52-68 peptides bound to I-A^b molecules were replaced by other peptides. The number of CD4$^+$CD8$^-$ NK1.1$^-$ T cells per thymus in B2L A$^{0/0}$Ii$^{0/0}$ and H3 A$^{0/0}$Ii$^{0/0}$ was 3.6 times and 1.8 times higher than that in A$^{0/0}$Ii$^{0/0}$ respectively, whereas the number in B2H A$^{0/0}$Ii$^{0/0}$ was comparable to that in A$^{0/0}$Ii$^{0/0}$ which lack MHC class II expression (*Table I*). The ratio of the number of CD4$^+$CD8$^-$NK1.1$^-$ T cells to that of CD4$^+$CD8$^-$ NK1.1$^+$ T cells, which would be a good indicator to assess the degree of CD4$^+$ T-cell differentiation directed by I-A^b/Eα52-68 complex because the similar number of CD4$^+$CD8$^-$NK1.1$^+$ T cells was observed in these mice analyzed at 6 weeks old, agreed with this (*Table I*). Lymph node CD4$^+$ T cells from B2L A$^{0/0}$Ii$^{0/0}$ and H3 A$^{0/0}$Ii$^{0/0}$ responded well to B6 spleen cells expressing wild-type I-A^b molecules, but did not show any response to spleen cells prepared from B2H A$^{0/0}$Ii$^{0/0}$ as well as those from syngenic cells. These observations are consistent with the recent reports showing that CD4$^+$ T cells positively selected by a single ligand recognize other peptides bound to the same MHC class II molecules but are tolerant to the selecting ligand [3-7]. However, neither the LN CD4$^+$ T cells from B2H A$^{0/0}$Ii$^{0/0}$ nor those from A$^{0/0}$Ii$^{0/0}$ showed any proliferation to B6 spleen cells, indicating a lack of the LN CD4$^+$ T cells differentiated in the context of I-A^b/Eα52-68 complex in B2H A$^{0/0}$Ii$^{0/0}$.

Taken together, these results clearly show that CD4$^+$ T cells were selected to mature on I-A^b/Eα52-68 complex in B2L A$^{0/0}$Ii$^{0/0}$ and H3 A$^{0/0}$Ii$^{0/0}$ with relatively low expression of this complex in the thymus, whereas CD4$^+$ T cells with any affinity for this ligand could not survive thymic selection in B2H A$^{0/0}$Ii$^{0/0}$ where I-A^b/Eα52-68 complexes were expressed in the thymus at higher level than that in B2L A$^{0/0}$Ii$^{0/0}$ and H3 A$^{0/0}$Ii$^{0/0}$. Since the only difference among these transgenic mouse lines is the expression level of I-A^b/Eα52-68 complex, our findings provide *in vivo* evidence that the cell-surface density of a given MHC class II/peptide complex in the thymus plays a crucial role in the determining the fate of CD4$^+$ T cells.

To assess the effect of the expression level of I-A^b/Eα52-68 complex on CD4$^+$ T-cell differentiation more directly, CD4$^+$ T cells were analyzed phenotypically and functionally in A$^{0/0}$Ii$^{0/0}$ expressing both B2L and B2H transgenes (B2L B2H A$^{0/0}$Ii$^{0/0}$). The proportion of CD4$^+$CD8$^-$ NK1.1$^-$ T cells in the thymus from B2L B2H A$^{0/0}$Ii$^{0/0}$ was much less than that from B2L A$^{0/0}$Ii$^{0/0}$ littermate. Consistent with this, lymph node CD4$^+$ T cells from B2L B2H A$^{0/0}$Ii$^{0/0}$ showed less robust proliferative response to B6 spleen cells than that from B2L A$^{0/0}$Ii$^{0/0}$. These observations indicate that the frequency of CD4$^+$ T cells selected to mature on I-A^b/Eα52-68 complex in the thymus from B2L B2H A$^{0/0}$Ii$^{0/0}$ markedly decreases as compared with that from B2L A$^{0/0}$Ii$^{0/0}$. It is unlikely that higher expression of I-A^b/Eα52-68 complex in the thymus of B2L B2H A$^{0/0}$Ii$^{0/0}$ decreases the efficiency of positive selection it-self. Our results thus strongly suggest that I-A^b/Eα52-68 complex, being affected by its cell-surface density in the thymus, can serve as negatively selecting ligand as well as positively selecting ligand *in vivo*. Our findings that the expression level of a given MHC class II/peptide complex in the thymus dramatically affects thymic selection thus suggest that a window of TCR affinity for the complex to survive positive and negative selection is considerably narrow as was suggested by Alam *et al.* [8] on the affinity of TCRs for MHC class I/peptide complexes.

Different from the case with B2H A$^{0/0}$Ii$^{0/0}$, however, a small but a definite number of CD4$^+$CD8$^-$ T cells were found to be selected to mature on I-A^b/Eα52-68 complex in B2L B2H A$^{0/0}$Ii$^{0/0}$. The expression of I-A^b/Eα52-68 complex in thymic medulla in B2H A$^{0/0}$Ii$^{0/0}$ is 5-10 times higher than that in B2L A$^{0/0}$Ii$^{0/0}$, whereas the difference in the expression level in thymic cortex between these two lines appears to be much less

Table I. Summary of three lines of transgenic mice expressing I-A^b molecules covalently bound to Eα52-68

	B2L $A^{0/0}Ii^{0/0}$	H3 $A^{0/0}Ii^{0/0}$	B2H $A^{0/0}Ii^{0/0}$	$A^{0/0}Ii^{0/0}$
Expression of I-A^b /Eα52-68 complex on spleen cells	+	++	++++	-
Expression of I-A^b /Eα52-68 complex in the thymus				
cortex	+	±	++	-
medulla	+	±	++++	-
The percentage of $CD4^+$ $CD8^-$ NK1.1^- thymocytes to total thymocytes lacking NK1.1 expression	1.9 ± 0.3%	1.4 ± 0.4%	0.5 ± 0.1%	0.5 ± 0.1%
The total number of $CD4^+$ $CD8^-$ NK1.1^- thymocytes per thymus (x 10^4)	458 ± 134	227 ± 29	130 ± 56	128 ± 48
The ratio of the number of $CD4^+$ $CD8^-$ NK1.1^- thymocytes to that of $CD4^+$ $CD8^-$ NK1.1^- thymocytes	11.6 ± 3.4	6.4 ± 2.7	2.7 ± 0.7	3.1 ± 0.4

than that in thymic medulla. In addition, several lines of evidence have indicated that epithelial cells in thymic cortex mediate positive selection, and bone marrow-derived cells and epithelial cells in thymic medulla mediate negative selection. Therefore, it is suggested that the ratio of the expression of a given MHC/peptide complex in thymic cortex for that in thymic medulla is a 'really' critical parameter to determine the fate of T cells directed by this ligand *in vivo*, which could explain the difference in $CD4^+$ T-cell differentiation between B2H $A^{0/0}Ii^{0/0}$ and B2L B2H $A^{0/0}Ii^{0/0}$.

In summary, we have shown that a single MHC class II/peptide complex, being affected by its expression level in thymic cortex and medulla, can serve as both positively and negatively selecting ligand for $CD4^+$ T cells *in vivo*, using transgenic mouse lines expressing this complex at different levels in the thymus. These transgenic mouse lines would be good tools to investigate the interaction of TCRs with a given MHC/peptide complex in thymic selection and facilitate biochemical analysis to reveal molecular mechanism undergoing positive and negative selection.

References

1. Hogquist KA, Jameson SC, Heath WR, Howard JL, Bevan MJ, Carbone FR. T cell receptor antagonistpeptides induce positive selection. *Cell* 1994; 76: 17-27.
2. Ashton-Rickardt PG, Banderia A, Pelaney JR, Van Kaer L, Pircher HP, Zinkernagel RM, Tonegawa S. Evidence for a differential avidity model of T cell selection in the thymus. *Cell* 1994; 76: 651-63.
3. Fukui Y, Ishimoto T, Utsuyama M, Gyotoku T, Koga T, Nakao K, Hirokawa K, Katsuki M, Sasazuki T. Positive and negative $CD4^+$ thymocyte selection by a single MHC class II/peptide ligand affected by its expression level in the thymus. *Immunity* 1997; 6:401-10.
4. Ignatowicz L, Kappler J, Marrack P. The repertoire of T cells shaped by a single MHC/peptide ligand. *Cell* 1996; 84: 521-9.
5. Miyazaki T, Wolf P, Tourne S, Waltzinger C, Dierich A, Barois N, Ploegh H, Benoist C, Mathis D. Mice lacking H2-M complexes, enigmatic elements of the MHC class II peptide-loading pathway. *Cell* 1996; 84: 531-41.
6. Martin WD, Hicks GG, Mendiratta SK, Leva HI, Ruley HE, Van Kaer L. H2-M mutant mice are defective in the peptide loading of class II molecules, antigen presentation, and T cell repertoire selection. *Cell* 1996; 84: 543-50.
7. Fung-Leung WP, Surh CD, Liljedahl M, Pang J, Leturcq D, Peterson PA, Webb SR, Karlsson L. Antigen presentation and T cell development in H2-M-deficient mice. *Science* 1996; 271: 1278-81.
8. Alam SM, Travers PJ, Wung JL, Nasholds W, Redlpath S, Jameson SC, Gascoigne NRJ. T-cell-receptor affinity and thymocyte positive selection. *Nature* 1996; 381: 616-20.

4 • HLA in medicine

The role of MHC class II molecules in susceptibility and resistance to type I diabetes mellitus

H.O. McDevitt

Departments of microbiology and immunology, and medicine, Stanford University School of Medicine, Fairchild bldg D345, Stanford, California 94605, USA

Beginning with the demonstration by Lilly that susceptibility and resistance to Gross virus induced leukemia in mice [1] was determined by the genotype of the major histocompatibility complex (MHC), there has been a growing body of evidence showing that MHC genes play a major role in determining inherited susceptibility to a wide variety of diseases. The demonstration that genes in the I region, now designated as the class II region of the MHC, determined the ability to mount an immune response to several synthetic polypeptides [2] led to the hypothesis that MHC genes might play an important role in diseases in which the immune response was required either to prevent the disease, as in infections, or in the pathogenesis of the disease, as in autoimmune syndromes [3]. In the ensuing years, it was found that susceptibility to more than twenty diseases, many of them thought to be autoimmune diseases, was determined by MHC genotype [4]. This list included several diseases not previously thought to be autoimmune in nature, including juvenile onset, type I, insulin dependent diabetes mellitus (IDDM) [4].

IDDM is a complex autoimmune disease for which susceptibility is determined by both environmental and genetic factors. The inheritance of susceptibility is polygenic, and genes in the MHC appear to be the strongest genetic factors [5]. Because of the influence of numerous [15-20] as yet uncharacterized genes unlinked to the MHC, MHC genotype is a necessary but not sufficient predisposing genetic factor.

Although MHC linked genetic control of specific immune responses, and close associations and specific linkage of MHC alleles with specific diseases have been known for more than twenty years, the precise molecular mechanisms by which MHC class I and class II genes influence susceptibility to various autoimmune diseases is still poorly understood.

The striking associations of IDDM with particular HLA genotypes, and the availability of a very similar spontaneous model of IDDM in the non-obese diabetic (NOD) mouse, coupled with rapidly developing knowledge of the autoantigenic targets of the diabetogenic process, makes IDDM a prime candidate for attempts to understand how MHC genes affect the pathogenesis of autoimmune disease.

MHC associations with IDDM

Extensive studies of MHC class I and class II genotype in patients with IDDM, analysis of restriction fragment length polymorphisms, and extensive sequencing of MHC class II alleles in man, the NOD mouse and the BB rat has indicated a primary role for HLA DQ alleles in man, and I-A alleles in the NOD mouse. Type I diabetes is most strongly associated with DQβ and I-Aβ alleles which encode a neutral amino acid (serine, alanine, or valine) at position 57 on both chromosomes [6]. DQβ and I-Aβ alleles encoding aspartic acid at position 57 are strongly associated with resistance to IDDM, with variation apparently due to the sequence of other residues in the DQ alpha and beta chains. Studies in many different populations have revealed several exceptions to this general finding, and have shown that polymorphisms in the DQα chain, elsewhere in the DQβ chain, and in the DR1β chain, play an important and sometimes critical modifying role [6,7].

Despite these modifying influences, the above mentioned polymorphism in DQβ and I-Aβ at position 57 appears to be the single strongest polymorphism determining susceptibility or resistance to IDDM. It therefore furnishes a convenient starting point for attempting to understand the mechanism of actions of MHC class II alleles in autoimmunity.

Effect of MHC class II genes in IDDM

Several lines of evidence indicate that IDDM susceptible MHC class II alleles support a predominant Th1 T cell response to islet cell antigens, contributing to an inflammatory process that ultimately results in destruction of beta cells in the islets of Langerhans. Among the findings supporting this conclusion (cited in [6]), perhaps the most striking is the demonstration by Katz *et al.* [8], that T cells from a TCR transgenic mouse expressing a diabetogenic TCR can transfer IDDM when these cells are cultured under conditions promoting a Th1 phenotype, and fail to transfer IDDM when these cells are cultured in the presence of IL-4 to promote development of a Th2 phenotype. Studies with NOD mice lacking expression of MHC class I molecules [9-11] have clearly shown that T cells restricted to MHC class I, presumably CD8+ T cells, are required for the development of insulitis and IDDM. These findings suggest that initiation of the diabetic process requires CD8+ cytotoxic T cells. Because the strongest MHC association with IDDM is with MHC class II genotype, and because a number of studies have shown that diabetes can be transferred with CD4 T cell clones [8,12], it would appear that the primary allele specific MHC association with IDDM is the class II association.

The studies referred to above indicate that in susceptible individuals, MHC class II alleles support a process of autoantigen presentation and subsequent T cell response that results in a predominant Th1 inflammatory T cell response, leading to β islet cell destruction. On the other hand, IDDM resistant MHC class II alleles, in an individual otherwise genetically susceptible to IDDM at the other non-MHC loci, lead to the development of a Th2 response to islet cell autoantigens. While this may result in the production of autoantibody to these antigens, the Th2 cells, by producing IL-4, IL-10 and perhaps TgFβ, prevent the development of an inflammatory destructive lesion in the islets of Langerhans. Several studies ([13], and references summarized in [13]) have shown that introduction into NOD embryos of I-A α/β genes or Aβ genes encoding aspartic acid at position 57 in the β chain decreases or completely prevents the development of IDDM in these transgenic mice.

Transgenic NOD mice expressing the Aβ position 57 aspartic acid positive $A\beta^d$ allele develop IDDM at a much lower incidence than non-transgenic litter mates. However, purified spleen T cells from recently diabetic $A\beta^d$ transgenic animals are very ineffective at transferring diabetes to irradiated young male NOD recipients. This is unlike their non-transgenic littermates, which transfer diabetes with 80-90% efficiency. Addition of NOD.$A\beta^d$ purified spleen T cells to diabetogenic NOD spleen T cells results in partial and occasionally complete suppression of transfer of IDDM [14] (see *Table I*). This result is compatible with the concept that T cells in the transgenic animal have a much greater proportion of Th2-like T cells than in non-transgenic littermates. This hypothesis requires confirmation by blocking this suppression with monoclonal antibodies to IL-4 and IL-10 (*Table II*), but is compatible with the other results cited above indicating that Th1 cells transfer IDDM, while Th2 cells with the same T cell receptor are incapable of transferring IDDM.

Table I. Transgenic T cells prevent adoptive transfer of diabetes

	% recipients diabetic		
Cells transferred	**Exp. 1**	**Exp. 2**	**Exp. 3**
10^7 diabetic cells alone	100 (10)	90 (10)	90 (10)
Diabetic cells + Tg T cells	30 (9)	73 (15)	25 (8)
Diabetic cells + non-Tg T cells	89 (9)	91 (11)	86 (7)

Irradiated recipients were reconstituted as described. Numbers in parentheses indicate number of animals per group. In Exps. 1 and 2, 4 million T cells were added to total spleen cells from diabetic mice. In Exp. 3,10 million T cells were added, Tg. transgenic. *P* values for Exps. 1, 2, and 3 are 0.053, 0.53, and 0.057, respectively.

Table II. Transfer of diabetes in NOD and NOD. $A\beta^d$ transgenic mice

Donor	**Recipient**	**% Transfer IDDM**
NOD	NOD	80 - 90%
NOD.$A\beta^d$	NOD	10 - 15%
NOD.$A\beta^d$	NOD.$A\beta^d$ + anti - IL- 4 anti - IL-10 anti - TGFβ	?

In summary, the principal effect of IDDM susceptible class II MHC alleles is to support a predominant Th1 response to islet cell autoantigens, while IDDM protective alleles lead to a predominant Th2 response to these antigens. This conclusion, which still requires further experimental confirmation, then leads to the following question: How do the sequence polymorphisms differing between susceptible and resistant IDDM alleles induce their phenotypic effects?

Possible mechanisms of action of IDDM susceptible and resistant MHC class II molecules

The factors which determine the development of Th1 and Th2 phenotypes in CD4(+) T cells are complex and only partially understood. The density of MHC/peptide complexes on the surface of antigen presenting cells [15], the nature of the antigen presenting cell, the TCR affinity/avidity for the peptide/MHC complex, interaction between co-stimulatory molecules [16], and the probable effect of other, background, non-MHC linked genes [17] all may play a role in determining the outcome of this developmental process. In addition, it is quite possible and even likely that structural differences in MHC class II molecules can result in the selection of different T cell receptor repertoires. The possible mechanisms of action of MHC class II alleles in the differential induction of Th1 and Th2 islet cell specific immune responses are listed below, in an undoubtedly incomplete listing:

1. Binding and presentation of different immunodominant peptide epitopes of islet cell antigens.
2. Increased/decreased affinity of these peptides for MHC class II.
3. Resultant increase/decrease in peptide/MHC stability.
4. Longer/shorter half life of peptide MHC complexes on the cell surface.
5. Selection of different TCR repertoires.

It should be noted that possibilities 2, 3, and 4 could result either from binding of a different peptide by susceptible or resistant alleles, or from differences in configuration of the same peptide due to differences in the structure of the susceptible and resistant alleles. In addition, mechanisms 1-4 are not mutually exclusive with mechanism 5. Both types of mechanisms could be operative and play important roles in the development of autoimmunity in IDDM.

There is already evidence which indirectly supports the concept that susceptible and resistant alleles bind and present different peptide epitopes from islet cell autoantigens. Rammensee *et al.* eluted peptides from purified HLA DR 04 molecules. Peptides eluted from HLA DR 0405 (DR B1 position 57-serine) bound peptides which predominantly expressed aspartic acid or glutamic acid at position p9 in the peptide [18]. In contrast, HLA DR 0401(DR B1 position 57 aspartic acid) bound peptides with alanine, serine or glutamine at position p9. These results are presumably due to the fact that in the absence of aspartic acid at position 57, a conserved arginine at DRα 79 is free to interact with negative charges in the carboxy terminus of the bound peptide. In position 57 aspartic acid positive alleles, asp 57 forms a salt bridge with the conserved arginine at alpha 79, so that the arginine is not free to interact with residues in the bound peptide [19]. Further evidence comes from studies by Kwok *et al.* [20] in analyzing the peptides bound by cells expressing DQ8 and DQ9. These HLA DQ alleles are identical in sequence except at position 57 in the β chain. DQ8 encodes alanine, and DQ9 encodes aspartic acid. These two DQ alleles show striking differences in binding selected peptides with either a negative or a positive charge at the carboxy terminus of the peptide.

The other possible mechanisms listed above have not yet been subjected to direct experimental test. Additional mechanisms have also been postulated. Nepom [21] and others [13] have suggested that competition between susceptible and resistant alleles for binding a critical diabetogenic peptide might be the basis for the observed results. In the latter case, the peptide bound by the resistant allele would presumably not induce an immune response but would be prevented from binding to the susceptible allele. Studies in IDDM families suggest that this is not the case. Thus, DQB1 0602 (a strongly resistant IDDM allele) positive siblings of diabetics rarely develop diabetes, although they can produce high titers of autoantibodies to several islet cell antigens. This finding indicates that resistant alleles binding islet cell peptides are capable of inducing an immune response which does not result in destruction of islets of Langerhans, a result which is more compatible with differential induction of an inflammatory versus a protective T cell response.

Future directions

In recent years, evidence in both the NOD mouse and in man has identified a number of autoantigens which are the target of both antibody and T cell responses in diabetic patients and in NOD mice. There is as yet no definitive evidence that any one of these antigens is the "critical" autoantigen responsible for the striking MHC restrictions seen in susceptibility to IDDM in man and the NOD mouse. However, three of these antigens - glutamic decarboxylase (GAD), insulin, and heat shock protein 60 kD have been shown to be capable of down-regulating the autoimmune process when injected parenterally in aqueous solution in pre-diabetic NOD mice (references in [6]). In addition, the first detectable immune responses to islet cell antigens are specific for GAD and insulin [6,22]. For these reasons, these antigens are leading candidates for an important role in initiating the diabetogenic process, and for being responsible for the observed MHC restriction.

With the availability of candidate autoantigens, it becomes possible to employ each of them to subject the mechanisms listed above to direct experimental test. This can be done in wild type NOD mice, and in NOD mice expressing resistant I-A transgenes. Similar studies can be carried out in NOD mice expressing susceptible and resistant HLA DQ alleles. Thus, NOD mice expressing the α/β chains of HLA DQ8, DQ7, and DQ6, as well as I-A transgenic mice, can be used to survey T cell clones and T cell hybridomas for their specificity for peptides of GAD 65 kD, insulin, and heat shock protein 60. Ideally, these studies should be carried out utilizing T cell clones or T cell hybridomas that develop spontaneously in untreated NOD mice and NOD transgenics. If this is not possible, immunization with these antigens by a variety of routes can be used to assess the immunodominant peptide epitopes of these islet cell autoantigens.

This would permit a direct test of whether susceptible and resistant MHC class II alleles bind different immunodominant peptide epitopes of islet cell autoantigens. Regardless of whether these resistant or susceptible alleles bind different or the same peptide epitopes, these peptides can be used to test the density of peptide/MHC complexes on the cell surface, the stability of these peptide/MHC complexes, and their half life on the cell surface. Systematic analysis of each of these parameters should advance our understanding of how susceptible and resistant alleles exert their effects. It should also be possible, using these peptide epitopes, to develop methods to compare the T cell receptor repertoires induced in NOD mice expressing IDDM susceptible and resistant alleles. All of these experimental approaches, taken together, offer the possibility of understanding the molecular basis for MHC mediated suseptibility to IDDM, a result which may serve as a paradigm for the role of class II MHC alleles in susceptibility to many other autoimmune diseases.

References

1. Lilly F. The histocompatibility-2 locus and susceptibility to tumor induction. *Natl Cancer Inst Monogr* 1966; 22: 631.
2. McDevitt HO, Tyan ML. Genetic control of the antibody response in inbred mice. Transfer of response by spleen cells and linkage to the major histocompatibility (H-2) locus. *J Exp Med* 1968; 128 (1): 1-11.
3. Grumet FC, Coukell A, Bodmer JG, Bodmer WF, McDevitt HO. Histocompatibility (HL-A) antigens associated with systemic lupus erythematosus. A possibile genetic predisposition to disease. *N Engl J Med* 1971; 285 (4): 193-6.
4. Svejgaard A, Platz P, Ryder LP. HLA and disease 1982: A survey. *Immunol Rev* 1983; 70: 193-218.
5. Vyse TJ, Todd JA. Genetic analysis of autoimmune disease. *Cell* 1996; 85: 311-8.
6. Tisch R, McDevitt HO. Insulin dependent diabetes mellitus. *Cell* 1996 ; 85: 291-7.
7. Cucca F, Lampis R, Frau F, Macis D, Angius E, Masile P, Chessa M, Cao A, Deviriliis S, Congia M. The distribution of DR4 haplotypes in Sardinia suggest a primary association of type I diabetes with DRB1 and DQB1 loci. *Hum Immunol* 1995; 43: 301-8.
8. Katz JD, Benoist C, Mathis D. T helper cell subsets in insulin dependent diabetes. *Science* 1995 ; 268: 1185-8.
9. Katz JD, Wang B, Haskins K, Benoist C, Mathis D. Following a diabetogenic T cell from genesis through pathogenesis. *Cell* 1993 ; 74: 1089-100.
10. Serreze, DV, Leiter EH, Christianson GJ, Greiner D, Roopenian DC. Major histocompatibility complex I deficient NOD-β2m null mice are diabetes and insulitis resistant. *Diabetes* 1994 ; 43: 505-9.

11. Wicker LS, Leiter EH, Todd JA, Renjilian RJ, Peterson E, Fischer PA, Podolin PL, Zijlstra M, Jaenisch R, Peterson LB. β2-microglobulin deficient NOD mice do not develop insulitis or diabetes. *Diabetes* 1995 ; 43: 500-4.
12. Haskins K, McDuffie M. Acceleration of diabetes in young NOD mice with a CD4 islet-specific T cell clone. *Science* 1990 ; 249: 1433-5.
13. Quartey-Papafio R, Lund T, Chandlker P, Picard J, Ozogbe P, Day S, Hutchings PR, O'Reilly L, Kioussis D, Simpson E, Cooke A. Aspartate at position 57 of nonobese diabetic I-A^{g7} β-chain diminishes the spontaneous incidence of insulin-dependent diabetes mellitus. *J Immunol* 1995 ; 154: 5567-75.
14. Singer S, Tisch R, Yang XD, McDevitt HO. An $A\beta^{d}$ transgene prevents diabetes in nonobese diabetic mice by inducing regulatory T cells. *Proc Natl Acad Sci USA* 1993 ; 90: 9566-95.
15. Pfeiffer C, Stein J , Southwood S, Ketelaar H, Sette A, Bottomly K. Altered peptide ligands can control CD 4 T lymphocyte differentiation *in vivo*. *J Exp Med* 1995 ; 181: 1569-74.
16. Lenschow DJ, Ho SC, Sattar H, Rhee L, Gray G, Nabavi N, Herold KC, Bluestone JA. Differential effects of anti-B7-1 and anti-B7-2 monoclonal treatment on the development of diabetes in the nonobese diabetic mouse. *J Exp Med* 1995 ; 181: 1145-55.
17. Scott B, Liblau R, Degermann S, Marconi LA, Ogata L, Caton AJ, McDevitt HO, Lo D. A role for non-MHC genetic polymorphism in susceptibility to spontaneous autoimmunity. *Immunity* 1994 ; 1: 73-82.
18. Ramensee HC, Friede T, Stevanovic S. MHC ligands and peptide motifs: first listing. *Immunogenetics* 1995 ; 41: 178-228.
19. Stern LJ, Brown JH, Jardetzky TH, Urban R, Strominger JL, Wiley DC. Crystal structure of the human class II MHC protein HLA DR1 complexed with an influenza virus peptide. *Nature* 1994 ; 368: 215-23.
20. Kwok WW, Nepom GT, Raymond FC. HLA-DQ polymorhpisms are highly selective for peptide binding interactions. *Immunology* 1996 ; 156: 2171-7.
21. Nepom GT. A unified hypothesis for the complex genetics of HLA associations with IDDM. *Diabetes* 1990 ; 39: 1153-7.
22. Tisch R, Yang XD, Singer SM, Liblau RS, Fugger F, McDevitt HO. Immune response to glutamic acid decarboxylase correlates with insulitis in nonobese diabetic mice. *Nature* 1993 ; 366: 72-5.

Antigens recognized by T lymphocytes on human tumors

T. Boon, B.J. Van den Eynde, P. Van der Bruggen

Ludwig Institute for Cancer Research, Brussels Branch, 74, avenue Hippocrate, UCL 74.59, B-1200 Brussels, Belgium
Cellular Genetics Unit, Université Catholique de Louvain, B-1200 Brussels, Belgium

Tumor-specific cytolytic T lymphocytes (CTL) have been obtained in several human tumor types, mainly in melanoma. By using a genetic approach based on the transfection of genomic or cDNA libraries, the genes encoding a number of human tumor antigens have been cloned. In most instances, this has led to the identification of antigenic peptides presented by tumors on various HLA class I molecules. On the basis of their pattern of expression, these antigens can be classified in three groups. Antigens of the first group are encoded by genes that are expressed in many tumor cells but are silent in normal adult tissues except testis. The second group consists of differentiation antigens. Antigens of a third group are unique to individual tumors and result from mutations occurring in genes that are expressed in most normal tissues.

Tumor specific shared antigens

Three families of genes that appear to code for highly specific tumor antigens have been identified so far, namely the MAGE, BAGE and GAGE genes [1-4]. These genes are frequently expressed in a wide range of tumor types such as melanoma, lung carcinoma, sarcoma, bladder carcinoma but very rarely in other tumor types such as brain tumors, rehal carcinoma and leukemia (*Table I*) [2, 5-7]. The only normal tissues where expression of these genes has been observed are testis and placenta [2]. Starting from CTL clones obtained by stimulating lymphocytes with an autologous melanoma cell line, seven antigens encoded by MAGE-1, MAGE-3, BAGE and GAGE have been identified [3, 4, 8-12].
For these seven antigens, both the presenting HLA molecule and the antigenic peptide have been completely defined (*Table II*). More than 60 % of Caucasian melanoma patients bear one of the presently defined antigens encoded by MAGE, BAGE and GAGE. For other cancers such as lung cancer, head and neck cancer and bladder cancer, the frequencies range from 40 % to 28 %. It appears increasingly unlikely that immunization of patients against one of these antigens will cause harmful immunological side-effects due to the expression of the relevant gene in testis. First this expression appears to occur in germ-line cells, more precisely spermatocytes and spermatogonia [13]. A similar observation has been made with the mouse equivalent of a MAGE gene by *in situ* hybridization [14]. Because these germ-line cells do not express MHC class I molecules, gene expression should not result in antigen expression [15]. These conclusions are further strengthened by immunization studies carried out with mouse tumor antigen P815A, which is encoded by a gene that is also expressed only in testis. After immunization with P815 tumor cells, which carry this antigen, male mice produced a strong CTL response. No inflammation of the testis was observed in the following months and the fertility of these mice was normal [40].
A new mode of origin for antigens that are also tumor-specific shared antigens, has been described recently [16]. Here, a gene that is ubiquitously expressed, namely N-acetyl-glucosaminyltransferase V (GnTV), contains an intron which itself appears to carry near its end a promoter that is activated only in melanoma cells. This atypical activation occurs in more than 50 % of melanomas. It produces a message containing a new open reading frame, which codes for the antigenic peptide in its intronic part.
Recently, we have identified a new antigen recognized by CTL on a kidney tumor. This antigen was found to be encoded by a previously unknown gene that we called RAGE [17]. This gene is silent in normal tissues except

Table I. Expression of genes MAGE-1,-3, BAGE, GAGE, and RAGE in tumor samples[a]

Histological type	Percentage of tumors positive for MAGE-1	MAGE-3	BAGE	GAGE-1,2	RAGE-1
Melanomas					
primary lesions	16	36	8	13	2
metastases	48	76	26	28	5
Non Small Cell Lung Carcinomas	49	47	4	19	0
Head and Neck tumors	28	49	8	19	2
Bladder carcinomas	22	36	15	12	5
Sarcomas	14	24	6	25	14
Mammary carcinomas	18	11	10	9	1
Prostatic carcinomas	15	15	0	10	0
Colorectal carcinomas	2	17	0	0	0
Renal carcinomas	0	0	0	0	2
Leukemias and lymphomas	0	0	0	1	0
Testicular seminomas	4/6	3/6	1/6	5/6	0/3

a. Expression was measured by RT-PCR on total RNA using primers specific for each gene.

retina, and is expressed in a small proportion of tumors, mainly in sarcomas, bladder tumors and melanomas *(Table I)*. Since most retinal cells do not express MHC class I molecules, this antigen is probably tumor-specific, although the formal proof of this will require the identification of the retinal cell type that expresses RAGE. The antigenic peptide recognized by the CTL has been identified. It is presented by HLA-B7 *(Table II)*.

Differentiation antigens

The observation that autologous CTL can be generated readily against differentiation antigens present on normal melanocytes as well as melanoma cells was unexpected. Four genes encoding melanoma differentiation antigens have been identified: tyrosinase, Melan-A/Mart-1, gp100 and gp75 [18-23]. Most of the identified antigenic peptides are presented by HLA-A2, but other HLA-peptide combinations have been found [22-31]. One tyrosinase peptide is presented by HLA-DR4 to CD4 T cells [27].

A tyrosinase peptide presented by HLA-A2 presents an interesting post-translational modification. An asparagine residue is transformed into an aspartic acid residue, presumably because the asparagine was glycosylated and subsequently deglycosylated by an enzyme which removed the aminogroup with the glycan [32].

There is concern for the potential side-effects of active or passive immunization against melanoma differentiation antigens. Not so much for the skin, where vitiligo due to the destruction of melanocytes might occur, but for the retina where melanocytes are present in the choroid layer. However, vitiligo has been associated with good prognoses in melanoma and also with adoptive transfer of TILs, without noticeable eye lesions [28, 30, 33, 34]. Carefully devised immunotherapy trials based on these antigens therefore seem permissible.

Antigens specific for individual tumors

Point mutations also generate antigens recognized on melanoma by autologous CTL. As was seen with the mouse antigens induced by mutagens, the mutations are located in the region coding for the antigenic peptide, enabling it to bind to the MHC molecule or generating a new epitope. A very interesting example is the point mutation of cyclin-dependent kinase 4 [35], which prevents this protein from binding to p16, thereby increasing the probability of its binding to the cyclin molecule and phosphorylating Rb, so that the E2F transcription factor is released and activates genes required for entry into the S phase of the cell cycle. This is clearly a mutation which is both antigenic and oncogenic. The oncogenic

Table II. Tumor-specific antigens shared by different tumors

Gene	Normal expression	MHC	Peptide	Position	Reference
MAGE-1	testis	HLA-A1	EADPTGHSY	161-169	8
		HLA-Cw16	SAYGEPRKL	230-238	9
MAGE-3	testis	HLA-A1	EVDPIGHLY	168-176	10
		HLA-A2	FLWGPRALV	271-279	12
		HLA-B44	MEVDPIGHLY	167-176	11
BAGE	testis	HLA-Cw16	AARAVFLAL	2-10	3
GAGE-1/2	testis	HLA-Cw6	YRPRPRRY	9-16	4
RAGE-1	retina	HLA-B7	SPSSNRIRNT	11-20	17
GnTV (atypical transcript)	none	HLA-A2	VLPDVFIRC	38-64	16

potential of this mutation is underscored by the observation that one out of 28 other melanomas that were tested carried the same mutation. The amino-acid change generated by this mutation enables the peptide to bind to the HLA-A2 presenting molecule.

Another interesting point mutation produces a new antigenic peptide which, remarkably, is partially encoded by the 5' end of an intron [36]. In this instance, the mutation generates a new epitope. A recent report describes an antigenic peptide produced by a mutation in the ß-catenin gene, which codes for a cell surface adhesion molecule. This mutation creates an anchor residue enabling the peptide to bind to HLA-A24 [37].

Point mutations may also create tumor antigens by directly altering an HLA molecule: we recently observed that autologous CTL directed against a human renal cell carcinoma recognized an HLA-A2 molecule that was altered as a result of a point mutation changing one amino acid in the alpha-2 helix [38].

Some of the tumor antigens that we have mentioned are in early stages of clinical study. There is little doubt that the coming years will witness a large number of clinical trials involving peptides, proteins and recombinant defective viruses. It appears that responses have been obtained in some melanoma patients immunized with a MAGE-3 peptide presented by HLA-A1 [39]. It is our hope that the careful study of the lymphocytes and the tumor cells of these patients will produce a rich harvest of additional antigens and a better understanding of what constitutes an effective anti-tumor response.

References

1. Van der Bruggen P, Traversari C, Chomez P, Lurquin C, De Plaen E, Van den Eynde B, Knuth A, Boon T. A gene encoding an antigen recognized by cytolytic T lymphocytes on a human melanoma. *Science* 1991; 254: 1643-7.
2. De Plaen E, Arden K, Traversari C, Gaforio JJ, Szikora JP, De Smet C, Brasseur F, van der Bruggen P, Lethé B, Lurquin C, Brasseur R, Chomez P, De Backer O, Cavenee W, Boon T. Structure, chromosomal localization and expression of twelve genes of the MAGE family. *Immunogenetics* 1994; 40: 360-9.
3. Boël P, Wildmann C, Sensi ML, Brasseur R, Renauld JC, Coulie P, Boon T, Van der Bruggen P. BAGE, a new gene encoding an antigen recognized on human melanomas by cytolytic T lymphocytes. *Immunity* 1995; 2: 167-75.
4. Van den Eynde B, Peeters O, De Backer O, Gaugler B, Lucas S, Boon T. A new family of genes coding for an antigen recognized by autologous cytolytic T lymphocytes on a human melanoma. *J Exp Med* 1995; 182: 689-98.
5. Brasseur F, Marchand M, Vanwijck R, Hérin M, Lethé B, Chomez P, Boon T. Human gene MAGE-1, which codes for a tumor rejection antigen, is expressed by some breast tumors. *Int J Cancer* 1992; 52: 839-41.

6. Brasseur F, Rimoldi D, Liénard D, Lethé B, Carrel S, Arienti F, Suter L, Vanwijck R, Bourlond A, Humblet Y, Vacca A, Conese M, Lahaye T, Degiovanni G, Deraemaecker R, Beauduin M, Sastre X, Salamon E, Dréno B, Jäger E, Knuth A, Chevreau C, Suciu S, Lachapelle M, Pouillart P, Parmiani G, Lejeune F, Cerottini JC, Boon T, Marchand M. Expression of MAGE genes in primary and metastatic cutaneous melanoma. *Int J Cancer* 1995; 63: 375-80.
7. Weynants P, Lethé B, Brasseur F, Marchand M, Boon T. Expression of MAGE genes by non-small-cell lung carcinomas. *Int J Cancer* 1994; 56: 826-9.
8. Traversari C, Van der Bruggen P, Luescher IF, Lurquin C, Chomez P, Van Pel A, De Plaen E, Amar-Costesec A, Boon T. A nonapeptide encoded by human gene MAGE-1 is recognized on HLA-A1 by cytolytic T lymphocytes directed against tumor antigen MZ2-E. *J Exp Med* 1992; 176: 1453-7.
9. Van der Bruggen P, Szikora JP, Boël P, Wildmann C, Somville M, Sensi M, Boon T. Autologous cytolytic T lymphocytes recognize a MAGE-1 nonapeptide on melanomas expressing HLA-Cw*1601. *Eur J Immunol* 1994; 24: 2134-40.
10. Gaugler B, Van den Eynde B, Van der Bruggen P, Romero P, Gaforio JJ, De Plaen E, Lethé B, Brasseur F, Boon T. Human gene MAGE-3 codes for an antigen recognized on a melanoma by autologous cytolytic T lymphocytes. *J Exp Med* 1994; 179: 921-30.
11. Herman J, Van der Bruggen P, Luescher I, Mandruzzato S, Romero P, Thonnard J, Fleischhauer K, Boon T, Coulie PG. A peptide encoded by human gene MAGE-3 and presented by HLA-B44 induces cytolytic T lymphocytes that recognize tumor cells expressing MAGE-3. *Immunogenetics* 1996; 43: 377-83.
12. Van der Bruggen P, Bastin J, Gajewski T, Coulie PG, Boël P, De Smet C, Traversari C, Townsend A, Boon T. A peptide encoded by human gene MAGE-3 and presented by HLA-A2 induces cytolytic T lymphocytes that recognize tumor cells expressing MAGE-3. *Eur J Immunol* 1994; 24: 3038-43.
13. Takahashi K, Shichijo S, Noguchi M, Hirohata M, Itoh K. Identification of MAGE-1 and MAGE-4 proteins in spermatogonia and primary spermatocytes of testis. *Cancer Res* 1995; 55: 3478-82.
14. Chomez P, Williams R, De Backer O, Boon T, Vennström B. The SMAGE gene family is expressed in post-meiotic spermatids during mouse germ cell differentiation. *Immunogenetics* 1995; 43: 97-100.
15. Haas GG Jr, D'Cruz OJ, De Bault LE. Distribution of human leukocyte antigen-ABC and -D/DR antigens in the unfixed human testis. *Am J Reprod Immunol Microbiol* 1988; 18: 47-51.
16. Guilloux Y, Lucas S, Brichard VG, Van Pel A, Viret C, De Plaen E, Brasseur F, Lethé B, Jotereau F, Boon T. A peptide recognized by human cytolytic T lymphocytes on HLA-A2 melanomas is encoded by an intron sequence of the N-acetylglucosaminyltransferase V gene. *J Exp Med* 1996; 183: 1173-83.
17. Gaugler B, Brouwenstijn N, Vantomme V, Szikora JP, Van der Spek CW, Patard JJ, Boon T, Schrier P, Van den Eynde BJ. A new gene coding for an antigen recognized by autologous cytolytic T lymphocytes on a human renal carcinoma. *Immunogenetics* 1996; 44: 323-30.
18. Brichard V, Van Pel A, Wölfel T, Wölfel C, De Plaen E, Lethé B, Coulie P, Boon T. The tyrosinase gene codes for an antigen recognized by autologous cytolytic T lymphocytes on HLA-A2 melanomas. *J Exp Med* 1993; 178: 489-95.
19. Coulie PG, Brichard V, Van Pel A, Wölfel T, Schneider J, Traversari C, Mattei S, De Plaen E, Lurquin C, Szikora JP, Renauld JC, Boon T. A new gene coding for a differentiation antigen recognized by autologous cytolytic T lymphocytes on HLA-A2 melanomas. *J Exp Med* 1994; 180: 35-42.
20. Kawakami Y, Eliyahu S, Delgado CH, Robbins PF, Rivoltini L, Topalian SL, Miki T, Rosenberg SA. Cloning of the gene coding for a shared human melanoma antigen recognized by autologous T cells infiltrating into tumor. *Proc Natl Acad Sci USA* 1994; 91: 3515-9.
21. Bakker ABH, Schreurs MWJ, de Boer AJ, Kawakami Y, Rosenberg SA, Adema GJ, Figdor CG. Melanocyte lineage-specific antigen gp100 is recognized by melanoma-derived tumor-infiltrating lymphocytes. *J Exp Med* 1994; 179: 1005-9.
22. Cox AL, Skipper J, Chen Y, Henderson RA, Darrow TL, Shabanowitz J, Engelhard VH, Hunt DF, Slingluff CL Jr. Identification of a peptide recognized by five melanoma-specific human cytotoxic T cell lines. *Science* 1994; 264: 716-9.

23. Wang RF, Robbins PF, Kawakami Y, Kang XQ, Rosenberg SA. Identification of a gene encoding a melanoma tumor antigen recognized by HLA-A31-restricted tumor-infiltrating lymphocytes. *J Exp Med* 1995; 181: 799-804.
24. Wölfel T, Van Pel A, Brichard V, Schneider J, Seliger B, Meyer zum Büschenfelde KH, Boon T. Two tyrosinase nonapeptides recognized on HLA-A2 melanomas by autologous cytolytic T lymphocytes. *Eur J Immunol* 1994; 24: 759-64.
25. Robbins PF, El-Gamil M, Kawakami Y, Rosenberg SA. Recognition of tyrosinase by tumor-infiltrating lymphocytes from a patient responding to immunotherapy. *Cancer Res* 1994; 54: 3124-6.
26. Brichard VG, Herman J, Van Pel A, Wildmann C, Gaugler B, Wölfel T, Boon T, Lethé B. A tyrosinase nonapeptide presented by HLA-B44 is recognized on a human melanoma by autologous cytolytic T lymphocytes. *Eur J Immunol* 1996; 26: 224-30.
27. Topalian SL, Rivoltini L, Mancini M, Markus NR, Robbins PF, Kawakami Y, Rosenberg SA. Human CD4+ T cells specifically recognize a shared melanoma-associated antigen encoded by the tyrosinase gene. *Proc Natl Acad Sci USA* 1994; 91: 9461-5.
28. Kawakami Y, Eliyahu S, Delgado CH, Robbins PF, Sakaguchi K, Appella E, Yannelli JR, Adema GJ, Miki T, Rosenberg SA. Identification of a human melanoma antigen recognized by tumor-infiltrating lymphocytes associated with *in vivo* tumor rejection. *Proc Natl Acad Sci USA* 1994; 91: 6458-62.
29. Kawakami Y, Eliyahu S, Sakaguchi K, Robbins PF, Rivoltini L, Yannelli JR, Appella E, Rosenberg SA. Identification of the immunodominant peptides of the MART-1 human melanoma antigen recognized by the majority of HLA-A2-restricted tumor infiltrating lymphocytes. *J Exp Med* 1994; 180: 347-52.
30. Kawakami Y, Eliyahu S, Jennings C, Sakaguchi K, Kang X, Southwood S, Robbins PF, Sette A, Appella E, Rosenberg SA. Recognition of multiple epitopes in the human melanoma antigen gp100 by tumor-infiltrating T lymphocytes associated with *in vivo* tumor regression. *J Immunol* 1995; 154: 3961-8.
31. Castelli C, Storkus WJ, Maeurer MJ, Martin DM, Huang EC, Pramanik BN, Nagabhushan TL, Parmiani G, Lotze MT. Mass spectrometric identification of a naturally processed melanoma peptide recognized by CD8 + cytotoxic T lymphocytes. *J Exp Med* 1995; 181: 363-8.
32. Skipper JCA, Hendrickson RC, Gulden PH, Brichard V, Van Pel A, Chen Y, Shabanowitz J, Wölfel T, Slingluff CL Jr, Boon T, Hunt DF, Engelhard VH. An HLA-A2-restricted tyrosinase antigen on melanoma cells results from posttranslational modification and suggests a novel pathway for processing of membrane proteins. *J Exp Med* 1996; 183: 527-34.
33. Bystryn JC, Darrell R, Friedman RJ, Kopf A. Prognostic significance of hypopigmentation in malignant melanoma. *Arch Dermatol* 1987; 123: 1053-5.
34. Richards JM, Mehta N, Ramming K, Skosey P. Sequential chemoimmunotherapy in the treatment of metastatic melanoma. *J Clin Oncol* 1992; 10: 1338-43.
35. Wölfel T, Hauer M, Schneider J, Serrano M, Wölfel C, Klehmann-Hieb E, De Plaen E, Hankeln T, Meyer zum Büschenfelde KH, Beach D. A p16INK4a-insensitive CDK4 mutant targeted by cytolytic T lymphocytes in a human melanoma. *Science* 1995; 269: 1281-4.
36. Coulie PG, Lehmann F, Lethé B, Herman J, Lurquin C, Andrawiss M, Boon T. A mutated intron sequence codes for an antigenic peptide recognized by cytolytic T lymphocytes on a human melanoma. *Proc Natl Acad Sci USA* 1995; 92: 7976-80.
37. Robbins PF, El-Gamil M, Li YF, Kawakami Y, Loftus D, Appella E, Rosenberg SA. A mutated ß-catenin gene encodes a melanoma-specific antigen recognized by tumor infiltrating lymphocytes. *J Exp Med* 1996; 183: 1185-92.
38. Brändle D, Brasseur F, Weynants P, Boon T, Van den Eynde B. A mutated HLA-A2 molecule recognized by autologous cytotoxic T lymphocytes on a human renal cell carcinoma. *J Exp Med* 1996; 183: 2501-8.
39. Marchand M, Weynants P, Rankin E, Arienti F, Belli F, Parmiani G, Cascinelli N, Bourlond A, Vanwijck R, Humblet Y, Canon JL, Laurent C, Naeyaert JM, Plagne R, Deraemaeker R, Knuth A, Jäger E, Brasseur F, Herman J, Coulie PG, Boon T. Tumor regression responses in melanoma patients treated with a peptide encoded by gene MAGE-3. *Int J Cancer* 1995; 63: 883-5.
40. Uytenhove C, Godfraind C, Lethé B, Amar-Costesec A, Renauld JC, Gajewski TF, Duffour MT, Warnier G, Boon T, Van den Eynde B. The expression of mouse gene *P1A* in testis does not prevent safe induction of cytolytic T cells against a P1A-encoded tumor antigen. *Int J Cancer* 1997, in press.

Strategies and future of HLA matching in organ transplantation

G. Opelz, T. Wujciak, J. Mytilineos, S. Scherer

Department of Transplantation Immunology, University of Heidelberg, Im Neuenheimer Feld 305, D-69120 Heidelberg, Germany

That HLA matching improves the outcome of cadaver kidney and heart transplants has been proven beyond any doubt [1-3]. However, there is no uniform agreement on how this knowledge can or should be utilized for the improvement of future transplantations. Different strategies for the allocation of cadaver kidneys have been adopted in different parts of Europe, where HLA matching is emphasized especially by the Eurotransplant organization, whereas the transplant policies in Scandinavia and Southern Europe place little emphasis on matching. In the United States, nationwide kidney sharing for the purpose of obtaining well matched transplants is restricted to the 6-antigen matched category. In heart transplantation, because the limit of cold ischemic preservation is about 4-5 hours, only few attempts have been made to obtain better matches through regional organ sharing. Based on the Collaborative Transplant Study experience, we would like to review our current knowledge concerning the impact of HLA matching on graft outcome, the influence of HLA-driven organ allocation, and the potential for improving the results further by employing molecular HLA typing techniques.

Methods

The Collaborative Transplant Study (CTS) was initiated in 1982. Currently, more than 300 kidney transplant centers, 100 heart and 60 liver transplant centers in 43 countries are participating. More than 150 000 kidney transplants, 20 000 heart or lung transplants, 9 000 liver transplants and 2 000 pancreas transplants have been registered.

HLA matching in cadaver kidney transplantation

The overall association of matching for the HLA-A,-B and -DR loci with cadaver kidney graft survival is illustrated in *Figure 1*. In our experience, the influence of the 3 loci is additive, whereby the strength is declining from HLA-DR to HLA-B to HLA-A. The difference in impact among the 3 loci, however, is not sufficiently great to require a differential weight assignment for the loci. For the practical purposes of matching, the simple addition of the number of mismatches at each locus is sufficient. We have been unable to confirm reports on the superiority of defining certain HLA mismatches as "permissible" [4].

HLA matching and kidney allocation

If kidneys are allocated to patients on the waiting list strictly according to the degree of HLA matching, one discriminates against patients with rare HLA phenotypes. Donor kidneys (which have a "normal" phenotype distribution) are usually allocated to recipients with

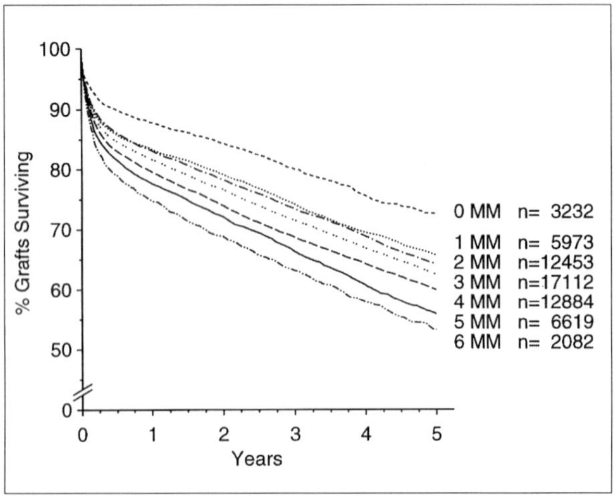

Figure 1. Association of the number of HLA-A,-B,-DR mismatches with outcome of first cadaver kidney transplants. Weighted regression p<0.0001. Numbers of patients studied in each mismatch category are indicated.

relatively frequent phenotypes. Donors with rare phenotypes are (by definition) rare, and recipients with rare phenotypes therefore accumulate on the waiting list and wait for prolonged periods of time. This has been a recurring topic of discontent, and many clinicians have requested that HLA matching be dropped altogether as an allocation criterion in favor of the waiting time. We developed a computer algorithm which considers both the HLA match, the HLA phenotype (and thus the likelihood of a patient to receive a good match), and the waiting time. This algorithm, termed "XCOMB", eliminates the main criticism against an HLA-driven organ allocation: the accumulation of patients with rare HLA phenotypes, especially members of racial minorities. The resulting HLA match distribution is still sufficiently good to achieve a substantial improvement in the overall transplant survival rate [5].

Figure 2 illustrates the results of a computer simulation in which the effect of kidney allocation according to the XCOMB model was compared with random allocation. The simulation was carried out based on the CTS data for transplants performed from 1986 to 1993. Over a 9 year simulated follow up period, allocation according to XCOMB results in a gain of approximately 6 000 function years for every 10 000 patients transplanted. The transplant results obtained in patients with or without immunosuppression with cyclosporine are plotted for comparison. Although a similar gain as that achievable with XCOMB can be attributed to the use of cyclosporine, it is evident that the cyclosporine effect diminishes over time whereas the HLA matching effect of XCOMB increases. In other words, the longer the follow up, the greater the relative advantage of the XCOMB allocation model. As evident from the numbers of patients studied, the XCOMB allocation simulation was based entirely on recipients treated with cyclosporine. Thus, the improvement effect achievable with XCOMB is not an alternative to the use of cyclosporine but rather an additional tool to further improve the transplant outcome in patients receiving optimal immunosuppression.

HLA and heart transplantation

An update on the CTS results of HLA matching in heart transplantation is shown in *Figure 3*. The correlation of matching with graft survival is statistically highly significant (regression p<0.0001). However, the survival curves for transplants with 3-6 HLA mismatches do not separate as clearly as those for the corresponding groups of kidney transplant recipients *(Figure 1)*. A possible explanation for this result is that heart transplant recipients receive higher doses of immunosuppressive drugs than kidney recipients. Stronger immunosuppression may in part overcome the effect of HLA mismatches. Although one might speculate that the effect of matching would be similarly reduced if kidney

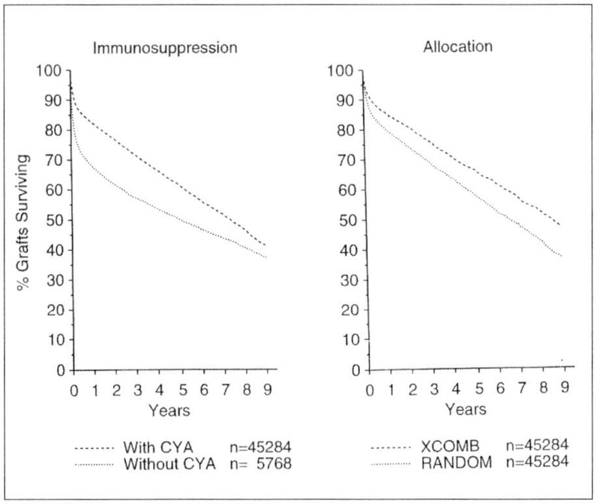

Figure 2. Comparison of improvement effect achieved with immunosuppression using cyclosporine with the additional improvement achievable by kidney allocation according to the XCOMB allocation method.

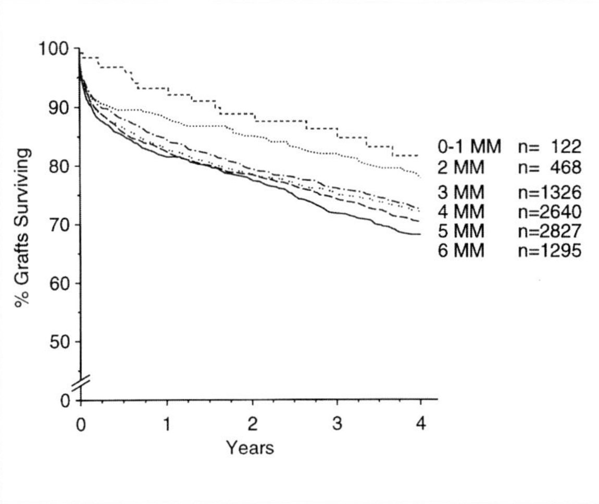

Figure 3. Correlation of number of HLA-A,-B,-DR mismatches with survival of first heart transplants. Weighted regression p<0.0001. 538 patients categorized as "poor risks" at the time of transplantation were excluded.

transplant recipients received higher doses of immunosuppression, it is important to point out the deleterious side effects of increased immunosuppression, most notably the higher incidence of posttransplant lymphomas [6]. A recent analysis of CTS data showed a cumulative rate of lymphomas 5 years post transplantation of 5% in heart recipients as compared to a 1% rate in kidney recipients. In both types of recipients, lymphomas were associated with a very high death rate of >50% during the first year following the diagnosis. In addition, preliminary data suggest that other fatal tumors also occur at a higher frequency in heart transplant recipients than in kidney recipients.

Although the retrospective data show that good HLA compatibility is associated with better graft outcome in heart transplantation, the preservation time limit of 4-5 hours makes it difficult to prospectively apply HLA matching for heart transplantation. Nevertheless, our computations suggest that a limited exchange on a regional basis would result in a significant improvement of the transplant success rate [3].

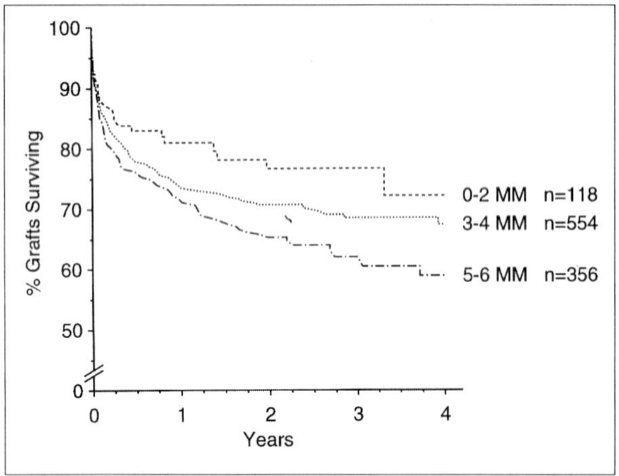

Figure 4. Association of number of HLA mismatches with outcome of pancreas transplants. Combined kidney and pancreas grafts were analyzed. Insulin-free survival was used as endpoint. Weighted regression p<0.04.

HLA matching and pancreas transplantation

Reports on HLA matching in pancreas transplantation have been inconsistent and variable. This may in part be attributable to the relatively small numbers of patients that were analyzed. In addition, the overall results of pancreas transplantation have increased substantially during the last 10 years due to technical improvements. For transplants performed from 1991 to 1995, the CTS data show a moderate but statistically significant improvement effect of HLA matching on graft outcome *(Figure 4)*.

HLA matching and liver transplantation

The situation is similar to that in pancreas transplantation because the overall results have improved in recent years and the patient numbers available for analysis are relatively small. For transplants performed from 1990 to 1995, the CTS data do not show evidence for improved graft outcome with good HLA compatibility *(Figure 5)*.

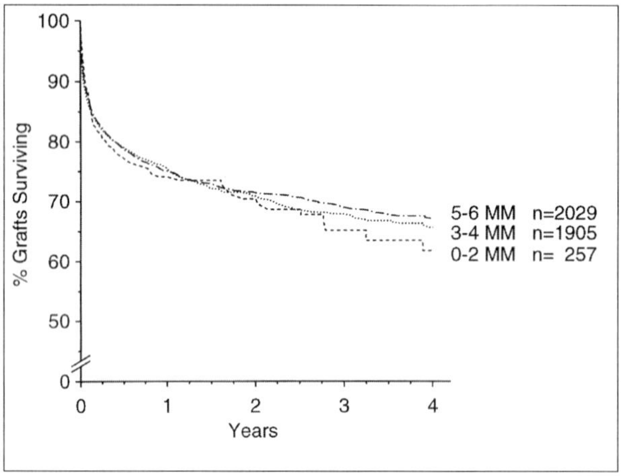

Figure 5. Analysis of HLA-DR mismatches in liver transplantation. No significant HLA matching effect was observed.

Impact of molecular HLA typing technology

The clinical correlations of HLA matching with kidney, heart and pancreas transplantation shown in *Figures 1-4* are most likely underestimations of the true HLA matching effect. Many HLA-DR typings were shown to be incorrect when retrospective DNA typing was performed, and the correlation of graft outcome with HLA matching improved when the incorrect typings were corrected [7]. A current update of the CTS project on DNA typing in cadaver kidney transplantation is provided in *Figure 6.* All transplants in this analysis were reported to the CTS study center as having 0 HLA-DR mismatches based on serological typing. Retrospective DNA typing, however, revealed that 26% of the transplants in fact were DR mismatched. The graft survival rate of "truly" matched and mismatched grafts differed significantly (p<0.0001). Introduction of the rapid PCR-SSP typing technique for HLA-DRB should allow the elimination of these typing errors in the future.

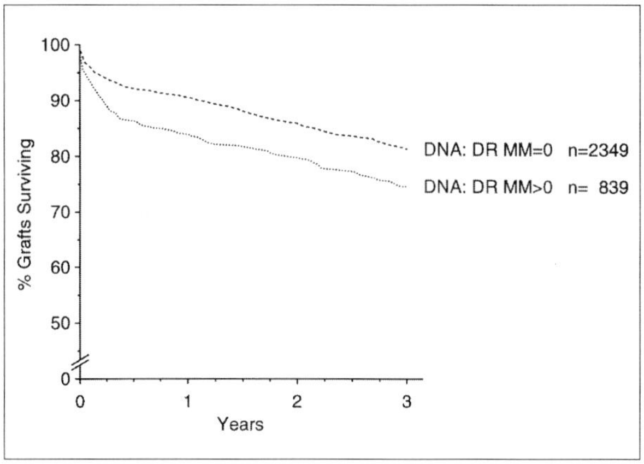

Figure 6. Analysis of first cadaver kidney transplants reported to have 0 HLA-DR mismatches based on serological typing. Retrospective DNA typing revealed an HLA-DR mismatch in 26% of the transplants. The survival rate of DR-mismatched grafts was significantly lower (log rank p<0.0001).

DNA results on HLA-DR "splits" and HLA-DP

Work currently in progress indicates that, whereas matching in primary kidney transplantation for the DR specificities DR1-DR10 is sufficient, consideration of the "split" specificities DR11-DR18 improves the correlation of matching with graft outcome in retransplants. Grafts that had no HLA DR mismatch according to DNA typing for both the "broad" specificities DRB1-DRB10 and the "split" specificities DRB11-DRB18 survived at a rate of 74±2% at 3 years. 105 transplants that were matched by the "broad" definition but showed evidence of a mismatch according to the "split" definition had a significantly lower 3-year survival rate of 68±4% (p=0.04). Likewise, matching for HLA-DP did not appear to have an influence on graft outcome in first cadaver kidney transplants, however, there was a significant impact on retransplants, where 316 transplants with no HLA-DP mismatch had an 83±2% survival rate at 1 year, compared with a rate of 76±2% for 646 grafts with 1 HLA-DP mismatch and 74±3% for 253 grafts with 2 HLA-DP mismatches (regression p<0.02). These results are very promising and suggest that further improvements in cadaver kidney allocation will be possible once DNA typing techniques are widely practiced for the typing of cadaver donors.

References

1. Opelz G, Wujciak T. Cadaver kidneys should be allocated according to the HLA match. *Transplant Proc* 1995; 27:93-9.
2. Zhou YC, Cecka JM. Effect of HLA matching on renal transplant survival. In: Terasaki PI, Cecka JM eds. *Clinical Transplants 1993.* Los Angeles: UCLA Tissue Typing Laboratory, 1994:499-510.
3. Opelz G, Wujciak T for the Collaborative Transplant Study. The influence of HLA compatibility on graft survival after heart transplantation. *N Engl J Med* 1994; 330:816-9.
4. Maruya E, Takemoto S, Terasaki PI. HLA matching: identification of permissible HLA mismatches. In: Terasaki PI, Cecka JM eds. *Clinical Transplants 1993.* Los Angeles: UCLA Tissue Typing Laboratory, 1994:511-20.
5. Wujciak T, Opelz G. A proposal for improved cadaver kidney allocation. *Transplantation* 1993; 56:1513-7.
6. Opelz G. Henderson R. Incidence of non-Hodgkin lymphoma in kidney and heart transplant recipients. *Lancet* 1993; 342:1514-6.
7. Opelz G, Mytilineos J, Scherer S, Dunckley H, Trejaut J, Chapman J, Middleton D, Savage D, Fischer G, Bignon JD, Bensa JC, Albert E, Noreen H. Survival of DNA HLA-DR typed and matched cadaver kidney transplants. *Lancet* 1991; 338:461-3.

Transplantation of hematopoietic stem cells from HLA matched unrelated donors

J.A. Hansen, E.W. Petersdorf, J. Pei, E. Mickelson, P.J. Martin, C. Anasetti

Fred Hutchinson Cancer Research Center, and
Department of Medicine, University of Washington School of Medicine, 1124 Columbia, Seattle, WA 98104, USA

Hematopoietic stem cell transplants from normal matched donors are potentially life saving for patients with fatal inherited or acquired diseases, including hematological malignancies [1]. Stem cells sufficient for transplantation can be obtained from bone marrow, from the umbilical cord of newborn infants, and by mobilization in peripheral blood with growth-factors followed by apheresis. Transplantation of peripheral blood stem cells (PBSC) and umbilical cord blood stem cells (UCB) has begun only recently, and there is only preliminary data available about the relative advantages of these products as alternatives to conventional marrow. The basic principle, however, remains the same. Hematopoietic stem cells have the capacity for continuous renewal and for generating committed progenitors which are capable of replenishing the mature functional cells that constitute the blood and immune systems. Engraftment of stem cells from normal donors can correct genetic abnormalities and can rescue patients from high-dose cytotoxic therapy. Stem cell grafts containing immunologically mature donor T cells can also provide a potent graft-versus-leukemia (GVL) effect, which significantly reduces the risk of post-transplant relapse [2]. The successful transplantation of marrow and hematopoietic stem cells, however, is strongly constrained by the need for HLA matching of the donor and recipient, and by the necessity of controlling graft-versus-host disease (GVHD) [3-6].

A few patients lacking an HLA identical sibling may be able to find an acceptable donor within their extended family by looking for a haploidentical relative who fortuitously shares HLA antigens. Cases such as this have been informative in revealing the significance of HLA incompatibility [3, 4]. However, success is limited by the degree of HLA mismatching. Results of haploidentical transplants are acceptable when mismatching is limited to one HLA-A, B or DR antigen, a situation which occurs infrequently [5, 6]. For the majority of patients lacking an HLA identical sibling, an HLA matched unrelated volunteer is the only alternative source of normal stem cells [6-9].

Unrelated donor registries

The extensive polymorphism of the HLA system has necessitated the establishment of large registries of HLA typed donors currently numbering more than 2.8 million worldwide. The US marrow donor registry, known as the National Marrow Donor Program (NMDP), is a network of more than 106 donor centers and 70 transplant centers, some of which are located in countries outside of the US [10, 11]. The main coordinating center is located in Minneapolis, MN. As of April 30, 1996, the NMDP registry had grown to more than 2.1 million HLA-A, B typed volunteers, including 760,499 donors (35%) typed for HLA-A, B and DR *(Figure 1)*. The racial composition of the NMDP donor registry is 75% Caucasian, 9.0% African American, 8.2% Hispanic, 5.9% Asian, 1.5% Native American, and 0.7% other *(Figure 2)*. From the beginning of NMDP operations in 1987, a total of 24,844 preliminary donor searches have been submitted, and 15,171 have gone on to formal searches with requests for confirmatory or high resolution HLA typing. During May, 1995, there were 475 new preliminary searches and 259 new formal searches submitted. More than 4,400 unrelated donor transplants have been facilitated by NMDP *(Figure 3)*, currently at a rate of approximately 85 transplants per month.

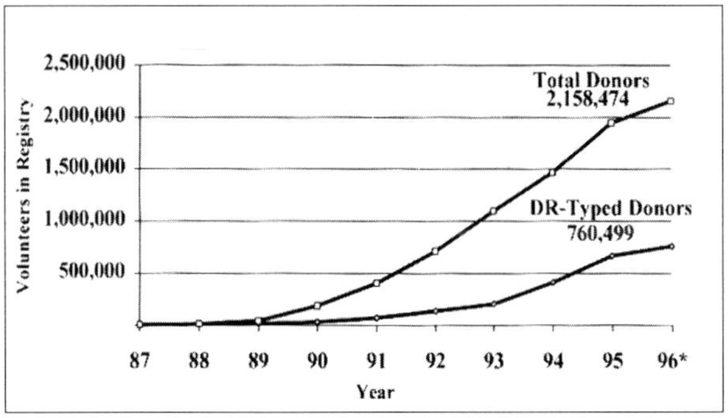

Figure 1. NMDP Donor Registry showing cumulative annual growth of HLA-A,B and HLA-A,B,DR typed volunteer donors.

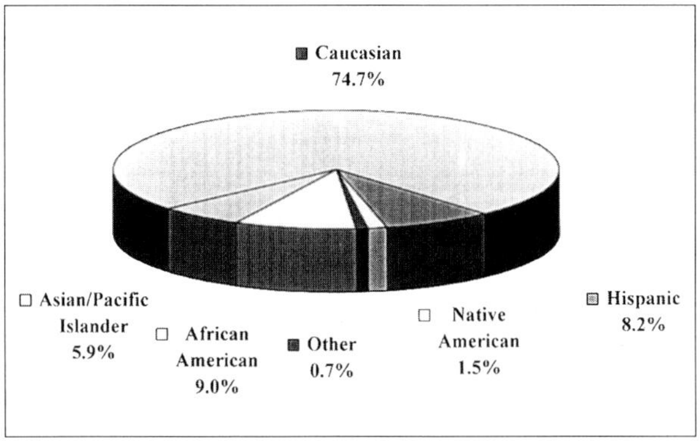

Figure 2. Percentage of volunteer marrow donors in the NMDP registry by racial origin.

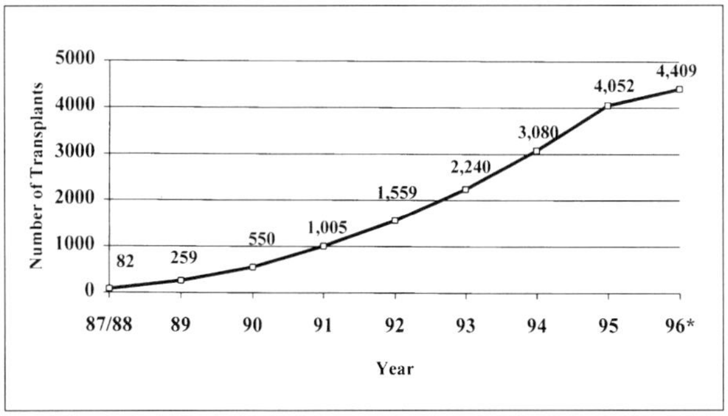

Figure 3. Cumulative annual growth in the number of unrelated donor marrow transplants facilitated through the NMDP.

Searching for an unrelated donor

The overall chance of finding an HLA-A, B and DR matched donor at the time of an initial search was 71% as of April 30, 1996, a significant improvement from 1990 (32%) and 1993 (54%) *(Table I).* Success of matching, however, varies according to the racial origin of the patient. In 1995 the chance of finding at least one HLA-A, B, DR identical donor at initial search was 72% for Caucasians, 59% for Hispanics, 49% for Asians and 24% for African Americans. Once a potential HLA match has been identified, the additional time required to complete high resolution and confirmatory HLA typing, and finalize the medical screening and counseling of the donor, can become a critical problem for patients with certain unstable diseases such as aplastic anemia, myelodysplasia or acute leukemia. Some of this delay may be minimized by the establishment of centralized repositories for donor DNA to expedite the testing necessary for final donor matching.

HLA typing and donor matching

Standard methods for HLA typing and donor matching based on phenotyping are limited in detecting genetic variants, many of which can be recognized by T cells [12-14]. Individual HLA alleles can only be identified using DNA or cDNA -based typing methods. Many clinical laboratories have adapted DNA technology for defining DRB and DQB alleles, and an increasing number of laboratories are applying high resolution typing to the class I HLA-A, B and C genes [15, 16]. Matching for HLA-A and B at our Center is still based on serology, but matching for DR and DQ requires identification of alleles. Final donor selection criteria also depends on patient age. Patients up to the age of 55 years are required to have a donor identical for HLA-A, B and DRB1. If this can not be achieved, patients <36 years may be transplanted from a donor differing by no more than one HLA-A, B or DR *minor* mismatch. An HLA-A or B *minor* mismatch is defined as two antigens that belong to the same crossreactive group or *CREG.* An HLA-DR *minor* mismatch is defined as two haplotypes that differ for a pair of distinct DRB1 alleles that encode the same DR specificity (DR1, 15{2}, 16{2}, 17{3}, 18{3}, 4, 11{5}, 12{5}, 13{6} 14{6} or 10); for example, 0401 and 0404. Donors who are phenotypically matched for HLA-A, B and DR will not necessarily be matched for DRB1 alleles. We have reviewed high resolution HLA typing data for patients studied at our Center and observed that the chance of achieving allele matching at the DRB1 locus was 40% if there was a single HLA-A, B, DR identical donor available. The chance of matching for DRB1 increased to 65% if there were 2 HLA-A, B, DR identical donors and 95% if there were 5 donors available [17].

Table I. Number of HLA-A, B and DR typed donors, number of donor searches, and chance of finding an HLA-A, B and DR match at the time of initial search

Year	Number of DR-typed donors	Total preliminary searches	Preliminary searches with at least one HLA-A, B, DR identical match
1990	43,995	2,472	32%
1991	91,189	3,067	36%
1992	151,253	3,552	41%
1993	234,850	3,930	54%
1994	438,572	4,280	62%
1995	666,252	5,266	69%
1996*	760,499	1,999	71%

*as of April 30, 1996.

Significance of matching for HLA alleles

To determine the significance of matching for DRB1 alleles we analyzed the results of 364 HLA-A,B,DR identical unrelated donor transplants [18]. All patients received non-T cell depleted marrow and cyclosporine plus methotrexate for GVHD prophylaxis. Matching for DRB1 was defined by PCR/SSOP. The probability of clinically severe grades III-IV acute GVHD was 48% for DRB1 matched and 70% for DRB1 mismatched transplants (p= < .01). The relative risk of grade III-IV acute GVHD for DRB1 mismatching was 1.7 (95% CI, 1.2-2.5) and the relative risk of transplant-associated mortality was 1.5 (95% CI, 1.0-2.2). More recently we have analyzed the effect of matching for both DRB1 and DQB1 in 449 HLA-A,B,DR identical transplants [19]. Three-hundred-thirty (74%) of the cases were matched for both DRB1 and DQB1, 48 (11%) were mismatched only for DRB1, 41 (9%) were mismatched only for DQB1, and 25 (6%) were mismatched for both DRB1 and DQB1 *(Table II)*. The probability of grades III-IV acute GVHD was lowest in transplants matched for both DRB1 and DQB1 (37%) and greatest in cases mismatched for both DRB1 and DQB1 (60%) *(Table III)*. The probability of severe GVHD was 56% in transplants mismatched only for DQB1 and 50% in transplants mismtched only for DRB1. The effect of DQB1 mismatching on risk of GVHD was significant when analyzed in a univariable Cox model with matching *(Table III)*. These data suggest that matching for DQB1 alleles is just as important as matching for DRB1 alleles.

Table II. Mismatching for HLA-DRB1 and DQB1 alleles among HLA-A, B, DR identical unrelated donor transplants

		DRB1 identical	DRB1 nonidentical	Total
DQB1	identical	335 (74%)	48 (11%)	383
	nonidentical	41 (9%)	25 (6%)	66 (15%)
	total	366	73 (17%)	449

Table III. Effect of mismatching for DRB1 and DQB1 alleles among HLA-A, B, DR identical unrelated donor transplants on the probability of grade III-IV acute GVHD

DRB1 *matched*	probability of grade III-IV acute GVHD	
DQB1 *matched*, n=325	38%	p=.02, RR= 1.9[a]
DQB1 *mismatched*, n=41	56%	
DRB1 *mismatched*		
DQB1 *matched*, n=48	50%	
DQB1 *mismatched*, n=25	60%	

[a]p-value for the univariable Cox Model; RR, indicates relative risk. When stratified for DRB1 match status the overall hazard of DQB1 allele mismatching gave a relative risk of 1.6 (p= .02).

In contrast to the increased risk of acute GVHD associated with mismatching for DRB1 and DQB1 alleles, we have not observed an increase in GVHD in unrelated donor transplants with a known *minor mismatch* for HLA-A or B. In an analysis of 333 patients transplanted from an unrelated donor for CML, 30 cases were incompatible for an HLA-A or B minor mismatch [18]. The incidence of grades III-IV acute GVHD was 33% in this group compared to 38% in patients matched for HLA-A, B and DRB1. It is unknown if mismatching for class I alleles will increase the risk of GVHD.

Graft failure or rejection after transplantation of unmodified T cell-replete marrow from an unrelated donor occurs in approximately 1% to 6% of cases [20, 21]. We have used direct DNA sequencing to retrospectively identify alleles of the HLA-A, B and C loci in a group of 21 consecutive graft failure patients [22]. Comparing the graft failure group with case matched controls in whom graft failure did not occur, we have shown that the overall rate of mismatching for HLA-A,B and C was increased in the graft failure group. The overall incidence of mismatching for HLA-A, B or C alleles was 90% in graft failure patients compared to 55% in controls and the incidence of mismatching for HLA-C (alone or in combination with mismatching for HLA-A and B) was 71% in graft failure patients compared to 33% in controls. The relative risk of mismatching for HLA-A or B alleles was 3.1 (LRT p = .09) and the relative risk of mismatching for HLA-C alleles was 4.0 (LRT p = .04)(*(Table IV)*. These data indicate the HLA-C locus can function as a transplantation antigen. The mechanism of graft failure in these patients, however, is not known. Previous studies have suggested that alloreactive cytotoxic T-lymphocytes (CTL) may mediate graft rejection [13], but it has also been shown that class I molecules, including HLA-C, can function as ligands for receptors on NK cells [23, 24]. NK cells have been implicated as effector cells in hybrid resistance and the rejection of hematopoietic stem cells [25, 26].

Table IV. Graft failure in unrelated donor transplants mismatched for class I HLA-A, B or C alleles

Allele mismatch	Relative risk	95% CI	p-value[a]	p-value (LRT)
HLA-A or B	3.1	(.8, 13)	.11	.09
HLA-C	4.0	(1.1, 15)	.04	.03

[a]multivariate conditional logistic regression analysis.

Role of functional assays in donor selection

Following the introduction of DNA-based typing and high resolution matching for HLA alleles, the question has remained whether functional tests measuring the responses of helper T cells or CTL might further improve donor selection by identifying genetic differences between donor and recipient, or differences in the immune response potential of the donor, which are not adequately measured by simply matching for HLA alleles. It has also been hypothesized that measuring functional responses might be helpful in selecting donors when an optimal match is not available. It has been generally assumed that the mixed lymphocyte culture (MLC) assay, which primarily measures T cell activation in response to class II DR, DQ and in some cases DP disparity, should predict for GVHD [27-29]. However, in a retrospective analysis of 435 unrelated donor transplants we have found that MLC reactivity, in contrast to allele matching for DRB1, does not predict for clinically severe grades III-IV acute GVHD, even among HLA-A,B,DR identical transplants [30]. Further analysis of this data also demonstrated that the MLC assay was not a strong predictor of DRB1 matching, presumably because of the variable effect of unrecognized DQ and DP disparity on the MLC. Nevertheless, these results indicated that MLC testing did not contribute to final donor selection and for this reason we have abandoned the MLC as a test for histocompatibility matching.

To determine whether the responses of T cells to class II disparity could be measured in a more meaningful way if precursor frequences were determined, we have analyzed IL-2 secreting helper T cell precursor (HTLp) responses in a limiting dilution assay and correlated HTLp frequencies with the risk of acute GVHD after unrelated marrow transplantation. Among 48 patients who engrafted and survived at least 30 days after transplantation, a nonparametric test suggested that the HTLp index was positively correlated with GVHD grade ($p = 0.1$), but the relationship was not sufficiently strong to predict the risk of acute GVHD [31]. We also tested whether the risk of acute GVHD after unrelated marrow transplantation correlates with the number of donor cytolytic T cell precursors (CTLp) specific for alloantigens of the host. Among 39 patients who engrafted and survived for at least 24 days after transplantation, donor anti-host CTL frequencies ranged from 0 to 388 per 1.0×10^6 PBL (mean, 70.5 per 10^6 PBL) [31]. No correlation was found, however, either between the donor anti-host CTLp frequency and the severity of GVHD ($p>0.75$) or between CTLp frequency and the onset time of GVHD ($p>0.25$). These results suggested that the role of HTL and CTL in mediating GVHD has not been clearly settled, and that measuring the activity of donor HLTp and CTLp reactions to a specific patient is not useful in predicting the risk of GVHD in unrelated donor transplants. A positive correlation between CTLp frequencies and risk of GVHD has been reported by some investigators [32], whereas others have reported no significiant correlation [33, 34].

Unrelated donor transplants for patients with chronic myeloid leukemia (CML)

The gold standard for determining the optimal outcome of stem cell transplants from normal donors has been the HLA genotypically identical sibling. When patients with chronic myeloid leukemia (CML) are transplanted in chronic phase from an HLA identical sibling, the probability of surviving 3 years approaches 80-90% when transplants are performed early in the course of disease [35]. However, the initial studies of unrelated donor transplants for chronic phase CML reported 2 year disease-free survival rates of only 36% to 45% [36-38]. We have analyzed the results of first unrelated donor transplants performed for 332 CML patients at our Center: 204 were in chronic phase, 78 in accelerated phase, 18 in second chronic phase and 32 in blast phase [20]. The median age of the patients was 36.1 years (range, 5 to 55) and the median age of the donors was 38.5 (19.0 to 57.). The median duration of disease prior to transplant was 21.4 months. Patients received non-T cell depleted marrow cells following cyclophosphamide and total body irradiation, and methotrexate and cyclosporine were given for GVHD prevention. A majority of the cases, 250 (75%), were identical with their donor for HLA-A,B,DRB1, and the remaining cases were incompatible for one HLA-A or B *minor mismatch* (n= 29, [9%]), at least one HLA-DR *minor* mismatch (n= 45, [14%]), or incompatible for 2 loci (n= 6, [2%]). The frequency of clinically severe grades III-IV acute GVHD was 37% for HLA identical transplants, 34% for HLA-A or B *minor mismatches,* and 61% for any DRB1 mismatch. The frequency of clinical extensive chronic GVHD was 63% for HLA identical transplants, 57% for HLA-A or B *minor mismatches,* and 70% for any DRB1 mismatch. The probability of survival at 3 years was 55% for patients transplanted in chronic phase, 40% for accelerated phase, 32% for second chronic phase and 7% for blast phase. The probability of relapse was 7% for chronic phase, 14% for accelerated phase, 17% for second chronic phase, and 56% for blast phase. A multivariable analysis was performed to identify risk factors for acute and chronic GVHD, relapse and survival. The major hazards for survival were advanced stage disease (transplantation in blast phase) and older patient age. Mismatching for DRB1 alleles was a significant hazard for acute but not chronic GVHD. There was no detectable effect of mismatching for DRB1 on relapse or survival among all CML patients; however, when only chronic phase patients were included in the multivariable analysis, mismatching for DRB1 was shown to significantly decrease the probability of survival. Incompatibility for HLA-A or B *minor mismatches* had no measurable effect in this study. The use of a female donor was associated with a greater risk of acute GVHD, and the use of a parous female donor was associated with an increase in chronic GVHD. Among patients in CP *<50 years old* transplanted from an *HLA matched* donor *<1 year* from diagnosis, the probability of surviving 3 years was 74% compared to 56% for patients *<50 years* transplanted from an *HLA matched* donor *>3 years* from diagnosis (p= .012) and 40% for patients *<50 years* transplanted from an HLA *mismatched* donor *>3 years* from diagnosis (p= .006). These results demonstrate that HLA-matched unrelated donor transplants performed early in the course of CML (within one year from diagnosis) can achieve survival rates that approach the favorable results observed for transplants from HLA-identical siblings.

Acknowledgments
This work was supported by grants AI33484, CA18029, CA15704 and a grant from the Friends of Allison Atlas Foundation. We are very grateful for the data provided by the US National Marrow Donor Program (NMDP).

References

1. Thomas ED. The Nobel lectures in immunology. The Nobel Prize for physiology and medicine, 1990. Bone marrow transplantation - past, present and future. *Scand J Immunol 1994;* 39:339-45.

2. Martin PJ, Hansen JA, Storb R, Thomas ED. Human marrow transplantation: an immunological perspective. *Adv Immunol* 1987; 40:379-438.
3. Beatty PG, Clift RA, Mickelson EM, *et al.* Marrow transplantation from related donors other than HLA-identical siblings. *N Engl J Med* 1985: 313:765-71.
4. Anasetti C, Amos D, Beatty PG, *et al.* Effect of HLA compatibility on engraftment of bone marrow transplants in patients with leukemia or lymphoma. *N Engl J Med* 1989: 320:197-204.
5. Anasetti C, Beatty PG, Storb R, *et al.* Effect of HLA incompatibility on graft-versus-host disease, relapse and survival after marrow transplantation for patients with leukemia or lymphoma. *Hum Immunol* 1990: 29:79-91.
6. Anasetti C, Hansen JA. Bone marrow transplantation from HLA-partially matched related donors and unrelated volunteer donors. In: Forman SJ, Blume KG, Thomas ED, eds. *Bone Marrow Transplantation.* Boston: Blackwell Scientific Publ ,1994: 665-79.
7. Anasetti C, Etzioni R, Petersdorf E, Martin PJ, Hansen JA. Marrow transplantation from unrelated volunteer donors. *Ann Rev Med* 1995: 46:169-79.
8. Hansen JA, Clift RA, Thomas ED, Buckner CD, Storb R, Giblett ER. Transplantation of marrow from an unrelated donor to a patient with acute leukemia. *N Engl J Med* 1980; 303:565-7.
9. Beatty PG, Hansen JA, Thomas ED, *et al.* Marrow transplantation from HLA-matched unrelated donors for treatment of hematologic malignancies. *Transplantation* 1991: 2:443-6.
10. McCullough J, Hansen J, Perkins H, Stroncek D, Bartsch G. The National Marrow Donor Program: how it works, accomplishments to date. *Oncology* 1989; 3: 63-74.
11. Stroncek D, Bartsch G, Perkins HA, Randall BL, Hansen JA, McCullough J. The National Marrow Donor Program. *Transfusion* 1993; 33:567-77.
12. Choo SY, Fan L, Hansen JA. Allelic variations clustered in the antigen binding sites of HLA-Bw62 molecules. *Immunogenetics* 1980; 37: 108-13.
13. Fleischhauer K, Kernan NA, O'Reilly RJ, Dupont B, Yang SY. Bone marrow-allograft rejection by T lymphocytes recognizing a single amino acid difference in HLA-B44. *N Engl J Med* 1990; 323: 1818.
14. Hansen JA, Mickelson EM, Choo SY, *et al.* Clinical bone marrow transplantation: donor selection and recipient monitoring. In: Rose NR, DeMacario EC, Fahey JL, Friedman H, Penn GM, eds. *Manual of Clinical Laboratory Immunology. Am Soc Microbiology,* 1992: 850-66.
15. Petersdorf EW, Stanley JF, Martin PJ, Hansen JA. Molecular diversity of the HLA-C locus in unrelated marrow transplantation. *Tissue Antigens* 1994; 44: 93.
16. Petersdorf EW, Hansen JA. A comprehensive approach for typing the alleles of the HLA-B locus by automated sequencing. *Tissue Antigens* 1995; 46: 73.
17. Anasetti C, Hansen JA. Effect of HLA incompatibility in marrow transplantation from unrelated and HLA-mismatched related donors. *Transfus Sci* 1994; 15:221-30.
18. Petersdorf EW, Longton GM, Anasetti C, Martin PJ, Mickelson EM, Smith AG, Hansen JA. The significance of HLA-DRB1 matching on clinical outcome after HLA-A, B, DR identical unrelated donor marrow transplantation. *Blood* 1995; 86: 1606.
19. Petersdorf EW, Longton GM, Anasetti C, Mickelson EM, Smith AG, Martin PJ, Hansen JA. Definition of HLA-DQ as a transplantation antigen. *Proc Natl Acad Sci USA* 1997 (in press).
20. Hansen JA, Gooley T, Clift R, Petersdorf EW, Martin PJ, Anasetti C. Unrelated donor marrow transplants for patients with chronic myeloid leukemia. *Blood* 1995; 86: 479a.
21. Sierra J, Storer B, Hansen JA, Martin PJ, Petersdorf EW, Appelbaum FR, Bryant E, Chauncey TR, Sale G, Sanders JE, Storb R, Sullivan KM, Anasetti C. Unrelated donor marrow transplantation for acute leukemia: beneficial effect of increased marrow cell dose (submitted).
22. Petersdorf EW, Longton GM, Anasetti C, Mickelson EM, McKinney SK, Smith AG, Martin PJ, Hansen JA. Association of HLA-C disparity with graft failure after marrow transplantation from unrelated donors. *Blood* 1997 (in press).
23. Colonna M, Spies T, Strominger JL, Ciccone E, Moretta A, Moretta L, Pende D, Viale O. Alloantigen recognition by two human natural killer cell clones is associated with HLA-C or a closely linked gene. *Proc Natl Acad Sci USA* 1992; 89: 79-83.
24. Lanier LL, Gumperz JE, Parham P, Melero I, Lopez-Botet M, Phillips JH. The NKB1 and HP-

3E4 NK cell receptors are structurally distinct glycoproteins and independently recognize polymorphic HLA-B and HLA-C molecules. *J Immunol* 1995; 154: 3320.

25. Cudkowicz G, Bennett M. Peculiar immunobiology of bone marrow allografts II. Rejection of parental grafts by resistant F1 hybrid mice. *J Exp Med* 1971; 134: 1513.
26. Kiessling R, Hochman PS, Haller O, Shearer GM, Wigzell H, Cudkowicz G. Evidence for a similar or common mechanism for natural killer cell activity and resistance to hemopoietic grafts. *Eur J Immunol* 1977; 7: 655.
27. Bach FH, Hirschhorn K. Lymphocyte interaction: a potential histocompatibility test *in vitro. Science* 1964; 143: 813-4.
28. Rodey GE, Bortin MM, Bach FH, Rimm AA. Mixed leukocyte culture reactivity and chronic graft versus host reactions (secondary disease) between allogeneic H-2k mouse strains. *Transplantation* 1974: 17: 84-8.
29. Dupont B, Hansen J, Yunis EJ. Human mixed-lymphocyte culture reaction: genetics, specificity, and biological implications. *Adv Immunol* 1976: 23: 107-202.
30. Mickelson EM, Longton G, Anasetti C, Petersdorf E, Martin PJ, Guthrie LA, Hansen JA. Evaluation of the mixed lymphocyte culture (MLC) assay as a method for selecting unrelated donors for marrow transplantation. *Tissue Antigens* 1996; 47:27-36.
31. Pei J, Martin PJ, Longton G, Masewicz S, Mickelson E, Petersdorf E, Anasetti C, Hansen JA. Evaluation of pretransplant donor anti-recipient cytotoxic and helper T lymphocyte responses as correlates of acute graft-versus-host disease and survival after unrelated marrow transplantation (submitted).
34. Kaminski E, Hows J, Man S, Brookes P, Mackinnon S, Hughes T, Avakian O, Goldman JM, Batchelor JR. Prediction of graft versus host disease by frequency analysis of cytotoxic T cells after unrelated donor bone marrow transplantation. *Transplant* 1989; 48:608-13.
33. Fontaine P, Langlais J, Perreault C. Evaluation of *in vitro* cytotoxic T lymphocyte assays as a predictive test for the occurence of graft vs host disease. *Immunogenetics* 1991; 34:222-6.
34. Van Els CACM, Bakker A, Zwinderman AH, Zwaan FE, van Rood JJ, Goulmy E. Effector mechanisms in graft-versus-host disease in response to minor histocompatibility antigens. I. Absence of correlation with cytotoxic effector cells. *Transplant* 1990; 50:62-6.
35. Clift RA, Buckner CD, Thomas ED, Bensinger WI, Bowden R, Bryant E, Deeg HJ, Doney KC, Fisher LD, Hansen JA, Martin P, McDonald GB, Sanders JE, Schoch G, Singer J, Storb R, Sullivan KM, Witherspoon RP, Appelbaum FR. Marrow transplantation for chronic myeloid leukemia. A randomized study comparing cyclophosphamide and total body irradiation with busulfan anc cyclophosphamide. *Blood* 1994; 84: 2036-43.
36. Kernan NA, Bartsch G, Ash RC, Beatty PG, Champlin R, Filipovich A, Gajewski J, Hansen JA, Henslee-Downey J, McCullough J, McGlave P, Perkins HA, Phillips GL, Sanders J, Stroncek D, Thomas ED, Blume KG. Analysis of 462 transplantations from unrelated donors facilitated by the National Marrow Donor Program. *N Engl J Med* 1993; 328: 593.
37. McGlave PB, Beatty P, Ash R, Hows JM. Therapy for chronic myelogenous leukemia with unrelated donor bone marrow transplantation: results in 102 cases. *Blood* 1990; 75: 1728.
38. Spencer A, Szydlo RM, Brookes PA, Kaminski E, Rule S, van Rhee F, Ward KN, Hale G, Waldmann H, Hows JM, Batchelor JR, Goldman JM. Bone marrow transplantation for chronic myeloid leukemia with volunteer unrelated donors using *ex vivo* or *in vivo* T-cell depletion: major prognostic impact of HLA class I identity between donor and recipient. *Blood* 1995; 86: 3590.

HLA associated diseases
A summary of the 12th International Histocompatibility workshop component

E. Thorsby

Institute of Transplantation Immunology, The National Hospital, University of Oslo, Pilestredet 32, 0027 Oslo, Norway

The 12th International Histocompatibility Workshop (12th IHWS) marks an anniversary in that it is almost 30 years since Amiel first reported an HLA association to a disease [1]. He found that Hodgkin's disease occurred more frequently in individuals carrying the HLA antigen 4C (later B5 + B35 + B18). This and other findings led to an extensive hunt for other HLA associated diseases. The list of such diseases now includes more than 500 entries [2]. For many of them the HLA associations are weak and may be fortuitous. For others, the HLA associations are so strong that they no doubt are a result of a direct involvement of one or more HLA complex genes in the pathogenesis of the disease.

A major question is: which HLA complex genes are primarily involved? Some of those encoding the peptide-presenting HLA molecules, or some of the many other more than 200 genes in the HLA complex? Or a combination? The problem is the strong linkage disequilibrium (or non-random association) which exists between genes in the HLA complex, which creates great difficulties when trying to establish which of the HLA genes are primarily involved, as discussed elsewhere [3].

International collaboration through IHWS's have been very important in addressing this question since HLA gene linkage disequilibria vary between populations and ethnic groups. Thus, comparing the HLA associations to a disease in different populations greatly facilitates identifying the HLA gene(s) being primarily involved (compare for example narcolepsy; see later).

Several diseases were extensively studied at the 12th. IHWS. It is impossible to give a full account of all the activities and results in a brief summary like this. In several cases the analysis also had not been finished. The reader is instead referred to the separate summary articles in the *Workshop Book.* Here just some "highlights" will be given, together with some comments and discussion of future challenges in this field.

The diseases studied during the 12th IHWS may be subdivided into diseases directly caused by microbiological or extrinsic agents, and those caused by a response to autoantigens; *i.e.* autoimmune diseases.

Diseases directly caused by microbiological/extrinsic agents

HIV disease

(chairman: R. Winchester)

The study group had studied 363 cases (all Caucasians) mainly with respect to HIV disease progression. The following main findings were made:

Development of opportunistic infections	
Protection:	A32, DRB1*13, DQA1*0103, DQB1*0603 B27
Accelerating:	A24, B35, Cw4 DRB1*03, DQB1*0201 B39

Development of Kaposi's sarcoma	
Protection:	B8, DRB1*03
Accelerating:	A30

Interestingly, a fast progression of HIV disease associated with B35 was also found during the 11th IHWS, while fast disease progression associated with the B8, DR3, DQ2 haplotype has previously been reported by several others. However, the number of patients studied at the 12th IHWS is small, and the results need to be confirmed in a larger series of patients.

HTLV-1 carriers/disease
(chairman: S. Sonoda)
119 HTLV-1 carriers and 250 patients with HTLV-1 disease had been studied. Some differences in HLA distributions among the groups were found. The reader is referred to the separate summary report.

Allergic disorders
(chairmen: M. Blumenthal/A. Ruffilli)
The analysis had not been completed at the workshop meeting. Preliminary data from sib-pair analysis suggested linkage between HLA and mite sensitivity and possibly also between HLA and asthma.

Rheumatic fever
(chairmen: J.E. Khalil/C. Goldberg)
The trigger here is an infection with streptococci. However, rheumatic fever may be due to an immune response to a cross-reactive myocardial antigen, and the disease may therefore more belong to the group of autoimmune diseases.

299 patients and 478 controls had been studied in five different populations. In some populations, HLA associations were seen, but the overall analysis did not reveal a consistent trend. However, more analyses will be performed (see the separate summary report).

Autoimmune diseases

Juvenile chronic arthritis (JCA)
(chairmen: C. Stavropoulos/A.M. Prieur)
This is a very heterogeneous disease, consisting of several different sub-types. This may be one reason that previous studies have revealed strong, but rather complex HLA associations. This study group had collected as many as 1562 JCA patients with a large number of patients in the various sub-types of the disease. The analysis had not been completed at the workshop meeting, but the results should provide new and important information concerning primary HLA associations in the various sub-types of JCA (see the separate summary report).

Autoimmune hepatitis
(chairman: L. Fainboim)
These studies included 188 adult and 130 pediatric patients. Among adult patients from Argentina and Mexico an increase of the DRB1*04, DQB1*0302 haplotype was found. Among pediatric patients from Argentina and Brazil an association to the DRB1*1301, DQB1*0603 haplotype was found, and a weaker association to DRB1*0301. Studies in Mexico suggested that the association to DRB1*1301 might be the strongest in this disease.

Graves disease
(chairmen: G. Semana/N. Farid)
This study group had carefully divided their patients into those without and those with accompanying other autoimmune diseases. In the former disease group (218 patients), an increase of the A1, B8, DRB1*03 haplotype was found (as in previous studies), while there was a significant decrease of A2 and DRB1*07. In the latter disease group (n=63), most patients also had IDDM, and the same HLA associations as in IDDM were found (see later).

Narcolepsy
(chairmen: G. Mueller-Eckhardt/E. Mignot)
At least two forms of this disease seem to exist. Most patients belong to the "sporadic" form, which previously has been found strongly associated to the DRB1*1501, DQA1*0102, DQB1*0602 haplotype. A minor form of the disease shows familial clustering, and here no strong HLA associations have previously been demonstrated.

Previous studies had suggested that narcolepsy might be more strongly associated to DQA1*0102, DQB1*0602 (*i.e.* DQ6), than DRB1*1501 (DR2) [4]. To further study this, patients were carefully selected to be DRB1*1501 negative and/or DQB1*0602 negative. A summary of the results obtained appears from *Table I.*

The results clearly demonstrate the value of studying disease associations in different ethnic groups (the linkage disequilibrium between DRB1*1501 and DQB1*0602 is almost complete among Caucasians and Japanese, but less complete in Blacks). From the data one may conclude that even though few patients have been studied (there are few "true" narcolepsy patients who are DRB1*1501 and/or DQB1*0602 negative) "sporadic" narcolepsy is in all probability primarily associated to DQB1*0602; *i.e.* the DQ(α1*0102, β1*0602) heterodimer. Secondly, "sporadic" narcolepsy is among the most strongly HLA associated diseases known. Thirdly, since the disease is so strongly associated to a particular peptide-presenting DQ molecule, an autoimmune pathogenesis of the disease is likely, but remains to be established.

Table I. Narcolepsy patients being either DRB1*1501 and/or DQB1*0602 negative

1501	0602	N
	Caucasians (24)	
+	-	0
-	+	5
-	-[1]	19[2]
	Blacks (35)	
+	-	0
-	+	33
-	-	2

1. 7:0601, 0603 or 0604.
2. Many familial cases.

Insulin-dependent diabetes mellitus (IDDM)

(chairmen: S. Caillat-Zucmann / J.F. Bach)

This disease was extensively studied also as part of the 11th IHWS [5]. In the 12th IHWS as many as 2438 patients and 2550 healthy controls had been included. The three main aims were: (1) What is the influence of DR4 subtypes on susceptibility or protection ; (2) what are the HLA associations in non-DQ2 non-DQ8 patients and (3) what are the HLA associations to autoantibody production or age of onset of IDDM.

It is impossible to give a comprehensive summary of the very interesting data obtained from this huge material. The reader is instead referred to the separate summary report. The data from the 12th IHWS support and extend, however, the results obtained at the 11th IHWS [5] as well as recent data from others [6-10] and will in the following be considered together.

Table II lists the DQ and DR4 molecules which are most strongly associated with IDDM susceptibility in most populations, and a tentative order of hierarchy. The reason that the DQ heterodimer DQ(α1*0301, β1*0201), is listed at the top is that (1) the strongest IDDM susceptibility in most populations is found for DR3, DQ2/DR4,DQ8 heterozygotes, who can encode this heterodimer in *trans* position of the corresponding DQA1 and DQB1 genes; (2) in Orientals, particularly Chinese, strong association of IDDM susceptibility is found for DR3,DQ2/DR9,DQ9 heterozygotes, who may encode the same DQ heterodimer in *trans* position [6] and (3) in Blacks and some Caucasians in the Mediterranean area there is a strong IDDM association with the same DQ heterodimer, but here encoded in *cis* position (together with various DR molecules; see [3]). The IDDM susceptibility associated with the DQ(α1*0301, β1*0201) heterodimer, as well as with DQ(α1*0301, β1*0302) is, however, strongly dependent on the accompanying DR4 subtype. At the 12th IHWS the DR4 subtypes DR(α,β1*0405, 0402 and 0401) were found associated with susceptibility, while DR(α,β1*0406, 0403 and 0404) were associated with protection (see later).

It was reported at the workshop meeting that in Basques, two different DR3, DQ2 haplotypes were found; B18, DR3, DQ2 and B8, DR3, DQ2. IDDM susceptibility was more strongly associated with the former than the latter haplotype, indicating an influence of other genes (B18?, genes in the HLA class III region?) on the DR3, DQ2 associated susceptibility. This may also explain why DR3, DQ2 confers different degrees of IDDM susceptibility in various populations (high in Basques, lower in Northern Europe). It should be noted,

Table II. Some DQ and DR4 molecules being significantly associated with IDDM susceptibility

DQ molecules	Hierarchy*
DQ(α1*0301, β1*0201)	1
DQ(α1*0301, β1*0302) (=DQ8)	2
DQ(α1*0501, β1*0201) (=DQ2)	3
DQ(α1*0301, β1*0401) (=DQ4)	4
DQ(α1*0301, β1*0303) (=DQ9)	4
DQ(α1*0401, β1*0402) (=DQ4)	4
DR4 sub-types	
DR(α,β1*0405)	1
DR(α,β1*0402)	2
DR(α,β1*0401)	3

* Average strength of association, based on data from many different populations.

however, that it has not been established whether DR3 or DQ2 (or any other HLA complex gene) is primarily associated with IDDM susceptibility on this haplotype, but by inference from the known DQ associated susceptibility, DQ2 is believed by most to be the candidate.

The three DQ heterodimers giving the lowest predisposition (two different variants of DQ4, and DQ9) turned up in many non-DQ2 non-DQ8 IDDM patients and may be mainly responsible for the IDDM susceptibility in this minor group of patients. It cannot be excluded, however, that the susceptibility associated with these DQ heterodimers is instead conferred by some other genes on the same haplotype.

Also *protection* against development of IDDM is associated both with some DQ and DR4 molecules. Some of the most important are listed in *Table III*. Here the protection sometimes is dominant (=D); i.e. when present these DQ or DR4 molecules overrule the IDDM susceptibility associated with any accompanying DQ or DR4 molecules.

Table III. Some DQ and DR4 molecules being significantly associated with protection against IDDM

DQ molecules	Hierarchy
DQ(α1*0102, β1*0602) (=DQ6)	1 (D)*
DQ(α1*0301, β1*0301) (=DQ7)	3
DQ(α1*0501, β1*0301) (=DQ7)	3
DQ(α1*0201, β1*0201)	3
DR4 sub-types	
DR(α,β1*0406, 0403)	1 (D)
DR(α,β1*0404)	3

* D=dominant protection.

Taken together, HLA associated predisposition to develop IDDM appears to be the net effect mainly of the *combination* of DQ or DR molecules carried by an individual, where some DQ and DR4 molecules appear to be most important. Maximum IDDM *susceptibility* is associated with DQ(α1*0301, β1*0201), when present together with DR(α,β1*0405). In contrast, maximum *protection* is associated with DQ(α1*0102, β1*0602) and DR(α,β1*0403 or 0406), and is dominant over susceptibility. Other combinations of DQ and DR molecules are "in between", with a degree of susceptibility, protection or neutrality depending on the particular combination.

The interaction between some DQ and DR4 molecules is intriguing. Based on some studies on peptide-binding motifs of various DR4 sub-types, we suggest that DR4 sub-types may confer different degrees of protection, DR(α,β1*0403 and 0406) being the most protective, while DR(α,β1*0405) is least if at all protective. Thus, IDDM susceptibility may be mainly determined by some DQ molecules, while other DQ and some DR4 molecules may confer different degrees of protection (see Undlien *et al.,* in this volume).

Almost 800 patient sera were analysed for five different IDDM related autoantibodies. Such antibodies were found more frequently in patients having DR-DQ genotypes associated with the strongest susceptibility; *i.e.* DQ2/DQ8 or DQ8/X. Similarily, age of onset seemed to be lower in patients carrying high-risk compared to those with more low-risk DR-DQ genotypes (*i.e.* DR3/4 or 4/4 compared to other genotypes).

Comments and future challenges

Taking the 12th IHWS studies together with many other recent studies on HLA and disease associations, one is left with the following tentative conclusions.

Some normal peptide-presenting HLA molecules are primarily involved

This seems to be the case for IDDM and narcolepsy, but also for ankylosing spondylitis, rheumatoid arthritis, coeliac disease and others (see [3]). However, exceptions exist, such as congenital adrenal hyperplasia and hemochromatosis, where the primary associations are to some other genes in the HLA complex, or to some closely linked genes (see [3]).

For many other diseases, it remains to be established whether the primary association is also to some peptide-presenting HLA molecules. In such studies, it is important to note that several different HLA molecules may be involved because they share a particular pocket in their peptide-binding cleft, which may be decisive for their ability to bind a particular peptide

[11,12]. By focusing more on common peptide-binding motifs it may be possible to resolve complex HLA associations (as in IDDM).

The mechanism behind the direct involvement of normal peptide-binding HLA molecules may be: (1) thymic effects of the involved HLA molecules on the selection of the T cell receptor repertoire; (2) preferential binding and presentation to T cells of some relevant antigen-derived peptides by these HLA molecules, or both. In order to study this, identification of the peptide-binding motifs of the involved HLA molecules would be most helpful, as would identification of the antigenic epitope which is initially recognized. Here identification of the peptide-binding motifs may be used to identify the latter. If the involved HLA molecules cause the disease associations by preferentially binding some relevant antigen-derived peptides (a concept for which there exists some good experimental evidence), one may speculate whether HLA associated disease susceptibility and protection may involve "competing" immune responses, such as Th1 versus Th2 in the case of IDDM (a concept for which there exist some other good experimental evidence; see for example McDevitt in this volume).

A primary involvement of the peptide-presenting HLA molecules may also explain why it is more difficult to find consistent HLA associations in diseases where microbiological or extrinsic agents are directly causing the disease, compared to autoimmune diseases. In the former case it would probably be better, in many cases, to look primarily for protection rather than susceptibility to given HLA molecules. More important, however, microbiological or other extrinsic agents (allergens, etc.) will consist of many different antigens and corresponding epitopes, which demonstrate extensive antigenic heterogeneity between strains, etc. An immune response may therefore involve many different peptide-presenting HLA molecules, which may differ in various geographic areas. In contrast, fewer antigens and epitopes are candidate autoantigens, and may show much less antigenic heterogeneity. If an autoimmune response is caused by molecular mimicry between an extrinsic triggering and a target autoantigenic epitope, this would further reduce the number of candidate autoantigenic epitopes which may be initially recognized in the autoimmune response. Thus, it should be more easy to find HLA associations in autoimmune diseases, and here primarily to susceptibility, which is also the case.

The HLA associated genetic predisposition is often the net result of a combination of HLA molecules

The typical example is IDDM, where both susceptible and protective DR and DQ molecules are known. This should be taken more into consideration in future studies of HLA associated diseases. For example, the effector mechanisms in some primarily HLA class II associated diseases most probably also involve CD8+ T cells, and thus also HLA class I molecules. By carefully matching patients and controls for the established disease associated HLA molecules, one may identify contributions also by other HLA molecules.

Influence of other HLA complex genes remains to be established

Several studies have been carried out on a possible influence of TAP or LMP polymorphisms on disease susceptibility, for example in IDDM. Most if not all of the found associations have turned out to be secondary to associations to HLA molecules, caused by linkage disequilibrium (see [3]). However, more studies are needed, in particular studies of contributions by other HLA complex genes, for example those in the class III region (complotypes, etc.). Again, since some primary HLA associations have now been established, it is possible to "freeze" patients and controls for the involved HLA molecules, which should enable detection of contributions by other HLA complex genes, which are not caused by linkage disequilibrium.

Influence of non-HLA genes and environmental factors remains to be established

Even though HLA genes represent the strongest genetic predisposition in many of these diseases, like IDDM, we know that non-HLA genes and environmental factors also play a major role. For many diseases some HLA genes are almost necessary for disease development, but they are not sufficient. Only very few individuals carrying DQ(α1*0102, β1*0602) will ever develop narcolepsy. These additional genetic and environmental factors are largely unknown and need to be identified.

Conclusion

The disease studies at the 12th IHWS added much to our knowledge of the primary HLA associations in several diseases. Taken together with other available evidence, the data support the concept that in many

HLA associated diseases some normal peptide-presenting HLA molecules are responsible for the genetic predisposition, and thus involved in the pathogenesis.

This adds a new dimension to the whole HLA field. For long HLA typing has been used to identify individuals at high risk to develop given diseases, but mainly for diagnostic purposes (e.g. B27 typing in the diagnosis of ankylosing spondylitis). Such use of HLA typing will continue to be of use. However, given present knowledge of the structure and function of HLA molecules, combined with modern molecular biology methods to identify peptide-binding motifs of HLA molecules, etc., we should shortly be able to unveil the mechanisms how the HLA molecules are involved in causing susceptibility or protection. With this knowledge at hand, identification of individuals at high risk should be used more to prevent or halt disease development. This may be a major part of the clinical application of HLA in the near future.

Acknowledgments
I wish to thank all participants in the HLA and disease component, in particular the chairmen, for all their efforts and for sharing with me their preliminary results. They are not, however, responsible for my interpretation of their results.

References

The reader is referred to the individual summary reports by the disease component chairmen (in volume I).

1. Amiel JC. Study of the leucocyte phenotypes in Hodgkin's disease. In: Cùrtoni ES, Mattiùz PL, Tosi RM eds. *Histocompatibility Testing 1967.* Copenhagen: Munksgaard, 1967.
2. Tiwari JL, Terasaki PI. HLA and disease associations. New York: Springer Verlag, 1985.
3. Thorsby E. HLA-associated disease susceptibility. Which genes are primarily involved? *The Immunologist* 1995; 3 : 51-8.
4. Mignot E, Lin X, Arrigoni J, Macaubas C, Olive F, Hallmeyer J, Underhill P, Guilleminault C, Dement WC, Grumet FC. DQB1-0602 and DQA1-0102-(DQ1) are better markers than DR2 for narcolepsy in Caucasian and Black Americans. *Sleep* 1994; 17 : 560-7.
5. Rønningen KS, Spurkland A, Tait BD, Drummond B *et al.* HLA class II associations in insulin-dependent diabetes mellitus among Blacks, Caucasoids and Japanese. In: Tsuji K, Aizawa M, Sasazuki T eds. *HLA 1991,* vol 1. Oxford : Oxford University Press, 1992; 713-22.
6. Huang H-S, Peng JT, She JY, Zhang LP, Chao CK, Liu KH, She JX. HLA-encoded susceptibility to insulin-dependent diabetes mellitus is determined by *DR* and *DQ* genes as well as their linkage disequilibria in a Chinese population. *Hum Immunol* 1995; 44 : 210-9.
7. Caillat-Zucman S, Garchon HJ, Timsit J, Assan R, Boitard C, Djilali-Saiah I, Bougners P, Bach JF. Age-dependent HLA genetic heterogeneity of type 1 insulin-dependent diabetes mellitus. *J Clin Invest* 1992; 90 : 2242-50.
8. Cucca F, Lampis R, Frau F, Macis D, Angius E, Masile P, Chessa M, Frongia P, Silvetti M, Cao A, De Virgiliis S, Congia M. The distribution of DR4 haplotypes in Sardinia suggests a primary association of type 1 diabetes with DRB1 and DQB1 loci. *Hum Immunol* 1995; 43 : 301-8.
9. Van der Auwera B, Van Waeyenberge C, Schuit F, Heimberg H, Vandewalle C, Gorus F, Flament J. DRB1*0403 protects against IDDM in Caucasians with the high-risk heterozygous DQA1*0301-DQB1*0302/DQA1*0501-DQB1*0201 genotype. Belgian Diabetes Registry. *Diabetes* 1995; 44 : 527-30.
10. Yasunaga S, Kimura A, Hamaguchi K, Ronningen KS, Sasazuki T. Different contribution of HLA-DR and -DQ genes in susceptibility and resistance to insulin-dependent diabetes mellitus (IDDM). *Tissue Antigens* 1996; 47 : 37-48.
11. Wucherpfennig KW, Strominger JL. Selective binding of self peptide to disease-associated major histocompatibility complex (MHC) molecules: a mechanism for MHC-linked susceptibility to human autoimmune diseases. *J Exp Med* 1995; 181 : 1597-601.
12. Zerva L, Cizman B, Mehra NK, Alahri SK, Murali R, Zmijewski CM, Kamoun M, Monos DS. Arginine at position 13 or 70-71 in pocket 4 of HLA-DRB1 alleles is associated with susceptibility to tuberculoid leprosy. *J Exp Med* 1996; 183 : 829-36.

Summary

Summary of the 12th International Histocompatibility Workshop and Conference

W. Bodmer

Imperial Cancer Research Fund, University of Oxford, Institute of Molecular Medicine, John Radcliffe Hospital, Headington, Oxford OX3 9DU, UK

In contributing this my seventh HLA Workshop summary, I am sad that some of the key players of previous workshops are no longer with us, namely Ruggero Ceppellini, Fleming Kissmeyer-Nielson and Hilliard Festenstein. Bernard Amos who started them off, and Rose Payne with whom Julia and I started studying the HLA system and who has attended every previous workshop, were also unfortunately not able to be present this time.

This is the second of the HLA Workshops to be held in France and mirrors the first, organised in 1972 by Jean Dausset, in having a major emphasis on anthropology. The spirit of collaboration, of exchange of materials and reagents and of technology transfer continues into the 32nd year since the workshops started. This time there is an even greater diversity and number of participating laboratories and populations throughout the world which have been studied. Computers which, in a primitive form, provided the analyses that first defined the HLA system now permeate all our activities, including communications. Nearly all laboratories, more than 240 world-wide, were inter-connected, for example, by E-mail. There are, of course, often problems with the data handling and analysis and this workshop was no exception. However, John Clayton and his colleagues from Toulouse worked extremely hard to provide some analysis in time for the meeting. While some laboratories still carried out serological tests, the overwhelming emphasis was on DNA analysis using a variety of techniques. These have progressed from restriction fragment-length polymorphism testing in previous workshops to oligonucleotide annealing for detecting specific sequence differences and now, in this workshop, the first application of the ARMS3 mismatch technique. This was used especially widely for the first time for DNA analysis of the HLA-A, B and C polymorphisms. Since the ARMS technique associates pairs of nucleotide differences on the same molecule, so long as the variants to be detected are not too far apart to produce a PCR product, this technique does not have the problem of distinguishing coupling and repulsion heterozygotes which is common to those techniques, for example, using oligonucleotide annealing which detect one, or a small cluster of basepair differences at a time. Sequence-based typing has a role to play, mainly in the identification of new variants.

For the future, large-scale inexpensive DNA typing will, in my view, depend on automation that by-passes the use of gel separation, for example, by direct identification of a PCR product in a multi-well plate, or perhaps in a few more years time, by the use of very high density computer-like chips containing tens of thousands of oligonucleotides.

Serology and HLA expression

Monoclonal antibodies and serological analysis still have a key role to play in studying the expression of HLA-gene products. Essentially all products are now detectable by specific monoclonal antibodies, but there are still relatively few antibodies for polymorphic determinants, especially of the class I specificities. The polymorphic antibodies are particularly valuable for studying the expression of polymorphic determinants, for example, on tumours and antibodies that work on paraffin sections would be extremely valuable. They are also useful in the study of T-cell restricted reaction patterns.

There are useful monoclonal antibodies for Bw4 and Bw6. Furthermore, the complex patterns of class I monoclonal antibodies can now be analysed following the same approaches that have been used for some years for the identification of class II serological epitopes. For example, as described in Renee Fauchet's summary, there are two monoclonal antibodies that react to the combination of B7, 27, 42, 54, 55, 56, 67, 73 and 81. This pattern is associated with alanine (A) at position 69, glutamine (Q) or lysine (K) at position 70 and alanine at position 71. This fits in with the fact that T (threonine) should be the consensus at position 69 for the B-locus, while it is (A), at the A-locus, and with the pattern of reaction of B46, which combines B and C locus specificities and has arginine at position 69, in common with all C locus alleles.

The serology has helped to define new haplotype combinations and, in combination with the DNA analysis, has uncovered the intriguing A24 non-expressing mutations. These seem to be found with higher frequency in some populations, such as perhaps in Northern Ireland, but this pattern is entirely consistent with an occasional increase in frequency of a mutation by chance, namely due to random genetic drift. There are many sites within the gene which can render it non-expressing, and under most circumstances this is most unlikely to be accompanied by any selective disadvantage. Given known rates of mutation, therefore, it is hardly surprising if occasional non-expressing variants do increase in frequency in particular populations.

Monoclonal antibodies, of course, pick up serological determinants, whose direct relevance for T-cell reactivity is not clear. It would be interesting, though technically demanding, to accumulate data on T-cell restriction patterns, and so HLA epitopes, for a range of antigens that might be considered important, either in infectious pathogens or with respect to auto-immunity.

Anthropology

The phylogenetic trees constructed using HLA gene frequency data in 1972 were already quite informative. The range of data, however, collected this time was very much greater. Julia Bodmer and colleagues' organisation of the anthropological work ensured that samples were collected based on sound criteria concerning the location, history and anthropological information available on the population itself, while also ensuring that details of the birthplace of individuals and their forebears fitted in with the definition of a population. Much further analysis will be required to reap this rich harvest of data, which includes great detail at the DNA level for variation at most of the HLA genes over a range of more than a hundred populations. These included populations in areas previously hardly studied, such as across the wide expanses of Asia, from Russia through to China, and a much wider representation of African populations, so important for establishing the origin of *Homo sapiens*. In some cases there was enough local detail to establish inter-relationships, for example, amongst the Celtic populations of Britain, and to show their marked differences from other European populations, such as the Italians on the one hand, and the distinctiveness of the Sardinian population on the other. Studies of the Jewish populations suggested that the A26 B38 haplotype reflected their common origins, while the new information on African populations indicated gradients of gene frequency change from North to South, as has been found in Europe. Amongst these was B53, raising inevitably a question as to the consistency of its association with malaria. Further studies, perhaps also using other markers than HLA, will help to distinguish the effects of acculturation from genetic admixture.

The resolution of the ARMS technique enabled a much more detailed study of the extraordinary range of "splits" of HLA-A2. As Julia Bodmer pointed out, whereas the overall A2 frequency seems remarkably constant throughout the world, this hides a considerable measure of variation in the frequencies of A2 splits. Somewhat similar stories can be told for other such variations on a theme, including, for example, B15 and DRB1 *14. Julia Bodmer has raised the question as to whether the number of T-cells that have been identified against flu which are A2 restricted is simply a matter of chance or ascertainment bias. Perhaps there are dominant epitopes such as A2 and B15, which are needed for effective resistance to key pathogenic determinants. The continuing war game between host and pathogen then leads to selection of variants around the theme both in the host, hence the A2 variants, for example, and in the pathogen. It is important to emphasise that it is epitopes of HLA molecules, presumably with respect to T-cell recognition, that are selected for in the battle between host and pathogen not alleles as such, which are combinations of epitopes. The apparent conservation of alleles between species is really a conservation of tried and trusted epitopes for peptide binding.

Recombination and linkage disequilibrium

For a given recombination fraction, linkage disequilibrium, which is the population association between alleles on the same haplotype, is largely dependent on time. The complement of this is that, for a given time of separation, it is the actual recombination fraction which generally determines the extent of linkage disequilibrium. Of course, as often pointed out before, a relatively rapid increase in the frequency of a haplotype due to selection for one of its component alleles can lead to anomalies, and explains the so-called extended haplotypes, while localised drift effects can also lead to unexpectedly strong associations. These are all effectively examples of time differences affecting linkage disequilibrium. It is only selective interactions between the effects of alleles on the same haplotype that can lead to the long term maintenance of linkage disequilibrium even for relatively larger recombination fractions.

This Workshop, for the first time, produced a detailed genetic map of the HLA region giving recombination fractions for 11 markers spread more or less uniformly from one end to the other. An extensive body of data, organised and analysed by Mogens Thomsen and Bill Klitz, showed a greater variation in recombination fractions within the HLA region than had previously been expected. The markers included micro-satellite variants as well as variants at the HLA loci themselves. The 77 recombination events analysed showed some intervals in which there appeared to be a marked excess of the female over the male recombination fraction, a phenomenon variably observed throughout the human genome. There were also at least two regions suggesting the existence of recombination hotspots, namely recombination fractions which clearly exceeded the average level expected from the physical length of the interval measured in basepairs. One of these, between DP and DQB1, clearly explains the general lack of linkage disequilibrium between DP alleles and alleles at other HLA loci and also probably explains the extraordinary lack of linkage disequilibrium between alleles at the two TAP loci. Another may exist in the region between HLA A and HLA B. Patterns of recombination should help to interpret linkage disequilibrium data and enhance their use for measuring the time of separation of different population groups.

New genes

The HLA region, summarised again by John Trowsdale and Duncan Campbell, continues to be populated with newly discovered genes, especially now it is all cloned into YACs and cosmids and well on the way to being sequenced. The class II region appears to be more or less completely characterised. The greatest surprise there is the role of DMA and DMB in class II processing and their equally distant relationship to class I and class II genes. The main source of new genes still seems to be in the interval between class I and class II, while there appear to be many gaps still to be filled in the class I region. The particular surprises are the discovery of a cluster of olfactory receptors, and the MICA and related class I-like genes which are β2-microglobulin associated. There is evidence that one or more of these maps more than one megabase telomeric to HLA-A while maintaining strong linkage disequilibrium with HLA- A alleles [1]. The fact that β2-microglobulin knock-out mice show evidence of haemachromatosis-like symptoms is therefore intriguing in suggesting that it may be one or more of these genes, apparently outside the HLA region as currently defined, and yet class I-like, which accounts for the association between HLA-A3 and haemachromatosis [2]. There are clearly many surprises here still to be uncovered.

Another surprising observation is the apparent homology between the HLA region on chromosome 6p21.3 and a region on chromosome 9q33-34, as outlined by Inoko and others. There exists a series of homologous genes including heat-shock proteins, a homeobox gene, a notch homologue, a TAP, LMPs, a collagen gene and a retinoid receptor in the same order in these two regions. It will be fascinating to see how far back in evolution these homologies go and to what extent they apply to other genes at these locations on chromosomes 6 and 9.

HLA and cancer and other functional studies

A collaborative study on the expression of HLA on tumours using monoclonal antibodies was, for the first time, a component of this workshop, organised by Garrido and colleagues. A good deal of variation in expression was observed in a variety of tumours using both immunohistology on sections and FACS analysis of isolated tumour cells and tumour derived cell lines. The data confirmed the now widely supported view that much reduction or loss of HLA class I expression can be found on a variety of tumours and probably reflects escape from immune attack. The mechanisms for escape include mutations in the TAP protein and in transcription factors regulating expression. DNA analysis on cell lines, as well as the use of monoclonal antibodies against polymorphic determinants, of which as already mentioned there are far too few, show that haplotype loss, presumably due to non-disjunction or somatic recombination, is a relatively common mechanism affecting expression of individual HLA determinants. Binding studies on normal cells carried out in parallel with those on tumours showed patterns of specificity of the monoclonal antibodies that did not always match those which had been claimed. This emphasises the importance of characterising the patterns of reactivity of monoclonal antibodies in binding assays before they are used for tumour expression studies.

Bodmer and his colleagues have pointed out the strong correlation between the mismatch repair status of colorectal carcinomas and the occurrence of β2-microglobulin mutations leading to reduced or complete absence of HLA class I expression [3]. Since mismatch repair deficiency gives rise, potentially, to many mutations in proteins that can be targets in tumours for immune recognition, this supports the view that changes in HLA class I expression do reflect escape from immune attack. Another piece of evidence to support this view comes from Ferrone's analysis of a specific A2 mutation leading to loss of A2 expression in a tumour.

Kärre summarised the evidence that NK cells may attack tumours lacking class I expression, raising the frequently asked question as to the balance between specific T-cell attack against tumours expressing novel determinants and the relevant HLA class I restriction elements, versus NK activity against tumours that have escaped T-cell specific attack through loss of HLA expression. It seems likely that tumour immune response is a relatively late event, so that any effects of NK cells would have to be at a late stage when there is a large tumour load and therefore at a time when the NK effects are unlikely to be sufficient to limit tumour growth significantly. Furthermore, mechanisms for escape from NK attack, for example, through loss of gamma interferon responsiveness which has frequently been described, can be selected for secondarily.

The variety of mechanisms by which HLA expression can be affected by mutations selected for in tumours parallels the extraordinary variety of mechanisms by which viruses contrive to escape the immune response, as summarised by Ploegh. Similarly, the complexity of regulation of HLA class II expression, outlined by Bernard Mach, provides many opportunities for selection for mutations affecting class II expression. These complex regulatory mechanisms, however, always seems to me to pose the question of where does it all start. "Big fleas have little fleas upon their backs to bite them and little fleas have lesser fleas and so on ad infinitum". Does the regulatory process trace a pathway all the way back to the distribution of proteins in the cytoplasm of the fertilised egg?

The remarkable scheme by which the invariant chains and the DMA/B heteropolymer co-operate to aid the delivery of specific peptides to class II molecules was outlined by Hidde Ploegh in his Ceppellini lecture (see *Figure 1*). The clue was the discovery of the invariant chain derived clip peptide in the peptide binding grove of the HLA class II molecules in mutant cells that lack functional DMA/B heteropolymers. This clip peptide is part of the invariant chain, whose association with class II has until now remained mysterious. It is cleaved from the rest of the molecule by cathepsin S. The DMA/B heteropolymer then somehow catalyses the exchange between the clip peptide and a specific peptide in the class II molecule groove. Though the structural analysis is proceeding well, as shown by Garboczi's description of the tri-molecular complex of T-cell receptor, peptide and class I molecule, there is still some way to go before detailed structural interactions between these various molecules and the way they achieve their purpose can be fully understood.

It has long been known that the trophoblast does not express normal HLA A,B and C molecules and been suggested that this may be a major basis for the survival of the foetus as an allograft [4]. More recently Ellis and McMichael and others showed that, under certain circumstances, HLA G is expressed on some trophoblasts and now Arnes-Villena has described the very limited polymorphism for the HLA-G gene. This is consistent with its role as a peptide restricter but without giving rise to the strong allograft responses associated with conventional HLA class I polymorphism. Now, following an earlier suggestion by Bodmer [5], Rodriguez and co-workers have confirmed how readily interferon gamma can switch on HLA class I functional expression in the villous trophoblast. Without this, these important cells would be dangerously exposed to virus attack.

The strange way in which NK cells act, involving specific inhibition by class I products and a human receptor whose mouse homologue seems to function rather differently, were described by Lanier. This network of interactions between NK cells and HLA polymorphic determinants is strangely reminiscent of the Jerne network hypothesis. There is still some way to go before the full implications of NK activity are understood, including its normal role (perhaps as a primary relatively non-specific alternative response to pathogens), the significance of the negative control by HLA polymorphic determinants, and the role of NK killing of cells which lack surface HLA-A, B and C expression, both in normal tissues and more especially in tumours.

Disease association

The majority of the studies on HLA and disease were confirmatory of previously observed associations. Further delving into the IDDM association did suggest a role for DRB1.0405, in addition to the DQ associations. The mouse models, so elegantly analysed by McDevitt, showed the likely complexity of the real biological situation and the difficulty in identifying specific T-cell targets that can explain the auto-immune deficiency, though a role for the DQ α/β heterodimer was very nicely confirmed.

Unwanted infection influenced the development of auto-immunity in the mice. It thus appears that it may be the spectrum of responses with respect to the level of expression, affinity and avidity in the T-cell response repertoire which is influenced by the HLA and H2 polymorphisms. Whether auto-immune disease develops or not may then depend on some form of threshold effect. These ideas, which are based on discussions with Hugh McDevitt and Helen Bodmer, can also explain why auto-immune diseases seem to be increasing in frequency so much in modern western society, whose people's immune systems are no longer put to work to the same extent to counteract infectious pathogens. As the parasite load decreases, the risk of the T-cell activity threshold being exceeded leading to auto-immune disease, increases. This form of antigenic competition was something that we observed in our earliest field studies of the Pygmy populations carried out with Cavalli-Sforza in the late 1960s. We were never able to detect significant reactions to maternal HLA antisera in spite of clear evidence of many samples being collected from young mothers with many offspring, the most recent of which was often under one year old. The Pygmies were full of parasites - their filaria were well preserved by the lymphocyte freezing conditions. The maternal allo antisera discovered by Rose Payne and Jon van Rood, and which were the basis for the original definition of the HLA polymorphism, may thus, like auto-immune disease, be products of the low parasite load of modern western society. The immune system perhaps obeys the rule that "Satan makes work for idle hands to do".

Conclusions

As has been emphasised by Julia Bodmer and others, the huge body of data collected in the course of this workshop leaves much to be analysed. There is a need for the future to ensure continuity by building a databa-

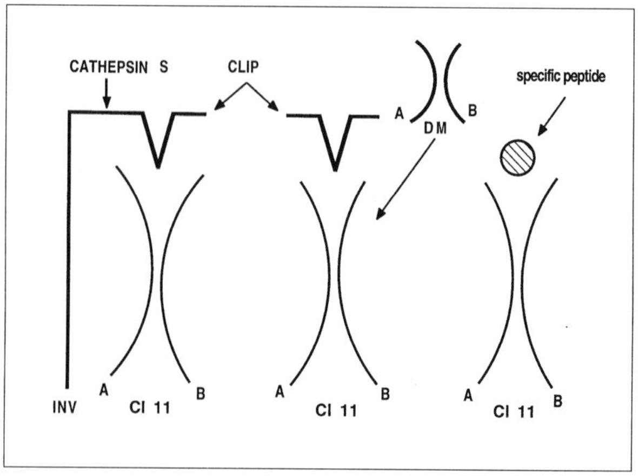

Figure 1. HLA class 11 peptide loading.

se that can continually be added to, and which is widely accessible. The anthropological studies can be extended to the use of other markers and so make a major contribution to the Human Genome Diversity Programme, a relationship which has already been initiated. In particular, interest will centre on the distribution of polymorphisms for new class I genes, for DMA and B , for the TAPS and LMPs, for TNF variants and the NK receptor, as well as for the olfactory genes, the mysterious class I related MICA and B and other genes. To this list can be added the minor histocompatibility determinants described by Els Goulmy, including finally the identification of the H-Y antigen.

This workshop has once again demonstrated the huge extent to which the HLA community collaborates internationally and the major results that come from working together in this way. We owe our thanks to Dominique Charron (chairman), Renée Fauchet (executive organizer), Anne Cambon-Thomsen, John Clayton, Ike Schreuder, Julia Bodmer and the many others who contributed to the enormous output of this workshop. The effectiveness of the collaboration once again ensured that there was a consensus to continue with a 13th workshop under a United States of America West Coast grouping led by John Hansen.

Julia Bodmer summarised the achievements of the 11th Workshop in Japan in 1991 with her haiku
" In studying our differences we come together".
Her haiku for this workshop is
"Having studied our differences we realise how much we all share".

References

References for this summary are contained in the main body of the two workshop conference volumes. Thus, only a few specific references, not otherwise covered, are given as follows.

1. Feder JN, Gnirke A, Thomas W, Tsuchihashi Z, Ruddy DA, Basava A, Dormishian F, Domingo Jr R, Ellis MC, Fullan A, Hinton LM, Jones NL, Kimmel BE, Kronmal GS, Lauer P, Lee VK, Loeb DB, Mapa FA, McClelland E, Meyer NC, Mintier GA, Moeller N, Moore T, Morikang E, Prass CE, Quintana L, Starnes SM, Schatzman RC, Brunke KJ, Drayna DT, Risch NJ, Bacon BR, Wolff RK. A novel MHC class I-like gene is mutated in patients with hereditary haemochromatosis. *Nature Genet* 1996; 13: 399.
2. Rothenberg BE, Voland JR. β2m Knockout mice develop parenchymal iron overload: a putative role for class I genes of the major histocompatibility complex in iron metabolism. *Proc Natl Acad Sci USA* 1996 ; 93: 1529-34.
3. Branch P, Rowan A, Bicknell DC, Bodmer WF, Karran P. Immune surveillance in colorectal carcinoma. *Nature Genet* 1995; 9 : 231-2 .
4. Barnstable CJ, Bodmer WF. Immunology and the fetus. *Lancet* 1978 ; i: 326.
5. Bodmer WF, Immunogenetics: chairman's introduction. The evolution and function of the HLA system. *Immunology* 1989; 2 (suppl) : 33-5.

Symposium communications

HLA Diversity

HLA typing and sequencing

Function of HLA

Transplantation biology and medicine

HLA and diseases

Symposium contributions were selected and reviewed by a panel of experts and the 12th IHWC European Committee

The Organising Committee greatly acknowledges the contribution of the following persons in selecting and reviewing the symposium communications

Albert E.
Alcalay D.
Altmann D.M.
Amoroso A.
Arnaiz-Villena A.
Auffray C.
Begovich A.
Bensussan A.
Bignon J.-D.
Blumenthal M.
Bodmer J.G.
Boitard C.
Bontrop R.
Buelow R.
Bunce M.
Busson M.
Caillat-Zucman S.
Cambon A.
Campbell R.D.
Carpenter C.
Charron D.
Claas F.H.J.
Clayton J.
Clerget-Darpoux F.
Colonna M.
David C.
Du Toit E.
Dufossé F.
Dupont B.
Duquesnoy R.J.
Eliaou J.F.
Erlich H.
Fauchet R.
Fernandez-Vina M.
Ferrara G.
Ferrone S.
Garrido F.
Gebuhrer L.
Geraghty D.E.
Gill T.J.
Goldmann S.F.
Goulmy E.
Hämmerling G.J.
Hanau D.
Hauptmann G.
Hors J.
Houssin D.
Inoko H.
Juji T.
Kalil J.
Kreis H.
Krensky A.
Lahoz C.
Lanier L.
Le Petit J.
Lebouteiller P.
Lechler R.
Lepage V.
Levy D.
Lopez-Larrea C.
Madrigal A.
Maeda H.
Marsh D.G.
Masucci M.G.
Mayr W.
Mazilli M.
McMichael A.
Mooney N.
Moretta L.
Morris P.
Natali P.
Neefjes J.
Olerup O.
Opelz G.
Oudshoorn M.
Parham P.
Peltre G.
Petersdorf E.
Piazza A.
Pinet V.
Pontarotti P.
Raffoux C.
Richiardi P.
Rubinstein P.
Sanchez-Mazas A.
Sasazuki T.
Sasportes M.
Schreuder I.
Semana G.
Sinnott P.
Soulillou J.-P.
Spies T.
Stastny P.
Suciu-Foca N.
Svejgaard A.
Tait B.D.
Terasaki P.
Teyton L.
Thorsby E.
Tilanus M.
Tongio M.
Toubert A.
Trowsdale J.
van Rood J.J.
Wassmuth R.
Wernet P.

HLA
Diversity

HLA diversity of alleles and haplotypes

Contents

• HLA diversity of alleles and haplotypes

Recombination hot spots in the HLA region of chromosome 6: refinement of localization using microsatellite markers

M.M. Barmada, N.L. Delaney, W.B. Bias, B.J. Schmeckpeper

Immunogenetics Laboratories, Johns Hopkins University School of Medicine, 2041E Monument Street, Baltimore, MD 21205-2222, USA

Using human chromosome 6p specific microsatellite markers we have further analyzed 28 caucasian families in which recombinant individuals had been previously identified by serologic (HLA-A, B, C, DR, and DQ), protein (F13A1, BF), or enzyme (GLO1) typing. Nine microsatellite markers (F13A01, D6S89, D6S285, D6S461, D6S105, D6S265, TNFα, DQCAR, D6S291) were analyzed in these families. The addition of microsatellite data to the serologic, enzyme, and protein polymorphism data has allowed us to fine map the recombination breakpoints in these families, and to identify potential «hotspots» for recombination.

Figure 1 shows the map we derived for this region of human chromosome 6p from composites of genetic and physical maps from the Genome Database, the Cooperative Human Linkage Consortium, and published sources [1]. Although some loci were only roughly placed (*e.g.* D6S265 somewhere between HLA-A and HLA-C), the composite map allowed us to order our loci, establish haplotypes, and thus more easily delineate the breakpoints of the recombination events in each individual. We decided against traditional methods of map building using our dataset because of the problem of ascertainment bias: families were selected based on the presence of recombinant individuals, thus enriching our population for recombination events, and inflating all subsequent calculations of map distance based upon this population. For this reason, a composite map was constructed and used in all subsequent analyses. Note that, because of their proximate locations, the serologic

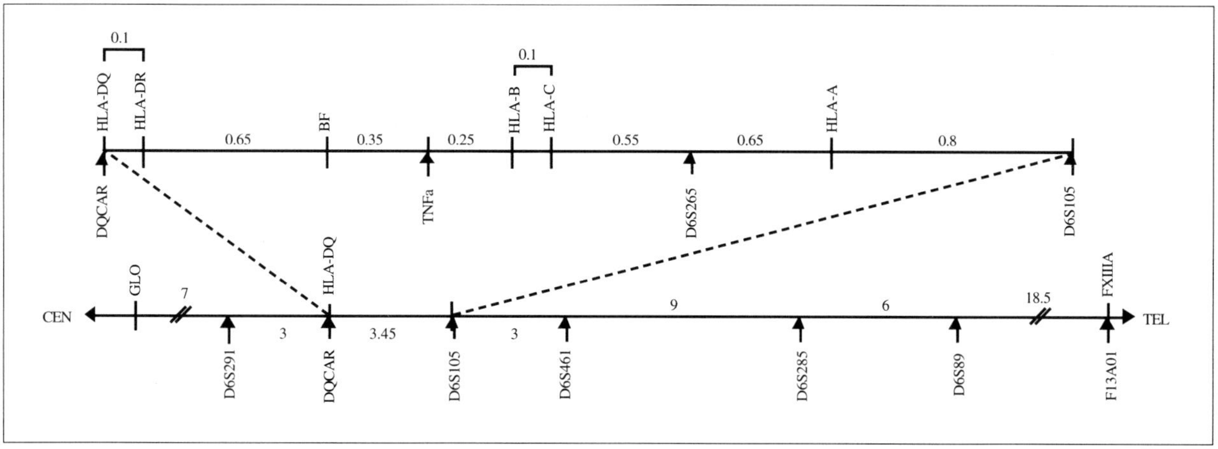

Figure 1. Genetic map of human chromosome 6p as deduced from multiple overlapping maps from the Genome Database (GDB), Cooperative Human Linkage Consortium (CHLC), and published sources [1]. Positions of microsatellite markers are estimated from data in GDB and CHLC. Microsatellite loci are indicated by arrows below the line. Distances are in centimorgans (cM).

Table I. Observed data by sex

Interval	Recombinant meioses				Nonrecombinant meioses			
	paternal	maternal	χ^2	p-value[1]	paternal	maternal	χ^2	p-value[1]
F13[2] - D6S89	14,01	14,26	0,0046	ns	57,79	64,49	0,6949	ns
D6S89 - D6S285	3,78	5,21	0,3900	ns	54,35	64,46	1,5851	ns
D6S285 - D6S461	3,69	6,12	0,9611	ns	47,44	53,05	0,5930	ns
D6S461 - D6S105	1,50	3,31	0,9892	ns	48,14	51,61	0,2340	ns
D6S105 - HLA-A	0,02	2,06	2,0168	ns	71,21	69,19	0,0588	ns
HLA-A - D6S265	0	0,93	0,9321	ns	73,93	67,82	0,5506	ns
D6S265 - HLA-C	3,00	3,75	0,1492	ns	70,43	62,40	1,0324	ns
HLA-C - HLA-B	0	0,05	0,0526	ns	89,43	77,35	1,8870	ns
HLA-B - TNFα	0	0,13	0,1316	ns	70,76	82,52	1,6750	ns
TNFα - Bf	0,09	0,22	0,0788	ns	46,93	56,62	1,6588	ns
Bf - HLA-DR	0,16	0,23	0,0232	ns	43,10	56,60	3,2190	ns
HLA-DR - DQ[3]	0,02	0,04	0,0036	ns	73,48	75,40	0,0490	ns
DQ[3] - D6S291	2,03	7,67	4,1450	0,0418	60,47	55,43	0,4580	ns
D6S291 - GLO	2,70	6,03	1,8395	ns	39,55	44,07	0,4635	ns
Totals	**31**	**50**	**7,2200**	**0,01**	**847**	**881**	**1,3121**	**ns**

[1]ns = Not Significant ($p \geq 0.05$)
[2]F13 = abbreviation for interval including F13A01 (F13A microsatellite) and FXIIIA (F13A protein polymorphism)
[2]DQ = abbreviation for interval including DQCAR and HLA-DQ

marker HLA-DQ and the microsatellite marker DQCAR (which are separated by only ~1.5 Kbp [2]) were merged into one locus (DQ) for subsequent interval analysis under the assumption that no recombination would occur between these two markers. Similarly, the interval between the protein polymorphism FXIIIA and the microsatellite marker F13A01 was ignored, and these loci merged (F13).

HLA serology, enzyme, and protein polymorphism typings were carried out by standard methods [3]. Microsatellite data were generated using fluorescently labeled PCR primers. The PCR products were separated on 6% polyacrylamide gels in the ABI 373A Automated DNA Sequencer, and semi-automated genotyping accomplished using GENESCAN™ (version 1.2.2-1) and GENOTYPER™ (version 1.1) software packages. The genotyping analysis (GENOTYPER™ allele assignment) was done in duplicate, and, where discrepancies arose (either between the two typings, or in establishing haplotypes) gels and/or amplifications were repeated. Controls on each gel included two CEPH reference individuals (1331-02, 1347-02), internal lane sizing standards (GS350, Perkin-Elmer), and No DNA controls.

Table I presents the results of haplotyping and recombination breakpoint assignment in our dataset. Fractional values come from averaging the number of informative meioses over regions of homozygosity. Parent-of-origin effects were considered when analyzing the data, leading to the observation that recombination events were more common on the maternal haplotypes, reflected by a cumulative χ^2 value of 7.22, p=0.01, 1 d.f. This is not unexpected since it has been previously shown that many portions of the human genetic map are larger in female meiotic events than in male meiotic events [4]. Comparatively, no significant deviations from expected were noted when analyzing the nonrecombinant paternal and maternal meioses. When the data from Table 1 were used to calculate the genetic distance between each interval, we obtained higher than expected values for almost every interval (see *Table II*), likely due to ascertainment bias. However, χ^2 analysis shows that the difference between calculated and expected map distances is only significant in two of the fourteen tested intervals: D6S265 - HLA-C, and DQ - D6S291.

The lack of available data on physical distances between microsatellite loci on our genetic map increased the difficulty of searching for recombination hotspots

Table II. Recombination intensity

Interval	Calculated map distance [1]	Expected map distances [2]	χ^2	p-value [3]	Recombination intensity [4]
F13 - D6S89	19,74	18,50	0,0834	ns	**0,91**
D6S89 - D6S285	7,08	6,00	0,1958	ns	**0,91**
D6S285 - D6S461	8,99	9,00	0,0000	ns	**0,63**
D6S461 - D6S105	4,61	3,00	0,8601	ns	**0,99**
D6S105 - HLA-A	1,46	0,80	0,5460	ns	**1,62**
HLA-A - D6S265	0,71	0,65	0,0051	ns	**0,96**
D6S265 - HLA-C	4,90	0,55	34,3546	$< 10^{-6}$	**8,25**
HLA-C - HLA-B	0,04	0,10	0,0376	ns	**0,40**
HLA-B - TNF α	0,11	0,25	0,0839	ns	**0,40**
TNFα - Bf	0,19	0,35	0,0688	ns	**0,35**
Bf - HLA-DR	0,38	0,65	0,1161	ns	**0,35**
HLA-DR - DQ	0,04	0,10	0,0375	ns	**0,36**
DQ - D6S291	7,73	3,00	7,4613	<0.01	**2,11**
D6S291 - GLO	9,57	7,00	0,9428	ns	**0,74**
Totals	**65,54**	**49,95**	**4,8643**	**0,0274**	**1,00**

[1]Map Distances (cM) calculated using following formula:

$$cM = \left[\frac{1}{4}\ln\left(\frac{1+2\theta}{1-2\theta}\right)\right] \times 100 \quad \text{where } \theta \text{ is the recombination fraction}$$

[2]Expected map distances (cM) obtained from composites of genetic maps (linkage, CEPH, recombination) of chromosome 6p (GDB, Johns Hopkins University), and physical maps of HLA [1]

[3]ns = Not Significant ($p \geq 0.05$)

[4]Recombination intensity calculated as follows: [6]

$$RI = \frac{R_i / L_i}{R_C / L_C}$$

The following definitions apply:
R_i = recombination in the interval in question
L_i = physical length of interval in question
R_C = recombination in the control interval
L_C = physical length of control interval

because it required us to make assumptions about the physical distances between loci. When we assumed that the correspondence between genetic distance and physical distance was 1 cM (centimorgan) = 1 Mbp on the composite map [5], we were able to make a rough estimate of the measure of recombination in each test interval as compared to the control interval (i.e. the entire map).

The estimate of the recombination in a test interval as compared to the recombination in a control interval is termed the recombination intensity [6], and allows the identification of potential recombination hotspots. By definition, recombination intensity over all intervals equals 1. Values of recombination intensity less than 1 indicate a lack of recombination in the test interval, while values greater than 1 indicate an abundance of recombination events or a recombination «hotspot». However, this distinction still does not give a specific value above which the recombination intensity must fall to have the test interval classified as a true recombination hotspot. For the purposes of this analysis, we have chosen only those regions which exhibit a recombination intensity ≥ 2 and a statistically significant deviation from the expected map distance estimate. *Table II* presents the calculation of recombination intensity in our families.

Two regions meet these criteria. The first, D6S265 - HLA-C, exhibits an extraordinarily high recombination intensity value. With genetic/physical distances as stated in *Figure 1*, the recombination intensity in this region approaches 8.25, with a χ^2 statistic of 34.3546 for the calculated map distance ($p<0.001$). Parent-of-origin analysis (data not shown) shows that recombination intensity is increased in both paternal and maternal meiotic events. This hotspot has been previously reported [7].

The second hotspot falls between DQ and D6S291, in the region of the TAP genes, and has been described by many groups [8,9], and recently sequenced [6]. In our dataset, the statistical evidence is not as strong as that for the D6S265 - HLA-C hotspot. However, when parent-of-origin effects are analyzed, the recombination intensity in this region on the maternal haplotypes reaches 2.9, while the recombination intensity on the paternal haplotypes is 1.1 (data not shown). This parent-of-origin effect can be predicted from analysis of paternal and maternal meiotic events as shown in *Table I,* where significance is only achieved in this interval ($\chi^2 = 4.145$, $p<0.05$).

A third potential hotspot may exist in the D6S105 - HLA-A interval. Like the hotspot in the TAP genes, this hotspot also exhibits parent-of-origin effects in it's expression. Recombination intensity on the maternal haplotypes approaches 2.6, while recombination intensity in this region on the paternal haplotypes is a surprisingly low 0.04 due to the lack of paternal recombination events in this small dataset (data not shown). Additional data are required to define this interval as a recombination hotspot. This hotspot, unlike the other two we identified, has not been previously reported.

References

1. Campbell RD, Trowsdale J. Map of the human MHC. *Immunol Today* 1993 ; 14 : 349-52.
2. Macaubas C, Hallmayer J, Kalil, J Kimura A, Yasunaga S, Grumet FC, Mignot E. Extensive polymorphism of a $(CA)_n$ microsatellite located in the HLA-DQA1/DQB1 class II region. *Hum Immunol* 1995 ; 42 : 209-20.
3. Nikaein A. *American Society for Histocompatibility and Immunogenetics Laboratory Manual, 3rd ed.* Lenexa : American Society for Histocompatibility and Immunogenetics, 1994.
4. NIH/CEPH Collaborative mapping group. A comprehensive genetic linkage map of the human genome. *Science* 1992 ; 258 : 67-86.
5. Donis-Keller H, Green P, Helms C, Cartinhour S, Weiffenbach B, Stephens K, Keith TP, Bowden DW, Smith DR, Lander ES, Botstein D, Akots G, Rediker KS, Gravius T, Brown VA, Rising MB, Parker C, Powers JA, Watt DE, Kauffman ER, Bricker A, Phipps P, Muller-Kahle H, Fulton TR, Ng S, Schumm JW, Braman JC, Knowlton RG, Barker DF, Crooks SM, Lincoln SE, Daly MJ, Abrahamson J. A genetic linkage map of the human genome. *Cell* 1987; 51 : 319-37.
6. Cullen M, Erlich H, Klitz W, Carrington M. Molecular mapping of a recombination hotspot located in the second intron of the human TAP2 locus. *Am J Hum Genet* 1995 ; 56 : 1350-8.
7. Thomsen M, Neugebauer M, Arnaud J, Borot N, Sevin A, Baur M, Cambon-Thomsen A. Recombination fractions in the HLA system based on the data set «Provinces Françaises»: Indications of haplotype-specific recombination rates. *Eur J Immunogenet* 1994 ; 21 : 33-43.
8. Carrington M, Colonna M, Spies T, Stephens JC, Mann DL. Haplotypic variation of the transporter associated with antigen processing (TAP) genes and their extension of HLA class II region haplotypes. *Immunogenetics* 1993 ; 37 : 266-73.
9. Powis SH, Tonks S, Mockridge I, Kelly AP, Bodmer JG, Trowsdale J. Alleles and haplotypes of the MHC-encoded ABC transporters TAP1 and TAP2. *Immunogenetics* 1993 ; 37 : 373-80.

Comprehensive sequence analysis of HLA-DQA1 and -DQB1 alleles and characterization of DRB1-QAP-DQA1-DQB1 haplotypes

S. Yasunaga[1], A. Kimura[2], T. Sasazuki[1]

1 Department of Genetics, Medical Institute of Bioregulation, Kyushu University, Fukuoka 812-82, Japan
2 Department of Tissue Physiology, Division of Adult Diseases, Medical Research Institute, Tokyo Medical and Dental University, Tokyo 101, Japan

It is well known that both α chain and β chain of HLA-DQ are highly polymorphic [1]. However the polymorphisms outside the hypervariable region (exon 2) were not fully examined so far. To further clarify the polymorphisms in the DQ genes, we determined the nucleotide sequences of full length cDNA, spanning from the leader sequence to the stop codon, from 15 DQA1 alleles and 15 DQB1 alleles (*Table I*). We identified several new DQ alleles which had identical exon 2 sequence and were different in other exons.

Table I. B-lymphoblastoid cell lines from which nucleotide sequence of DQ alleles were determined

DQA1 allele	cell line	DQB1 allele	cell line
DQA1*0101	KAS116	DQB1*0501	KAS116
DQA1*01021	EMJ	DQB1*0502	KAS011
DQA1*01022	KAS011	DQB1*05031	EK
DQA1*0103	E4181324	DQB1*06011	E4181324
DQA1*0104	EK	DQB1*0602	AMAI
DQA1*0105	AK93007	DQB1*0603	OMW
DQA1*0201	MOU	DQB1*0604	EMJ
DQA1*0301	BOLETH	DQB1*0609	AK93022
DQA1*0302	DKB	DQB1*0201	VAVY
DQA1*0303	YT	DQB1*0202	MOU
DQA1*0401	SPACH	DQB1*0301	AMALA
DQA1*05011	VAVY	DQB1*0302	BOLETH
DQA1*05013	BM16	DQB1*03032	DKB
DQA1*0503	AMALA	DQB1*0401	YT
DQA1*0601	LUY	DQB1*0402	SPACH

On the basis of the sequence analyses, a comprehensive PCR-based oligotyping system for the DQA1 gene was established. In this system, a region spanning from exon 3 to exon 4 of DQA1 gene was first analyzed by PCR-SSOP (sequence specific oligonucleotide probe) method [2]. Secondly, a region spanning from the promotor region to exon 1 and a region within exon 2 of DQA1 gene were analyzed to distinguish some DQA1 alleles. We then characterized DRB1-QAP(DQA1 promoter)-DQA1-DQB1 haplotypes (*Table II*) of B-lymphoblastoid cell lines homozygous for HLA and healthy unrelated Japanese and Norwegian populations. DRB1, DQB1 and QAP alleles were typed as previously described [3, 4]. These haplotypes were assigned on the basis of known linkage disequilibria.

Table II. DRB1-QAP-DQA1-DQB1 haplotypes characterized in this study

DRB1	QAP	DQA1	DQB1
0101/0102/0103	1.1	0101	0501
1001	1.3	0105	0501
1401/1405/1407	1.3	0104	05031/0502
1501	1.2	01021	0602
1302	1.4	01021	0604/0609
1601/1602	1.2	01022	0502
1502	1.2	0103	06011
08032	1.4	0103	06011
1301	1.3	0103	0603
0701	2.1	0201	0202/03032
0401/0403/0406	3.1	0301	0302
0401/0407	3.1	0303	0301
0405	3.1	0303	0401
0410	3.1	0303	0402
0901	3.2	0302	03032
0301	4.1	05011	0201
1101/1201	4.1	05013	0301
1402/1403/1406	4.1	0503	0301
0801/0802/0302	4.2	0401	0402
08032/12021	4.2	0601	0301

DQA1*0101 was different from DQA1*0104 at codon 2 (GGC vs GAC), codon -4 (CCC vs CCT), codon -7 (GTG vs ATG) in exon 1 and at codon 199 (ACC vs GCC) in exon 4, although they had identical sequences in exon 2 and exon 3. On the other hand, a new allele, DQA1*0105, was identical to DQA1*0104 in exon 1 (except codon -4) and to DQA1*0101 in exon 4. As shown in *Table II*, DQA1*0101 was linked to QAP 1.1, whereas DQA1*0104 and *0105 were linked to QAP 1.3. In contrast, DQA1*0101 and *0105 were linked to DQB1*0501, whereas DQA1*0104 was linked to DQB1*0502 or *05031. Accordingly DQA1*0105 was suggested to be generated by homologous recombination of DQA1*0104 (5' side) and DQA1*0101 (3' side). Of note was that DQA1*0101, *0104 and *0105 were linked to different DRB1 alleles.

DQA1*0302, which was different from DQA1*0301 by a polymorphism in codon 160 (GAT vs GCT) in exon 3, was split to DQA1*0302 and DQA1*0303 by the difference in the leader sequence (exon 1). DQA1*0302 carried ACG (Thr) at codon -6 and was associated with DRB1*0901-QAP 3.2-DQB1*03032 haplotype, whereas DQA1*0303 had ATG (Met) at codon -6 and was linked to DRB1*0401 or *0407-QAP 3.1- DQB1*0302 haplotypes, DRB1*0405-QAP 3.1- DQB1*0401 haplotype, and DRB1*0410-QAP 3.1-DQB1*0402 haplotype. It should be noted that the QAP3.1-DQA1*0303 was linked to different DRB1 and DQB1 alleles, suggesting that the DQA1 locus was more conserved than the DRB1 and DQB1 loci.

As for DQA1*0101/*0104/*0105 and DQA1*0301/0302/*0303, we could find polymorphisms of DQA1 gene outside of exon2, that correspond to QAP polymorphisms or linked DRB1 and DQB1 alleles. However in case of DQA1*01021 and DQA1*0103, QAP polymorphism did not correspond to DQA1 polymorphism. From the analogy of QAP1-DQA1*0101 subtypes and QAP3-DQA1*03 subtypes described above, there might be polymorphisms in the other regions of the DQA1 gene in these alleles.

In conclusion, we have extensively analyzed the polymorphisms in the DQ genes and characterized further the class II haplotypes. Our study suggests that the organization of DR-DQ haplotypes may have been generated in the early stage of human lineage.

References

1. Marsh SGE, Bodmer JG. HLA class II region nucleotide sequences, 1995. *Tissue Antigens* 1995 ; 45 : 258-80.
2. Yasunaga S, Kimura A, Hamaguchi K, Rønningen KS, Sasazuki T. Different contribution of HLA-DR and -DQ genes in susceptibility and resistance to insulin-dependent diabetes mellitus (IDDM). *Tissue Antigens* 1996 ; 46 : 37-48.
3. Kimura A, Sasazuki T. Eleventh International Histocompatibility Workshop reference protocol for the HLA DNA typing technique. In: Tsuji K, Aizawa M, Sasazuki T, eds. *HLA 1991 : Proceedings of the eleventh International Workshop and Conference.* Vol 1. Oxford : Oxford University Press, 1992 : 397-419.
4. Haas JP, Kimura A, Andreas A, Hochberger M, Keller E, Brunler G, Bettinotti MP, Yao Z, Nevinny-Stickol C, Sierp G, Sasazuki T, Albert ED. Polymorphism in the upstream regulatory regions of DQA1 genes and DRB1, QAP, DQA1, DQB1 haplotypes in the German population. *Hum Immunol* 1994 ; 39 : 31-40.

RT-PCR amplification of the complete coding region of HLA-DQB1. Molecular cloning of the new DQB1*0612 allele

C. Vilches[1], J.M. García-Pacheco[2], R. de Pablo[1], S. Puente[3], M. Kreisler[1]

1 Servicio de Inmunología, Clínica Puerta de Hierro, San Martín de Porres 4, 28035 Madrid, Spain
2 Unidad de Inmunología, Hospital do Meixoeiro, Vigo, Spain
3 Servicio de Medicina Tropical, Hospital Carlos III, Madrid, Spain

During the oligotyping analysis of the HLA-DQB1 locus in the Bubi population from Equatorial Guinea, an anomalous PCR-SSO reactivity pattern was observed, which suggested the presence of a new allelic variant differing from DQB1*0609 and *06051 around polymorphic codon 70. The PCR-SSO variant was detected in 2% of Bubi individuals from Equatorial Guinea, in apparent association to DRB1*1301.
In order to characterize the new allelic variant an RT-PCR method seemed the best experimental approach. However, analysis of the scientific literature showed that, surprisingly, PCR had never been used to amplify the whole coding region of a DQB1 allele. Furthermore, almost all class II alleles reported in recent years are not complete sequences but gene fragments [1,2](*Figure 1*).

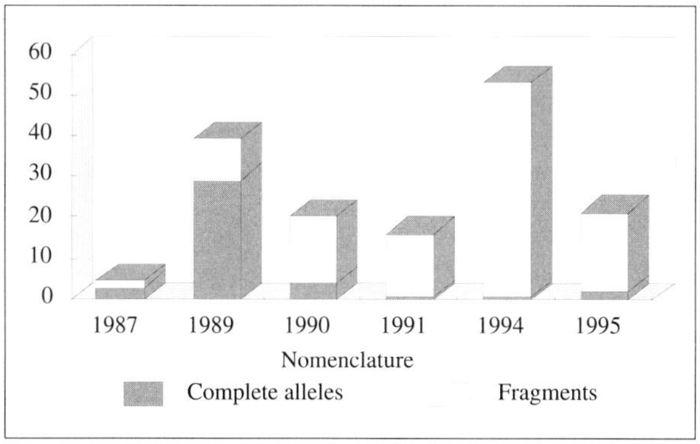

Figure 1. Number of newly recognized HLA class II alleles (DRB1+DQB1+DQA1) in the last reports of the WHO Nomenclature Committee for factors of the HLA System [1].

This apparent paradox is due to the fact that recently recognized HLA class II alleles have often been obtained from the same PCR-products used for oligotyping, which usually consist of a segment of the most polymorphic exon 2. Given that polymorphic positions exist in other exons of DQB1 [2], we decided to analyse the complete primary structure of the new variant. With this purpose, we designed two PCR primers recognizing the untranslated regions of DQB1 [3]. With these primers, we amplified the whole coding region of DQB1 from cDNA of the cell in which the PCR-SSO variant had been found. After molecular cloning of the PCR-product and nucleotide sequencing, two different alleles were identified, their sequences corresponding to the already known DQB1*03032 and to a new allele (*EMBL X96420*) which received the official DQB1*0612 name in March 1996.

DQB1*0612 displays extensive similarity with DQB1*0604, *06051 and *0609, but differs from them at codon 70 ('GGG' vs 'AGG'), in which it equals other DQB1 alleles including *0602 and *0603. DQB1*0609 is in fact identical to the hereby described allele, except for this aforementioned change. DQB1*0604 and *06051 differ from *0612 by additional single changes at codons 30 and 14, respectively (*Table I*).
It is worth noting that DQB1*0612 shares with *0604 an 'A' change at codon 130 (exon 3) not present in any other DQB1 allele. Given that no sequence information <on their third exons of DQB1*0609 and *06051 is

Table I. Nucleotide sequence alignment of DQB1*0612 with related alleles. DQB1*0602 and *0603 have been included to illustrate their identity to *0612 at codon 70. Only those codons in which the compared alleles differ from one another are shown. Dashes indicate identity to DQB1*0501

DQB1*	9	14	27	30	48	57	70	86	87	91	130
0501	TAC	CTG	GTG	CAC	CGG	GTT	GGG	GCG	TAC	CTG	CGG
0602	-T-	A--	---	T--	--C	-A-	---	---	-T-	T--	---
0603	---	A--	--A	---	--C	-A-	---	---	-T-	T--	---
0604	---	A--	--A	---	---	---	A--	-G-	---	---	-A-
06051	---	---	--A	T--	---	---	A--	-G-	---	---	***
0609	---	A--	--A	T--	---	---	A--	-G-	---	---	***
0612	---	A--	--A	T--	---	---	---	-G-	---	---	-A-

available, it cannot be ascertained which of the three alleles (DQB1*0604, *06051 or *0609) is in fact more closely related to DQB1*0612.

In conclusion, our results indicate that DQB1 alleles can be specifically amplified by the described RT-PCR method, which permits the characterization of their complete coding region. Since sequence polymorphism of unknown fuctional significance exists in most exons of this locus, the partial `sequences obtained with methods analysing only exon 2 can lead to ambiguities in nomenclature and typing. We thus consider that complete characterization of HLA class II alleles should be encouraged.

References

1 Bodmer JG, Marsh SGE, Albert ED, *et al.* Nomenclature for factors of the HLA system, 1995. *Tissue Antigens* 1995: 46: 1-18.
2 Marsh SGE, Bodmer JG. HLA Class II region nucleotide sequences, 1995. *Tissue Antigens* 1995: 46: 258-80.
3 Vilches C, García-Pacheco JM, de Pablo R, Puente S, Kreisler M. Complete coding region of the new HLA-DQB1*0612 allele, obtained by RT-PCR. *Tissue Antigens* 1997, in press.

Sequencing of a new HLA-DR4 allele with an unusual residue at position 88 that does not seem to affect T cell allorecognition

L. Gebuhrer[1], N. Adami[2], F. Javaux[1], A.C. Freidel[1], M. Jeannet[2], H. Betuel[1], J.M. Tiercy[2]

1 Établissement de transfusion sanguine de Lyon, 1-3, rue du Vercors, 69342 Lyon, France
2 Transplantation Immunology Unit, Hôpital Cantonal, Geneva, Switzerland

It is not exceptional to encounter new HLA alleles identified by unorthodox hybridization patterns observed during low and/or high resolution oligotyping with sequence-specific oligonucleotides (SSO) or when serology does not match the oligotyping result. One of the best examples is locus DRB1, where allelic subtypes [1] are caracterized by a combination of a limited number of residues located in three hypervariable (HPV) regions of exon 2.

Routine HLA-DR low resolution oligotyping of a female French Caucasoid volunteer bone marrow donor from the Lyon Registry led to the identification of an apparently homozygous DR11 cell. After amplification with DR generic primers DRBP1 and DRBP2 [2,3] the following alleles were identified: DRB1*1101, DRB3*0202, and DRB4*01. This donor was however typed by serology, using local alloantisera as DR4, DR11,DR52, DR53, DQ7, DQ8. Analysis of DR4 subtypes by PCR-SSP (Dynal kit) revealed an amplification pattern typical for DRB1*0404. Altogether, these observations strongly suggested that this DR4 allele was caracterized by an exon 2 sequence that differed in either one of the two segments to which our DRB generic primers correspond.

We have therefore amplified genomic DNA from this donor with primers GH46 and CRX37 [4], cloned and sequenced the entire exon 2 amplified DNA in both orientations. The sequence of this new allele, now referred to as DRB1*0423, reveals that this DR4 subtype differs from DRB1*0404 by a single nucleotide at codon 88, resulting in a Ser to Arg exchange (*Figure 1*). Indeed, this mutation was precisely located at the very 3'end of our DRB generic right hand primer [2,3], thereby preventing amplification of this allele. If other 3' primers had been used (*Figure 1*), *e.g.* 11th IHW primers [5], or generic PCR-SSP primers [6], this DR4 variant would have gone undetected by any of the DR typing procedures currently in use. From family genotyping analysis, the complete PCR/SSO-oligotyping of this DR4 haplotype is: A*68011-B*4402-Cw*0704-DRB1*0423-DRB4*0103-DQA1*0301-DQB1*0302-DPB1*0601.

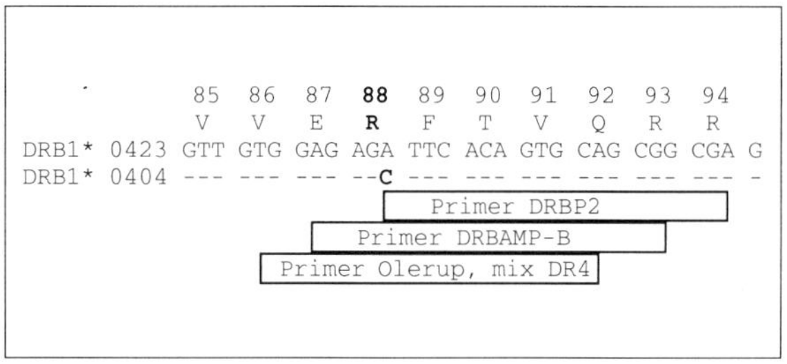

Figure 1. Position of the single nucleotide difference in codon 88 between DRB1*0423 and DRB1*0404, and of different DRB 3'end primers [3,5,6] used for DR generic typing.

In order to evaluate the functional role of the residue 88 exchange, the response of MAG cells and of heterozygous DRB1*0404 cells was tested in a cellular HTC typing against three irradiated DRB1*0404 HTCs from the 9th IHW, as well as DRB1*0401, 0402, and 0403 HTCs. As effector cells, MAG as well as four other DRB1*0404 cells, and non-DR4 cells (positive controls) were used.

Strong proliferative responses (>50%) are induced when MAG cells are cultured in the presence of DRB1*0401,

Table I. MLC response of MAG (DRB1*0423) to DRB1*04 HTCs

	Irradiated stimulating cells				
	9W1405	9W1401	9W1406	Rat	9W1001
DRB1	0404	0404	0404	0401	0402
DQB1	0302	0302	0302	0301	0302
DPB1	0201,1301	0301,0601	2001	0401	0401
Responder +					
MAG (0423) #	35	18	26	96	70
DRB1*0404 §	32	24	42	100	89
pos.control	80	87	84	104	76

+ results as % SRR
# MAG: DRB1*1101,0423 - DQB1*0301,0302 - DPB1*0101,0601
§ mean of 4 heterozygous DRB1*0404 cells

0402 (*Table I*) or 0403 (not shown) cells. This contrasts with the low proliferation (18-35%) of MAG induced by all DRB1*0404 HTCs.This low response could be accounted for by the DP incompatibilities. It is interesting to note that the lowest response was induced by the one DRB1*0404 HTC that shares one DP antigen (DPB1*0601) with MAG. DRB1*0404 effector cells gave very similar responses (24-42%) as compared to MAG cells. Altogether these results suggest that DRB1*0423 cells behave like DRB1*0404 cells in cellular assays. Therefore the difference in residue 88 may not significantly affect T cell allorecognition, possibly due to its location at the far end of the a-helix flanking the peptide binding site.

*The name DRB1*0423 was officially assigned by the WHO Nomenclature Committee in January 1996, following the agreed policy in Bodmer and co-workers (1995). The nucleotide sequence data reported in this paper have been submitted to the EMBL database and have been assigned the accession number Z68503.*

References

1. Bodmer JG, Marsh SGE, Albert ED, Bodmer WF, Bontrop RE, Charron D, Dupont B, Erlich HA, Mach B, Mayr WR, Parham P, Sasazuki T, Schreuder GMT, Strominger J, Svejgaard A, Terasaki PI. *Tissue Antigens* 1995; 46: 1-18.
2. Tiercy J-M, Goumaz C, Mach B, Jeannet M. *Transplantation* 1991; 51: 1110-1114.
3. Cros P, Allibert P, Mandrand B, Tiercy JM, Mach B. *Lancet* 1992; 340: 870-873.
4. Scharf StJ, Griffith RL, Erlich HA. *Hum Immunol* 1991; 30: 190-201.
5. Kimura A, Sasazuki T. Eleventh International Histocompatibility Workshop reference protocol for the HLA DNA typing technique. In: Tsuji K, Aizawa M, Sasazuki T, eds. *HLA 1991.* Oxford: Oxford University Press, 1992, vol. 1: 397-419.
6. Olerup O, Zetterquist H. *Tissue Antigens* 1992; 39: 225-235.

Two new alleles of the HLA-B22 group in Japanese

M. Bannai[1], Kat. Tokunaga[2,3], H. Tanaka[3], L. Lin[3], Kas. Tokunaga[4], T. Juji[3]

[1] Japanese Red Cross Tokyo Metropolitan Blood Center, 1-26-1, Kyonan-cho, Musashino-shi, Tokyo 180, Japan
[2] Department of Human Genetics, University of Tokyo, Japan
[3] JRC Central Blood Center, Japan
[4] JRC Fukuoka Blood Center, Japan

HLA-B22-group alleles in Japanese subjects were determined using PCR-single-strand conformation polymorphism (SSCP) and sequence analyses.
Five different B22 alleles, B*5401, B*5501, B*5502, B*5601 and B*5602, have been identified by means of nucleotide sequencing to date [1]. Among them, B*5401 and B*5502 were detected in the cDNA of Oriental subjects. B*5501 and B*5601 were detected in the cDNA of Caucasian subjects, whereas B*5602 was detected in that of an Australian Aborigine. For the Japanese population, no alleles encoding B22-group antigens other than B54 [1] have thus far been identified.
Five different B22 split antigens, B54, B55.1, B55.2, B56 and B22N, have been detected in Japanese [2-4]. Among them, B55.2 and B22N are rare antigens. Serologically typed allele frequencies of B54, B55 (B55.1) and B56 in Japanese were reported to be 8.27%, 2.63% and 0.78%, respectively [2].
In this study, we analyzed the alleles which encode various B22 group antigens in Japanese and found two new alleles in genomic DNA extracted from peripheral blood samples that were positive for the rare B22 split antigens.

Methods

Two-step PCRs and SSCP analysis were performed essentially according to the methods described previously [5,6]. In the first PCR, 0.8kb fragments including exon 2, intron 2, and exon 3 were amplified. In the second PCR, exon 2 and exon 3 were amplified separately using 1/100 diluents of the first PCR products as templates. In the present study, the primer BEX2-1 (5'-GAGGTATTTCTACACCGCCA) was used instead of the primer BEX2-2 or BEX2-4 described in a previous report [6]. Exon 2 and exon 3 fragments amplified in the second PCRs were separately analyzed using an SSCP method. Electrophoresis was carried out in 10% polyacrylamide gel (acrylamide: bisacrylamide = 49: 1, without glycerol), and the electrophoretic temperature was 30 °C for both exon 2 and exon 3.
Genomic DNAs extracted from samples of peripheral blood collected from 18, 10, and 4 Japanese individuals that were positive for B54, B55 (B55.1), and B56 antigens, respectively, were analyzed using the SSCP method. Genomic DNAs from two and five Japanese individuals positive for the rare antigens B55.2 and B22N, respectively, were also analyzed.
The DNA samples which gave different SSCP patterns were further analyzed by direct sequencing [6,7]. Each exon 2 or exon 3 fragment from different B22-group alleles was obtained by the second PCR and both sense and antisense strands of the fragments were sequenced.

Results and discussion

In the SSCP analysis of exon 2, three different banding patterns were identified: one common to all B55.1-, B56-, and B55.2-positive samples, one common to all B54-positive samples, and one common to all B22N-positive samples. In the SSCP analysis of exon 3, four different patterns were identified: one common to all B54- and B55.1-positive samples, one common to all B56-positive samples, one common to all B55.2-positive samples, and one common to all B22N-positive samples. In the SSCP analysis of both exons 2 and 3, we discriminated five different B22-group alleles. Each separate allele was identified from the samples positive for each separate B22-serological split antigen. For each antigen-positive sample, exon 2 and exon 3 fragments showed identical SSCP-banding patterns.
Sequence analysis revealed that the alleles encoding B55.1 and B56 antigens were B*5502 and B*5601, respectively. The alleles encoding the two rare antigens, B55.2 and B22N, were found to be previously undefined alleles. Amino acid sequences predicted from the nucleotide sequences in the $\alpha1$ (exon 2) and $\alpha2$ (exon 3) domains of the B22-group alleles are shown in *Figure 1* together with those for B*5502 as a consensus sequen-

α1-domain (1-90)

Allele	9	11	12	24	32	41	45	46	52	63	66	67	69	70	71	74	76
B*5502	Y	A	M	A	Q	A	E	E	I	N	I	Y	A	Q	A	D	E
B*5401	-	-	-	-	-	-	G	-	V	-	-	-	-	-	-	-	-
B*5501	-	-	-	-	-	-	-	-	-	-	-	-	-	-	-	-	-
B*5601	-	-	-	-	-	-	-	-	-	-	-	-	-	-	-	-	-
B*5602	-	-	-	-	-	-	-	-	-	-	-	-	-	-	-	-	-
B55.2	-	-	-	-	-	-	-	-	-	-	-	-	-	-	-	-	-
B22N	-	-	-	-	-	-	-	-	-	-	-	-	-	-	-	-	-
B*1501	-	-	-	-	-	-	M	A	-	E	-	S	T	N	T	Y	-
B*4601	-	-	-	-	-	-	M	A	-	E	K	-	R	-	-	-	V
B*0705	-	S	V	S	-	-	-	-	-	-	-	-	-	-	-	-	-
B*4002	H	S	V	T	L	T	K	-	-	E	-	S	T	N	T	Y	-

α2-domain (91-182)

Allele	95	97	103	114	116	131	152	156	163	177	178	180
B*5502	W	T	L	N	L	S	V	L	T	E	T	Q
B*5401	-	-	-	-	-	-	-	-	-	-	-	-
B*5501	-	-	-	-	-	-	E	-	-	-	-	-
B*5601	-	-	-	-	-	-	-	-	L	-	-	-
B*5602	L	R	-	-	-	-	-	-	L	-	-	-
B55.2	L	S	V	-	Y	R	-	-	-	-	-	-
B22N	L	R	V	D	S	-	E	W	L	-	-	-
B*1501	L	R	V	D	S	-	E	W	L	-	-	-
B*4601	L	R	V	D	S	-	E	W	L	-	-	-
B*0705	L	S	V	-	Y	R	E	R	E	D	K	E
B*4002	L	S	V	-	Y	R	-	-	E	-	-	-

Figure 1.
Amino acid sequences predicted from nucleotide sequences of B22-group alleles. The sequences for the α1 and α2 domains of each allele are compared with those for B*5502. Only differences in the sequences are indicated. Identical sequences are enclosed by rectangles.

ce. The B55.2 allele had a unique sequence in the α2 domain. The 5'-half sequence of the α2 domain was identical to that of B*0705, B*2707, B*4002, B*4005 and B*4801, while the 3'-half sequence was identical to that of B*5401 and B*5502. For the B22N allele, the entire α2 sequence was identical to that of B*1501, B*1508, B*1511, B*1515 and B*4601.

All B55, B56 and B22N alleles had identical α1 sequences except that the B22N allele had a synonymous nucleotide substitution in codon 31. All other sequence differences among these alleles were observed in the α2 domain. The amino acid sequences predicted from the nucleotide sequence of the B*5502 and B55.2 alleles differ by five amino acid residues from position 95 to position 131, the entire region of which is predicted to be located in the β-sheet. The sequences of the B*5601 and B22N alleles differ by seven amino acid residues, predicted to extend through the β-sheet to the α-helix. The sequences of the B22N and B56 alleles have the same substitution compared with those of the B55 alleles at position 163, T to L, which is predicted to be located in the α-helix. The presence of this amino acid residue leucine at position 163 in B56 and B22N may be related to the fact that some B22 antisera can be used to discriminate B56 and B22N from B55 and B54.

References

1. Hildebrand WH, Madrigal JA, Little AM, Parham P. HLA-Bw22: a family of molecules with identity to HLA-B7 in the α1-helix. *J Immunol* 1992;148:1155-62.
2. Akaza T, Imanishi T, Fujiwara K, Tokunaga K, Yashiki S, Fujiyoshi T, Sonoda S, Juji T. HLA alleles and haplotypes of Japanese population. *MHC and IRS* 1994;1 (suppl):219-26.
3. Tokunaga K, Kagawa Y, Fujisawa U, Yoshinari M. *Ishoku Jpn J Transplantation* 1983;17:501-3.
4. Higurashi T, Kurata T. *Transplantation Now* 1991;4 (suppl 2):78-81 (in Japanese).
5. Bannai M, Tokunaga K, Lin L, Kuwata S, Mazda T, Amaki I, Fujisawa K, Juji T. Discrimination of human HLA-DRB1 alleles by PCR-SSCP (single-strand conformation polymorphism) method. *Eur J Immunogenet* 1994;21:1-9.
6. Bannai M, Tokunaga K, Lin L, Ogawa A, Fujisawa K, Juji T. HLA-B40, B18, B27, and B37 allele discrimination using group-specific amplification and SSCP method. *Hum Immunol* 1996; 46 : 907-13.
7. Bannai M, Tokunaga K, Lin L, Park MH, Kuwata S, Fujisawa K, Juji T. A new HLA-DR11 DRB1 allele found in a Korean. *Hum Immunol* 1994;39:230-2.

The natural history of a microsatellite located in the HLA DQ region

E. Mignot, C. Macaubas, L. Jin, J. Hallmayer, A. Kimura, F.C. Grumet

Stanford Center for Narcolepsy, 701 Welch Road, suite 2222, Palo Alto, CA 94304, USA

Microsatellite sequences are very polymorphic stretches of di- or more nucleotide repeats that widely distributed within the human genome. These genetic markers are intensively used in human genetics but a good understanding of the mutational mechanism that generate such diversity lags far behind their application as genetic markers for gene mapping studies. Microsatellite alleles usually differs from each other by an even number of repeats, suggesting that mutation at this level process by expansion or contraction of single repeat units, presumably as the result of replication slippage [1].

In a previous publication, we have characterized the polymorphism of a CA repeat sequence located 1 to 2 kb telomeric to DQB1, between DQA1 and DQB1 [2]. More than 10 alleles were found at the level of this loci, all of which were tightly associated with specific DQB1 alleles. The location of this marker within the HLA class II region makes this CA repeat loci very interesting to study. First, a large number of sequencing information is available in the flanking area of the CA repetitive sequence within the DQA1 and DQB1 coding sequence. This allows for the direct comparison of sequence evolution patterns within the HLA and the microsatellite repetitive sequence using a phylogenetic approach. Second, this region of the genome is uniquely important for genetic predisposition to a large number of human disorders, most of which are autoimmune in nature. The typing of this marker in various HLA class II associated disorders can thus be used to further our understanding of these associations and to study the value of microsatellite marker typing for association studies.

DQCAR allelic diversity in specific haplotypes is dependent on the size of individual DQCAR alleles

The linkage disequilibrium pattern of 14 DQCAR alleles was established using 941 samples oligotyped at the DRB1, DQA1 and DQB1 level. Samples included unrelated subjects from Japan, Papoua New Guinea, African Americans and Caucasians, 10th WS cell lines and patients with various Class II associated diseases [2,3].

The most striking finding of this study was the discovery that DQCAR variation differed greatly between DQ1 and non DQ1 haplotypes. Almost all DQ1 samples shared a single DQCAR allele (DQCAR 103). In contrast, non DQ1 haplotypes displayed a large amount of additional DQCAR variation, with for example up to 5 alleles in association with DQB1*0202 (*Figure 1*).

In order to assess the importance of microsatellite allelic size in the generation of DQCAR allelic diversity, frequent DQA1-DQB1 combinations were selected and the number of DQCAR alleles observed surimposed on each haplotype (*Figure 1*). The selection of these haplotypes allowed us to examine the influence of microsatellite repeat size on allelic diversity within a single DQA1/DQB1 environment, thus excluding the confounding effect of cross overs in the region of interest.

The conclusion of these studies was that as the total size of the microsatellite increases, more DQCAR alleles were observed in individual haplotypes, thus strongly suggesting increased mutation rates with increased CA repeat microsatellite sizes [2]. DQCAR 99, the shorter DQCAR allele observed in our survey, was found exclu-

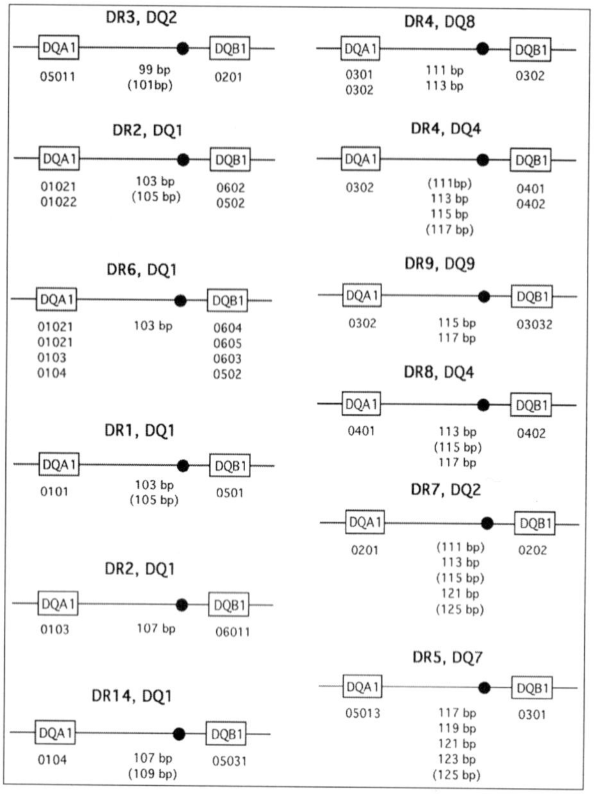

Figure 1. DQCAR polymorphisms observed in a selected set of DQB1/DQA1 haplotypes. DQA1/DQCAR/DQB1 haplotypes were ordered by increasing DQCAR sizes. Only frequent haplotypic combinations in various ethnic groups are included. Rare DQCAR allelic combinations are between parenthesis.

sively in association with the DRB1*0301, DQA1*05011, DQB1*0201 haplotype. In 167 individuals with this haplotype, DQCAR 99 was observed in all but one individual (DQCAR 101). A similar striking result was observed with DRB1*0101, DQA1*0101, DQB1*0501 or DRB1*1501, DQA1*0102, DQB1*0602 and DQCAR 103. Of 373 samples of various ethnic groups (African Americans, Caucasians, Chinese, New Guineans and Japanese) with DQA1*0102 and DQB1*0602, all but one were DQCAR 103 positive; this last sample was DQCAR 105. In contrast, haplotypes bearing DQCAR alleles longer than DQCAR 111 displayed a lot of additional diversity (*Figure 1*). DRB1*0701, DQB1*0201, DQB1*0202 for example very frequently carried either DQCAR 113 or DQCAR 121 and more rarely other alleles such as DQCAR 111, 115 or 125 (*Figure 1*).

DQCAR typing in selected HLA class II associated disorders

We also explored the value of DQCAR typing in a few selected HLA Class II associated disorders (celiac disease, narcolepsy, insulin-dependent diabetes mellitus [IDDM] and corticosensitive idiopathic nephrotic syndrome [INS]) [4]. Caucasian patients with celiac disease and DR3,DQ2 (n=36) or narcolepsy and DR15,DQ6 (n=65) were selected because of their association with HLA haplotypes bearing short DQCAR alleles, DQCAR 99 and DQCAR 103 respectively (*Figure 2*). Japanese patients with IDDM and DR4,DQ4 (n=25) and Caucasian patients with INS and DR7, DQ2 (n=31) were also selected since these haplotypes carry several large DQCAR alleles (*Figure 2*). Our hope was that INS or IDDM patients could carry only one of the several DQCAR alleles known to be associated with these haplotypes in the general population. This would have suggested the existence of a previously undetected disease-specific polymorphism in the region (class II related or not).
The results clearly demonstrated that high resolution class II typing was a better marker than DQCAR [4]. In Celiac Disease and narcolepsy, all subjects carried a single DQCAR alleles as in controls with the same haplotype (DQCAR 99 and DQCAR 103 respectively). In IDDM and INS, several DQCAR alleles were observed in association with the susceptibility haplotypes (*Figure 2*), as found in the control population [2,4].

Phylogenetic studies of HLA DQB1 and DQCAR

An alternative approach to the study of individual DQCAR allele mutation rates was developed using a phylogenetic approach [3]. In this study, a phylogenetic tree of fourteen common DQB1 alleles was reconstructed based upon the aligned complete coding sequence obtained from the EMBL data library [3]. Superimposed on this DQB1 tree, we estimated the number of DQCAR alleles observed in each branch in a total of 2,140 chromosomes (*Figure 3*).
The interest of this approach is that it is possible to evaluate the effect of branch length and thus evolutionary time on DQCAR allelic diversity in each individual branches. In this direction, it is expected that DQCAR lineages associated with old DQB1 alleles would have had more evolutionary time to develop additional muta-

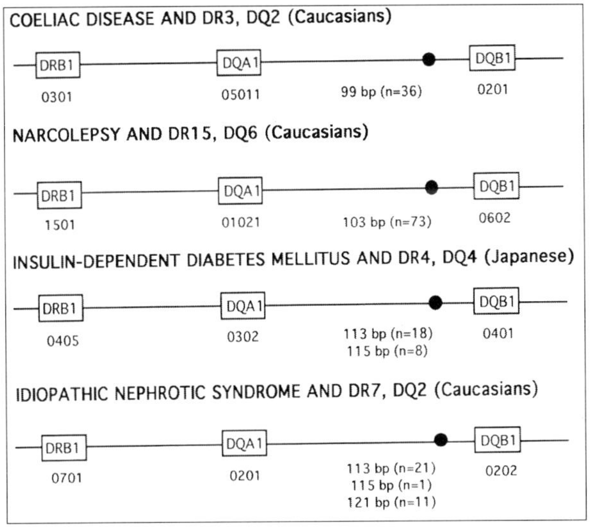

Figure 2. DRB1, DQA1, DQCAR, DQB1 haplotypes observed in four HLA class II associated disorders. Data included is reported for patients with celiac disease and DR3, DQ2 (n=36), narcolepsy and DR15, DQ6 (n=65), insulin-dependent diabetes mellitus and DR4, DQ4 (n=25), corticosensitive Idiopathic Nephrotic Syndrome and DR7, DQ2 (n=31). The number under parenthesis are the number of haplotypes observed with a given DQCAR allele in each group. For details on haplotype assignments, see [2]. Similar haplotypes were observed in control subjects of the same ethnic groups [2,4].

tions and thus would be associated with a larger number of DQCAR alleles. Since DQCAR is located 1-2 kb away from DQB1, the existence of cross overs between DQCAR and DQB1 is likely to be negligible in a large sample of individuals over long periods of evolutionary time. In fact, we never observed an unexpected DQCAR allele in all the samples typed to date, for example a DQCAR 103 allele in a non DQ1 haplotypes in several thousand individuals typed to date.

The surprising result of this approach was that branch length had only a modest influence on DQCAR diversity (*Figure 3*) when compared to mean DQCAR allele size in each branch. DQB1*06011, for example, is a relatively old allele by evolutionary standards but all 206 samples tested displayed only a single allele. In contrast, DQB1*0202, a very recent HLA DQ allele, displayed a large number of alleles. This result suggest that the mutation rates drastically drops with microsatellite sizes smaller than 12 CA repeats.

Additional sequence diversity can be found within individual allele microsatellite sequences

One of the most surprising result of this study was the almost absolute monomorphism of the DQCAR 103 allele in a large number of DQ1 positive samples in 5 distinct ethnic groups. In 652 haplotypes total, only three DQCAR 105 alleles were observed, all other being DQCAR 103 positive. In order to further our understanding of this lack of variation, we PCR amplified, cloned and sequenced various DQCAR size alleles in a representative subset of workshop cell lines (data not shown).

DQCAR sequencing results were very informative to explain the lack of DQCAR polymorphism in DQ1 haplotypes. In all the low variation DQ1 haplotypes (i.e DQCAR 103 and 107 alleles), the stretch of CA was interrupted by a C to A mutation, thus leading to a short CA repeat stretches flanking a triple A sequence. In the DRB1*1501, DQCAR 103, DQB1*0602 haplotypes for example, the polymorphic area of the sequence was: CA(GA)2(CA)5AA(CA)8(GA)4. The CA to AA change in the middle of the CA repeat sequence reduces the longer uninterrupted sequence of the DQCAR allele associated with DQB1*0602 to 8 repeats, thus making it now the shorter microsatellite sequence of all DQCAR alleles and explaining the extreme monomorphism of this lineage (*Figure 3*). In contrast, all DQCAR mutating alleles in the non DQ1 lineage had relatively longer perfect CA repeat sequences. In the DRB1*0701, DQCAR 121, DQB1*0202 haplotype for example the sequence was (CA)22GCAA(GA)5, thus bearing a very long stretch of 22 CA uninterrupted repeats [2].

Other sequence changes were also observed in the flanking area of the microsatellite where CA to GA conversions were frequently observed. In the DQCAR 103 allele associated with DQB1*0603 or DQB1*0604 for example, the polymorphic sequence was CA(GA)2(CA)5AA(CA)9(GA)3 instead of CA(GA)2(CA)5AA(CA)8(GA)4 for DQB1*0602, thus suggesting a GA to CA change that extended the CA repeat sequence. These results suggest that sequence polymorphisms within individual microsatellite alleles that may influence the mutation rate of each allele are frequently observed even when alleles have the same size.

Conclusion

These results have important consequences for association and linkage studies using microsatellite markers. The rela-

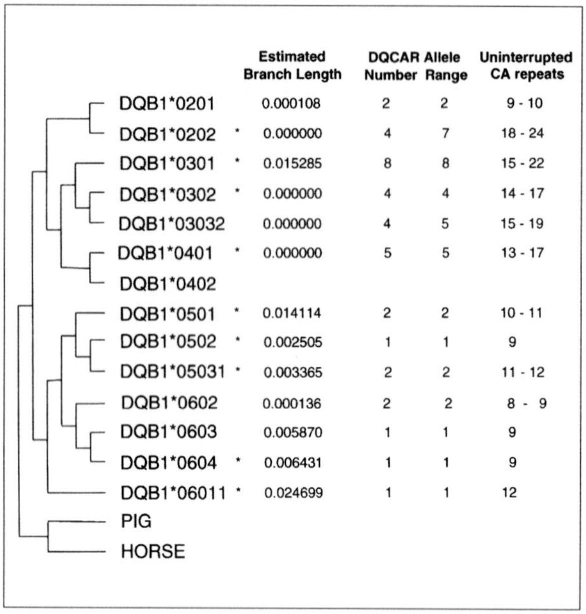

Estimated Branch Length
DQCAR Allele Number Range
Uninterrupted CA repeats
DQB1*0201 0.000108 2 2 9 - 10
DQB1*0202 * 0.000000 4 7 18 - 24
DQB1*0301 * 0.015285 8 8 15 - 22
DQB1*0302 * 0.000000 4 4 14 - 17
DQB1*03032 0.000000 4 5 15 - 19
DQB1*0401 * 0.000000 5 5 13 - 17
DQB1*0402
DQB1*0501 * 0.014114 2 2 10 - 11
DQB1*0502 * 0.002505 1 1 9
DQB1*05031 * 0.003365 2 2 11 - 12
DQB1*0602 0.000136 2 2 8 - 9
DQB1*0603 0.005870 1 1 9
DQB1*0604 * 0.006431 1 1 9
DQB1*06011 * 0.024699 1 1 12
PIG
HORSE

Figure 3. Estimated branch lengths, numbers and ranges of DQCAR alleles and numbers of uninterrupted CA repeats observed for each DQB1 allele. A phylogeny of fourteen DQB1 alleles presented in our samples was reconstructed based upon the aligned coding sequences of these alleles. Genetic distances were estimated using Kimura's two parameter model [3]. Several other measures of genetic distances were used and all gave identical results in term of the topology of the phylogeny obtained using Neighbor-joining method (see 3 for details). The tree was rooted by including pig and horse DQB sequences. Both MEGA and TDRAW were used in the analysis. Stars indicate the appearance of a new branch (new derivative), as witnessed by the existence of a unique nucleotide change to the allele. The branch lengths of all external lineage were estimated using synonymous substitution rates based on the full length sequences [3]. The number of DQCAR alleles number observed in association with each branch was estimated by typing 167 haplotypes with DQB1*0201, 125 subjects with DQB1*0202, 200 haplotypes with DQB1*0301, 157 haplotypes with DQB1*0302, 152 haplotypes with DQB1*03032, 212 haplotypes with DQB1*0401, 216 haplotypes with DQB1*0402, 124 haplotypes with DQB1*0501, 55 haplotypes with DQB1*0502, 53 haplotypes with DQB1*05031, 373 haplotypes with DQB1*0602, 39 haplotypes with DQB1*0603, 61 haplotypes with DQB1*0604, 206 haplotypes with DQB1*06011. The range of DQCAR alleles observed indicate the number of CA multiples separating the shorter and the longer DQCAR allele observed in linkage with this DQB1 allele. The number of estimated uninterrupted CA repeats was estimated from DQCAR allele sequencing data (data not shown).

tively high mutation rates of these markers may limit their use for association studies, as examplified in our study with DQCAR in the HLA region and INS or IDDM. The existence of additional sequence polymorphisms within same-size-microsatellite alleles could be used to increase the informativeness of these markers for linkage and association studies for many CA repeat loci. It is also clear from these studies that individual microsatellite alleles have drastically different mutation rates even within a single locus. This may have important consequences for disease-microsatellite markers studies. Indeed, disease mutations that occur in linkage with short microsatellite alleles should have more chance to maintain linkage disequilibrium with this allele for long periods of evolutionary time (e.g. DQCAR 103 and narcolepsy/DQB1*0602). In contrast, disease mutations that would occur in linkage with large microsatellite alleles could result in more complex patterns of association if the disease mutation is old in evolutionary term. In this case, an association with several large alleles of adjacent 2 bp sizes might be frequently observed.

Acknowledgments

This study is funded by NIH grants NS23724 and 33797 to E. Mignot.

References

1. Weber JL. Informativeness of human (dC-dA)n.(dG-dT)n polymorphisms. *Genomics* 1990; 7: 524-30.
2. Macaubas C, Hallmeyer J, Kalil J, Grumet FC, Mignot E. Extensive polymorphism of a (CA)n microsatellite located in the HLA-DQA1/DQB1 class II region. *Hum Immunol* 1995; 42(3): 209-20.
3. Jin L, Macaubas C, Hallmeyer J, Kimura A, Mignot E, Tracking the evolutionary history of a microsatellite locus located in the HLA DQA1/DQB1 class II region: a phylogenetic approach. In: Masatoshi N, Naoyuki T, eds. Current Topics on Molecular Evolution. *Proceedings of the Bionational Workshop on Molecular Evolution*, Japan, August 1995. Philadelphia: Institute of Molecular Evolutionary Genetics Pennsylvania State University, 1995: 79-87.
4. Mignot E, Kimura A, Abbal M, Thorsby E, Lin X, Voros A, Macaubas C, Bouissou F, Sollid LM, Cambon-Thomsen A, Yasunga S, Grumet FC. DQCAR polymorphisms in three selected HLA Class II associated diseases. *Tissue Antigens* 1995; 46: 299-304.

Microsatellites in the HLA central region are markers of HLA conserved extended haplotypes

S. D'Alfonso[1], N. Cappello[2], C. Carcassi[3], M.E. Fasano[2], P. Momigliano-Richiardi[1,4]

[1] Dipartimento di Scienze Mediche, Università Torino, Via Solaroli 17, 28100 Novara, Italy
[2] Dipartimento Genetica, Biologia e Chimica medica, Università Torino, Torino, Italy
[3] Cattedra di Genetica Medica, Università Cagliari, Cagliari, Italy
[4] Centro CNR Immunogenetica e Oncologia Sperimentale, Torino Italy

Microsatellites are widely used as genetic markers because of their ubiquitous distribution in the genome and their high polymorphism. Several microsatellite loci have been detected in the HLA region. We focussed our interest to the central HLA region spanning from TNF to HSP70 loci. Microsatellites in this region include TNFa, TNFb, TNFc, TNFd, and TNFe [1], K11A [2], R2A [3], and D6S273 [4]. The map position of these loci is detailed in reference [5]. While alleles at the TNFa-e loci have been already characterized in different populations and in homozygous cell lines [1], no information is available concerning the population distribution of alleles at the latter three loci.

A panel of 98 healthy North Italian unrelated individuals was analysed for 4 of the above microsatellite loci, namely TNFa, R2A, K11A and D6S273. Detected alleles and their gene frequencies are reported in *Table I.*

All tested individuals had been previously typed for polymorphisms spanning the region from HLA-A to DP and including classical HLA class I and class II as well as complement, TNFB, TNFA promoter and HSP70-1 loci [6,7].

Interestingly several significant associations were detected between alleles at the TNFa, R2A, K11A and D6S273 microsatellite loci and «marker alleles» of previously described [8] extended conserved haplotypes. The strongest associations were between markers of the: (1) B8-DR3 haplotype and microsatellite alleles TNFa2, K11A-151, D6S273-140, (2) B18-DR3 and TNFa1, K11A-159, D6S273-130, (3) B57-DR7 and D6S273-136, (4) B13-DR7 and TNFa7, K11A-157, D6S273-130, (5) B50-DR7 and TNFa5, R2A-132, K11A-147, D6S273-128, (6) B7-DR15 and TNFa11, (7) B44-DR7 and TNFa7. These results suggested that a specific allele at each microsatellite is preferentially present in each of the above conserved haplotypes. To test this hypothesis the frequency of alleles at each microsatellite locus was separately examined in individuals carrying the whole string of marker alleles from HLA-B to DR characterising each associated extended haplotype. A panel of ninteen B18-DR3 positive Sardinians was also included in this analysis. In most cases one allele for each microsatellite was identified in all or most individuals with the same conserved haplotype, behaving as an haplospecific marker. Such microsatellite allele was therefore assumed to be carried by the conserved haplotype (*Table II*). When possible, this assignement was confirmed by family segregation or in homozygous cell lines. In a few instances (boxed in *Table II*) the indicated microsatellite allele or combination of alleles was found only and in all individuals carrying a given haplotype. *Table III* shows the frequency of the "haplospecific" microsatellite allele among individuals carrying the above 7 conserved haplotypes. Strikingly, in most cases 100% of the individuals carrying the whole string of markers of a conserved haplotype also carried the proposed haplospecific microsatellite allele. For the TNFa locus this holds true for all the haplotypes. For D6S273, only 2 (1 B57-DR7 and 1 B44-DR7) out of 75 individuals did not carry the expected haplospecific allele. Respectively 17% and 13% of the individuals did not carry the haplospecific R2A and K11A allele. The absence of the expected microsatellite allele can be best explained by a mutation event since in every case it was the only discrepancy from the expected combination of alleles characterizing the conserved haplotype from HLA-B to DR (*Table II*). The mutations appeared to be randomly distributed among the different haplotypes, with a slightly higher rate for B7-DR15 and B44-DR7, and to affect mostly the R2A and K11A microsatellite

Table I. Frequencies of alleles at TNFa , K11A, R2A and DS6273 loci in the Italian population

TNFa		K11A		R2A		D6S273	
ALLELE	FREQUENCY[a] (N=91)	ALLELE	FREQUENCY[a] (N=91)	ALLELE	FREQUENCY[a] (N=92)	ALLELE	FREQUENCY[a] (N=98)
a1	0.027	145	0.016	108	0.006	120	0.005
a2	0.229	147	0.033	112	0.006	128	0.033
a3	0.011	149	0.065	116	0.006	130	0.088
a4	0.055	151	0.161	118	0.011	132	0.148
a5	0.076	153	0.210	120	0.035	134	0.263
a6	0.114	155	0.161	122	0.214	136	0.329
a7	0.115	157	0.094	124	0.123	138	0.033
a8	0.011	159	0.139	126	0.097	140	0.099
a9	0.016	161	0.034	128	0.194	BLANK	0.0001
a10	0.152	163	0.044	130	0.171		
a11	0.124	BLANK[b]	0.042	132	0.084		
a12	0.000			134	0.034		
a13	0.059			136	0.006		
BLANK	0.009			138	0.006		
				BLANK	0.011		
XW9075 cell line typing: a2		XW9075 cell line typing: 153		XW9075 cell line typing: 128		XW9075 cell line typing: 134	

[a]Maximum likelihood estimates
[b]The presence of a blank allele has been evidenced in one family
Microsatellite typing: amplification fragments were analysed on an AB1 373A sequencer using the GENESCAN program and GS350tamra as a size standard. PCR primers and conditions have been previously described for TNFa [1], K11A [2], D6S273 [4]. R2A primers: 5'ATTTGCATAGCAATCACCTT3', 5'ACAGAGTGAGACTCCAGCTC3' R2A PCR profile was: 94° 30 sec, 55° 30 sec, 72° 1 min, 1.0 mM $MgCl_2$ on a 480 Perkin Elmer PCR thermal cycler

Table II. Markers of the HLA central region in 7 HLA conserved extended haplotypes

Kb	0	220	223	223	224		253	283	283-453	53		53-678	1253
Haplotype	HLA B	TNF a	NcoI-RFLP	TNF c	TNFA -308	TNFA -238	R2A	K11A	D6S273	HSP70-1 -120	+190	Complotype	HLA-DR
B8-DR3	8	2	1	1	2	G	122	151	140	C	C	SC01	3 (17.1)
B18-DR3	18	1	2	2	1	A	122	159	130	C	C	F1C30	3 (17.2)
B57-DR7	57	2	2	2	1	A	130	155	136	A	G	SC61	7 (7.2)
B13-DR7	13	7	2	1	1	G	130	157	130	C	C	SC31	7 (7.2)
B50-DR7	50	5	1	1	2	G	132	147	128	C	C	S07C21	7
B7-DR15	7	11	2	1	1	G	128 ?	153 ?	136	A	G	SC31	1501
B44-DR7	44	7	2	1	1	G	130 ?	151 ?	132 ?	A	G	FC31	7 (7.1)

The DR TaqI-RFLP alleles are reported in brackets.
Microsatellite alleles, or combination of alleles, present only and in all the indicated haplotypes are boxed.
? = tentative assignements.

Polymorphism references:
Microsatellites: TNFa [1], TNFc [1], K11A [2], R2A [3], D6S273 [4],
Nucleotide substitutions: TNFA -308 (Ref. n°2 in [5], this volume); TNFA -238 [7]; NcoI-RFLP (Ref. n°3 in [5], this volume); HSP70-1 -120 +190 [6].

Table III. Phenotypic frequency of the haplospecific microsatellite alleles (see *Table II*) among individuals carrying the indicated HLA extended haplotypes

LOCUS	HAPLOTYPE								
	B8-DR3 (N = 14)	B18-DR3 (Italy, N=6)	B18-DR3 (Sardinia, N=19)	B57-DR7 (N = 10)	B13-DR7 (N = 7)	B50-DR7 (N=3)	B7-DR15 (N=10)	B44-DR7 (N=6)	TOTAL[a] (N=75)
TNFa	1.00	1.00	1.00	1.00	1.00	1.00	1.00	1.00	1.00
R2A	0.83	0.83	1.00	0.87	0.71	1.00	0.67	0.60	0.83
K11A	0.83	1.00	0.94	0.78	1.00	1.00	0.56	0.67	0.87
D6S273	1.00	1.00	1.00	0.90	1.00	1.00	1.00	0.83	0.97

For each haplotype the frequency of the microsatellite haplospecific alleles is calculated among individuals carrying the complete set of alleles characterising the indicated haplotype, conserved over the B-DR interval.
[a]: Cumulative frequency of microsatellite haplospecific alleles in the 7 extended haplotypes

loci. This should be confirmed in a different population. However, the most striking observation is the overall unexpected stability of these microsatellites that can thus be considered as markers, and in some cases very specific markers, of conserved haplotypes. This confirms and extends what previously reported for the TNFa1 allele and the B18-DR3 haplotype [9] and shows that stability is not restricted to a particular microsatellite or to a particular allele. Stability has been shown to be induced by the presence of internal point mutations that could decrease the rate of slippage of the polymerase and therefore mutation [10]. However the present data, which refer to different loci and different haplotypic combinations, are unlikely to be accounted for by such mechanism.

Acknowledgement
This work was supported by "MURST 60%".
Authors thank Dr Marco Colonna, Basel Institute for Immunology, for providing sequences of microsatellites.

References

1. Udalova IA, Nedospasov SA, Webb GC, Chaplin DD, Turetskaya RL. Highly informative typing of the human TNF locus using six adjacent polymorphic markers. *Genomics* 1993; 16: 180-6.
2. Colonna M, Ferrara GB, Strominger J, Spies T. Hypervariable microsatellites in the central MHC class III region. In: Tsuji K, Aizawa M, Sasazuki T eds. *HLA 1991.* Oxford: Oxford University Press, 1992: 179-80.
3. Colonna M, Spies T, Strominger J, Ciccone E, Moretta A, Moretta L, Pende D, Viale O. Alloantigen recognition by two human natural killer cell clones is associated with HLA-C or a closely linked gene. *Proc Natl Acad Sci USA* 1992; 89: 79-83.
4. Martin M, Mann D, Carrington M. Recombination rates across the HLA complex: use of microsatellites as a rapid screen for recombinant chromosomes. *Hum Mol Genet* 1995; 4: 423-8.
5. D'Alfonso S, Pociot F, Berrino M, Momigliano Richiardi P. Association analysis of a new intragenic TNFA polymorphism with TNFα quantitative production. In: Charron D, ed. *Genetic Diversity of HLA: functional and medical implication*, vol. II. Sèvres: EDK, 1997.
6. D'Alfonso S, Cappello N, Borelli I, Mazzola G, Peruccio D, Giordano M, Cascino I, Tosi R, Momigliano R. HLA supratypes in an Italian population. *Immunogenetics* 1994; 39: 114-20.
7. D'Alfonso S, Momigliano Richiardi P. A polymorphic variation in a putative regulation box of the TNFA promoter region. *Immunogenetics* 1994; 30: 150-4.
8. Christiansen FT, Witt CS, Dawkins RL. Questions in marrow matching: the implications of ancestral haplotypes for routine practice. *Bone Marrow Transplant* 1991; 8: 8386-9.
9. Crouau-Roy B, Bouzekri N, Carcassi C, Clayton J, Contu L, Cambon-Thomsen A. Strong association between microsatellites and HLA-B, DR haplotype (B18-DR3): implication for microsatellite evolution. *Immunogenetics* 1996; 43 :255-60.
10. Kunst CB, Warren ST. Cryptic and polar variation of the fragile X repeat could result in predisposing normal alleles. *Cell* 1994; 77: 853-61.

HLA-DRB1*1124: the missing link between HLA-DRB1*1101 and HLA-DRB1*1115?

S. Moser, M. Petrasek, I. Faé, G.F. Fischer

Department of Blood Group Serology, University of Vienna, Waehringer Guertel 18-20, A-1090 Vienna, Austria

Nucleotide sequencing analysis of HLA-DRB1 alleles has revealed a much larger number of alleles as appreciated by serological or cellular assays: More than 130 HLA-DRB1 alleles [1] differ from each other at the nucleotide level whereas all of them give rise to only 18 serological specificities. The distribution of the number of alleles per serological specificity is non-random. While only one allele has been described for the DR7 specificity, other specificities comprise more subtypes. More than 20 alleles, *e.g.*, encode the DR11 specificity. Analyses of the sequences could help in addressing questions as to the mechanisms involved in the generation of the polymorphism. We found, sequentially, two novel HLA-DRB1*11 alleles which are highly related to HLA-DRB1*1101. HLA-DRB1*1115 has been described previously [2], the sequence of HLA-DRB1*1124 will be reported in this paper [3].
All samples have been typed at low resolution by SSO-LBT typing [4]. Both individuals, carrying either the HLA-DRB1*1115 or the *1124 alleles, were typed as HLA-DRB1*01,*11. Therefore it was possible to selectively amplify exon 2 of HLA-DRB1*11 alleles for sequencing analysis using primers DRBAMP-3 [5] and DRBAMP-3i (5'-CTC GCC iCT GCA CiG TiA AGC-3'). After precipitation an aliquot was cycle sequenced [6] using a DyeDeoxy Terminator Cycle Sequencing Kit (Applied Biosystems, Foster City, CA) according to the recommendations of the supplier. Both strands were sequenced with sequencing primers DRBAMP-3 and DRBAMP-B [5] at empirically optimised concentration. After phenol/chloroform purification and ethanol precipitation, the sequencing product was resuspended in formamide buffer and loaded onto a 6% polyacrylamide gel containing urea at a concentration of 8.3M. The electrophoresis was performed on an automated DNA sequencer (373A DNA Sequencer, Applied Biosystems, Foster City, CA).
We have observed a rare HLA-DR11 variant segregating in a family of Turkish origin [2]. The sequence of exon 2 was very similar to that of HLA-DRB1*1101 with a difference in two nucleotides giving rise to a two amino acid exchange at codons 37 and 38. While in HLA-DRB1*1101 alleles the amino acids tyrosine (Y in the single letter amino acid code) and valine (V) are encoded there, HLA-DRB1*1115 contains a triplett coding for aspartic acid (D) and leucine (L).
Then this DL motif has been found in no other HLA-DRB1 allele. It is, however, present in the HLA-DRB5 *0101 allele. The HLA-DRB5 locus is commonly found in DR2 and rarely in DR1 haplotypes [7,8]. Thus it seemed tempting to speculate that a gene conversion event could have led to the generation of the HLA-DRB1*1115 allele: Codons 37 and 38 are identical between the HLA-DRB1*1115 and the HLA-DRB5*0101 alleles. However, when compared with other alleles of the HLA-DRB1 locus, this stretch is unique and defines a novel allele. Thus the HLA-DRB5 could have acted as a «donor» in a gene exchange event.
Interestingly, we encountered during the 1995 German cell exchange study another novel HLA-DRB1*11 variant, which has been in the meantime officially named HLA-DRB1*1124. Its nucleotide sequence differed from both the HLA-DRB1*1101 and HLA-DRB1*1115 sequences in one nucleotide. HLA-DRB1*1124 showed a G to T exchange in codon 37 as compared to HLA-DRB1*1101 therefore encoding aspartic acid instead of tyrosin. Apart from this nucleotide the sequence of HLA-DRB1*1124 is identical to HLA-DRB1*1101. Similarly the sequence of the novel allele is identical to HLA-DRB1*1115 except a T to G exchange at codon 38, where HLA-DRB1*1124 encodes valin and HLA-DRB1*1115 encodes leucin.
Thus the existence of the HLA-DRB1*1124 allele could indicate that the generation of the HLA-DRB1*1115 took place as a series of point mutations, where an HLA-DRB1*1101 allele was converted to an HLA-DRB1*1124 allele by a T to G mutation at codon 37. Subsequently a G

```
                                            20                                      30  31                      37
DRB1*1115     G TCT GAG TGT CAT TTC TTC AAT GGG ACG GAG CGG GTG CGG TTC CTG GAC AGA TAC TTC TAT AAC CAA GAG GAG GAC
DRB1*1124     - --- --- --- --- --- --- --- --- --- --- --- --- --- --- --- --- --- --- --- --- --- --- --- --- ---
DRB1*1101     - --- --- --- --- --- --- --- --- --- --- --- --- --- --- --- --- --- --- --- --- --- --- --- --- T--
DRB5*0101     - -A- --G --- --- --- --- --C --- --- --- --- --- --- --- --- C-- --- G-- A-- --- --- --- --- --- ---

              38      40                          47          50                                      60
DRB1*1115     TTG CGC TTC GAC AGC GAC GTG GGG GAG TTC CGG GCG GTG ACG GAG CTG GGG CGG CCT GAT GAG GAG TAC TGG AAC
DRB1*1124     G-- --- --- --- --- --- --- --- --- --- --- --- --- --- --- --- --- --- --- --- --- --- --- --- ---
DRB1*1101     G-- --- --- --- --- --- --- --- --- --- --- --- --- --- --- --- --- --- --- --- --- --- --- --- ---
DRB5*0101     --- --- --- --- --- --- --- --- --- -A- --- --- --- --- --- --- --- --- --- --C -CT --- --- --- ---

                                          70                                      80                    86
DRB1*1115     AGC CAG AAG GAC TTC CTG GAA GAC AGG CGG GCC GCG GTG GAC ANC TAC TGC AGA CAC AAC TAC GGG GTT GGT G
DRB1*1124     --- --- --- --- --- --- --- --- --- --- --- --- --- --- --- --- --- --- --- --- --- --- --- --- -
DRB1*1101     --- --- --- --- --- --- --- --- --- --- --- --- --- --- --- --- --- --- --- --- --- --- --- --- -
DRB5*0101     --- --- --- --- --- --- --- --- --- --C --- --- --- --- --- --- --- --- --- --- --- --- --- --- -
```

Figure 1. Compiles parts of the sequences of exon 2 of HLA-DRB1*1115, *1101 *1124 and HLA-DRB5*0101 alleles. At codons 37 and 38 HLA-DRB5*0101-characteristic sequences are found in the HLA*1115 allele. Dashes indicate identical nucleotides.

to T mutation at codon 38 of an HLA-DRB1*1124 allele gave rise to the HLA-DRB1*1115 allele.

Both novel alleles are extremely rare variants in our population. We have found them only once in more than 200 HLA-DRB1*11 haplotypes as defined by sequencing analysis. Nevertheless the increasing number of alleles, some with sequence motifs not characteristic for HLA-DRB1 but rather HLA-DRB5 alleles as e.g. HLA-DRB1*1115, has implications for high resolution tissue typing. If one intends to identify all known polymorphic sites with oligonucleotide probes, the number of probes required will increase that much, that it seems almost impracticable to perform a «complete» typing. Probably nucleotide sequencing will become more and more the method of choice to struggle with the vast polymorphism of HLA-DRB1 alleles.

References

1. Bodmer JG, Marsh S, Albert ED, Bodmer WF, Bontrop RE, Charron D, Dupont B, Erlich HA, Mach B, Mayr WR, Parham P, Sasazuki T, Schreuder G, Strominger JL, Svejgaard A, Terasaki PI. Nomenclature for factors of the HLA system, 1995. *Tissue Antigens* 1995; 46:1-18.
2. Fischer GF, Faé I, Petrasek M, Haas H, Mayr WR. An HLA-DR11 variant (HLA-DRB1*1115) segregating in a family of Turkish origin. *Tissue Antigens* 1995; 45: 143-4.
3. The nucleotide sequence data reported in this paper will appear in EMBL under the accession number Z50746. The name listed for this sequence has been officially assigned by the WHO Nomenclature Committee in July 1995. This follows the agreed policy that, subject to the conditions stated in the most recent nomenclature report [1], names will be assigned to new sequences as they are identified. List of such new names will be published in the following WHO Nomenclature Report.
4. Fischer GF, Faé I, Petrasek M, Moser S. A combination of two distinct *in vitro* amplification procedures for DNA typing of HLA-DRB and -DQB 1 alleles. *Vox Sang* 1995; 69: 328-35.
5. Tsuji K, Aizawa M, Sasazuki T. HLA 1991. Oxford: Oxford University Press, 1992: 411.
6. Craxton M. Linear amplification sequencing, a powerful method for sequencing. Methods: a companion to Methods in Enzymology. *Meth Enzymol* 1991; 3: 20-26.
7. Campbell RD, Trowsdale J. Map of the human MHC. *Immunol Today* 1993; 14: 349-52.
8. Fischer GF, Faé I, Pickl WF. The HLA-DRB6*0201 allele of a pseudogene commonly associated with HLA-DR2 specificities is present in an HLA-DRB1*0101-DRB5*0101 haplotype. *Immunogenetics* 1993; 37: 285-7.

Characterization of a new HLA-B allele (B*3702) generated by an intronic recombination event

J.L. Vicario, S. Santos, E. Trompeta, J.L. Mèrino, A. Balas

Laboratory of Histocompatibility, Regional Transfusion Centre, Menendez Pelayo 65, 28009 Madrid, Spain

Routine serological HLA typing of a Syrian-Spanish family revealed a Bw4-associated HLA-B blank antigen showing Mendelian segregation together with the haplotype A1,Cw2,DR11,DQ7 (a father from Syria and one of his children, cells #5958641 and #1958125). A more extensive serological analysis was done by using additional polyclonal and monoclonal antibodies (mAb) (One-Lambda BL-60 and LM172 plates) as well as the 12th International Workshop class I mAb plate. Both cells showed no conclusive typing reactions with sera towards HLA-B27 and HLA-B37 antigens. Two mAb, PAMELA (B27,44,38) and FAY (B13,27,37,47), were able to recognize this antigen. The great majority of reagents against B37 showed negative reactions, while positive results were more frequently observed with anti-B27 sera (*Table I*).

Full length cDNA was amplified after reverse transcription of 2 μg of cytoplasmic RNA by using the HLA-B specific 5p2/3UTB primer combination [1]. Several clones derived from two different amplifications were fully sequenced in both senses for both individuals. Comparison of the consensus sequence with all other HLA-B published sequences showed a new HLA-B allele, confirming, as serologically predicted, the greatest relationship to HLA-B37 and HLA-B27 genes [2] (*Figure 1*). Based on the exon 2 sequence similarity to B*3701, this new allele has been officially designated B*3702 [3].

B*3702 is identical in exon 2 to B*3701 [4], which codes for the HLA-B37 antigen that was well characterized in the Sixth International Workshop. In contrast, proteins derived from B*3702 and B*3701 differ in 9 amino acids at alpha 2 (7 residues), and in transmembrane and cytoplasmic domains. Exons 3 to 8 are identical between B*3702 and a number of HLA-B27 subtypes (all except Oriental HLA-B27 subtypes B*2704, B*2706, and B*2707, the Caucasian B*2709 allele, B*27053, and B*2710) [2,5-7]. B*3702 alpha 1 domain differs from those of B*2701, B*2702, B*2703, B*2705, and B*2708 in 9, 11, 9, 8, and 12 residues, respectively [8]. In spite of the fact that polymorphism in

Table I. Serological reaction pattern of two B*3702 cells

Serum	Specificity	#5958641+	#1958125+
CTM 56	B27	6	4
FGR 1020	B27	1	1
FRE 8292	B27,47	8	8
*PAMELA	B27,44,38	8	8
*EMILY	B7,DT,27,42,55,56,67	1	1
*FAY	B13,27,37,47	8	8
*JANICE	B27	1	1
*ISABEL	B40,27	1	1
*VICKI	B37	1	1
X9306	B27	6	6
X4928.AO	B37	1	1
820470	B37	1	1
PROBOST	B37	6	6
*12W046	B27,7,22,42,73	1	1
*12W050	B7,27,55,67,DT,OL7X48	1	1
*12W063	B17,27,63	8	1

+ HLA class I typing for #5958641: A1,A30 Cw2,Cw7 B57,B*3702 Bw4; #1958125: A1,A2 Cw2,Cw5 B44,B*3702 Bw4; * Monoclonal Antibodies.

HLA class I leader peptide, alpha 3, transmembrane and cytoplasmic domains is extremely limited, the mosaicism found in B*3702 strongly suggests that this new allele could be derived by homologous recombination at the intron 2 region between the B*3701 gene and some of the following B27 subtypes: B*2701,02,03,052,08 (*Figure 1*). However, sequencing analysis of the 5'-regulatory region, and introns 1 and 2 from alleles involved in this genetic event would be necessary in order to demonstrate such hypothesis. This evolutionary mechanism has been previously suggested in the origin of other HLA class I alleles [9].

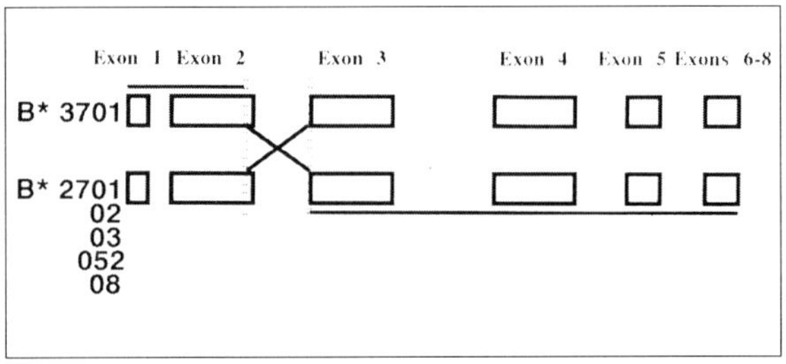

Figure 1. Generation of HLA-B*3702. GenBank accession number U31971.

B*3702 is not recognized by either B27 or B37 monospecific reagents, which would mainly identify residues at alpha 1 (Lysine 94) and alpha 2 (Serine 123) domains, respectively. Sera detecting both B27 and B47 would also target B*3702, probably through the sequence HQD (138-140) in the alpha 2 domain. The B7,22,27,42,67 epitope is further confirmed to be located at the alpha 1 domain in the sequence AQTDRE (95-100). The right serological or molecular definition for B*3702 would be of great importance when allogeneic responses were to be considered. Lastly, B*3702 differs from the most common Caucasoid B*27 allele (B*2705) in the structure of the peptide-binding pockets B (4 residues) and C (2 residues), and therefore the capability to present immunogenic peptides associated with ankylosing spondylitis and reactive arthritis would be apparently affected.

Acknowledgments

This work was supported by grants 90/1257 and 91/0245 from the Fondo de Investigaciones Sanitarias, Ministry of Health, Spain.

References

1. Zemmour J, Little A, Schendel DJ, Parham P. The HLA-A,B "negative" mutant cell line C1R expresses a novel HLA-B35 allele, which also has a point mutation in the translation initiation codon. *J Immunol* 1992; 148: 1941-8.
2. Arnett KL, Parham P. HLA class I nucleotide sequences, 1995. *Tissue Antigens* 1995; 45: 217-57.
3. Bodmer JG, Marsh SGE, Ekkehard DA, Bontrop RE, Charron D, Bodmer WF, Dupont B, Erlich HA, Mach B, Mayr WR, Parham P, Sasazuki T, Schreuder GMT, Strominger J, Svejgaard A, Terasaki PI. Nomenclature for factor of the HLA system, 1995. *Tissue Antigens* 1995; 46: 1-18.
4. Ennis PD, Zemmour J, Salter RD, Parham P. Rapid cloning of HLA-A,B cDNA by using the polymerase chain reaction: Frequency and nature of errors produced in amplification. *Proc Natl Acad Sci USA* 1990; 87: 2833-7.
5. Lopez de Castro JA. HLA-B27 and HLA-A2 subtypes: structure, evolution and function. *Immunol Today* 1989; 10: 239-46.
6. Choo SY, Fan Li-an, Hansen JA. A novel HLA-B27 allele maps B27 allospecificity to the region around position 70 in the alpha 1 domain. *J Immunol* 1991; 147: 174-80.
7. Del-Porto P, D'Amato M, Fiorillo MT, Tuosto L, Piccolella E, Sorrentino R. Identification of a novel HLA-B27 subtype by restriction analysis of a cytotoxic gamma delta T cell clone. *J Immunol* 1994; 153: 3093-100.
8. Hildebrand WH, Domena JD, Shen SY, Marsh SG, Bunce M, Guttridge MG, Darke C, Parham P. The HLA-B7Qui antigen is encoded by a new subtype of HLA-B27 (B*2708). *Tissue Antigens* 1994; 44: 47-51.
9. Holmes N, Parham P. Exon shuffling *in vivo* can generate novel class I MHC antigens. *EMBO J* 1985; 4: 2849-54.

Analysis of the molecular epitopes of anti-HLA antibodies using a computer program, OODAS. Object Oriented Definition of Antibody Specificity

M.C.N.M. Barnardo, M. Bunce, M. Thursz, K.I. Welsh

Nuffield Department of Surgery, Oxford Radcliffe Hospital, OX3 7LJ Oxford, UK

Antibodies reactive with HLA molecules are regularly found in the serum of patients awaiting organ allografts. These antibodies, which constrain the selection of HLA non-identical donors, are most often formed in response to previous transplants, blood transfusion and pregnancy although spontaneous production is described [1]. For many years anti-HLA immunoglobulin (Ig) has been detected by lymphocytotoxicity of serum against a panel of HLA typed cells and more recently by ELISA using solubilized or secreted HLA. Traditionally, the data obtained from these tests has been analysed using two by two statistical analysis of antigens with the reactivity pattern [2] or visual inspection of the raw data by an experienced serologist.

These methods have been shown to be relatively robust, however, there are drawbacks associated with their use. The statistical method compares the presence and absence of each antigen in both the positive and negatively reacting panel cells and assigns a probability value. The antigen associated with lowest p value is considered to contain an epitope of some Ig in the serum. The cells containing this antigen are removed from the data set and the analysis is repeated. This iterative process is continued until the p values are no longer significant. The list of antigens with significant p values constitutes the specificities of the anti-HLA Ig. Such analysis is not ideal for a number of reasons. First, the specificity definition is restricted to those antigens which are present in the panel, ie no information can be gathered on other alleles which may form part of a cross-reactive group with the commoner alleles. For example, an antibody reacting to the broad A10 specificity may be identified as anti A25 and A26. If A66 is not present in the panel then there will be no indication that this also contains an epitope specific for the Ig. Second, this analysis cannot indicate whether a multispecific serum contains one antibody against a 'public' epitope or several 'private' antibodies. Last, in the case of public antibodies, the p values for the less common alleles may not be significant due to low numbers.

The other common method, that of visual assessment, can solve the above problems but is time consuming and requires an experienced serologist to apply learnt rules of cross-reactivity to predict reactivity against antigens not present in the panel.

We have combined the benefits of these two methods of analysis: the automation of a computerized statistical algorithm with the molecular basis for Ig reactivity and cross-reactivity, ie the amino acid sequences, in the development of a computer program for anti-HLA antibody analysis. Data from a program based on a similar approach have been described by Park *et al.* [3] and this program was applied to analyze screening using extremely large cell panels (approximately 7000 cells). Laundy *et al.* [4] have also published work involving the analysis of HLA screening data using the amino acid sequences in which 2x2 tests were performed without the use of a computer. We present data here which demonstrate the utility of this methodology with a low panel size (typically 40 cells) and it's ability to predict specificities absent from the panel which may be tested in further screening.

The OODAS program

OODAS has been developed using the object-oriented programming language, SmallTalk (Digitalk) and is PC compatible. The known sequences of HLA class I alleles are resident in the program and these can be updated. The screening data is imported as tab delimited text with HLA phenotypes/genotypes in the form of

Table I. The analysis of data from the anti-HLA screening of 16 sera: a comparison of the results of 3 different analysis methods, visual interpretation, computerised χ^2 program (Saxon Euro) and OODAS, an amino acid based χ^2 program . The specificities obtained by each method are listed together with the specificities missed with respect to the visual interpretation method. The final column lists the specificities predicted by OODAS which were not obtained by either of the other methods

	Visual	χ^2 (Saxon)		OODAS		
	Specificities	**Specificities**	**missed**	**Specificities**	**missed**	**extras**
1	A23, 24, B44	A23, 24, B44		A23, 24, B44		
2	A23, 24, 32, Bw4	Bw4, A23, 24	A32	A23, 24, 25, 32, Bw4		A25
3	A23, 24, 25, 32, Bw4	Bw4, A24	A23, 25, 32	A23, 24, 25, 32, Bw4		
4	A1, 2, 23, 24	NS*	A1, 2, 23, 24	A2, 23, 24, 1, 36		A36
5	B8	B8		B8		
6	B57	B57		B57, 58		B58
7	B51, 52, 35, 53	B51	B52, 35, 53	B35, 51, 52, 53, 58, 78		B58, 78
8	A3	A3		A3		
9	A2, 23, 24	A2, 23, 24		A2, 23, 24		
10	A1	A1		A1, 36		A36
11	A2, 28	A2, 28		A2, 28		
12	Bw4	Bw4		Bw4		
13	A1, 23, 24	A1	A23, 24	A1, 23, 24, 80		A80
14	A1, 2, 44	A2, 1, B44		A2, 1, B44		
15	B7, 13, 40, 44	B7	B13, 40, B44	B7, 13, 27, 40, 47, 48, 73, 81	B44	B27, 47, 48, 73, 81
16	A3, 11, Bw6	Bw6	A3, 11	NS*	A3, 11, Bw6	

*NS = not significant.

allelic nomenclature or antigen names. The program carries out a chi-square test for each amino acid at each position with reference to it's presence and absence in the positive and negative groups. Yates' correction is used automatically where applicable. The resultant allele or group of alleles of the same locus which contain the amino acid at a given position with the lowest p value are taken as a specificity of serum. In the case of more than one position sharing the same, lowest, p value the smallest group of alleles is taken as the specificity. A tail analysis is performed in which the cells containing any of these alleles are removed from the data set and the remainder is reanalyzed.

Methods

Sixteen sera with clear specificities were randomly selected from our transplant waiting list. Retrospective data from standard complement dependent cytotoxicity (CDC) plus dithiothreitol (DTT) reduction and extended post-complement incubation were analysed by the following three methods: (a) visual interpretation; (b) 2x2 tail analysis of antigen names (Saxon Euro) and (c) 2x2 tail analysis of amino acid sequences, OODAS *(Table I)*.

Results

In the 16 sera 43 antibody specificities were assigned (using medium resolution serological nomenclature including Bw4 and Bw6) by visual interpretation. The Saxon program found 25 out of 43 specificities to be significant and failed to assign 18 with respect to the visual method. Fifty-one specificities were found to be significant using the amino-acid based program OODAS. Sixteen specificities were discrepant between the visual and OODAS methods, 4 of the discrepancies were due to failure of the program to assign specificities obtained by visual interpretation and 12 were due to extra reactivity which OODAS predicted but were not identified by either of the two other methods. Three of the 4 specificities which were missassigned by OODAS

were also discrepant by the Saxon program. The results are summarised in the table.
7 of the 12 antibody specificities that were uniquely identified by OODAS were further tested by CDC and the results showed that 4 of these were positive as predicted. These were serum 1, A25; serum 10, A36 and serum 15, B27 and B47. The two putative B58 specificities were found to be negative as was serum 15 with B73. The antigens A80, B48, B78 and B81 were not tested due to lack of availability.

Discussion

Existing automated analyses of anti-HLA screening data rely on determining statistical correlations between antigens and their reactivity with sera. One of the problems with this method is the variability in the frequency of each HLA antigen in any population. Rare antigens are often not tested or appear in low numbers on a random selection of cell phenotypes. Because of this, rare antigens which form part of an antibody specificity which also includes more common ones may easily be missed due to non-significance. Reappraisal of the results by an experienced serologist is required to predict further reactivity in the serum based on the well-defined rules of cross reactivity groups. The coupling of these two methods can result in excellent specificity determination in many cases but this is time consuming and therefore costly. In developing OODAS we have attempted to address two issues. First, a practical one, to improve on the pre-existing methods thus saving the time which is spent either checking computer print-outs or characterizing antibodies by eye using the raw screening data; and second to utilize the extensive amino acid sequence data to make sense of antibody definition in terms of the molecular epitopes against which they react.
The results show that OODAS is at least as competent at defining anti-HLA specificities as the previous automated method employed. In fact OODAS identified 15 specificities which were not found to be significant by the Saxon program but were identified by visual interpretation. In the 2 sera where OODAS failed to identify the correct specificity (with respect to visual interpretation) Saxon also failed in 3/4 specificities. Moreover, OODAS identified 4 new specificities which were either not tested originally or were masked by other positive reactions.
At present most laboratories type for class I either by serology or medium resolution molecular methods [5]. When analysing the sequences of these antigens it is necessary to make a best guess assignment of antigen name to allele. In a predominantly Caucasoid population such as we have in Oxford, the best guess is usually the allele ending in 01, but obviously in some large allele groups, such as B15, other alleles are also used. Ideally, the sequences of the exact alleles present would be utilized in order to best define epitopes and this is now possible with high resolution typing by SSP. Primers can be designed to specicifically amplify any allele and high resolution SSP sets are being developed by several groups.
This study is based on a small number of sera which already have defined patterns of reactivity. Our aim is to carry on testing the program using many more such sera in order to build up a data set upon which we can base assumptions about the molecular targets to which antibodies react and to continue to develop OODAS to incorporate these rules.

References

1. Lenhard V, Diehm H, Romer W, Rauterberg EW, Kownatzki E, Roelcke D. A «spontaneous» cold-reactive IgM antibody with anti HLA-B8 specificity in a patient with multiple sclerosis. *Immunobiol* 1982; 160: 382-91.
2. Van Rood JJ, D'Amaro J, Doetjes RS, Steen GVD. The role of the computer in a histocompatibility laboratory. *Tissue Antigens* 1972; 2: 196-201.
3. Park MS, Lau M, Geer LI, Terasaki PI. International sera exchange analyses in relation to DNA sequences: summary report from 1990-1994. In: Terasaki PI, Cecka JM eds. *Clinical Transplants 1994.* Los Angeles: UCLA Tissue Typing Laboratory, 1995: 489-508.
4. Laundy GJ, Bradley BA. The predictive value of epitope analysis in highly sensitized patients awaiting renal transplantation. *Transplantation* 1995; 8: 1207-13.
5. Bunce M, O'Neill CM, Barnardo MCNM, Krausa P, Browning MJ, Morris PJ, Welsh KI. Phototyping: comprehensive DNA typing for HLA-A, B, C, DRB1, DRB3, DRB4, DRB5 and DQB1 by PCR with 144 primer mixes utilizing sequence-specific primers (PCR-SSP). *Tissue Antigens* 1995; 46: 355-67.

HLA-DP detected by serology

M.M. Tongio, E. Van Den Berg Loonen, J.D. Bignon, D. Chandanayingyong, A. Dormoy, T. Eiermann, W. Marshall, M.S. Park, G.M.T. Schreuder

Établissement de Transfusion Sanguine, 10, rue Spielmann, BP 36, 67065 Strasbourg Cedex, France

The polymorphism of the HLA-DP region was originally described using the Primed Lymphocyte Typing (PLT) technique, as no specific anti-DP serological reagents were available. Nevertheless, anti-DP monoclonal antibodies (Mabs) of either murine [1-6] or human [6-8] origin have occasionally been described as has been the existence, mainly in multiparous women, of alloantisera reacting with DP alloantigens [9-11]. Analyses of the specificities of these antibodies were far from giving clear cut results, since the tests were based on reactivities with cell lines typed by PLT for a limited number of DP specificities (DP1 to DP6). More recently, molecular biology has shown the polymorphism of HLA-DP to be more extended than expected and 68 alleles have now been described. All these alleles result from combinations of variable sequences located in six hypervariable regions, a characteristic unique to HLA-DP where no allele specific sequence exists. The question has thus been raised as to how man and mouse recognize HLA-DP antigens. Our present study relating to this problem was performed by determining the reactivities of anti-DP Mabs and allosera with a panel of cells DP typed by molecular biology and carrying not only the most common DP specificities but also specificities less frequently represented in the population.

DP monoclonal antibodies

The Terra Nova Company (Memorial University of Newfoundland, St John's, NF Canada A1C 5S7) whose aim is to develop anti-DP Mabs provided 23 Mabs, while a further 7 Mabs were donated by Workshop participants. A total of 29 Mabs were products of murine hybridomas and one was of human origin (12w622). Mabs were studied by flow cytometry in three laboratories using a total of 25 EBV cell lines (FRA MYE, GER GOL) and 20 peripheral B lymphocyte suspensions (FRA-BIG). The following alleles were examined : DPA1*01, 0201, 0202, DPB1*0101, 0201, 0202, 0301, 0401, 0402, 0501, 0601, 0901, 1001, 1101, 1301, 1401, 1501, 1701, 1901, 2001, 2301 and 3401. Origins of the Mabs and their specificities as defined both by the laboratories providing the Mabs and the AHS#18 participating laboratories are given in *Table I.* Whereas no Mab recognized an allele specific DP antigen, these antibodies recognized epitopes located on the DPα chain (M:31, R:50) or on the DPβ chain (FV:35-36, DE:55-56, DED:55-57, DEE:55-57, DEAV:85-87, GPM:85-87). Certain Mabs reacting with the DPB DE or DEE epitopes also recognized the 57-58 DE epitope present on the DR11 allele.

DP human allosera

In parallel, 67 allosera mainly obtained from placentas and preselected for DP analysis were provided by M.S. Park. These were studied using the lymphocytotoxicity NIH technique with 141 EBV cell lines (FRA-MYE, THA-DCH, USA-TER, HOL-ROO) and 140 peripheral B lymphocyte suspensions (FRA-MYE, HOL-BRL, FRA-BIG, THA-DCH, USA-TER, HOL-ROO). The following DP alleles were examined : DPA1*01, 02, 0301, 0401, DPB1*0101, 0201, 0202, 0301, 0401, 0402, 0501, 0601, 0801, 0901, 1001, 1101, 1301, 1401, 1501, 1601, 1701, 1801, 1901, 2001, 2101, 2201, 2301, 2601, 2801, 3001, 3101, 3201, 3401. Only 26 sera having an r value for DP higher than 0.6 with either peripheral B or EBV cells were retained and given in *Table II.* While no human alloserum recognized an allele specific DP antigen, these sera recognized epitopes located on the DPα chain (1 case) or on the DPβ chain (YA:35-36, DED:55-57, DE:55-56, DEAV:84-87). Many sera also contained additional DR and/or DQ antibodies.

Table I. Study of DP monoclonal antibodies

mAb	Isotypes	Announced specificity	Specificity found	rvalue
M67	IgG1	DP monomorphic	Monomorphic	
M68	IgG 2b	DP monomorphic	Monomorphic	
AN87	IgG1	DP	Monomorphic	
M116	IgG1	DPA:31:M(01,0,04 chains)	DPA*0103(NT0104,0301,0401)	1.00
M114	IgG1	DPA:31:M(01,03,04 chains)	DPA*0103(NT0104,0301,0401)	1.00
M118	IgG1	DPA:50:R(02,04 chains)	DPA*0201,0202,(NT0401)	0.96
M121	IgG1	DPA1:50:R(02,04 chains)	DPA*0201,0202,(NT0401)	0.94
M122	IgG1	DPA1:50:R(02,04 chains)	DPA*0201,0202,(NT0401)	0.88
M70*	IgG2a	DPA1:50:R(02,04 chains)	DPA*0201,0202,(NT0401)	0.88
12W623*	IgM	DPA1*02	Too weak	
M77*	IgG1	DPB1:11:L+35-36:FV	DPB1:11:L+35-36:FV	0.75
M117	IgG1	DPB1:11:L+35-36:FV	DPB1:55-57:DED	1.00
M111	IgG1	DPB1:55-57:DED+ DRB1:57-58:DE	DPB1:55-57:DED	1.00
AL/DP234*	IgG1	DP9	DPB1:55-57 DEDweak	1.00
M119	IgG2	DPB1:55-57:DED+ DRB1:57-58:DE	DPB1:55-57:DED	1.00
M60	IgG2b	DPB1:55-56:DE+ DRB1:57-58:DE	DPB1:55-56:DE+ DRB1:57-58:DE	0.80
12W622*	IgM	DPB2.1+3+4.2+8+9+10+14	DPB1:55-56:DE	1.00
M73	IgG1	DPB1:55-56:DE+ DRB1:57-58:DE	DPB1:55-56:DE	1.00
M58*	IgG2a	DPB1:55-56:DE+ DRB1:57-58:DE	DPB1:55-56:DE+ DRB1:57-58:DE	1.00
M75	IgM	DPB1:55-56:DE+ DRB1:57-58:DE	Negative	
M106	IgG2b	DPB1:55-57 DEE+ DRB1:57-58:DE	DPB1:55-57 DEE+ DRB1:57-58:DE	1.00
M66*	IgG1	DPB1:84-87:DEAV	DPB1:84-87:DEAV	1.00
M126	IgG1	DPB1:84-87:DEAV	DPB1:84-87:DEAV	0.90
12W624*	IgG2a	DP1,DP3,DP5	DPB1:84-87:DEAV ?	0.89
M120	IgG2	DPB1:85-87:GPM	DPB1:85-87:GPM	1.00
M125	IgM	DPB1:85-87:GPM	DPB1:85-87:GPM	0.82
12W625*	IgG2a	DP2,4+	DPB1:85-87:GPM	0.94
M123	IgM	DPB1:84-87:GGPM	Too weak	
M124	IgM	DPB1:84-87:GGPM	Too weak	
13.3.B4*	IgG3	DP2+4	Too weak	

* 12w623 (PLM10, ref [2]) ; AL/DP234 (ref [4]) ; 12w622 (MP8, ref [6]) ; 12w624 (AL/DP143 ref [4]) ; 12w625 (DP11.1 ref [1]) ; 13.3.B4 (ref [3]). Mabs provided by Terra Nova start with M. M70, M77, M58, M66 have previously been reported in reference [5].

Table II. Study of the DP alloantisera

Serum Number	DP epitope (and DR/or DQ specificity) recognized by : Peripheral B lymphocytes (n=140)		EBV cell lines (n=141)	
9023	DPB1:35-36 YA	r=0.80	DPB1:35-36 YA	r=0.65
9031	DPB1:55-57 DED	r=0.72	DPB1:55-57 DED	r=0.78
9046	DPB1:55-57 DED	r=0.83	DPB1:55-57 DED	r=0.73
9056	DPB1:55-57 DED	r=0.88	DPB1:55-57 DED	r=0.76
9033	DPB1:55-57 DED	r=0.57	DPB1:55-57 DED	r=0.68
9037	DPB103+14+17	r=0.48	DPB1:55-57 DED+DR11	r=0.80
9036	DPB1:55-57 DED+DPB*1001	r=0.81	DPB1:55-57 DED+DPB1*1001	r=0.72
9032	DPB1:55-57 DED+DR11	r=0.84	DPB1:55-57 DED+DR11	r=0.71
9038	DPB1:55-57 DED+DR11	r=0.81	DPB1:55-57 DED+DR11	r=0.76
9043	DPB1:55-57 DED+DR11	r=0.60	DPB1:55-57 DED+DR11	r=0.53
9035	DPB1:55-57 DED+DR7	r=0.68	DPB1:55-57 DED+DR7	r=0.73
9039	DPB1:55-57 DED+DR4	r=0.77	DPB1:55-57 DED+DR4	r=0.64
9044	DPB1:55-57 DED+DR13	r=0.36	DPB1:55-57 DED+DR13+DQ6	r=0.61
9034	DPB1:55-57 DED+DR4+DR9	r=0.85	DPB1:55-57 DED+DR4+DR9	r=0.65
9084	DPB1:55-57 DED+DR53	r=0.81	DPB1:55-57 DED+DR53	r=0.84
9029	DPB1:55-57 DED+DQ3+DQ4	r=0.65	DPB1:55-57 DED+DQ3+DQ4	r=0.54
9030	DPB1:55-57 DED+DQ4	r=0.78	DPB1:55-57 DED+DQ4+DR4	r=0.78
9042	DPB1:55-57 DED+DQ2	r=0.65	DPB1:55-57 DED+DQ2+DR9	r=0.67
9041	DPB1:55-57 DED+A2	r=0.64	DPB1:55-57 DED+A2	r=0.45
9073	DPB1:55-56 DE+DR11	r=0.83	DPB1:55-56 DE+DR11	r=0.58
9040	DPB1:84-87 DEAV	r=0.71	DPB1:84-87 DEAV	r=0.52
9080	DPB1:84-87 DEAV	r=0.87	DPB1:84-87 DEAV	r=0.67
9081	DPB1:84-87 DEAV	r=0.66	DPB1:84-87 DEAV	r=0.56
9082	DPB1:84-87 DEAVDP3neg	r=0.75	DPB1:84-87 DEAV	r=0.43
9083	DPB1:84-87 DEAV	r=0.72	DPB1:84-87 DEAV	r=0.64
9024	DPA10201+0202	r=0.95	DPA10201+0202	r=1.00

According to these data, it appears that contrary to T cell clones which recognize individual DP alloantigens, DP antibodies (Mabs and allosera) recognize DP epitopes shared by several DP specificities located either on the DPα or on the DPβ chain. The same conclusion was reached by G. Mueller-Eckhardt from studies of DP allosera using the MAILA technique, also within the framework of this Workshop (personal communication). As noted above, most of the DP epitopes recognized are located around positions 31 and 50 on the DPα chain or positions 55-56, 55-57 and 84-87 on the DPβ chain. However one Mab and one alloantiserum recognized epitopes located on the β sheets of the DPβ chain (35-36:FV and YA respectively). It must be mentionned that most of the murine Mabs previously published in the literature were included in this work. Some of these were too weak to allow analysis by flow cytometry (12w623[2], 12w624[4], 13.3.B4[3]), whereas the specificities of others were in agreement with our results (AL/DP234[4], M58[5], M66[5], M70[5]). Furthermore, the Mab 12w625[1] previously reported to recognize a DPα chain epitope sensitive to interactions between DPα and its polymorphic DPβ partner was classified here as recognizing the DPB GPM epitope. Mab 77[5], described as recognizing epitopes located on the β sheets of the DPβ chain (11:L, 35-36FV), behaved more specifically with peripheral B lymphocytes (one missing reaction : FRA-BIG) than with EBV cell lines (4 weak false positive reactions [FRA-MYE]). Thus the question remains open as to the epitope (or peptide) reacting with this antibody. Considering the previously published human antibodies, the specificities of some human Mabs could be interpreted as anti-DP DEAV for Mabs TrB50 and TrE11 [8], as anti-DP:DE for Mab MP8 [6] and DP:DE + DR:DE for Mab MP4 [6]. Also two alloantisera described in 1989 by Colonna *et al.* [7] were reanalysed in the light of the current knowledge of DP and their reactivities attributed respectively to DEAV (WT) and GPM (BUT).

This work leads us to the conclusion that monoclonal antibodies reliably recognize some DP epitopes and are therefore suitable for studies of DP epitope expression on the cell surface. On the other hand, DP alloantibodies may develop more frequently than previously thought. Mueller-Eckhardt *et al.* [11] in particular found an incidence of 9.7% DP positive sera in a prospective series of unselected sera from pregnant women. Since these alloantibodies are directed against epitopes present on many different DP alleles and are often mixed with anti-DR and DQ antibodies, their reactivity may easily be considered as aspecific. Nevertheless their clinical importance in organ and in HLA-DP incompatible bone marrow transplantation might not be negligible and should be further investigated.

References

1. Young JAT, Lindsay J, Bodmer JG, Trowsdale J. Epitope recognition by a DPα chain-specific monoclonal antibody (DP11.1) is influenced by the interaction between the DPα chain and its polymorphic DPβ chain partner. *Hum Immunol* 1988; 23:37-44.
2. Maeda H, Hirata R, Hitomi Y, Tohyama H. A polymorphic monoclonal antibody, PLM10, that reacts with B-cell lines carring HLA-DPw1, DPw5 and DP «Cp63». *Tissue Antigens* 1988; 33:421-4.
3. Viken HD, Gaudernack G, Thorsby E. Characterization of a monoclonal antibody recognizing a polymorphic epitope mainly on HLA-DPw2 and DPw4 molecules. *Tissue Antigens* 1989; 34:250-9.
4. Inoko H, Bodmer JG, Heyes JM, Drover S, Trowsdale J, Marshall WH. W.T.1. Joint Report of the Transfectant/Monoclonal antibody component. In : Tsuji K, Aizawa M, Sasazuki T, eds. *HLA 1991,* vol. 1. Oxford : Oxford Science Publications, 1991: 919-30.
5. Marshall WH, Drover S, Mervart H, Younghusband HB, Liu H. Production of a series of monoclonal antibodies to polymorphisms of HLA-DP. In Tsuji K, Aizawa M, Sasazuki T, eds. *HLA 1991*, vol. 2. Oxford : Oxford Science Publications, 1991: 415-7.
6. Klohe E, Pistillo MP, Ferrara GB, Goeken NE, Greazel NS, Karr RW. Critical role of HLA-DRβ1 residue 58 in multiple polymorphic epitopes recognized by xenogeneic and allogeneic antibodies. *Hum Immunol* 1992; 35:18-28.
7. Colonna M, Tanigaki N, Tosi R, Ferrara GB. Serological detection and molecular localization of allelic HLA-DP supertypic epitopes. *Eur J Immunol* 1989; 19:433-40.
8. Kolstad A, Hannestad K. A supertypic HLA-DP specificity defined by two human-human hybridoma antibodies (TrB50; TrE11). *Hum Immunol* 1989; 25:247-56.
9. Johnson AH, Park MS, Bodmer JG, Kennedy L, Marsh S, Ferrara GB, Bratlie A, Goldmann S, Jakobson BK, Mervart H, Mueller-Eckhardt G, Svejgaard A, Thorsby E, Tsuji K. In : Dupont BO ed. *Immunobiology of HLA*, vol. I. New York : Springer-Verlag, 1989: 286-8.
10. Park MS, Takenouchi T, Terasaki PI, Tonai R, Barbetti A. HLA-DP region complexity by CDC, RFLP, and cellular assays. In : Dupont BO ed. *Immunobiology of HLA,* vol. II. New York : Springer-Verlag 1989, 311-4.
11. Mueller-Eckhardt G, Kiefel V, Tlusty A, Scholten J, Schmidt A, Mueller-Eckhardt C. Incidence and specificity of HLA-DP antibodies in pregnancy sera. *Hum Immunol* 1990; 29:166-74.

Identification of an HLA-Cw2/Cw4 hybrid allele in four individuals from Papua New Guinea

A.M. Little[1,2], A. Mason[1], S.G.E. Marsh[2], P. Parham[1]

1. Departments of Structural Biology, Microbiology and Immunology, Stanford University, Stanford, CA, USA
2. Anthony Nolan Research Institute, The Royal Free Hospital, Pond Street, Hampstead, London NW3 2QG, UK

HLA class I polymorphism in eleven unrelated Papua New Guineans has been studied. Ten of the individuals are from two cultural groups, the Kwoma (KWO) and Iatmul (IAT) and the eleventh individual is from Madang (MAD). HLA-A, B and C serological typing was performed on peripheral blood lymphocytes using 10th International Histocompatibility Workshop (IHW) antisera. HLA-A, B and C DNA typing was performed using the 12th IHW HLA class I SSP ARMS-PCR typing kit. HLA-A and B types assigned by serology and DNA typing agree (*Table I*). In contrast, HLA-C DNA typing results were discordant with serological data in particular over the assignments of Cw2 and Cw4. Individuals KWO011, KWO010 and KWO006, typed for Cw*04 by DNA typing but the Cw4 antigen was not identified by serology. Morover, individuals KWO010, KWO001 and IAT003 who typed as Cw2 by serology were not assigned the Cw*02 DNA type (*Table I*).

To investigate the discrepancy between serology and DNA typing the HLA-C alleles from the eleven individuals were further defined. HLA-C alleles were amplified from cDNA as described previously [1,2], by the polymerase chain reaction (PCR) using HLA-C specific primers: 5'CLSP-23: 5'-CCGCGTCGACTCAGATTCTCCCAGACGCCGAGATGC-3' which anneals immediately upstream to, and includes the initiation codon, and 3'UTC: 5'-CCGCAAGCTTTCGGGGAGGGAACACAGGTCAGTGTGGGGAC-3', which anneals in the 3' untranslated region of HLA-C. *Sal*I and *Hind*III sites, which are underlined, were incorporated to facilitate subcloning into the m13 vector.

DNA sequencing [1,2] confirmed the results obtained from DNA typing by finding the presence of the Cw*0401, Cw*0304, Cw*12022 and Cw*1502 alleles (*Table I*). In addition a novel HLA-C allele was identified in four of the five individuals from the Kwoma cultural group. This allele which has been assigned the name Cw*0403[1], is most similar in structure to HLA-Cw*0401 and is predicted to react with the primer mixes specific for Cw*0401 in the SSP ARMS-PCR typing kit. HLA-Cw*0403* is a hybrid allele, composed of sequences found in both HLA-Cw*0401 and Cw*02. There are 10 nucleotide differences between HLA-Cw*0401 and Cw*0403, 9 are found in exon 2 and 1 is located in exon 5 (*Table II*). We postulate that Cw*0403 was derived through recombination between an ancestor of Cw*0401 and Cw*0201 or Cw*02022 (*Figure 1*). A subsequent point mutation at nucleotide 979 (G to A) in the ancestral Cw*0401 gave rise to Cw*0401.

Seven of the 9 nucleotide substitutions in exon 2 are non-synonymous resulting in six amino acid differences between Cw*0401 and Cw*0403 at positions 9, 11, 14, 16, 21 and 49 (*Table II* and *Figure 2*). Of these six amino acid differences, only residue 9 in the B pocket of the peptide binding site is predicted to directly interact with a peptide ligand. The substitution of a bulky tyrosine residue in Cw*0403 for a serine in Cw*0401 at residue 9 may cause a difference in the repertoire of peptides which bind to Cw*0401 and Cw*0403 molecules. However, comparison of the peptide motifs for HLA-Cw*0401 with other C molecules which possess a tyrosine at residue 9 [3] demonstrated that both tyrosine and serine residues allow binding of peptides with proline at position 2 which interacts with pocket B.

1. The sequence of the Cw*0403 allele has been deposited with the Genome Sequence Data Base and has the accession number L540559. The name Cw*0403 was offially assigned by the World Health Organization (WHO) Nomenclature Committee in December 1995.

Table I. HLA-C type of eleven Papua New Guineans by serology, DNA typing and sequencing

Cell Line	Serology	HLA-C type by DNA typing	HLA-C alleles
IAT002	A11 B13,61 Cw4	ND[1]	Cw*0401, Cw*0304
IAT003	A11,24 B61 Cw2,'-'	Cw*1502	Cw*1502
IAT004	A11 B39,61 Cw'-'	Cw*1201/02, Cw*1502	Cw*12022,Cw*1502
IAT008	A11 B13 Cw4	ND	Cw*0401
IAT009	A11,24 B61 Cw2,'-'	ND	Cw*1502
KWO001	A24 B61,62v Cw2,?w4	Cw*1502, Cw*04	Cw*1502, Cw*0403
KWO005	A24 B13 Cw9	Cw*0304	Cw*0304
KWO006	A24 B13,62 Cw9	Cw*0304, Cw*04	Cw*0304, Cw*0403
KWO010	A11,34 B27,62v ?Cw2,'-'	Cw*1201/02, Cw*04	Cw*0403, Cw*12022
KWO011	A24 B13,62 Cw9	Cw*0304, Cw*04	Cw*0304, Cw*0403
MAD001	A11 B13 Cw4	ND	Cw*0401

[1]ND = not done.

These results predict that the peptide binding properties of Cw*0403 and Cw*0401 will not be globally different, although it is possible that the difference at residue 9 could discriminate the binding of certain antigenic peptides to either the Cw*0401 or Cw*0403 molecule. Both Cw*0401 and Cw*0403 express the identical inhibitory epitope for Natural Killer cells (residues 77 to 80) [4,5], therefore from what we know about NK cell interaction with HLA-C we do not expect these antigens to behave differently.

Cw*0403 was sequenced from four individuals, each of whom typed differently by HLA-C serology. Two individuals, KWO010 and KWO001, who typed blank for one C antigen, typed as Cw2 for the second C antigen. The Cw2 reactivity can be explained by the hybrid nature of the Cw*0403 allele which has a segment in common with Cw2. Indeed of the 6 amino acid differences which distinguish Cw*0403 from Cw*0401 serine 16 is unique to Cw2 and Cw*0403 and likely a critical residue for the epitope recognised by alloantisera reactive with Cw2. KWO001 cells also had weak reactivity with sera reactive with Cw4, whereas KWO010 cells did not. The other two Cw*0403 positive individuals typed neither for Cw2 nor Cw4. Both individuals, KWO006 and KWO010, typed as Cw9 by serology and possessed Cw*0304 as their second allele. In conclusion, the serological properties of the product of the Cw*0403 allele are poorly defined.

The presence of different Cw*04 subtypes in the Kwoma and Iatmul populations may reflect the action of random drift or selection. Although the size of the

Table II. Nucleotide and amino acid differences between Cw*0401 and Cw*0403

					EXON 2					EXON 5
Nucleotide	98	102	103	105	112	118	126	134	218	979
Cw*0401	C	A	T	C	T	G	G	G	A	A
Cw*0403	A	C	G	T	C	A	A	A	C	G
Amino Acid	9	10	11		14	16	18	21	49	327
Cw*0401	S	T	S		W	G	G	R	E	M
Cw*0403	Y	T	A		R	S	G	H	A	V
					α1					TM

Nucleotides are numbered from the start of exon 1. Amino acids are numbered from the begining of the a1 domain. a1 is the a1 domain. TM is the transmembrane domain.

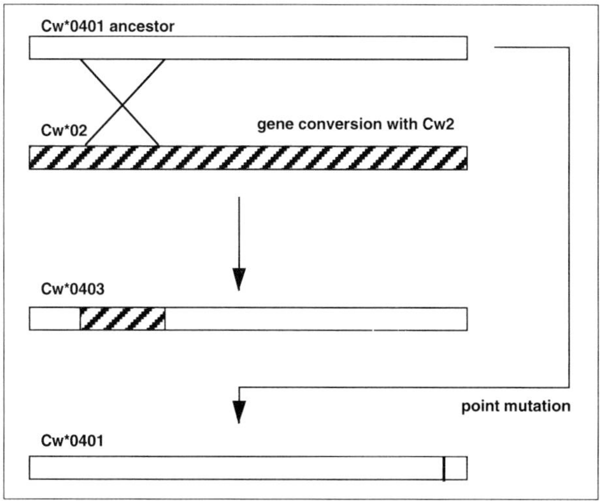

Figure 1. Cartoon depicting a possible mechanism for the generation of Cw*0403 from a Cw*0401 ancestral allele and a Cw*02 allele.

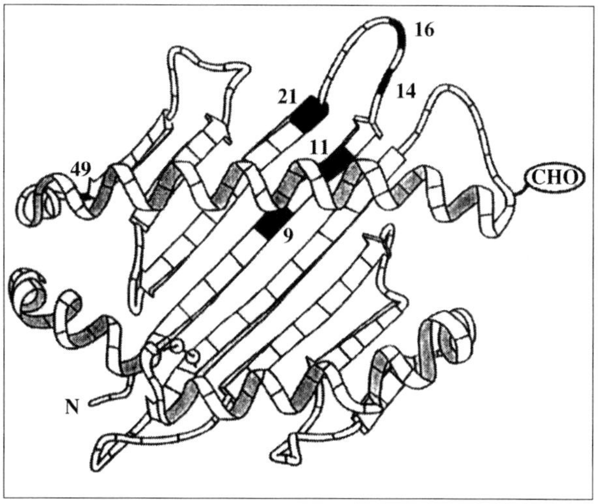

Figure 2. Ribbon diagram of the a1 and a2 domains of the HLA class I molecule showing six amino acid differences between HLA-Cw*0403 and Cw*0401.

segment involved in the recombination event which generated Cw*0403 is large (between 121 to 215 nucleotides), we do not expect the effect on function to be significant. Therefore the formation of Cw*0403 which may function identically to Cw*0401 would not be deleterious and so would not be selected against. Alternatively any subtle difference between the function of Cw*0403 and Cw*0401 may have been advantageous for the Kwoma and thus this antigen could have been positively selected at the expense of the Cw*0401 antigen in the Kwoma population. Although both the Kwoma and Iatmul populations inhabit the Coastal region of Papua New Guinea; the Kwoma group reside in an area abutting on the Highland region, which has different vegetation and climate from the region inhabited by the Iatmul. It is therefore possible that the two populations have been exposed to different local pathogens.

The Cw*0403 allele is not unique to the PNG population although its distribution may be restricted to Asian, Oceanic populations. Since this study was completed, Mike Bunce in England has shown that the Cw*0403 allele is not present in 604 British Caucasians. However he has found it in one Pakistani family who typed weakly as Cw2 and Cw4 by serology. Cw*0403 has also been found in a Thai individual by E. D. Albert's group.

Acknowledgements

We thank Jim Mason, Anthropology Department, Stanford University; the organisers and the Papua New Guinean carvers involved in the development of the Papua New Guinea Sculpture Garden, Stanford University and Drs. Carolyn Cooper and Stewart Cooper for phlebotomy and help in establishing cell lines. This research was supported by grant GM28428 from the NIH.

References

1. Domena JD, Little AM, Madrigal JA, Hildebrand WH, Johnston-Dow L, du Toit E, Bias WB, Parham P. Structural heterogeneity in HLA-B70, a high frequency anigen of black populations. *Tissue Antigens* 1993; 42: 509-17.
2. Little AM, Parham P. HLA class I gene and protein sequence polymorphism. In: Dyer P, Middleton D, eds. *Histocompatibility Testing: a practical approach.* Oxford: IRL Press at Oxford University Press, 1993; 159-90.
3. Falk K, Rotzschke O, Grahovac B, Schendel D, Stevanovic S, Gnau V, Jung G, Strominger JL, Rammensee HG. Allele-specific peptide ligand motifs of HLA-C molecules. *Proc Natl Acad Sci USA* 1993; 90: 12005-9.
4. Colonna M, Borsellino G, Falco M, Ferrara GB, Strominger JL. HLA-C is the inhibitory ligand that determines dominant resistance to lysis by NK1- and NK2-specific natural killer cells. *Proc Natl Acad Sci USA* 1993; 90: 12000-4.
5. Colonna M, Brooks EG, Falco M, Ferrara GB, Strominger JL. Generation of allospecific natural killer cells by stimulation across a polymorphism of HLA-C. *Science* 1993; 260: 1121-4.

A new HLA C locus sequence (HLA Cw*0403) identified in a Thai individual

D. Chandanayingyong[2], Z. Yao[1], A. Volgger[1], M. Sirikong[2], K. Longta[2], E.D. Albert[1]

1 Labor fur Immungenetik, Kinderpoliklinik der LMU, Munchen, Germany
2 Department of Transfusion Medicine, Faculty of Medicine Siriraj Hospital, Mahidol University, 10700 Bangkok, Thailand

In the framework of the 12th International Histocompatibility Workshop, the DNA from a Thai individual (DCH-HLA-730) was sequenced for the HLA C locus and a novel sequence appeared which corresponds in the second half of exon 2 and the entire exon 3 to that of Cw*0401, but which has in the beginning of exon 2 a sequence which corresponds to that of Cw*02. The same sequence has been identified by Parham *et al.* (*elsewhere in this volume*).

Materials and methods

The sample of genomic DNA used for sequencing is from cell DCH-HLA-730 with the typing HLA-A2, A11.1, B62, B46, Bw6, DR16, DR12.

Sequencing. PCR amplification: based on the available HLA C locus sequencences [1], we constructed two primers for the amplification of the HLA C locus promoter region. The 5' sided primer (5'-GAGGCCTGGTGTAG-GAGAAGAC-3') is located in the 5' untranslated region and the 3' sided primer (CTB) (5'-TCGTGGCG-TCGCTGTCGAACCT-3') is placed in the intron 1 of the HLA C locus.

Exon 2 and exon 3 sequencing was performed using primers described by Cereb *et al.*, 12th International Technical Handbook (*elsewhere in this volume*). The PCR amplification programme includes 30 cycles with denaturation at 96°C for 30 seconds, annealing at 57°C for one minute and extension at 72°C for one minute. Sequencing was performed using purified PCR products and a dideoxy-terminator cycle sequencing kit from Applied Biosystems (Foster City, California, USA). As described previously [2]. The amplification primers were also used as sequencing primers in the forward and reversed directions.

Results

The sequence line up for the promoter, exon 1, exon 2 and exon 3 for the alleles Cw*0201, *0401 and *0403. It can be seen that in the beginning of exon 2 of the new sequence there are four base exchanges characteristic for Cw*02. In exon 1, the sequence of the novel allele is again identical to that of Cw*0401 (although the difference is only one base exchange). As far as the promoter sequence is concerned, one observes, that from position -1 to -299 the sequence of the novel allele is identical to that of Cw*0401. In positions -22 and -210 this sequence is different from that of Cw*0201. Surprisingly however, in position -300 the new allele carries a G, which is present in the consensus and in Cw*0201. These results indicate, that most likely a conversion-like mechanism has created the new allele. The surprising difference in promoter position -300 may be due to a point mutation (*Table I*).

References

1. Summers CW, Hampson VJ, Taylor GM. HLA class I non-coding nucleotide sequences, 1992. *Eur J Immunogenet* 1993, 20: 201-40.
2. Yao Z, Volgger A, Scholz S, Albert ED. Sequence polymorphism in the HLA-B promoter region. *Immunogenetics* 1995, 41: 343-53.

Table I. Sequence line-up of promoter exon 1, exon 2 and exon 3 of Cw*0201, Cw*0401 and Cw*0403. Note, that the consensus for exon 1 to exon 3 is a C-locus consensus, while the consensus to the promoter sequence is an HLA-A, B, C consensus

Promotor							
	-376	-370	-360	-350	-340	-330	-320
Consensus	GTTTC*	TCAGACAGCT	CCTGGGCCAA	GA*CTCAGGG	AGACATT**G	AGACAGAGC*	GCTTGGCACA
Cw*0201		--------A-	---T-----G	--*------C	-C---G-GT-	-C-A---*T*	------TGT-
Cw*0401		--------A-	---T-----G	--*------C	-C---G-GT-	-C-A---*T*	------TGT-
Cw*0403		--------A-	---T-----G	--*------C	-C---G-GT-	-C-A---*T*	------TGT-
	-310	-300	-290	-280	-270	-260	-250
Consensus	GGAGCAGAGG	GGTCAGGGCG	AAGTCCCAGG	GCCCCAGGCG	TGGCTCTCAG	GGTCTCAGGC	CCCGAA*GGC
Cw*0201	----A-----	-A-----A--	----------	T---GG-CG-	*---------	----------	*T-C--*--G
Cw*0401	----A-----	AA-----A--	----------	T---GG-CG-	*---------	----------	*T-C--*--G
Cw*0403	----A-----	-A-----A--	----------	T---GG-CG-	*---------	----------	*T-C--*--G
	-240	-230	-220	-210	-200	-190	-180
Consensus	T*GTGTATGG	ATTGGGGAGT	CCCAGCCTTG	*G*GATTCCC	CAACTCCGC*	*******AGT	TTCACTTCTT
Cw*0201	CC----C--C	-C-------G	-G-C--G---	A-*-----T-	--C*---C**	****CTG---	----------
Cw*0401	CC----C--C	-C-------G	-G-C--G---	G-*-----T-	--C*---C**	****CTG---	----------
Cw*0403	CC----C--C	-C-------G	-G-C--G---	G-*-----T-	--C*---C**	****CTG---	----------
	-170	-160	-150	-140	-130	-120	-110
Consensus	***CTCCCAA	CCTGTGTCGG	GTCCTTCTAT	CCTGGATACT	CATGACGCGG	CCCCAGTTCT	CACTCCCATT
Cw*0201	***-------	----C-----	--------*-	----A-----	---------T	-----A---C	----------
Cw*0401	***-------	----C-----	--------*-	----A-----	---------T	-----A---C	----------
Cw*0403	***-------	----C-----	--------*-	----A-----	---------T	-----A---C	----------
	-100	-90	-80	-70	-60	-50	-40
Consensus	GGGTGTCGGG	TTTCTAGAGA	AGCCAATCAG	TGTCGCGTCG	GTCCCTGTTC	TAAAGTCCCC	ACGCACCCAC
Cw*0201	----------	*---------	----------	C---T-CG-A	-----G----	----------	-GT-------
Cw*0401	----------	*---------	----------	C---T-CG-A	-----G----	----------	-GT-------
Cw*0403	----------	*---------	----------	C---T-CG-A	-----G----	----------	-GT-------
	-30	-20	-10				
Consensus	CGGGACTCAG	ATTCTCCCCA	GACGCCGAGG	ATG			
Cw*0201	-C------G-	----------	---------*	---			
Cw*0401	-C--------	----------	---------*	---			
Cw*0403	-C--------	----------	---------*	---			
Exon 1 ->							
Consensus	ATGCGGGTCA	TGGCGCCCCG	AACCCTCCTC	CTGCTGCTCT	CGGGGGCCCT	GGCCCTGACC	GAGACCTGGG
Cw*0201	----------	----------	-------a--	----------	----a-----	----------	----------
Cw*0401	----------	----------	-------a--	----------	----a-----	----------	----------
Cw*0403	----------	----------	-------a--	----------	----a-----	----------	----------
Consensus	CCGG						
Cw*0201	--t-						
Cw*0401	----						
Cw*0403	----						

Table I. (continued)

Exon 2 ->		81	91	101	111	121	131
Consensus	TCCCA	CTCCATGAGG	TATTTCTACA	CCGCCGTGTC	CCGGCCCGGC	CGCGGGGAGC	CCCGCTTCAT
Cw*0201	-----	----------	----------	----t-----	-------a--	-----a----	---a------
Cw*0401	-----	----------	-------c--	-at-------	-t--------	----------	----------
Cw*0403	-----	----------	----------	----t-----	-------a--	-----a----	---a------
	141	151	161	171	181	191	201
Consensus	CGCAGTGGGC	TACGTGGACG	ACACGCAGTT	CGTGAGGTTC	GACAGCGACG	CCGCGAGTCC	GAGGATGGAG
Cw*0201	----------	----------	----------	----c-----	----------	----------	a--agg----
Cw*0401	----------	----------	----------	----c-----	----------	----------	a--agg----
Cw*0403	----------	----------	----------	----c-----	----------	----------	a--agg----
	211	221	231	241	251	261	271
Consensus	CCGCGGGCGC	CGTGGATAGA	GCAGGAGGGG	CCGGAGTATT	GGGACCGGGA	GACACAGATC	TTCAAGACCC
Cw*0201	-------gc-	gc---g-g--	----------	----------	----------	--------ag	-a----cg--
Cw*0401	-------a--	-----g-g--	----------	----------	----------	--------ag	-a----cg--
Cw*0403	----------	-----g-g--	----------	----------	----------	--------ag	-a----cg--
	281	291	301	311	321	331	341
Consensus	ACACACAGAC	TGACCGAGAG	AGCCTGCGGA	ACCTGCGCGG	CTACTACAAC	CAGAGCGAGG	CCGG
Cw*0201	-gg-------	--------t-	-a--------	-a--------	----------	----------	----
Cw*0401	-gg-----g-	--------t-	-a--------	-a--------	----------	----------	a---
Cw*0403	-gg-----g-	--------t-	-a--------	-a--------	----------	----------	a---
Exon 3		351	361	371	381	391	401
Consensus	GTCTCA	CACCCTCCAG	AGGATGTATG	GCTGCGACGT	GGGGCCGGAC	GGGCGCCTCC	TCCGCGGGTA
Cw*0201	------	----------	--------c-	--------c-	------c---	----------	----------
Cw*0401	------	----------	-------t--	--------c-	----------	----------	----------
Cw*0403	------	----------	-------t--	--------c-	----------	----------	----------
	411	421	431	441	451	461	471
Consensus	TGACCAGTAC	GCCTACGACG	GCAAGGATTA	CATCGCCCTG	AACGAGGACC	TGCGCTCCTG	GACCGCGGCG
Cw*0201	--------c-	----------	----------	----------	----------	----------	------c---
Cw*0401	-a------t-	----------	----------	----------	--------t-	----------	------c---
Cw*0403	-a------t-	----------	----------	----------	--------t-	----------	------c---
	481	491	501	511	521	531	541
Consensus	GACACGGCGG	CTCAGATCAC	CCAGCGCAAG	TGGGAGGCGG	CCCGTGTGGC	GGAGCAGCTG	AGAGCCTACC
Cw*0201	-----a----	----------	----------	----------	------a---	-------tg-	----------
Cw*0401	----------	----------	----------	----------	------a---	--------g-	----------
Cw*0403	----------	----------	----------	----------	------a---	--------g-	----------
	551	561	571	581	591	601	611
Consensus	TGGAGGGCAC	GTGCGTGGAG	TGGCTCCGCA	GATACCTGGA	GAACGGGAAG	GAGACGCTGC	AGCGCGCGG
Cw*0201	--------ga	----------	----------	----------	----------	----a-----	---------
Cw*0401	----------	----------	----------	----------	----------	----------	---------
Cw*0403	----------	----------	----------	----------	----------	----------	---------

Sequence analysis of the HLA class I introns uncovers systematic diversity

R. Blasczyk, J. Wehling

Department of Internal Medicine, Division of Hematology and Oncology, Bloodbank, Virchow-Klinikum, Humboldt-Universität zu Berlin, Augustenburger Platz 1, 13353 Berlin, Germany

The existence of introns, interrupting the coding regions of nuclear genes, is a typical feature of genomic DNA in higher eukaryotes. Introns are usually much longer than exons and are responsible for the major part of structural genes. In HLA class I genes two third of the gene are made up by intron sequences [1]. Little is known about the function of introns. They might play a role in alternative splicing processes [2]. There is also evidence that the introns contain stretches of regulatory sequences modulating the transcriptional activity [3]. One of the most remarkable theories attributes the provision of stem-loop potential to the introns of polymorphic systems [4].

In the field of Immunogenetics little attention has been paid to introns. Most researchers have focused on mRNA analysis to encompass the limitations related to the investigation of genomic DNA, i.e. the handling of large DNA fragments and the problems associated with the numerous pseudogenes. Due to these features, introns are more considered as foes than friends. Little is known about the structure of the HLA class I introns. The large introns, located between the typing relevant polymorphic exons, appear to complicate PCR based sequencing approaches.

The primary concern of this study was to take advantage of intron sequences for sequencing based typing strategies [5]. The 1st through 3rd intron of the HLA-A and B gene were sequenced in almost all serological groups and most of their subtypes. The alignment of the intron sequences showed a remarkable diversity which is extremely beneficial for setting up PCR based typing strategies. Additionally, the intron sequences are useful for evolutionary studies, delivering further insights into the genetic relationship between different alleles and the mechanisms involved in the diversification of HLA.

Materials and methods

A total of 48 cell lines mostly from the 10th Histocompatibility Workshop and 195 PCR typed clinical samples were investigated, representing almost all serologic specificities and most of their subtypes. For template preparation, PCR amplification was performed haplotype specific by the use of group or allele specific primer combinations located in the 5' flanking region and the 1st through 4th exon [6]. The resulting PCR products carried the intron of interest of a single allele flanked by exon sequences.

The introns were sequenced in both directions using nested exon-located sequencing primers. Sequencing reactions were done as described elsewhere [6]. In brief, genomic DNA was amplified in a 100 µl volume, using 10 pmol biotinylated 3' or 5' primer. Single stranded templates were generated by magnetic beads technique (Dynal) and sequenced with Sequenase® dye terminator chemistry. Electrophoresis and analysis of the sequences were performed on an automatic DNA sequencer (Applied Biosystems 373A, software version 1.2.1).

Results and discussion

The structural features of the HLA-A and B introns 1-3 are summarized in *Table I.* In both genes the variability was highest in intron 1 and lowest in intron 3. The GC content of the introns 1 and 2 was exceptionally high. This is concordant with the class I coding regions which have their greatest GC content in the 5' part of the gene [7].

Table I. Structural features of the HLA-A and B introns 1-3

		Size	GC content (%)	Variability (%)
	Intron 1	129 - 130 bp	76,2	14,6
HLA-A	**Intron 2**	239 - 241 bp	72,2	9,6
	Intron 3	579 - 601 bp	55,2	6,2
	Intron 1	128 - 129 bp	77,5	11,7
HLA-B	**Intron 2**	243 - 248 bp	74,4	7,7
	Intron 3	570 - 573 bp	55,1	6,8

Beside multiple gene specific sequence motifs mainly in the 3rd intron, the HLA-A and B introns exhibited a remarkably systematic diversity which was group specific rather than allele specific. With the exception of the A*30 and A*74 groups, showing individual sequence motifs for A*3002 and A*7403, no differences were found between serologically undefined variants. The diversification of the introns has stopped on the level of the serologically detectable variability. The diversity reflected the ancestral relationship of the HLA alleles. The phylogenetic tree of the HLA-A introns 1-3, constructed by the use of the neighbour-joining algorithm, separated the sequences in six families corresponding to the ancestral HLA-A lineages defined on the basis of the coding regions *(Figure 1)* [8].

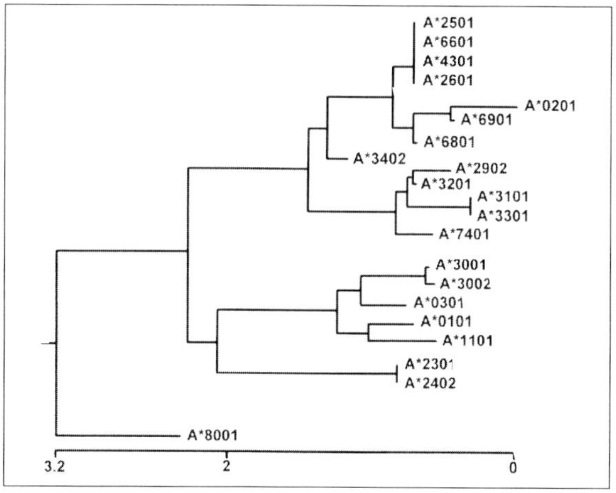

Figure 1. Phylogenetic tree of the HLA-A introns 1-3 using the neighbour-joining algorithm. The sequences are divided into six families corresponding to the ancestral HLA-A lineages A1/3/11/30, A2/28, A9, A10, A19 and A*8001, which have been defined on the basis of the coding sequences.

The intronic polymorphism, reflecting the serologically defined variability, is extremely beneficial for setting up PCR based typing systems. In particular, sequencing based typing strategies will benefit from intron-restricted priming for amplification and sequencing. The complete analysis of the polymorphic exons and the determination of *cis/trans* linkages of sequence motifs are facilitated using group specific intron motifs as priming sites.
The striking conservation of the introns within each serological group suggests that point mutations have been negatively selected. This finding could be explained by the evolutionary pressure on base order, promoting the potential to extrude single-strand stem-loops from supercoiled duplex DNA (fold pressure) [4]. This pressure is believed to be important for recombination but has been overridden in polymorphic systems by the evolutionary protein pressure to encode an optimal amino acid sequence. This may have caused a shifting of the stem-loop potential to intron sequences. It has also been suggested that conversion between different class I sequences is facilitated by regions of strong homology, stabilizing the pairing of variable regions [9]. Therefore, homologous intron sequences could enhance gene conversion activity. The remarkable clustering of CpG islands in the 1st and 2nd intron points in the same direction. It has been proposed that CpG islands may be directly involved in the exchange of short stretches of DNA during unequal crossing-over events [10]. These observations provide strong evidence that the introns substantially contribute to the recombinational potential of class I genes.

Acknowledgment

This work was supported by a grant from the Wilhelm Sander-Stiftung.

References

1. Malissen M, Malissen B, Jordan BR. Exon/intron organization and complete nucleotide sequence of an HLA gene. *Proc Natl Acad Sci USA* 1982; 79: 893-7.
2. Moreau P, Carosella E, Teyssier M, Prost S, Gluckman E, Dausset J, Kirszenbaum M. Soluble HLA-G molecule: an alternatively spliced HLA-G mRNA form candidate to encode it in peripheral blood mononuclear cells and human trophoblasts. *Hum Immunol* 1995; 43: 231-6.

3. Ganguly S, Vasavada HA, Weissmann SM. Multiple enhancer-like sequences in the HLA-B7 gene. *Proc Natl Acad Sci USA* 1989; 86: 5247-51.
4. Forsdyke DR. Stem-loop potential in MHC genes: a new way of evaluating positive Darwinian selection? *Immunogenetics* 1996; 43: 182-9.
5. Blasczyk R, Wehling J, Weber M, Salama A. Sequence analysis of the 2nd intron revealed common sequence motifs providing the means for a unique sequencing based typing protocol of the HLA-A locus. *Tissue Antigens* 1996; 47: 102-10.
6. Blasczyk R, Hahn U, Wehling J, Huhn D, and Salama A. Complete subtyping of the HLA-A locus by sequence-specific amplification followed by direct sequencing or single- strand conformation polymorphism analysis. *Tissue Antigens* 1995; 46: 86-95.
7. Arnett KL, Parham P. HLA class I nucleotide sequences, 1995. *Tissue Antigens* 1995; 46: 217-57.
8. Lawlor DA, Zemmour J, Ennis PD, Parham P. Evolution of class I MHC genes and proteins: from natural selection to thymic selection. *Annu Rev Immunol* 1990; 8: 23-63.
9. Kourilsky P. Genetic exchanges between partially homologous nucleotide sequences: possible implications for multigene families. *Biochimie* 1983; 65: 85-93.
10. Jaulin C, Perrin A, Abastado JP, Dumas B, Papamatheakis J, Kourilsky P. Polymorphism in mouse and human class I H-2 and HLA genes is not the result of random independent point mutations. *Immunogenetics* 1985; 22: 453-70.

An entropy-based measure of allelic association (linkage disequilibrium)

H. de Solages, D. Ramsbottom, B. Crouau-Roy, J. Clayton

CNRS UPR 8291, Centre d'immunopathologie et de génétique humaine, Hôpital Purpan, avenue de Grande Bretagne, 31300 Toulouse, France

Many parameters has been proposed to measure allelic association (AA), but most are arbitrary and none of them provide an answer to basic questions. E.g. one cannot say if the AA rate is greater in such or such population, or between loci A and B or between C and D. Most tests of AA are designed only for 2-locus problems, and their level of significance is not known.

Using the concept of entropy

The same formula $H = -\sum_{i=1}^{N} p_i \log_2 p_i$ is used in thermodynamics as a measure of disorder and in communication sciences as the amount of information, p_i being the probability for a particule or a character to be in state n° i. [1]

In our population genetics context, the possible states for a locus (or a set of loci) are the possible alleles (or haplotypes). The p_i are then the allelic [2] or the haplotypic frequencies. The entropy H of a set of loci (or a locus) is the pertinent measure of the uncertainty about the corresponding haplotype (or allele). H is the mean information we get when typing one individual.

- The haplotypic frequency of a population is maximum when there is no allelic association. This global maximum is the only local maximum.
- This maximum of haplotypic entropy is the sum of allelic entropies of each locus. Thus the difference between this maximum and the real entropy measures the order contained in this allelic association. More generally, the difference between the sum of entropies calculated for subsets of loci and the real entropy measures the order contained in the association between the subsets. This difference is called mutual information.

Mutual information is the amount of statistically redondant information contained in the typing of all loci about the others. It's calculated as $\sum_{\text{all loci } L} H(L) - H(\text{set of loci})$.

When there are only 2 loci in the set, mutual information is the mean amount of in mation contained in one locus about the other.

Methods

A set of loci, an experimental procedure determining alleles, and a sample are supposed given and fixed for the whole *Methods* text.

Computing 3 statistics

We used the expectation-maximization algorithm [3] to estimate the maximum likelihood. In our case, this algorithm does not usually compute the real maximum likelihood but reaches a saddle point. But the same algorithm and a standardized starting point are used for all samples, thus providing a *function f* of the sample.

Once the haplotypic structure pseudo-maximizing the likelihood is computed, we compute its mutual information, and the Pearson statistic (" χ^2 "). Taking the log-likelihood into account, we thus have 3 statistics computed at this point.

Testing allelic association

Any measure *f* of a phenomenon provides a test of its existence. The power of such a test is an indication of how relevant an index of the phenomenon this *f* is.

For computational reasons, we only studied subsets (*Table I*) of our set of 9 loci (See *Material* below.). For each such subset, all hypotheses for organizing loci into associated groups are tested.

We compare the results of the tests based on the 3 studied functions *f* of haplotypic structure regarded as AA index : log-likelihood, mutual information, Pearson statistic.

For each such hypothesis, we simulate at least 200 samples *s* from the data s_{obs} under this hypothesis, phenotypes for loci 1 and 3 being drawn, without replacement, from the same individual whenever 1 and 3 are assumed to be associated. So the simulated samples have the same size as the real one, and the same sub-haplotypic frequencies (corresponding to those subsets of loci supposed completely associated).

For each such simulated sample *s*, we compute *f*(*s*). All these values give us an empirical distribution of *f* under this hypothesis. If $f(s_{obs})$ belongs to the upper portion α

Table II. List of hypotheses NON rejected, according to the 3 methods

	Likelihood	Mutual information	Pearson
Basques	no hypothesis	(A) (B) (A D6S265) (B MIB) (A B) (DQA) (A DRB1 DQA DQB) (B) (DRB1 DQA DQB) (TNFa DQCAR) (DRB1 DQA DQB DQCAR) (TNFa) (DRB1 DQA DQB TNFa) (DQCAR)	42 hypotheses
Sardinians	(A) (B) (A) (B DQA) (A) (B DRB1 DQA DQB)	(A) (B) (DQA) (A) (B DQA) (A DQA) (B) (A B) (DQA) (A) (B DRB1 DQA DQB) (A DRB1 DQA DQB) (B)	65 hypotheses

E.g. "(DRB1 DQA DQB) (TNFa DQCAR)" refers to the hypothesis that DRB1 DQA DQB and TNFa DQCAR form 2 completely associated sets of loci, with no association between them. No-association hypotheses (*e.g.* "[A B]") are not rejectable and have been excluded.

of this distribution, then the null hypothesis (no association between the subsets of loci) is rejected with a type I error of α. This is classical statistics.

Table I. List of sets of loci studied

A B
A D6S265
B DRB1
B TNFa
B MIB
DRB1 DQCAR
DRB1 TNFa
DQA DQB
DQA DQCAR
DQB DQCAR
A B DQA
B TNFa DRB1
A B D6S265 MIB
A B DRB1 DQA DQB
DRB1 DQA DQB DQCAR
DRB1 DQA DQB TNFa DQCAR

Material

Forty five unrelated healthy French Basques, whose origins were checked for 3 generations, have been typed for HLA classical loci, serologically or molecularly, depending on the locus. Four microsatellites markers were also used: 1 near HLA A (D6S265), 1 near TNF (TNFa), 1 near DQ (DQCAR), and MIB. Their alleles have been determined by PCR-SSO. Fifty three unrelated healthy Sardinians have been typed for the same 9 loci.

Results

The log-likelihood test is slightly better than the one based on mutual information, and both are far better than Pearson test *(Table II)*. For 2-point haplotypes, log-likelihood and mutual information methods are equivalent.

Discussion and conclusion

That likelihood-based test is better than mutual information-based test means that " mutual information " does not measure the discriminating power of the information contained in the data. Maybe another entropy-based quantity would have the same property for sets of more than 2 loci. Possibly, the fact that the EM algorithm does not reach the maximum likelihood lowers the mutual information-based test power.

However that may be, as far as *measuring* is concerned, mutual information is a measure, while Pearson statistic is only an index, and log-likelihood is intrinsically bound to the present experimental constraints (only phenotypes are available), not only to the allelic association phenomenon. Comparing mutual information for different populations and difference sets of loci makes sense.

An AA between 3 loci with no AA in any pairs *is* perfectly possible. Our multi-point approch can measure such a phenomenon.

Acknowledgements

We thank Cédric Souchon, who wrote the main computer program.

References

1. Yaglom AM, Yaglom IM. *Probabilité et information*. Paris : Dunod, 1959.
2. Lewontin RC. The apportionment of human diversity. *Evol Biol* 1972 ; 6 : 381-98.
3. Dempster AP, Laird NM, Rubin DB. Maximum likelihood from incomplete data *via* the *EM* algorithm. *J Roy Stat Soc B* 1977 ; 39 : 1-22

Uniparental isodisomy of chromosome 6 discovered during a search for an HLA identical sibling

M.C. Bittencourt[1], M.A. Morris[2], J. Chabod[1], A. Gos[2], B. Lamy[1], F. Fellmann[3], S.E Antonarakis[2], E. Plouvier[4], P. Hervé[1], P. Tiberghien[1]

1 Établissement de Transfusion Sanguine de Franche-Comté, 1, boulevard Fleming, BP 1937, 25020 Besançon Cedex, France
2 Division of Medical Genetics, Geneva University Hospital, Switzerland
3 Laboratoire de Cytogénétique, CHU Besançon, France
4 Service de Pédiatrie, CHU Besançon, France

Uniparental disomy (UPD) was defined theoretically in 1980 [1] as the inheritance of two copies of a given parental chromosome from only one parent. Two subtypes of UPD can be established: *heterodisomy* occurs when the inheritance of genetic material is from both chromosomes of a parental pair, with mainteinance of a heterozygous state; *isodisomy* is present when two copies of the same parental chromosome are inherited, a condition with increased risk for recessive disorders due to homozygosity. Both forms of UPD can cause disorders related to imprinting. The reported cases of UPD involving various chromosomes are usually associated with deleterious effects (for review [2]).We describe the fortuitous detection of a paternal chromosome 6 isodisomy.

The patient is a nine year-old girl, with β thalassaemia major, confirmed by haemoglobin electrophoresis. No phenotype abnormalities were noted in the physical examination. Isodisomy of chromosome 6 was discovered after HLA typing of the patient and her family, searching a potential donor for an allogeneic bone marrow transplantation (BMT). HLA class I typing of all family members was performed using the standard microlymphocytotoxicity test. HLA class II typing was performed by hybridization with sequence-specific oligonucleotides after polymerase chain reaction DNA amplification for DRB1, DQB1 and DPB1 loci. HLA typing results of the family and segregation analysis showed that the patient was homozygous for one of the paternal haplotypes with no inheritance of a maternal haplotype (*Figure 1*). The other siblings had normal inheritance of both maternal and paternal HLA haplotypes.

Furthermore, additional genotypes were obtained for the patient and her parents at five highly-informative micro-

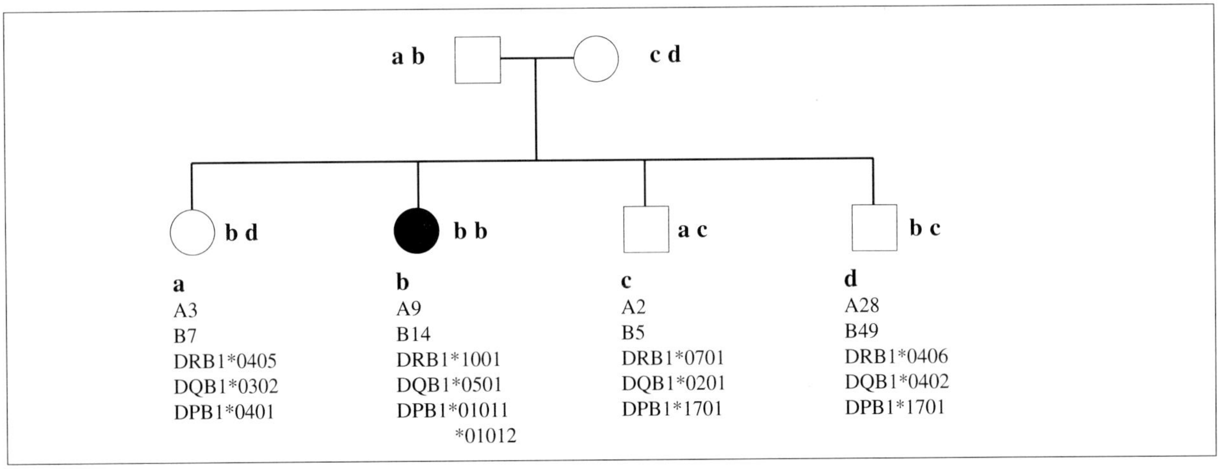

Figure 1. HLA typing of the family. The patient is represented by a solid symbol. The haplotypes were deduced by segregation analysis and are indicated by arbitrary lower-case letters.

Table I. Microsatellite polymorphism genotyping of chromosome 6 and seven other autosomes

	Chromosome 6					chr. 1	chr.5	chr.7	chr. 11	chr.12	chr. 15	chr.19
	SCA1 (6 p)	HLA superlocus (6 p)	TNFa (6 p)	TNFb (6 p)	D6S1009 (6 q)	D1S436	D5S351	D7S507	D11S1985	D12S79	GABRA	APOC2
father	1 2	1 2	1 3	2 3	1 2	1 4	3 4	2 3	1 2	1 2	1 3	1 2
child	2 2	2 2	3 3	3 3	1 1	1 3	2 4	1 2	1 3	2 3	2 3	1 3
mother	3 3	3 4	1 2	1 2	3 3	2 3	1 2	1 1	3 4	2 3	2 2	3 4

satellite polymorphisms from chromosome 6 (6p and 6q) as well as from seven other autosomes *(Table I)*. Phenotyping of erythrocyte markers (for which the genes are located on chromosomes 1, 4, 7, 18, 19 and 22) was performed (data not shown). The results of these analysis are entirely compatible with a paternal isodisomy of chromosome 6 with normal biparental origin of the other chromosomes. A motherhood probability superior to 99.9% could be established - BAYES theorem.

As expected with a paternal isodisomy of chromosome 6, mixed leukocyte cultures revealed that the patient's cells did not stimulate paternal responder cells and that the patient's cells were, however, capable of responding to the father's cells (data not shown).

Reported cases of paternal isodisomy of chromosome 6 are associated with deficiency of the fourth component of complement [3] and with agenesis of pancreatic β cells and consequent diabetes mellitus [4]. Karyotype analysis of the patient and C4 levels were normal and there is no evidence of diabetes mellitus. The β-thalassaemia trait was found in both parents. Microsatellite analysis excluded the possibility of uniparental isodisomy also at chromosome 11, which contains the β-globin locus [5].

We believe this is the first reported case of paternal isodisomy of chromosome 6 with no apparent side-effects. Maternal isodisomy of chromosome 6 in a renal transplant patient with no other genetic abnormality was recently reported [6]. Uniparental disomy hypothetically results in a pathology only when it produces homozygosity for a recessive mutation or for imprinted genes [2]. These combined findings suggest that there is no imprinting of genes on maternally and paternally derived chromosomes 6. The fortuitous detection of chromosome 6 UPD in a β-thalassaemia patient indicates that some cases of UPD may go undetected in the population. However, chromosome 6 is an intensively-studied chromosome - because of HLA typing - and the fact that this is the first such fortuitous detection of paternal UPD confirms the rarity of this condition. Lastly, the results of HLA typing and mixed lymphocyte cultures suggest that the risk of graft-*vs*-host reaction associated with the use of the father for BMT could be acceptable.

References

1. Engel E. A new genetic concept: Uniparental disomy and its potential effect, isodisomy. *Am J Med Genet* 1980; 6: 137-43.
2. Cassidy SB. Uniparental disomy and genomic imprinting as causes of human genetic disease. *Environ Mol Mutagen* 1995; 25 (suppl 26): 13-20.
3. Welch TR, Beischel LS, Choi E, Balakrishnan K, Bishof NA. Uniparental isodisomy 6 associated with deficiency of the fourth component of complement. *J Clin Invest* 1990; 86: 675-8.
4. Abramowicz MJ, Andrien M, Dupont E, Dorchy H, Parma J, L Durpez J, Ledley FD, Courtens W, Vamos E. Isodisomy of chromosome 6 in a newborn with methylmalonic acidemia and agenesis of pancreatic beta cells causing diabetes mellitus. *J Clin Invest* 1994; 94: 418-21.
5. Beldjord C, Henry I, Bennani C, Vanhaeke D, Labie D. Uniparental disomy: a novel mechanism for Thalassemia major. *Blood* 1992; 80: 287-9.
6. Vandenbergloonen EM, Savelkoul P, Vanhooff H, Vaneede P, Riesewijk A, Geraedts J. Uniparental maternal disomy 6 in a renal transplant patient. *Hum Immunol* 1996; 45 1: 46-51.

Anthropology today: contribution of HLA

Contents

• Anthropology today: contribution of HLA

Diversity of HLA class I genes in northern and southern Chineses

X. Sun[1], Y. Sun[2], X. Gao[3*]

1 Guangzhou Second Hospital, Guangzhou, China
2 China-Japan Friendship Hospital, Beijing, China
3 Human Genetics Group, the Australian National University, GPO Box 334, Canberra, ACT 2601, Australia
* Corresponding author

In our previous studies of serological HLA typing [1, 2] and molecular typing for HLA class II genes [3, 4] phylogenetic analysis based on HLA gene frequencies divided Chinese populations into two major groups namely northern and southern Chinese groups. Though both groups shared common features identifying their Chinese background significant differences were observed between them. The characteristics and the magnitude of such genetic differences may not be simply explained by genetic drift and geographic isolation. They may also reflect different origins of the ancient northern and southern gene pools before the Chinese nationality was formed as well as constant genetic inputs from other sources in the Chinese history. In the present report we extended our investigation to HLA class I genes to investigate previously unknown polymorphisms at the nucleotide sequence level.

Study populations and methods

Two populations representing northern and southern Chinese were examined. The samples included 67 randomly chosen unrelated donors from Beijing in northern China and 102 unrelated individuals from Guangzhou in southern China. DNA typing was based on PCR and SSO (sequence-specific oligonucleotide) technologies. The typing protocols recently developed in the Australian National University [5] were able to completely discriminate HLA class I alleles and genotypes. Briefly, the HLA class I gene from exon 2 through exon 3 was selectively amplified using locus-specific intronic primers for HLA-A, B or C. PCR products were dot-blotted on membranes and hybridised with a panel of SSOs (45 for A, 100 for B and 50 for C typing). SSO hybridisation patterns were interpreted on the basis of known class I sequences. Novel alleles predicted from unusual SSO patterns were subjected to the sequencing analysis.

Results and discussion

A total of 18 HLA-A, 36 B and 19 C alleles were found in the two Chinese populations. In addition, three novel B and one novel C SSO patterns were observed in the southern Chinese group. Gene frequencies of these alleles in the two populations are shown in *Table I.*

In the HLA-A locus A2 showed extraordinary heterogeneity in both groups with six subtypes identified in DNA typing including A*0201, 0203, 0205, 0206, 0207 and 0210. In both populations A*0201, though being the most common A2 type, was well outnumbered by the combined frequency of other A2 subtypes. A*0203 was predominantly found in southern Chinese. All the other serological specificities were each represented by a single DNA-defined subtype in these populations. On the single-allele basis A*1101 replaced A2 as the most common A allele in southern Chinese with a gene frequency doubling that of the northern group ($p<0.0001$).

In the HLA-B locus 28 and 29 HLA-B alleles were detected in the northern and southern populations respectively. Fifteen alleles were found in either population. B*4001 and 4601 were the most common B alleles in the north and south respectively. At the resolution level equivalent to serological typing eight B antigens showed significant divergence in the two groups including B44, B48, B52 and B61 confined to the north, and B38, B46, B58 and B75 (B*1502) confined to the south. Nine out of 19 serological specificities detected in more than one case harboured further subtypes. Some of the antigens previously showing no difference in Chinese populations were found in this study to be different subtypes in different groups. For instance, B7 and B55 were

Table I. Gene frequencies (gf) of HLA-A, B and C alleles in northern (n=67) and southern (n=102) Chineses

Allele	gf(N)	gf(S)	p	Allele	gf(N)	gf(S)	p
A*0101	.037	.010	ns	A*2301	.075	.005	ns
A*0201	.187	.128	ns	A*2402	.149	.152	ns
A*0203	.008	.098	<.001	A*2601	.082	.020	<.0025
A*0205	.000	.005	ns	A*2901	.000	.015	ns
A*0206	.048	.040	ns	A*3001	.090	.005	<.0001
A*0207	.067	.093	ns	A*3101	.037	.000	<.025
A*0210	.000	.005	ns	A*3201	.022	.000	ns
A*0301	.045	.029	ns	A*3303	.030	.054	ns
A*1101	.164	.338	<.0001	A*6801	.022	.000	ns
B*0702	.015	.000	ns	B*3901	.008	.020	ns
B*0705	.000	.020	ns	B*4001	.129	.130	ns
B*0801	.008	.005	ns	B*4002	.046	.000	<.01
B*1301	.053	.100	ns	B*4006	.038	.005	ns
B*1302	.076	.015	<.005	B*4402	.030	.000	<.05
B*1501	.053	.015	ns	B*4403	.030	.005	ns
B*1502	.015	.110	<.001	B*4601	.068	.155	<.025
B*1511	.000	.005	ns	B*4801	.053	.000	<.005
B*1518	.023	.005	ns	B*5001	.000	.005	ns
B*1525	.000	.020	ns	B*5101	.053	.055	ns
B*1527	.000	.005	ns	B*5201	.061	.005	<.01
B*2704	.008	.025	ns	B*5401	.038	.045	ns
B*2705	.008	.005	ns	B*5501	.008	.000	ns
B*3501	.053	.025	ns	B*5502	.000	.015	ns
B*3505	.000	.005	ns	B*5601	.000	.005	ns
B*3701	.046	.015	ns	B*5701	.008	.000	ns
B*3801	.008	.015	ns	B*5801	.023	.085	<.05
B*3802	.008	.060	<.05	B*6701	.015	.000	ns
				B*?	.023	.020	ns
C*0102	.100	.184	ns	C*0704	.015	.005	ns
C*02022	.015	.005	ns	C*0801	.114	.158	ns
C*0302	.023	.077	<.05	C*0802	.008	.000	ns
C*0303	.068	.010	<.01	C*1202	.061	.031	ns
C*0304	.114	.117	ns	C*1203	.023	.031	ns
C*0401	.100	.056	ns	C*1402	.023	.041	ns
C*0501	.015	.000	ns	C*1502	.046	.020	ns
C*0602	.121	.036	<.0025	C*1505	.000	.015	ns
C*0701	.015	.005	ns	C*1601	.008	.000	ns
C*0702	.136	.199	ns	C*04new	.000	.010	ns

gf(N) and gf(S) are gene frequencies of northern and southern Chinese populations respectively. Gene frequencies were calculate by direct gene counting. ? represents undecided alleles.

represented exclusively by B*0702 and 5501 in the north and by B*0705 and 5502 in the south; B*1301 and 1302 were predominantly detected in southern and northern Chinese respectively.

In the HLA-C locus 18 and 16 HLA-C alleles were detected in the northern and southern Chinese groups respectively. In addition, an unusual SSO pattern was identified in two southern Chinese donors. Five serological specificities were found to have DNA-defined subtypes. Three alleles, C*0302, 0303 and 0602 showed significant variation between the two populations. In previous serological studies HLA-C was marked by high frequencies of "blanks" due to unsophisticated serology.

Table II. HLA class I haplotypes showing positive linkage disequilibrium in northern and southern Chinese populations

Haplotype	rD(n)	rD(s)	Haplotype	rD(n)	rD(s)
A*0101-B*3701	0.56	1.00	B*0702-C*0702	1.00	
A*0203-B*3802		0.78	B*0705-C*1505		1.00
A*0207-B*4601	0.51	0.75	B*1301-C*0304	0.82	0.92
A*1101-B*2704		1.00	B*1302-C*0602	1.00	1.00
A*2901-B*0705		1.00	B*1502-C*0401		0.94
A*3001-B*1302	0.87		B*2704-C*1202		0.80
A*3303-B*5801	1.00	0.87	B*3701-C*0602	1.00	1.00
			B*3801-C*1203		1.00
A*0101-C*0602	0.75	1.00	B*3802-C*1202		1.00
A*0203-C*0702		0.74	B*4006-C*0801		1.00
A*0207-C*0102	0.47	0.72	B*4601-C*0102	1.00	0.89
A*1101-C*1202	0.70	1.00	B*4801-C*0801	1.00	
A*2901-C*1505		1.00	B*5401-C*0102	0.59	0.67
A*3001-C*0602	0.86		B*5801-C*0302	1.00	1.00
A*3303-C*0302	1.00	0.87	B*6701-C*0702	1.00	

rD(n) and rD(s) are relative values in northern and southern Chinese populations respectively. rD values are presented in the range of 0.00~1.00 with rD 1.00 as the maximum linkage strength of the haplotype in the population.

Linkage disequilibrium (value) between the three HLA class I gene loci was tested. The haplotypes having positive values in the two populations are shown in *Table II*. Comprehensive DNA typing allowed us to identify stronger and more accurate linkage relationships between class I loci. Most antigens showing multiple linkage relationships with antigens of other loci were found in this study to be different subtypes on the haplotypes. As expected the strongest linkage relationship was observed between HLA-B and C. Several three-locus haplotypes can also been deduced from this analysis including A*0101-C*0602-B*3701, A*0203-C*0702-B*3802, A*0207-C*0102-B*4601, A*1101-C*1202-B*2704, A*2901-C*1505-B*0705, A*3001-C*0602-B*1302 and A*3303-C*0302-B*5801.

This study was designed as a pilot project to investigate previously unknown HLA class I subtypes in two representative Chinese populations. HLA subtypes within a serological group were generated by gene mutation and normally contain minor nucleotide variation [6]. Most subtypes have comparatively shorter history and are confined to particular human groups, therefore being more informative in anthropological analyses. The DNA typing results from this study provided further genetic evidence to the hypothesis based on multiple genetic markers including HLA that the contemporary Chinese nationality may have two parallel origins in northern and southern China [2]. Gene flow due to diffusing mating between the two ancient gene pools has resulted in the frequency gradient of some polymorphic markers penetrating the latitude. Meanwhile, other markers especially those with lower frequencies remain confined to their original regions. Furthermore, both the northern and southern gene pools were constantly contributed by genetic inputs from different sources in the history. The alleles and haplotypes detected in this study can be classified into two categories: the ones shared by both northern and southern populations and the ones confined to either population. While the alleles and haplotypes in the former category reflect the common Chinese background the ones in the latter category may provide valuable information in tracing the origins of northern and southern Chinese and the sources of historical genetic inputs into the ancient gene pools. However, the full interpretation of these data requires more comprehensive population studies and the global picture of HLA distributions.

Comprehensive DNA typing for HLA class I genes also has important implications for unrelated-donor-bone-marrow transplant (UDBMT). For instance, in the HLA-B locus more than one third of the serological specificities detected in Chinese were further split in DNA typing. Predicted from the population data the main trouble makers in the HLA-B serological matching for Chinese donor-recipient pairs would be B7, B13, B38, B44, B60 and B75. In the HLA-A locus particular attention should be paid to a single antigen A2 since A2 is the only serological specificity with DNA-defined subtypes in both northern and southern Chinese. Due to the high frequency and tremendous heterogeneity of A2 in Chinese, 40% of the donor-recipient pairs thought to be matched by serology for HLA-A would be mismatched.

Conclusions

Complete DNA typing for HLA class I genes revealed previously unknown genetic differences between northern and southern Chinese. The present results support the hypothesis that multiple origins were involved in the arising of the Chinese nationality. The data presented in this report also have important implications for clinical medicines.

References

1. Sun YP, Lee J, Gao XJ, Song CX, Li SL, Shi QX, Li ZX. HLA antigens in Chinese populations. In Aizawa M ed. *HLA in Asia-Oceania 1986*. Sapporo : Hokkaido University Press, 1986: 502-10.
2. Lee TD, Zhao TM, Mickey R, Sun YP, Lee G, Song CX, Cheng DZ, Zhou MS, Ding SQ, Cheng DX, Song FJ, Lee PY, An JB, Mittal KK. The polymorphism of HLA antigens in the Chinese. *Tissue Antigens* 1988 ; 32 : 188-208.
3. Gao XJ, Sun YP, An JB, Fernandez-Vina M, Qiu JN, Lin L, Stastny P. DNA typing for HLA-DR, -DQ and -DP alleles in a Chinese population using the polymerase chain reaction (PCR) and oligonucleotide probes. *Tissue Antigens* 1991 ; 38: 24-30.
4. Sun YP, Gao XJ, An JB, Stastny P, Serjeantson SW. HLA class II polymorphisms in five Chinese populations detected by polymerase chain reaction and sequence-specific oligonucleotide probes. In Tsuji K, Aizawa M, Sasazuki T eds. *HLA 1991,* vol. 2. Oxford : Oxford Science Publications, 1992 : 237-240.
5. Gao XJ, Serjeantson SW. Heterogeneity in HLA-DR2-related DR, DQ haplotypes in eight populations of Asia-Oceania. *Immunogenetics* 1991; 34: 401-7.
6. Parham P, Lawlor DA, Lomen CE, Ennis PD. Diversity and diversification of HLA-A, B, C alleles. *J Immunol* 1989 ; 142 : 3937-50.

High resolution molecular typing of HLA-A and HLA-B in three South American Indian tribes

M.A. Fernandez-Vina, A.M. Lazaro, C.Y. Marcos, C.J. Nulf, V.M. Fish, J.E. McGarry, E.H. Raimondi, P. Stastny

Department of Internal Medicine, UT Southwestern Medical Center, 5323 Harry Hines boulevard, Dallas, TX 75235, USA
PRICAI, Buenos Aires, Argentina

The colonization of the American continent by Paleo Indians seems to date 11,000 to 40,000years [1, 2]. The descendants of the early founders then populated the continent by southward migrations. In addition, it has been suggested that migrations from Oceania to the South-American subcontinent have occurred [2]. The relatively accurate determination of the colonization time span, the identification of putative ancestors in Asia and Oceania and the state of the isolation of many tribes of native American Indians (Amerindians), provide a unique opportunity for the study of genetic polymorphism and the effects of selective forces acting on them.

Several studies of the population distribution of HLA alleles in native Americans have shown limited HLA polymorphism [3]. HLA-class I antigens determined by serology and DNA-sequencing studies [4, 6] have shown that few allelic lineages are present in the Amerindian HLA gene pools. In spite of these findings several subtypes, exclusively found in indigenous inhabitants of the Americas, have been characterized. So far, 11 HLA-A and 46 HLA-B alleles, including those observed in the present study, have been found in individuals with native American ancestry. Of these, 7 HLA-A and only 10 HLA-B alleles have been observed in other ethnic groups [6]. Thus, HLA-B locus presents a larger number of alleles exclusively found in Amerindians. The majority of the novel HLA-B alleles were found in South American aboriginals [4, 6], thus it has been suggested that this locus is evolving rapidly in the tribes from this region [4, 6].

In this report we present results of the distribution of HLA-A and B alleles in 3 South American Indian tribes from northeast Argentina, determined by high resolution molecular typing of HLA-A and B loci. These methodologies allowed us to identify previously unidentified alleles whose nucleotide sequences were subsequently determined. These studies included unrelated individuals of the Toba, Wichi and Pilaga tribes from the Gran Chaco area. The study of HLA-class II alleles has been reported previously [7]. Molecular typing of HLA-A locus of 138 individuals of the Toba (n=84), Wichi (n=44) and Pilaga (n=10) tribes from the Province of Formosa, Argentina, showed that only seven alleles with "probable indigeneous origin" were present in these populations. These alleles belong to five allelic lineages which can be recognized by serological typing which include HLA-A2, A9, A11, A68 and A31. The gene frequencies of these alleles are shown in the figure. Other groups of alleles defined by DNA-sequence homology and/or serological cross-reactivity, which are common in other populations were virtually absent in these tribes or had low frequencies (A*0101, 0301, 2601 and 2901 as A-NI in the *Figure 1*).

The alleles A*0201, A*2402, A*68012 and A*31012 found in studies of other American Indians tribes [4, 5] were commonly detected in the Argentinian tribes *(Figure 1)*. The alleles A*2403 and A*0219 have not been found in other Indian tribes analyzed so far. In fact, A*0219 was initially identified by its unusual hybridization pattern. We determined the nucleotide sequence of exons 2 and 3 of this allele and found that it is identical to A*0201 in exon-2 and in the first segment of exon-3 while the other part of exon-3 is identical to A*2402. A*2403 was another HLA-A allele frequently observed. This allele was originally described in samples of Caucasoid and Oriental ancestry [8]. In addition to those frequent alleles, A*1101 was observed in only one individual.

Oligonucleotide typing of HLA-B locus alleles showed the presence of 22 American Indian alleles. Their gene frequencies are shown in the *Figure 1*. These included several subtypes of the 6 evolutionary lineages or serological groups (B5, B15, B35, B39, B40 and B48) of HLA-B alleles found in Amerindians. We detected 3 variants of HLA-B39, 5 of HLA-B15 and 2 of HLA-B5 (B*5101 and B*52012). All these alleles have been identified in previous studies of American Indian populations [4, 5]. In the HLA-B40 group, in addition to B*4002 and B*4004 we identified the novel allele B*4009. We observed 6 subtypes of HLA-B35, 3 of which have been found in other Amerindian tribes [4, 5]and we observed 3 novel subtypes B*35092 and B*3518, which seem to be evolutionary related, and B*3519. HLA-B48 was the sixth HLA-B lineage present in the Argentinian Indians. In addition to B*4801 and B*4802, previously found in Amerindians, we identified the novel subtype B*4803.

In the Toba tribe we observed 20 alleles of possible Amerindian origin; the newly described allele B*4803 was the most frequent HLA-B allele in this tribe (gf=0.1810); followed by B*1507, B*5201 and B*4002. The relatively larger number of HLA-B alleles and the lack of a highly predominant one, resulted in a very low frequency of homozygosity (F=0.0911). In the Wichi tribe, 12 of the 13 HLA-B alleles have possible Amerindian origin. Eleven of them had gene frequencies ranging from 0.0326 to 0.2500. The newly described allele, B*3519 was the most frequent allele at this locus, followed by B*4002, B*3903 and B*4803. The frequency of homozygosity at HLA-B locus (F=0.1497) was low in the Wichi tribe as well. We observed 4 HLA-A and 14 HLA-B alleles in the small number of individuals studied of the Pilaga tribe. In spite of this limited sample size, the Pilaga Indians presented HLA-A and B allelic frequencies similar to those observed in Toba Indians. Interestingly, both tribes belong to the same linguistic group. In spite of the overlap of many alleles found in Toba and Wichi tribes we observed some differential representations of alleles of HLA-A and B loci. In our previous study of the same tribes [7] we observed 10 DRB1 and 7 DPB1 alleles of presumed Amerindian origin including the novel allele DRB1*0417.

The analysis of linkage disequilibria showed associations of some HLA-A subtypes with multiple HLA-B alleles. For example A*0201 had associations with B*1507, B*3519 and B*4801 and A*68012 was associated with B*4803, B*4004 and B*3903. The newly identified allele A*0219 was in strong linkage disequilibrium with B*5201. In general, alleles of HLA-B (the most polymorphic locus) had unique associations with alleles of the HLA-A and DRB1 loci, and most of them were not absolute. The exception was B*3519 which showed significant associations with DRB1*0417 and DRB1*0404. The 3 loci haplotypes A*0201-B*1507-DRB1*0411, A*0201-B*4801-DRB1*0802, and A*0219-B*5201-DRB1*0403 were restricted to the Toba tribe. The haplotypes A*0201-B*3519-DRB1*0417 and A*68012-B*4803-DRB1*1406 were observed in both tribes.

The reduced allelic variation in the HLA system of American Indians probably reflects the limited size and/or genetic diversity of the founding populations. DNA sequencing of HLA- class I alleles of American Indians supports the concept of limited polymorphism since only 4 and 6 allelic lineages of HLA-A and B, respectively, have been detected [4, 6]. However, the restriction of the polymorphism of HLA-class I loci seems to vary in different parts of the continent. While few alleles have been found in North American Indian tribes, the indigenous South American populations seem to be richer in subtype variation. This allelic diversity is more notorious in HLA-B and it has been suggested that this locus is evolving rapidly in the South-American subcontinent [4, 5]. The number of novel alleles found in the present study is consistent with this hypothesis. Even though the patterns of allelic distributions for HLA-A, B and DRB1 loci were similar in the 3 indigenous tribes reported here, these loci showed remarkable differences in the degree of polymorphism and in the emergence of new alleles. Heterozygous advantage conferred by overdominant selection has been invoked as a factor for maintenance of the MHC polymorphism [9, 10]. The highest variabilty of MHC proteins is found in residues pointing to the peptide-binding region [10]. Most of the novel alleles identified in this study differ from their putative progenitors in residues located in the peptide-binding specificity pockets. In these populations with limited HLA founder polymorphism inbreeding is quite common. The high frequency of many of the novel alleles suggests that they have been positively selected, perhaps to enlarge the peptide binding repertoire of these

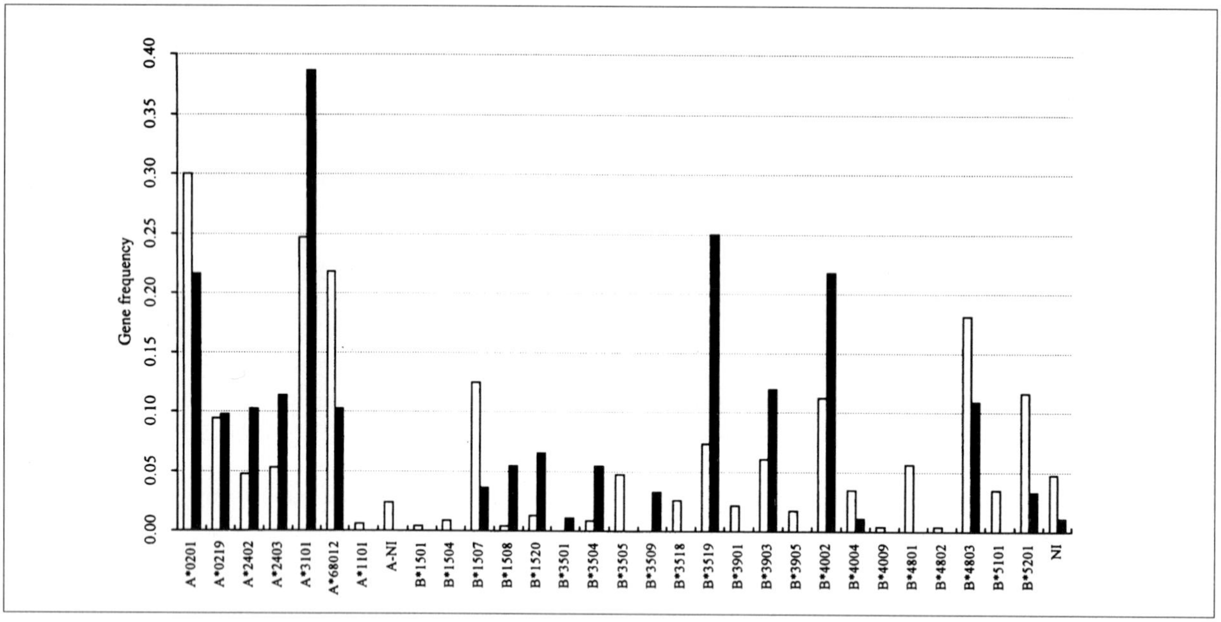

Figure 1. Gene frequency of HLA-A and HLA-B alleles in Toba (open bars) and Wichi (hatched bars) Indians from North-East Argentina. Gene frequencies of alleles of non-aboriginal origin were pooled and are shown as NI.

populations. The allelic distribution of HLA-A and HLA-B loci as well as DRB1, DQA1 and DQB1 fits with the overdominant selection model (heterozygous advantage). Characterization of HLA allelic distributions in other Amerindian tribes and their putative ancestor populations by DNA-based procedures may help to further delineate the relationship among tribes and to depict their migrations. The knowledge of such relationships may prove useful to depict the evolutionary forces operating on the generation and maintenance of HLA polymorphism.

References

1. Cavalli-Sforza LL, Piazza A, Menozzi P, Mountain J. Reconstruction of humanevolution: bringing together genetic, archaeological, and linguistic data. *Proc Natl Acad Sci USA* 1988; 85:6002-6.
2. Salzano FM, Callegari-Jacques SM. South American Indians. A case study in evolution. New York: Oxford University Press, 1988.
3. Kostyu DD, Amos DB. Mysteries of the Amerindians. *Tissue Antigens* 1981; 17:111-23.
4. Belich MP, Madrigal JA, Hildebrand WH, *et al.* Unusual HLA-B alleles in two tribes of Brazilian Indians. *Nature* 1992; 357:326-9.
5. Watkins DI, McAdam SN, Liu X, *et al.* New recombinant HLA-B alleles in a tribe of South American Amerindians indicate rapid evolution of MHC class I loci. *Nature* 1992; 357:329-33.
6. Parham P, Ohta T. Population biology of antigen presentation by MHC class I molecules. *Science* 1996; 272:67-74.
7. Cerna M, Falco M, Friedman H, *et al.* Differences in HLA class II alleles of isolated South American Indian populations from Brazil and Argentina. *Hum Immunol* 1993; 37:213-20.
8. Little AM, Madrigal JA, Parham P. Molecular definition of an elusive third HLA-A9 molecule: HLA-A9.3. *Immunogenetics* 1992; 35:41-4.
9. Takahata N, Nei M. Allelic genealogy under overdominant and frequency-dependent selection and polymorphism of major histocompatibility complex loci. *Genetics* 1990; 124:967-78.
10. Hughes AL, Nei M. Pattern of nucleotide substitution at major histocompatibility complex class I loci reveals overdominant selection. *Nature* 1988: 335:167-70.

HLA class I alleles in three sympatric West African ethnic groups

D. Modiano[1], G. Luoni[1], V. Petrarca[1], M. De Luca[2,3], S.G.E. Marsh[3], M. Coluzzi[1], J.G. Bodmer[3], G. Modiano[4]

1 Institute of Parasitology, University La Sapienza, Roma, Italy
2 Department of Cellular Biology, University of Calabria, Arcavacata di Rende, Italy
3 Tissue Antigen Laboratory, Imperial Cancer Research Fund, London, UK
4 Department of Biology, University Tor Vergata, Roma, Italy

A phylogenetic analysis was carried out with HLA markers on three sympatric West African ethnic groups, Mossi, Rimaibé and Fulani. The population samples studied live in a rural Savanna area about 35 kms north-east of Ouagadougou, Burkina Faso. The Fulani are well differentiated from the Mossi and Rimaibé, since the former are nomadic pastoralists with non-Negroid features of possible caucasoid origin [1], while the latter are Sudanese Negroid populations with a long tradition of sedentary farming in sub-Saharan savannas [2]. Closer to the Mossi in terms of ethnic origin, the Rimaibé have adopted most of the Fulani's socio-cultural habits, having been their slaves. The increasing tendency of the Fulani to settle and converge with the habits of sedentary populations determined stable sympatric and even syntopic conditions in our study area.

The genetic analysis of these three ethnic groups was promoted in the context of a parasitological study on the susceptibility to malaria whose results showed consistent interethnic differences between the Mossi-Rimaibé group on one side and Fulani on the other side ([3], and Modiano *et al.*, in preparation).

Materials and methods

HLA class I typing

DNA extracted from the blood samples has been typed for HLA class I with the "Amplification Refractory Mutation System" (ARMS/PCR) technique [4]. Since the available European data have been obtained by serological techniques, it has been necessary to transform our data in terms of antigenic frequencies according with the nomenclature for factors of the HLA system [5].

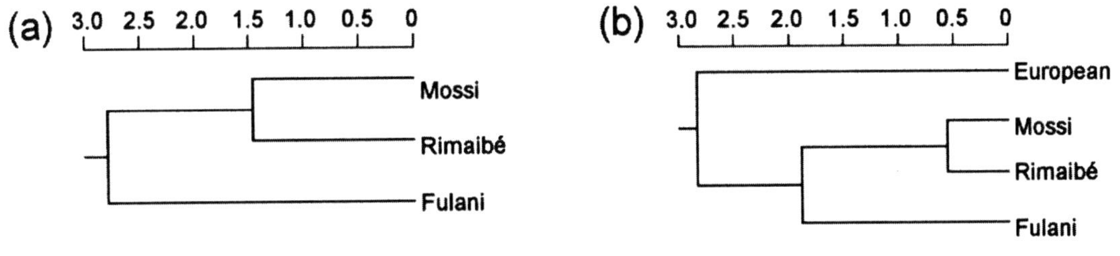

(a)

	Mossi	Rimaibé	Fulani
Mossi	0.000		
Rimaibé	1.463	0.000	
Fulani	2.913	2.663	0.000

(b)

	European	Mossi	Rimaibé	Fulani
European	0.000			
Mossi	2.946	0.000		
Rimaibé	3.035	0.553	0.000	
Fulani	2.531	1.895	1.883	0.000

Figure 1. UPGMA dendrograms (above) from matrixes of chord distances (below), between three West African ethnic groups (a) and comparison with the Europeans [7] (b).

Table I. Allele frequencies of HLA A,B and Cw in random samples of unrelated subjects (11-76 years old) from three ethnic groups of Burkina Faso. Sample sizes are between parentheses. The solid arrows indicate the 15 alleles which show significant difference(s) among the frequencies in the three ethnic groups. The 27 alleles not found in any of the three samples were excluded from the *Table*

ALLELES	Mossi (53)	Rimaibé (47)	Fulani (49)
→ A*01	0.04717	0.031915	0.132653
A*02	0.037736	0	0
A*0201	0.066038	0	0
A*0201/04/06/09/10/11	0.04717	0.138298	0.05102
A*0202	0.037736	0.053191	0
A*0203	0	0.010638	0
A*0205/08	0.009434	0.042553	0.091837
A*0205/08/14	0.009434	0	0
A*0207	0	0	0.010204
A*03	0.028302	0.021277	0.020408
A*23	0.09434	0.170213	0.132653
→ A*24	0	0.010638	0.081633
A*2601	0.009434	0.010638	0
A*2601/02/04/4301	0.009434	0	0
A*2601/03/04	0	0 010638	0
→ A*29	0	0.010638	0.102041
→ A*30	0.132075	0.106383	0.010204
A*31	0.009434	0	0.020408
→ A*3201	0.037736	0	0.081633
A*33	0.084906	0.12766	0.132653
A*3402	0.066038	0.021277	0.030612
A*34/66	0.009434	0.021277	0.010204
A*3601	0.037736	0.010638	0.020408
A*68	0	0.042553	0
A*6801	0.09434	0.053191	0.030612
A*6802	0.04717	0.085106	0.020408
A*6901	0.018868	0	0
A*7401	0.066038	0.021277	0.010204
A*8001	0	0	0.010204
→ B*07	0.028302	0.106383	0.091837
B*08	0.018868	0	0
B*14	0.009434	0	0.030612
B*1501/1502/1508/1511/1512/1514/1515/1519/1520	0.009434	0	0
B*1503/4802	0.056604	0.138298	0.061224
B*1503/4802/4003	0.009434	0	0.010204
B*1509/10/18	0.04717	0.010638	0.040816
B*1513/16/17	0	0.021277	0
B*1516/1517	0.009434	0	0
B*18	0.028302	0.042553	0.020408
B*27	0.009434	0	0.081633
B*27/7301	0.009434	0	0.020408
B*35	0.09434	0.170213	0.081633
→ B*3701	0	0	0.122449
B*38/39/6701	0.009434	0	0
→ B*4001	0	0	0.040816
B*4101	0.018868	0.010638	0
→ B*4201	0.132075	0.095745	0
B*44	0.018868	0.031915	0.020408
B*4501	0.056604	0.010638	0.010204
B*4802	0	0	0.020408

Table I. (continued)

ALLELES	Mossi (53)	Rimaibé (47)	Fulani (49)
B*4802/1503	0	0.010638	0
B*5001	0	0.010638	0.020408
B*51/52	0.066038	0.042553	0.071429
B*51/52/7801	0.018868	0.021277	0.030612
→ B*5301	0.188679	0.202128	0.061224
B*5301/35	0.018868	0.021277	0.020408
B*57	0.04717	0	0
B*5801	0.056604	0.042553	0.061224
B*73	0.009434	0	0
→ B*7801	0.028302	0.010638	0.081633
→ CW*02	0.113208	0.095745	0.22449
CW*0302	0.018868	0.010638	0.020408
CW*0302/0304	0.009434	0	0
CW*0303	0	0	0.010204
CW*0304	0.037736	0.021277	0.061224
→ CW*04	0.226415	0.255319	0.071429
CW*0501	0.009434	0.021277	0.010204
→ CW*0602	0.04717	0.074468	0.153061
CW*0701/02/03	0.113208	0.148936	0.173469
CW*0704	0	0	0.010204
CW*08	0.037736	0.010638	0.020408
CW*1201/02	0	0.010638	0.010204
CW*1203	0.009434	0.042553	0
CW*1301	0.009434	0	0
CW*14	0.009434	0 021277	0
CW*15	0.028302	0.021277	0
CW*1601	0.179245	0.159574	0.214286
→ CW*1701	0.150943	0.106383	0.020408

Analysis

For the few alleles with a sufficiently high frequency, Hardy-Weinberg equilibrium was tested and no significant deviations from expected genotypic ratios were observed. From matrixes of genetic distances UPGMA (unweighted pair-group method arithmetic averages) dendrograms were obtained. The genetic distances were expressed in terms of chord distances [6], because of their previous use in the HLA literature.

Results and discussion

The frequencies of HLA class I alleles are shown in *Table I.* There were 15 alleles with at least one interethnic statistically significant difference with chi-square test. In 14 out of 15 alleles the Mossi and Rimaibé frequencies turned out to be very similar, but different from those of Fulani. Only for the B*07 allele Fulani and Rimaibé were similar but different from Mossi. It is worth pointing out the findings about B*3701 and B*5301 alleles. The former, not found in the Mossi and Rimaibé, is present at a relatively high frequency in the Fulani and is not a typical negroid allele; conversely the B*5301 allele, a typical negroid marker, was found in the Fulani sample at a much lower frequency than in the Mossi and Rimaibé. The UPGMA dendrogram *(Figure 1a)* confirms the difference between Mossi-Rimaibé group and Fulani, being the latter in a different cluster from that of Mossi and Rimaibé. Since Fulani's ethnic origin is believed to be Caucasoid, we compared the allelic frequencies of our three populations with those of Europeans *(Figure 1b).* The values of the genetic distances show that Fulani are not as far from Europeans as Mossi and Rimaibé are. These data show that Fulani are well differentiated from Mossi and Rimaibé and, as already suggested in literature [7], they are also more similar to Caucasoids than other sub-Saharan African populations.

References

1. Stenning DJ. The pastoral Fulani of Northern Nigeria. In: Gibbs JL ed. *People of Africa.* University of Minnesota, 1965.
2. Skinner EP. *The Mossi of the Upper Volta.* Stanford, California : Stanford University Press, 1964.
3. Modiano D, Petrarca V, Sirima BS, Nebié I, Diallo D, Esposito F, Coluzzi M. *Plasmodium falciparum* malaria in sympatric ethnic groups of Burkina Faso, West Africa. *Parasitologia* 1995; 37: 255-9.
4. Sadler AM, Petronzelli F, Krausa P, Marsh SGE, Guttridge MG, Browning MJ, Bodmer JG. Low resolution DNA typing for HLA-B using sequence-specific primers in allele - or group - specific ARMS/PCR. *Tissue Antigens* 1994; 44: 148-54.
5. Bodmer JG, Marsh SGE, Ekkehard D, Bodmer WF, Bontrop RE, Charron D, Dupont B, Erlich HA, Mach B, Mayr WR, Parham P, Sasazuki T, Schreuder GMT, Strominger JL, Svejgaard A, Terasaki PI. Nomenclature for factors of the HLA system, 1995. *Tissue Antigens* 1995; 46: 1-18.
6. Cavalli-Sforza LL, Edwards AWF. Phylogenetic analysis: models and estimation procedure. *Am J Hum Genet* 1967; 19: 233-57.
7. Allsopp CEM, Harding RM, Taylor C, Bunce M, Kwiatkowski D, Anstey N, Brewster D, McMichael AJ, Greenwood BM, Hill AVS. Interethnic genetic differentiation in Africa: HLA class I antigens in the Gambia. *Am J Hum Genet* 1992; 50: 411-21.

HLA-A2 alleles in north east Asian populations

Y. Ishikawa[1], K. Tokunaga[1,2], J.M. Tiercy[3], K. Kashiwase[1], H. Tanaka[1], J. Liu[4], T. Akaza[1], K. Tadokoro[1], N.O. Chimge[5], G.J. Jia[4], T. Juji[1]

1. Japanese Red Cross Central Blood Center, 4131 Hiroo Shibuya Ky, Tokyo, Japan
2. Departement of Human Genetics of Tokyo, Tokyo, Japan
3. Transplantation Immunology Unit, Centre Medical, Geneva, Switzerland
4. Harbin Red Cross Blood Center, Harbin, China
5. National Center of Anthropology, Ulaanbaatar, Mongolia

HLA-A2 is a common antigen in most human populations. It is a highly polymorphic antigen, and eighteen alleles have been identified to date. However, only a few antigen specificities can be distinguished using a serological method. We have already reported that A*0201, A*0206, A*0207 are common and A*0203 and A*0210 are rare alleles in Japanese [1]. In Caucasian, however, most A2s are encoded by A*0201 [2]. We have developed a PCR-SSOP (sequence specific oligonucleotide probe) method which can be used to distinguish HLA-A2 alleles (A*0201-A*0217) and for typing of a large number of samples. Using this method, we determined A2 alleles in north east Asian populations to study the allelic distribution.

Materials and methods

Blood samples were collected from healthy Japanese (n=114), Chinese (Korean [n=100], Manchurian [n=100]), Mongolian (n=100) and Buryat (n=100) donors and typed by serological microcytotoxicity method. Then genomic DNAs were prepared from the A2-positive samples using QIAamp Blood Kit (QIAGEN, CA, USA), after red cell lysis. The genomic DNAs were PCR amplified with A2-specific primers (1), and the amplified fragments were analyzed using 22 oligonucleotide probes designed on exons 2 and 3 (see AHS#2 report in these proceedings). Samples typed as A*0201 or A*0207 based on the analysis of the exons were further analyzed for exon 4 using 2 additional probes after amplification with A2-exon 4 specific primers [1], because the sequences of exons 2 and 3 of A*0201 and A*0209 and of A*0207 and A*0215N are identical.

Results

A total of six alleles, A*0201, A*0202, A*0203, A*0205, A*0206 and A*0207, were detected in this study *(Table I)*. In all populations, A*0201 and A*0206 were the most frequent A2 alleles, accounting for 50-60% and 20-35%, respectively, of the A2 alleles. These alleles did not exhibit any strong associations with other loci. A*0207 was detected at relatively high frequency in Japanese, Korean and Manchurian and was also detected in Buryat and Mongolian. In Japanese, A*0207 was strongly associated with Cw*0102-B*4601-DRB1*0803 (5/9). This association, however, was infrequent in Manchurian (0/11), Korean (1/5) and Buryat (1/4). In Buryat and Mongolian, the frequency of A*0205 was higher than that of A*0207. The A*0205 was strongly associated with Cw6-B50-DR7 (5/8, 5/11) in both of these populations, A*0203 occurred at a relatively high frequency in Manchurian and at low frequency observed in Buryat, Mongolian and Korean. The allele was associated with B52 and DRB1*1404 (5/6).

Table I. Distribution of HLA-A2 alleles among various ethnic groups

Allele	Mongolian	Buryat	Chinese		Japanese
			Man	Korean	
	n=100	n=100	n=100	n=100	n=115
A*0201	15.0	21.0	17.0	20.0	10.6
A*0202	--	0.5	--	--	--
A*0203	1.0	--	4.0	1.0	--
A*0205	4.0	5.5	0.5	--	--
A*0206	7.5	3.5	8.0	6.0	8.4
A*0207	1.0	1.0	5.5	3.0	4.0
total	28.5	31.5	35.0	30.0	23.0

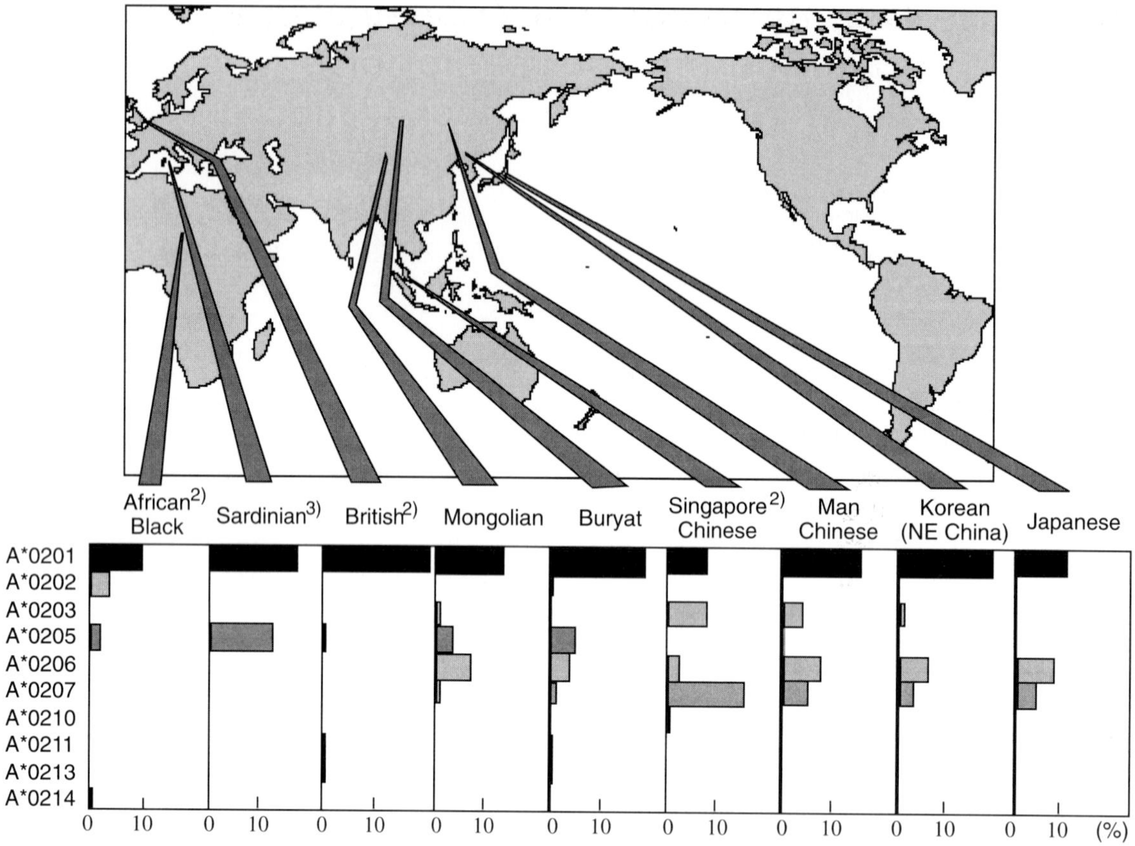

Figure 1. Distribution of HLA-A2 alleles among various ethnic groups.

Discussion

Figure 1 shows A2 allele frequencies determined in this study and ones reported elsewhere. Krausa *et al.* [2] have reported that the most common A2 allele in Caucasian and African Black is A*0201 and that they detected A*0206 and A*0207 in Singapore Chinese but not in Caucasian or African Black. A*0205 was found in Buryat and Mongolian as a common allele, but not in Korean or Japanese in our study. A*0205 was also not detected in Singapore Chinese [2], but has been detected in African Black [2] and Sardinian [3] at relatively high frequency. These findings suggest that A*0206 and A*0207 are shared in East Asian populations and that A*0205 is widely distributed in Eurasia and Africa.

HLA-A2 is common in most populations. Based on the results of this study, however, it is clear that the allele or subtype frequencies differ among populations.

References

1. Ishikawa Y, Tokunaga K, Kashiwase K, Akaza T, Tadokoro K, Juji T. Sequence-based typing of HLA-A2 alleles using primer with an extra base mismatch. *Hum Immunol* 1995; 42: 315-8.
2. Krausa P, Brywka M III, Savage D, Hui KM, Bunce M, Ngai JLF, Teo DLT, Ong YW, Barouch D, Allsop CEM, Hill AVS, McMichael AJ, Bodmer JG, Browning MJ. Genetic polymorphism within HLA-A*02: significant allelic variation revealed in different populations. *Tissue Antigens* 1995; 45: 223-31.
3. Carcassi C, Krausa P, Bodmer J, Contu L, Browning M. Characterization of HLA-A*02 subtypes in the Sardinian population. *Tissue Antigens* 1994; 46: 391-3.

HLA class I alleles typed by PCR-ARMS in Greenlanders of Eskimo origin

N. Grunnet[1], *R. Steffensen, K. Varming, C. Jersild*

Regional Centre for Blood Transfusion and Clinical Immunology, Aalborg Hospital, PO Box 561, 9100 Aalborg, Denmark
1 Present address: Tissue typing laboratory, Department of Clinical Immunology, Aarhus University Hospital, Skejby, Denmark

In the anthropology component of the 12th International Histocompatibility Workshop, we had studied a group of 43 unrelated, randomly selected Inuits, born in Greenland with residence in Denmark. Samples were collected in 1990 from the Inuits and from a group of 30 healthy, unrelated random Danes, to point out possible ethnic differences.

We characterized HLA-A, -B and -Cw alleles by polymerase chain reaction by use of a amplification refractory mutation system (PCR-ARMS), detectable by sequence specific primers from XII International Workshop [1]. Due to the complexity of the HLA class I system a total of 82 PCR-ARMS reactions are necessary to obtain a resolution of HLA-class I : 32 primer mixes identified the A locus, 27 primer mixes identified the B locus and 23 primer mixes identified the Cw locus.

In addition, we also performed HLA-A*02 subtyping using nested PCR-technique primers from XII International Workshop [2] and HLA-A9 subtyping by primers distributed by Dynal.

Results

The gene frequencies for the two investigated populations are given in table 1.

The Danish population shows a typical Caucasian pattern where the most frequent alleles are A*02, A*01 and A*03; B*44, B*07, B*08 and B*35; Cw*07 and Cw*03.

Among the Inuits the most prevalent HLA-A, -B and -Cw alleles are: A*24 and A*02 representing 81.4 per cent of the HLA-A gene frequencies (see *table I*); the most common HLA-B alleles found are B*27, B*40, B*15 and B*48, together representing 58.1 per cent of the HLA-B gene frequencies; at HLA-Cw, Cw*03, Cw*02, Cw*04, Cw*07 and Cw*08 are found most commonly, where Cw*02 and Cw*03 together account for 55.8 per cent of the HLA-Cw gene frequencies.

Significant differences ($p<0.05$) are observed in 10 specificities *(table II)*, where the most prominent differences are the extremely increased frequency of A*2402 (57 versus 13.3 per cent) and the decreased frequency of Cw*07 (12.8 versus 38.3 per cent) in Inuits compared to Danes.

Moreover the A*02 subtypes have a different distribution among the Inuits compared to Danes. A*0201 is presumably the only A*02 variant represented in the Danish population, but in Inuits both A*0201 and A*0206 are very frequent. The HLA-A9 genomic subtyping showed no polymorfism at all in either of the two populations due to the fact that A*2402 was the only detected allele in A24 positive individuals.

Discussion

Although a limited number of samples are studied and the vast majority of the Inuits in this study comes from the Western part of Greenland, where a mixture of Caucasian genes are presumed to be more common, this HLA class I allele frequency analysis shows a high level of genetic diversity between Inuits and Danes.

The present study of HLA class I typing performed by PCR-ARMS confirmed previous serological results, well established during the Eleventh International Workshop [3, 4]. In addition this study describes several new alleles in the Inuit population, indicating DNA typing to have a superior resolution thus enabling identification of subtypes. In addition, typing of samples can be performed with a similar precision on historical and freshly obtained samples.

Our study demonstrates that Inuits share some HLA

Table I. Gene frequencies (%) of HLA-class I alleles

HLA-A	Inuits (n=43)	Danes (n=30)	HLA-B	Inuits (n=43)	Danes (n=30)	HLA-Cw	Inuits (n=43)	Danes (n=30)
*01	4.7	16.7	*51	8.1	5	*01	1.2	3.3
*0201	11.6	25	*07	7	13.3	*02	17.4	8.3
*0206	12.8	0	*08	8.4	13.3	*03	38.4	16.7
*03	3.5	13.3	*44	4.7	18.3	*04	14	10
*23	1.2	0	*15	14	5	*05	2.3	5
*2402	57	13.3	*57	0	3.3	*06	0	8.3
*25	0	3.3	*27	17.4	8.3	*07	12.8	38.3
*34	0	1.7	*35	11.6	11.7	*08	11.6	0
*11	3.5	5	*37	0	1.7	*12	1.2	3.3
*29	1.2	3.3	*39	1.2	3.3	*14	0	1.7
*30	0	1.7	*40	15.1	15	*15	0	3.3
*31	0	1.7	*47	1.1	1.7	*16	1.2	1.7
*32	0	1.7	*48	11.6	0			
*33	0	1.7						
*68	4.7	11.7						

Most common HLA alleles in Inuits are underlined.

Table II. HLA-allelogene frequencies (%) of significant difference in Inuits

Allele	Inuits (n=43)	Danes (n=30)	p-value *
Increased frequency			
HLA-A			
*0206	12.8	0	0.005
*2402	57	13.3	< 0.001
HLA-B			
*48	11.6	0	0.008
HLA-Cw			
*03	38.4	16.7	0.007
*08	11.6	0	0.008
Decreased frequency			
HLA-A			
*01	4.7	16.7	0.03
*19	1.2	10	0.04
HLA-B			
*44	4.7	18.3	0.02
HLA-Cw			
*06	0	8.3	0.02
*07	12.8	38.3	< 0.001

* p-value using Fisher exact test, two-sided.

class I genetic pattern with North American Indians in agreement with the HLA class I and II genetic affinities earlier reported [5, 6] and this fits well with their known interrelationship. Furthermore there seems to be some connection to Oriental populations due to the fact that A*0206 was first decribed as an allele among Singapore Chinese people [7].

References

1. Reference manual for HLA Class I SSP ARMS-PCR typing kit prepared by: Tissue Antigen Laboratory, Imperial Cancer Research Fund, 44, Lincoln's Inn Fields, London WC2A 3PX, United Kingdom, 1995.
2. Reference manual for HLA-A*02 SSP ARMS-PCR subtyping kit prepared by: Tissue Antigen Laboratory, Imperial Cancer Research Fund, 44, Lincoln's Inn Fields, London WC2A 3PX, United Kingdom, October 1995.
3. Lindblom B, Svejgaard A. HLA genes and haplotypes in the Scandinavian populations. In: Tsuji K, Aizawa M, Sasazuki T, eds. *HLA 1991*. Oxford : Oxford Science Publication, 1992: 651-5.
4. Lamm LU, Graugaard B, Grunnet N, Schroeder ML. HLA types in Eskimos. In: Tsuji K, Aizawa M, Sasazuki T, eds. *HLA 1991*. Oxford: Oxford Science Publication, 1992: 689-90.
5. Williams RC, Troup GM, Nelson JL, Kostyu DD, McAuley JE, Pettitt DJ, Knowler WC, Templin DW, Mickelson EM, Hansen JA, Hoy W. Report of the North American Indian anthropology section. In: Tsuji K, Aizawa M, Sasazuki T, eds. *HLA 1991*. Oxford: Oxford Science Publication, 1992: 683-5.
6. Grunnet N, Steffensen R, Jersild C. Increased frequency of HLA-DRw14b(w6)-associated RFLP in Greenlanders of Eskimo origin. *Tissue Antigens* 1991: 37 : 127-9.
7. Krausa P, Brywka III M, Savage D, Hui KM, Bunce M, Ngai JLF, Teo DLT, Ong YW, Barouch D, Allsop CEM, Hill AVS, Mcmichael AJ, Bodmer JG, Browning MJ. Genetic polymorphism within HLA-A*02: significant allelic variation revealed in different populations. *Tissue Antigens* 1995: 45 : 223-31.

Application of SSP/ARMS to HLA class I loci in Samoans

L.D. Severson, D.E. Crews, R.W. Lang

The Ohio State University, 333 West 10th avenue, 2060 Graves Hall, Columbus, 43210 1239 Ohio, USA

Islands of the South Pacific provide an excellent opportunity for migration studies. The period of human occupation is short, averaging about 2,000 years (range approximately 3,300 - 500 years). In addition, the islands are isolated so there is little difficulty in projecting back from present occupants to the first settlers. Lastly, at one time there were no prior populations on the islands with which migrants could genetically mix. We are particularly interested in the widely accepted "Fast Train Model" hypothesis for Polynesian settlement. According to this model, the earliest Polynesians carried a culture known as Lapita, characterized by red slip pottery with dentate design. This culture complex is believed to have first appeared in the Philippines and eastern Indonesia. Linguistic evidence suggests that the Lapita people belonged to the Austronesian language family which is rooted in Taiwan and S. China. A major migration of Austronesian speakers left the Philippines, reaching New Guinea about 3,500 B.C. From this migration, a subgroup which formed the Oceanic speakers moved to the area of New Britain / New Ireland by 3,000 B.C. From this area, a group migrated southeast through the Melanesian Islands reaching Fiji by 1,500 B.C. Part of this group moved on to Tonga and Samoa around 1,300 B.C., giving rise to the Polynesians. A central element in the "Fast Train Model" is that there was little genetic mixing between the Lapita people and Papuan populations already present in Melanesia. Most Lapita sites in Melanesia are found on the coasts of larger islands and on small offshore islands, supporting the hypothesis that the interiors of these islands were already inhabited. When the Lapita reached Polynesia, these islands were uninhabited, thus they became the founding population. In addition to the linguistic and archaeological evidence, this model has been supported by serologic HLA studies [1].

Recently the "Fast Train Model" has been challenged by analysis of mtDNA from Polynesians. The predominant mtDNA lineage group found in 96% of Polynesians is the 9 bp Asian-specific deletion [2]. However, 4% of modern day Polynesians carry a mtDNA lineage which appears to be of Melanesian origin. In the oldest skeletal remains from Fiji, Tonga, and Samoa, the 9 bp deletion is absent suggesting that the first settlers of Polynesia were Melanesian [3]. Clearly this is a question that must be explored using additional nuclear loci. The recently developed SSP/ARMS technique for HLA class I provides an opportunity to address this question.

Material and methods

Sample

DNA samples were obtained from 264 American Samoan residents of the island of Tutuila. Individuals with non-Samoan surnames were excluded. Details of the population and sample have been published previously [4].

HLA typing

At present 24 individuals have been typed for HLA-A, B, and C using the class I sequence specific primers (SSP) amplification refractory mutation system (ARMS) polymerase chain reaction (PCR) protocol of the 12th International Histocompatibility Workshop [5-8]. Kits containing the primer mixes were provided by the Imperial Cancer Research Fund. DNA samples were amplified in PCR volumes of 19.5 µl overlaid with mineral oil. The protocol was modified for adaptation to a Hybaid TR thermocycler using 0.6 ml thin wall PCR tubes. Glycerol was added to the reaction and annealing temperatures in the standard protocol were adjusted to 67 °C, 62 °C and 55 °C.

Statistical methods

Allele frequencies were determined by the gene counting method. These frequencies then were used to compare with published HLA frequencies from other Polynesian and Melanesian populations [1]. HLA-A and HLA-B were used, but HLA-C was not included because allele frequencies were not available for all of the populations. Fst and genetic distances were determined by R-matrix analysis using SAS/IML. Fst represents the reduction in heterozygosity of a population due to random genetic drift.

Results

Table I shows allele frequencies for the American Samoan population. HLA-A locus results indicate high frequencies of HLA-A02, A1101, A2402, and A3401. HLA-B locus results indicate high frequencies of HLA-B40 and B5501. HLA-C locus results indicate high frequencies of HLA-Cw0101, Cw03, and Cw07.

Table I.

Locus A Allele	Freq.	Locus B Allele	Freq.	Locus C Allele	Freq.
02(1,4,6,9)	.07	13(1,2)	.04	01(1,2)	.20
0207	.02	15(9,10,18)	.02	0302	.03
0203	.04	1521	.02	0303	.03
02	.02	35(1-8)	.02	0304	.13
11(1,2)	.13	38(1,2)	.04	03	.03
24(2,3)	.17	39(11,13,21, 3-7)	.02	04(1,2)	.08
26(1,2,4)	.02			07(1,2,3)	.10
2603	.04	40(11,12)	.11	08(1,2,3)	.05
3401	.11	40(2,4,5,6)	.11	1203	.03
6802	.02	4007	.02	15(1-3,5)	.08
null	.22	4801	.04	1601	.03
uncert.	.13	5401	.02	null	.13
		55(1,2)56(1,2)	.20	uncert.	.13
		null	.15		
		uncert.	.17		

null = no amplification;
uncertain = positive amplification but unable to determine specific allele.

Fst values for all of the populations compared are as follows: Papua New Guinea Coast 0.094, New Caledonia 0.080, Fiji-Nadi 0.061, Hawaii 0.051, Tokelau 0.109, Marquesa 0.043, Western Samoa 0.052, New Zealand Samoan 0.032, and American Samoa 0.084. Average Fst for all populations is 0.067.

The first three eigenvalues of the R matrix which describe approximately 84% of the variation in allele frequencies are as follows: Papua New Guinea Coast (-0.277, -0.144, 0.057), New Caledonia (-0.186, 0.209, 0.105), Fiji-Nadi (-0.011, -0.049, -0.050), Hawaii (-0.075, 0.031, 0.112), Tokelau (0.043, -0.185, 0.103), Marquesa (0.362, -0.090, 0.062), Western Samoa (-0.094, -0.007, -0.061), New Zealand Samoa (-0.108, -0.157, 0.035), and American Samoan (-0.184, -0.130, -0.078)

Discussion

The American Samoan allele frequencies correspond well with previously published HLA frequencies for Western Samoans and New Zealand Samoans [9,10], suggesting that the preliminary sample is representative of the native Samoans on Tutuila. Analysis of the first three eigenvalues indicates a relatively closer affinity among the three Samoan populations, Fiji, and Hawaii. Papuan New Guinea Coast and New Caledonia are more distantly related, and are found together along the third axis, while the Marquesas are most distantly related to the Melanesian populations. These results appear to confirm the genetic distances predicted by the "Fast Train Model." The Polynesian populations tend to show closer affinity to each other than the Melanesian populations. While Fiji is found in the outermost region of Melanesia, it is near the Samoan Islands and significant admixture among these populations is expected. The Marquesas are among the farthest outlying Polynesian Islands, and therefore are predicted to show the least affinity with the Melanesian populations.

These preliminary results appear to support the "Fast Train Hypothesis." However, additional considerations must be incorporated in subsequent analysis when the entire American Samoan population has been typed. The weighted effective population sizes should be used in the R-matrix calculations. It is known that significant population size differences exist among these islands, and when relatively larger populations are weighted equally with smaller populations, they appear to possess greater genetic variation. The addition of Class II loci and the use of haplotype frequencies will more fully reflect the genetic structure of the populations.

Acknowlegements

We wish to thank Dr. Paul Sciulli for assistance with the genetic distance analysis. This presentation was funded in part by the Hughes Memorial Fund, The Ohio State University and Immune Response Corporation. The American Samoan fieldwork was supported by a seed grant from the Ohio State University Office of Research.

References

1. Serjeantson SW. HLA genes and antigens. In : Hill AVS, Serjeantson SW, eds. *The Colonization of the Pacific: a genetic trail.* Oxford : Clarendon Press, 1989: 120-73.
2. Sykes B, Leiboff A, Low-Beer J, Tetzner S, Richards M. The origins of the Polynesians: an interpretation from mitochondrial lineage analysis. *Am J Hum Genet* 1995 ; 57: 1463-75.
3. Hagelberg E, Clegg JB. Genetic polymorphisms in prehistoric Pacific Islanders determined by analysis of ancient bone DNA. *Proc R Soc Lond* 1993 ; 252(1334): 163-70.
4. Crews DE, Bindon J, Kamboh M. Apolipoprotein polymorphisms and phenotypic variability in American Samoans: preliminary data. *Am J Hum Biol* 1993 ; 5: 39-48.
5. Browning MJ, Krausa P, Rowan A, Bicknell DC, Bodmer JG, Bodmer WF. Tissue typing the HLA-A locus from genomic DNA by sequence-specific PCR: comparison of HLA genotypes and surface expression on colorectal tumor cell lines. *Proc Natl Acad Sci USA* 1993 ; 90: 2842-5.
6. Bunce M, Welsh KI. Rapid DNA typing for HLA-C using sequence-specific primers (PCR-SSP): identification of serological and non-serologically defined HLA-C alleles including several new alleles. *Tissue Antigens* 1993 ; 43: 7-17.
7. Krausa P, Moses J, Bodmer WF, Bodmer JG, Browning MJ. HLA-A locus alleles identified by sequence specific PCR. *Lancet* 1993 ; 341: 121-2.
8. Krausa P, Bodmer JG, Browning MJ. Defining the common subtypes of HLA A9, A10, A28 and A19 by use of ARMS/PCR. *Tissue Antigens* 1993 ; 42: 91-9.
9. Crosier PS, Douglas R. The distribution of HLA in a Polynesian population - Western Samoans. *Tissue Antigens* 1976 ; 8:173-80.
10. Booth PB, Faoagali JL, Kirk RL, Blake MN. HLA types, blood group, serum protein and red cell enzyme types among Samoans in New Zealand. *Hum Heredity* 1977 ; 27: 412-23.

Typing and characterization of B60/B61 split in the Korean population

K.W. Lee, Y.S. Kim, H.C. Cho

Department of Clinical Pathology, Hallym University, 445 Gil-Dong, Kangdong-Ku, Seoul 134-701, Korea

HLA-B40 is the most frequently found HLA-B family in the Korean population (13.4%) [1]. It can be divided into two serologic specificities, B60 and B61. However, serologic discrimination is limited by lack of B61 mono-specific alloantisera and cross reactivity of sera defining B60 and B61. This ambiguity is particularly evident in samples reacting strongly to all B60 and B61 specific alloantisera but not to any other HLA-B specific sera in the typing tray [2]. In our experience, about 1% of Korean sample exhibit this type of reaction pattern. Although these samples were tentatively assigned as putative B60/B61 heterozygotes, correct assignment of B40 subtypes for these samples is still not clear. The purpose of this study was to establish an efficient typing system for discrimination of B60 and B61.

Results and discussion

PCR-SSP is known to be a very specific and fast typing system for HLA typing [3]. Two sets of SSP were used in this study: 60-5': CCA CTC CAT gAg gTA TTT CC and 60-3': CTC CAA CTT gCg CTg ggA for B60 specific gene amplification (678 bp); 61-5', CgC CAC gAg TCC gAg gAA and 61-3': TCC CAC TTg CgC Tgg gT for B61 specific gene amplification (549 bp). To monitor PCR quality, each PCR tube contained internal control primers amplifying exon 15 of the adenomatous polyposis coli gene (256 bp). Amplification conditions and cycle reactions were performed as described by Bunce et al [4]. This PCR-SSP system was applied to 24 samples (B60-12; B61-12) exhibiting standard serologic reaction patterns and to 39 samples exhibiting the putative B60/B61 heterozygous reaction pattern in a commercial typing tray (OT-72, One Lambda, USA) containing four different B40 specific alloantisera.

Using the PCR-SSP system described above, clear discrimination of B60 and B61 was possible in all B40 positive samples in this study (Figure 1). Results obtained from 24 samples exhibiting standard serologic patterns were consistent with serology. Among the 39 putative B60/B61 heterozygous samples, however, only 29 samples were B60/B61 heterozygotes (74.4%). Among the rest five were B60 homozygotes (12.8%) and five were B61 homozygotes (12.8%). Based on this result, alloantisera defining B60 and B61 in the typing tray appeared to exhibit false positive reactivity.

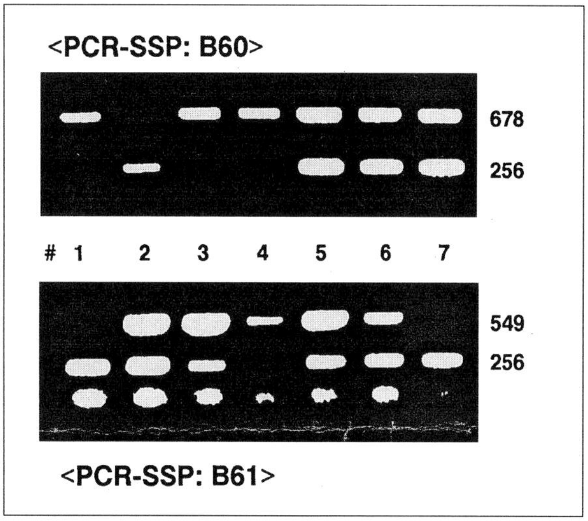

Figure 1. B60 (top photo) and B61 (bottom photo) specific gene amplification patterns. The size of B60 (678 bp), B61 (549 bp) and internal control (256 bp) fragments are indicated. Lane 1, B60 positive control; lane 2, B61 positive control; lane 3-7, B60/B61 putative heterozygous samples. Samples in lane 3-6 were revealed as B60/B61 heterozygotes while a sample in lane 7 was revealed as a B60 homozygote by the PCR-SSP method described in this study.

Conclusion

PCR-SSP is an excellent method for clear discrimination of B60 and B61, and thus, useful in accurate and consistent assignment of these two types. This system will be specifically useful in populations exhibiting a high frequency of putative B60/B61 heterozygote based on serologic reaction patterns.

References

1. Imanish T, Akaza T, Kimura A, Tokunaga K, Gojobori T. Allele and haplotype frequencies for HLA and complement loci in various ethnic groups. In: Tsuji K, Aizawa M, Sasazuki T, eds. *HLA 1991, Proceedings of the Eleventh International Histocompatibility Workshop and Conference*. Oxford: Oxford University Press, 1992:1065-220.
2. Crawford L, Tonai R, Cabacungan C, Hardy S, Terasaki PI. Correction of B*40 complex serologic typing by DNA based assays. *Hum Immunol* 1995;44 (suppl):43.
3. Olerup O, Zetterquist H. HLA-DR typing by PCR amplification with sequence-specific primers (PCR-SSP) in 2 hours: an alternative to serological DR typing in clinical practice including donor-recipient matching in cadaveric transplantation. *Tissue Antigens* 1992;39:225-35.
4. Bunce M, Fanning GC, Welsh KI. Comprehensive, serologically equivalent DNA typing for HLA-B by PCR using sequence specific primers (PCR-SSP). *Tissue Antigens* 1995;45:81-90.

HLA polymorphism in Iraqi Jews

S. Orgad, R. Kelt, Y. Moskovitz, E. Gazit

Tissue Typing Laboratory, Sheba Medical Center, Ramat Gan, Israel

The ancient history of the Jewish people was greatly influenced by three great disasters, which culminated in the exile of most of the Jews from Israel. The first exile of the 10 tribes of Israel took place in 753 BC. The fate of these 10 tribes is unknown but it is believed that some settled in Mesopotamia, today Iraq. After the destruction of the first Temple in 586 BC the tribes of Judah and Benjamin were exiled to Babylon. It is possible that they mixed with the descendants of the first exile. These exiles uprooted whole families, who have settled in areas of Iraq where they neither mixed nor intermarried with the local Arab population. First cousin marriages were as high as 25% [1]. As this trend is now changing and since 130 000 Iraqi Jews returned to Israel in 1951, it is important to study the HLA system of this group while we still can.

The origin of Ashkenazi and North African Jews

The origin of Ashkenazi and North African Jews can be traced to the third great exile which occurred after the distraction of the second Temple in 70 AD. This exile continued in several waves. First, only war prisoners were exiled across the Alps to France and Germany. Later whole families were exiled, and they dispersed around the Roman Empire and the Mediterranean, mainly in Italy, Spain and North Africa. In 1492, the Spanish Inquisition caused all the unconverted Jews to be expelled from Spain.. These Sephardi (Spanish in Hebrew) Jews were dispersed throughout Europe and North Africa.

The Moroccan Jews

Jewish communities existed in North Africa before the destruction of the second Temple by the Romans in 70 AD. Additional migration waves into and out of North Africa throughout the ages and especially after the expulsion of Jews from Spain, contributed to the fact that north African Jews cannot be regarded as one distinct group [2].

The return of Jews to Israel

The return of Jews to Israel in considerable numbers began over 100 years ago. This process was dramatically accelerated after the Holocaust and with the establishment of the State of Israel, when whole communities of Jews from all over the Diaspora returned to Israel. The Israeli Jewish population comprises today a mosaic-like composition of various groups who came from many different countries, yet they claim descent from a common ancient background. These groups were scattered all over the world and were separated from each other, with almost no communication for 80-100 generations. Each group was exposed to a different environment and to the surrounding population. They differ in physiognomy, life style and language but they kept their religion, prayers and customs. Strict religious rules and social isolation prevented them from mixing with the local population and prevented a large scale inflow of novel genes. It provides a unique opportunity for a study of the Jewish groups and a comparison to the host population using histocompatibility antigens as genetic tools.

Materials and methods

We have studied 113 randomly selected Iraqi Jews, whose parents and grandparents were all born in Iraq. HLA-DR was tested in 99 individuals by PCR-SSP method. Class I was studied in 72 people by serology and PCR-ARMS using local antisera and 12WS DNA primers. We compared HLA gene frequencies of Iraqi Jews with that published for Moroccan and Ashkenazi Jews [3] and with Iraqi Arabs [4, 5].

Results

The genotype frequencies of HLA -A, -B, -C, and DRB1* are summarized in *Table I.* HLA antigens gene frequencies of Iraqi Jews were compared using two by two tables with Iraqi Arabs, Ashkenazi and Moroccan Jews. The comparison between the Iraqi Jews and Arabs revealed that seven of 9 DRB1* antigens and 7 of 27 class 1 antigens were significantly different. p (Pearson's) values were: HLA-A1, A11 p=0.02, A30 p=0.005, A33 p=0.002, B8, B12, and B15 p= 0.04. DRB1*01 p= 0.0022, B1*02 p=< 0.00001, B1*03 p= 0.01, B1*05 p< 0.00001, B1*06 p< 0.00001, B1*07 p=0.008. The frequency of eight of 36 class I and 3 of 12 DRB1* antigens were significantly different when Iraqi and Ashkenazi Jews were compared. HLA-A2 p=0.02, A11, A30 p=0.004, A26 p=0.003 HLA-B13 p=0.01, B14, B44 p= 0.03, B38 p=0.005, DRB1* 01 p= 0.0001, DRB1*02 p, 0.00001, and DRB1*10 p= 0.003. The differences between Iraqi and Moroccan Jews were much smaller. Only 3 class I and 2 DRB1* antigens were significantly deviant: HLA-A30 p= 0.04, B52 p=0.001, B35 p=0.005, DRB1*02 p= 001 and DRB1*07 p=0.0002.

Table II gives the significant calculated haplotype frequencies and D values based on population data. Linkage disequilibrium (p<0.01) occurred for (A2-B57), (A11-B51), (A11-B49), (A24-B18), (A26-B38), (A29-B7), (A29-B38), (A29-B41) ,(A31-B13), (A33-B14), (A- Blank-B14), and *Table III* those of (p<0.05) for haplotypes (A1-B8), (A2-B51), (A2-B53), (A2-B44), (A2-B18), (A3-B51), (A24-B38), (A26-B40), (A26-B50), (A26-B53), (A30-B13), (A33-B13), (A32-B57), (A86-B45)

Discussion

Genetic studies have shown that several rare genetic diseases are found in relatively high frequency among specific groups of Jewish communities. In Babylonian (Iraqi) Jews there are few genetic defects which are characteristic to this group, such as thalassaemia, hemoglobin H, and G6PD deficiency , which is in frequency of 25% in Iraqi Jews. These defects are absent in local non-Jewish populations, almost absent in Ashkenazi Jews and is present in low frequency in North African Jewish groups [1]. Genetic disorders typical of Ashkenazi Jews include Nieman-Pick, Tay-Sacks, Gaucher, familial dysautonomia and pentosuria syndromes. Glycogen storage disease type III, ataxia telangiectasia [6] and congenital deafness [7] are particular to Moroccan Jews. However, FMF (familial mediterranean fever) is prevalent in Jews

Table I. HLA antigens frequencies (%) of Iraqi Jews

HLA- A	HLA-B	HLA-B	HLA-C	HLA-DRB1	
A1 23	B7 4.0	B51 6.0	Cw1 0.7	B1*01	3.0
A2 15	B8 3.6	B52 0.0	Cw2 3.6	B1*02	4.7
A3 8.7	B13 6.5	B53 4.0	Cw3 3.6	B1*03	6.3
A11 11.8	B14 6.0	B40 2.0	Cw4 16.0	B1*04	10.0
A23 0.0	B18 6.0	B22 0.7	Cw5 2.8	B1*07	6.3
A24 1.0	B27 0.7		Cw6 6.4	B1*08	1.6
A25 0.0	B35 15.0		Cw7 6.4	B1*09	0.0
A26 4.0	B37 0.0		Cw8 11.8	B1*10	6.3
A29 6 0	B38 6.5		Cw12 8.0	B1*11	26.0
A30 8.8	B39 0.0		Cw13 0.7	B1*12	3.0
A31 2.0	B41 4.0		Cw14 0.7	B1*13	18.0
A32 2.8	B42 0.0		Cw15 1.4	B1*14	7.0
A33 1.4	B44 12.6		Cw17 3.6	Blank	7.8
A34 0.7	B45 1.4				
A68 4.0	B49 3.6				
A69 0.7	B50 4.0				

Table II. Significant (p<0.01). Calculated haplotypes frequency and D values. Based on population data x 10^4 (n=72)

Haplotypes	HF	D values
A2 -B57	211	181
A11-B51	259	200
A11-B49	274	232
A24-B18	334	271
A26-B38	196	164
A29-B7	199	170
A29-B38	193	156
A29-B41	274	246
A31-B13	136	122
A33-B14	139	131
A Blank-B14	133	117

Table III. Significant (p<0.05). Calculated haplotypes frequency and D values. Based on population data x 10^4 (n=72)

Haplotype	HF	D value
A1-B8	263	182
A2-B51	-88	-159
A2-B53	-88	-159
A2-B44	498	319
A2-B18	241	161
A3-B51	189	145
A24-B38	246	175
A26-B40	66	57
A26-B50	125	101
A26-B53	126	101
A30-B13	181	130
A33-B13	65	56
A32-B57	66	60
A68-B45	67	61

from North Africa, Iraq and Turkey [8]. These variances between the Jewish groups are apparent also in their histocompatibility genes.

Iraqi Jews, like Moroccan Jews, were characterized by a high frequency of A1 and a lower prevalence of A2. A26 is markedly over expressed in Ashkenazi Jews and was found in much lower frequency both in Iraqi and Moroccan Jews

We have observed significant variability in 8 of 36 HLA class I and 3 of 10 class II antigens between the Iraqi Jews compared to the Ashkenazi Jews. The HLA of Moroccan Jews varied only in 3 of 36 class I and 2 of 10 class II antigens. This suggests greater genetic similarities between the Iraqi and Moroccan Jews than between Iraqi and Ashkenazi Jews. However, compared to the Iraqi Arabs , there is a significant disparity in 7 of 27 class I and in 6 of 8 class II antigens.

Some of the most common haplotypes among the Caucasoid (A1-B8), (A2- B12), were found to be present in low frequency ($p<0.05$) for the Iraqi Jews. However, the A26-B38 ancestral haplotype, was in a significant linkage disequilibrium also in the Iraqi Jews. HLA-B57 which in Ashkenazi Jews is in linkage disequilibrium with A1 was association with A2 in Iraqi Jews. The linkage of haplotypes (A2-B57), (A11-B51), (A11-B49), (A24-B18), (A29-B38), (A29-B41) ,(A31-B13), (A33-B14) is characteristic of Iraqi Jews.

The three Jewish ethnic groups compared here show similar but not identical antigen frequency which suggests that they belong to the same genetic stock, forged with time and isolation, certain genetic forces such as founder effect, high intra-familial marriages and selection of influx of genes through proselytes. Taken together these results suggest that HLA antigens are useful in the analysis of Jewish population. Although the Iraqi were separated from other Jewish groups for many generations, they still share antigens frequencies with Moroccan Jews, suggesting a common genetic origin. The heterogeneity between Iraqi and Ashkenazi Jews is admissible considering their dissemination during the past 20 centuries. They were exposed to genetic processes such as the bottleneck phenomenon, genetic drifts, specific selective pressures or even admixture with other gene pools.

References

1. Sheba C. Gene frequencies in Jews. *Lancet* 1970; i: 1230-1.
2. Bonne-Tamir B *et al. Am J Phys Enthrop* 1978; 49:465-72.
3. Roitberg Tambur A *et al. Tissue Antigens* 1995; 46:104-10.
4. Jabbar AAR. *Disease Markers* 1993; 11(4): 161-70.
5. Ollier W *et al. Tissue Antigens* 1985; 25: 87-95.
6. Levin S *et al. Isr J Med Sci* 1967; 3: 397-410.
7. Winter S, Dar H. *Isr J Med Sci* 1967; 3:894-8.
8. Gazit E, Orgad S, Pras M. *Tissue Antigens* 1977; 9:273-5.

MHC haplotypes including eight microsatellites in French Basques and in Sardinians

D. Ramsbottom[1], C. Carcassi[2], H. de Solages[1], M. Abbal[3],
B. Crouau-Roy[1], J. Clayton[1], A. Cambon-Thomsen[1], L. Contu[2]

1. Centre d'Immunopathologie et de Génétique Humaine (CIGH), CNRS UPR 8291, CHU Purpan, 31300 Toulouse, France
2. Universita di Cagliari, Catedra di Genetica Medica, Via San Giorgio 12, 09124 Cagliari, Italy
3. Laboratoire d'Immunologie, CHU Rangueil, 31400, Toulouse, France

Basques and Sardinians are genetically quite distinct from other European populations [1]. Basques are characterised by a very specific language and are probably the most direct descendants of the earliest post-Neanderthal settlers of Europe. They preceded the arrival of Neolithics 7 000 years ago and were present in a larger area than presently (south-western France and north-eastern Spain). Sardinia was the first Mediterranean island with a human settlement at least 10 000 years ago. Some genetic similarities between Basques and Sardinians support the hypotheses that the first settlers of Sardinia were pre-Neolithic; the island was then the target of several waves of invasions from various Mediterranean regions. Both populations have been the subject of a number of studies regarding HLA region serological and molecular markers over the years [2, 3] and especially during International Histocompatibility Workshops. Sardinians followed by Basques have the highest frequencies in the world of the extended haplotype HLA-A30, B18, BFF1, C4A3, C4BQ0, DRB1*0301, DQA1*0501, DQB1*0201 whereas the two populations have quite different of other HLA alleles and haplotypes, each distribution showing a characteristic pattern. The aim of our study was to supplement the HLA markers with various polymorphic microsatellites spanning the HLA region in order to better study the associations of the microsatellite polymorphisms with HLA alleles as previously described for some of them [4] and to estimate the value of such markers in population studies as compared to HLA. Microsatellites are formed by tandemly repeated short DNA sequences (1-6 nucleotides, most frequently 2) and are distributed throughout the genome. As a matter of fact microsatellites of the HLA region were previously used in population studies [5] but rarely a series of them in conjunction with HLA class I and II. It is especially interesting to investigate these associations (1) on HLA haplotypes shared by these populations (probably the most ancient haplotypes) in view of evaluating the stability of the various microsatellites [6] and (2) in haplotypes frequent in these populations and rare elsewhere as a unique source of such haplotypes.

Samples of populations, markers and methods

Eighty-five unrelated healthy French Basques and 102 unrelated healthy Sardinians (whose origins were checked for 3 generations) were analysed. The same samples were used in previous studies.

HLA typing was done by serology for HLA-A and B and by PCR-SSO according to 11th or 12th workshop protocols for HLA-DRB1, DQA1 and DQB1.

Microsatellites were analysed using 200ng of genomic DNA amplified by polymerase chain reaction (PCR) in a total volume of 20 µl using 0.5U of Taq DNA polymerase. The 8 microsatellites used were the following dinucleotide repeats TNFa, b, c, d and e in the vicinity of TNF genes [7], DQ CAR between DQA and DQB, 1-2 kb telomeric to DQB1 [8], D6S265 centromeric to HLA-A [9] and MIB, 20 kb centromeric to HLA-B [10]. The PCR products were analysed for length polymorphism on an Applied 373 DNA sequencer. In addition a di-allelic Nco1 restriction fragment in the first intron of TNFB (TNF n) was also analysed as previously described [5]. The primers used for microsatellite PCR were as described in references [7-10] as well as the nomenclature used for microsatellite polymorphisms (allele number or number of basepairs).

Allele and haplotype frequencies were estimated by a maximum likelihood estimator using an estimation-

Table I. Combined classical HLA markers and MHC microsatellite haplotypes in Basques and Sardinians

	BASQUES			SARDINIANS		
	Freq.	Support intervals	Test Stat	Freq.	Support intervals	Test Stat.
MHC class I region						
*A - **D6S265** - B - **MIB***						
1 - 4 - 17 - 6	0.078	0.027 - 0.147	21.52			
30 - 4 - 18 - 1	0.067	0.026 - 0.136	19.43	0.113	0.053 - 0.193	39.52
29 - 7 - 44 - 3	0.064	0.013 - 0.143	20.15			
11 - 5 - 27 - 4	0.044	0.013 - 0.103	20.15			
2 - 7 - 17 - 7				0.037	0.011 - 0.087	14.42
24 - 4 - 18 - 1	0.042	0.011 - 0.100	7.96	0.019	0.000 - 0.059	2.54
2 - 7 - 18 - 9				0.019	0.000 - 0.059	3.11
1 - 4 - 8 - 9	0.022	0.003 - 0.069	11.97	0.019	0.003 - .0059	14.05
TNF microsatellite haplotypes						
b - a - n - c - d - e						
4 - 7 - 2 - 1 - 3 - 3	0.094	0.034 - 0.174	inf.	0.190	0.003 - 0.059	inf.
4 - 11 - 2 - 1 - 3 - 3	0.089	0.038 - 0.168	inf.	0.113	0.053 - 0.193	inf.
5 - 2 - 2 - 2 - 4 - 3	0.072	0.012 - 0.142	inf.	0.038	0.010 - 0.089	19.2
4 - 11 - 2 - 1 - 3 - 3	0.054	0.010 - 0.120	9.46			
4 - 10 - 2 - 1 - 3 - 3	0.012	0.000 - 0.054	1.84	0.167	0.096 - 0.256	inf.
5 - 1 - 2 - 2 - 4 - 3	0.049	0.015 - 0.124	inf.	0.113	0.053 - 0.193	inf.
1 - 2 - 2 - 2 - 4 - 1				0.074	0.024 - 0.144	inf.
5 - 6 - 1 - 1 - 3 - 3	0.019	0.001 - 0.069	inf.	0.560	0.016 - 0.116	inf.
MHC class II region						
*DQA- **DQCAR** - DQB*						
501 - 1 - 201	0.189	0.108 - 0.288	49.28	0.198	0.128 - 0.288	inf.
201 - 10 - 303	0.100	0.040 - 0.180	28.56	0.038	0.011 - 0.087	25.09
201 - 1 - 201	0.078	0.000 - 0.147	2.97	0.010	0.001 - 0.043	inf.
102 - 3 - 602	0.056	0.015 - 0.125	12.60	0.028	0.006 - 0.073	inf.
102 - 3 - 502				0.149	0.078 - 0.228	inf.
501 - 11 - 301	0.067	0.016 - 0.136	26.88	0.113	0.053 - 0.193	inf.
3 - 6 - 302	0.044	0.013 - 0.102	8.32	0.113	0.053 - 0.193	inf.
101 - 3 - 501	0.047	0.011 - 0.110	10.40	0.094	0.044 - 0.164	inf.

When Test Statistic is >5 the presence of the haplotype is very likely — - inf. = infinite — - Microsatellite loci are in bold character

maximisation algorithm. Support intervals and a statistic which tests the hypothesis of non existence of the haplotype were calculated in each case as described in [6].

Results and discussion

Some of the markers could not be explored on the totality of the samples, so that the sample size varies according to the marker at the time of the present analysis. The number of individuals studied for all markers and thus taken into account for the haplotype analyses was 45 in Basques and 53 in Sardinians. Microsatellites appeared to be very stable and both classical HLA haplotypes and microsatellite haplotypes were found strongly associated across the MHC. As the sample size made difficult the estimation of frequencies of 13 point haplotypes some specific combinations of markers (3 to 5) were chosen for estimation of their haplotype frequencies. Considering these haplotypes in overlapping combinations of markers allowed in certain cases to merge them in order to re-construct the most probable extended haplotypes. Results show that the same extended haplotype is the most frequent in both populations with a frequency roughly twice higher in Sardinians than in Basques: A30, D6S265 [4], B18, MIB1, TNF b5, a1, c2, n2, d4, e3, DR3, DQA1*0501, DQ CAR1, DQB1*0201. The fact that the same TNF microsatellites were found on this B18, DR3 haplotype in both populations has already been discussed [6] and points to the stability of such markers in this conserved haplotype. It is interesting to note that this is also the case for other microsatellites. However some microsatellites on other haplotypes had alleles with less strong linkage disequilibrium. DQ CAR alleles allowed to split some DQA-DQB combinations. The next most frequent haplotypes were different in the two populations, with some overlaps. One very frequent in the Basques and not found in Sardinians is: HLA-A29, D6S265 [7], HLA-B44, MIB3, TNF b4, a7, n2, c1, d3, e3, DR7, DQA*0201, DQ CAR 1, DQB1*0201. The frequencies of the most frequent three to five point haplotypes in the two populations are presented in *Table I,* grouped according to the region of the MHC and with markers ordered according to their relative mapping on the chromosome: class I (HLA-A, D6S265, HLA-B, MIB); central TNF region (TNF b, a, n, c, d, e); class II with DQA, DQ CAR and DQB. A higher number of class I, TNF and class II region haplotypes had a frequency over 2% among the Basques. Sardinians were more homogeneous, except for the TNF region markers. The marked isolation of these populations, more pronounced for Sardinians than for Basques, correlates with a somewhat restricted HLA polymorphism with characteristic haplotypes. The difference in haplotype distribution between the two populations was more significant for TNF markers than for class II, then class I region markers. These results are in agreement with the hypotheses of an ancient common origin for a part of these two populations, each of them being then diversified through their independent history. Such a study also shows the practical use of microsatellites in population studies as good markers of HLA haplotypes.

Acknowledgements

D. Ramsbottom had an EU fellowship "Human Capital and Mobility". The authors wish to acknowledge the technical assistance of R. Jambou and M.L. Sorignet. This work was supported by EU "HCM" grants: Biological history of European populations: ERBCHBGCT 920090 and 920032, Conseil régional Midi-Pyrénées : 9407538 and an INSERM/AFS grant N° 5FS5

References

1. Cavalli-Sforza LL, Piazza A. Human genomic diversity in Europe: a summary of recent research and prospects for the future. *Eur J Hum Genet* 1993; 1: 3-18.
2. Contu L, Arras M, Carcassi C, La Nasa G, Mulargia M. HLA structure of the Sardinian population: a haplotype study of 551 families. *Tissue Antigens* 1992; 40: 165-74.
3. Martinez-Laso J, De Juan D, Martinez-Quiles N, Gomez-Casado E, Cuadrado E, Arnaiz-Villena A. The contribution of HLA-A,-B,-C and -DR,-DQ DNA typing to the study of Spaniards and Basques origins. *Tissue Antigens* 1995; 45: 237-45.
4. Jongeneel CV, Briant L, Udalova I, Sevin A, Nedospasov SA, Cambon-Thomsen A. Extensive genetic polymorphism in the human tumor necrosis factor region and relation to extended HLA haplotypes. *Proc Natl Acad Sci USA* 1991, 88: 9717-21.
5. Crouau-Roy B, Briant L, Pociot F, Stavropoulos C, Cambon-Thomsen A, Clayton J. Tumor necrosis factor microsatellites in four European populations. *Hum Immunol* 1993, 38: 213-6.
6. Crouau-Roy B, Bouzekri N, Carcassi C, Clayton J, Contu C, Cambon-Thomsen A. Strong association between microsatellites and an HLA-B, DR haplotype (B18, DR3): implication for the evolution of the microsatellites. *Immunogenetics* 1996; 43: 255-60.
7. Nedospasov SA, Udalova IA, Kuprash DV, Turetskaya RL. DNA sequence polymorphism at the human tumor necrosis factor (TNF) locus. Numerous TNF/lymphotoxin alleles tagged by two closely linked microsatellites in the upstream region of the lymphotoxin (TNF-b) gene. *J Immunol* 1991; 147: 1053-9.
8. Macaubas C, Hallmayer J, Kalil J, Kimura A, Yasunga S, Grumet F C, Mignot E. Extensive polymorphism of a (CA)n microsatellite located in the HLA-DQA1/DQB1 region. *Hum Immunol* 1995; 42: 209-20.
9. Weissenbach J, Gyapay G, Dib C, Vignal A, Morissette J, Millasseau P, Vaysseix G, Lathrop M. A second generation linkage map of the human genome. *Nature* 1992; 359: 794-801.
10. Grimaldi MC, Clayton J, Pontarotti P, Cambon-Thomsen A, Crouau-Roy B. A new highly polymorphic microsatellite in linkage disequilibrium with HLA-B. *Hum Immunol* 1996; 51: 89-94.

Anthropological study of west Algerian population

S. Benhamamouch[1], A. Boudjemaa[1], S. Djoulah[1, 2], I. Le Monnier de Gouville[2], K. Bessaoud[3], J. Hors[2], A. Sanchez-Mazas[4]

1 Institute of Biology, Molecular Biology and Genetics, Es senia University, Oran, Algeria
2 LNH, Department of Immunology, INSERM U93, Centre Hayem, Hôpital Saint-Louis, 1, avenue Claude Vellefaux, 75475 Paris Cedex 10, France
3 Department of Epidemiology and Statistics, INESM, Oran, Algeria
4 Laboratory of Genetics and Biometry,University of Geneva, Geneva, Switzerland

The aim of the work was to extend our previous study [1] to a large sample in the framework of the XIIth International Histocompatibility Workshop and perform genetic distance analysis with 12 Mediterranean populations.

Material and methods

HLA-DRB1 and DQB1 alleles were determined using PCR-SSO INNO-LIPA HLA typing tests (Innogenetics NV, Zwijnaarde, Belgium) based on reverse hybridization. Amplified biotinylated DNA material was hybridized with specific oligonucleotide probes immobilized as parallel lines on membrane-based strips. After hybridization, streptavidin labeled with alkaline phosphatase was added and bound to any biotinylated hybrid previously formed. Incubation with BCIP/NBT chromogen resulted in a purple/brown precipitate.

Subjects

Blood samples were obtained from 99 unrelated healthy Algerian volunteers, with documented family origin and their grand parents being born in Oran region. All were 20-50 years old and had their origins in Western Algeria (latitude 35°40' North, longitude 0°40' West).

Statistical analysis

Allele and haplotype frequencies were estimated by a maximum likelihood method algorithm using the program package Arlequin (Excoffier, Schneider and Kuffer, personal communication). Genetic distances (defined as $D_{xy} = \frac{1}{2}\sum|x_i - y_i|$, where x_i and y_i are the frequencies of the ith allele in populations x and y, respectively, and k is the size of the frequency vector, were computed as for previous HLA data analyses [2]. A set of 12 population samples from Mediterranean area was considered [3-6].
The mean genetic distance matrix computed over loci DRB1 and DQB1 was used for a principal coordinate analysis, using the local program Ancoo GB Geneva.

Results and discussion

A total of 32 DRB1, and 19 DQB1 alleles were recognized. HLA-DRB1, DQB1 alleles frequencies estimated in the West Algerian population are displaid in *Table I* and haplotypes frequencies in *Table II*. The following alleles were observed at a level of > 10% : DRB1*0301, DRB1*0701, DQB1*0201, DQB1*0301 and two haplotypes emerged as : DRB1*0301-DQB1*0201 (13.6%) and DRB1*0701-DQB1*0201 (10.8%).

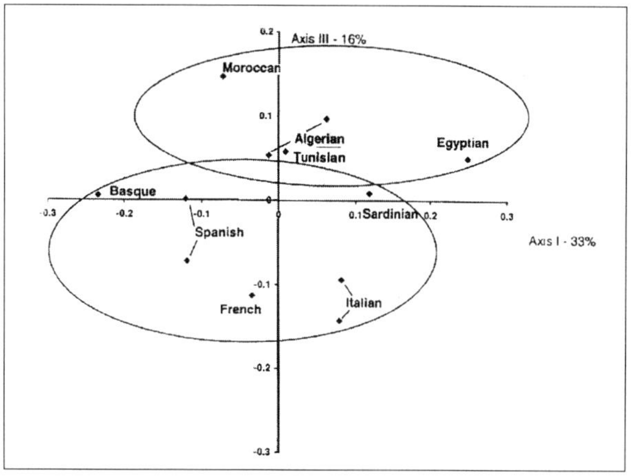

Figure 1. Principal coordinate analysis for 12 Mediterranean population samples tested for DRB1 and DQB1 polymorphism. Axis I (33%) and III (16%). The axis II (22%, not shown) only separates the Sardinian population from the others.

The DRB1 and DQB1 frequency distributions found in the Algerians from Oran are close to that observed in two other populations of Algerians from Algiers [4, 7] although some differences are observed between the two samples (in particular, a lower DRB1*1501 and a higher DQB1*0201 frequency in the former population). These haplotypes are also the most frequent in the recently typed Moroccan population from Souss-Agadir [6], Algerians from Algiers [4, 7] and Tunisians [5].

Table I. DRB1 and DQB1 allele frequencies in the West Algerian sample (N=99)

DRB1 Allele	Frequency (%)	DQB1 Allele	Frequency (%)
0301	15.2	0201	30.1
0701	13.6	0301	18.4
1101	8.6	0602	7.0
0402	8.1	0501	6.8
1502	6.6	0302	6.0
1302	4.5	0604	5.2
1001	3.5	0502	4.0
1104	3.5	0601	4.0
1301	3.5	0603	3.5
0405	3.0	0503	2.6
1501	3.0	0402	2.0
1102	2.5	0303	1.5
1601	2.5	0609	1.0
0103	2.0	0102	0.5
0403	2.0	0304	0.5
1303	2.0	0401	0.5
0101	1.5	0607	0.5
0102	1.5	0608	0.5
0406	1.5	Blank	0.4
0901	1.5		
1402	1.5		
0302	1.0		
0801	1.0		
1109	1.0		
1401	1.0		
1602	1.0		
0404	0.5		
0803	0.5		
1103	0.5		
1304	0.5		
1310	0.5		
1504	05		
Blank	0		

Table II. DRB1-DQB1 haplotype frequencies in the West Algerian sample (N=99)

DRB1-DQB1 haplotypes	Frequency (%)
0301-0201	13.6
0701-0201	10.8
1101-0301	7.1
0402-0302	4.5
1502-0602	4.0
1001-0501	2.5
1102-0301	2.5
1302-0604	2.5
1104-0301	2.5
1502-0601	2.0
1501-0602	2.0
0101-0501	1.5
0402-0201	1.5
0405-Blank	1.5
0901-0201	1.5
1101-0502	1.5
1301-0604	1.5
1601-0502	1.5
0103-0501	1.5
0701-Blank	1.2
0402-Blank	1.1
0102-0501	1.0
0302-0201	1.0
0402-0301	1.0
0403-0302	1.0
0406-0301	1.0
0701-0303	1.0
1301-0301	1.0
1301-0603	1.0
1302-0609	1.0
1303-0603	1.0
1401-0503	1.0
1402-0301	1.0

The observed (obs.) heterozygosity almost reach the maximum values expected (max. exp.) for each allelic set (DRB1 : obs. 0.93 max. exp. 0.96 for 31 alleles; DQB1 : obs. 0.85 max. exp. 0.94 for 18 alleles in the Oranese).

Genetic comparisons with other Mediterranean populations (*Figure 1*) reveal that Algerians (from Oran and Algiers) are intermediate between the Moroccans and the Egyptians [8] and close to the Tunisians. This is in agreement with an east to west geographic differentiation, which is also visible among the southern Europeans included in the analysis (lower cluster). Overall, the genetic distance analysis presented in *Figure 1* is very close to a geographic projection of the studied populations around the Mediterranean Sea.

Acknowledgments

We would like to thank the French-Algerian cooperation project (CMEP 93 MEN 241b) supporting the study, the Algerian volunteers (University students and laboratory staff) for their participation in this work, and M Nobili for helpful management of the Workshop database. The statistical analysis study has been supported by grants CMEP (France), and FNRS 3100-039847.93 (Switzerland).

References

1. Djoulah S, Sanchez-Mazas A, Khalil I, Benhamamouch S, Degos L, Deschamps I, Hors J. HLA-DRB1, DQA1 and DQB1 DNA polymorphisms in healthy Algerian and genetic relationships with other populations. *Tissue Antigens* 1994; 43: 102-9.
2. Dard P, Sanchez-Mazas A, Tiercy JM, Magzoub M, Verduyn W, Goumaz C, Jeannet M, Pellegrini B, Excoffier L, Langaney A. Joint report : HLA-A, -B, and DR differentiations among North and West African populations. In: Tsuji K, Aizawa M, Sasazuki T eds. *HLA 1991,* vol. 1. Oxford: Oxford University Press, 1992; 632-6.
3. Imanishi T, Tatsuya A, Kimura A, Tokunaga K, Gojobori T. Allele and haplotype frequencies for HLA and complement loci in various ethnic groups. In: Tsuji K, Aizawa M, Sasazuki T eds. *HLA 1991*, vol. 1. Oxford: Oxford University Press, 1992; 1065-220
4. Arnaiz-Villena A, Benmamar D, Alvarez M, Diaz-Campos N, Verala P, Gomez-Casado E and Martinez-Laso. HLA allele and haplotype frequencies in Algerians, relatedness to Spaniards and Basques. *Hum Immunol* 1995; 43: 259-68.
5. Hmida S, Gauthier A, Dridi A, Quillivic F, Genetet B, Boukef K, Semana G. HLA class II gene polymorphism in Tunisian. *Tissue Antigens* 1995; 45: 63-8.
6. Izaabel H, Sanchez-Mazas A, Caillat-Zucman S, Beaurin G, Akhayat O, Bach JF, Garchon HJ. Three DRB1-DQA1-DQB1 haplotypes account for 45% of total haplotype frequencies in Moroccan from the Souss Area. *Hum Immunol* 1996; 47:57 (P 300).
7. Reviron D, Andre M, Cantaloube JF, Baignini P, Chicheportiche C, Mercier P. Polymorphisme HLA-DRB1 dans la population algérienne originaire d'Alger. *Rev Fr Transfus Hemobiol* 1993; 36: 509-16.
8. El Chenawi F, Djoulah S, Abbas F, Abdel N, Laperrière J, Hors J, Charron D, Sanchez-Mazas A. HLA class II DRB1 and DQB1 polymorphisms in the Egyptian population of Siwa. *Hum Immunol* 1996; 47:142 (P 772).

Distribution of HLA-A-B-DRB1 haplotypes in five ethnic groups in North-East Asia

H. Tanaka[1], K. Kashiwase[1], Y. Ishikawa[1], K. Tokunaga[1,2], E. Sideltseva[3], G.J. Jia[4], M.H. Park[5], T. Akaza[1], K. Tadokoro[1], T. Juji[1]

1 Japanese Red Cross Central Blood Center, 4131 Hiroo Shibuya Ku, Tokyo 150, Japan
2 Department of Human Genetics, University of Tokyo, Japan
3 Immunogenetic Research Center, Civil Health Service, Angarsk, Irkutsk, Russia
4 Harbin Blood Center, Harbin, China
5 Department of Clinical Pathology, Seoul National University Hospital, Seoul, Korea

The distribution of HLA alleles and haplotypes in various ethnic groups have been reported up to date. The purpose of the present study was to determine the HLA-A, B antigens and DRB1 alleles in unrelated subjects of five ethnic groups, Chinese (Northern Han, Man, Northern Koreans), Southern Koreans, and Buryat in northeast Asian (*Figure 1*) and analyze the distribution of HLA-A-B-DRB1 haplotypes.

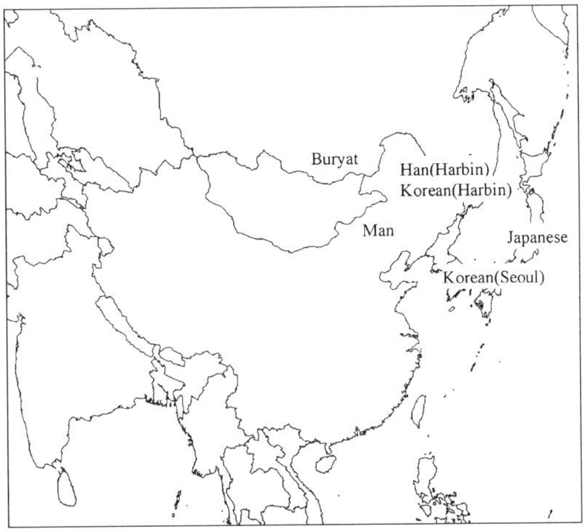

Figure 1. Map of residing areas of five ethnic groups and Japanese.

Materials and methods

HLA-A, B antigens and DRB1 alleles in 923 healthy unrelated subjects including 570 Chinese (197 Northern Han, 172 Man, 201 Northern Koreans) living near Harbin city, 212 Southern Koreans, and 141 Buryat have been typed. All subjects were typed for HLA-A and B antigens using a standard microcytotoxicity method. For typing of HLA-DRB1 alleles, PCR-microtiter plate hybridization (PCR-MPH) low- and high- resolution typing plates were used [1, 2]. For the confirmation of alleles typed by PCR-MPH, PCR-single strand conformation polymorphism (PCR-SSCP) method was used [3]. The frequencies of HLA-A-B-DRB1 haplotypes were calculated from phenotype data using the program previously developed [4] for the 11th International Histocompatibility Workshop (11th IHW).

Results and discussion

Table I presents the distribution of HLA-A-B-DRB1 haplotypes observed at frequencies of more than 2% in some of the ethnic groups. Several common haplotypes were shared among Japanese, Northern Koreans and Southern Koreans. The most common haplotype in Japanese, A24-B52-DRB1*1502, was observed in both Northern Koreans (2.2%) and Southern Koreans (1.5%) with relatively high frequencies [5, 6]. In both Northern and Southern Koreans, the most common haplotype was A33-B44-DRB1*1302. This haplotype was second most common in Japanese (4.8%), and also common in Northern Han [5, 6]. Other three common haplotypes in Japanese, A24-B7-DRB1*0101, A24-B54-DRB1*0405 and A2-B46-DRB1*0803, were observed in both Northern and Southern Koreans with frequencies of >0.5%. Two haplotypes, A33-B17-DRB1*1302 and A33-B44-DRB1*0701, however, observed with more than 2% in Northern and Southern Koreans were rare in Japanese. The former type was the second most common haplotype in Buryat (3.5%).

A30-B13-DRB1*0701 was the most frequent haplotype in Northern Han (4.0%) and Man (5.8%), and also observed in Korean populations. A2-B13-DRB1*0701 was the most frequent haplotype in Buryat (4.6%) and less frequently observed in Man (0.6%), but it was rare in the other four ethnic groups. These two haplotypes carrying HLA-B13 were rare in Japanese but frequently observed in various

Table I. Common HLA-A,-B,-DRB1 haplotypes in six East-Asian populations

A- B-DRB1	Buryat (n=141)	Man (n=172)	N. Han (n=197)	Korean (N. China) (n=201)	Korean (n=212)	Japanese* (n=1216)
24- 7-0101				1.7	3.3	4.0
2-61-1501		2.9	0.6			0.5
24-52-1502				2.2	1.4	8.6
24-61-0401	2.5					
2-70-0401	2.1			0.7		
24-54-0405	1.3	1.2		0.9	1.2	3.1
11-62-0406		1.7		2.5	0.7	1.2
24-60-1101			2.0			
2-13-1202		3.0	2.0	2.0	1.2	0.6
33-17-1302	3.5		0.8	2.5	2.6	
33-44-1302			2.0	3.5	5.1	4.8
24-61-1401	2.1					
2-52-1404		2.3				
2-13-0701	4.6	0.6				
30-13-0701		5.8	4.0	1.7	2.4	
23-44-0701	2.5					
33-44-0701				2.5	3.0	
2-50-0701	2.8					
2-46-0803			0.8	0.7	1.4	2.2
2-51-0901	2.5	0.6	0.7		1.3	0.7
2-75-0901		2.3	1.4			

*: Data from 11th Japan HLA Workshop [5].

ethnic groups in Europe [7]. Another B13-carrying haplotype, A2-B13-DRB1*1202, was observed in five ethnic groups except for Buryat.

In Buryat, two HLA-A-C-B-DR-DQ haplotypes possessing the same class II haplotype, A2-Cw7-B70-DR4-DQ7 and A24-Cw10-B61-DR4-DQ7, were frequently observed [8]. Latter type was commonly observed in Inuit (Eskimo) and South Amerindians [7]. In the present study, A2-B70-DRB1*0401 and A24-B61-DRB1*0401 were observed in Buryat, at the frequency of 2.5%. Thus, it is suggested that DR4 antigen carrying by above two haplotypes is encoded by DRB1*0401.

Consequently, similarities as well as heterogeneities among these East Asian populations have been revealed in terms of HLA-A-B-DRB1 haplotypes.

References

1. Kawai S, Maekawajiri S, Tokunaga K, Juji T, Yamane A. A simple method of HLA-DRB typing using enzymatically amplified DNA immobilized probes on microtiter plate. *Hum Immunol.* 1994; 41: 121-6.
2. Kawai S, Maekawajiri S, Tokunaga K, Miyamoto M, Akaza T, Juji T, Yamane A. HLA-DRB typing using PCR-MPH (microtiter plate hybridization). *MHC and IRS* 1994; 1 (suppl) : 121-5.
3. Bannai M, Tokunaga L, Lin L, Kuwata S, Mazda T, Amaki I, Fujisawa K, Juji T. Discrimination of human HLA-DRB1 alleles by PCR-SSCP (single strand conformation polymorphism) method. *Eur J Immunogenet* 1994; 21: 1-9.
4. Imanishi T, Akaza T, Kimura A, Tokunaga K, Gojobori T. Estimation of allele and haplotype frequencies for HLA and complement loci. In: Tsuji K *et al.* eds. *HLA 1991,* vol. 1. Oxford: Oxford University Press, 1992: 76-9.
5. Akaza T, Imanishi T, Fujiwara K, Tokunaga K, Yashiki S, Fujiyoshi T, Sonoda S, Juji T. HLA alleles and haplotypes of Japanese population. *MHC and IRS* 1994; 1(suppl): 219-26.
6. Tokunaga K, Imanishi T, Takahashi K, Juji T. On the origin and dispersal of East Asian populations as viewed from HLA haplotypes. In: Akazawa T, Szathmary EJ eds. *Prehistoric Mongoloid Dispersals.* Oxford: Oxford University Press, 1996: 187-97.
7. Imanishi T, Akaza T, Kimura A, Tokunaga K, Gojobori T. Allele and haplotype frequencies for HLA and complement loci in various groups. In: Tsuji K *et al.* eds. *HLA 1991*, vol. 1. Oxford: Oxford University Press, 1992: 1065-220.
8. Tokunaga K, Sideltseva EW, Tanaka H, Uchikawa C, Nieda M, Sideltsev VV, Zhuravleva E, Imanishi T, Itoh K, Akaza T, Takahashi K, Khalturin V, Alexeev LP, Juji T. Distribution of HLA antigens and haplotypes in the Buryat population of Siberia. *Tissue Antigens* 1995; 45: 98-102.

Are the Trobrianders emigrants of South-East Asia ?

M. Nagy, H. Zimdahl, C. Krüger, P. Anders, M. Kayser, L. Roewer, W. Schiefenhövel[1]

Institute of Forensic Medicine/Charite, Hannoversche Strasse 6, 10115 Berlin, Germany
1 Humanethologie I D MPG, Andechs ,Germany

The colonization of the West Pacific has been much examined with linguistic, archaeological, and anthropological evidence increasingly being supplemented by genetic data early with serological studies [2] and later on with DNA typing [1,3-6,8-10].
Two major prehistoric migration stages are thougt to have occured in this area. First, beginning approximately 50 000 years ago ancient hunting and gathering groups are believed to have emigrated to Melanesia. Second, Austronesian speaking horticultural groups with advanced voyaging technology entered New Guinea about 2 000 to 3 000 years BC. So, New Guinea mainland and the surrounding islands are settled with two fundamentally different populations, classed according to their linguistic affiliations «Papuan» and «Austronesian». Papuans are spread throughout most of New Guinea, whereas the Austronesian speakers live mainly on some islands in the north and east of New Guinea and on the mentioned region of the Northern coast *(Figure 1)*. The most surprising fact is that Austronesian languages are not confined to Melanesia but are spoken by people living so far away as Taiwan, Easter Island, New Zealand and Madagascar. The relative unity of Austronesian languages in Melanesia can be attributed to a relatively small time span of separation.
In the seventies, German human ethologists were looking for a traditional island population in the West Pacific for their anthropological investigations. In this

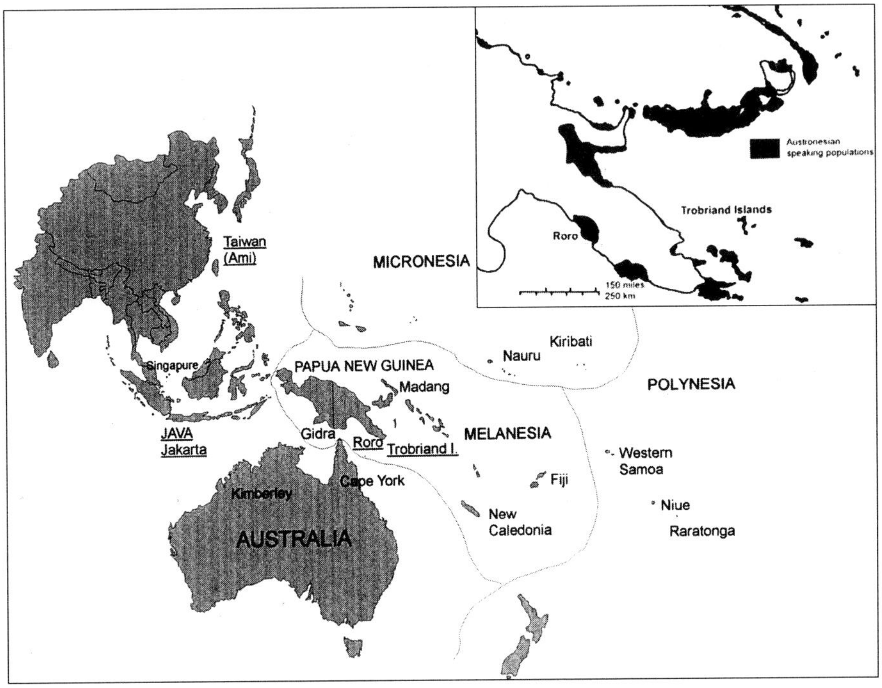

Figure 1. Geographical locations of studies and published populations in Asia-Oceania and Austronesian language groups in Melanesian (studied populations are underlined).

Table I. HLA-DRB1 and -DPB1 allele frequencies in three populations of Asia-Oceania

	Allele frequency[1] and standard error[2] (%) in populations[3]						
DRB1 allele	***TROB N = 81***	***RORO N = 26***	***JAVA N = 58***	***DPB1 allele***	***TROB N = 81***	***RORO N = 26***	***JAVA N = 58***
0101	0.0	0.0	0.9±0.8	**0101**	0.6±0.6	2.1±2.1	1.7±1.2
1501	0.0	0.0	1.7±1.2	**0201**	0.6±0.6	8.3±4.0	2.6±1.5
1502	7.4±2.1	23.1±5.8	14.6±3.3	**0202**	0.0	0.0	7.8±2.5
1601	0.0	1.9±1.9	0.0	**0301**	0.0	0.0	5.2±2.2
1602	4.3±1.6	21.2±5.7	1.7±1.2	**0401**	1.2±0.8	12.5±4.8	20.7±3.8
0301	0.0	0.0	1.7±1.2	**0402**	0.0	2.1±2.1	4.3±1.9
0401	0.0	3.8±2.6	0.0	**0501**	97.6±1.2	70.8±6.6	13.8±3.2
0403	12.3±2.6	9.6±4.1	0.8±0.8	**0901**	0.0	0.0	0.9±0.8
0404	0.6±0.6	0.0	0.0	**1301**	0.0	0.0	21.6±3.8
0405	5.6±1.8	3.8±2.6	2.6±1.5	**1401**	0.0	2.1±2.1	1.7±1.2
0406	0.0	0.0	1.7±1.2	**1501**	0.0	0.0	0.9±0.8
1101	6.2±1.9	1.9±1.9	2.6±1.5	**1701**	0.0	0.0	0.9±0.8
1201	0.6±0.6	3.8±2.6	0.0	**1901**	0.0	0.0	0.9±0.8
1202	1.8±1.0	0.0	53.4±4.6	**26012**	0.0	0.0	0.9±0.8
13	0.0	0.0	1.7±1.2	**2801**	0.0	0.0	12.1±3.0
1401	8.7±2.2	3.8±2.6	0.0	**3101**	0.0	2.1±2.1	2.6±1.5
1404	0.6±0.6	0.0	3.4±1.7	**05/38**	0.0	0.0	1.7±1.2
1407	0.6±0.6	0.0	0.0				
1408	0.6±0.6	3.8±2.6	0.0				
0701	0.0	0.0	8.6±2.6				
0803	32.1±3.7	9.6±4.1	0.9±0.8				
0810	0.6±0.6	0.0	0.0				
0901	17.9±3.0	13.5±4.7	1.7±1.2				
1001	0.0	0.0	1.7±1.2				

N = Number of typed unrelated individuals.

1) Allele frequencies were calculated by direct counting.

2) Standard errors were computed as the square root of the variance of a binomial distribution [f(1-f)/2N], where f represents the frequency and N the number of individuals tested.

3) TROB =Trobriand Islanders, RORO =Papua New Guinean Lowlanders, JAVA =Javaneses.

time cultural change led to fundamental social and economical changes on islands like Nauru, Majuro and the Salomon islands. The people on the small Trobriand island Kaileuna still adhered to life style and customs described by early ethnographers, living in wooden houses thatched with pandanus and sago leaves, subsisting by planting yams, fishing, gathering and exchanging ceremonial valuables by voyaging [7].

In this study, we have compared genetic findings in the different areas of Melanesia in order to test the hypothesis that the likely origin of the Austronesian odyssey was South-East Asia and we were particularly interested in the genetic relationship of two distinct Austronesian culture and language groups with the Austronesian arrival: the Trobriand islanders east of New Guinea and the Roro people living on the Southern coast of the mainland approximatly 150 kms west of Port Moresby. We have examined nucleotide sequence polymorphisms at the DRB1, DQA1, DQB1 and DPB1 loci in Trobriand, Roro, Ami (results not shown because of the small number of samples) and Javanese populations, using SSO-, SSP- and sequencing based typing described in the 12th Workshop protocol.

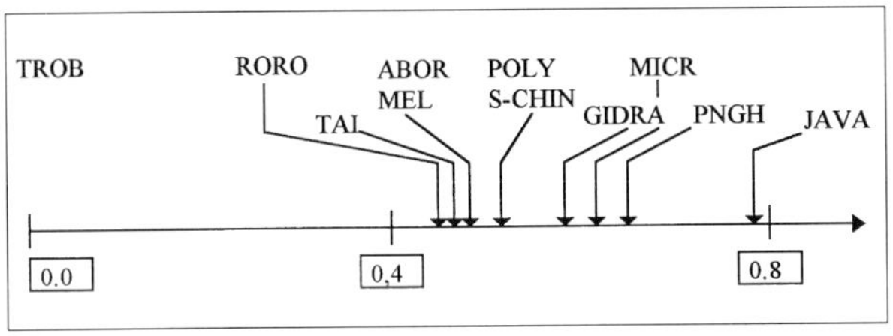

Figure 2. Genetic distances between Trobriand Islanders and studied and published populations of Asia-Oceania (DRB1-Locus).
TROB = Trobriand Islanders; RORO = Papua New Guinean Lowlanders, Austronesian; JAVA = Javaneses. S-CHIN = Singapore Chineses [3]; TAI = Taiwan Aborigines [4]; MEL = Melanesians [6]; PNGH = Papua New Guinean Highlanders [6]; MICR = Micronesian[6]; POLY = Polynesian [6]; ABOR = Australian Aborigines [6]; GIDRA = Papua New Guinean Lowlanders, Non-Austronesian [9].

Results and discussion

HLA-DRB1 and -DPB1 allele frequencies in three ethnic groups are given in *Table I*. The main features are:

1. The number of different HLA alleles segregating the populations is relatively small with a total of only 16 allels being discovered at the DRB1 locus and 4 respectively 7 different alleles in Trobriand islanders and Roro peoples being found at the DPB1 locus. Especially the results of the DPB1 analysis - 98% of the Trobriand samples carry the Asian DPB1 allele *0501 (Buyi 52%, Japanese 39.0%, Singapore Chinese 48.1% [3] - provide evidence of the South-east Asian origin of Trobriand islanders. This lack of diversity may probably reflect a limited genetic diversity of the founding population followed by population explosion with no subsequent gene flow from the periphery and/or the effect of drift would have reduced the number of alleles in the population [2].
2. Because genetic data of complete families were not available, class II haplotypes were inferred from the analysis of linkage disequilibrium patterns of alleles in homozygous and heterozygous individuals. The DRB1-DQA1-DQB1 haplotypes of the Trobriand islanders and Roro were the same as those commonly seen in Asia. The most common haplotype found in the Trobriand samples is with 32% DRB1*0803-DQA1*0103-DQB1*0601 the same as in Australian East Cape York aborigines (29%) [6] representing that the Trobriander and Cape York aborigines may considered to have the same origin. In Japanese and Korean populations this haplotype is one of the three most common haplotypes.[3,8] The shared most common haplotype of DRB1*1202-DQA1*0601-DQB1*0301 in Javanese and Micronesian populations found by GAO and SERJEANTSON [6] could be confirmed.
A DRB1*15021-DQB1*0502 and a DRB1*0901-DQB1*0601 haplotype was also seen in Trobriand and Roro samples which have not been detected in other populations.
3. There was no significant discordance of genotype frequencies from their Hardy-Weinberg expectations (Goodness of Fit-Test for the most frequent genotypes).
4. The genetic distances showed in *Figure 2* and *3* were computed from allele frequencies according to

$$D_{xy} = 1/2 \sum_{i=1}^{k} |f_{xi} - f_{yi}|$$

where f_{xi} and f_{yi} are the allelic frequencies observed in populations x and y, respectively, and k is the total number of alleles. The results demonstrate the shortest distance between the two Austronesian speaking populations -the Trobriand and Roro people -although this distance of 0.45 in *Figure 2* is relatively high, which can be attributed to a relatively long time span of separation and independent development of these two populations. Otherwise the present data show that the Trobriand islanders are genetically closer to Aboriginal Australians and Taiwanese than to the Nonaustronesian speaking Papuans from the New Guinea Highlands and Lowlands.

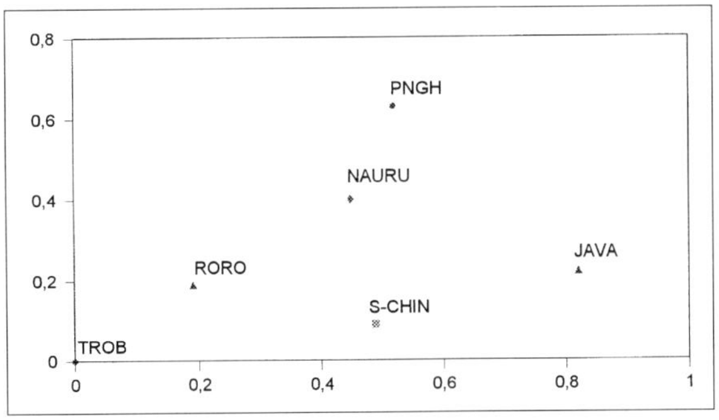

Figure 3. Genetic distances between studied and published populations of Asia-Oceania (DPB1-Locus).
TROB = Trobriand Islanders; RORO = Papua New Guinean Lowlanders, Austronesian; JAVA = Javaneses.
S-CHIN = Singapore Chineses [3], PNGH = Papua New Guinean Highlanders[3], NAURU = Micronesians [1].

The very short distance of 0.39 between the Austronesian Roro's and the Nonaustronesian speaking Gidra [9] population confirmed that the linguistic difference is not reflected in genetic distance. This suggests that although the Roro remain a distinct cultural unit there has been genetic admixture with neighbouring Lowland groups. This is also known from oral history. There should be considerable exchange of marriage partners between different linguistic neighbours so that the linguistic differences do not necessarily act as a barrier to gene flow.

Nevertheless the Trobriand population seems to be characterized by the allele repertoire of the colonizing population - possibly South-East Asian -, by relatively strong geographic isolation coupled with some degree of selection and genetic drift up to the last generations. From 150 investigated Trobriand islanders - we had collected genealogical data down to the third generation - only five of them stated that one of their parents or grand parents originated from outside the Trobriand islands in spite of the exchanging system over hundreds of kilometers to islands like Woodlark, Dentrecasteaux and more remote islands by voyaging. Those genetic findings coincide with the opinion of the Trobriand islanders that there is no reason to leave their rich and lovely islands.

Y-chromosomal and especially mt-DNA studies of the Trobriand and Roro people together with HLA analysis of other distinct populations of Asia-Oceania especially Taiwan aborigines will give further information on the real scenario which happened on the Trobriand and other islands during the colonization of the Pacific up to present time.

Acknowledgements

The field survey among the Trobriand and Roro people was supported by the Chiang Ching-Kuo Foundation of Taiwan.

We thank Erika Hagelberg for helpful comments and discussions. Thanks are due, most especially, to the people of Trobriand and Roro villages for their cooperation in providing the blood samples for testing.

References

1. Easteal S, Voorhoeve AH, Zimmet P, Serjeantson SW. RFLP-defined HLA-DP polymorphism in four ethnic groups. *Hum Immunol* 1989 ; 25 : 169-79.
2. Hill VS, Serjeantson SW. The colonization of the Pacific. A genetic trail. Oxford: Oxford Clarendon Press, 1989.
3. Tsuji K, Aizawa M, Sasazuki T. Ethnic code No. 20202, 40101, 40104, 40204 and 40421. *HLA 1991.* Oxford : Oxford University Press, 1992 : 1169.
4. Kobayashi K, Atoh M, Suzuki H, Oshima K, Young CD, Huang KY, Zon YH, Sekiguchi S. A study of HLA distribution among Taiwan Aborigines. In : Tsuji K, Aizawa M, Sasazuki T eds. *HLA 1991.* Oxford : Oxford University Press, 1992 : 679-80.
5. Bhatia K, Doran T, Roberts M, Prasad M, Kimura A, Dunckley H, Beck HP, Witt C, Varney M, Sullivan J, Koki G, McCluskey J, Tait B, Sadler N, Kabintik S, Woodfield G. Genetic variation in populations of the South-west Pacific. In : Tsuji K, Aizawa M, Sasazuki T eds. *HLA 1991.* Oxford : Oxford University Press, 1992 : 641-3.
6. Gao X, Serjeantson SW. Analysis of 2600 HLA-DR, DQ haplotypes in Asia-Oceania. In : Tsuji K, Aizawa M, Sasazuki T eds. *HLA 1991.*Oxford: Oxford University Press, 1992 : 229-32.
7. Schiefenhövel W, Uher J, Krell R. Im Spiegel der Anderen. München: Realis Verlags-GmbH, 1993.
8. Hashimoto M, Kinoshita T, Yamasaki M, Tanaka H, Imanishi T, Ihara H, Ichikawa Y, Fukunushi T. Gene frequencies and haplotypic associations within the HLA region in 916 unrelated Japanese individuals. *Tissue Antigens* 1994 ; 44 : 166-73.
9. Yoshida M, Ohtsuka R, Nakazawa M, Juji T, Tokunaga K. HLA-DRB1 frequencies of Non-Austronesian-Speaking Gidra in South New Guinea and their genetic affinities with Oceanian populations. *Am J Phys Anthropol* 1995 ; 96 : 177-81.
10. Melton T, Peterson R, Redd AJ, Saha N, Sofro ASM, Martinson J, Stoneking M. Polynesian genetic affinities with Southeast Asian populations as identified by mtDNA analysis. *Am J Hum Genet* 1995 ; 57 : 403-14.

A comparison of HLA-DRB1 and -DQB1 alleles in three Lebanese villages reproductively isolated by geography and religion

W.B. Bias[1], N. Nuwayri-Salti[2], W.H. Wood[1], B. Cissell[1], S. Berger[1], B.J. Schmeckpeper[1]

1 Immunogenetics Laboratories, Johns Hopkins University School of Medicine, 2041 East Monument Street, Baltimore MD 21205-2222, USA
2 American University of Beirut, Beirut, Lebanon

Until recently, the societies of the Middle East have been differentiated on the basis of religion rather than economics. These historic customs have had a profound influence on present social patterns. Until the last few decades, Lebanon has been a peasant society primarily residing in small agricultural villages. In these rural societies, loyalities to clan, village, and sect continue to be of primary importance in virtually all spheres of activity. Of special interest for this study are the marriage customs. In general, marriages occur outside the conjugal family but are endogamous within the extended family. Within societies of remote villages, marriage is prohibited with members of other sects. Especially favored are patrilateral parallel cousin marriages, *i.e.*, those in which a male marries his father's brother's daughter [1]. As in all societies, historic customs such as these become blurred with migrations to urban areas and a degree of exogamy becomes acceptable.

The social structure of Lebanese villages presented an opportunity to determine the magnitude of differences in HLA allele frequencies between small populations derived from a single parental ethnic population but reproductively isolated by religious customs for several centuries. In order to minimize gene flow, the villages were selected to be relatively distant geographically, as well *(Figure 1)*. Our hypothesis was that the village populations originated from the same gene pool, but inbreeding and random genetic drift would result in considerable variation in the frequencies of shared alleles and/or the occurrence of "village specific" alleles.

The experimental design was to obtain test samples from 50 nuclear families comprised of both parents and two children in each of three villages. The parents would represent the «random» sample. The children of each mating would permit haplotype assignments (not reported here). The villages selected were Kafar Zubian (KZ), pop. 6,000 Maronite Christians; Niha el Shouff (NS), pop. 4,200 Druze Muslims; and Yohmor (YH), pop. 3,000 Shia Muslims [2]. KZ has been reproductively isolated since the 16th century, NS since the10th century, and YH since the late 16th to early 17th century [2]. Actual numbers of families from whom blood samples were obtained were 51 in KZ, 46 in NS, and 50 in YH, each with the requisite two offspring. Lymphocytes were isolated in the American University, Beirut (AUB)

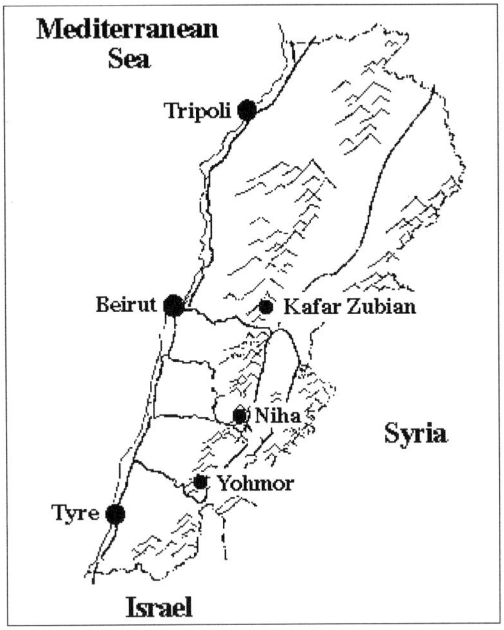

Figure 1. Map of Lebanon showing relative geographic positions of the villages of Kafar Zubian, Niha el Shouff, and Yohmor.

laboratory of NN-S, frozen in liquid nitrogen (LN) until transported in LN to Johns Hopkins. Unfortunate difficulties in transport both in Lebanon and internationally resulted in a loss in viability of most cells and failure of a few samples to amplify in PCR. Consequently, no class I typing was carried out and no cell lines initiated. The final data base consisted of 93 parental samples from KZ, 59 from NS, and 81 from YH. A portion of each sample was retained in the AUB laboratory from which it may be possible to initiate cell lines and/or do DNA-based class I typing at a later date. This report and two posters presented at these proceedings, together, describe the results of class II typing using the 12IHWS SSOP protocols for DRB1, DRB3, DRB4, DRB5, DQB1 and DPB1.

A total of 36 previously reported DRB1 alleles were represented in the three villages. KZ had 24, NS had 25, and YH had 22 alleles. The most frequently shared alleles were DRB1*0701, *1104, *1101, accounting for 35% of KZ, 52% of NS, and 55% of YH alleles. All three villages shared 15 of the 36 alleles, but differed in frequencies. Five alleles were shared by two villages, while the remaining 16 alleles were found in only one village. An unusual allele, DRB1*1112, was observed in 4/118 alleles of the NS parental samples and in 9/62 alleles of 31 non-parental volunteer donors from this village. It was not observed in KZ nor YH. DRB1*1112 was described by Baxter-Lowe in a single sample of unknown ethnic origin (AC#L23988). The DRB1 alleles and their distribution are shown in *Table I*.

Table II shows the distribution of DQB1 alleles in the three village populations. Twelve alleles were observed in KZ, 11 in NS, and 13 in YH. As expected from DR/DQ linkage disequilibrium, four DQB1alleles, DQB1*0301, *02XX, *0501, and *0302, accounted for 77% of all alleles in all villages.

Goodness-of-fit to Hardy-Weinberg equilibrium was calculated for both DRB1 and DQB1. Therewas no deviation from expectation for either locus in any of the three villages. For DRB1: $\chi^2 = 37.39$ (62 df), p = 0.9944 for KZ; $\chi^2 = 29.44$ (46 df), p = 0.9726 for NS; and $\chi^2 = 54.25$ (51 df), p = 0.3517 for YH.

Similarly, for DQB1: $\chi^2 = 26.27$ (31 df), p = 0.7083 for KZ; $\chi^2 = 18.19$ (23 df), p = 0.7474 for NS; and $\chi^2 = 41.50$ (34 df), p = 0.1763 for YH.

Genetic distance between the villages was calculated using the formula [3]:

$$D = \sqrt{1 - \sum_{j=1}^{n} \sqrt{p_{Aj}\, p_{Bj}}}$$

D = Genetic distance
p Aj = frequency of allele j in population A
p Bj = frequency of allele j in population B

Genetic distance will range from 0 to 1.0, with 0 expected within a randomly breeding single population and a

Table I. Frequencies of DRB1 alleles

Alleles	KZ (n=186)	NS (n-118)	YH (n=162)
A. Alleles occurring in all three villages			
1104	**0.2366**	**0.1696**	**0.1296**
1101	**0.0699**	**0.1017**	**0.1667**
0701	**0.0430**	**0.0932**	**0.1975**
1001	**0.0054**	**0.1525**	**0.0556**
0102	0.0968	0.0254	0.0309
03011	0.0914	0.0169	0.0741
0402	0.0215	0.0254	0.0864
0403	0.0914	0.0254	0.0432
0404	0.0161	0.0169	0.0247
1301	0.0323	0.0339	0.0123
1302	0.0161	0.0508	0.0185
1303	0.0161	0.0678	0.0123
1401	0.0269	0.0339	0.0432
1501	0.0054	0.0085	0.0123
1502	0.0161	0.0085	0.0432
B. Alleles occurring in two villages			
0101	0.0430	0.0	0.0062
0401	0.0376	0.0085	0.0
1305	0.0161	0.0	0.0062
1404	0.0323	0.0085	0.0
1601	0.0	0.0085	0.0123
C. Alleles occurring in one village			
0405	0.0323	0.0	0.0
0406	0.0	0.0085	0.0
0407	0.0054	0.0	0.0
0408	0.0	0.0	0.0062
0410	0.0	0.0085	0.0
0801	0.0	0.0424	0.0
0804	0.0108	0.0	0.0
0810	0.0	0.0254	0.0
1102	0.0	0.0	0.0062
1103	0.0	0.0169	0.0
1112	0.0	0.0339	0.0
1201	0.0161	0.0	0.0
1311	0.0	0.0	0.0062
1318	0.0	0.0	0.0062
1414	0.0	0.0085	0.0
1602	0.0215	0.0	0.0

Table II. Frequencies of DQB1 alleles

Alleles	KZ (n=186)	NS (n-118)	YH (n=162)
0301	**0.3883**	**0.4508**	**0.3171**
02XX	**0.1596**	**0.1066**	**0.2073**
0501	**0.1489**	**0.1639**	**0.0976**
0302	**0.0798**	**0.0492**	**0.1463**
0305	0.0585	0.0246	0.0183
0503	0.0585	0.0410	0.0427
0603	0.0319	0.0328	0.0183
0502	0.0213	0.0246	0.0122
0402	0.0160	0.0492	0.0244
0601	0.0160	0.0082	0.0427
0604	0.0160	0.0492	0.0244
0602	0.0053	0.0	0.0061
03032	0.0	0.0	0.0427

maximum of 1.0 between two populations with no shared alleles. The results of these calculations using DRB1 and DQB1 are as follows:

KZ - NS: DRB1 = .5182; DQB1 = .1503

KZ - YH: DRB1 = .4454; DQB1 = .2104

NS - YH: DRB1 = .4149; DQB1 = .2628

The lower genetic distance estimates for DQB1 result from fewer alleles, most of which are shared at that locus.

These comparisons of DRB1 allele frequencies in three Lebanese village populations show that a single highly polymorphic locus can demonstrate whether relatively small populations are in Hardy-Weinberg equilibrium. They also can provide reasonable estimates of the effects of inbreeding, drift, or gene flow.

The authors wish to express their gratitude for the support of the Ministry of Public Health of Lebanon in facilitating the field work in the villages visited for this study.

References

1. Alamuddin, Nura S, Starr, Paul D. Crucial bonds. Marriage among the Lebanese Druze. Delmar NY: Caravan Books, 1980.
2. Boutros MA. Introduction to Lebanon. The Encyclopedia of the Lebanese cities and villages, 1979.
3. Cavalli-Sforza LL, Bodmer WF. The genetics of human populations. San Francisco: W.H. Freeman and Co, 1971.

HLA class II and Gm markers in Ethiopian Oromo and Amhara populations

M. Fort [1], J.M. Dugoujon [2], G. Scano [3], E. Ohayon [1], M. Abbal [1], G.F. De Stefano [3]

1 Service d'Immunologie, CHU Rangueil, 1, avenue Jean Poulhes, 31403 Toulouse Cedex 4, France
2 Centre d'Immunopathologie et de Génétique Humaine, CNRS UPR 8291, Toulouse, France
3 Department of biology, Roma University, Italy

The Ethiopian populations tested for the anthropology component of the 12th International Histocompatibility Workshop consisted of 83 Oromo and 98 Amhara.
In Ethiopia, the currently population seems to have resulted from a large intermixing during the last three millennia, among different populations such as Mediterranean, Sudanic, Oriental, Semitic and Cushitic. Despite this, two ethnic groups emerge : Amhara and Oromo, representing 38% and 35% of the Ethiopian population.
Amhara descend from South-Arabia Semitic conquerors. They live in the central and western part of the country and are essentially agriculturists. Their language belongs to the Semitic division of the Afro-Asiatic family. Most of them are Christians and monogamy prevails.
Oromo represent an important group among Cushitic people. Their language is part of the Cushitic branch of the Afro-Asiatic language family. They were naturally nomads and became sedentary agriculturists because of the admixture with Amhara and other ethnic groups. Therefore, the Oromo of the Western and Northern regions have become either Muslims or Christians and those living in the southern part of the country are pagans.

Materials and methods

The blood samples were collected in the Arssi province. All individuals, their parents and grandparents belonged to the corresponding ethnic group.
HLA class II typing was performed using PCR-SSO technic and IgG Gm typing using passive inhibition of hemagglutination.

Results and discussion

Among the Gm observed haplotypes : Gm*1,17;..;5*, Gm*1,17;..;5,6,10,11,14, and Gm*1,17;..;5,6,11,24 are characteristic of sub Saharian African populations. They represent 55 % of the whole haplotypes. Three other haplotypes: Gm*1,17;..;21,28, Gm*3;23;5* and Gm*3;..;5* are commonly found in Caucasoid and Mediterranean populations. The Gm*1,17;..;10,11, 13,15,16 haplotype, frequent in some East Asian populations but rare in Near East and India, is present only in Oromo population at a frequency of 1,52%.
HLA class II DRB1, DQB1, and DQA1 allele frequencies are reported in *Figure 1*. They were compared with our local reference panel of 1300 volunteer bone marrow donors from South of France. Both studied Ethiopian populations differ of the Caucasoid reference population with a decrease of DRB1*11 ($p<0.001$) and an increase of DRB1*13 ($p<0.01$). DRB1*08 is significantly increased only in Amhara, ($p<0.02$). The most interesting feature is found in DRB1*08 and DRB1*13 subtypes. About 90 % of the DRB1*08 subtypes are DRB1*0804 and 70 % of DRB1*13 are DRB1*1302 in both populations. Missing alleles is DRB1*09 in both population and DRB1*12 only in Amhara.
A borderline DRB1*01 allele frequency difference exists between Oromo and Amhara ($p<0.05$). A corresponding difference is found on DQB1*0501 and DQA1*0101/0104 allele frequencies ($p<0.05$) which are well known to be in linkage disequilibrium with DRB1*01.
The high frequency of DQB1*0604 and DQB1*0605 compared to our Caucasoid population ($p<0.001$ in both groups) is consistent with the linkage desequilibrium of the major DRB1*13 subtype *i. e.* DRB1*1302.
No additional difference at the DQA1 locus is observed. According to previously described associations in various populations, we defined the putative haplotypes of the three-locus HLA class II region : DRB1-DQA1-DQB1.

Table I. Three-locus HLA class II haplotype frequencies (HF)

Oromo					Amhara					French reference population				
DRB1	**DQA1**	**DQB1**	**n**	**HF**	**DRB1**	**DQA1**	**DQB1**	**n**	**HF**	**DRB1**	**DQA1**	**DQB1**	**n**	**HF**
7	201	201	31	**0,1867**	7	201	201	38	**0,1938**	11	501	301	22	**0,1358**
301	501	201	16	**0,0961**	1	101/4	501	24	**0,1224**	7	201	201	20	**0,1234**
4	3	302	15	**0,0903**	1302	102	604	20	**0,1021**	2	102	602	18	**0,1111**
1302	102	604	15	**0,0903**	301	501	201	16	**0,0816**	4	3	302	16	**0,0987**
2	102	602	14	**0,0843**	804	501	301	15	**0,0765**	301	501	201	15	**0,0925**
1302	102	605	11	**0,0662**	2	102	602	14	**0,0714**	1	101/4	501	13	**0,0802**
1	101/4	501	9	**0,0542**	4	3	302	11	**0,0561**	1301	103	603	10	**0,0617**
2	102	603	6	**0,0361**	1302	102	605	11	**0,0561**	2	102	502	7	**0,0432**
4	3	201	6	**0,0361**	2	102	603	7	**0,0357**	4	3	301	7	**0,0432**
4	3	402	5	**0,0301**	10	101/4	501	6	**0,0306**	801	401	402	5	**0,0308**

Figure 1. Allele frequencies.

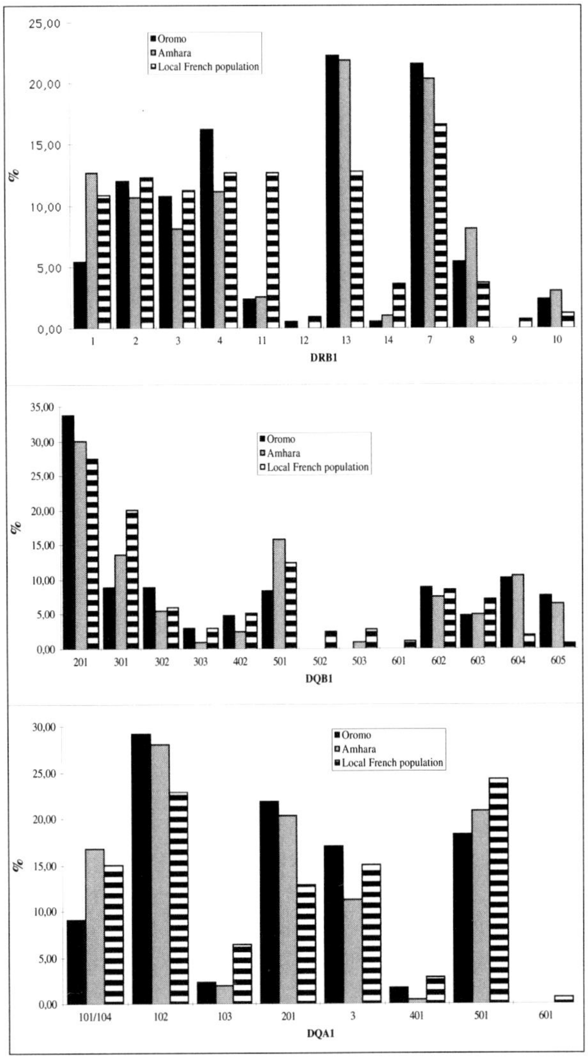

Among the ten more frequent haplotypes (*Table I*), DRB1*07-DQA1*0201-DQB1*0201 is the main one and is typical of these populations. In the same way, the high frequency of DRB1*1302-DQA1*0102-DQB1*0604 or 0605 is characteristic of Amhara and Oromo. The DRB1*11-DQA1*0501-DQB1*0301 haplotype usually frequent in caucasoid and negroid populations is weakly represented in Ethiopians.

In respect to the number of HLA haplotypes, the Amhara population is more homogeneous than the Oromo one (23 haplotypes versus 28). Two unexpected haplotypes:DRB1*0301-DQA1*0201-DQB1*0201 and DRB1*0804-DQA1*03-DQB1*0201 are reported in the Oromo group.

Such a greater genetic diversity among the Oromo population seems to be related to their migration and mixing tendency. This is in good agreement with their larger geographical distribution and way of life.

It would be interesting to calculate genetic distances between both populations and others submitted to the XIIth International Histocompatibility Workshop.

HLA class II anthropological study in the Polish population from Wielkopolska

*M. Jungerman[1], A. Sanchez-Mazas[2], P. Fichna[3], R. Ivanova[4], D. Charron[4,5], J. Hors[4], S. Djoulah**

1 Institute of Human Genetics, Polish Academy of Sciences, Strzeszynska 32, 60-479 Poznan, Poland
2 Laboratory of Genetics and Biometry, Department of Anthropology and Ecology, University of Geneva, Switzerland
3 Institute of Pediatrics, Academy of Medicine, Poznan, Poland
4 LNH, Department of Immunology, Saint-Louis Hospital, Paris, France
5 INSERM U396, Paris, France
*Address for correspondence: LNH, Centre Hayem, Hôpital Saint-Louis
1, avenue Claude Vellefaux, 75475 Paris Cedex10, France

Previous genetic distance analyses of HLA-A and -B polymorphisms suggest that European populations differentiate into a northern and a southern group [1]. According to these data, the Polish appear to be genetically close to their geographic neighbours Slovak and Ukrainian, which also speak an Indo-European Slavic language.
We thus selected a random sample of Polish individuals to analyze the SSP polymorphism of DRB1, DQA1 and DQB1 loci. We present here the allele estimated for this population, as well as a preliminary comparison to other Europeans.

Materials and methods

Subject studies

DNA was isolated for a total of 99 healthy individuals originating from Wielkopolska (51°3'-53° North, 15°-18°30' East), which is a historic province located in mid-western Poland. It covers an area of approximately 45,000 square kilometres inhabited by 5,5 million people, which represent about 14% of the whole area and population of Poland. The largest city of the province is Poznan. It was Wielkopolska when the state of Poland was brought to life, on the turn of the 9th century. Since then, some migrations took place, especially from neighbouring Germany.

HLA typing

HLA DRB1 and DQB1 alleles were determined by INNO-LIPA HLA typing tests (Innogenetics NV, Zwijnaarde, Belgium) based on the reverse hybridization principle [2].
For HLA-DQA1 typing, we used the DNA PCR-SSO method. The SSO probes were 3' end labelled (DIG-11-ddUTP) [3].

Statistical analysis

Allele and haplotype frequencies were estimated by a maximum likelihood method algorithm using the program package ARLEQUIN (Excoffier, Schneider and Kuffer, personal communication). Genetic distances (defined as $D_{xy} = \frac{1}{2}\sum\left|x_i - y_i\right|$, where x_i and y_i are the frequencies of the ith allele in populations x and y, respectively, and k is the size of the frequency vector [4] were computed as for previous HLA data analyses [5]. A set of 16 population samples from all parts of Europe was considered (see legend for *Figure 1*). The following subset of currently known HLA alleles was taken into account for the genetic distance analysis.
The mean genetic distance matrix computed over loci DRB1, DQA1, and DQB1 was used for a principal coordinate analysis, using the local program Ancoo (Roessli *et al.*, personal communication).

Results and discussion

Allele frequencies

HLA-DRB1, DQA1 and DQB1 allele frequencies estimated in the Polish population are presented in *Table I*. The mean genetic distances computed over loci DRB1, DQA1 and DQB1 indicate that the Polish population from Wielkopolska is close to the French and the Danes, followed by the Czech, the Basques, the German and the Spanish.
The first 3 principal axes represent 69% of the total variance. The first axis (39%) mainly differentiates the northern and western European populations (Polish, Danes, German, French, Czech, Spanish and Basques) from the south-eastern European populations (Italian, Rumanian, Croatian, Bulgarian and Sardinian) and the

Table I. DQB1, DQA1 and DRB1 allele frequencies in the Polish population from Wielkopolska (N=99)

Allele	Frequency	Allele	Frequency
DQB1*0201	0.1786	DRB1*1501	0.1616
DQB1*0602	0.1693	DRB1*0701	0.1212
DQB1*0501	0.1526	DRB1*0101	0.0959
DQB1*0301	0.1268	DRB1*0301[1]	0.0757
DQB1*0302	0.0992	DRB1*1301	0.0707
DQB1*0603	0.0797	DRB1*1101	0.0657
DQB1*0402	0.0454	DRB1*0104	0.0404
DQB1*0601	0.0404	DRB1*0401	0.0354
DQB1*0303	0.0303	DRB1*0806	0.0252
DQB1*0304	0.0202	DRB1*1303	0.0252
DQB1*0502	0.0151	DRB1*1601	0.0252
DQB1*0305	0.0051	DRB1*1307	0.0202
DQB1*0503	0.0051	DRB1*0406	0.0151
DQB1*0604	0.0051	DRB1*0413	0.0151
BLANK	0.0271	DRB1*0801	0.0151
		DRB1*1104	0.0151
DQA1*0501	0.2171	DRB1*1502	0.0151
DQA1*0102	0.1877	DRB1*0103	0.0101
DQA1*0101	0.1707	DRB1*0403	0.0101
DQA1*0301	0.1206	DRB1*0407	0.0101
DQA1*0201	0.1173	DRB1*0414	0.0101
DQA1*0103	0.0997	DRB1*0901	0.0101
DQA1*0401	0.0454	DRB1*1001	0.0101
DQA1*0502	0.0051	DRB1*1103	0.0101
BLANK	0.0364	DRB1*1106	0.0101
		DRB1*1201	0.0101
		DRB1*1503	0.0101
		DRB1*1504	0.0101
		DRB1*0304	0.0051
		DRB1*0402	0.0051
		DRB1*0419	0.0051
		DRB1*0805	0.0051
		DRB1*1102	0.0051
		DRB1*1107	0.0051
		DRB1*1202	0.0051
		DRB1*1203	0.0051
		DRB1*1401	0.0051
		DRB1*1407	0.0051
		BLANK	0

[1]DRB1*03011: 0.0657; DRB1*03012: 0.0051; DRB1*0301 not subtyped: 0.0051.

Gypsies. According to the second axis (18%), a main differentiation is observed for Sardinians, on one hand, and Gypsies, on the other hand. The peculiar segregation of the Gypsies supports the hypothesis of their eastern (probably Indian) origin. The second axis also segregates Polish and Danes from the other western and northern populations. The third axis (12%) separates Basques and Spanish, on one hand, and Germans, on the other hand, the latter being related to the French and Polish.

The present results show that the Polish population from Wielkopolska is genetically related to geographically neighbouring populations (northern and central Europeans), rather than to other Balto-Slavic speakers (Czech, Bulgarian, Croatian). The highest variance component (39%) seems to be related to a south-eastern/north-western European differentiation, as it has been observed for many other genetic systems, and explained by the demic diffusion of Neolithic farmers, some 10'000 years ago [9], for a review. On the other hand, the populations belonging to a same linguistic family (Italic family including French, Spanish, Italian, Sardinian, and Rumanian, Germanic family including German and Danish, Slavic family including Polish, Bulgarian, Czech, Croatian) are genetically heterogeneous, and the distinct linguistic families (all belonging to the Indo-european phylum, except the Basque) overlap. The Basque is a linguistic isolate possibly related to North Caucasian [9], and present some peculiar genetic traits, as for many polymorphisms. However, they are not as distant here, genetically, as the geographically isolated Sardinians are from other Europeans. Thus, geographic rather than linguistic boundaries are detectable by HLA class II data analysis in Europe.

Acknowledgements

We would like to thank the Poznan volunteer blood donors for their participation in this work. This study was supported by FNRS (Switzerland) grant 3100-039847.93 INSERM and GREG. S.Djoulah is recipient of a grant BFA/95/6748 from CMEP.

References

1. Imanishi T, Tatsuya A, Kimura A, Tokunaga K, Gojobori T. Allele and haplotype frequencies for HLA and complement loci in various ethnic groups. In: Tsuji K, Aizawa M, Sasazuki T, eds. HLA *1991*, vol 1. Oxford: Oxford University Press, 1992: 1065-220.
2. Buyse I, Decorte R, Baens M, Cuppen H, Semana G, Emonds M P, Marynen, Cassiman JJ. Rapid DNA typing of class II HLA antigens using the polymerase chain reaction and reverse dot blot hybridization. *Tissue Antigens* 1993; 41: 1-14

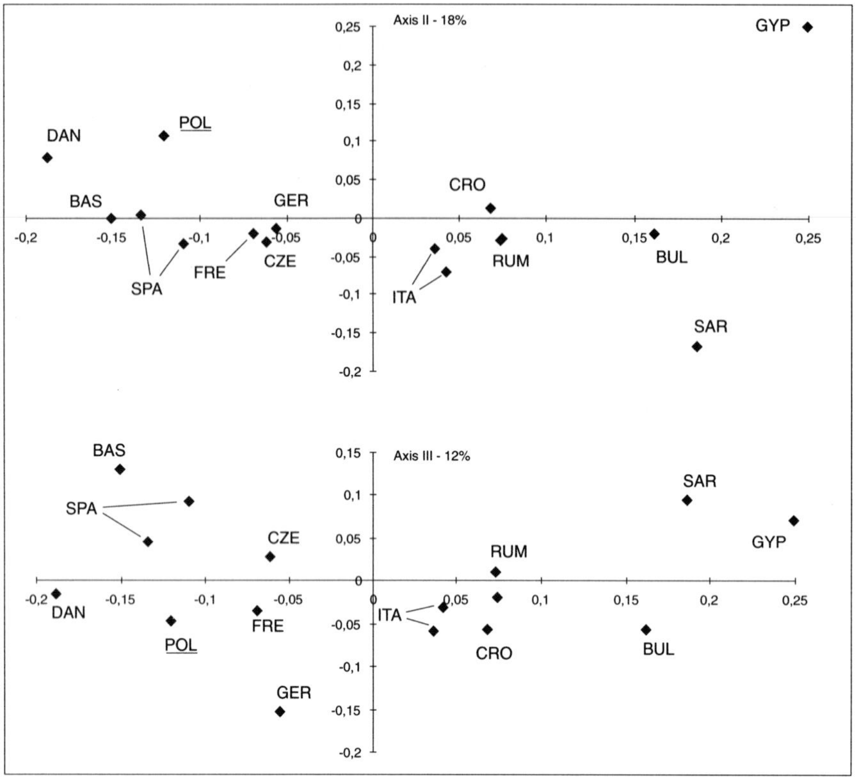

Figure 1. Principal coordinate analysis for 16 European population samples tested for DRB1, DQA1, and DQB1 polymorphisms.
Top: axe I (horizontal) and II (vertical); bottom: axes I (horizontal) and and III (vertical).
POL: 99 Polish from Wielkopolska (present study); BUL: 100-116 Bulgarian [7]; CRO: 141 Croatian [8], CZE: 99 Czech [9], DAN: 53-55 Danes [1], FRE: 171-180 French [1], GER: 88-90 German [1], ITA: 284-492 Italian [1] and 99-100 Italian [10], RUM: 51-73 Rumanian [1] and 83-76 Rumanian [11], SAR: 91 Sardinian [1], SPA: 154-166 Spanish [1] and 176 Spanish [12], BAS: 80 Spanish Basques [12], GYP: Spanish Gypsies [13].

3. Neveny-Stickel C, Bettinotti M, AndreasA, Hinz Peter M, Schmitz G, Albert ED. Non radioactive HLA class II typing using polymerase chain reaction and digoxigenin 11-2'3'. *Hum Immunol* 1991; 31: 7-13.
4. Powell JR, Levene H, Dobzhanski T. Chromosomal polymorphism in Drosophila pseudoobscura used for diagnosis of geographic origin. *Evolution* 1972; 26: 553-9.
5. Grundschober C, Sanchez-Mazas A, Excoffier L, Langaney A, Jeannet M, Tiercy JM. HLA-DPB1 DNA polymorphism in the Swiss population: linkage disequilibrium with other HLA loci and population genetics affinities. *Eur J Immunogenet* 1994; 21: 143-57.
6. Cavalli-Sforza LL, Menozzi P, Piazza A. The history and geography of human genes. Princeton-New Jersey: Princeton University Press, 1994.
7. Ivanova R, Naounova E, Lepage V, Djoulah S, Yordanov Y, Loste M N, Charron D. HLA-DRB1, DQA1, DQB1 DNA polymorphism in the Bulgarian population. *Tissue Antigens* 1996; 47: 122-6.
8. Grubic Z, Unec R, Naipal A, Kastelan A, Giphart M J. Molecular analysis of HLA class II polymorphism in Croatians. *Tissue Antigens* 1996; 46: 122-6.
9. Cerna M, Fernandez-Vina M, Ivaskova E, Stasny P. Comparison of HLA class II allleles in Gypsy and Czech populations by DNA typing with oligonucleotide probes. *Tissue Antigens* 1992; 39: 111-6.
10. D'Alfonso S, Cappello N, Mazzola G, Cornaglia M. Frequencies of HLA class II alleles in Piedmont (Northern Italy). *Gene Geogr* 1994; 8: 55-66.
11. Reed E, Ho E, Lupu F, McManus P, Vasilescu R, Foca-Rodi A, Suciu-Foca N. Polymorphism of HLA in the Romanian population. *Tissue Antigens* 1992; 39: 8-13.
12. Martinez-Laso J, De Juan D, Martinez-Quiles N, Gomez-Casado E, Cuadrado Arnaiz-Villena A. The contribution of the HLA-A, -B, -C, and -DR, -DQ DNA typing to the study of the origins of Spaniards and Basques. *Tissue Antigens* 1995; 45: 237-45.
13. De Pablo R, Vilches C, Moreno ME, Rementeria M, Solis R, Kreisler M. Distribution of HLA antigens in Spanish Gypsies: a comparative study. *Tissue Antigens* 1992; 40: 187-96.

HLA class II DR and DQ typing in New South Wales Australian Aborigines. A novel DRB1 allele: DRB1*8Taree

J. Trejaut, N. Duncan, W. Greville, S. Boatwright, C. Kennedy, J. Moses, H. Dunckley

Molecular Genetics, Tissue Typing, NSW Red Cross Blood Transfusion Service, 153 Clarence Street, Sydney 2000, Australia

Previous HLA class II studies of Australian Aborigines comprise carefully chosen populations to avoid samples with admixture from non-Aboriginal peoples. These studies suggested that on the basis of generic HLA class II typing, the polymorphism from one Aboriginal population to another was limited [1]. However with HLA class II subtyping, this polymorphism was found to be greater and there was geographical variation across inland and Northern Australia [1-3]. Regions such as New South Wales (NSW) and Victoria have not been investigated for the reason mentioned above. In this study, we have used polymerase chain reaction-restriction fragment length polymorphism (PCR-RFLP) to examine the HLA-DRB1, -DRB3, -DRB4, -DRB5, -DQA1 and -DQB1 genes in 140 present day NSW Australian Aborigines which showed a high level of Caucasoid admixture. Statistical analysis was then used to derive the haplotypic profile of a putative pre-European contact Aboriginal population. A novel DR8 allele is also described.

Results and discussion

Frequencies of putative haplotypes are given in *Table I* where haplotype frequencies are also given for an English Caucasian population comprising 177 random individuals [4]. The Aborigines shared many alleles with the Caucasian group indicating a high level of Caucasian admixture. After determination of the haplotypic structure of the present day Australian Aboriginal population [P(H)] and favouring the English Caucasians [P(B)] as the most likely population from which the genes introduced were derived, Bernstein's formula {m=[P(H)-P(B)]/[P(A)-P(B)]} [5] (where P() represents the haplotype frequency, and "m" the coefficient of admixture) was applied to determine the genetic structure of a putative pre-European contact NSW Australian Aboriginal population [P(A)].

The HLA profile of a probable NSW Aboriginal population was characterized and showed a more restricted range of alleles *(Table I)*. Twenty two out of the 25 DRB1 alleles initially defined were retained, giving 38 haplotypes of Australian Aboriginal ancestry compared with 49 in the present day Aboriginal population. This indicates there is at least 78% admixture. Significant allele frequency differences of this putative Aboriginal population compared with Aboriginal groups in other parts of Australia were revealed [1-3]. The most common allele DRB1*08032 (gene frequency=17.5%) was not seen as frequently as in other Aboriginal populations (26-33%) DRB1*1501 (13.2%) was common in the putative NSW Aboriginal population and has been seen previously in the Cape York (5.0%) and the Central Desert (0.7%) populations, but not the Kimberley and Yuendumu regions. DRB1*0404 (6.7%) is seen at a low frequency in the Cape York and Kimberley regions (3.9% combined) but not in the Yuendumu and Central Desert areas. DRB1*1407 (9.5%) and DRB1*1414 (6%) have previously been described only in the Central Desert Aboriginal population (2.3% and 2.9% respectively). Genetic drift rather than different waves of migration could be the cause of this genetic variability with other Australian Aboriginal groups.

A novel PCR-RFLP pattern, locally designated DRB1*8Taree, was observed. The nucleotide sequence of the second exon of DRB1 was determined by automated DNA sequencing, which showed DRB1*8Taree was different to DRB1*08032 from codons 57 to 60. This suggests there was a segmental transfer *(Figure 1)* from a common Australian Aboriginal allele, DRB1*1408 (codons 57 to 60), to another common Australian Aboriginal allele, DRB1*08032, to generate

Table I. HLA-DRB, -DQA1, and -DQB1 putative haplotype frequencies in pre-European contact NSW Australian Aborigines

Haplotypes				Present day Australian Aborigines n=140	Caucasians[@] n=177	Putative pre-European Contact Australian Aborigines
DRB1	-DRB3/4/5	-DQA1	-DQB1	P(H)	P(B)	P(A)
*0101		*0101/4	*0501	3.6	10.2	-
*0103		*0101/4	*0501	-	2.3	-
*0301	*0101	*0501	*0201	10.2	9.6	5.6
*0301	*0201/2	*0501	*0201	1.2	3.1	-
*0401	*0101	*0301	*0301	0.4	4.0	-
*0401	*0101	*0301	*0302	0.4	8.2	-
*0403	*0101	*03#	*0301	-	1.7	-
*0403	*0101	*03#	*0302	-	5.1	-
*0404	*0101	*0301	*0402	1.1	-	2.0
*0404	*0101	*0301	*0302	1.5	-	2.7
*0404	*0101	*0301	*0301	1.1	-	2.0
*0405	*0101	*0301	*0402	0.4	-	0.7
*0405	*0101	*03#	*0302	-	2.0	-
*0408	*0101	*0301	*0301	0.4	-	0.7
*0408	*0101	*0301	*0401	1.1	-	2.0
*0408	*0101	*0301	*0402	1.1	-	2.0
*0410	*0101	*0301	*0402	2.4	-	4.3
*0701	*0101	*0201	*0201	7.7	10.5	-
*0701	*0101	*0201	*0302	0.7	0.6	0.5
*0701	*0101	*0201	*0303	1.5	2.3	-
*0801		*0401	*0402	0.4	1.7	-
*0802		*0103	*0601	0.4	-	0.7
*08032		*0103	*0601	9.4	-	16.8
*08032		*0103	*0503	0.4	-	0.7
*8Taree		*0103	*0601	0.7	-	1.2
*0901	*0101	*0301	*0303	1.1	1.4	0.1
*1101	*0202	*0501	*0304	0.4	-	0.7
*1101	*0202	*0501	*0301	0.4	4.0	-
*1102/3	*0201/2	*0501	*0301	-	1.4	-
*1201	*0202	*0501	*0402	0.4	-	0.7
*1201	*0201	*0501	*0402	0.4	-	0.7
*1201	*0101	*0501	*0402	0.4	-	0.7
*1201	*0101	*0501	*0301	1.1	0.6	1.2
*1202	*0101	*0501	*0402	0.4	-	0.7
*1301	*0101	*0103	*0603	1.4	2.0	-
*1301	*0301	*0103	*0603	0.4	-	0.7
*1302	*0301	*0102	*0604	2.8	2.5	1.7
*1302	*0301	*0102	*0603	0.7	-	1.2
*1302	*0301	*0103	*0604	0.7	-	1.2
*1401	*0201	*0101/4	*0503	3.1	2.3	2.5
*1405	*0202	*0101/4	*0503	1.1	-	2.0
*1407	*0202	*0101/4	*0503	4.2	-	7.5
*1407	*0201	*0101/4	*0503	1.1	-	2.0
*1408	*0202	*0101/4	*0503	2.4	-	4.3
*1414	*0202	*0101/4	*0503	3.1	-	5.5
*1414	*0201	*0101/4	*0503	0.3	-	0.5
*1501	*0101	*0102	*0602	10.0	14.1	-
*1501	*0101	*0102	*0603	7.0	-	12.5
*1501	*0101	*0102	*0601	0.4	-	0.7
*1502	*0101	*0102	*0601	4.9	-	8.8
*1502	*0101	*0102	*0602	0.4	-	0.7
*1502	*0102	*0101	*0501	0.4	-	0.7
*1502	*0101	*0102	*0603	0.4	-	0.7
*1502	*0102	*0103	*0601	0.4	0.6	-
Others				-	10.0	-

@ Data from British Caucasians taken from reference [4].

Not defined; $P_i(A)=100*[[P_i(H)-mP_i(B)]/(1-m)]/\Sigma_{1 \text{ to } n}[[P_i(H)-mP_i(B)]/(1-m)]$; i=1 to n; m=coefficient of admixture.

		57			60							67
DRB1*0101	CCT	GAT	GCC	GAG	TAC	TGG	AAC	AGC	CAG	AAG	GAC	CTC
DRB1*08032	---	AGC	---	---	---	---	---	---	---	---	---	A--
DRB1*1408	---	---	--G	---	C--	---	---	---	---	---	---	---
DRB1*8Taree	---	---	--G	---	C--	---	---	---	---	---	---	A--

Figure 1. Possible intragenic recombination to generate DRB*8Taree from DRB1*08032 and DRB1*1408. Except for codons 57 to 60, DRB*8Taree is identical to DRB1*08032.

DRB1*8Taree with the following haplotypic arrangement: DRB1*8Taree-DQA1*0103-*DQB1*0601.

Conclusion

This study has shown there is value in examining populations with admixture. The results obtained here have given a haplotypic profile of a putative NSW Aboriginal population which shows differences with other Aboriginal populations. This contributes to a better understanding of the settlement of the Aboriginal populations in Australia.

Note

*DRB1*0815 has been officially assigned to DRB1*8 Taree by the WHO nomenclature committee in July 1996. The accession number assigned by Gen Bank is U6 3802.*

References

1. Gao X, Veale A, Serjeantson SW. HLA class II diversity in Australian Aborigines: unusual HLA-DRB1 alleles. *Immunogenetics* 1992; 36: 333-7.
2. Gao X, Serjeantson SW. Analysis of 2600 HLA-DR, DQ haplotypes in Asia-Oceania. In: Tsuji K, Aizawa M, Sasazuki T eds. *HLA 1991. Proceedings of the Eleventh International Histocompatibility Workshop and Conference,* vol. 2. Oxford: Oxford Science Publication, 1992 : 229-32.
3. Lester S, Cassidy S, Humphreys I, Bennett G, Hurley CK, Boettcher B, Mc Cluskey J. Evolution in HLA-DRB1 and major histocompatibility complex class II haplotypes of Australian Aborigines. Definition of a new DRB1 allele and distribution of gene frequencies. *Hum Immunol* 1995; 42: 154-60.
4. Doherty DG, Vaughan RW, Donaldson PT, Mowat AP. HLA DQA, DQB and DRB genotyping by oligonucleotide analysis: distribution of alleles and haplotypes in British Caucasoids. *Hum Immunol* 1992; 34:53-63.
5. Williams RC, McAuley JE. HLA class I variation controlled for genetic admixture in the Gila river Indian community of Arizona: a model for the Paleo-Indians. *Hum Immunol* 1992; 33: 39-46.

HLA class II variation and linkage disequilibrium in nine Amerindian and three African American populations from Colombia. Results of *Expedicion Humana*

E.A. Trachtenberg[1], H.A. Erlich[1], J. Hollenbach [2], G. Keyeux [3], J. Bernal [3], W. Klitz [2]

1 Children's Hospital Oakland Research Institute, 747 52nd Street, Oakland, California 94609-1809, USA and Department of Human Genetics, Roche Molecular Systems, Alameda CA, USA
2 Department of Integrative Biology, University of California, Berkeley, CA, USA
3 Instituto de Genetica Humana, Facultad de Medicina, Pontificia U. Javeriana, Bogota, Colombia

A summary of the HLA class II variation (DRB1-DQA1-DQB1-DPB1) in nine Amerindian and three African American populations from six geographically distinct regions of Colombia is presented with DRB1-DPB1 linkage disequilibrium analysis on seven of the populations. As expected from anthropological, genetic and HLA analyses of other Amerindian and African groups, the number of different class II alleles and haplotypes in the Colombian Amerindians is markedly reduced in comparison with the very high degree of class II allelic and haplotypic variability found in the neighboring Colombian African populations. Several novel DRB1-DQB1 haplotypes in both the Colombian Amerindians and Africans, and a new DQB1*0203 allele in one Colombian African population were identified. The overall linkage disequilibrium values from seven populations, including six Amerindian and the Colombian African Providencia population, indicated significant disequilibrium between DRB1 and DPB1, and strong haplotype associations in the class II region of these populations. This molecular analysis of HLA class II alleles and linkage disequilibrium analysis of haplotypes of the Colombian Amerindian and neighboring Colombian African populations provides insights on ancestral relationships between these and other native populations and aids in the study of HLA allelic and haplotypic evolution.

HLA class II variability

PCR/SSOP characterization and analysis of HLA class II loci (DRB1-DQA1-DQB1-DPB1) were performed on samples from 227 unrelated individuals from the Kogui (Sierra Nevada), Ijka (Sierra Nevada), Sikuani (Eastern Plains), Ingano (Amazonas), Coreguaje (Amazonas), Nukak (Eastern Amazonas), Waunana (Pacific), Embera (Pacific) and Tule (NW Pacific Coast) Colombian Amerindian populations, as recently described [1]. In addition, 80 samples from the Cauca (Pacific), Choco (North Pacific Coast) and the Providencia (Caribbean island) Colombian African populations were also analyzed, as reported recently [2]. All samples were collected and analyzed under the auspices of the *Gran Expedicion Humana* (U. Javeriana, Bogota, Colombia).

In the Colombian Amerindian groups, DR2 (DRB1*1602), DR4 (DRB1*0407, *0404, *0403 and *0411), DR6 (DRB1*1402) and DR8 (DRB1*0802) comprise >95% of all DRB1 alleles. There is an absence of DR3 in all populations, and alleles from the DR1, DR7 and DR9 serogroups are either very rare or absent. Finding the great diversity of DR4 alleles is in striking contrast to the marked reduction in representation of other DRB1 alleles in these groups. The allelic distribution differed significantly among the nine Amerindian populations. Geographically isolated populations, such as the Kogui, Coreguaje and Nukak, have only 4-5 DRB1 alleles, and the other six populations carry between 7-10 of the 20 different DRB1 alleles found in total. Each population has one or two very common DRB1 allele(s) (f=~0.22-0.65) and DRB1-DQA1-DQB1 haplotype. Traces of Caucasian and African alleles were found at very low frequencies in a few populations, and were attributed to admixture. At the DPB1 locus, DPB1*0402 (f=0.28-0.82), *1401 (f=0.03-0.45) and *3501 (f=0.03-0.27), are the three most prevalent alleles, with one of these alleles maintained as the predominant (f>0.26) DPB1 allele in each population. In contrast, the three Colombian African populations exhibit a great diversity of class II haplotypes, including DRB1 alleles from each serological class and a novel DQB1*02 allele (*0203). The novel DQB1*0203 allele differs from DQB1*0201 by a second base substitution

(C→A) at codon 57, converting alanine to aspartic acid. Several novel class II haplotypes were identified in both the Amerindian and African American populations. Analysis of the HLA class II variability in these extraordinary populations is of value to clinical and anthropological studies, and may serve to pinpoint the exact African origins of the Colombian African populations, who arrived via slave ships from Africa during the last ~500 years.

HLA class II haplotypes in Colombian Amerindians and Colombian Africans

The 500 kb of DNA between the DR and DP loci is a useful interval for indicating the dynamic interaction between recombination and linkage disequilibrium. Here we examine the Colombian African Providencia population and six Amerindian populations, including the Coreguajes, Sikuani, Ijka, Kogui, Tule, and Waunana, each of which have at least 25 individuals or 50 sampled haplotypes. DRB1-DPB1 haplotypes were estimated using standard MLE procedures [3]. A chi square-based statistic, Wn, which ranges from 0 to +1 [4] was used to measure the overall (global) disequilibrium between the two loci. The statistical significance of overall disequilibrium was measured with the chi square testing (using the G test) of the two locus haplotype frequencies of DRB1 and DPB1. Many rare alleles greatly boost the degrees of freedom making the test generally conservative. Only in the case of the highly polymorphic Colombian African samples were rare alleles (those seen only one or two times) combined into a single class before testing. The degree of disequilibrium in individual haplotypes was measured with the normalized disequilibrium parameter, D', which ranges between -1 and +1.

In each of the seven populations significant positive disequilibrium was present for several haplotypes, often reaching the maximum possible value (+1) in which an allele at one locus is found only in association with a single allele at a second locus *(Table I)*. Differences in haplotypic associations may reflect the evolution of different groups of DR4 alleles in the Colombian Amerindian groups. Three of the Colombian Amerindian populations share the DRB1*0411-DPB1*0402 haplotype in linkage disequilibrium, occurring at a higher frequency in the Coreguajes (0.24), and at lower but similar frequencies in the Waunana (0.13) and Tule (0.09) populations. The DRB1*0403 allele is also found in strong disequilibrium with DPB1*0402 in the Tule (0.20) and Ijka (0.07). A strong DRB1*0404-DPB1*0501 association was found in the Coreguajes group. Similarly, the DRB1*0407-DPB1*1401 haplotype is shared at widely different frequencies in the Ijka (0.07), Tule (0.11), Kogui (0.38) and Sikuani (0.85) groups. However, DRB1*0407 was found in strong association with DPB1*0401 in the Waunana (0.05), and with DPB1*3501 in the Kogui (0.24). Both DPB1*1401 and DPB1*3501 are in strong linkage disequilibrium with DRB1*0407 in the Kogui, a finding which supports our hypothesis that DPB1*3501 could have arose from the putative parental DPB1*1401 independently in the Colombian Amerindian groups [1].

Table I. The more common DRB1-DPB1 haplotypes in linkage disequilibrium in six Colombian Amerindian populations and one Colombian African population

Population	DRB1	DPB1	D'	Haplotype frequency	Total with haplotypes significant D' (f>0.05)
Coreguajes	0411	0402	0.55	0.24	0.60
	0404	0501	0.61	0.21	
	0802	1401	0.70	0.15	
Sikuani	1402	0402	0.75	0.38	0.85
	1602	0402	1.0	0.38	
	0407	1401	1.0	0.85	
Ijka	0403	0402	1.0	0.07	0.64
	0802	0402	0.60	0.50	
	0407	1401	0.47	0.07	
Kogui	0802	0402	0.98	0.13	0.87
	1402	0402	0.70	0.12	
	0407	1401	0.57	0.38	
	0407	3501	0.75	0.24	
Tule	0403	0402	0.66	0.20	0.52
	0411	0402	1.0	0.09	
	1402	0401	0.44	0.07	
	0407	1401	0.77	0.11	
	0410	1401	1.0	0.05	
Waunana	0407	0401	0.72	0.05	0.18
	0411	0402	1.0	0.13	
Providencia (Colombian African)	0101	0401	0.70	0.05	0.21
	0301	0402	0.58	0.10	
	1503	0201	0.51	0.05	

Analysis of DRB1-DPB1 associations also help to illustrate the power of HLA haplotypic associations in interpreting anthropological relationships. For example, the DRB1*0802 allele is in very strong linkage disequilibirum with DPB1*0402 in the Ijka (0.50) and Kogui (0.13) populations, which are closely related geographically and thought to be related historically. DRB1*0802 is also found very strongly associated with DPB1*1401 in the Coreguaje (0.15) population, which is not geographically or historically close to the Ijka or Kogui groups. Similarly, DRB1*1402-DPB1*0402 is in very strong disequilibrium in the Sikuani (0.38) and Kogui (0.12) populations, but DRB1*1402 is in association with DPB1*0401 in the Tule, which is geographically in the northwest of Colombia, remote from the more eastern Sikuani or northeastern Kogui populations. Further analysis of the HLA haplotypic associations, in relationship with known anthropological data, will aid both the genetic and anthropological interpretations of the distribution of the class II alleles and haplotypes in these Colombian populations.

The proportion of all haplotypes in strong positive disequilibrium was greater than 0.50 in all of the Amerindian populations except the Waunana, which had a proportion of more common haplotypes in positive disequilibrium of 0.18. At the other extreme, in the Kogui with a proportion of 0.87, all haplotypes were in strong positive disequilibrium. The Wn values for disequilibrium between DRB1 and DPB1 was significant in all cases, ranging from 0.53 in the Waunana, 0.56 in the Tule, 0.62 in the Kogui, 0.76 in the Ijka, 0.77 in the Sikuani, 0.71 in the Coreguaje, to 0.77 in the Sikuani. In contrast, the Wn values for these loci in Caucasians is only 0.32.

The extreme disequilibrium between DR-DQ has been recognized for many years. More recently, population data has become available to measure disequilibrium between the DR-DQ region and DPB1. Begovich *et al.* [5] and Klitz *et al.* [4] reported measurable levels of disequilibrium between DRB1 and DPB1 in a Caucasian sample, and Trachtenberg *et al.* [6] made similar observations in the native Ecuadorian Cayapa people. Very significant levels of overall disequilibrium between DRB1 and DPB1 was observed in the Amerindian samples examined here. In the Kogui, which have the lowest levels of polymorphism with only three and four DRB1 and DPB1 alleles, respectively, nearly all sampled haplotypes are in strong population level association. The Colombian African Providencia population, with its characteristically high class II polymorphism and variability, also demonstrated significant overall disequilibrium between DRB1 and DPB1, albeit at a lower level than seen in several of the Amerindian groups. The evidence permits the conclusion of strong population level haplotype associations occurring across the HLA class II region in these populations.

Acknowledgments

The authors would like to thank the peoples of Colombia for participating in the Expedicion Humana, *C. Rodas for her assistance in sample collection and DNA extractions, and Janel Noble for sequencing. This work was supported in part by a grant from the NIH to HAE (#HL47170-02), from the NIH to WK (GM32359), and by the Expedicion Humana, Instituto de Genetica Humana, Pontificia Universidad Javeriana, Bogota, Colombia.*

References

1. Trachtenberg EA, Keyeux G, Bernal J, Rhodas C, Erlich HA. Analysis of HLA class II (DRB1-DQA1-DQB1-DPB1) alleles and DR-DQ haplotypes in nine Amerindian populations from Colombia. Results of *expedicion humana*: part I. *Tissue Antigens* 1997, in press.
2. Trachtenberg EA, Keyeux G, Bernal J, Noble J, Erlich HA. Analysis of HLA class II alleles in three African American populations from Colombia using the PCR/SSOP: identification of a novel DQB1*02 (*0203) allele. Results of the *expedicion humana*: part I. *Tissue Antigens* 1997, in press.
3. Baur MP, Danilovs J. Population analysis of HLA-A, B, C, DR and other genetic markers. In: Terasaki PI, ed. *Histocompatibility Testing 1980.* Los Angeles : University of California, 1980 : 955-68.
4. Klitz W, Stephens JC, Grote M, Carrington M. Discordant patterns of linkage disequilibrium of the peptide-transporter loci within the HLA class II region. *Am J Hum Genet* 1995; 57.
5. Begovich AB, McClure GR, Suraj VC, *et al.* Polymorphism, recombination and linkage disequilibrium within the HLA class II region. *J Immunol* 1992; 148:249.
6. Trachtenberg EA, Klitz W, Rickards O, De Stefano GF, Erlich HA. Analysis of HLA class II linkage disequilibrium and haplotype evolution in the Cayapa Indians of Ecuador. *Am J Hum Genet* 1995; 57:415-24.

Molecular analysis of HLA class II polymorphism on the island of Hvar-Croatia

Z. Grubic[1], R. Zunec[1], V. Kerhin[1], E. Cecuk[1], D. Kastelan[1], I. Martinovic[2], M. Bakran[2], B. Janicijevic[2], P. Rudan[2], A. Kastelan[1]

1 Tissue Typing Laboratory, University Hospital Zagreb, Kispatic street 12, YU-10000 Zagreb, Croatia
2 Institute for Anthropological Research, Zagreb, Croatia

As part of the anthropology component of the 12th International Histocompatibility Workshop a total of 104 randomly chosen autochtonous inhabitants of the island of Hvar were studied for class II polymorphism.
The purpose of this study is to continue our previous work on class I and class II polymorphism in Croatian population [1,2] as well as in populations of Dalmatian Islands [3].
The island of Hvar belongs to the group of Middle Dalmatian Islands, Republic of Croatia. The island has a total of about 11500 inhabitants, living in 24 settlements. Considering the geographic configuration, ethnohistorical and socio-cultural characteristics the insular population can be divided into the subpopulations of western and eastern regions of the island [4].

Material and methods

The western subpopulation consisted of 58 individuals living in three different villages at the western part of island while eastern subpopulation consisted of 46 individuals living in three different villages at the eastern part of island. These samples represent 3.9% and 7.1% of the inhabitants, respectively.
The DRB1, DRB3, DRB4, DRB5, DQA1 and DQB1 gene polymorphism was analysed by PCR-SSOP method using 12th International Histocompatibility Workshop primers and probes.
The allele frequencies were estimated by the maximum likelihood method. Probable two- and three- locus haplotypic associations were assigned on the basis of known linkage disequilibria. The allele and probable haplotype frequencies were calculated separately for the western and eastern region of the island. The significance of differences was evaluated using chi-square while Fisher's exact test was used if any value in a 2x2 table was less than five.

Results and discussion

Most of the HLA allele frequencies are quite similar between the western and eastern subpopulation. However, some differences are observed. In *Table I*, the allele frequencies that show differences between the western and eastern subpopulation are listed.
Significant differences are observed for DRB1*0701, DQA1*0201 and DQB1*0603 alleles that are more frequent in eastern subpopulation.
At the DRB1 locus four rare alleles are found: *0411, *1110, *1113, *1310. At the DQB1 locus three rare alleles are found: *0607, *0304 and *0305. None of these alleles have been previously found in Croatians [5].
Analysis of haplotypic associations revealed a great diversity. Thirty-four and 38 distinct haplotypes have been identified in the eastern and in the western subpopulation, respectively.
Table II shows the thirteen most represented haplotypic associations for western and eastern subpopulations. Among common haplotypes, significant difference is found for DRB1*0101-DQA1*0101-DQB1*0501 which is more frequent at the western part of the island. In addition, significant difference is found in the occurence of two rare haplotypes: DRB1*0101-DQA1*0102-DQB1*0501; DRB1*1501-DQA1*0102-DQB1*0604. Interestingly, in both subpopulations, DRB1*0701 is always found with DQA1*0201 but with two different DQB1 alleles: *0201 and *0303. Six different rare haplotypes have been found either on the the western or on the eastern part of the island *(Table III)*.
The observed difference in distribution pattern of HLA class II alleles and haplotypes between the western and eastern region of the island confirms previous ethnohis-

Table I. Frequency of selected HLA class II alleles-Island of Hvar

Allele	West (N=116) %	East (N=92) %
DRB1*0101	14.7	6.5
1501	11.3	7.6
1601	8.1	3.3
1301	2.4	8.7
0701	3.6	13.0
DQA1*0101	12.9	6.5
0103	5.1	11.9
0201	3.6	13.0
DQB1*0501	15.5	8.7
0603	2.6	9.8
0201	11.2	18.4

Table II. The most represented DRB1-DQA1-DQB1 haplotypic associations-Island of Hvar

Haplotype DRB1	DQA1	DQB1	West (N=116) %	East (N=92) %
0101	0101	0501	12.1	3.3
0101	0102	0501	0	4.4
1501	0102	0602	6.0	6.5
1501	0102	0604	4.4	0
1601	0102	0502	8.6	3.3
0301	0501	0201	9.5	8.7
0401	0301	0303	4.4	2.2
1101	0501	0301	9.5	8.7
1104	0501	0301	7.6	6.5
0701	0201	0201	1.7	5.4
0701	0201	0303	1.7	5.4
1301	0103	0603	0.8	5.4
1303	0501	0301	4.4	2.2

Table III. Unusual DRB1-DQA1-DQB1 haplotypic associations-Island of Hvar

Haplotype			Region	
DRB1	DQA1	QB1	W	E
1501	0102	0502	1	1*
1501	0103	0502	1	0
1101	0501	0302	1	0
1301	0103	0607	1	2
1305	0102	0603	1	0
1306	0103	0607	1	0

* No of occurence.

toric, sociocultural and biological division of the insular population into two major subpopulation groups. This paper offers further evidence that HLA polymorphism can be utilised to distinguish between the subpopulations originating from the same ethnic groups, living within the extremely restricted geographic area.

References

1. Kastelan A, Kerhin-Brkljacic V, Hors J, Brkljacic LJ, Macasovic P. The distribution of HLA antigens and genes in the Yugoslav population. *Tissue Antigens* 1974; 4: 69-74.
2. Cuccia M, Astolfi P, Gyodi E, Kastelan A, Papasteriades C, Salerno A, Suciu-Foca N, Veratti A. HLA in five populations of souther Europe. In: Tsuju K, Aizawa M, Sasazuki T, eds. *HLA 1991. Proceedings of Eleventh International Histocompatibility Workshop and Conference,* vol. 1. Oxford: Oxford University Press, 1992: 655-6.
3. Cambon-Thomsen A, Sommer E, Sevin A, Chaventre A, Borot N, Ohayon E, Rudan P. HLA polymorphism in Olib and Silba populations. *Coll Antropol* 1989; 2: 311-23.
4. Rudan P, Roberts DF, Sujoldzic A, Macarol B, Smolej N, Kastelan A. Geography, ethnohistory and demography of the island of Hvar. *Coll Antropol* 1982; 6:47-67.
5. Grubic Z, Zunec R, Naipal A, Kastelan A, Giphart MJ. Molecular analysis of HLA class II polymorphism in Croatians. *Tissue Antigens* 1995; 46: 293-8.

Mitochondrial DNA (mtDNA) variation and HLA genetics studies in the French population

R. Ivanova[1,2], S. Djoulah[1,3], F. Schächter[4], M.N. Loste[1], J. Hors[1], E. Naoumova[5], L. Excoffier[6], A. Sanchez-Mazas [6], J. Dausset[4], V. Lepage[1], D. Charron[1]

1 Laboratoire d'Immunologie, Hopital Saint-Louis, 1, avenue Claude Vellefaux, 75475 Paris Cedex 10, France
2 INSERM U396, Hopital Saint-Louis, Paris, France
3 INSERM U93, Hôpital Saint-Louis, Paris, France
4 CEPH, Fondation J. Dausset, 75010, Paris, France
5 Division of Clinical and Transplantation Immunology, Medical University, Sofia, Bulgaria
6 Laboratoire de Génétique et Biométrie, Département d'Anthropologie de l'Université de Genève, Suisse

The molecular nature and type connection of mtDNA and the extraordinary polymorphism of HLA genetic system are powerful markers for anthropological studies.This is the report of a population genotyped for both nuclear HLA (DRB1, DRB3, DRB4, DRB5, DQA1, DQB1, DPB1) markers and mtDNA polymorphisms.

Material and methods

Subjects

DNA extracted from 151 French individuals randomly selected was used for HLA class II typing. Among them, 83 subjects were characterised for mtDNA variation.

PCR-RFLP

We used the Expand Long PCR System to amplify 15649 bp of closed circular duplex mtDNA [1]. The remaining 920 bp of the genome were amplified using second step PCR in standard conditions with a set of specific primers.

Each PCR segment was screened with 6 restriction endonucleases : Hpa I, Bam HI, Hae II, Msp I, Ava II, Hinc II. The resulting fragments were resolved by electrophoresis in agarose or Polyacrylamid gels depending on the expected size of the restriction fragments and visualised by ethidium bromide staining and UV induced fluorescence.

HLA typing

PCR-SSO reverse dot blot was performed to define 122 DRB, 25 DQB1 and 59 DPB1 alleles using 32, 21 and 24 probes respectively. PCR-SSO classical dot blot was used to define 8 DQA1 alleles with 14 probes.

Results and discussion

Restriction enzyme patterns

The present study investigates the RFLP mtDNA variation of 83 French individuals characterized with a set of 6 endonucleases.

The 83 French tested were monomorphic for Hpa I , which corresponds to the published mtDNA sequence [2]. Two morphs Bam HI -1 and Bam HI -3, two morphs Msp I and two Hae II were observed in our samples. Digesting with Hinc II, 7 different patterns were defined and using Ava II, 6 morphs were found in the tested samples (*Table I*).

Table I. mtDNA types and their frequencies in 83 French individuals

Type#		N	Frequencies (%)
1-2	(2-1-1-1-1-2)	59	71
1-9	(2-1-1-1-1-9)	1	1.2
1-10	(2-1-1-1-1-10)	1	1.2
6-2	(2-1-2-1-1-2)	6	7.2
18-2	(2-3-1-4-9*-2)	3	3.6
28-2	(2-1-1-4-1-2)	1	1.2
36-2	(2-1-1-1-13-2)	1	1.2
47-9	(2-1-1-1-3-9)	1	1.2
57-5	(2-3-1-4-13-5)	1	1.2
75-2	(2-1-1-4-9*-2)	3	3.6
81-2	(2-1-1-1-27-2)	1	1.2
1-new Fr	(2-1-1-1-1-18^{Fr})	1	1.2
1-18^{Fr}	(2-1-2-1-1-2)	1	1.2
New Fr-2	(2-1-2-4-1-Fr)	1	1.2
New Fr-2	(2-1-1-1-Fr-2)	1	1.2
New Fr-2	(2-1-1-4-Fr-2)	1	1.2

Enzyme morphs are listed in the order Hpa I, Bam HI, Hae II, Msp I, Ava II and Hinc II.

mtDNA types

Sixteen mtDNA types have been identified in the French sample. As already reported elsewhere for European populations, the mtDNA type-1, 71% in our sample, is the most frequent. The next in frequency is type 6 (7.2%), which is separated from type 1 by a single mutation. The types 18-2 and 75-2 were observed in our sample with frequencies 3.6%. Types 6-2 and 18-2 are characteristic of southern European populations[3].
Five new types were identified.

HLA haplotypes frequencies

In our study we investigated the polymorphism of seven HLA class II loci (HLA-DRB1, DRB3, DRB4, DRB5, DQA1, DQB1, DPB1) for 151 individuals. The most common combinations with significant delta values ($p<10^{-3}$) concerning DRB1*-DQA1*-DQB1* haplotypes are shown in *Table II.*

Table II. The most frequent significant delta values ($p < 10^{-3}$) HLA-DRB1 - DQA1 - DQB1 haplotypes in 151 French population

DRB1*1501-DQA1*0102-DQB1*0602 :
DRB1*1301-DQA1*0103-DQB1*0603
DRB1*0101-DQA1*0101-DQB1*0501

DRB1*1501-DQA1*-0102-DQB1*0602 (associated with HLA-B7, Cw15 - data not shown); DRB1*0101-DQA1*0101-DQB1*0501 were found among the four most frequent out of 22 highly conserved MHC ancestral haplotypes revealed from the analysis of 829 unrelated haplotypes [4].

The data of highly polymorphic and unlinked genetic system as nuclear HLA class II genes (nDNA) and mtDNA variations are useful to define the genetic profile of the French population.

References

1. Paul R, Santucci S, Saunteres A, Desnuelle C, Paquts-Flucklinger, V. Rapid mapping of mitochondrial DNA deletions by large-fragment PCR. *Trends Genet* 1996 ; 12 : 131-2.
2. Anderson S, Bankier AT, Barrell BG, de Bruijn MHL, Coulson AR, Drouin J, Eperon IC, Nierlich DP, Roe BA, Sanger F, Shreier PH, Smith AJH, Staden R, Yong IG. Sequence organization of the human mitochondrial genome. *Nature* 1981; 290 : 457-465.
3. Graven L, Passarino G, Semino O, Boursot P, Santachiara-Benerecetti AS, Langaney, A, Excoffier L. Evolutionary correlation between control region sequence and RLFP diversity pattern in the mitochondrial genome of a Senegalese sample. *Mol Biol Evol* 1995;12:334-45.
4. Degli-Esposti MA, Abraham LJ, Witt C, Cameron PU, Zhang WJ, Christiansen FT, Dawkins RL. Ancestral haplotype are conserved population haplotypes with a unique MHC structure. In *HLA 1991 Proceedings of the Eleventh International Histocompatibility Workshop and Conference.* Oxford : Oxford University Press, 1992.

HLA
Diversity

New HLA region genes and markers TNF and Complement

Contents

Transcribed genes from the distal Major Histocompatibility Complex (MHC) class I region

J.R. Gruen[1], S.R. Nalabolu[2], T.W. Chu[1, 2], C. Bowlus[3], W.F. Fan[5], V.L. Goei[1], H. Wei[7], R. Sivakamasundari[1], Y.C. Liu[2], H.X. Xu[2], S. Parimoo[6], G. Nallur[2], R. Ajioka[4], H. Shukla[8], P. Bray-Ward[2], J. Pan[2], J. Ahn[1], J. Choi[4], S.M. Weissman[2, 3]

1. Departments of Pediatrics, Yale University School of Medicine, 295 Congress Avenue, New Haven CT 06510, Connecticut, USA
2. Genetics, Yale University School of Medicine, New Haven, Connecticut, USA
3. Internal Medicine, Yale University School of Medicine, New Haven, Connecticut, USA
4. Division of Hematology/Oncology, University of Utah School of Medicine, Salt Lake City, Utah, USA
5. Human Genome Center, Lawrence Livermore National Laboratory, Livermore, California, USA
6. Johnson and Johnson, Skin Biology Research Center, Stillman, New Jersey, USA
7. Biogen, 14 Cambridge Center, Cambridge, Massachusetts, USA
8. SmithKline Beecham Pharmaceuticals, King of Prussia, Pennsylvania, USA

The Major Histocompatibility Complex (MHC) has been defined as the region of chromosome six which contains the genes for the MHC class I and class II surface antigens. However, linkage disequilibrium and extended haplotypes covering the class I genes may extend considerably further telomeric beyond HLAF, and even through the adjacent histone gene cluster and the distal marker D6S105 [1]. While the gene content of the class II and class III adjacent regions of the MHC has been extensively explored by several groups [2], the gene content of the extended class I region has been less broadly investigated. Our laboratories have used the technique of cDNA selection to detect additional transcripts and genes derived from the region of the MHC beginning proximal to the TNF cluster and extending beyond the telomeric histone cluster. Large portions, but perhaps not all, of this region are also gene dense, and the genes in the region represent a partial interspersion of genes of several structurally distinct families as well as a number of single copy genes [3, 4].

The method and general usefulness of cDNA selection have been discussed elsewhere [5] and the approach has been used to identify mutant genes in a number of positional cloning projects. The approach can be very sensitive and detect even very rare transcripts. Obviously one cannot detect mRNAs for genes not represented in the input cDNA libraries. Therefore the approach would probably miss genes expressed only in special locations such as the retina or adrenal cortex not well represented in the mix of cDNA libraries used in our selection. Short transcripts represent a smaller target for selection and therefore are likely to be less well represented in the mixture of selected cDNA fragments. The method of cloning involves cleavage of fragments with EcoR1 followed by size selection, and therefore cDNAs containing multiple EcoR1 sites will be biassed against. The cDNA selection method will in general not distinguish between true genes and well preserved pseudogenes and most, but not all, of the potential transcript encoding sequences we have found in the MHC have been confirmed to represent true genes either because they represent the sole genomic template for a transcript, or because they contain introns and are not part of a family of duplicated sequences within the MHC. Finally, to avoid the abundance of class I genes and pseudogenes we have generally ruled out inserts with homology to known class I genes and in the process may have eliminated some new transcripts [6]. With these caveats, the approach so far has uncovered over 60 transcripts from the MHC region that were not previously detected or assigned to this chromosomal locus, as well as confirming the presence of most of the transcripts noted by others.

The class II and class III regions of the MHC are known to contain several genes such as heat shock proteins that are broadly expressed in a range of cell types and presumably function in general aspects of cell metabolism. The distal MHC includes a number of such genes including: Ran, a GTP binding protein involved in macromolecular transport in and out of the nucleus; B30.7, the probable homologue of yeast RNA polymerase I 13.7 kD subunit; the human TRAM protein ; the myelin oligodendrocyte glycoprotein; a cluster of histone genes; 1-8U, an interferon induced protein of unknown function; and the human analogue of the *S. cerevisiae* GCN20 protein. This last protein is of interest because its action is relatively well understood in yeast, where it regulates a kinase that in turn mediates translational regulation by nutrient starvation. An analogous system has not been analyzed in animal cells, but the similarity of the yeast and human protein suggest that at least some of the biochemical aspects of the pathway may be preserved in higher cells.

Mating preferences in mice are controlled in part through genes linked to the MHC, and this effect is mediated through olfaction. There is also a provocative suggestion that there may be MHC linked mating type preference in humans. Presumably, the MHC linked genes in mice must control the type of odorant produced by the mouse in order to account for the observed phenomena. Study of the genes so far identified in the MHC do not provide any substantial clue as to which, if any, might be involved in production of allele specific odors. It is curious, however, that the distal end of the MHC proper contains olfactory receptor-like genes, at least some of which seem to contain intact coding regions [7].

Another family of genes is interspersed with the distal class I genes. These genes contain sequences at their C-terminal coding region that are substantially homologous to the 100 or so carboxy-terminal amino acids of butyrophilin. Butyrophilin itself is encoded in the distal portion of the extended MHC and is a protein that is a presumptive milk-fat-globule membrane protein. At least five other genes have been identified in the MHC that show sufficient homology to butyrophilin to be considered members of the same "butyrophilin box" family of proteins. Curiously several of these other proteins show structural features such as zinc finger sequences and acidic domains that suggest they may function as transcription factors. Some are broadly expressed in tissues, but one is expressed preferentially in muscle tissue with expression also in spleen but not other organs of the immune system.

In addition to the known genes of the MHC that function in the immune system, we have studied six other structurally unrelated genes that are expressed preferentially in one or another organ or cell type of the immune system. These include a B cell specific diubiquitin, a lymph node specific mRNA, a thymus specific transcript, the above mentioned muscle and spleen specific transcript, and two genes from the TNF region of the MHC [4]. The latter two genes are the human homologue of the murine B144 gene described some years ago on the basis of a partial cDNA sequence, and a gene we term 1C7. Both of these genes show remarkable patterns of splicing.

The 1C7 gene was originally detected as a short fragment selected by DNA from a 200 kb YAC that contained the TNF cluster and the *MIC A* gene. This cDNA fragment was then used to detect an extended cDNA from an oligo-dT primed human spleen cDNA library. Most of the cDNA was encoded by a DNA template lying just centromeric to the TNF cluster. However, the 5' exon was not encoded in the original selecting YAC but rather in DNA from an adjacent telomeric YAC. This places the 5' exon at least 100 kb telomeric to the remainder of the template. The intron between the first exon and the remainder of the gene includes at least 7 transcribed genes, containing transcription units running in both directions relative to the 1C7 transcript. In addition, the 5' exon gave considerably stronger signals on RNA blots than did the remainder of the 1C7 cDNA, suggesting that there are other transcripts sharing this same 5' exon. These are currently under investigation.

The human B144 transcript is about 700 bases long and is very abundantly expressed in the U937 cell line. The B144 RNA actually represents a complex mixture of alternatively spliced forms of RNA using alternative 5' exons. At present we recognize eight exons that contribute in various combinations to the B144 transcript family. There appear to be 3 alternative 5' exons and a total of as many as 50 alternative forms of the RNA, a number of which are present at relatively similar levels of abundance in U937 cells. Jurkat T cells also express a similar complex mixture of B144 transcripts although their absolute levels are lower than in the U937 cells. Among the spliced forms are some that use the highly unusual GA sequence as the first two bases of the 5' splice site intronic sequences, rather than the common GT or the occasionally used GC. Although putative homologies can be seen between potential reading frames of B144 and other proteins, direct evidence is needed as to which, if any, peptides are translated *in vivo* from B144 RNA before speculation about the function of the gene is warranted. At any rate the number of additional genes in the MHC that function in the immune system increase the difficulty of assigning weak QTL's (quantitative trait loci) for autoimmune diseases to specific genes within the MHC.

References

1. Raha-Chowdhury R, Bowen DJ, Burnett AK, Worwood M. Allelic associations and homozygosity at loci from HLA-B to D6S299 in genetic haemochromatosis. *J Med Genet* 1995; 32:446-52.
2. Campbell RD, Trowsdale, J. Map of the human MHC. *Immunol Today* 1993; 14:349-52.
3. Gruen JR, Nalabolu SR, Chu TW, Bowlus C, Fan WF, Goei VL, Wei H, Sivakamasundari R, Liu YC, Xu HX, Parimoo S, Nallur G, Ajioka R, Shukla H, BrayWard P, Pan J, Weissman SM. A transcription map of the major histocompatibility complex (MHC) class I region. *Genomics* 1996; 36: 70-85.
4. Nalabolu SR, Shukla H, Nallur G, Parimoo S, Weissman SM. Genes in a 220 kb region spanning the TNF cluster in human MHC. *Genomics* 1996; 31:215-22.
5. Parimoo S, Kolluri R, Weissman, SM. cDNA selection from total yeast DNA containing YACs. *Nucleic Acids Res* 1993; 21: 4422-3.
6. Vernet C, Boretto J, Mattei MG, Takahashi M, Jack, LJ, Mather IH, Rouquier S, Pontarotti P. Evolutionary study of multigenic families mapping close to the human MHC class I region. *J Mol Evol* 1993; 37:600-12.
7. Fan, WF, Liu YC, Parimoo S, Weissman, SM. Olfactory receptor-like genes are located in the human major histocompatibility complex. *Genomics* 1995;27:119-23.

Nucleotide sequence determination of the 237 kb segment around the HLA-B and -C genes and gene evolution of the MHC

N. Mizuki[1, 2], H. Ando[3], M. Kimura[1], S. Ohno[2], S. Miyata[1], M. Yamazaki[4], H. Tashiro[4], K. Watanabe[4], A. Ono[4], S. Taguchi[4], K. Okumura[5], K. Goto[1,2], M. Ishihara[1,2], T. Shiina[1], A. Ando[1], T. Ikemura[6], H. Inoko[1] *

1 Department of Genetic Information, Division of Molecular Life Science, Tokai University School of Medicine, Bohseidai, Isehara, Kanagawa 259-11, Japan
2 Department of Ophthalmology, Yokohama City University School of Medicine, 3-9 Fukuura, Kanazawa-ku, Yokohama, Kanagawa 236, Japan
3 Shonan Red Cross Blood Center, 1837 Aiko, Atsugi, Kanagawa 243, Japan
4 Bioscience Research Laboratory, Fujiya Co, Ltd, 228 Soya, Hadano, Kanagawa 257, Japan
5 Bioscience Laboratory, Mie University School of Bioresource, 1515 Kamihama- cho, Tsu, Mie 514, Japan
6 Department of Evolutional Genetics, National Institute of Genetics, 1111 Yata, Mishima, Shizuoka 411, Japan
* Corresponding author

The human leukocyte antigen (HLA) gene complex is located on the short arm of chromosome 6 within 6p21.3 and covers an about 4 Mb (4,000 kb) segment. There are presently 19 HLA or HLA-like expressed genes, more than 80 non-HLA expressed genes and 25 pseudogenes or gene fragments localized within the HLA region [1]. It is notable that many non-HLA genes involved or not involved in the immune response are located in the HLA region, although the function of most of these genes still remains uncertain. In this paper, in order to clarify the genomic structure of the uncharacterized class I region and to identify new genes involved in the development of HLA-associated diseases, the genomic sequence of a YAC (Y109) clone covering the 237 kb segment around the HLA-B and -C genes was determined and 5 novel genes designated as NOB (new organization associated with HLA-B) were identified. Further, we will present evidence that the HLA region on chromosome 6 and the 9q33-34 region on chromosome 9 likely arose as a result of an ancient duplication and discuss on the origin and evolution of the MHC.

Results and discussion

Cosmid contig of the Y109 YAC clone

A YAC clone, Y109 was isolated from a YAC library constructed from the B cell line, CGM1, using HLA class I specific primers *(Figure 1)* [2]. Y109 was partially digested with the restriction enzyme EcoR I and subcloned into the pWE15 cosmid vector. By screening the obtained cosmid clone library using the human Alu-repeat or genomic sequence as a probe, 316 cosmid clones containing human genomic DNAs in their inserts were isolated. These cosmid clones were completely digested with EcoR I followed by Southern hybridization using these EcoR I fragments as probes and could be assembled into a single contig.

Nucleotide sequence analysis

The nucleotide sequences of 7 representative overlapping cosmid clones in a cosmid contig were determined by the shot gun method, covering the 237 kb segment around the HLA-B and -C genes on chromosome 6. The 236,822 bp long sequence was determined by the redundancy of 6.4. This region was confirmed to contain the four previously known genes, MICA, HLA-17, HLA-B and HLA-C *(Figure 1)*. All 6 exons of the MICA gene were identified and the complete genomic sequence of the MICA gene was determined. The MICA gene spanning a 11,720 bp stretch of DNA was located 46,445 bp centromeric of the HLA-B gene. The orientation of the MICA gene was opposite to that of the HLA-B gene, facing each other in a head to head fashion. The distance between the HLA-B and -C genes could be exactly determined to be 81,247 bp long. This is close to the previous estimate (85 kb) roughly calculated based on pulsed field gel electrophoresis analysis. It is interesting to note that the nucleotide sequence of the downstream region of the HLA-B gene spanning about 39 kb, was highly homologous to that downstream of the HLA-C gene spanning about 33 kb, with more than 80 % nucleotide identity, suggesting segmental duplication including the MHC class I gene.

Homology search

Homology searches of the nucleotide sequences represented by these 7 cosmid clones against the up-to-date DNA database were carried out using FASTA and BLAST. The significantly homologous region to the P5-1 cDNA sequence was observed 1.3 kb centromeric of the HLA-17 pseudogene *(Figure 1)*. The nucleotide identity was 75.4 % over the coding sequence of the P5-1 cDNA clone. It was supposed to be a new member of the P5 multicopy family and designated as P5-8 gene. Similar to other P5 genes, the P5-8 gene is also located next to one of the HLA class I genes, HLA-17 pseudogene. One DHFR processed pseudogene was found to be 7 kb centromeric of the HLA-B gene and was designated DHFRP (DHFR pseudogene) *(Figure 1)*. The segment 7 kb centromeric of the HLA-C gene showed high homology to the human ribosomal protein L3 (RPL3) cDNA *(Figure 1)*. This sequence is not identical, but has 94.6 % nucleotide identity and 91.7 % amino acid identity with the human RPL3 cDNA sequence, suggesting that it is not a functional RPL3 gene but a pseudogene. This sequence was termed RPL3-Hom.

RT-PCR analysis and 5 new genes (NOB : new organization associated with HLA-B) detected by Northern blot analysis

The 237 kb sequence was also analyzed for coding probability and exon-intron structure, using the coding recognition module (CRM) of Grail, Grail II. In this way, 64 regions which gave "excellent", "good" or "marginal" by Grail II analysis and/or where coding sequences were predicted by homology search, were identified. RT-PCR was carried out using mRNAs from B cells, T cells and monocytes as templates and PCR was also performed using DNAs isolated from skin, kidney, duodenum and eye cDNA libraries as templates. As a result, 5, 4, 13, 15, 14, 24 and 3 transcripts (32 in total) were successfully amplified from B cells, T cells, monocytes, skin, kidney, eye and duodenum, respectively by this analysis.

In order to confirm the results of the RT-PCR analysis, Northern blot analysis was performed using the genomic fragments, from which the transcripts were detected by RT-PCR. Thus so far 5 new genes (NOB1-5) have been identified. A transcript of 10 kb detected ubiquitously in a large variety of tissues was mapped about 2 kb upstream of the MICA gene and this gene was designated as NOB1 *(Figure 1)*. From the NOB3 gene spanning the 45 kb region next to NOB1 *(Figure 1)*, 7 kb, 1.4 kb, 1.2 kb and 0.9 kb transcripts were identified in skeletal muscle. A 1.1 kb transcript was detected in pancreas from the NOB2 gene located between NOB1 and P5-8. A similar 7 kb transcript was also identified in skeletal muscle from the NOB5 gene upstream of HLA-C, but NOB3 and NOB5 did not show any homology to each other. The NOB4 gene, expressed specifically in placenta with a 6 kb transcript, was identified to be about 30 kb telomeric of the HLA-C gene *(Figure 1)*.

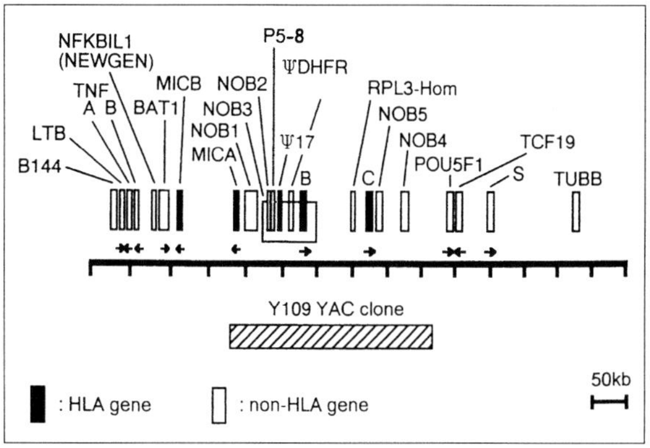

Figure 1. Gene organization of the HLA class I region subjected to nucleotide sequencing which spans the 237 kb region cloned by a YAC clone, Y109.

The 237 kb cosmid contig which was derived from a YAC clone, Y109 encoding the HLA-B and -C regions were determined for the nucleotide sequence by the shot gun method. The NOB (new organization associated with HLA-B)1-5 genes were newly identified in this study. The POU5F1 gene is also called, OCT3.

Table I. Gross similary of genes on 6p21.3 and those on 9q33-34

6p21.3 (HLA region)		9q33-34	
gene / locus	physical location	gene / locus	physical location
VARS2 (valyl-tRNA synthetase)	6p21.3	VARS1 (valyl-tRNA synthetase)	9
HSP70 (heat shock protein 70)	6p21.3	Bip(Ig heavy chain binding protein) GRP78 (glc-regulated protein)	9q33-34.1
C2, C4A, C4B	6p21.3	C5	9q33
TNX (tenascin-x)	6p21.3	HXB (tenascin C)	9q32-34
PBX2 (homeobox oncogene)	6p21.3	PBX3 (homeobox oncogene)	9q33-34
INT3 (Notch homologue)	6p21.3	TAN1 (Notch1)	9q34.3
TAP(ABC transporter)	6p21.3	ABC2 (ABC2 transporter)	9q33-34
LMP(LMP subunits of proteasome)	6p21.3	Z (z subunit of proteasome)	9q33-34
NAT(RING3 : homeotic gene)	6p21.3	NAT / RING3 homologue	9
COL11A2(collagen XIα2 chain)	6p21.3	COL5A1(collagen Vα1 chain)	9q34.2-34.3
RXRB (retinod x receptor β)	6p21.3	RXRA (retinod x receptor α)	9q34

Gross similarity of the HLA region on chromosome 6 and the 9q33-34 region on chromosome 9, and the evolution of the MHC

Through the analyses of the gene organization of the HLA region, we have noticed that the so far 11 genes including the HSP70 gene in the HLA region (6p21.3) have homologous related genes or sequences in the 9q33-34 region of chromosome 9 *(Table I)*. This linkage similarity between two sets of the gene region on chromosomes 6 and 9 may reflect a part of the paralogous chromosomal segments, indicating that these two regions were brought on and generated by segmental genome duplication during the process of gene evolution, probably before the appearance of the MHC genes. The HSP70 protein has the ability to bind peptide as chaperon molecule as observed in HLA antigen and the high dimensional conformation of HSP70 is very similar to that of HLA molecule with a large cleft surrounded by two α helixes which accommodates peptide and called peptide binding domain. Based on this similarity, it is tempting to speculate that the MHC gene was generated by assembly of the peptide-binding domain from the HSP70 gene in the ancestral syntenic group after the process of the duplication. Further, it is of great interest that in the midst of the 9q33-34 region, the ABO gene which determines the tissue type of red blood cell was located, possibly corresponding to the HLA genes which determine the tissue type of white blood cell in the 6p21.3 region. It can be hypothesized that these similar gene organization inserted by tissue type controlling genes, the ABO and HLA genes between the chromosome 9q33-34 and HLA regions confers upon the organism the selective advantage and reflect some adaptation under selective pressures.

Conclusion

We have determined the 236,822 bp nucleotide sequence including the MICA, HLA-B and HLA-C genes, and have identified so far 5 novel genes, NOB1-5 as well as the P5-8, DHFRP and RPL3-Hom genes. The two segments (about 40 kb) downstream of the HLA-B and HLA-C genes showed high sequence homology to each other, suggesting that segmental genome duplication including the MHC class I gene must have occurred during the evolution of the MHC. The HLA region on chromosome 6 and the 9q33-34 region on chromosome 9 contain at least 11 pairs of evolutionary related genes thought to have originated by duplication.

References

1. Campbell RD, Trowsdale J. Map of the human MHC. *Immunol Today* 1993 ; 14 : 349-52.
2. Imai T, Olson, MV. Second-generation approach to the construction of yeast artificial-chromosome libraries. *Genomics* 1990 ; 8 : 297-303.

MIC-A allelic variants

N. Fodil[1], L. Laloux[2], V. Wanner[1], P. Pellet[2], G. Hauptmann[1], T. Spies[3], I. Theodorou[2], S. Bahram [4]

1 Centre de Recherche d'Immunologie et d'Hématologie, 4, rue Kirschleger, 67085 Strasbourg Cedex, France
2 Laboratoire d'Immunologie Cellulaire et Tissulaire, Hôpital Pitié-Salpêtrière, 83, boulevard de l'Hôpital, 75651 Paris Cedex 13, France
3 Fred Hutchinson Cancer Research Center, Seattle, USA
4 J Basel Institute for Immunology, Grenzacherstrasse 487, Postfach, CH-4005 Basel, Switzerland

The classical major histocompatibility complex class I (MHC-Ia) molecules are highly polymorphic membrane bound glycoproteins that present endogenously derived peptide antigens to the αβ T-cell receptor of CD8+ T cells. They are represented in humans by the HLA-B, A and C molecules. In contrast, the so-called nonclassical or MHC-Ib genes (*i.e.* HLA-E, F and G) are almost invariant and, with the possible exception of HLA-G, do not play a discernible role in antigen presentation. However, despite this dramatic functional dichotomy, MHC-Ia and Ib molecules share a great degree of structural homology suggesting their recent divergence from a common ancestor late in speciation.

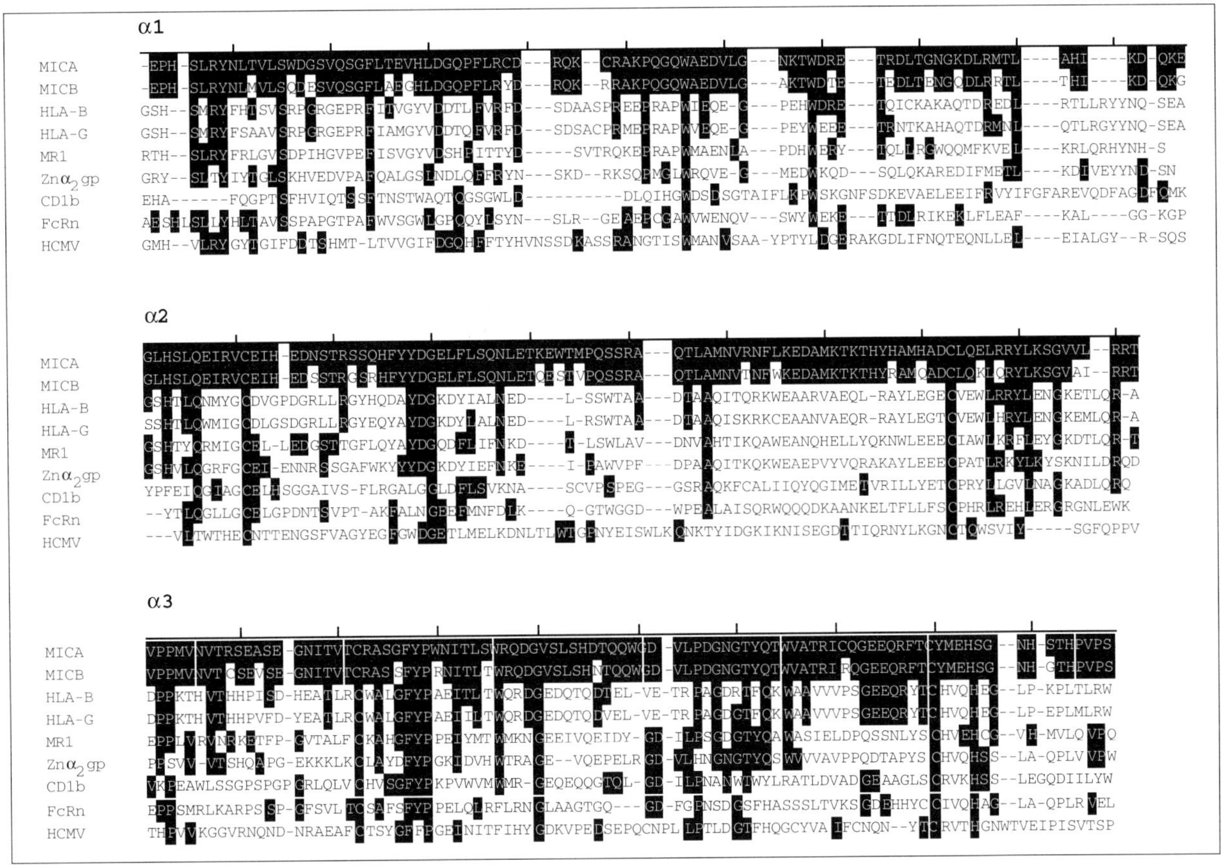

Figure 1. MICA and MICB are distant members of the MHC-I family of molecules.

Percent Similarity

2	3	4	5	6	7	8	9	10	11	12	13	14	15	16		
86.5	22.3	24.5	23.4	24.5	23.4	21.9	24.7	19.1	13.9	15.0	15.3	14.6	22.6	13.5	1	MICA
	23.0	23.0	23.0	23.0	22.6	21.9	24.7	18.0	13.5	15.0	16.1	13.9	22.6	13.9	2	MICB
		85.8	83.2	76.3	76.6	82.5	35.1	22.1	16.8	16.4	14.6	14.6	31.9	16.4	3	HLA-A*0201
			86.5	78.8	82.5	82.8	35.8	24.0	16.1	16.8	15.0	16.1	33.0	15.7	4	HLA-B*2702
				76.6	79.6	81.8	35.1	23.2	17.2	16.4	14.2	14.6	31.1	16.4	5	HLA-C*0301
					73.7	77.7	35.8	25.1	17.2	16.1	15.0	15.7	28.9	18.2	6	HLA-E
						78.8	35.1	25.5	16.8	16.8	15.3	17.5	31.1	16.1	7	HLA-F
							35.4	23.2	18.2	17.2	16.1	15.3	31.9	16.4	8	HLA-G
								27.3	24.0	19.9	19.9	17.7	32.6	13.7	9	MR1
									19.1	18.7	18.0	21.0	24.3	12.4	10	FcRn
										62.1	58.1	54.5	19.6	10.8	11	CD1a
											62.1	56.7	20.0	11.2	12	CD1b
												50.9	19.3	10.4	13	CD1c
													18.5	10.1	14	Cd1d
														11.5	15	Zn$\alpha_2$gp
															16	HCMV

Figure 2. Percent similarity of MICA and MICB within the MHC-I and MHC-I like molecules.

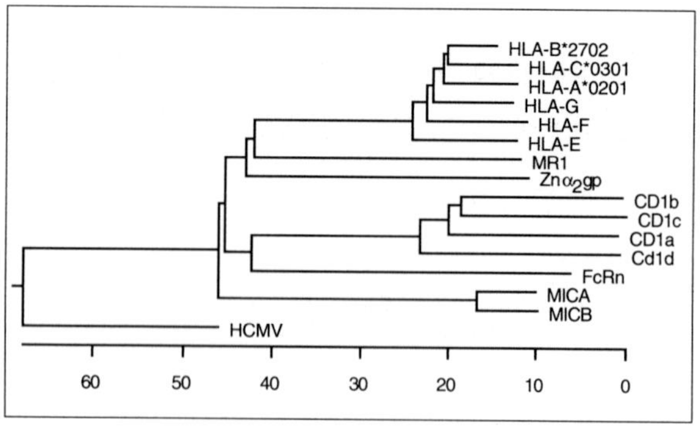

Figure 3. Phylogenetic tree.

In addition to these well known HLA genes, the human MHC harbors a second lineage of MHC-I genes [1-4]. The *MICA* and *MICB* (MHC class *I* chain-related) genes in this family are the most divergent MHC-I genes identified to date and are conserved throughout mammalian evolution *(Figure 1, 2* and *3)*. *MICA* and *MICB* expression is restricted mainly to cells of epithelial and fibroblastic origin. Their absence from the mouse genome, mirrored by the reciprocal lack of murine MHC-Ib genes in other mammals, suggests that *MICA* and *MICB* may be functional homologues of the murine MHC-Ib genes.

A hallmark of the MHC-Ia molecules is their extraordinary level of polymorphism, which enables them to collectively present an almost infinite range of peptide antigens to T cells. More than 150 alleles are known for HLA-B, close to 70 for *HLA-A* and almost 40 for *HLA-C*. In this context, parallel study of MIC polymorphism may shed light on their function in the immune system. As part of a comprehensive effort to unravel the degree of *MICA* and *MICB* polymorphism, we have been able to identify eleven new alleles for *MICA* which differ by a total of 22 amino acid substitutions [5]. Thus, the total number of *MICA* alleles identified to date is 16. Understanding the nature of selective forces driving MIC polymorphism is clearly our immediate goal.

Acknowledgments

We thank Susan Gilfillan and Marco Colonna for critical reading of this manuscript. Work in Strasbourg was supported by Association Française contre les Myopathies and Sidaction. Basel Institute for Immunology was founded and is supported by F. Hoffmann-La Roche Ltd, Basel, Switzerland.

References

1. Bahram S, Bresnahan M, Geraghty DE, Spies T. A second lineage of mammalian major histocompatibility complex class I genes. *Proc Natl Acad Sci USA* 1994; 91:6259-63.
2. Bahram S, Mizuki N, Inoko H, Spies T. Nucleotide sequence of the human MHC class I *MICA* gene. *Immunogenetics* 1996; 44: 80-1.
3. Bahram S, Spies T. Nucleotide sequence of a human MHC class I *MICB* cDNA. *Immunogenetics* 1996; 43: 230-3.
4. Bahram S, Spies T. The MIC gene family. *Res Immunol* 1996; 147: 328-33.
5. Fodil N, Laloux L, Wanner V, Pellet P, Hauptmann G, Mizuki N, Inoko H, Spies T, Theodorou I, Bahram S. Allelic repertoire of the human MHC class I *MICA* gene. *Immunogenetics* 1996; 44: 351-7.

Interlocus sequence analysis of the PERB11 gene family: implication for rapid diversification to different functions

C. Leelayuwat[1,2], S. Gaudieri[1], J. Mullberg[3], D. Cosman[3], R. Dawkins[1]

1 The Centre for Molecular Immunology and Instrumentation, The University of Western Australia, Perth, Western Australia, 6001 Australia
2 Department of Clinical Immunology, Faculty of Associated Medical Sciences, Khon Kaen University, Khon Kaen, 40002 Thailand
3 Immunex Research and Development Corporation, Seattle, Washington 98101, USA

PERB11 or MIC is a gene family belonging to the Immunoglobulin supergene family. It possesses multiple copies at least five of which are located in the MHC [1, 2]. The putative amino acid sequences of the PERB11.1 (MICA) and PERB11.2 (MICB) molecules are approximately 30% identical to MHC Class I molecules, neonatal IgG Fc receptor (FcRn) and Zinc-alpha2-glycoprotein. The PERB11.1 and PERB11.2 genes are located approximately 60 and 140 kb centromeric of HLA-B, respectively [1-3]. Although the functions of the PERB11 gene family have yet to be unravelled, it is most likely that immunological and transport processes are involved.

Results and discussions

In order to understand the functions of the PERB11 gene family, we have produced anti-peptide antibodies against the PERB11 molecules [4]. In addition, we have developed an approach based upon comparative analysis of DNA and protein sequences. We have sequenced three members of the PERB11 gene family; PERB11.1, PERB11.2 and PERB11.4. Sequence analysis includes the PERB11.1 sequences derived from 5 MHC ancestral haplotypes, two PERB11.2 sequences and the PERB11.4 sequence derived from the 57.1 MHC ancestral haplotype (HLA-A1, Cw6, B57,BfS, C4A6, C4B1, DRB1*0700, DQB1*03032). The allelic and interlocus differences of the PERB11 sequences are shown in *figure 1*. It can be seen that the most divergent domain is the transmembrane region when PERB11.1 and PERB11.2 are compared. The putative PERB11.2 protein sequence lacks all the potential glycosylation sites existing in the alpha-1 and alpha-2 domains of PERB11.1. It can also be seen that the allelic as well as interlocus differences include the presence and absence of glycosylation sites *(Figure 1)*. PERB11.1 derived from 8.1 (HLA-A1, Cw7, B8,BfS, C4AQ0, C4B1, DRB1*0301, DQB1*0201) possesses a nucleotide insertion in the transmembrane region resulting in a frameshift and an immature stop codon. This leads to a putative truncated molecule lac-

Table I. Percent identity of different domains amongst different members of the PERB11 gene family

	PERB11.1-18.2 (percent identity)											
	signal peptide		alpha-1 domain		alpha-2 domain		alpha-3 domain		transmembrane		cytoplasmic tail	
	protein 23aa	DNA 69nt	protein 85aa	DNA 255nt	protein 95aa	DNA 285nt	protein 93aa	DNA 279nt	protein 44aa	DNA 132nt	protein 42aa	DNA 126nt
PERB11.1-57.1	ND	ND	97,6	99,2	97,9	98,9	ND	ND	ND	ND	ND	ND
PERB11.1.7.1	ND	ND	97,6	98,4	96,8	98,6	ND	ND	ND	ND	ND	ND
PERB11.1-8.1	ND	ND	97,6	98,4	96,8	98,6	94,6	97,8	*	*	ND	ND
PERB11.1-46.1	ND	ND	96,5	98,4	95,8	98,2	ND	ND	ND	ND	ND	ND
PER11.2-IMX	73,9	82,6	83,5	92,0	85,3	92,3	90,3	95,7	56,8	74,2	ND	ND
PERB11.2-57.1	ND	ND	83,5	91,4	82,1	90,2	ND	ND	ND	ND	85,7	90,5
MICB	73,9	82,6	82,4	91,4	85,3	92,3	91,4	96,4	59,0	75,0	88,1	92,0
PERB11.4-57.1	ND	ND	74,1	84,7	*	*	ND	ND	ND	ND	ND	ND

```
SIGNAL PEPTIDE

PERB11.1-18.2     MGLGPVFLLLAGIFPFAPPGAAA
MICA              -----------------------
MICB              ----R-L-F--VA------A---
PERB11.2(IMX)     ----R-L-F--VA------A---

ALPHA1 DOMAIN

PERB11.1-18.2     EPHSLRYNLTVLSWDGSVQSGFLTEVHLDGQPFLRCDRQKCRAKPQGQWAEDVLGNKTWDRETRDLTGNGKDLRMTLAHIKDQKE
PERB11.1-57.1     -------------G---------A-------------------------------------------------------------
PERB11.1-7.1      -----------------------A-----------Y-------------------------------------------------
PERB11.1-46.1     -----P-----------------A-----------Y-------------------------------------------------
PERB11.1-8.1      -----------------------A-----------Y-------------------------------------------------
MICA              -------------------------------------------------------------------------------------
MICB              ---------M---Q-E-------A-G---------Y----R--------------A----T--E---E--Q---R--T------G
PERB11.2(IMX)     ---------M---Q---------A-G---------Y----R--------------A----T--E---E--Q---R--T------G
PERB11.2-57.1     ---------M---Q---------A-G---------Y----R--------------A----T--E---E--Q---R--T------G
PERB11.4-57.1     G----H-------------------G--------LFN---G--GSR-----A---AE---T--E---E--Q---RA--Y--G--G

ALPHA2 DOMAIN

PERB11.1-18.2     GLHSLQEIRVCEIHEDNSTRSSQHFYYDGELFLSQNLETKEWTMPQSSRAQTLAMNVRNFLKEDAMKTKTHYHAMHADCLQELRRYLKSGVVLRRT
PERB11.1-57.1     -----R---------------------------------E--------------------------------------------------------
PERB11.1-7.1      ---------------------------------------E---V-------------------------------------------E--------
PERB11.1-46.1     ---------------------------------------E---V-------------------------------------------E-S------
PERB11.1-8.1      ---------------------------------------E---V-------------------------------------------E--------
MICA              ------------------------------------------------------------------------------------------------
MICB              ----------------S---G-R----------------Q-S-V-------------T--W-----------R--Q-----K-Q-------AI---
PERB11.2-IMX      ----------------S---G-R----------------Q-S-V-------------T--W-----------R--Q-----K-Q-------AI---
PERB11.2-57.1     ----------------S---G-R----------------Q-S-V-----X-----D-T--W-G---------R-HE-----K-Q-------AI-X-

                            ↓ FRAMESHIFT
PERB11.4-57.1     A--------G---RKPAAPGALGIPTLMGSSSSLSTWRLRKGQYPSPPELRPLL*

ALPHA3 DOMAIN

PERB11.1-18.2     VPPMVNVTRSEASEGNITVTCRASGFYPWNITLSWRQDGVSLSHDTQQWGDVLPDGNGTYQTWVATRICQGEEQRFTCYMEHSGNHSTHPVPS
PERB11.1-8.1      ------------------------S---R--I-T-----------------------------------R-----------------------
MICA              ---------------------------------------------------------------------------------------------
MICB              --------C--V------------S---R----T----------N-----------------------R-----------------G------
PERB11.2-IMX      -------IC--V------------S---R----T----------N-----------------------R-----------------G------

TRANSMEMBRANE REGION

PERB11.1-18.2     GKVLVLQSHWQTFHVSAVAAAAIFVIIIFYVRCCKKKTSAAEGP

                                      ↓ FRAMESHIFT
PERB11.1-8.1      --------------------GCCYFCYYYFLCPLL*
MICA              --------------------------------------------
MICB              --------QRTD-PYVSA-MPCFVI---LC-P------------
PERB11.2-IMX      --A-----QRTD-PYVSA-MPCFVI---LC-P------------

CYTOPLASMIC DOMAIN

PERB11.1-18.2     ELVSLQVLDQHPVGTSDHRDATQLGFQPLMSDLGSTGSTEGA
MICA              ------------------------------------------
MICB              ---------------G-----A---------AT---------
PERB11.2-57.1     --V------G-----A---------AT--------T
```

Figure 1. Amino acid comparison of the PERB11 gene family. The comparison between different haplotypes of the PERB11.1 gene reveals several polymorphic sites giving rise to different alleles of the gene. The 8.1 haplotype shows a high degree of polymorphism in the transmembrane region, where a single base insertion at the DNA level has resulted in an early termination site. Inter-locus comparison of the PERB11 gene family reveals a high degree of diversity amongst the three members; PERB11.1, PERB11.2 and PERB11.4. The most divergent domain is the transmembrane region when PERB11.1 and PERB11.2 are compared. The number of shared amino acids between PERB11.2 and PERB11.4 in the alpha 1 domain is greater than that shared by PERB11.1 and PERB11.2 suggesting a closer relationship between the two gene sequences. PERB11.4 has an early termination signal in the alpha 2 domain. Dashes indicate identity and an asterisk indicates a stop codon. Potential glycosylation sites are boxed. The differences in glycosylation sites are found in both allelic and interlocus comparisons.

king the cytoplasmic portion. The 8.1 MHC ancestral haplotype is associated with several diseases [5-7]. The relevance of this finding to disease development associated with this haplotype is currently under investigation.

Table I compares percent identity at both DNA and protein levels of different domains of PERB11.1 derived from 18.2 (HLA-A30, Cw5, B18,BfF1, C4A3, C4BQ0, DRB1*0301, DQB1*0201) versus PERB11.1 from four MHC ancestral haplotypes, three PERB11.2 sequences and one PERB11.4. The allelic differences in the alpha-1 and alpha-2 domains of PERB11.1 is low ranging from 2.1 to 4.2 % at the protein level and 0.8 to 1.8% at the DNA level. In contrast, the differences of the same domains between PERB11.1 and PERB11.2 at the protein level is much higher ranging from 14.7 to 17.9% with a low degree of differences at the DNA level ranging from 7.7 to 9.8%. Like MHC class I molecules, the alpha-3 domain is the most conserved domain (~90% at amino acid and 95% at DNA) when PERB11.1 and PERB11.2 are compared. It appears that the molecules have diverged more at the protein than at the DNA level. The result suggests that PERB11.1 and PERB11.2 may bind different ligands leading to different functions. Indeed, there may be extremely diverse as suggested by the recent claim that so called HLA-H which is closely related to the PERB11 family may be involved in the pathogenesis of haemochromatosis [8].

Conclusion

We have described here a comparative genomic analysis of the PERB11 gene family which suggests that the two members of the gene family, PERB11.1 and PERB11.2, have diverged rapidly at the protein level leading to diverse functions. This approach can be used to identify protein regions and motifs that would be useful for antibody production to further characterise the functions of the gene family.

Acknowledgments

We would like to thank David Townend, Gerhard Saueracker, Louise Taylor and Laila Gizzarelli for their technical assistance. This work was supported by the Australian National Health and Medical Research Council and the Immunogenetics Research Foundation. Publication number 9622 of the Centre for Molecular Immunology and Instrumentation, The University of Western Australia, The Institute for Molecular Genetics and Immunology, Departments of Clinical Immunology, Royal Perth Hospital and Sir Charles Gairdner Hospital.

References

1. Leelayuwat C, Townend DC, Degli-Esposti MA, Abraham LJ, Dawkins RL. A new polymorphic and multicopy MHC gene family related to nonmammalian class I. *Immunogenetics* 1994; 40: 339-51.
2. Bahram S, Bresnahan M, Geraghty DE, Spies T. A second lineage of mammalian major histocompatibility complex class I genes. *Proc Natl Acad Sci USA* 1994; 91: 6259-63.
3. Bahram S, Spies T. Nucleotide sequence of a human MHC class I MICB cDNA. *Immunogenetics* 1996; 43: 230-3.
4. Leelayuwat C, Hollingsworth P, Pummer S, Lertmemongkolchai G, Thom G, Mullberg J, Witt C, Kaufman J, Cosman D, Dawkins R. Antibody reactivity profiles following immunisation with diverse peptides of the PERB11 (MIC) family. *Clin Exp Immunol* 1997 (in press).
5. Degli-Esposti MA, Andreas A, Christiansen FT, Schalke B, Albert E, Dawkins RL. An approach to the localization of the susceptibility genes for generalised myasthenia gravis by mapping recombinant ancestral haplotypes. *Immunogenetics* 1992; 35: 355-64.
6. Degli-Esposti MA, Abraham LJ, McCann V, Spies T, Christiansen FT, Dawkins RL. Ancestral haplotypes reveal the role of the central MHC in the immunogenetics of IDDM. *Immunogenetics* 1992; 36: 345-56.
7. Cameron PU, Mallal SA, French MAH, Dawkins RL. Central MHC genes between HLA-B, complement C4 confer risk for HIV-1 disease progression. In: Tsuji K, Aizawa M, Sasazuki T eds. *HLA 1991*, vol 2. New York: Oxford University Press, 1992: 544-7.
8. Feder JN, Gnirke A, Thomas W *et al.* A novel MCH class I - like gene is mutated in patients with hereditary haemochromatosis. *Nature Genet* 1996; 13: 399-408.

MHC class I chain-related gene-A (MIC-A) polymorphism

C.J.T. Visser[1], D. Charron[1], R. Tamouza[1], Z. Tatari[1], E.H. Rozemuller[2], M.G.J. Tilanus[2]

1 Laboratory of Immunology and Histocompatibility, INSERM U 396, Saint-Louis Hospital,
1, avenue Claude Vellefaux, 75475 Paris Cedex 10, France
2 Department of Pathology, University Hospital, Heidelberglaan 1, 3584 CX Utrecht, The Netherlands

Human Leucocyte Antigen (HLA) molecules are very polymorphic. Based on their function, HLA class I and class II molecules can be discriminated, both presenting antigens to T-lymphocytes leading to an immunologic responce of these cells. The class I (HLA-A, -B and -C) and class II (HLA-DR, -DQ, -DP) gene families are located in distinct 1600- and 900-kb regions at the telomeric and centromeric sides of the MHC, respectively. They flank a 1000-kb central region occasionally called the class III region. Spies *et al.* [1] reported the existence of at least 19 genes with still unrevealed function in this central region.

Following this line of research, Bahram *et al.* [2] described the cloning and characterization of MICA and, more recently, MICB [3] genes. Leelayuwat *et al.* [4] reported the finding of a genomic probe located approximately 60 kb centromeric of HLA-B, which they called PERB11. It happened to be that Bahram and Leelayuwat most probably found the same gene [5].

In these papers it was demonstrated that these genes have an amino acid sequence structure characteristic for HLA class I genes but have an unusual intron-exon structure. Moreover, up to five MIC genes (MICA-MICE) were discovered in the MHC. In contrast to the classical HLA class I genes, MICA genes have been found to be restrictedly expressed in epithelial cells mostly, whereas no expression could be detected in B- or T-lymphocytes.

The MICA gene has also been reported to be polymorphic [2,4]. However, until now, only seven (partial) MICA allele nucleotide sequences have been submitted to Genbank or EMBL databases. Moreover, of these published sequences, only two MICA sequences do not contain unresolved heterozygous nucleotide bases. In the present paper, polymorphism of MICA exon 3 nucleotide sequences are reported in 41 cell lines, using fully automated sequencing based typing (SBT).

Materials and methods

Polymerase chain reaction (PCR)

Most cell lines reported in this paper were HLA typing cell lines obtained from ECACC. DNA samples were also obtained directly from ECACC or isolated from these cell lines using standard procedures. Cell lines having names starting with B27 were a generous gift from dr. R. Tamouza (Paris, France). For MICA exon 3 PCR, forward (5'-TTCGGGAATGGAGAAGTCACTGC-3') and reverse (5'-GGAAAATCAGGACACGATGTGCC-3') primers were selected in homologous intron areas based on sequences submitted to the Genbank database by Leelayuwat *et al.* [4]. Using the NCBI-BLAST internet server, these oligonucleotide sequences were tested for specificity for MICA. PCR was performed in an PE9600 or PE2400 Thermocycler (Perking Elmer), using Taq-polymerase (Perking Elmer or ATCG; 5 U/ml). PCR samples were stored at 4°C until used. Integrity, purity and size of the PCR products (5 μl/sample) were checked on ethidium bromide-containing 2% agarose gels. Forward primers were tailed with a -21M13 sequence, whereas reverse primers were tailed with the M13RP1 sequence in order be able to directly sequence the obtained PCR products using the non-radioactive Taq-FS sequencing kit (ABI/Perking Elmer) according to the suppliers instructions. All PCR-products were sequenced both in forward- and reverse direction. Sequence products were run on ABI 737 or ABI 377 automated sequencers and data were collected by the respective ABI-Prism/Perking Elmer Data Extraction Programs running on Power Macintosh computers.

Table I. MICA exon 3 putative polymorphism

Polymorphic positions																		Cell line	Cloned	MICA typing
59	81	109	115	118	130	161	196	212	226	229	230	253	262	268	271	281	287			(artificial names)
G	C	C	A	G	G	C	A	A	C	G	C	C	G	G	G	G	C	Consensus		
																		CHI013		MICA-A
																		MT48		MICA-A
																		LAF		MICA-A
																		DKB		MICA-A
																		Jurkat		MICA-A
																		PAR		MICA-A
																		SPO010		MICA-A
																		MCF7		MICA-A
		G												A				LUY		MICA-B
		G												A				JHAF	x	MICA-B
		G												A				EHM-allele	x	MICA-B
		G												A				BOB (2)		MICA-B
		G												A				BOB (3)		MICA-B
					A		G						A					LWAGS	x	MICA-C
					A		G						A					MZO70782		MICA-C
					A		G						A					T47D		MICA-C
		G												A	A			KAS116 (1)	x	MICA-D
		G												A	A			KAS116 (2)		MICA-D
					A								A					WJR076		MICA-E
					A								A					BM16		MICA-E
					A								A					HOM-2		MICA-E
					A								A					ZR75-1		MICA-E
					A								A					WDV		MICA-E
					A								A					WT24		MICA-E
					A								A					B2709	x	MICA-E
	T	G												A				MANIKA	x	MICA-F
														A				JO528239		MICA-G
														A				OLL	x	MICA-G
A					A									A				EHM-allele	x	MICA-H
		s												r				BT549		A/B
					r								r					B2701		A/E
					r								r					B2705		A/E
					r								r					B2708		A/E
					r								r					WBD001088		A/E
					r								r					THOMA		A/E
					r								r					GRE,G		A/E
					r								r					SK-BR3		A/E
					r								r					CTM195341		A/E
					r								r					LS40		A/E
					r								r					AVE,G		A/E
					r								r					IHL,AD031		A/E
	y	s			r								r	r				B2703		E/F
														r				B2707		A/G
														r				KNE		A/G
r		s			r								r	r				EHM	x	B/H

Data analysis
Data analysis was performed on Power Macintosh computers using the ABI-Prism Perking Elmer Sequence Analysis (version 2.1.1)- and Sequence Navigator (version 1.0.1) software. In addition, a number of sequences has been analyzed using the MS-DOS compatible programs HETERO, ALLELE and POLALL similar to HLA-DPB sequencing based typing [6].

Cloning
Heterozygous sequences and sequences exhibiting new polymorphic positions were cloned using the Stratagene pCR-Script™ SK(+) blunt-end cloning kit according to the suppliers instructions. Plasmids were isolated from the bacteria using the Miniprep Express™ Kit (BIO 101, Vista, CA, USA) according to suppliers instructions. These plasmids were used directly for sequencing as described above for PCR products.

Results

Sequencing of MICA exon 3 DNA samples from 41 different cell lines resulted in 25 homozygous and 16 heterozygous sequences as summarized in *Table I* (cell lines BOB and KAS116 have been typed from two different DNA samples). Individual alleles of these 16 heterozygous sequences could be deduced from the homozygous sequences. Subsequent cloning confirmed the seven homozygous nucleotide sequences (from which only the consensus sequence has been published previously [4]) and resolved the heterozygous sequence of cell line EHM resulting in another new MICA exon 3 allele. Additionally, 12 other cell lines (not shown) demonstrate heterozygous sequences that could not be deduced from the known homozygous sequences; the individual alleles still have to be resolved by cloning.
Translation of the eight MICA exon 3 alleles results in seven putative protein sequences (*Table II*). Due to a silent nucleotide substitution at position 81, the MICA-F allele appears to have an identical protein translation when compared with the MICA-B allele.

Conclusions and discussion

In the present paper seven new MICA exon 3 nucleotide sequences are reported using a fully automated sequencing based typing (SBT) approach. Being a rather new technique, from these experiments it can be concluded that a routinely performed SBT protocol (such as performed in several HLA-typing laboratories) can be implemented on the typing of "new gene" alleles without major adaptations. Now we are able to deal with 36 samples from DNA to sequence analysis in only 36 hours. The automation of data collection and the substitution of the radiolabelled nucleotides or primers with fluorescent dyes have resulted in a fast, safe and convenient way of SBT, generating data with the highest possible resolution.
From our results it can be concluded that MICA exon 3 is the most polymorphic exon of the MICA gene, although the extent of polymorphism probably will be no more than 10-15 homozygous sequences. From preliminary experiments in our laboratory (not shown) and from results published [2,4] it can be concluded that exon 2 has also polymorphic positions, although most probably to a lesser extend than exon 3. Therefore, combinatorial polymorphism of exon 3 and exon 2 data will result in additional MICA alleles. Moreover, cloning experiments that currently are performed in our laboratory will resolve a number of heterozygous ambiguity sequences, resulting in even more MICA homozygous sequences. However, due to silent mutations, not all variations in nucleotide sequences will be reflected in different amino acid sequences. It is our estimate now, that the number of MICA alleles will be around 15. Preliminary experiments on MICA mRNA expression in our laboratory are confirming the absence of expression in T- and B-lymphocytic cells and the presence in epithelial cells as reported previously [2,4], and also expression in several epithelial tumor cell lines.
The exon-homology of the MICA gene with classical HLA class I molecules, the polymorphism in exon 2 and 3 and its dissimilar expression pattern are pointing to a functional role that is related to, but will probably be quite different from the classical HLA class I molecules. Since the MICA gene is located close to HLA-B and since HLA-B (sub)types have been associated with various diseases, it may be interesting to investigate linkage between HLA-B (sub)types and the various MICA alleles.

Table II. MICA exon 3 putative protein sequences

Consensus	**GLHSLQEIRV**	**CEIHEDNSTR**	**SSQHFYYDGE**	**LFLSQNLETE**	**EWTVPQSSRA**	**50**
MICA-A	....	....	....	....	....	50
MICA-B	....	.........K	....	....	...M......	50
MICA-C	....	....	....	....	...M......	50
MICA-D	....	....	....	......V...	....	50
MICA-E	....	....	....	....	...M......	50
MICA-G	....	....	....	....	....	50
MICA-H	....	....	....	......V...	....	50

Consensus	**QTLAMNVRNF**	**LKEDAMKTKT**	**HYHAMHADCL**	**QELRRYLESG**	**VVLRRT**	**96**
MICA-A	....	....	....	....	......	96
MICA-B	....	....	....	.......K..	......	96
MICA-C	....	.....V....	....	.......K..	......	96
MICA-D	....	....	....	.........S	I.....	96
MICA-E	....	....	....	.......K..	......	96
MICA-G	....	....	....	.........S	......	96
MICA-H	....	....	....	.........S	......	96

References

1. Spies T, Bresnahan M, Strominger JL. Human major histocompatibility complex contains a minimum of 19 genes between the complement cluster and HLA-B. *Proc Natl Acad Sci USA* 1989; 86: 8955-8.
2. Bahram S, Bresnahan M, Geraghty DE, Spies T. A second lineage of mammalian major histocompatibility complex class I genes. *Proc Natl Acad Sci USA* 1994; 91: 6259-63.
3. Bahram S, Spies T. Nucleotide sequence of a human MHC class I MICB cDNA. *Immunogenetics* 1996; 43: 230-3.
4. Leelayuwat C, Townend DC, Degli-Esposti MA, Abraham LJ, Dawkins RL. A new polymorphic and multicopy MHC gene family related to nonmammalian class I. *Immunogenetics* 1994; 40: 339-51.
5. Leelayuwat C, Townend DC, Degli-Esposti MA, Abraham LJ, Dawkins RL. Idem. Erratum. *Immunogenetics* 1995; 41: 174 .
6. Rozemuller EH, Bouwens-Rombouts AGM, Bast EJEG, Tilanus MGJ. Assignment of HLA-DPB alleles by computerized matching based upon sequence data. *Hum Immunol* 1993; 37: 207-12.

Characterisation of the G15 gene located between the class II region and the C4 genes in the human MHC

B. Aguado, R.D. Campbell

MRC Immunochemistry Unit, Department of Biochemistry, Oxford University, South Parks Road, Oxford OX1 3QU, UK

Characterisation of a 150kb segment of DNA located between the class II region and the complement C4 genes in the class III region of the human MHC, has revealed that it contains at least eight genes: NOTCH-3, G18, PBX-2 (G17), RAGE, G16, G15, G14 and G13. NOTCH-3, the human counterpart of the mouse mammary tumor gene *int*-3, encodes a member of the Notch family of transmembrane proteins; PBX-2 is a multicopy gene that encodes a homeodomain-containing protein with extensive similarity to PBX-1, which is involved in acute pre-B-cell leukemias; RAGE is the gene for the receptor of advanced glycosylation end products of proteins, a member of the immunoglobulin superfamily of cell surface molecules; and G13 contains a leucine zipper, bZip domain, which is conserved in many transcriptional factors including the cyclic AMP-response element binding (CREB) protein family (for review see [1]). In this report we describe the initial characterisation of the G15 gene which shows homology with the 1-acyl-*sn*-glycerol-3-phosphate acyltransferase (lysophosphatidic acid acyl transferase; LPAAT) from bacteria and yeast.

LPAAT is the enzyme that converts lysophosphatidic acid (LPA) into phosphatidic acid (PA). LPA (1-acyl-*sn*-glycero-3-phosphate) is formed in the endoplasmic reticulum (ER) membrane from glycerol 3-phosphate through the action of glycerolphosphate acyltransferase (GPAT). LPA consists of a glycerol backbone with a fatty acyl chain at the *sn*-1 position, a hydroxyl group at the *sn*-2 position and a phosphate group at the *sn*-3 position. LPA is then further acylated by LPAAT to yield PA, the precursor of all glycerolipids. PA can either be hydrolyzed to yield diacylglycerol (DAG) or, alternatively, be converted to CDP-DAG for the synthesis of more complex phospholipids in the ER, from which they are transported to different subcellular compartments (see references in [2]).

Nucleotide sequence of G15

The G15 gene, which is localised ~260kb telomeric of the DRA gene, is a single copy gene as defined by comparative analysis of genomic and cosmid Southern blots. Northern blot analysis of RNA from the cell lines U937 (promonocytic leukemia), Molt4 (T-cell leukemia) and Raji (Burkitt lymphoma) revealed that the G15 gene encodes a 2.1kb mRNA. Screening of a U937 cDNA library, using two cosmids (D3A and E91) as probes, resulted in the isolation of 22 clones. Characterisation of these clones by restriction enzyme mapping revealed that pG15-3B contained a full-length cDNA insert of ~2.1kb [3]. Both strands of this cDNA were sequenced by the dideoxy chain termination method after cloning random sonicated fragments in the size range 300-1000bp by blunt end ligation into SmaI-cut M13mp18.

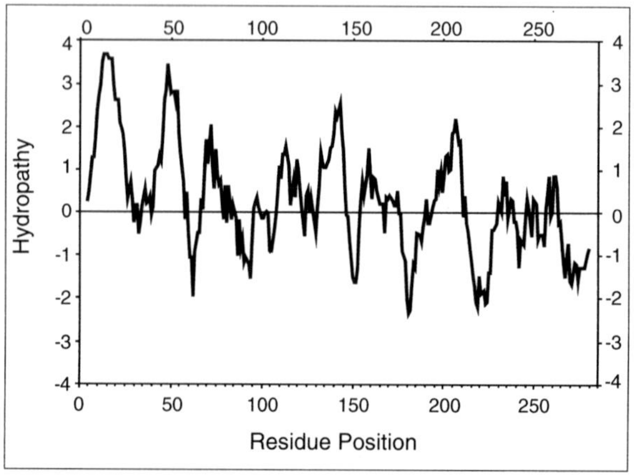

Figure 1. Hydrophobicity profile of G15 generated using the PepWindow program from the GCG package.

2051bp were determined with a degeneracy of 9.0. This clone contained a poly(A) signal AATAAA 17bp upstream of a 21bp poly(A) tail.

Translation of the DNA sequence in 6 phases revealed a single long ORF which was predicted to encode a polypeptide of 283 amino acids and with a predicted molecular weight of ~31.7kDa. The hydrophobicity plot of G15 is shown in *Figure 1* indicating that the G15 gene encodes a hydrophobic protein. At the N-terminus there are two potential signal sequences and there are 5 or 6 potential membrane spanning regions, suggesting that G15 could be a transmembrane protein.

G15 database search

A search of the SWISSPROT databases using the FastA program in the software package of the University of Wisconsin Genetics Computer Group (GCG) [4] with the G15 protein sequence revealed homology with the entire sequence of LPAAT from different bacteria (*Haemophilus, Salmonella, Escherichia,* and *Neisseria*) and from yeast (*Saccharomyces*). Using the BestFit program from the GCG package, G15 was shown to be related to the LPAAT from *Saccharomyces cerevisiae* (30.88% identity and 54.44 % similarity) [5], from *Haemophilus influenzae* (30.41% identity and 56.66% similarity) [6], from *Salmonella typhimurium* (28.09% identity and 51.24% similarity) [7], from *Escherichia coli* (27.68% identity and 51.24% similarity) [8], and from *Neisseria gonorrhoeae* (24.89% identity and 47.21% similarity) and *Neisseria meningitidis* (24.03% identity and 47.64% similarity) [9] *(Table I)*. Multiple sequence aligment of these sequences (PileUp program from the GCG package) shows that they are highly related and the corresponding dendrogram indicates the relationships *(Table II)*.

Table I. Percentage of amino acid identities (ID) or similarities (SIM) between the complete sequence of G15 and LPAATs from different organisms: human (G15), *Saccharomyces cerevisiae* (Sacc.Cer.), *Haemophilus influenzae* (H.Influ.), *Salmonella typhimurium* (S.Typhi.), *Escherichia coli* (E.Coli), *Neisseria gonorrhoeae* (N.Gono.) and *Neisseria meningitidis* (N.Menin.). BestFit scores were obtained from the GCG package

% ID \ SIM	G15	Sacc.Cer.	H.Influ.	S.Typhi.	E.Coli	N.Gono.	N.Menin.
G15	—	30.88	30.41	28.09	27.68	24.89	24.03
Sacc.Cer.	54.44	—	29.83	33.05	31.38	26.55	23.69
H.Influ.	56.66	51.26	—	60.41	61.66	21.49	20.17
S.Typhi.	51.24	56.48	78.75	—	93.87	22.08	21.25
E.Coli	51.24	55.23	79.16	96.73	—	21.66	20.83
N.Gono.	47.21	51.86	43.42	44.58	43.75	—	97.65
N.Menin.	47.64	49.80	43.42	44.16	43.33	98.82	—

Table II. Dendrogram or tree representation of clustering relationships of LPAAT from different species generated using the PileUp program in the GCG package

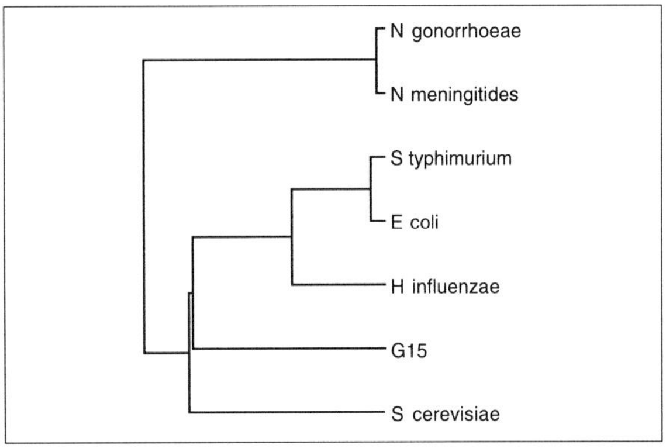

Expression of G15 in insect cells using the baculovirus system

To characterise the G15 gene product, the protein was expressed in Spodoptera frugiperda (Sf) 21 insect cells infected with baculovirus (Autographa californica Nuclear Polyhedrosis Virus) kindly provided by Dr. A. Alcami (Sir William Dunn School of Pathology, University of Oxford). To remove the 3' and 5' flanking sequences of G15, in order to express only the coding sequence under the control of the polyhedrin promoter, a PCR copy of the ORF was generated using oligonucleotide primers, ligated into the plasmid pBluescript KS^{+} and several clones were sequenced. The insert of one clone, that did not include any PCR errors was excised, and ligated to the baculovirus transfer vector pAcCL29.1, kindly provided by Dr. I. Jones (NERC Institute of Virology and Environmental Microbiology, Oxford) to yield pG15Bac. Sf21 cells were cotransfected with BacPACK6 DNA (Clontech) and pG15Bac, using lipofectin, to create G15 recombinants. After the cotransfection and the first plaque assay, ten clones were isolated and plaque purified four times. At this stage, pulse-label experiments were done to detect expression of G15 and the results using two of the clones are shown in *Figure 2*.

G15 was not secreted into the medium *(Figure 2)* in contrast to the control AcB15R, the soluble interleukin-Iß receptor of vaccinia virus expressed in insect cells using the baculovirus system (kindly provided by Dr. A. Alcami) [10]. Analysis of the labeled cell extracts showed that the wild type baculovirus contained the polyhedrin protein (P) not present in the polyhedrin negative recombinants G15 or AcB15R. Specific proteins of 26 and 28kDa were detected in G15 recombinants that were not present in cell extracts obtained from AcB15R or wild type viruses *(Figure 2)*. The expected molecular weight for G15 is ~31.7kDa including the signal peptide. The SigCleave program in the GCG package predicts two signal peptides, one that would be cleaved after amino acid 22, and the second after amino acid 58. The 26 and 28kDa forms of G15 found in insect cells could be explained by the processing of G15 after both of these potential cleavage sites *(Figure 2)*. However, as the G15 protein could be aberrantly processed in insect cells, whether G15 is processed after either or both of these two potential cleavage sites in mammalian cells will be checked by immunoprecipitation or Western blot analysis of mammalian cell lines.

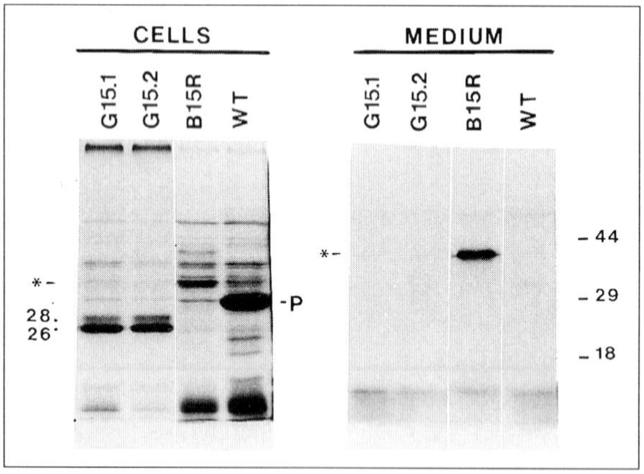

Figure 2. Expression of G15 protein in baculovirus infected insect cells. Sf21 cells infected with wild type baculovirus (WT), AcB15R (B15R) or G15 recombinants (G15.1, G15.2) were pulse labeled with ^{35}S-Trans-label from 24 to 27 hours post-infection, and proteins present in cells and in the medium were analyzed by SDS-PAGE and visualized by autoradiography. The proteins and the molecular size markers are indicated in kDa. The positions of the polyhedrin protein (P) and the IL1βR protein of vaccinia virus (*) are shown.

Conclusion

The novel gene G15 encodes a 283 amino acid protein with a predicted molecular weight of ~32kDa which contains putative transmembrane segments. The polypeptide shows homology with the enzyme LPAAT from *Saccharomyces cerevisiae, Haemophilus influenzae, Salmonella typhimurium, Escherichia coli, Neisseria gonorrhoeae* and *Neisseria meningitidis*. G15 is a very hydrophobic cellular protein and is most likely to be a transmembrane protein. The synthesis of phospholipids occurs on the cytosolic side of the ER membrane where each enzyme in the pathway is an integral membrane protein of the ER with its active site facing the cytosol, where all the intermediates required for phospholipid assembly are located. We have expressed G15 in insect cells using the baculovirus system and work is in progress to demonstrate by enzymatic assays whether G15 is the human LPAAT and to identify the cellular localisation of the enzyme in mammalian cell lines by immunofluorescence.

References

1. Aguado B, Milner CM, Campbell RD. Genes of the MHC class III region and the functions of the proteins they encode. In: Browning M, McMichael A, eds. *HLA/MHC: genes, molecules and function.* Oxford, UK: Bios Scientific Publishers Ltd, 1996: 39-75.
2. Jalink K, Hordijk PL, Moolenaar WH. Growth factor-like effects of lysophosphatidic acid, a novel lipid mediator. *Biochim Biophys Acta* 1994; 1198: 185-96.
3. Kendall E, Sargent CA, Campbell, RD. Human major histocompatibility complex contains a new cluster of genes between the HLA-D and complement C4 loci. *Nucleic Acids Res* 1990; 18: 7251-7.
4. Pearson WR, Lipman DJ. Improved tools for biological sequence comparison. *Proc Natl Acad Sci USA* 1988; 85: 2444-8.

5. Nagiec MM, Wells GB, Lester RL, Dickson RC. A suppressor gene that enables *Saccharomyces cerevisiae* to grow without making sphingolipids encodes a protein that resembles an *Escherichia coli* fatty acyltransferase. *J Biol Chem* 1993; 29: 22156-63.
6. Fleischmann RD, Adams MD, White O, Clayton RA, Kirkness EF, Kerlavage AR, Bult CJ, Tomb JF, Dougherty BA, Merrick JM, McKenney K, Sutton G, Fitzhugh W, Fields C, Gocayne JD, Scott J, Shirley R, Liu LI, Glodek A, Kelley JM, Weidman JF, Phillips CA, Spriggs T, Hedblom E, Cotton MD, Utterback TR, Hanna MC, Nguyen DT, Saudek DM, Brandon RC, Fine LD, Fritchman JL, Fuhrmann JL, Geoghagen NSM, Gnehm CL, McDonald LA, Small KV, Fraser CM, Smith HO, Venter JC. Whole-genome random sequencing and assembly of *Haemophilus influenzae* Rd. *Science* 1995; 269: 496-512.
7. Luttinger AL, Springer AL, Schmid MB. A cluster of genes that affects nucleoid segregation in *Salmonella typhimurium. New Biol* 1991; 7: 687-97.
8. Coleman J. Characterization of the *Escherichia coli* gene for 1-acyl-sn-glycerol-3-phosphate acyltransferase (plsC). *Mol Gen Genet* 1992 ; 232: 295-303.
9. Swartley JS, Balthazar JT, Coleman J, Shafer WM, Stephens DS. Membrane glycerophospholipid biosynthesis in *Neisseria meningitides* and *Neisseria gonorrhoeae*: identification, characterization, and mutagenesis of a lysophosphatidic acid acyltransferase. *Mol Microbiol* 1995; 18: 401-12.
10. Alcami A, Smith GL. A soluble receptor for interleukin-1ß encoded by vaccinia virus: a novel mechanism of virus modulation of the host response to infection. *Cell* 1992; 71: 153-67.

Tissue specific expression and variable alternative splicing of the *LST1* gene in the TNF region

A. de Baey[1,2], B. Fellerhoff [2], S. Maier [2], E.D. Albert [3], E.H. Weiss[2]

1 Department of Dermatology, University of Munich, Germany
2 Institute for Anthropology and Human Genetics, University of Munich, Richard-Wagner-Straße 10/1, 80333 Munich, Germany
3 Immunogenetics Laboratory, Children's Policlinic, University of Munich, Germany

Extensive studies of the central MHC (class III) which is be well conserved between species, has revealed a high density of genes encoding proteins involved in immune functions. In particular the tumor necrosis factor (TNF) locus, located about 250 kb centromeric of HLA-B and 350 kb telomeric of the class III complement genes, encodes the cytokines TNF-α, TNF-β (lymphotoxin α) [1] and lymphotoxin β (LT-β) [2] which play an important role as inflammatory mediators. Four kb upstream from the *LTB* gene and about 26 kb telomeric from the *G1* gene [3] the human homologue of the mouse *B144* gene - leucocyte specific transcript 1, LST1 - has been identified [4] *(Figure 1)*. The previous report has decribed a cDNA, pLST1, of 636 bp length, which allowed the identification of four exons and three introns. The polymorphic microsatellites TNFd and TNFe [5] are located in intron three of LST1 and a polymorphic Pvu II restriction site (ADB) 260 bp downstream of the polyadenylation signal has been analysed in detail [6]. LST1 mRNA, which is about 800 nt in size, is expressed constitutively in T cell and macrophage cell lines, and at low levels in human tonsilla, lung, and liver. In monocytic cell lines transcription can be strongly enhanced by interferon-γ (IFN-γ). Comparison of the deduced protein sequence of this human cDNA with the published mouse B144 sequence [7] did not allow the identification of a long common open reading frame. In order to characterize the complex LST1 expression pattern we isolated additional full-length cDNA clones from a human and a mouse macrophage cell line, and identified several different LST1 mRNA species.

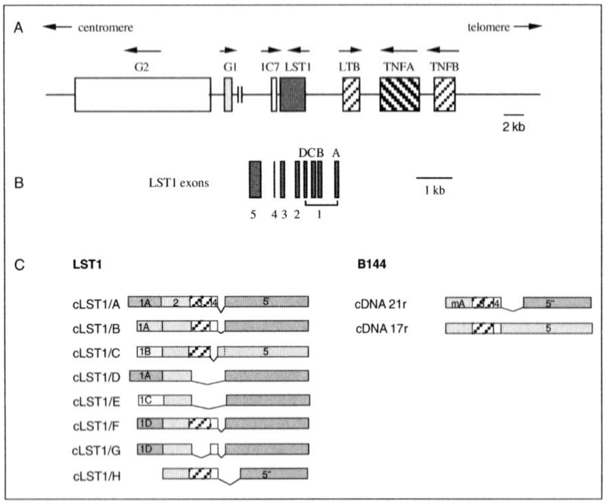

Figure 1. (A) Schematic diagram of the human TNFB-LST1 region. Arrows indicate the transcriptional orientation of the genes. (B) Exon-intron structure of LST1. (C) Splice variants of *LST1* and *B144* show differential usage of exons and transcription initiation sites.

Results and discussion

Using a modified RACE technique to ensure complete reverse transcription of 5' ends we isolated four different alternatively spliced cDNA clones. By comparison with the genomic sequence, which was derived from the cosmid cah5 containing the entire TNF region and about 12 kb sequence upstream of LTB [8], seven exons and four introns spanning a total of 2.7 kb were identified. Each of the LST1 splice junction sequences conforms to the eukaryotic splice consensus sequence (AG/GT). Whereas exons 2 was contained in all alternatively spliced cDNAs the transcription initiation site varied and accordingly three exons 1 (A-C) are utilized in U937 cells. The LST1 cDNA matches a number of cDNA sequences from the fetal liver and spleen library submitted by the Washington University-Merck expressed sequence tag (EST) project. This data base revealed four further LST1 splice variants and a new transcription initiation site with exon 1D.

Alternative splicing could lead to five different protein isoforms (97 aa, 83aa, 66 aa, 54 aa, and 28 aa). The 97-aa polypeptide contains a hydrophobic aminoterminus (exon 3) that possibly acts as a membrane-anchoring domain and that is absent in the 54 aa polypeptide which potentially represents a soluble form.

RT-PCR revealed a constitutive transcription of four LST1 splice variants in monocytes and peripheral blood lymphocytes (PBL). Whereas apart from lung tissue, in all other tissues tested, only the long LST1 isoform, LST1/A, is transcribed. The expression of similar transcripts in U937 cells and lung tissue may be due to the high number of macrophages in the lung. In the cervix carcinoma cell line HeLa, the T cell line MT2, and in B-LCL-cells no constitutive nor an IFN-γ inducible LST1 expression was observed.

In contrast to TNF-α which is mainly expressed in macrophages, and only at low levels in T cells too, the neighbouring genes *TNFB* and *LTB* show a T cell specific expression. *LST1* again, similar to *TNFA* is predominantly transcribed in macrophages and only at low levels in T cells. The low LST1 mRNA production in T cells could be explained by the vicinity of the enhancer of the LT-β gene encoded on the opposite strand possibly resulting in a "leaky" transcription of *LST1*. Therefore, we conclude that *LST1* most likely has a macrophage specific regulation. IFN-γ not only stimulates LST1 transcripts but also affects their splicing pattern, resulting in U937 cells in a preferential expression of transcripts lacking exon 3 and which encode the putatively soluble forms. In contrast, in T cells stimulation leads to the preferential production of the long LST1 isoform encoding the 97-aa polypeptide.

Sequence determination of the 10 kb DNA segment upstream of LTB that contains *LST1* allowed us to localize the recently identified cDNA 1C7 just 3' of *LST1* [9]. This gene is in opposite orientation and contains the ADB polymorphism.

The function of *LST1* is not known so far. It is suggestive to speculate that *LST1* might have a specific role in cell signalling regulating inflammatory responses.

References

1. Dunham I, Sargent CA, Trowsdale J, Campbell RD. Molecular mapping of the major histocompatibility complex by pulsed-field gel electrophoresis. *Proc Natl Acad Sci USA* 1987; 84: 7237-41.
2. Browning JL, Ngam-Ek A, Lawton P, DeMarinis J, Tizard R, Chow EP, Hession C, O'Brine Greco B, Foley S F, Ware CF. Lymphotoxin ß, a novel member of the TNF family that forms a heteromeric complex with lymphotoxin on the cell surface. *Cell* 1993; 72: 847-56.
3. Olavesen, MG, Thomson W, Cheng J, Campbell RD. *Proceedings of the 11th International Histocompatibility Workshop.* Oxford:Oxford University Press, 1993: 190-3.
4. Holzinger I, de Baey A, Messer G, Kick G, Zwierzina H, Weiss EH. Cloning and genomic characterization of *LST*1: a new gene in the human *TNF* region. *Immunogenetics* 1995; 42: 315-22.
5. Udalova IA, Nedospasov SA, Webb GC, Chaplin D D, Turetskaya RL. Highly informative typing of the human TNF locus using six adjacent polymorphic markers. *Genomics* 1993; 16: 180-6.
6. De Baey A, Holzinger I, Scholz S, Keller E, Weiss E H, Albert E. Pvu II polymorphism in the primate homologue of the mouse B144 (Lst-1). *Hum Immunol* 1995; 42: 9-14.
7. Tsuge I, Shen FW, Steinmetz M, Boyse EA. A gene in the H2S:H2D interval of the major histocompatibility complex which is transcribed in B cells and macrophages. *Immunogenetics* 1987; 26: 378-80.
8. Messer G, Spengler U, Jung MC, Honold G, Bloehmer K, Pape GR, Riethmüller G, Weiss EH. Polymorphic structure of the tumor necrosis factor (TNF) locus: an NcoI polymorphism in the first intron of the human TNFβ gene correlates with a variant amino acid in position 26 and a reduced level of TNF-β production. *J Exp Med* 1991; 173: 209-19.
9. Nalabolu SR, Shukla H, Nallur G, Parimoo S, Weissman SM. Genes in a 220 kb region spanning the TNF cluster in the human MHC. *Genomics* 1996; 31: 215-22.

Association analysis of a new intragenic TNFA (tumor necrosis factor alpha) polymorphism with TNFα quantitative production

S. D'Alfonso[1], F. Pociot [2], M. Berrino[3], P. Momigliano-Richiardi[1-4]

1 Dipartimento di Scienze Mediche, Universita di Torino, Via Solaroli 17, 28100 Novara, Italy
2 Steno Diabetes Center , Gentofte, Denmark
3 Dipartimento di Genetica Biologia e Chimica Medica, Universita di Torino, Torino, Italy
4 Centro CNR Immunogenetica ed Oncologia Sperimentale, Torino, Italy

Genes encoding tumor necrosis factor alpha (*TNFA*) and beta (*TNFB*) map tandemly in the HLA class III region. Several polymorphisms have been described in the TNF region including dimorphisms as well as microsatellites as shown in *Figure 1*. Some of these polymorphisms may be involved in TNFα expression which has been shown to be associated with HLA haplotypes. In particular, the secretory capacity in LPS stimulated monocytes has been associated with markers within the TNF region, namely NcoI -RFLP polymorphism in the TNFB first intron [3] and microsatellites TNFα and TNFβ located in the 5' region of the *TNFB* gene [6]. However, these sequences are not located in regulatory regions of the *TNFA* gene. Thus it is possible that they are not directly involved in the regulation of TNFα expression but are in linkage disequilibrium with polymorphic variations in the TNFA regulatory sequences. Contrary to expectation, no association was detected between TNFα production and two diallelic polymorphisms at positions -308 and -238 of the TNFA promoter [7,8]. Of the two further polymorphisms detected in the TNFA promoter, alleles at position -376 has the same population distribution as -238, while polymorphism at position -163 is scarsely informative [1].

We have recently described a new polymorphism in the first intron of *TNFA* gene [9]. The first intron is sometimes involved in gene expression regulation [10]. Therefore it was interesting to test whether this polymorphism is associated with TNFa production.

Materials and methods

PCR and SSO hybridization conditions

PCR primers: Sense oligo: 5'TGCACTTTGGAGTGATCGGC3'. Antisense oligo: 5'TTCCCGCTCTTTCTGTCTCA3' ; SSOs: 5'AAAAAAACATGGAGAAAG3' and 5'CTTTCTCCACGTTTTTTTC3', detecting respectively the A and G sequences.

PCR was performed in 25μl containing 20ng DNA, 10pmol each primer, and 0.5 U Taq DNA polymerase (Perkin Elmer), 2mM $MgCl_2$. The PCR profile included: 1' 95°C, 1' 55°C, 1' 72°C for 30 cycles, in a Perkin Elmer 480 Thermal cycler. Two μl of PCR product were spotted on a positively charged nylon membrane and hybridized with 0.5 pm/ml Digoxigenin-dUTP (Boehringer) labeled SSO at 46°C and 50°C respectively for "A" and "G" detecting SSOs. Two stringent washings were performed at 48°C and 52°C respectively for the "A" and "G" detecting SSOs. The membranes were visualized using an anti-digoxigenin alkaline phosphatase conjugate antibody and a luminogen alkaline phosphatase substrate, according to the manufacturer's instructions (Boehringer).

TNFα stimulation and quantitation

Monocytes from a panel of 78 Danish individuals were stimulated *in vitro* by LPS; TNFα production in the cell culture supernatant was quantified as previously described [6,7].

Statistical analysis

Gene frequencies were calculated by direct counting. The Mann Whitney test was used for testing differences of TNFα production between groups.

Results and discussion

The here analysed polymorphism consists of a G-A transition at position 4583 (according to the sequence number reported in Nedospasov *et al.*, 1986) in the first intron of the *TNFA* gene.

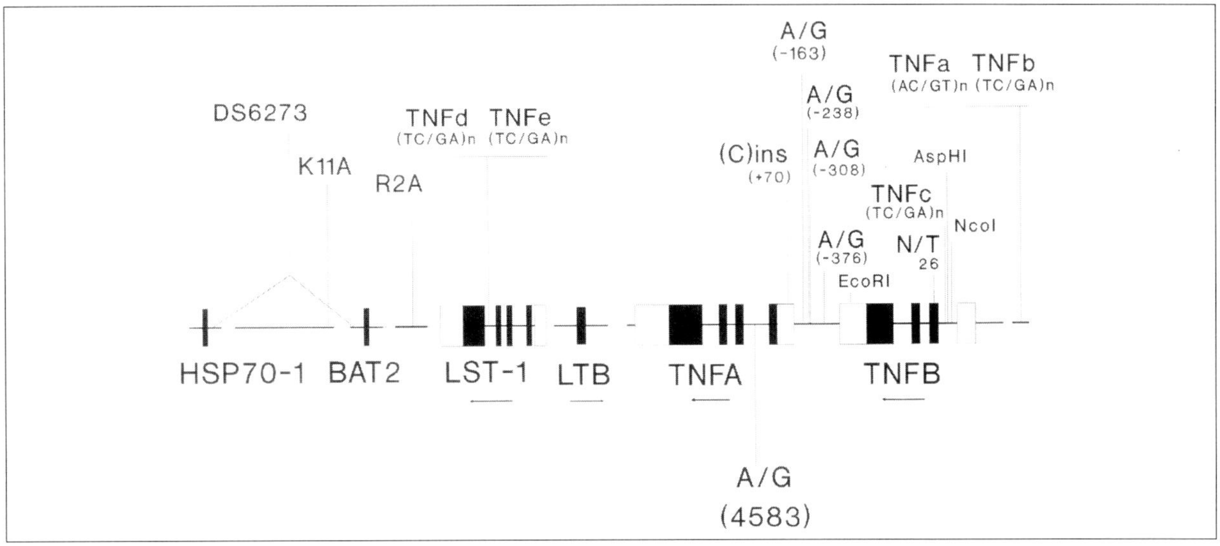

Figure 1. Polymorphisms in the TNF region.
Alternative nomenclature : TNFB = LTA; TNFA = TNF.
References:
Microsatellites: TNFa,b,c,d,e [Ref. 1 in D'Alfonso *et al.*, this volume];
K11A [Ref. 2 in D'Alfonso *et al.*, this volume]; R2A [Ref. 3 in D'Alfonso *et al.*, this volume]; D6S273 [Ref. 4 in D'Alfonso *et al.*, this volume].
A/G transitions in the TNFA promoter: positions -163 and -376 [1]; -308[2]; -238 [Ref. 7 in D'Alfonso *et al.*, this volume].
RFLP dimorphisms in the TNFB regions: NcoI [3]; AspHI [4]; EcoRI [3].
(C)ins: C nucleotide insertion at position +70 of TNFA 5' untranslated region [5].
N/T (26): Asparagin/ Threonin polymorphism at codon 26 of TNFB gene [3].
A/G (4583): polymorphism at position 4583 in the first intron of TNFA gene, decribed in this report.
The relative positions of the two microsatellite loci K11A and D6S273 are not defined.

The presence of the polymorphic sequence was tested by dot blot of the PCR amplified DNA fragment hybridized with sequence specific oligonucleotides (SSO).
The frequency of the two alleles was analysed in two European populations. In a panel of 102 HLA typed Italian random healthy individuals the following genotype frequencies were observed: GG = 0.74, AG = 0.24 , AA = 0.02. Gene frequencies of G and A alleles were 0.86 and 0.14. In a panel of 78 healthy Danish individuals the gene frequencies of G and A alleles were 0.90 and 0.10, similar to what observed in the Italian population. No individuals homozygous for the A allele were present. Both tested population were in Hardy-Weinberg equilibrium at this locus.
The association of this polymorphism with TNFα production was tested in the Danish sample previously characterized for TNFα secretory capacity upon LPS *in vitro* stimulation [6-8]. A/G heterozygous individuals showed a mean level of TNFα production higher than G/G homozygous individuals *(Table I)*. However this difference was not significant (p=0.222, Mann Whitney test).
The here tested polymorphism is the third polymorphism in putative TNFA regulatory regions that has been shown not to be associated with TNFα production. These data suggest that the variable production of TNFα associated with HLA is controlled by sequences outside the regulatory regions of the TNFA gene.

Table I. *In vitro* TNFα production by genotypes at position 4583 in the first intron of TNFA

Genotype	N°	Mean (±SD) Production (ng/ml)
A/G	15	3.2 ±0.95
G/G	63	2.9 ±1.16

Acknowledgement
This work was supported by "MURST 60%".

References

1. Hamann A, Mantzoros C, Vidal-Puig A, Flier JS. Genetic variability in the TNF-alpha promoter is not associated with type II diabetes mellitus (NIDDM). *Biochem Biophys Res Commun* 1995; 211: 833-7.
2. Wilson AG, Di Giovine FS, Blakemore AIF, Duff GW. Single base polymorphism in the human tumor necrosis factor alpha (TNFα) gene detectable by NcoI restriction of PCR product. *Hum Mol Genet* 1992; 1: 353.
3. Messer G, Spengler U, Jung MC, Honold G, Blomer K, Pape GR, Riethmuller G, Weiss EH. Polymorphic structure of the tumor necrosis factor (TNF) locus: an NcoI polymorphism in the first intron of the human TNF-β gene correlates with a variant amino acid in position 26 and a reduced level of TNF-β production. *J Exp Med 1991*; 173: 209-19.
4. Ferencik S, Lindemann M, Horsthemke B, Grosse-Wilde H. A new restriction fragment length polymorphism of the human TNFβ gene detected by Asp HI digest. *Eur J Immunogenet* 1992; 19: 425-6.
5. Brinkman B, Kaijzel E, Huizinga T, Giphart M, Breedveld F, Verweij C. Detection of a C-insertion polymorphism within the tumor necrosis factor alpha (TNFA) gene. *Hum Genet* 1995; 96:493.
6. Pociot F, Briant L, Jongenel CV, Worsaae H, Molvig J, Abbal M, Thomsen M, Nerup J, Cambon-Thomsen A. Association of tumor necrosis factor (TNF) and class II MHC alleles with the secretion of TNFα and TNFß by human mononuclear cells: a possible link to insulin-dependent diabetes mellitus. *Eur J Immunol* 1993; 23: 224-31.
7. Pociot F, Wilson AG, Nerup J, Duff GW. No independent association between a tumor necrosis factor-α promoter region polymorphism and insulin-dependent diabetes mellitus. *Eur J Immunol* 1993; 23: 3043-9.
8. Pociot F, D'Alfonso S, Compasso S, Scorza R, Momigliano Richiardi P. Functional analysis of a new polymorphism in the human TNF alpha gene promoter. *Scand J Immunol* 1995; 42: 501-4.
9. D'Alfonso S, Momigliano Richiardi P. A new intragenic polymorphism in the *TNFA* (tumor necrosis factor alpha) gene. *Immunogenetics* 1996; 44:321-2.
10. Palmiter R, Sandgren E, Avarbock M, Allen D, Brinster R. Heterologous introns can enhance expression of transgenes in mice. *Proc Natl Acad Sci USA* 1991; 88: 478-82.

Identification of new olfactory receptor genes located close to the human major histocompatibility complex

H. Gallinaro, C. Amadou, P. Avoustin, M.T. Ribouchon, C. Bouissou, F. Lapointe[1], P. Pontarotti, C. Ayer-Le Lièvre[1, 2]

CIGH-UPR 8291-CNRS, CHU de Purpan, 31, avenue de Grande Bretagne, 31300 Toulouse, France
1 Institut d' Embryologie Cellulaire, Nogent-sur-Marne, France
2 Present address: URA 1485 CNRS, 87025 Limoges, France

In the distal part of the human major histocompatibility complex region (MHC) only few genes or markers were identified. Our goal was to refine and extend the map beyong HLA-F region. Among the new genes we identified two genes bearing strong homology to olfactory receptor genes isolated from several species. Those genes were conserved between man and mouse and expressed as mRNA in mouse olfactory epithelium.

Mapping, conservation between man and mouse, characterisation

Numerous mouse anonymous probes were checked for their conservation in human genomic DNA digested by frequently-cutter restriction enzymes. Among those probes Leh89 and Tu42, isolated by microdissection of the mouse chromosome 17 hybridized on Southern blots of man or mouse DNA, displaying more complex pattern in mouse than in human *(Figure 1)*. So the two probes are conserved in human. Using several YACs, from CEPH library, overlapping the region between MOG and RFP genes, compared to genomic DNA, we demonstrated that both probes are located in this region. A more precise mapping of both genes was deduced from their position relative to identified markers beared by the various YACs *(Figure 2)*. The two genes are located in a 700 kb space telomeric to HLA-F

The mouse probe Leh 89 (1.7kb) allowed the isolation of a cosmid from the ICRF reference library containing the orthologous gene OLF89. Cosmid was sequenced. Comparison of both sequences OLF89 (human) and Olf89 (mouse) showed identies of 53% for the nucleic acids and 72% in amino acid sequences. However the hydrophobicity profile highlighted that a change in the human reading frame phase led to the loss of hydrophobic amino acids forming the fourth transmembrane domain (TM) *(Figure 3)*. Looking for similarity in database with the blast program [1] they showed strong similarities with olfactory receptor genes, a subfamily of seven transmembrane receptor genes.

The Tu42 clone (1.9kb) was sequenced. It contained the first 150 nucleotides of the mouse Olf42 gene but did not allow us to isolate by screening any full length mouse or human clone. Using specific PCR primers on the transmembrane domain II (TM II) and VI deduced from the just published human OR-like gene HSORLMHC [2], we amplified a 650 bp DNA fragment overlapping the coding sequence. This DNA fragment had been used as specific human probe OLF42 for

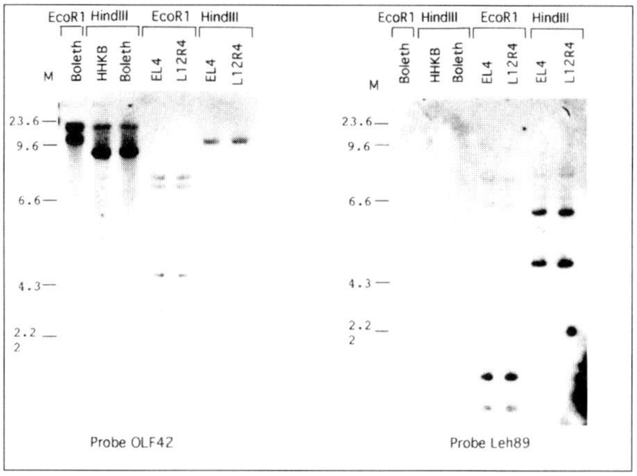

Figure 1. Hybridization of genomic DNA with human or mouse probes: *Left panel*: OLF42 probe was produced by PCR amplification of HSORLMHC sequence between positions 151 (TMII) and 778 (TMVI). *Right panel*: hybrization was with an 1.7 Kb EcoR1 fragment isolated from mouse chromosome 17. HHKB and Boleth: Human genomic DNA. EL4 or L12R4 DNA from C57/Bl6 mouse cell lines.

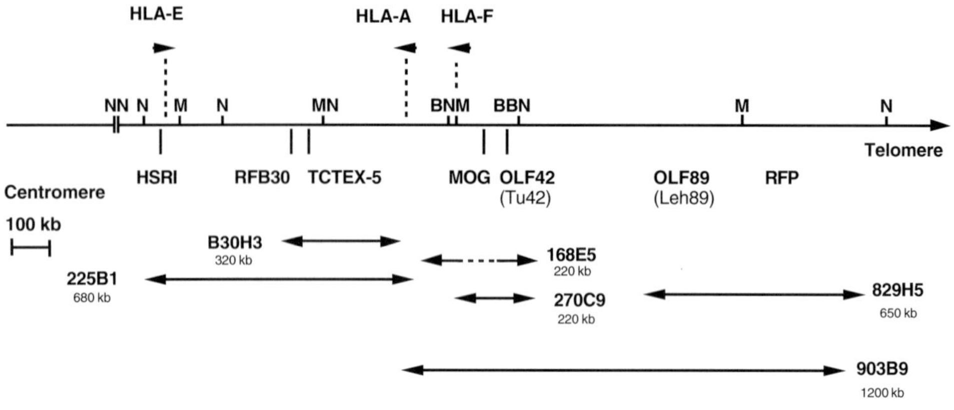

Figure 2. The positions of the studied YACs are indicated by double arrow. N, M, B, pointed to the respective site for NotI; MluI and BssHII restriction enzymes. Arrow heads showed the transcription sense for the HLA genes.

screening of the ICRF reference library produced cosmids. Comparison of the sequence with database indicated that the best similarity was with human HSORLMHC [2] and mouse Olf3 genes [3].

Other informations can be drawn from hybridization of probes OLF42, Tu42 and OLF89 onto filters bearing both genomic DNA and YACs located in this region *(Figure 4)*. The OLF42 probe revealed 4 bands of 15 kb, 5 kb, 2kb and 1 kb respectively in YAC DNA digested by Hind III *(Figure 4A)*, whereas the Tu42 probe which contained only the first 150 nucleotides revealed only 2 bands of 1 kb and 15 kb *(Figure 4B)*. The screening of ICRF library produced 5 cosmids. Digested with Hind III 4 cosmids shared a band around 15 kb revealed with OLF42 probe and one fifth cosmid showed 3 bands (1kb, 1.7 kb and 2.5kb)(data not shown). Together this suggests that there are likely two copies of the OLF42 gene in this region one containing one Hind III site and the other not. The OLF89 probe is single copy under stringent conditions in human as well as in mouse genomic DNA *(Figure 4C)*.

We described two new genes linked to the MHC with a strong homology with OR genes already described in several species or located on other human chromosomes (17 and 19). They were usually organized in clusters (see for review [4-6]). So it can bee also found other genes in this part of the genome.

Expression pattern of both genes

To check wether those genes are truly olfactory receptor genes, their expression pattern was studied by *in situ* hybridization of riboprobes, synthesized either from Leh89 (mouse Olf89) or human OLF42 probes, to coronal sections of mouse heads. The two anti-sens RNA probes revealed specific expression in the median zone of the olfactory organ. The labelled cells have morphology and localization similar to the olfactory neurons. A similar expression pattern was found both in adults and 18 day fœtus.

Polymorphism

To see if those genes can possess a polymorphism in the same order of magnitude as other genes of the MHC and if it can be establish an association with HLA haplotypes we first looked for polymorphism for both genes, in five individual different HLA haplotypes chosen in the 4AOHW cell line panel [7].

Using oligonucleotide pairs specific to each gene, we generated by PCR on each genomic DNA ten to twelwe clones and sequenced those. The OLF89 gene presented in all the analyzed individuals the same frameshift leading to the loss of the transmembrane domain IV. The sequences all together exhibited only one silent mutation. Thus we did not find any polymorphism for this gene.

More complex situation was found for the OLF42 gene.

OLF89 (Human)	MPLTNESHPE	........DR	........TS	...M..I.V.	...T...M.R	50
Olf89 (Mouse)	----------	EFILLGFANH	PWLELPLFVT	LLITYPMALM	GNIAIILVST	40
OLF89	..S..H....	...T......	....	........K.	..S.M..A..	100
Olf89	LDPRLYSPMY	FFLKNLSFLD	MCYTTSIVPQ	MLFNLGSSRK	TITYIGCVVQ	90
OLF89	..F.......	....	.......R..	....	....*FHRVAN*	150
Olf89	LYVFHIMGGT	ECLLLAIMSF	DRYVAICKPL	HYTLIMNQRV	CILSVSIMWL	140
OLF89	*WNNLCCLRGH*	*CHITIATVC-*	S......V..	......I...	..GS...T..	199
Olf89	TGVIFGFSEA	TLTLQLPLCG	TNKLDHLLCE	IPVLIKTACG	EKEFNELALS	190
OLF89	.....M.A..	........AS	..S..FK...	.K..K.....	........F.	249
Olf89	VVCIFILIVP	LCLILASYVN	IGCAVLRIKS	SEGRRKAFGT	CSSHLIVVSL	240
OLF89	....A.....	..P.S.S...	........G.	V..S......	.....N....	299
Olf89	FYGPGISMYL	QPSSLITRDQ	PKFMALFYAV	ITPTLNPFIY	TLRNKDVKGA	290
OLF89	LRN.V...SA	L.D.G	314			
Olf89	FKKLLRSI--	FS-SK	302			

Alignment of the amino-acid sequences of human and mouse receptor-like genes (OLF89) close to MHC

Figure 3. The part of the human OLF89 sequence where occurs the frame shift is indicated in italics. Only the amino acis which differ are indicated in human sequence.

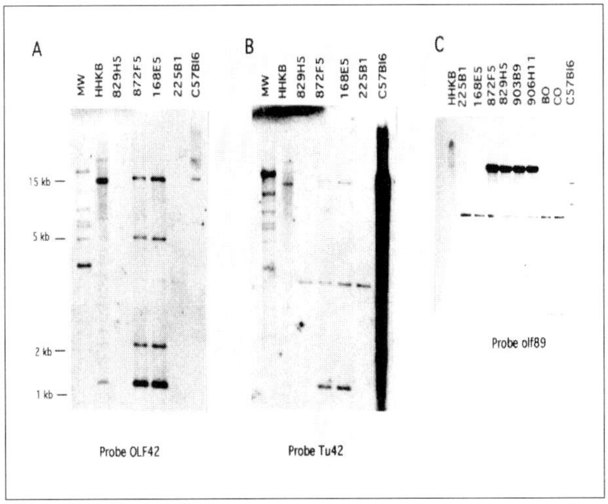

Figure 4. Hybridization of genomic DNA and YAC DNA with human OLF42 probe (A), mouse Tu42 probe (B) or mouse Olf89 probe (C).
HHKB: human genomic DNA; C57/Bl6: mouse genomic DNA . 225B1, 168E5, 872F5, 903B9, 906H11: YACs from man and located in the class I region. BO : ICRFy902B0736; CO : ICRFy903C00418 are two mouse YACs located in the distal part of the H-2 complex. Digestion was with HindIII.

First according to restriction profil of the sequences they can be classified in two sets. The first one contained a HindIII site and showed a very similar restriction pattern (OLF42A). The second (OLF42B) did not contained the HindIII site and showed a different restriction pattern but close to that of HSORLMHC. According to our conclusions about the two genes located in this region (first part), the alignment of the translation products was made on this basis *(Figure 5)*. First OLF42A sequences showed a clear polymorphism mainly localized in three domains: internal 2 and 3 (I2, I3) and external 3 (E3) domain. The I2 and E3 domains togeher with the TM III and IV are important for the fonction of those receptors specially for the specifity. Thus, such a polymorphism in OR sequences could reflect individual differences in odor sensitivity. For OLF42B, only the E3 domain showed a marked difference in the amino acids. From each set one consensus sequence can be drawn. Comparison in between showed that the more marked divergences are located in I2, I3 and E3 and also in TM IV and TM V. Comparison of OLF 42B with HSORLMHC suggested that it is very similar to HSORLMHC sequence with however scarce

```
          Tm2                    E 2                    Tm3
Consensus YFFLSNLSFL DLCFTISCVP GMLVNLWEPK KTIILLGCSV QFFIFLSLGT
9108-2    ---------- -----T---- Q------G-- ---SF-D--- -I--------
9109-6    ---------- ---------- ---------- ---------- ----------
9110-1    ---------- ---------- ---------- ---------- ----------
9108-1    ---------- ---------- R--------- ---------- ----------
9079-6    ---------- ---------- ---------- ---------- ----------

                                 I 2                    Tm4
Consensus TECILLTVMA FDRYMAIFKP LRHATIVHLC LCWQLASVAW VIGLVESVVQ
9108-2    ---------- L---V-VCQ- -HY---I-PR ---------- ----------
9109-6    ---------- ---------- ---------- ---------- ----------
9110-1    ---------- ---------- ---------- ---------- ----------
9108-1    ---------- ---------- ------A--- ---------- ----------
9079-6    ---------- -------CQ- -HY-----PL ---------- -MS-------

                     E 3                                Tm5
Consensus TPSTLRLPFC PHQQVDDFVC EVPALIRLSC EDTSYNEIQM AVASVFILAV
9108-2    -----QF-SV -DR-M----- ---------- ---------v --------v-
9109-6    -TIH------ ---------- ---------- ---------- ----------
9110-1    ---------- ---------- ---------- ---------- ----------
9108-1    ---------- ---------- ---------- ---------- ----------
9079-6    -----H---- -DR------- ---------- ---------L ----------

                                 I 3                    Tm6
Consensus PLSLILVSYG AIAWAVLRTN   KGQRKAFG TCSSHLTVVT LFYS  194 A.A.
9108-2    ---------- --T-----I- SA--R----- ---------- ----
9109-6    ---------- ----------*LP-------- ---------- ----
9110-1    ---------- ---------- C  -------- ---------- ----
9108-1    ---------- ---------- SA-------- ---------- ----
9079-6    ---------- ---------- SA-------- ---------- ----
```

Human OLF42 A

```
          Tm2                    E 2                    Tm3
Consensus YFFLS LSFL DLCFTTSCVP QMLVNLWGPK KTISFLGCSV QLFIFLSLGT
9109-3    -----D---- ---------- ---------- ---------- ----------
9026-2    -----N---- ---------- ---------- ---------- ----------
9026-1    -----D---- ---S------ ---------- ---------- ----------
9079-3     ----V---- ---------- ---------- ---------- ----------

                                 I 2                    Tm4
Consensus TECILLTVMA FDRYVAVCQP LHYATIIHPR LCWQLASVAW VMSLVQSIVQ
9109-3    ---------D ---------A ---------- ---------- ----------
9026-2    ---------- ---------- ---------- ---------- ----------
9026-1    ---------- ---------- ---------- ---------- ----------
9079-3    ---------- ---------- ---------- ---------- ----------

                     E 3                                Tm5
Consensus TPSTLHLPFC PHQQIDDF C EVPSLIRLSC GDTSYNEIQL AVSSVIFVVV
9109-3    --T-PP---- --------Y- ---------- ---------- ----------
9026-2    ---------- --------L- ---------- ---------- ----------
9026-1    ---------- --------L- ---------- ---------- ----------
9079-3    -T-------- --------Y- ---------- ---------- ----------

                                 I 3                    Tm6
Consensus PLSLILASYG ATAQAVLRIN SATAWRKAFG TCSSHLTVVT LFYS 194 A.A
9109-3    ---------- ---------- T--------- ---------- ----
9026-2    ---------- ---------- ---------- ---------- ----
9026-1    ---------- ---------- ---------- ---------- ----
9079-3    ---------- ---------- ---------- ---------- ----
```

Human OLF42 B

Figure 5. Comparative alignment of translation products deduced from the two human olfactory-like receptor genes. Numbers on the left designated the human cell lines with the 10IHW nomenclature.

differences. Polymorphism is higher than expected for neutral conditions if the gene is not under selection pressure, and mutation are mostly non synonymous.This study must be extent to the other HLA haplotypes to conclude about a relationship between polymorphism of OR genes and HLA haplotypes.

References

1. Altschul SF, Gish W, Miller W, Myers EW, Lipman DJ. *J Mol Biol* 1990 ; 215: 403-10.
2. Fan WF, Liu YC, Parimoo S, Weissman S. *Genomics* 1995; 7: 119-23.
3. Nef P, Hermans-Borgmeyer I, Artieres-Pin H, Beasley L, Dionne VE, Heinemann SF. *Proc Natl Acad Sci USA* 1992; 89: 8948-52.
4. Lancet D, Ben-Arie N, Cohen S, Gat U, Gross-Isseroff R, Horn-Saban S, Khen M, Lehrach H, Natochin M, North M, Seidmann E, Walker N. *Ciba Foundation Symposium* 1993; 179: 131-41.
5. Ben-Arie N, Lancet D, Taylor C, Khen M, Walker N, Ledbetter DH, Carrozzo R, Patel K, Sheer D, Lehrach H, North MA. *Hum Mol Genet* 1994; 3: 229-35.
6. Sullivan SL, Ressler KJ, Buck LB. *Mol Neurobiol* 1994; 75-84.
7. Degli-Esposti MA, Griffiths MS, Daly LN, Witt CS, Simons M, Carcassi C, Albert ED, Giphart MJ Dawkins RJ. *Hum Immunol* 1993; 38: 3-16.

HLA-G. Reproductive immunology

Contents

HLA-G surface expression in haematopoietic cells using a new monoclonal antibody BFL1

L. Amiot[1], B. Drénou [1], M. Onno[1], A. Bensussan[2], P. Le Bouteiller[3], G. Semana[4], B. Le Marchand[1], T. Lamy[1], R. Fauchet[1]

1 University laboratory for Hematology and Biology of Blood cells, JE DRED 287, University of Rennes I, Hôpital de Pontchaillou, rue Henri Le Guilloux, 35000 Rennes, France
2 INSERM U 448, Créteil, France
3 Inserm U 395, CHU Purpan, Toulouse, France
4 Center for Blood Transfusion, Rennes, France

HLA-G, a non classical HLA class I gene has a tissue specific expression on human extravillous cytotrophoblast [1], which lack major histocompatibility complex (MHC) class I classical antigens. As no HLA-G monoclonal antibodies were available. HLA-G protein was only detected by immunoprecipitation and immunohistochemistry with W6/32, a monomorphic anti-class I monoclonal antibody (mAb).

HLA-G gene can produce four alternatively spliced isoforms encoding bound-membrane proteins (G1: a full length transcript, G2 lacking α2 domain, G4 lacking α3 domain, G3 devoid of α2 and α3 domains) and two encoding soluble forms [2]. We have recently reported that HLA-G gene is transcribed in lymphocytes and is not detected at transcriptional level in CD34+ cells, polynuclear and monocytes [3]. No splicing patterns could be assigned to a particular cellular type or malignancy. In addition we have shown that the transcription is not a constitutive phenomenon since transcripts are not detected in some lymphocytes samples [4].

A new mAb BFL1 was recently produced by immunization of HLA B27/ human β2 microglobulin double transgenic mice with tranfected murine L cells expressing both HLA-G and human β2 microglobulin [5]. To approach the potential function of the different isoforms, we investigated HLA-G cell surface expression on normal and malignant hematopoietic cells by using BFL1 mAb. HLA-G transcription results previously studied by using RT-PCR assays were compared to those of HLA-G cell surface expression.

Material and methods

Cell lines

KG1a (CD34+ myeloblastic leukemia), Molt4 (T lymphoblastic leukemia), Raji, Daudi (Burkitt's lymphoma), Kas (Epstein Barr virus transformed B lymphoblastoid cells), Rex (T lymphoblastic cells), T2 (B-T hybridoma lacking TAP genes), U937 (monohistiocytic proliferation) were studied.

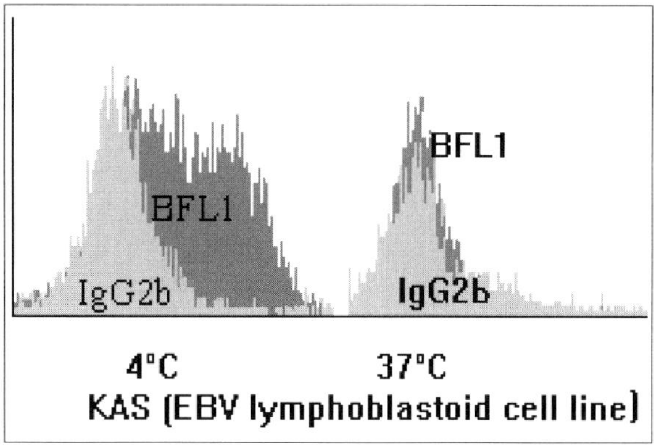

Figure 1. Induction of HLA-G expression by particular conditions on a EBV transformed lymphoblastoid cell line, KAS. The two cytometry graphs show on the left a BFL1 positivity on Kas maintained at 4°C and on the right a lack of HLA-G expression on the same cell line cultured at 37°C. IgG2b mAb is used as isotypic control.

Lymphoid cells

Four peripheral blood cells were studied as normal lymphoid cells. Four B chronic lymphocytic leukemia (B-CLL), two non Hodgkin lymphoma (B-NHL), two B acute lymphoblastic leukemia (B-ALL) were tested as malignant cells.

BFL1 mAb

BFL1 is an anti HLA-G monoclonal antibody of IgG2b isotype which identifies cell surface products on HLA-G expressing cell-lines: Jeg3, a choriocarcinoma derived cell line and HLA-G transfected cell lines. It immunoprecipitates a 39 kDa protein in HLA-G expressing cell lines [5]. The absence of recognition of classical HLA class I molecules demonstrated its specificity.

Reverse transcription and amplification

PolyA+ mRNAs were purified from 5.10^5 to 10^6 cells using Dynabeads (dT)25 (Dynal)

RT-PCR assays were performed by using specific primers located in exon 2 and in 3'UT region as previously described [6] and was followed by hybridization with exon-specific probes and sequencing assays.

Flow cytometry analysis

Cells were labeled by indirect immunofluorescence with BFL1. An IgG2b monoclonal antibody was used as isotypic control. After incubation with the first mAb and washing, the cells were incubated with F(ab')2 anti mouse IgG conjugated with DDAF. Fluorescence was read with a cytoron absolute (Ortho).

Results

HLA-G transcription and cell surface expression on cell lines

The results are summarized in *Table I*. Three cell lines (KG1a, Molt4, Raji) were used as negative controls. In the other cell lines, no HLA-G cell surface expression was detected in normal conditions although HLA-G mRNA isoforms were found.

	HLA-G mRNA forms encoding membrane-bound proteins	HLA-G cell surface expression
CELL LINES		
KG1a	-	-
Molt 4	-	-
Raji	-	-
T2	G1,G2,G3,G4	-
Rex	G1,G2,G3,G4	-
Kas	G1,G2,G3,G4	-
Daudi	G3	-
U937	G3	-
NORMAL CELLS		
PBL 1	G1,G2,G3,G4	-
PBL 2	G1,G2,G3	-
PBL 3	G1,G2	-
PBL 4	G1	-
B LYMPHOID MALIGNANCIES		
B-CLL 1	G1,G2,G3,G4	-
B-CLL 2	G1,G2,G3	-
B-CLL 3	G1,G2,G4	-
B-CLL 4	G1	-
B-NHL 1	G1,G2,G3,G4	-
B-NHL 2	G1	-
B- ALL 1	G1,G2,G3	-
B- ALL 2	G1,G3	-

Table I. HLA-G mRNA forms and cell surface expression on cell lines and lymphoid cells. Peripheral blood leukocytes (PBL), B chronic lymphocytic leukemia (B-CLL), B non Hodgkin lymphoma (B-NHL), B acute lymphoblastic leukemia (B-ALL). The different isoforms are designated as in the text

In particular conditions of temperature (4°C), a strong BFL1 positivity is observed on some lymphoid cell lines (Rex, Kas, T2) *(Figure 1)* whereas this reactivity disappears on the same cell lines maintained at 37°C.

HLA-G cell surface expression on normal and malignant lymphoid cells

The results are summarized in *Table I*. Several HLA-G mRNA isoforms could be observed in peripheral blood cells and malignant cells. G1 is the major form which is detected both in normal and in malignant cells. The isoforms patterns seem to be not correlated to a cellular subpopulation or a malignancy type. No BFL1 reactivity is found in both normal cells and various B tumoral cells.

Discussion and conclusion

Until now, trophoblast cells appear to be the unique cell type expressing HLA-G membrane protein [1]. Previous studies by using different anti-HLA-G mAb demonstrated that first trimester extravillous trophoblast cells express cell surface HLA-G protein. By contrast only intracellular HLA-G proteins are expressed in the villous cytotrophoblast [7]. HLA-G transcription was detected in various tissues and in lymphoid cells [3,6]. Flow cytometry analysis with BFL1 did not detect HLA-G product at the cell surface of various normal and malignant lymphoid cells. A dissociation is observed in lymphoid cells between mRNA isoforms expression and the non cell surface detection with BFL1. HLA-G expression at the cell surface of lymphoid cells may be regulated either at level of translation or molecule transport to the cell membrane. Translation of the alternate transcripts was not yet proven but is strongly suggested by the HLA-G expression induction in particular conditions. The appearance of BFL1 positivity on some cell lines maintained at 4°C before labeling suggest a stabilization of HLA-G molecule at the cell surface at low temperature. Like a non classical HLA class I gene, HLA-E [8], the instability of the HLA-G molecule may be due to a inefficient binding to the endogenous peptides which would be restored at low temperature. Since HLA-G membrane-bound forms are irregulary expressed, conditions of assembly, processing and intra cellular traffic of these molecules remain to be precised. On the other hand, as the HLA-G gene is able to produce soluble forms in lymphoid cells, we could speculate on its potential function in immunologic tolerance which should be investigated.

References

1. Kovats S, Main EK, Librach C, Stubbledine M, Fisher SJ, De Mars R. A class I antigen, HLA-G, expressed in human trophoblast. *Science* 1990; 248: 220-3.
2. Fujii T, Ishitani A, Geraghty DE. A soluble form of the HLA-G antigen encoded by a messenger ribonucleic acid containing intron 4. *J Immunol* 1994; 153: 5516-24.
3. Amiot L, Onno M, Renard I, Drénou B, Guillaudeux T, Le Bouteiller P, Fauchet R. HLA-G transcription studies during the different stages of normal and malignant hematopoiesis. *Tissue antigens* 1996; 47: 408-13.
4. Amiot L, Onno M, Drénou B, Le Marchand B, Lamy T, Semana G, Fauchet R. Distribution of HLA-G alternative mRNAs including soluble forms in normal lymphocytes and in lymphoid cell-derived leukemia. *Eur J Immunogenet* 1996; 23 (4): 311-20.
5. Bensussan A, Mansur IG, Mallet V, Rodriguez AM, Girr M, Weiss E, Brem G, Boumsell L, Gluckman E, Dausset J, Carosella E, Le Bouteiller P. Detection of membrane-bound HLA-G translated products with a specific monoclonal antibody. *Proc Natl Acad Sci USA* 1995; 92:10292-6.
6. Onno M, Guillaudeux T, Amiot L, Renard I, Drénou B, Hirel B, Girr M, Semana G, Le Bouteiller P, Fauchet R. *Hum Immunol* 1994; 41: 79-86.
7. Le Bouteiller P, Rodriguez AM, Mallet V, Girr M, Guillaudeux, T, Lenfant F. Placental expression of HLA class I genes. *Am J Reprod Immunol* 1996; 35: 216-25.
8. Ulbrecht M, Kellermann J, Johnson JP, Weiss EH. Impaired intracellular transport and cell surface expression of non polymorphic HLA-E: evidence for inefficient binding. *J Exp Med* 1992; 176: 1083-90.

The non classical HLA-G gene is transcriptionally inactive in immature CD34+ cells in spite of the CpG island hypomethylation

M. Onno, L. Amiot, N. Bertho, B. Drénou, R. Fauchet

University laboratory for Hematology and Biology of Blood cells
University of Rennes I, 2, avenue du Dr Léon Bernard, 35043 Rennes Cedex, France

Human leukocyte antigen G (HLA-G) gene is a non classical class I gene which codes for the only detected major histocompatibility complex antigen in fetal placental tissues: HLA-G is expressed at high levels in early gestation tissues as cytotrophoblast populations, and transcripts and proteins decline as the pregnancy progresses to term. Membrane bound and soluble proteins of HLA-G, expressed in a transfected cell line 721-221, are able to bind nonameric peptides derived from a variety of intracellular proteins [1]. HLA-G proteins may play a role in immune surveillance to recognize virally infected placenta cells. Morever, several studies show that HLA-G could decrease fetal and transfected cell susceptibility to natural killers and to large granular lymphocytes CD56+ CD16+ from decidual endometrial mother cell lysis.

Transcription studies show that the hematopoietic progenitors and the granulo-macrophagic lineages have an HLA-G negative phenotype and that several HLA-G mRNA forms are expressed in lymphocytes [2]. The

Table I. Analysis of CpG methylation level in PCR products. The status of methylation at CpG sites in CD2+ lymphocytes is compared to that assessed in CD34+ cells. The CpG sites are numbered according to the reference [10]

A) Promoter (Enh A/ICS 601-617; Enh B 682-692; CAAT 708-712; TATA 733-738; ATG 783)

CpG	390	428	494	512	523	543	573	596	598	634	659	663	715	718	721	723	744
CD34	P	P	P	M	M	P	P	P	P	P	P	P	P	P	P	P	P
CD2	P↗	P =	P =	M	P	M	P↗	P↗	P↑	P↑	P↑	P↘	P↗	P↑	P↑	P↑	P =

B) Exon 1 — Intron 1

CpG	801	823	842	853	863	880	889	891	915	921	930	937	939	942	954	958	976
CD34	P	P	P	P	P	P	P	P		P	P	P	0	0	0	0	0
CD2	P↗	P =	P↘	P↗	P↗	P↗	P↑	P↗	P	P↗	P↗	P↘	0	P	P	0	P

C) Exon 2

CpG	1010	1013	1016	1023	1028	1032	1034	1044	1052	1064	1070	1075	1082	1086
CD34	0	0	0	0	P	0	0	0	P	P	P	P	P	P
CD2	P	P	P	0	P	P	P	P	P↗	P↑	P↗	P↗	P↗	P↗

CpG	1091	1097	1102	1105	1111	1123	1125	1128	1132	1153	1176	1193	1227	1229	1247
CD34	P	P	P	P	P	P	P	P	P	P	P	P	P	P	P
CD2	P↗	P =	P =	P =	P =	P↘	P =	P↑	P =	P↗	0	P↗	P =	P↗	P↗

M: fully methylated CpG, P: partially methylated CpG, 0: unmethylated CpG, P ↗ : indicates a higher level of methylation, P ↑ : indicates a much higher level of methylation, P ↘ : indicates a lower level of methylation.

role and the function of HLA-G products in lymphocytes are not yet established. A HLA-G specific antibody is currently available to search for the presence of potential proteins in lymphocytes.

Both mechanistically and functionnally, the limited expression of HLA-G gene poses interresting problems. It appears that regulation of HLA class I genes is influenced by DNA methylation [3]. Several studies have tried to establish a relationship between the level of CpG island methylation in the HLA-G gene and its transcriptional activity. Methylation changes were mainly detected and localized by using Southern blot analyses with methylation-sensitive restriction enzymes. The trophoblast-derived human cell line Jar, which expresses no any HLA class I genes except HLA-E, exhibited methylated CpG islands in all HLA class I loci other than HLA-E [4]. After a 5'azacytidine demethylating agent treatment followed by cell cloning, these cells recover the HLA-G gene and other HLA class I genes transcription, and cell surface expression.

In the present report, we examined DNA methylation as a potential regulatory mechanism of HLA-G transcription in two cell types of the adult lymphomyeloid lineage: the CD2+ lymphocytes have low expression of transcripts while transcription is undetectable in CD34+ cells. The HLA-G gene contains a 1070 bp CpG island which covers the first three exons, including the transcription start [5]. We analyzed the methylation pattern of a 457 bp region in the 5'CpG island upstream from the transcription initiation site. This region includes exon 1, intron 1 and exon 2 sequences and contains 46 CpG sites. The methylation status of these CpG sites was established using bisulfite-treated genomic DNA sequencing [6]. Bisulfite treatment converts preferentially unmethylated cytosine (C) residues to uracyl. After amplification, C residues appear as thymine (T) in the PCR products and only methylated cytosine residues are amplified as C. DNA sequences were determined using an automated DNA sequencer. Direct sequencing of the PCR products provides the means of evaluating the level of methylation in genomic DNA on the electropherograms. Sequencing of cloned PCR products provide methylation maps of single DNA molecules.

Results

Analysis of CpG methylation level using direct sequencing of PCR products

The methylation level of the 46 CpGs for the two hematopoietic cells are compared on *Table I*. No CpG site appears to be fully methylated in the two DNAs. Several CpG sites are not methylated: 12 and 4 CpGs are found to be unmethylated in CD34+ cells and CD2+ lymphocytes respectively. There are several CpG dinucleotides, such as CpGs 939, 958, 1023 which are

Table II. Methylation of CpG sites in cloned PCR products derived from CD34+ cells (CD34) and CD2+ lymphocytes (CD2). Only methylation of exon 2 is shown. The CpG sites are numbered according to [10]. M: methylated CpG

	Exon 2																												
CpG	1010	1013	1016	1023	1028	1032	1034	1044	1052	1064	1070	1075	1082	1086	1091	1097	1102	1105	1111	1123	1125	1128	1132	1153	1176	1193	1227	1229	1247	Total
Clones																														
CD34-1													M	M	M	M	M									M				6
CD34-2																													M	1
CD34-3																													M	1
CD34-4																														0
CD34-5																														0
CD34-6																														0
Clones																														
CD2-1			M					M		M	M			M										M			M	M		8
CD2-2	M	M														M	M					M	M			M			M	8
CD2-3																											M	M		2
CD2-4																						M							M	2
CD2-5																								M						1
CD2-6								M																						1

demethylated in the two DNAs. In CD34+ cells, the unmethylated CpG dinucleotides are concentrated in the 3' part of intron 1 and in the 5' part of exon 2. In CD2+ lymphocytes, most CpG sites display a similar or higher amount of methylation that those in CD34+ cells. Four CpG sites, scattered all over the CpG island (CpG 842, CpG 937, CpG 1123, CpG 1176), are found to be less methylated that those in CD34+ cells. CpG 1176 is the unique CpG site which is methylated in CD34+ cells and totally demethylated in CD2+ lymphocytes.

Methylation analysis in cloned PCR products

Methylation of the 46 CpG sites was analyzed in 6 randomly cloned PCR products. The methylation patterns obtained in exon 2 are shown on *Table II*. The distribution of methylation is not uniform across the 46 CpG sites. The CD34+ cells clones display no methylation at any CpG site in exon 1, intron 1 (data not shown). In one clone (CD34-1), we detected 6 methylated CpG sites (CpG 1082 to CpG 1102 and CpG 1193) localized in the 3' part of exon 2. A single CpG (CpG 1247) located in the 3' part of exon 2 is methylated in 2 clones (CD34-2, CD34-3). The three other clones are completely demethylated. In CD2+ lymphocytes, the number of methylated CpG sites per clone range from 1 to 13 of 46 CpGs and a single molecule (CD2-1) is methylated in the domain close to the transcription initiation at the CpGs 823 and 842 in exon 1 and CpGs 889, 891 and 958 in intron 1 (data not shown).

Conclusion and discussion

Analysis of CpG methylation from PCR products showed that the CpG island of HLA-G gene is hypomethylated in HLA-G positive cells (CD2+) and in HLA-G negative cells (CD34+). Morever, in CD2+ lymphocytes, most CpG sites tend to maintain or increase methylation relative to those of the CD34+ cells which suggests that there is not a developmentally regulated demethylation of HLA-G gene during hematopoiesis. However, for the two hematopoietic cells, the clones have considerably different methylation patterns. It is correspondingly important that we consider how far methylation pattern is a clonal property of the target population and how far an unregulated event. If we can measure weakly surface HLA-G expression using monoclonal antibodies on the CD2+ cells, it will be possible to separate them by cell sorting into categories of different expression level and analyse methylation patterns independently.

The HLA-G gene is transcriptionally inactive in immature CD34+ cells in spite of a hypomethylation of the CpG island. Christophe and Pichon [7] have revived the debate on the relationship between DNA methylation and gene activity. They show that the repression of the bovine thyroglobulin gene is maintained in non-differentiating thyrocytes or if an enhancer element was lacking. The authors suggest that the negative effect of DNA methylation is maintained only under conditions where the complete set of transcription factors are activated in fully differentiated thyrocytes. Such a reversal of the negative effect of DNA methylation in conditions where transcription is optimally stimulated had been also observed in the transcription of the rat α-actin gene [8] and the Xenopus estrogen-inductible vitellogenin genes [9]. In the same way, our data suggest that repression of HLA-G gene in undifferentiated CD34+ cells may be maintained by the absence of specific activating factors and that methylation is not the mechanism of HLA-G transcriptional regulation in hematopoietic cells.

One could speculate that classical class I genes are regulated by establishing a specific methylation pattern in the CpG island allowing their continuous expression in somatic cells. HLA-G gene that appears to be expressed irregulary (unpublished observation) can hardly be controlled by changes in DNA methylation, since this would involve replication of the DNA at each time.

References

1. Lee N, Malacko AR, Ishitani A, Chen MC, Bajorath J, Marquardt H, Geraghty DE. The membrane-bound and soluble forms of HLA-G bind identical sets of endogenous peptides but differ with respect to Tap association. *Immunity* 1995; 3: 1-20.

2. Amiot L, Onno M, Renard I, Drenou B, Guillaudeux T, LeBouteiller P, Fauchet R. HLA-G transcription studies during the different stages of normal and malignant hematopoiesis. *Tissue Antigens* 1996; 47:408-13.
3. LeBouteiller P. HLA class I chromosomal region, genes, and products: facts and questions. *Crit Rev Immunol* 1994; 14: 89-130.
4. Boucraut J, Guillaudeux T, Alizadeh M, Boretto J, Chimini G, Malecaze F, Semana G, Fauchet R, Pontarotti P, LeBouteiller P. HLA-E is the only class I gene that escapes CpG methylation and is transcriptionally active in the trophoblast-derived human cell line JAR. *Immunogenetics* 1993; 38: 117-30.
5. Larsen F, Gundersen G, Lopez R, Prydz H. CpG islands as gene markers in the human genome. *Genomics* 1992; 13 : 1095-107.
6. Frommer M. McDonald L, Millar DS, Collis C, Watt F, Grigg GW, Molloy PL, Paul LP. A genomic sequencing protocol that yields a positive display of 5-methylcytosine residues in individual DNA strands. *Proc Natl Acad Sci USA* 1992; 89: 1827-31.
7. Christophe D, Pichon B. DNA methylation and gene activity: towards the end of the debate? *Mol Cell Endocrinol* 1994; 100: 155-8.
8. Yisraeli J, Adelstein RS, Melloui D, Nudel U, Yaffe D, Cedar H. Muscle-specific activation of a methylated chimeric actin gene. *Cell* 1986; 46: 409-16.
9. Gerber-Huber S, May F, Westley BR, Felber BK, Hosbach H, Andres AC, Ryffel GU. In contrast to other Xenopus genes the estrogen-inducible vitellogenin genes are expressed when totally methylated. *Cell* 1983: 33: 43-51.
10. Geraghty DE, Koller BH, Orr HT. A human major histocompatibility complex class I gene that encodes a protein with a shortened cytoplasmic segment. *Proc Natl Acad Sci USA* 1987; 84: 9145-9.

Interferon-γ rescues HLA class Ia cell surface expression in term villous trophoblast cells by inducing synthesis of TAP proteins

A.M. Rodriguez, V. Mallet, F. Lenfant, P. Le Bouteiller

INSERM U395, CHU Purpan, BP 3028, 31024 Toulouse Cedex, France

Human placental trophoblast cells that constitute the materno-fetal interface during pregnancy escape maternal alloimmune attack [1]. The different villous and extravillous trophoblast cell subpopulations have developed efficient regulatory mechanisms to prevent expression of most β2-microglobulin (β2m)-associated HLA class Ia heavy chains (HC) at their cell surface [2]. We previously reported the presence at low levels of HLA-A and HLA-B/C class Ia messages in villous cytotrophoblast cells and in the *in vitro*-differentiated syncytiotrophoblast purified from term placenta [3]. Thus, in addition to transcriptional control, post-transcriptional regulatory mechanisms are likely to operate in these trophoblast cells to prevent cell surface expression of these polymorphic, potentially harmful, glycoproteins. In this study, we first investigated whether the HLA class Ia transcripts detected in the villous trophoblast cells purified from term placenta could be translated and in which intracellular compartment they could be located. It is known that interferon-γ (IFN-γ) is a powerful HLA class Ia cytokine inducer, due to the presence of an "Interferon Consensus Sequence" in their promoter [4]. We thus examined whether a treatment of these trophoblast cells with IFN-γ was able to restore cell surface expression of these HLA class I molecules. As such IFN-γ treatment induces a significant expression of HLA class Ia at the cell surface, we finally analyzed whether HLA class Ia HC could be associated with peptide transporter TAP proteins.

Results and discussion

HLA class Ia HC are translated in both villous trophoblast cell subpopulations purified from term placenta

The technic of purification of villous cytotrophoblast cells and of *in vitro* differentiation of syncytiotrophoblast has been described elsewhere [3]. Absence of cell surface expression of HLA class Ia and HLA-G by cytotrophoblast cells was demonstrated by a flow cytometry analysis, using a panel of anti-HLA class I mAbs, including two recently described anti-HLA-G [5, 6]. By comparison, all of these mAbs labeled the trophoblast-derived JEG-3 control cell line, known to express both HLA-C and HLA-G [1]. Both W6/32 monomorphic anti-HLA class I and BFL.1 anti-HLA-G [6] fail to immunoprecipitate biotin-labeled cell surface proteins in either trophoblast cell subpopulation, confirming the absence of detectable membrane-bound HLA class Ia or HLA-G in both cytotrophoblast cells and syncytiotrophoblast. We next examined whether HLA class Ia transcripts, previously detected in cytotrophoblast cells and syncytiotrophoblast [2], were translated in proteins. Immunoprecipitation studies were carried out with different anti-HLA class I mAbs, using lysates from cytotrophoblast cells or syncytiotrophoblast metabolically labeled with [^{35}S]methionine-cysteine. Comparison was made with control cell lines known to express HLA class Ia (HHK) or HLA-G and HLA class Ia (JEG-3). Immunoprecipitates were analyzed by SDS-PAGE. W6/32 mAb immunoprecipitates two proteins of 45-kDa (HLA class Ia HC) and 39-kDa (HLA-G HC) from JEG-3 cell lysates and reveals a single 45-kDa band in the HHK lymphoblastoid control cell line. The same mAb immunoprecipitates two proteins of 45- and 40-kDa from cytotrophoblast cell lysates and a single 45-kDa species from syncytiotrophoblast. These data demonstrate that HLA class Ia and HLA-G messages are translated in the cytotrophobast cells whereas only HLA class Ia translated HC are present in syncytiotrophoblast. We noted that the apparent m.w. of the HLA-G protein in cytotrophoblast cells was 40-kDa instead of 39-kDa in JEG-3.

Translated HLA class Ia HC are retained in the endoplasmic reticulum (ER)

The maturation state of the intracellular HLA class I HC present in cytotrophoblast cells and syncytiotrophoblast was assessed by examining their susceptibility to digestion by Endoglycosidase H (Endo H). Such a treatment of the W6/32 immunoprecipitated class I HC from cytotrophoblast cells shifted the apparent m.w. of both 45- and 40-kDa species to smaller products, respectively down to 42 and 37-kDa. Similarly, the 45-kDa band immunoprecipitated from syncytiotrophoblast lysates was reduced in size by Endo H digestion and migrated with an apparent m.w. of 37-kDa. Such an increase in mobility on SDS-PAGE demonstrates that all HLA class I HC present in cytotrophoblast cells and syncytiotrophoblast from term placenta are Endo H sensitive. Therefore, it is likely that they are immature molecules retained into the lumen of the ER.

IFN-γ treatment induces appearance of Endo-H resistant HLA class Ia HC that reach the cell surface

We investigated whether a treatment with IFN-γ modified the maturation state of the intracellular HLA class I HC. Cytotrophoblast cells and syncytiotrophoblast were treated or not with IFN-γ for 24h, labeled with [^{35}S]methionine-cysteine, lysed and immunoprecipitated with the W6/32 mAb. Immunoprecipitated lysates were incubated or not with endo H and separated on SDS-PAGE. IFN-γ treatment induces appearance of mature Endo H resistant 45-kDa bands in both cell populations, as compared with cells untreated with IFN-γ which exclusively exhibit Endo H sensitive bands. Thus, after IFN-γ treatment, at least part of HLA class Ia HC become mature and are exported from the ER. We next examined whether the mature HLA class Ia HC detectable in cytotrophoblast cells after IFN-γ treatment could reach the cell surface. We performed a two-color immunofluorescence staining on cytotrophoblast cells treated or not with IFN-γ, using both W6/32 anti-HLA class I and JEG-13 anti-trophoblast marker mAbs. Whereas no binding of W6/32 occurs in untreated cells, part of them become W6/32 positive after IFN-γ treatment. These data were reproducible and confirmed by W6/32 immunoprecipitation of cell surface labeled biotinylated proteins. Therefore, these findings demonstrate that the cell surface expression of HLA class Ia molecules can be rescued on both trophoblast cell subpopulations by exposure to IFN-γ.

IFN-γ treatment induces both transcription and translation of TAP

We then investigated whether IFN-γ corrects the defect in cell surface expression of HLA class Ia HC in trophoblast cells by increasing the levels of MHC class I transcription or by another mechanism involving the antigen processing and TAP proteins in particular. A Northern blot analysis was performed on cytotrophoblast cells and syncytiotrophoblast, using locus-specific HLA class Ia, TAP1 and TAP2 DNA probes. Both trophoblast cell subpopulations express HLA-A and B/C transcripts. Treatment with IFN-γ slightly increased their levels. The level of HLA-G transcription in cytotrophoblast cells was not affected by the IFN-γ treatment. Both TAP1 and TAP2 mRNA that were almost undetectable in untreated cytotrophoblast cells and syncytiotrophoblast were clearly inducible in these two cell populations after treatment with IFN-γ. These results show that IFN-γ enhances synthesis of both TAP1 and TAP2 transcripts in villous cytotrophoblast and syncytiotrophoblast whereas it does not significantly increase the levels of the HLA class Ia messages. We then studied whether TAP transcripts were translated in proteins. Untreated or IFN-γ treated trophoblast cells were labeled with [^{35}S]-methionine-cysteine, immunoprecipitated with an anti-TAP1 mAb and analyzed by SDS-PAGE. As expected, a mutant T2 control cell line did not contain TAP1 proteins. TAP1 proteins were also undetectable in both untreated cytotrophoblast cells and syncytiotrophoblast. Following IFN-γ treament, the anti-TAP1 mAb co-immunoprecipitates 70- and 45-kDa bands, that correspond to the m.w. of TAP1 and HLA class Ia HC respectively, in both trophoblast cell subpopulations. These data are consistent with the mRNA study mentioned above and show that, after IFN-γ treatment, 45-kDa HLA class Ia HC become associated with TAP1 molecules in villous cytotrophoblast and syncytiotrophoblast.

Conclusion

We have shown that, in villous trophoblast cells purified

from term placenta, HLA class Ia HC are Endo H sensitive and thus retained in the ER. Following IFN-γ treament, export of these HC from the ER and their expression at the cell surface appear together with translation of TAP proteins. Thus, the constitutive absence of HLA class Ia cell surface expression in term villous cytotrophoblast and syncytiotrophoblast is likely to be due to a lack of transporter proteins that participate in the proper assembly in the ER. The same conclusion was recently drawn by Clover *et al.* [7] and Roby *et al.* [8]. Such a defect can be reversed by IFN-γ treatment. Stable cell surface expression of class I molecules requires association of HC with β2m and peptide ligand in the ER [9]. These three components are critical for the formation of mature class I complex and most class I molecules that are not fully assembled are instable and degraded. Part of the class Ia HC present in the ER of trophoblast cells are associated with β2m. This was demonstrated by the immunoprecipitation of 45-kDa proteins with the W6/32 mAb, known to only recognize HC associated with β2m [2]. Therefore, the β2m component is present in these cell types and can associate with the class I HC. Our data suggest that the availability of peptides in the ER is likely to be the limiting factor in the export and expression of HLA class Ia molecules in these trophoblast cells.

Acknowledgements

We thank Dr Jacques Arnaud and Dr Armand Bensussan for helpful discussions and Maryse Girr for her participation in part of the work. We thank Drs D. Bellet (Villejuif, France), M. B. Brenner (Boston, MA, USA), D. E. Geraghty (Seattle, WA, USA), H.T. Orr (Minneapolis, MN, USA), O. Fardel (Rennes France), B.L. Hsi (Nice France), H. L. Ploegh (Cambridge, MA, UK), P. Sanseau (London, UK) and R. Tampe (Martinsried) for their kind gifts of gene probes or Abs. This work was supported by INSERM, ARC and Conseil Régional Midi-Pyrénées. AMR was supported by a fellowship from Fondation Mérieux, VM by a fellowship from MESR; FL is a recipient of a post-doctoral fellowship from Société de Secours des Amis des Sciences.

References

1. Loke YW, King A. *Human implantation: cell biology and immunology.* Cambridge: Cambridge University Press, 1995.
2. Le Bouteiller P, Rodriguez AM, Mallet V, Girr M, Guillaudeux T, Lenfant F. Placental expression of HLA class I genes. *Am J Reprod Immunol* 1996 ; 35 : 216-25.
3. Guillaudeux T, Rodriguez AM, Girr M, Mallet V, Ellis SA, Sargent IL, Fauchet R, Alsat E, Le Bouteiller P. Methylation status and transcriptional expression of the MHC class I loci in human trophoblast cells from term placenta. *J Immunol* 1995 ; 154 : 3283-99.
4. Le Bouteiller P. HLA class I chromosomal region, genes and products : facts and questions. *Crit Rev Immunol* 1994 ; 14 : 89-129.
5. Lee N, Malacko AR, Ishitani A, Chen MC, Bajorath J, Marquardt H, Geraghty DE. The membrane-bound and soluble forms of HLA-G bind identical sets of endogenous peptides but differ with respect to TAP association. *Immunity* 1995 ; 3 : 591-600.
6. Bensussan A, Mansur IG, Mallet V, Rodriguez AM, Girr M, Weiss EH, Brem G, Boumsell E, Gluckman E, Dausset J, Carosella E, Le Bouteiller P. Detection of membrane-bound HLA-G translated products with a specific monoclonal antibody. *Proc Natl Acad Sci USA* 1995 ; 92 : 10292-1296.
7. Clover LM, Sargent IL, Townsend A, Tampé R, Redman CWG. Expression of TAP1 by human trophoblast. *Eur J Immunol* 1995 ; 25 : 543-8.
8. Roby KF, Gershon D, Hunt JS. Expression of the transporter for antigen processing-1 (Tap-1) gene in subpopulations of human trophoblast cells. *Placenta* 1996 ; 17 : 27-32.
9. Ortmann B, Androlewicz MJ, Cresswell P. MHC class I/b2-microglobulin complexes associate with TAP transporters before peptide binding. *Nature* 1994 ; 368 : 864-7.

Mhc-G and *-E* alleles in humans and primates

M. Alvarez[1], M. J. Castro[1], J. Martínez-Laso, E. Gómez-Casado, N. Díaz-Campos, G. Vargas-Alarcón, R. Alegre, P. Morales, A. Arnaiz-Villena

Department of Immunology, Hospital Universitario 12 de Octubre, Universidad Complutense, Carretara de Andalucia 28041, Madrid, Spain
1 The contribution by Miguel Alvarez and M. José Castro is equal and the order of authorship is arbitrary

The non-classical class I *Mhc-G* and *-E* genes have been supposed not to be as polymorphic as classical *Mhc-A*, *-B* and *-C* genes. However, 6 DNA *HLA-G* alleles (both with productive and non productive changes) have been described [1-4] (see *Table I*).

In addition, allelic diversity at *Mhc-G* locus has also been found in Chimpanzee, Orangutan and primates belonging to the Cercophitecidae family (Green Monkey, Rhesus Monkey and Cynomologous). However, *Mhc-G* polymorphism does not follow the classical pattern of three hypervariable regions per domain and exon 3 ($\alpha2$ domain) bears stop codons in all individuals of the *Cercophitecidae* family [1]. This suggests that primates (at least *Cercophitecidae*) may not use this molecule as an antigen presenting one to the clonotipic T-cell receptor and other (soluble?) isoforms may be the physiological important ones, particularly the isoform containing only the $\alpha1$ domain (G3).

There is a clear *trans*-species evolution of allelism and *Mhc-G* intron 2 show a typical conserved motif in all studied species which consists of a 23 base pair deletion between positions 161 and 183 [1].

With regard to *Mhc-E* molecules they also present a polymorphism [5] and new alleles have also been found (unpublished results). Both humans and primates show *Mhc-E* allelism with a polymorphism not limited to the three hypervariable regions (like *Mhc-G*). There is a strong pressure at the antigen binding side that only permit synonymous changes in all studied primates. This suggests that *Mhc-E* molecules are only able to bind a specific and limited antigens peptide repertoire [5]. *Mhc-E* molecules show a clear *trans*-species evolution [5] and two different primate species (Rhesus monkey and Cynomologous) bear the same allele regarding exon 2 and 3; this is the first example of objective *trans*-species evolution, if convergent evolution is discarded. In addition, it is very likely that *Mhc-G* sequences found in cotton-top tamarin [6] may be in fact *Mhc-E* sequences according to the presently available data (see dendrogram in *Figure 1*).

Acknowledgments

This work was supported by a Fondo de Investigaciones Sanitarias and a Fundación Ramón Areces grants.

References

1. Castro MJ, Morales P, Fernández-Soria V, Suárez B, Recio MJ, Alvarez M, Martín-Villa JM, Arnaiz-Villena A. Allelic diversity at the primate *Mhc-G* locus: exon 3 bears stop codons in all *Cercophitecinae* sequences. *Immunogenetics* 1996; 43:327-36.
2. Pook M, Woodcock J, Tessabehji M, Campbell RD, Summers C, Taylor M, Strachan T. Characterization of an expressible non classical class I *HLA* gene. *Hum Immunol* 1991; 32:102-9.

Table I. Number of alleles at Mhc-G and -E loci in primates

Human	Chimpanzee	Gorilla	Orangutan	Rhesus	Cyno
6(3)	2(0)	1(0)	4(0)	7(0)	7(0)
4(0)	2(2)	2(2)	1(0)	8(0)	5(0)

Data from [3], [1] and [5]. In parenthesis are numbers of non-productive alleles included in the total number, *i.e.*: synonymous DNA substitutions.

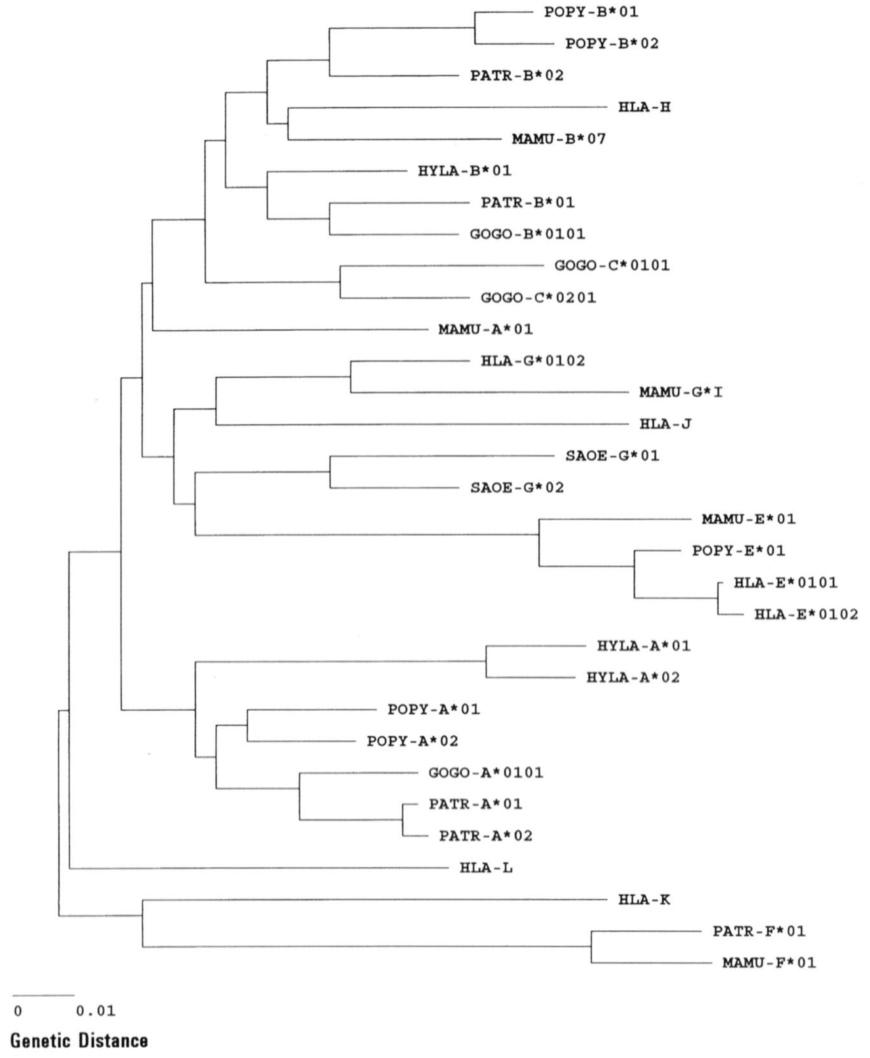

Figure 1. Neighbour joining dendrogram depicting the evolutive relationships among exon 2 and exon 3 of primate class I sequences [5].

3. Morales P, Corell A, Martínez-Laso J Martín-Villa J M, Varela P, Allende LM, Arnaiz-Villena A. Three new *HLA-G* alleles and their linkage disequilibria with *HLA-A*. *Immunogenetics* 1993; 38:323-31.
4. Yamashita T, Fujii T, Watanabe Y, Tokunaga K, Tadokoro K, Juji T, Taketani Y. Polymorphism of the *HLA-G* gene in Japanese. *Immunogenetics* 1997 (in press).
5. Alvarez M, Martínez-Laso J, Varela P, Díaz-Campos N, Gómez-Casado E, Vargas-Alarcón G, García de la Torre C, Arnaiz-Villena A. High polymorphism of *Mhc-E* locus in non-human primates: the same allele is found in two different species. *Tissue Antigens* 1997 (submitted).
6. Watkins D, Letvin N, Hughes A, Tedder T. Molecular cloning of cDNA that encode *Mhc* class I molecules from a new world primate *(Saguinus oedipus). J Immunol* 1990; 144:1136-43.

Cellular function of soluble HLA-G

Y. Mitsuishi, K. Miyazawa, A. Sonoda, P.I. Terasaki

UCLA Tissue Typing Laboratory, 950 Veteran Avenue, Los Angeles, CA 90095, USA

A non-classical HLA antigen, HLA-G, is expressed only on the extravillous cytotrophoblast in the placenta, especially during the first trimester of pregnancy [1,2]. HLA-G is much less polymorphic than HLA-A or B. It is well known that classical HLA-class I and class II antigens are not detected in the placenta, although HLA-C may be expressed. This observation may explain how the semiallogeneic fetus is tolerated by the maternal immunological system. However, the absence of classical HLA antigens cannot explain how the fetus can be protected from maternal NK killing or infections. A recent paper has shown that the soluble form of HLA-G (s-HLA-G) is secreted not only in the extravillous trophoblast but also in the syncytiotrophoblast where the membrane bound form of HLA-G (m-HLA-G) is not expressed [3]. The s-HLA-G may have synergistic or complementary effects with m-HLA-G. The mechanism of translation of s-HLA-G is similar to that of the CD1 molecule. Intron 4 is not spliced during transcription and translation terminates after the stop codon located at the beginning of intron 4 [4]. It has been observed that the choriocarcinoma cell line, Jeg-3 expresses m-HLA-G and secretes s-HLA-G. The HLA-G gene produces at least 4 distinct kinds of HLA-G proteins using complex alternative splicing mechanisms of mRNA transcription. G1 is the full length polypeptide, G2 is missing the $\alpha2$ domain, G3 is missing the $\alpha2$ and $\alpha3$ domains and G4 is missing $\alpha3$ [5,6]. Ishitani [5] has suggested that a homodimer of the G2 protein can function as a classical class II molecule.

A sense primer specific to 5'UTR of HLA-G and an antisense primer for intron 4 were used to amplify the s-HLA-G gene with cDNA obtained from the Jeg-3 cell line and from early-stage placentas. Several bands were identified in the sizing gel. Each band was excised, purified and ligated into a pCR3 vector. After sequencing with an ABI autosequencer, the cloned DNA products were transfected into CHO and Hela cell lines with lipofectine. Four s-HLA-G products (designated H, M, L and SL) have been identified. Two products, H and M, were identical to G1sol and G2sol, whereas L and SL showed the new alternative splicing patterns. L has only the $\alpha3$ domain while SL has only the $\alpha1$ domain. In the first week, most of the cells died *via* the G-418 selection process and 2-3 weeks later a few colonies formed. These colonies were transferred to new trays and cultured with G-418. Transfection of H and M has been confirmed with RT-PCR, immunoprecipitation and ELISA. However, confirmation of L and SL at the protein level still remains to be done. H, M and L were used for the following work.

We were interested to determine whether s-HLA-G interacted with T cells or NK cells in the placenta. To test this, supernatants (sup) containing s-HLA-G were added to several MLC and NK killing tests. Two kinds of supernatants were used; one from the Jeg-3 cell line and the other from the transfectants. Supernatants from K562 and non-transfected CHO or Hela cells cultured in the same FCS for the same time period were used as negative controls. A sandwich ELISA method with monoclonal w6/32 bound to the tray and OPD-conjugated sheep polyclonal $\beta2$m antibody, was used to detect secretion of s-HLA-G in the Jeg-3 and SB27 (a cell line secreting HLA-B27) supernatants as seen in *Table I*. However, only the H transfectant produced a protein detectable in this ELISA test (not shown). Detection requires $\beta2$m association and deletions of the $\alpha1$, $\alpha2$ and $\alpha3$ domains may preclude identification of the M, L, and SL products. Thus, the Jeg-3

Table I. ELISA assay for the soluble HLA-G

	Dilution		
	neat	1/10	1/100
PBS	0.04	-	-
K562 sup	0.05	0.05	0.04
Jeg-3 sup	0.84	0.12	0.04
SB27 sup	1.10	0.50	0.05

Table II. MLC inhibition test (cpm)

	S1/R2	S1/R1	S2/R1	S2/R2
JEG-3 sup	4207	2819	5922	2325
JEG-3 + K562 sups	6202	4091	9537	5498
K562 sup	46167	7356	77773	14149

Table III. NK killing inhibition test (1) (% cytolysis) E/T ratio = 50:1

	Fresh NK cells		Cultured NK cells	
	Exp 1	Exp 2	Exp 3	Exp 4
Media	68.5	53.3	36.0	53.1
K562 sup	64.1	49.7	47.4	55.5
Jeg-3 sup	58.7	45.6	25.8	22.0

Table IV. NK killing inhibition test (2) (% cytolysis) E/T ratio = 50:1

	Fresh NK cells		Cultured NK cells	
	Exp 1	Exp 2	Exp 3	Exp 4
Media	48.3	49.2	45.1	55.8
H sup	45.7	46.1	15.1	7.6
M sup	45.9	43.1	21.1	9.7
L sup	47.2	42.7	38.1	23.5

supernatant contains full-length s-HLA-G, and this was used for inhibition of MLC and NK killing.
Four stimulator/responder combinations were tested with supernatants from JEG-3, K562 (the negative control), and a 1:1 mixture as shown in *Table II*. The MLC was consistently inhibited by the JEG-3 supernatant (70-95%) and the inhibition was reduced by dilution with K562 supernatant. After 6 days of culture, blasts were detected by flow cytometry in the K562 supernatant groups, but no clear blast population was detected in cultures with Jeg-3 supernatant. Jeg-3 supernatants were collected after different durations of culture, and the inhibition rate varied among these different supernatants. However, the inhibition results did not correlate with the ELISA data, suggesting some forms of s-HLA-G other than the full-length polypeptide may inhibit. A preliminary experiment indicated that the MLC was strongly inhibited by supernatant from the H ($\alpha 1+ \alpha 2+ \alpha 3$) and M ($\alpha 1+ \alpha 3$) transfectants, but not by supernatant from L (only $\alpha 3$). This data is still preliminary and more data is necessary to confirm this observation.
NK cell killing tests were done using the microtray NK assay method [7]. Unequivocal inhibition of cytolysis on K562 targets in the presence of 20% supernatant from JEG-3 cultures was not observed when fresh NK cells were tested, but when the effectors were cultured for 5 days with Jeg-3 supernatant *(Table III)* or with supernatant from H, M or L transfectants *(Table IV)*, NK killing was blocked by 20-70%. This blocking is still not stable and should be confirmed by additional studies. Nevertheless, the results suggest a minimal requirement for the alpha 1 domain for effective inhibition.
The apparent capacity of s-HLA-G to block or inhibit function of alloreactive T-cells and NK cells suggests that HLA-G may serve an important protective function in the placenta in addition to its potential antigen presenting capability.

References

1. Geraghty D, Keller B, Orr H. A human major histocompatiblity complex class I gene that encodes a protein with a shortened cytoplasmic segment. *Proc Natl Acad Sci USA* 1987 ; 84 : 9145-9.
2. Kovats S, Main EK, Librach C, Stubblebine MF, Fisher SI, DeMars R. A class I antigen, HLA-G, expressed in human trophoblasts. *Science* 1990 ; 248 : 220-3.
3. Hirano Y, Ishitani A, Geraghty DE. The expression of HLA-G antigen in different human tissues and placentas at different stages of pregnancy. *J Nara Med Ass* 1994 ; 45 : 616-25.
4. Fujii T, Ishitani A, Geraghty D. A soluble form of HLA-G antigen is encoded by a messenger ribonucleic acid containing intron 4. *J Immunol* 1994 ; 153 : 5516-24.
5. Ishitani A, Geraghty D. Alternative splicing of HLA-G transcripts yeilds proteins with priminary structures resembling both class I and class II antigens. *Proc Natl Acad Sci USA* 1992 ; 89 : 3947-51.
6. Kirszenbaum M, Moreau P, Gluckman E, Dausset J, Carosella E. An alternative spliced form of HLA-G mRNA in human trophoblasts and evidence for the presence of HLA-G transcript in adult lymphocytes. *Proc Natl Acad Sci USA* 1994 ; 91: 4209-13.
7. Wang XM. Terasaki PI, Rankin G, Chia D, Zhong HP, Hardy S. A new microcellular cytotoxicity test based on calcein AM release. *Hum Immunol* 1993 ; 37: 264-70.

Polymorphisms of transporter associated with antigen processing (TAP) genes in recurrent spontaneous abortion

M. Saitoh[1], O. Ishihara[1], S. Takeda[1], K. Kinoshita[1], T. Nishimoto[2], S. Kuwata[3], R. Hirata[4], H. Maeda[4]

1 Deptartment of Obstetrics and Gynecology
2 BML Central Laboratory
3 Blood Transfusion Service, Tokyo University Hospital
4 Blood Transfusion Service, Saitama Medical School and Center, 1981 Tsujido, Kamoda Kawagoe, Saitama 350, Japan

The role of major histocompatibility complex (MHC) in reproductive immunology has been extensively studied since Komlos *et al.* [1] first reported increased HLA antigen sharing in the couples with a history of recurrent spontaneous abortion (RSA) compared with control couples. However, a lot of studies have reported about HLA compatibility between couples with RSA and controls with conflicting results. Since the MHC is the center of immunologic functions, this study has been conducted.

Surface expression of class I MHC molecules is dependent upon availability of the peptides which bind the MHC molecules in the endoplasmic reticulum. A peptide transporter, the transporter associated with antigen processing (TAP), plays an important role in maintaining adequate levels of the peptide. As the TAP genes are polymorphic, the allelic differences may play a role in the disease associated with MHC alleles by altering the peptides that bind class I MHC molecules. In addition, it is well known that TAP polymorphisms also affect the level of class I MHC expression, because mutations could influence the efficiency of the transport of peptides that would bind class I MHC.

Thus, TAP gene polymorphisms could have some impact on RSA by changes in the peptide processing pathway. The aim of the study is to investigate the immunogenetic background of patients with RSA in terms of polymorphisms of TAP genes.

Material and methods

Patients

The subjective cases are 38 women patients with RSA and 40 of their husbands as controls. In total, 78 cases were analyzed.

Methods

Genomic TAP1 and TAP2 were detected by PCR-RFLP method. After genomic DNAs were extracted from peripheral blood leukocyte, PCR amplifications were conducted for TAP1 in two regions and TAP2 in four regions. PCR cycles consisted of initial 2 minutes (min.) denaturation at 95 centigrade (°C) and combination of 30 cycles of 1 min. denaturation at 95°C, 1 min. annealing at 52°C, and 1 min. extension at 72°C, followed by 5 min. extension at 74°C. Genotypes of dimorphisms of TAP1 and TAP2 were detected by PCR-RFLP, using several restriction endonucleases as follows. TAP1-1 was detected by digestion with Sau3A, TAP1-2 with AccI, TAP2-1 with AccII, TAP 2-3 with RsaI, TAP2-2 with MspI and BfaI, respectively. As there was no appropriate restriction endonuclease for amino acid position 379, 565, 665 and 687, we have made mismatched upper primers to create the cutting sites for AccII, RsaI, MspI and BfaI, respectively. After the digestion, samples were subjected to electrophoresis in 12 % polyacrylamide gel. Digested fragments were visualized after staining with ethidium bromide.

Four possible TAP1 alleles were determined in a combination of two dimorphic sites at amino acid position (aa) 333 (Ile-Val) and aa 637 (Asp-Gly). As for TAP2 alleles, 8 possible TAP2 alleles were determined in a combination of 4 dimorphic sites at aa 379 (Val-Ile), at aa 565 (Ala-Thr), at aa 665 (Ala-Thr), at aa 687 (Gln-stop).

Results

The TAP gene frequencies are shown in *Table I.* When two possible combinations of alleles were found, we assigned the alleles in proportion to the respective allele frequencies. The highest allele frequencies of TAP1 in

Table I. The gene frequencies in both patients with RSA and their husbands

TAP1 allele (aa: 333-637)	total (%) n=78	patients (%) n=38	husbands (%) n=40
A (Ile-Asp)	134 (85.9)	64 (84.2)	70 (87.5)
B (Val-Gly)	18 (11.5)	9 (11.8)	9 (11.3)
C (Val-Asp)	1 (0.6)	1 (1.3)	0 (0)
D (Ile-Gly)	3 (1.9)	2 (2.6)	1 (1.3)

TAP2 allele (aa: 379-565-665-687)	total (%) n=76	patients (%) n=36	husbands (%) n=40
A (Val-Ala-Thr-Stop)	83 (54.6)	37 (51.4)	46 (57.5)
B (Val-Ala-Ala-Gln)	32.5 (21.4)	16 (22.2)	16.5 (20.6)
C (Ile-Ala-Thr-Stop)	20 (13.2)	9.5 (13.2)	10.5 (13.1)
D (Ile-Thr-Thr-Stop)	2.5 (1.6)	2 (2.8)	0.5 (0.6)
E (Val-Thr-Thr-Stop)	6.5 (4.3)	3.5 (4.9)	3 (3.8)
G (Val-Thr-Ala-Gln)	1 (0.7)	0.5 (0.7)	0.5 (0.6)
H (Ile-Ala-Ala-Gln)	6.5 (4.3)	3.5 (4.9)	3 (3.8)

aa: amino acid position, RSA: recurrent spontaneous abortion

Table II. Sharing of TAP1 and TAP2 genes between patients and their husbands

No. of shared TAP1 genes	couples n=35 (%)	expected n=35 (%)	r
0	0 (0)	0.9 (2.6)	n.s.
1	16 (45.7)	12.2 (35.0)	n.s.
2	19 (54.3)	21.9 (62.4)	n.s.

No. of shared TAP2 genes	couples n=33 (%)	expected n=33 (%)	r
0	9.5 (28.8)	6.8 (20.6)	n.s.
1	15.5 (47.0)	19.6 (59.4)	n.s.
2	8 (24.2)	6.6 (20.0)	n.s.

both patients and their husbands were seen in TAP1A category. The highest allele frequencies of TAP2 in both patients and their husbands were seen in TAP2A category. The allele frequencies between patients and their husbands had no significant differences.

The sharing of TAP genes between patients and their husbands were shown in *Table II*. The expected values in the shared TAP genes were calculated by TAP gene frequencies of husbands which served as controls. These sharing frequencies between couples were not significantly different from those of the expected values.

Discussion

A lot of studies have been conducted for HLA compatibility between couples with RSA and controls to evaluate a possible unfavorable immune mechanism(s) among women with RSA. However, a growing body of evidence suggests that this was not the case for RSA couples. Recently, a non-classic HLA class I gene, HLA-G, was revealed to be the only major histocompatibility complex antigen expressed on cytotrophoblasts of placenta with extremely low polymorphism [2]. This preferential expression in fetal tissues suggests that HLA-G products may play a specific role in embryonic development and/or fetomaternal immune response. However, the limited polymorphism of the gene seems to be difficult for the target of rejection mechanism in RSA. In contrast, the TAP genes are known to be polymorphic and the allelic differences may play a role in the disease association with MHC alleles by altering the peptides that bind class I MHC molecules. In this study, we therefore investigated whether TAP alleles in patients with RSA showed significant differences or preferential association of TAP.

The results of the study demonstrated no altered frequencies of TAP alleles in patients with RSA and their husband compared to a published control population [3-6, 8]. In addition, the frequencies of shared TAP1 and TAP2 alleles between the couples were not significantly different from those of controls.

In conclusion, there seems to be no direct involvement of TAP1 and TAP2 in the etiology of RSA.

References

1. Komlos L, Zanir R, Joshua H, Halbrecht I. Common HLA antigens in couples with repeated abortions. *Clin Immunol Immunopathol* 1977 ; 7 : 330-5.
2. Morales P, Corell A, Martinez-Laso J, Martin-Villa JM, Varela P, Paz-Artal E, Allende LM, Arnaiz-Villena A. Three new HLA-G alleles and their linkage disequilibria with HLA-A. *Immunogenetics* 1993 ; 38 : 323-31.
3. Kuwata S, Yanagisawa M, Saeki H, Nakagawa H, Etoh T, Tokunaga K, Juji T, Shibata Y. Polymorphisms of transporter associated with antigen processing genes in atophic dermatitis. *Allergy Clin Immunol* 1994 ; 3 : 565-74.
4. Cano P, Baxter-Lowe LA. Novel human TAP2*103 allele shows further polymorphism in the ATP-binding domain. *Tissue Antigens* 1995 ; 45 : 139-42.
5. Lee JE, Loflin PT, Laud PR, Lu M, Reveille JD, Lawlor DA. The human leukocyte antigen TAP2 gene defines the centrometric limit of melanoma susceptibility on chromosome 6p. *Tissue Antigens* 1996 ; 47 : 117-21.
6. Powis SH, Tonks S, Mockridge I, Kelly AP, Bodmer JG, Trowsdale J. Alleles and haplotypes of the MHC-encoded ABC transporters TAP1 and TAP2. *Immunogenetics* 1993 ; 37 : 373-80.
7. Ishihara M, Ohno S, Mizuki N, Yamagata N, Naruse T, Shiina T, Kawata H, Kuwata S, Inoko H. Allelic variations in the TAP2 and LMP2 genes in Behcet's disease. *Tissue Antigens* 1996 ; 47 : 249-52.
8. Moins-Teisserenc H, Semana G, Alizadeh M, Loiseau P *et al.* TAP2 gene polymorphism contributes to genetic susceptibility to multiple sclerosis. *Hum Immunol* 1995 ; 42 : 195-202.

HLA Diversity

Evolution of MHC. Ancient DNA

Contents

The MHC class I genes of the rhesus monkey: different evolutionary histories of MHC class I and II genes in primates

C. Shufflebotham, J.E. Boyson, L.F. Cadavid, J.A. Urvater, L.A. Knapp, A.L. Hughes[1], *D.I. Watkins*

Wisconsin Regional Primate Research Center and Department of Pathology and Laboratory Medicine, University of Wisconsin, 1220 Capitol Court, Madison, WI 53715, USA
1 Penn State University, University Park, PA 16802, USA

During evolution of the great apes and Old World primates, major histocompatibility complex (MHC) class II genes and their allelic lineages have been remarkably well preserved [1] and have evolved in a trans-specific fashion [2]. *HLA-A* and *-B* homologues have also been described in several different species of Old World primates and great apes, and at the *A* locus an allelic lineage is preserved between chimpanzees and humans [3-6]. As yet, *C* locus alleles have only been described in chimpanzees and gorillas [3, 7], and there is no evidence for a *C* locus in either the Old World primates, or the orangutans and gibbons. However, it has been suggested that the orangutan has two *HLA-B* locus homologues [8]. This has led to speculation that the *C* locus is a recent duplication of the *B* locus in great apes and humans. Since the ancestors of the rhesus monkey diverged from the lineage leading to humans approximately 35 million years ago, we examined the MHC class I loci of the rhesus monkey and compared them to their non-human primate and human counterparts to shed further light on the mechanisms of MHC class I evolution.

To determine the age of the MHC class I *C* locus and to examine the evolution of the *A* and *B* loci we cloned, sequenced and *in vitro* translated sixteen MHC class I cDNAs from two unrelated rhesus monkeys (*Macaca mulatta*) using both cDNA library screening and PCR amplification with several primer pairs. This analysis resulted in the isolation of five *A* locus alleles, ten *B* locus alleles and one *E* locus allele from the two monkeys (*Table I*). We then made trees comparing exon 2 of the rhesus and human *A* and *B* locus alleles (*Figure 1*). All of the rhesus monkey *A* locus alleles clustered outside the 6 different families of human *A* locus alleles, suggesting that there was no sharing of allelic lineages over the evolutionary distances separating humans and rhesus monkeys. Interestingly, some of the rhesus monkey *A* locus alleles (*Mamu-A*03, -A*05, -A*06* and *A*07*) clustered with exon 2 of other primate *A* and *B* locus alleles, indicating perhaps that these rhesus monkey *A* locus alleles were the product of an ancient segmental exchange event. Construction of gene trees spanning nucleotides 3 to 212 of exon 2 revealed a significant clustering of *Mamu-A*03, -A*05, -A*06* and *-A*07* with *HLA-H, Gogo-A*03, Popy-B*01, HLA-B*7901* (*Figure 2*). Interestingly, *Gogo-A*03* is a recombinant between the *A* and *H* loci [7, 9]. To explain this clustering one would have to propose several different recombination events to account for the presence of this stretch of nucleic acids on three different primate MHC class I loci. It is also possible that these alleles are the result of convergent evolution and selection for a particular function has maintained them in primate populations.

Like the rhesus monkey *A* locus alleles, the majority of the rhesus monkey *B* locus alleles clustered outside the other primate *B* locus alleles indicating that *B* locus allelic lineages are not shared between humans and rhesus monkeys. This is in sharp contrast to the *DRB1* and *DQB1* loci where trans-specific sharing of allelic lineages between humans and rhesus monkeys is seen [10]. It, therefore, appears that the MHC class I loci of primates are undergoing a continual process of segmental exchange and duplication and then expansion or deletion of their MHC class I loci. Since our data suggest that there are multiple *A* and *B* loci in the rhesus monkey, it is likely that rhesus monkey MHC class I haplotypes can differ in their complement of MHC class I loci in a manner similar to that seen at the primate MHC class II loci. This is quite different from the constancy of the number of classical MHC class I genes seen in human haplotypes.

We have, therefore, shown that the rhesus monkey MHC

Table I. Summary of all MHC class I cDNAs isolated from rhesus monkeys 84557 and 88090

Allele	Number of copies	Animal	Primer pair/s
*Mamu A*05*	2	84557	5'/ 3' MAS
[a]***Mamu A*06***	18	84557	5'/ 3' MAS AND 5' BETA 3 XHO/ 3' CLOC H3
Mamu A*07	21	84557	5'/ 3' MAS, 5' BETA 3 XHO/ 3' CLOC H3 AND 5' BETA 3 XHO/ 3' ALOC H3
Mamu B*01	6	84557	5'/ 3' MBS
*Mamu B*06*	6	84557	5'/ 3' MBS AND 5' BETA 3 XHO/ 3'BETA 2 H3
*Mamu B*07*	24	84557	5'/ 3' MBS, 5' BETA 3 XHO/ 3'BETA 2 H3 AND 5' BETA 3 XHO/ 3' ALOC H3
Mamu B*08	16	84557	5'/ 3' MBS, 5' BETA 3 XHO/ 3'BETA 2 H3, 5' BETA 3 XHO/ 3' CLOC H3 AND 5' BETA 3 XHO/ 3' ALOC H3
*Mamu B*09*	5	84557	5'/ 3' MBS, 5' BETA 3 XHO/ 3'BETA 2 H3 AND 5' BETA 3 XHO/ 3' CLOC H3
Mamu A*03	7	88090	cDNA library
Mamu A*04	2	88090	cDNA library
Mamu B*02	8	88090	cDNA library
Mamu B*03	2	88090	cDNA library
Mamu B*04	3	88090	cDNA library
*Mamu B*05*	5	88090	cDNA library
*Mamu B*11*	2	88090	cDNA library
*Mamu E*05*	16	88090	cDNA library

[a]Bold typing indicates MHC class I cDNAs encoding proteins with isoelectric focusing points identical to immunoprecipitated MHC class I molecules from PBLs (data not shown).

class I haplotype consists of at least one *HLA-A* homologue and at least two *HLA-B* homologues. We found no evidence for a *HLA-C* locus homologue, suggesting that the *C* locus in gorillas, chimpanzees and humans is of fairly recent origin.

References

1. Kasahara M, Klein D, Fan W, Gutknecht J. Evolution of the class II major histocompatibility complex alleles in higher primates. *Immunol Rev* 1990; 113: 65-82.
2. Klein J. Origin of major histocompatibility complex polymorphisms: The transspecies hypothesis. *Hum Immunol* 1987; 1: 155-62.
3. Lawlor DA, Ward FE, Ennis PD, Jackson AP, Parham P. HLA-A and B polymorphism predate the divergence of humans and chimpanzees. *Nature* 1988; 335: 268-71.
4. Mayer WE, Jonker M, Klein D, Ivanyi P, Van Seventer G, Klein J. Nucleotide sequences of chimpanzee MHC class I alleles: evidence for a trans-species mode of evolution. *EMBO J* 1988; 7: 2765-74.
5. McAdam SN, Boyson JE, Liu X, Garber TL, Hughes AH, Bontrop RE, Watkins DI. Chimpanzee major histocompatibility complex class I *A* locus alleles are related to only one of the six families of human *A* locus alleles. *J Immunol* 1995; 154: 6421-9.
6. Lawlor DA, Edelson BT, Parham P. Mhc-A locus molecules in pygmy chimpanzees: conservation of peptide pockets. *Immunogenetics* 199; 42: 291-5.
7. Lawlor DA, Warren E, Ward FE, Parham P. Gorilla class I major histocompatibility complex alleles: Comparison to human and chimpanzee class I. *J Exp Med* 1991; 174: 1491-507.
8. Chen ZW, McAdam SN, Hughes AL, Dogon AL, Letvin NL, Watkins DI. Molecular cloning of orangutan and gibbon MHC class I cDNA: The HLA-A and -B loci diverged over 30 million years ago. *J Immunol* 1992; 148: 2547-54.

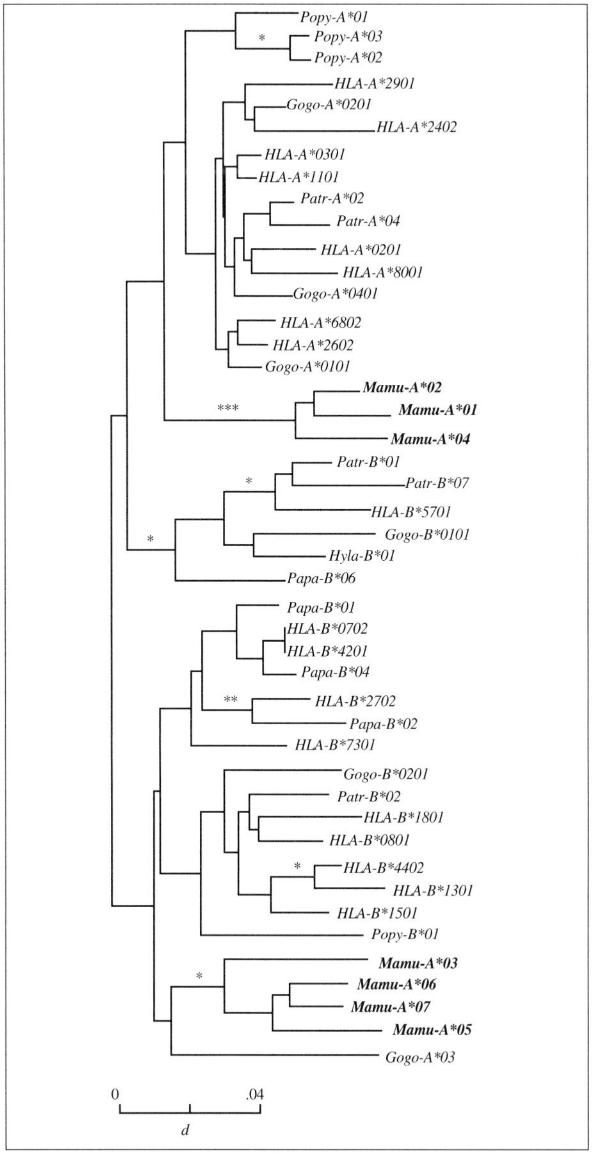

Figure 1. The rhesus monkey *A* locus alleles do not evolve in a trans-specific fashion. Phylogenetic tree of exon 2 constructed using the neighbor joining method, based on nucleotide substitutions per site (d), estimated by Jukes and Cantor's method. *P<0.05, **P<0.01 and ***P<0.001.

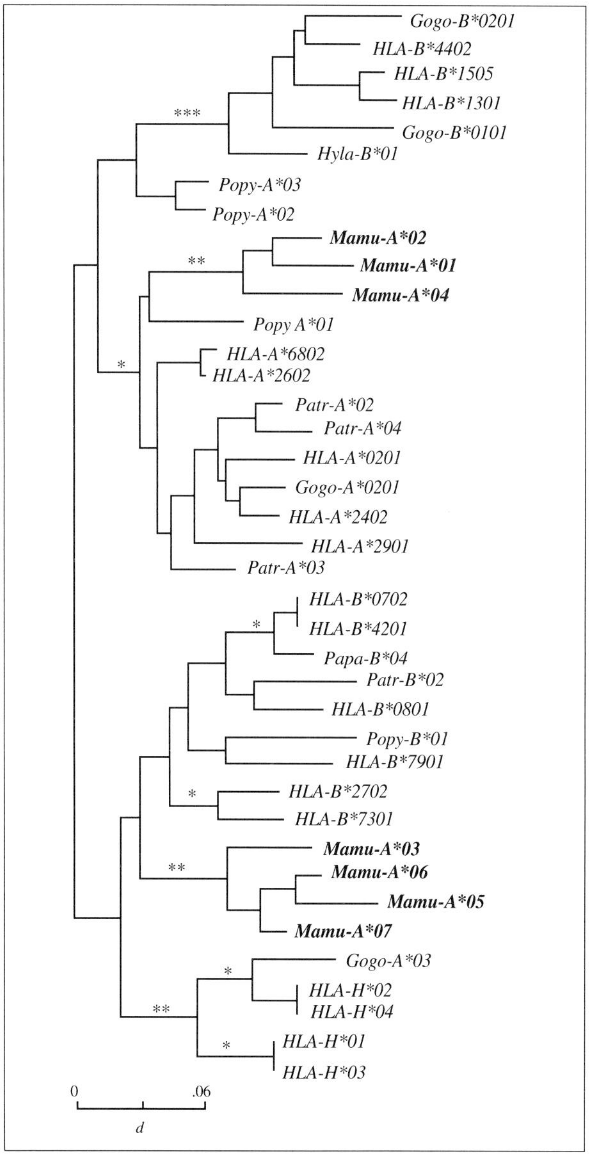

Figure 2. Unusual relationship among rhesus monkey *A* locus alleles and alleles of the *A*, *B*, and *H* loci. Gene trees were based on nucleotides 3 to 212 of exon 2. (Tree construction is as for *Figure 1*).

9. Watkins DI, Chen ZW, Garber TL, Hughes AL, Letvin NL. Segmental exchange between MHC class I genes in a higher primate: recombination in the gorilla between the ancestor of a human non-functional gene and an *A* locus gene. *Immunogenetics* 199; 34: 185-91.

10. Slierendregt BL, Van Noort JT, Bakas RM, Otting N, Jonker M, Bontrop RE. Evolutionary stability of transspecies major histocompatibility complex class II DRB lineages in humans and Rhesus monkeys. *Hum Immunol* 1992; 35: 29-39.

The HLA-B repertoire of the Warao Indians from Venezuela: novel and conserved alleles and the nature of HLA-B evolution in South America

M. Ramos, E. García, D. Barber, Z. Layrisse[1], J.A. López de Castro

Centro de Biología Molecular "Severo Ochoa", Consejo Superior de Investigaciones Científicas and Universidad Autonoma de Madrid, E-28049 Madrid, Spain
1 Centro de Medicina Experimental, Instituto Venezolano de Investigaciones Científicas, Caracas, Venezuela

Molecular analysis of HLA-B antigens in South American indians has revealed multiple new alleles, mainly in the HLA-B locus, not found in other populations [1]. Some of the issues raised by this phenomenon concern the extent to which this polymorphism is population-specific or shared by multiple tribes, and whether it reflects selection-driven evolution under pressure from the environmental pathogen load of their tropical habitat, or just genetic drift within the limited HLA repertoires of these populations. Addressing these questions requires extensive molecular analysis of the HLA class I alleles of aboriginal unmixed populations. In this study we have analysed the DNA coding sequence of the HLA-B alleles from the Warao indians of the Orinoco Delta in North-eastern Venezuela [2]. This population, which has until recently remained isolated and genetically unmixed, has a limited number of serologic HLA-B specificities *(Table I).*

Table I. HLA-B alleles in the Warao indians

HLA-B gene frequencies[a] Antigen	Frequency	**HLA-B alleles**	**Warao Cell lines**[b]
B35	0.10	Not done	
B39	0.09	B*3909	143.2
B51	0.31	B*5101	A70 and 437.3
B60	0.12	B*4002 (B61)[b]	143.2
B62	0.38	B*1501	OLGA[c]
		B*1504	A70
		B*1520	437.3 and OLGA[c]

[a] Data from [3].
[b] Cell lines: A70 (A31; B5, 62; Cw3); 143.2 (A24, 28; B39, B*4002; Cw3, 7); 437.3 (A2, 31; B51, 62; Cw3); OLGA (A31, B62, Cw3); LCL 143.2 was originally typed as B39, B60.
[c] Data from [4].

Full length cDNA clones corresponding to the HLA B alleles were obtained from three lymphoblastoid cell lines (LCL) of Warao individuals (*Table I*), and their sequence was determined as previously described [5]. HLA-B51 (*B* 5101*) was sequenced from two individuals, and the other alleles were sequenced from single individuals. LCL typing as HLA-B62 expressed three different alleles: *B*1504*, *B*1501* and *B*1520*. The multiplicity of alleles within single serologic specificities, also found in other tribes, emphasises the need for systematic molecular typing of HLA antigens in South American Indian populations.

The ethnic distribution of the HLA-B alleles found in the Warao falls into two categories (*Table II*). The first one is represented by *B*3909*, *B*1504* and *B*1520*. These alleles have been found in other South Amerindian tribes, but not outside South America. Thus, they may represent alleles of recent origin (*i.e.* 10.000 to 40.000 years) that arose early in the South American population. *B*3909* was first sequenced from the Warao [5]. This allele is identical to *B*39011* except for two consecutive nucleotides at codon 99 (A>C368 and C>T369) leading to a Tyr>Ser99 change in the gene product. This polymorphism suggests an origin by gene conversion, in which de putative donor gene was *Cw*0702*, also found in the Warao [5]. Residue 99 is located in the β-pleated sheet of the peptide binding site, and takes part in the D pocket, which interacts with residue 3 of bound peptides. This change is also likely to alter hydrogen bonding of peptide residue 2 in the B pocket. Four other HLA-B39 alleles have been described among South Amerindians: *B*3903*, *B*3905*, *B*3906* and *B*3907* [6, 7]. The amino acid changes of the corresponding gene products are spatially close to residue 99 [5]. This clustering strongly suggests that the diversification of HLA-B39 in South America was driven by selection, presumably to improve the antigen presenting capability of the limited

HLA class I repertoire of these populations, and was not just a result of genetic drift. This argues towards a significant role of the HLA-B locus in adaptation to the local habitat.

A more extensive molecular typing of South American indians must define to what extent the alleles found only in these populations are shared by multiple tribes. This will clarify the importance and rate of the HLA-B diversification in South America.

Table II. Ethnic distribution of the HLA-B alleles found in the Warao indians

Alleles in Warao (Venezuela)	Other Areas in South America	Outside South America
B*3909	Brazil	Not found
B*1504	Argentina Brazil Ecuador	Not found
B*1520	Argentina Brazil	Not found
B*1501	Argentina Ecuador Venezuela	North Amerindians Orientals Caucasians
B*5101	Brazil	North Amerindians Orientals Caucasians
B*4002	Argentina Ecuador	North Amerindians Orientals Caucasians

A second category of alleles is represented by *B*1501*, *B*5101* and *B*4002*. These alleles are found in other South American populations, as well as among North Amerindians, Orientals and Caucasians. Thus, they are old alleles that have remained unchanged. The apparently widespread persistence of these alleles in South America indicates that generation of new alleles has taken place without replacement of the parental ones imported by the founding population. The coexistence of new and old alleles in populations effectively increases their HLA repertoire, enabling them to deal more efficiently with pathogens. This is exemplified among Warao by the three HLA-B15 alleles found in this population.

In conclusion, the HLA-B repertoire in the Warao consists of alleles that have remained unchanged since they were imported in South America, and alleles that appear to have originated early among South Amerindians and are now widespread in the continent. This polymorphism has functional significance, as it can modulate antigen presentation. The number of alleles in the Warao is greater than suggested by serologic typing, and is a new example of the ongoing diversification and enlargement of the HLA-B allelic repertoire in South America.

Acknowledgements

This work was supported by grant SAF 94-0891 from the Plan Nacional de I+D to JALC, and by an institutional grant from the Fundación Ramón Areces to the CBMSO.

References

1. Parham P, Ohta T. Population bilogy of antigen presentation by MHC class I molecules. *Science* 1996; 272: 67-74.
2. Layrisse Z, Layrisse M, Heinen HD, Wilbert J. The histocompatibility system in the Warao Indians of venezuela. *Science* 1976; 194: 1135-8.
3. Layrisse Z, Heinen HD, Balbas O, García E, Stoikow Z. Unique HLA-DR/DQ associations revealed by family studies in Warao Amerindians. Haplotype and homozygosity frequeencies. *Hum Immunol* 1988; 23: 45-57.
4. Domena JD, Litttle AM, Arnett KL, Adams EJ, Marsh SG, Parham P. A small test of a sequence-based typing method: definition of the B*1520 allele. *Tissue Antigens* 1994; 44: 217-24.
5. Ramos M, Postigo JM, Vilches C, Layrisse Z, López de Castro JA. Primary structure of a novel HLA-B39 allele (B*3909) from the Warao Indians of Venezuela. Further evidence for local HLA-B diversification in South America. *Tissue antigens* 1995; 45: 401-4.
6. Watkins DI, McAdam SN, Liu X, Strang CR, Milford EL, Levine CG, Garber TL, Dogon AL, Lord CI, Ghim SH, Troup GM, Hughes AL, Letvin NL. New recombinant HLA-B alleles in a tribe of South American Amerindians indicate rapid evolution of MHC class I loci. *Nature* 1992: 357: 329-33.
7. Garber TL, Butler LM, Trachtenberg EA, Erlich HA, Rickards O, De Stefano G, Watkins DI. HLA-B alleles of the Cayapa of Ecuador: new B39 and B15 alleles. *Immunogenetics* 1995: 42: 19-27.

Functional and evolutionary considerations based on homology models of five distinct HLA-A alleles

G. Chelvanayagam, I.B. Jakobsen, X. Gao, S. Easteal

Human Genetics Group, John Curtin School of Medical Research, Australian National University, Mills Road Acton, Canberra, ACT 2601, Australia

On the basis of nucleotide sequence and parsimony analysis, HLA-A alleles can be divided into five distinct families (A2, A1/3/11/30, A9, A10, A19) derived from two ancient lineages [1]. An additional family (A80) is formed by the A*8001 allele which has been found in African populations and is difficult to classify into any of the existing five groups [2]. Interestingly, allele and haplotype frequency studies [3] show that the five allele families can be found in most global populations, although they may be represented by different subtypes in various ethnic groups. This raises the possibility that each family possesses a unique property, for example the ability to bind a set of mutually exclusive peptides, so that their simultaneous presence is selected for in current populations. To investigate this possibility, computer models for the antigen presenting domains of the five alleles A*1101, A*2402, A*3401, A*2901 and A*8001, from the A1/3/11/30, A9, A10, A19 and A80 families respectively, have been constructed and analysed. Models were based on the known structure of the A2 allele A*0201 [4].

Results and discussion

As a result of the high level of sequence identity between HLA-A alleles, the overall structure of the models resemble very closely the A*0201 template. Importantly, conserved residues (Tyr 7, Tyr 84, Thr 143, Trp 147, Tyr 159, Tyr 171) that form hydrogen bonds with the ends of the peptide appear to preserve this role, suggesting that peptides generally bind to HLA-A molecules in a canonical manner. Further, a general tendency for large residues to occur at positions 97 and/or 114 support an arched shape for the peptide backbone with principle anchor positions occurring at P2 and P9 of the peptide.

Anchor motifs have previously been defined for two of the alleles that are modelled here (see [5] for a review). A*1101 has been reported to have a preference for Val or Thr at P2 and Lys at P9 in comparison to Leu at P2 and Val at P9 in A*0201. Also, A24 alleles have been found to bind preferentially Tyr at P2 and Phe at P9. *Figure 1* illustrates the differences between the clefts of A*0201 and the model of A*1101. The figure also shows the peptide AVAAAAAAK modelled in the cleft and how, at a simplistic level, the amino acid exchanges of Phe 9 and Tyr 116 in A*0201 to Tyr 9 and Asp 116 in A*1101 facilitate the observed anchor residue preferences by forming pockets that complement size, shape and charge of the anchor residues. Similarly, in the A*2402 model, in complex with the peptide AYAAAAAAF (data not shown), residue exchanges with respect to A*0201 involving Tyr 9 and Leu 81 to Ser and Ala respectively, also help to accommodate the large bulk of the anchoring residues. Both Ser and Ala have small side-chains. Peptide anchor binding specificity can not be determined on the basis of these residues alone, however, and all polymorphic residues around the P2 and P9 binding sites must be considered. *Table I* illustrates the polymorphic residues that contribute to the P2 (B pocket [6]) binding site in the models.

Aside from the known motifs for A*1101 and A*2402, the models suggest possible P2 motifs for A*3401, A*2901 and A*8001. The P2 pocket of A*3401 is quite similar to that of A*1101 (*Figure 1*, *Table I*). A key difference involves residue Asn 63 which increases the volume of the pocket and reduces the negative charge around the pocket. This may allow a small variation in the canonical binding of the peptide N-terminal main-chain to compensate for changes in other positions of the cleft (*e.g.* Trp 156). Generally, however, the pocket would appear to support small residues with a branched side-chain, such as Thr. The P2 pocket of A*2901 is distinct from that of A*1101. In particular, Thr 9 dramatically increases the depth of the P2 pocket while Gln 63 involves a loss of a negative charge. The deep nature of the pocket is reminiscent of the P2 pocket of the A9 family, thus it is possible that A*2901 also binds Tyr or Glu at P2. The A*8001 P2 pocket is very similar to A*1101 and consequently it is expected that this allele will also bind Val, Thr or perhaps Leu in this pocket.

Table I. Polymorphic residues in the P2 pockets of the models

Model	9	63	66	67	70	99
A*1101	Y	E	N	V	Q	Y
A*2402	S	E	K	V	H	F
A*3401	Y	N	K	V	Q	Y
A*2901	T	Q	N	V	Q	Y
A*8001	F	E	N	V	Q	Y

Strikingly, polymorphic residues in the P9 (F pocket [6]) binding site *(Table II)* follow a distribution which identifies an overall preference for smaller aliphatic residues such as Val in A2 alleles, aromatic residues such as Phe in A9 alleles and large polar residues such as Lys, Gln or Tyr in most other alleles. These general preferences can be inferred by examining the models and the polymorphic residues of the P9 binding sites of alleles with known anchor residue motifs [5]. Alleles which display an overall similar binding pocket are expected to bind similar residues. The A30, A68 and A80 alleles show some deviation from the trend in *Table II*. Interestingly, all of these alleles are strongly represented in African populations and may represent intermediates between the three states A2, A9 and A1/3/11/10/19. Four other alleles also show minor deviations: A*0211, A*6901, A*2602 and A*2606.
Examination of the upper surfaces of the helices in the models, the putative T-cell receptor interface, reveals three surface motifs involving residues at the tail end of the $\alpha 1$ helix and the start of the $\alpha 2$ helix (*Figure 2*). The polymorphic residues in this region are illustrated in *Table III*. On the $\alpha 1$ helix, all the families share a common motif, with the exception of the A9 family, while on the $\alpha 2$ helix, all the families share a common motif, with the exception of the A2 family. Thus, the three surface motifs also distinguish the A2 and A9 families from each other and from all other alleles. If the polymorphism on the $\alpha 1$ and $\alpha 2$ helices are termed the A2/A2 motif in the A2 family and the A24/A24 motif in the A9 family, then all other alleles show an A2/A24 motif. The only exceptions to this are the alleles A*2501 and A*3201 which show the A24/A24 motif. Interestingly, no alleles show an A24/A2 motif. Non-polymorphic residues in the models that flank the residues in *Table III* help to enlarge the motif area. Other areas along the upper surface of the $\alpha 1$ and $\alpha 2$ helices generally appear quite diverse in family terms. Notable, however, are conserved residues (Lys 68, Ala 69, Gln 72, Arg 75, Gln 154, Gln 155) in the middle upper surface of both helices.

Table II. Polymorphic residues in the P9 pockets of the families

Family	74	77	80	81	95	116
A2	H	D	T	L	V/L	Y
A9	D	N	I	A	L	Y
A*6802	D	D	T	L	I	Y
A30	D	N/D	T	L	I	H
A*6801	D	D	T	L	I	D
A/1/3/11	D	N/D	T	L	I	D
A10	D	N/D/S	T	L	I	D
A19	D	N/D	T	L	I	D
A80	N	N	T	L	I	D

Table III. Polymorphic residues in the helix surface motif

		$\alpha 1$			$\alpha 2$	
Family	79	80	82	83	142	145
A2	G	T	R	G	T	H
A9	R	I	L	R	I	R
A1/3/11/(30)	G	T	R	G	I	R
A10	G	T	R	G	I	R
A19	G	T	R	G	I	R
A80	G	T	R	G	I	R

Conclusions

Close inspection of the allele frequency data show that almost all populations contain high counts of alleles

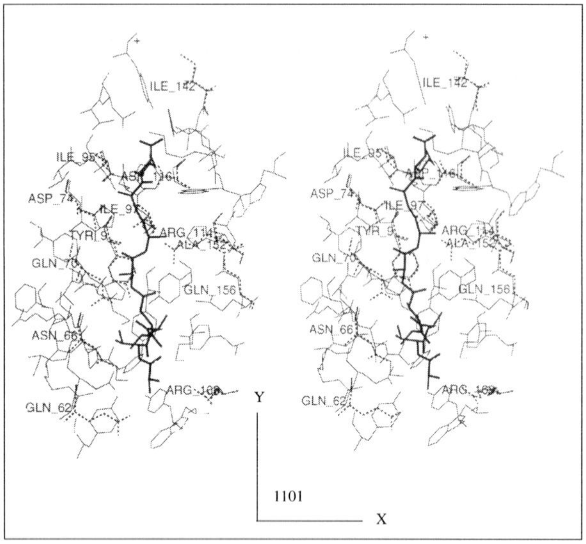

Figure 1. A stereo view of the A*1101 model. Residues show are those in the antigen binding cleft in complex with the peptide AVAAAAAAK. The model is superimposed onto the equivalent set of residues in A*0201. Residue types that differ are highlighted with those in A*1101 being dashed.

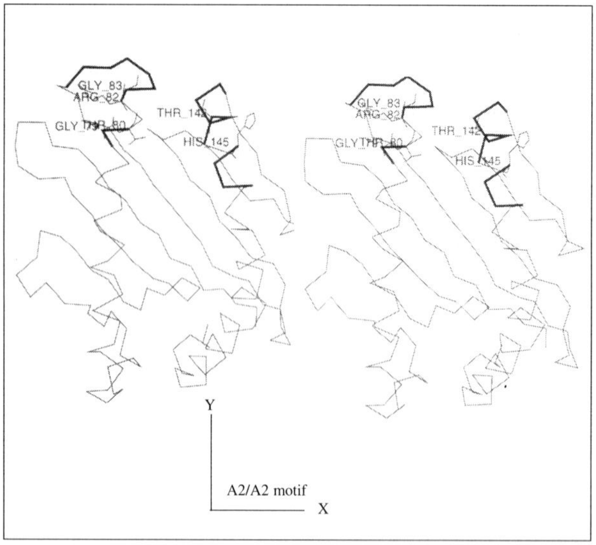

Figure 2. A stereo view showing the Cα trace of the peptide binding domains of A*0201 highlighting the putative A2/A2 surface motif. Polymorphic residues that form the motif are labelled. The motif can be extended to include conserved residues in the loops between strands 1 and 2 and between the α1 helix and strand 5.

from the A2, A9 and A1/3/11/(30) families, while generally only low counts from the other families. This is consistent with the functional groupings described above. Both P9 pocket specificity and the possible molecular recognition site fall into three general groups that match the A2, A9 and A1/A3/A11/(30) families. Thus, these functional sites may provide the molecular basis for the observed distribution of alleles. At the HLA-A functional level, this suggests that the A1/3/11/(30) family may have evolved from the A2 and A24 families and that the A10 and A19 families arose subsequently through genetic recombination. At the nucleotide level, polymorphic synonymous sites may provide evidence for convergent evolution of molecules towards similar function.

References

1. Lawlor DA, Warren E, Taylor P, Parham P. Gorilla class I major histocompatibility complex alleles: comparison to human and chimpanzee class I. *J Exp Med* 1991; 147: 1491-509.
2. Domena JD, Hilderbrand WH, Bias WB, Parham P. A sixth family of HLA-A alleles defined by HLA-A*8001. *Tissue Antigens* 1993; 42: 156-9.
3. Imanishi T, Akaza T, Kimura A, Tokunaga K, Gojobori T. Allele and haplotype frequencies for HLA and complement loci in various ethnic groups. *Proceedings of the 11th international histocompatibility workshop and conference, Yokohama, Japan, 1991.* Oxford, New York, Tokyo: Oxford University Press, 1992.
4. Bjorkman PJ, Saper MA, Samraoui B, Bennett WS, Strominger JL, Wiley DC. Structure of the human class I histocompatibility antigen HLA-A2. *Nature* 1987; 329: 506-11.
5. Rammensee HG, Friede T, Stevanovič S. MHC ligands and peptide motifs: first listing. *Immunogenetics* 1995; 41: 178-228.
6. Saper MA, Bjorkman PJ, Wiley DC. Refined structure of the human histocompatibility antigen HLA-A2 at 2.6Å resolution. *J Mol Biol* 1991; 219: 277-319.

Evolution of MHC-DRB genes in primates and related taxa as inferred from non-coding sequences

H. Kupfermann[1], W.E. Mayer[1], H. Tichy[1], J. Klein[1,2]

1 Max Planck Institute for Biology, Immunogenetics Department, Correnssstrasse 42, D-72076 Tübingen, Germany
2 Department of Microbiology and Immunology, University of Miami School of Medicine, Miami, FL 33101, USA

The evolutionary relationship between primates and other orders of eutherian mammals remains obscure in spite of extensive paleontological, morphological, biochemical, and molecular studies [6, 9]. Tree shrews (tupaias), chiropteras (bats), and insectivores have all been considered at one time or another to be the closest primate relatives. Primates can be subdivided into two suborders, the Prosimii and Anthropoidea [1]. The Prosimii are represented by tarsiers, lemurs and lorises whereas the Anthropoidea includes two infraorders, Catarrhini and Platyrrhini. The Catarrhini are Old World primates, apes and humans; the Platyrrhini are the New World primates which are divided into two families, Callitrichidae and Cebidae. The tree shrews of Southeast Asia are small, scansorial, squirrel-like mammals, that occupy a range of niches. On the basis of morphological features early investigators included the Tupaiidae in the order of Primates. Modern molecular analysis reveals, however, that the tree shrews form a distinct order, the Scandentia. The Chiropteras can be divided into two suborders: Megachiroptera (megabats) and Microchiroptera (microbats). The Megachiroptera are a uniform Old World group of large, vegetarian bats; the Microchiroptera are distributed worldwide and are predominantly insectivorous. The insectivores also have a worldwide distribution; they include such species as hedgehogs, shrew-mice, moles and tenrecs. In the present study, we have investigated the evolutionary relationships between these mammalian orders based on non-coding sequences of *DRB* genes.

Results and discussion

Non-coding sequences are suitable for the study of evolutionary relationships among mammalian orders because intron sequences are relatively free of selection pressure [2]. By contrast, certain exon sequences, for example exon 2 sequences of *Mhc* class II genes, may phylogenetically provide misleading information because their peptide binding region (PBR)-encoding sites evolve under the influence of balancing selection [4, 7]. The selection seems to favor certain substitutions over others and leads to their preferential incorporation into persisting allelic lineages.

In the present study, a combination of exon 4- and exon 5-specific primers was used to amplify part of exon 4 and the complete intron 4. The amplified products, which were each about 600 bp long, were sequenced and the sequences were then aligned. The alignment of the intron sequences required the introduction of several gaps to identify the homologous regions in the different orders as well as order-specific regions.

A neighbour-joining tree constructed from intron 4 data shows all primate (platyrrhine, catarrhine and prosimian) sequences forming their own branch apart from tree shrews, bats and insectivores; each of these other orders also forms a monophyletic group *(Figure 1)*. The bootstrap value of the branch leading to the Platyrrhini and Catarrhini is 100%, that leading to the prosimians is 75% and that leading to Primates 88%. Within each group the genetic distances are relatively short and the bootstrap values lie between 50% and 100%. The authenticity of these clusters is supported by the existence of several platyrrhine-, catarrhine- and prosimian-specific substitutions and indels. Some prosimian sequences, especially those of the African prosimians *Galago senegalensis* and *Galago moholi,* possess common indels and cluster together in the tree. The Asian prosimians *Perodicticus potto, Nycticebus cougang* and *Loris tardigradus* form a separate branch. In an earlier study *Lemur catta,* a prosimian from Madagascar, was reported to lack *Mhc-DRB* genes [8]. During this investigation, however, amplifications by

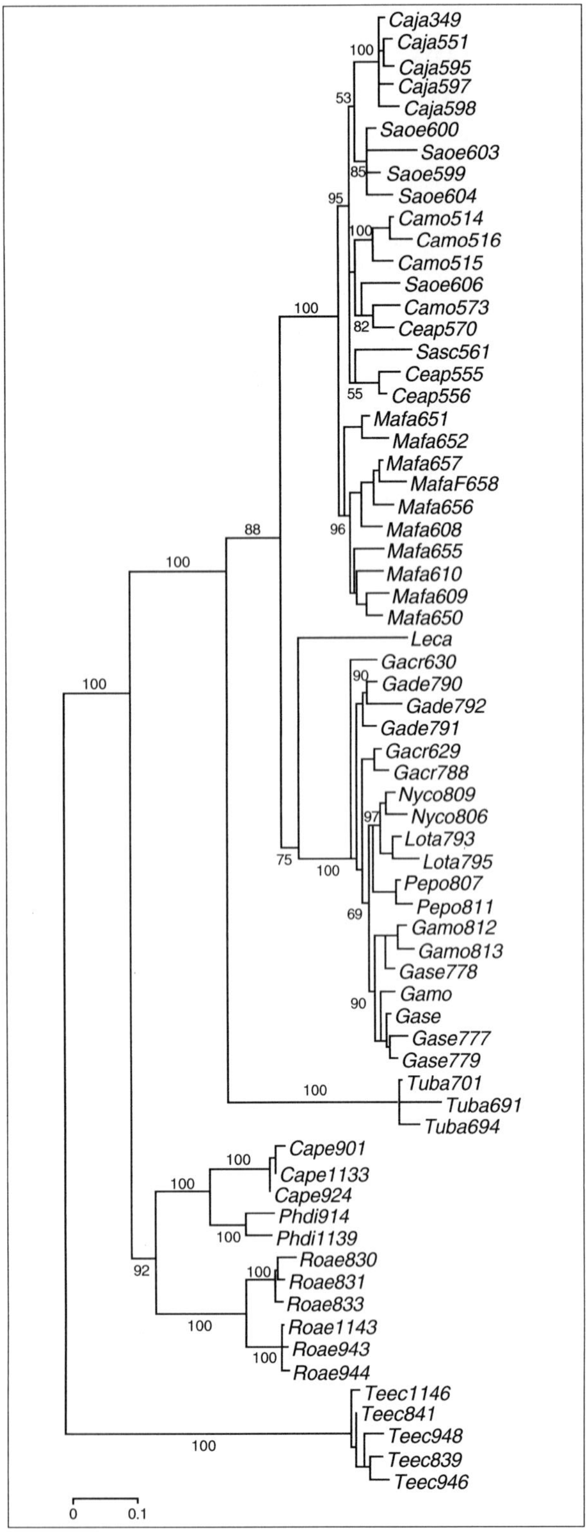

Figure 1. Phylogenetic tree of primates, tree shrews, chiropteras and insectivores intron 4 sequences (508 bp). The tree was constructed from genetic distances calculated by Kimura's two-parameter method, using the neighbour-joining algorithm. The number on each brach indicates the bootstrap probability in 500 replications.

the polymerase chain reaction (PCR) led to the identification of *Mhc-DRB* intron 4 (and also intron 5 and exon 6) indicating the presence of at least the 3' region of *DRB* genes in this species. The *Lemur* sequence is quite different from all other prosimian sequences and possesses a 70 bp deletion within intron 4. In the phylogenetic tree the lemur-specific sequence branches out from all the other prosimian sequences. Thus the phylogenetic analysis of the *Mhc-DRB* sequences supports the intraordinal relationship of the primates based on morphological and molecular data [1, 10].

There is no agreement concerning the closest living relative of primates. Based on molecular studies Dermoptera, Scandentia, Chiroptera and Lagomorpha have been proposed as candidates for this position [9]; based on morphological data, the Scandentia, Chiroptera and Dermoptera have been proposed to constitute a sister group of the primates [6]. Our analysis reveals the tree shrews to be more closely related to the primates than any other mammalian order. We amplified several alleles of one *Mhc-DRB* gene from *Tupaia balangerii.* After the exclusion of indels that are not alignable with the primate sequences, a high bootstrap value (100%) clearly supported the phylogenetic relationship between the Primates and the Scandentia. This result is consistent with morphological and some molecular data [9]. Whether bats are monophyletic or diphyletic is controversial [6, 9]. According to the 'flying primate hypothesis', Megachiroptera are more closely aligned with Primates than with Microchiroptera [3]. The hypothesis is supported by characteristics based on neural morphology, the metacarpophalangeal index and β-globin amino acid sequences [3, 5]. Analysis of Mega- and Microchiroptera species in this study supports the monophyletic status of the bats by a high bootstrap value of 92%. The position of the insectivores in the phylogenetic tree is consistent with them being an outgroup. The study thus demonstrated the usefulness of *Mhc* intron sequences in helping to resolve outstanding questions of vertebrate taxonomy.

References

1. Martin RD. Primate origins: plugging the gaps. *Nature* 1970; 363: 223-34.
2. Kimura M. The neutral theory of molecular evolution. Cambridge: Cambridge University Press, 1983.
3. Pettigrew JD. Flying primates? Megabats have advanced pathway from eye to midbrain. *Science* 1986; 231: 1304-6.
4. Hughes AL, Nei M. Pattern of nucleotide substitution at major histocompatibility complex class I loci reveals overdominant selection. *Nature* 1988; 335: 167-70.
5. Mindell DP, Dick CW, Baker RJ. Phylogenetic relationships among megabats, microbats, and primates. *Proc Natl Acad Sci USA* 1991; 90: 10322-6.
6. Novacek MJ. Mammalian phylogeny: shaking the tree. *Nature* 1992; 356: 121-5.
7. Takahata N, Satta Y, Klein J.Polymorphism and balancing selection at major histocompatibility complex loci. *Genetics* 1992; 130: 925-38.
8. Figueroa F, O'hUigin C, Tichy H, Klein J. The origin of the primate *Mhc-DRB* genes and allelic lineages as deduced from the study of prosimians. *J Immunol* 1994; 152: 4456-65.
9. Allard MW, McNiff BE, Miyamoto MM. Support for interordinal eutherian relationships with an emphasis on primates and their archonton relatives. *Mol Phyl Evol* 1996; 5: 78-88.
10. Shoshani J, Groves CP, Simons EL, Gunnell GF. Primate phylogeny: morphological vs molecular results. *Mol Phyl Evol* 1996; 5: 102-54.

Trans species polymorphism versus independent evolution of class II MHC sequence motifs

*M. Yeager, A.L. Hughes**

Department of Biology, 208 Mueller Laboratory, and Institute of Molecular Evolutionary Genetics,The Pennsylvania State University, University Park, PA 16802, USA
*Corresponding author

In addition to the striking amount of polymorphism observed at certain loci within the MHC, another remarkable feature of these loci is the presence of "trans species" polymorphism [1,2]; certain polymorphic allelic lineages have been maintained within related species, having been present in their common ancestor. For example, certain human alleles are more closely related to certain chimpanzee alleles than they are to other human alleles. Since there are orthologous loci among the different orders of placental mammals, it is possible to discern how long such polymorphism might be shared. Two alternative hypotheses have been given by Andersson *et al.* [3] and Lundberg and McDevitt [4]. The former group hypothesized that sharing of amino acid residues between human and bovine constituted a case of independent evolution at these residues rather than common ancestry. By contrast, the latter group concluded that shared polymorphic residues between human and mouse were due to 'direct descent of ancestral sequences rather than convergent evolution' [4].

Since theoretical studies have shown that there is an upper limit to how long such a polymorphism may been maintained [5], we addressed the question by examining the extent of three types of shared amino acid polymorphism between human *DRB* and *DQB* sequences and orthologous sequences from a number of mammalian orders whose divergence times have been estimated. We determined the extent of shared (1) single-amino acid residues, (2) two-amino acid motifs, and (3) three-amino acid motifs. In the case of two- and three-amino acid motifs, 'sharing' refers to, in a sliding window of six amino acids, positions that are polymorphic in both species and at which at least two identical motifs are present in both species. For example, at positions 84 and 85 of the *DQB* chain, the sequence motifs EV and QL occur in both human and chimpanzee. Likewise, for the three-amino motif test, at positions 53, 55, and 57 of the *DQB* chain, the sequence motifs QRV and LPA occur in both human and chimpanzee. We expected to find a much lower level of sharing of two- and three-amino acid motifs when sharing of polymorphism was due to independent evolution rather than to common ancestry because more complicated motifs are more likely to evolve convergently.

The results *(Figure 1A, B)* showed that there is a high proportion of shared polymorphic amino acid residues between human and other mammals, and that this proportion is high even in the very distantly-related species. However, the proportion of sharing rapidly decreases with time for the two- and three-amino acid motifs, particularly for *DQB*. We used logistic regression models to predict the rate of decline of sharing of amino acid motifs. Those models predicted that, after 80 million years of divergence, only about 30% of two- and three-amino acid motifs would be shared by *DRB* alleles, while only about 6% of two-amino acid motifs and 1% of three-amino acid motifs motifs would be shared by *DQB* alleles. By contrast, 73% of single amino acid residue polymorphisms at *DRB* were expected to be shared after 80 million years, and 43% of single amino acid residue polymorphisms at *DQB*.

These results agree with the hypothesis that sharing of polymorphic residues by mammals of different orders is more likely to be due to independent evolution [3] than to maintenance of an ancestral polymorphism [4]. The results showed a difference between *DQB* and *DRB* in that sharing of the two-and three-amino acid motifs appeared to decline less rapidly in the latter and perhaps even to rebound *(Figure 1A)*. *DRB* has duplicated independently in different mammalian species, and the

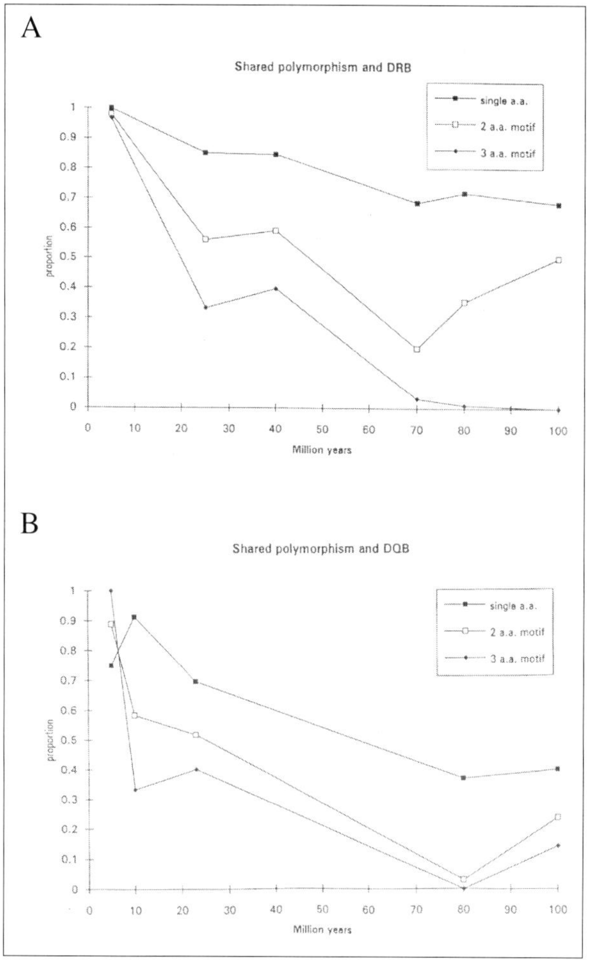

Figure 1. Proportion of single, two-, and three- shared polymorphic amino acid motifs in a sliding window of six between human and other mammals for (A) DRB and (B) DQB locus sequences. Sequences from the following species were compared with human sequences, and grouped into categories according to divergence times. DRB: chimpanzee, 5 million years ago (Mya); pigtail macaque, rhesus macaque, 25 Mya; capuchin, marmoset, owl monkey, squirrel monkey, titi monkey, 40 Mya; cow, red deer, dog, goat, horse, moose, pig, sheep, 80 Mya; mouse, 100 Mya. DQB: chimpanzee, 5 Mya; gorilla, 10 Mya, rhesus macaque, 25 Mya; cow, dog, pig, sheep, 80 Mya; mouse, rat, 100 Mya. All sequences were obtained from GenBank.

presence of multiple *DRB* loci should make it possible to preserve more of a species' ancient polymorphism. The apparent increase in sharing of the two amino acid motifs at *DRB* between 80 and 100 million years may actually represent convergent evolution, since given a long enough time more complicated motifs will have had time to evolve independently in different lineages.

References

1. Lawlor DA, Ward FE, Ennis PD, Jackson AP, Parham P. HLA-A, B polymorphisms predate the divergence of humans and chimpanzees. *Nature* 1988; 335: 268-71.
2. Mayer WE, Jonker D, Klein D, Ivanyi P, Van Seventer G, Klein J. Nucleotide sequence of chimpanzee MHC class I alleles: evidence for trans-species mode of evolution. *EMBO J* 1988; 7: 2765-74.
3. Andersson L, Sigurdardottir S, Borsch C, Gustafsson K. Evolution of MHC polymorphism: extensive sharing of polymorphic sequence motifs between human and bovine DRB alleles. *Immunogenetics* 1991; 33: 188-93.
4. Lundberg AS, McDevitt HO. Evolution of major histocompatibility complex class II allelic diversity: direct descent in mice and humans. *Proc Natl Acad Sci USA* 1992; 89: 6545-9.
5. Takahata N, Nei M. Allelic genealogy under overdominant and frequency-dependent selection and polymorphism of major histocompatibility complex loci. *Genetics* 1990; 124: 967-78.

The chimeric P5-1 sequence in the HLA class I region: gene or pseudogene?

N. Pomies[1], P. Pontarotti[1], R. Bontrop[2], B. Crouau-Roy[1]

1 CIGH , CNRS UPR 8291, CHU Purpan, avenue de Grande Bretagne, 31300 Toulouse, France
2 Biomedical primate Research Center, Ryswijh, The Netherlands

The human major histocompatibility complex (MHC) includes three types of class I MHC genes: (1) classical class I loci (HLA-A, -B, -C), which are highly expressed and polymorphic; (2) non classical class I loci, with much reduced expression and polymorphism; and (3) unexpressed class I pseudogenes [1-2]. Phylogenetic analysis suggests that both non-classical class I loci and pseudogenes arose by duplication of class I loci. 5' regulatory elements conserved in class I genes are not conserved in either non-classical class I genes or pseudogenes, but the former show evidence of purifying selection at nonsynonymous sites in coding regions that is lacking in the latter [3].

A putative coding sequence, the P5-1 sequence has been located telomeric to HLA-X in the class-I region [4]. This sequence is a chimeric transcript created by non homologous recombination between an MHC class I gene and an unrelated sequence [5] having the 5' class I sequence (including the promoter region, the first exon, and the half of the first intron) fused to an unrelated intron and a large exon (*Figure 1*). The unrelated sequence is present within the MHC class I region in multiple copies, defining the P5 family. Although this sequence, with an intact open reading frame (ORF), can be transcribed, spliced and polyadenylated, we do not know if it is functional. This article intends to define the quality of gene or pseudogene of the P5-1 sequence. Furthermore, the action of selection could be determined by comparing synonymous and substitutional changes in the P5-1 sequences at the intra and interspecies levels [6, 7]. On the assumption that it is a pseudogene, there should be a high overall level of nucleotide variation from person to person, with substitution rates in the first and second codon positions 10 times greater (nonsynonymous sites) than those in normal genes, but the rates in the third position (synonymous sites) should be similar.

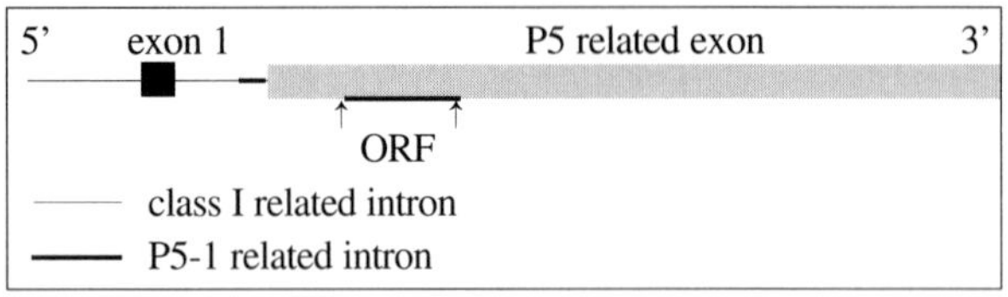

Figure 1. Schematic representation of the structure of the P5-1.

Material and methods

The P5-1 region (including the P5-1 related intron plus 420 bases of the P5-1 related exon whose ORF) was sequenced in 15 homozygote cell lines. These cell lines were selected on the basis of their HLA haplotypes and come from the panel of the 4th Asia Oceanic Histocompatibility Worshop (4 AOH [8]) or the 10th International Histocompatibilty Worshop (10 IHW). Two sets of primers have been used for the amplification, the couples P5-A / P5-B and P5-C / P5-D (P5-A: 5'-CCCGGAGGAGTAAATCTGCA-3'; P5-B : 5'-TCGTTCCTGTGCTCTGACATCCTC-3'; P5-C: 5'-ACAGCCTGAGAGAGAAGTAGGGCC-3'; P5-D: 5'- GCGGGTGAGAAGAGGAGTCCCC-3'). The PCR products were cloned into the PGEM vector and sequenced with dye terminator (Perkin Elmer). For each homozygote cell line, up to 5 clones have been sequenced to determine the consensus sequence for an HLA haplotype determined.

Results and discussion

A region consisting of 636 bases, including the P5-1 related intron and the 5' part of the P5-1 related exon, was sequenced to investigate the pattern of nucleotide substitution with particular emphasis on the number of synonymous and non-synonymous substitutions. The 15 different HLA haplotypes display a nearly identical sequence. On the 5' part of the P5-1 related exon before the ORF only three variations were observed and all are transitions: one substitution T→C in the nucleotide position 68 (numbered

5'CCCGGAGGAG	*TAAATCTGCA*	*CATATATTTA*	*ATTACAGATT*	ACAATTACAA	50
TCAAGGCAGA	AATGATC**T**CA	TTTTTACATT	ACAACTCTGG	AAAAGGCAAT	100
AGACTGAGAT	GCAAGTGTGC	CCCCAAGTGA	TGGGCAGAAG	GAGAGAAGGT	150
GTTTTGGATG	CATTCTAGAA	CACAGGTAAT	CTAAGGAGAG	TTGATCAAGG	200
CCGTGGAAGA	GTCCTCCAGC	CACTATTGGC	CATCAAAGGA	GTCCTCTGTG	250
TCCCAGGAAT	GGTCCTGCTT	TGGTGTCCCT	GGTGTGACCC	AT**C**ACCCGCT	300
GGGAACAGCC	TGAGAG**A**AGT	AGGGCCTCTG	CACCA<u>ATG</u>CT	GCTGAGGATG	350
TCAGAGCACA	GGAACGAGGC	CTTGGGAAA**T**	TACCTGGAAA	TGCGACTGAA	400
ATCTTCCTTC	CTGAGGGGTC	TGGGCTCTTG	GAAATCAAAC	CCTCTCAGGT	450
TGGGTGGCTG	GACGATTCTC	CTCACACTTA	CAATGGGACA	AGGGGAACCA	500
GGAGGCCCCC	AAGGGGATCC	CTGGGTTCCA	CACG**A**ACTCC	TCCTACCCTC	550
ATTGTGTGAC	AGCAGCCATG	CCTCCTCCTG	GGGATCAGGA	TCTATTACCT	600
GTGCCTGGAG	AGGAGGGGAC	TCCTCTTCTC	ACCCGC		636

Figure 2. Sequences of the P5-1 related intron and the 5' region of the P5-1 related exon. The intron is shown in italic letters. The codon ATG underlined is the hypothetical start codon. Observed substitutions are in bold.

according to that reported in *Figure 2*) in the individual 9016 (10 IHW; HLA-DR 16, -DQ 7, -B51, -A2), one C→T in the individual 9020 (10 IHW; QBL: HLA-DR 3, -DQ 2, -DP 2, -B 18, -A 26) in the nucleotide position 293 and one substitution A→G in the individual 10002N 4AOH (HLA-DR 1, -DQ 5, -B 14, -A 33.1) in the nucleotide position 317 (*Figure 2*). In the ORF, only two substitutions occur, one transversion (T→A) in the third codon position and one transversion (A→C) in the second codon position. These both transversions occur in the same individual 100059F 4AOH (HLA-DR9, -B46, -A2.2).

Given the great conservation observed for the P5 related exon within different human HLA haplotypes, we only examined the variations between human and two chimpanzees. The sequence is conserved between the two chimpanzees. Only few variations are observed between individuals of the two species. P5 related exon with the ORF will be examined in others lineages of Primates to better understand the molecular population genetics of this potential gene or pseudogene.

If P5-1 was a pseudogene, we expect to have a great number of variations, some stop codons and also insertions and deletions which are known to be abundant in the evolution of mammalian pseudogenes [9, 10]. Our molecular population genetic observations, with little substitutions on 636 bases sequenced, no insertions and deletions imply that P5-1 is highly conserved so probably not a pseudogene.

Acknowledgements

We greatly appreciate the technical assistance of R. Jambou.

References

1. Geraghty DE, Koller BH, Hansen, JA, Orr HT. The HLA class I gene family includes at least six genes and twelve pseudogenes and gene fragments. *J Immunol* 1992; 149: 1934-46.
2. Geraghty DE, Koller BH, Pei J, Hansen JA. Examination of four HLA genes and pseudogenes: common events in the evolution of HLA genes and pseudogenes. *J Immunol* 1992; 149: 1947-56.
3. Hughes AL. Origin and evolution of HLA class I pseudogenes. *Mol Biol Evol* 1995; 12: 247-58.
4. Vernet C, Ribouchon MT, Chimini G, Jouanolle AM, Sidibe I, Pontarotti P. A novel coding sequence belonging to a new multiple copy gene family mapping within the human MHC class I region. *Immunogenetics* 1993; 38: 47-53.
5. Avoustin P, Ribouchon MT, Vernet C, N'Guyen B, Crouau-Roy B, Pontarotti P. Non-homologous recombination within the major histocompatibility complex creates a transcribed hybrid sequence. *Mammalian Genome* 1994; 5: 771-6.
6. Kreitman M. Detecting selection at level of DNA. In: Selander RK, Clarks AG, Whittam TS eds. *Evolution at the molecular level.* Sunderland, MA: Sinauer Associates, 1991: 204-21.
7. Maynard Smith. Estimating selection by comparing synonymous and sustitutional changes. *J Mol Evol* 1994; 39: 123-8.
8. Abraham LJ, Marley JV, Cambon-Thomsen A, Crouau-Roy B, Dawkins RL, Giphart MJ. Microsatellite, restriction fragment-length polymorphism, and sequence-specific oligonucleotide typing of the tumor necrosis factor region. Comparisons of the 4AOHW cell panel. *Hum Immunol* 1993; 38: 17- 24.
9. Li WH. In: Nei M, Koehn RN, eds. *Evolution of duplicate genes and pseudogenes.* Sunderland, MA: Sinauer, 1983: 14-37.
10. Walsh JB. How often do duplicated genes evolve new functions? *Genetics* 1995; 139: 421-8.

Conserved sequence motifs create a pattern of MHC genetic diversification within primate DRB lineages

L.K. Gaur, G.T. Nepom, K.E. Snyder, J. Anderson, E.R. Heise

Molecular Biology laboratory, Puget Sound Blood Center, 921 Terry Avenue, Seattle WA 98104-1256, USA

The class II region of the major histocompatibility complex (MHC) is extensively polymorphic in man and several other species. This polymorphism is likely to confer immune protection within populations by permitting alteration in the specificity of the MHC combining site and the resulting repertoire of peptides bound [1]. Polymorphism is particularly pronounced in the second exon of the class II ß-chain genes which encode stretches of sequence motifs ("hypervariable regions") within the β domains which differ between allelic variants.

In order to analyze the generation and maintenance of these specific localized MHC polymorphisms, we have undertaken interspecies comparative studies among various nonhuman primates. Human and nonhuman primate MHC comparisons were performed using oligotyping methods, as well as second exon sequence analysis [2,3]. *Figure 1* shows an alignment of the three principal hypervariable regions from the ß-chain alleles for selected human and nonhuman primate DR genes. Several patterns of sequence relationships are evident among the human DRB1 alleles listed at the top of the *Figure 1*. Within the HVR_I segment, corresponding to codons 9-14, multiple different sequences are seen, and it is customary to use sequence alignments within the HVR_I segment as markers for allelic lineages. Although highly variable among alleles, however, human HVR_I sequences are often recapitulated in nonhuman primate sequences, some of which are listed in the *Figure 1*. As noted by other investigators [4,5], this conservation of presumed allelic lineages is consistent with a trans-species mode of inheritance, in which some of the specific polymorphisms in HVR_I are ancient, and represent conserved ancestral motifs.

HVR_{II} and HVR_{III} sequences are less variable than the HVR_I sequences among human DRB alleles; nevertheless, they too represent a limited set of highly conserved sequence variants which are present on multiple genes. The combination of different HVR_{I}, $_{II}$ and $_{III}$ segments creates a patchwork distribution of hypervariable regions which, by assorting in different combinations, creates a large degree of allelic diversity for the human DRB alleles.

Comparing these segmental diversification patterns among nonhuman primate sequences reveals some interesting relationships. First, although several HVR_I sequences are conserved between human and nonhuman primates, consistent with the trans-species mode of inheritance, many other HVR_I sequences are unique to the nonhuman primates. This could represent ancestral HVR_I sequences which failed to be maintained in modern human lineages or, alternatively, may represent the continued accumulation of HVR_I mutations among nonhuman primates subsequent to species diversification. HVR_{III} sequences, on the other hand, show quite limited additional sequence variation. In other words, there is more conservation in HVR_{III} between nonhuman primates and humans than of the other HVR segments. Closely related or identical nucleotide segments for HVR_{III} are found in multiple primate species, loci and individual alleles, suggesting that selective pressures for diversification in this segment may differ from those in HVR_I and HVR_{II}.

Using a sequence-specific oligonucleotide typing method, we evaluated the conservation of HVR_{III} segments on a large number of samples from macaques. Speçific DNA probes for human HVR_{III} sequences showed striking cross-reactive hybridization patterns with nearly 80% of the macaque genes tested. In contrast, cross-reactive hybridization patterns using human HVR_I probes recognized only between 20-30% of macaque

	HVR I						HVR II						HVR III							
AA position	9					14	26					31	67							74
HLA-DRB1*0101	TGG	CAG	CTT	AAG	TTT	GAA	TTG	CTG	GAA	AGA	TGC	ATC	CTC	CTG	GAG	CAG	AGG	CGG	GCC	GCG
HLA-DRB1*1001	GA-	G--	G--	---	---	--G	---	---	---	---	C--	G--	T--	---	---	-G-	---	--T	---	---
HLA-DRB1*0701	---	---	GG-	---	-A-	A-G	--C	---	---	---	CT-	T--	A--	---	---	G--	-C-	---	-G-	CA-
HLA-DRB1*1501	---	---	-C-	---	AGG	--G	--C	---	--C	---	-A-	T--	---	---	---	---	GC-	---	---	---
HLA-DRB1*0301	GA-	T-C	TC-	-C-	-C-	--G	-AC	---	--C	---	-A-	T--	---	---	---	---	-A-	---	-G-	CG-
HLA-DRB3*0101	GA-	-T-	-G-	---	-C-	--G	--C	---	--C	---	-A-	T--	---	---	---	---	-A-	---	-G-	CG-
HLA-DRB1*0401	GA-	---	G--	--A	CA-	--G	--C	---	--C	---	-A-	T--	---	---	---	---	-A-	---	---	---
HLA-DRB1*0103	---	---	---	---	---	---	---	---	---	---	---	---	A--	---	--A	G-C	GA-	---	---	---
HLA-DRB1*1601	---	---	-C-	---	AGG	--G	--C	---	--C	---	-A-	T--	T--	---	--A	G-C	---	---	---	---
HLA-DRB1*0402	GA-	---	G--	--A	CA-	--G	--C	---	--C	---	-A-	T--	A--	---	--A	G-C	GA-	---	---	---
HLA-DRB1*0801	GA-	T-C	TC-	-C-	GG-	--G	--C	---	--C	---	-A-	T--	T--	---	--A	G-C	---	---	---	CT-
HLA-DRB1*1102	GA-	T-C	TC-	-C-	-C-	--G	--C	---	--C	---	-A-	T--	A--	---	--A	G-C	GA-	---	---	---
HLA-DRB1*1201	GA-	T-C	TC-	-C-	GG-	--G	--A	---	--G	---	CA-	T--	---	---	--A	G-C	---	--C	---	---
HLA-DRB1*1301	GA-	T-C	TC-	-C-	-C-	--G	--C	---	--C	---	-A-	T--	A--	---	--A	G-C	GA-	---	---	---
HLA-DRB1*1403	GA-	T-C	TC-	-C-	-C-	--G	--C	---	--G	---	-A-	T--	---	---	--A	G-C	---	---	---	CT-
HLA-DRB5*0101	CA-	---	GA-	---	-A-	--G	--C	---	C-C	---	GA-	---	---	---	--A	G-C	---	--C	---	---
HLA-DRB1*1404	GA-	T-C	TC-	-C-	GG-	--G	--C	---	--C	---	-A-	T--	---	---	---	-G-	---	---	---	-A-
HLA-DRB1*1401	GA-	T-C	TC-	-C-	-C-	--G	--C	---	--C	---	-A-	T--	---	---	---	-G-	---	---	---	-A-
HLA-DRB1*1402	GA-	T-C	TC-	-C-	-C-	--G	--C	---	--G	---	-A-	T--	---	---	---	---	---	---	---	---
HLA-DRB1*0901	AA-	---	GA-	---	---	--G	-AT	---	C-C	---	G--	---	---	---	---	-G-	---	---	---	-A-
HLA-DRB1*0401	GA-	---	G--	--A	CA-	--G	--C	---	--C	---	-A-	T--	---	---	---	---	-A-	---	---	---
Paca-DRB1*13a	GA-	T-C	TC-	-CA	-C-	--G	--C	---	--C	---	-A-	T--	TA-	---	--A	G-C	GA-	---	---	---
Mane-DRB1*13a	GA-	T-C	TC-	-CA	-C-	--G	--C	---	--C	---	-A-	T--	A--	---	--A	G-C	GC-	---	---	---
Mane-DRB1*13b	GA-	T-C	TC-	-CA	-C-	--G	--C	---	--C	---	-A-	T--	A--	---	--A	G-C	GC-	---	---	---
Mane-DRB1*13d	GA-	T-C	TC-	-CA	-C-	--G	-AC	---	--C	---	-A-	T--	A--	---	--A	G-C	CA-	---	---	T--
HLA-DRB1*0301	GA-	T-C	TC-	-C-	-C-	--G	-AC	---	--C	---	-A-	T--	---	---	---	---	-A-	---	-G-	CG-
Mafa-DRB1*03a	GA-	T-C	TC-	-CA	-C-	--G	-AC	---	--C	---	-A-	T--	A--	---	---	---	-A-	---	---	CG-
Mane-DRB1*03b	GA-	T-C	TC-	-CA	-C-	--G	-AC	---	--C	---	-A-	T--	A--	---	---	---	-A-	---	---	CG-
Mafa-DRB1*04a	GA-	---	G--	--A	CA-	--G	-AC	---	--G	---	CA-	T--	---	---	--A	G-C	---	---	---	CGG
Mafa-DRB1*04b	GA-	---	G--	--A	CA-	--G	--C	---	--C	---	-A-	T--	T--	---	--A	G-C	---	---	---	-T-
Mane-DRB1*04a	GA-	---	G--	--A	CA-	--G	--C	---	--T	---	-A-	T--	A--	---	--A	G-C	GC-	---	---	---
Mane-DRB1*04b	GA-	---	G--	--A	CA-	--G	--C	---	--C	---	-A-	T--	A--	---	--A	G-C	---	---	---	-T-
Mane-DRB5*01a	AA-	---	GA-	---	-A-	--G	--C	---	C-C	---	GA-	---	A--	---	--A	G-C	---	---	---	---
Gaga-DRB*01	GA-	---	G--	---	CA-	--G	--C	---	--C	---	-A-	T--	A--	---	---	G--	GC-	---	---	---
HLA-DRB4*0101	GA-	---	GC-	---	-G-	--G	AAC	---	ATC	---	-A-	---	---	---	---	-G-	---	---	---	-A-
Mane-DRB4*04c	GA-	T-C	TG-	---	---	--G	AAC	---	ATC	---	-A-	T--	---	---	---	---	---	---	---	CA-
Mane-DRB4*04d	GA-	T-C	G--	---	---	--G	-AC	---	ATC	---	GT-	T--	---	---	---	---	---	---	---	-A-
Mane-DRB1*03e	GA-	T-C	TC-	-CA	-C-	--G	--C	---	--C	---	-A-	T--	T--	---	---	---	---	---	---	---
Mafa-DRB5*09a	AA-	---	GA-	---	---	--G	--C	---	C-C	---	GA-	---	A--	---	---	-G-	---	---	---	-A-
Mane-DRB3*02a	G--	--T	GC-	---	-CA	--G	--C	---	C-G	---	-A-	---	A--	---	---	-G-	GA-	---	---	CA-
Mane-DRB3*02b	G--	--T	GC-	---	-CA	--G	--C	---	C-G	---	-A-	---	A--	---	---	-G-	GA-	---	---	CA-
Paca-DRB4*05a	GA-	T-C	G--	---	---	--G	-AC	---	ATC	---	GT-	T--	TT-	---	---	---	-A-	---	A--	A--
HLA-DRB5*0101	CA-	---	GA-	---	-A-	--G	--C	---	C-C	---	GA-	---	---	---	--A	G-C	---	--C	---	---
Paca-DRB5*03a	AA-	---	AC-	---	GC-	--G	---	---	--C	---	CA-	T--	TA-	---	---	-G-	-C-	---	---	-A-
Paca-DRB5*03b	AA-	---	AC-	---	GC-	--G	---	---	--C	---	C--	T--	TA-	-C-	---	-G-	-C-	---	---	-A-
Mafa-DRB5*01a	CA-	---	-AA	---	GC-	--G	---	---	--G	---	-A-	---	---	---	---	---	---	---	A--	CA-
Mane-DRB1*03d	GA-	T-C	TC-	-CA	-C-	--G	--C	---	--C	---	-A-	T--	A--	---	---	G--	-A-	---	-A-	AA-
HLA-DRB6*0101	GA-	---	GC-	---	-G-	--G	-AC	---	A-C	---	-A-	---	A--	---	---	G--	-AT	---	-A-	AA-
Mane-DRB6*02a	GA-	---	GC-	---	-G-	--G	-AC	---	A-C	---	-A-	---	A--	---	---	G--	-A-	---	-A-	AA-
Mane-DRB6*02b	GA-	---	GC-	---	-G-	--G	-AC	---	A-C	---	-A-	---	A--	---	---	G--	--C	G--	-A-	AA-
Mane-DRB4*05a	GA-	T-C	G--	---	---	--G	--C	---	ATC	---	GT-	T--	TA-	---	---	---	---	---	---	---
Mane-DRB5*01b	AA-	---	GA-	---	-A-	--G	--C	---	C-C	---	-A-	---	TA-	---	---	---	-A-	---	---	---
Mane-DRB5*02a	AA-	---	GC-	---	GC-	--G	--C	---	--G	---	CA-	T--	TA-	---	---	---	---	---	---	---
Mane-DRB5*03a	AA-	---	AC-	---	GC-	--G	---	---	--C	---	CA-	T--	TA-	---	---	---	---	---	---	---
Mane-DRB6*03c	GA-	---	GG-	---	-C-	--G	-AC	---	C-G	---	CA-	T--	TA-	---	---	---	---	---	---	---
Mane-DRB?*ps01	GA-	T--	GC-	---	-G-	--G	--C	---	--C	---	-A-	T--	TA-	---	---	---	GC-	---	---	---
Mane-DRB6*pss01	GA-	T--	GC-	---	-G-	--G	-AC	---	A-C	---	AA-	---	***	***	***	***	***	***	***	***
Mane-DRB6*pss02	GA-	---	GC-	---	-G-	--G	-AC	---	A-C	---	-A-	---	***	***	***	***	***	***	***	***
Mafa-DRB6*pss01	GA-	---	GC-	--A	-A-	--G	-AC	--A	A-C	---	AA-	---	***	***	***	***	***	***	***	***
Mane-DRB6*pss03	GA-	---	GC-	---	-G-	A-G	-A-	---	A-C	---	-A-	---	***	***	***	***	***	***	***	***
Paca-DRB6*pss01	AA-	---	GC-	---	-G-	--G	-AC	---	A-C	---	AA-	---	***	***	***	***	***	***	***	***

Figure 1. HVR sequence alignments from the second exon of human and other primate DRB genes. Sequences are as previously reported [2,10]. Mane=*Macaca nemestrina*; Mafa=*M. fascicularis*; Paca=*Papio cynocephalus anubis*; Gaga=*Galago garnetti*.

sequences tested. It has previously been suggested, on the basis of the frequency of silent substitutions, that the HVR_{III} segment of DRB1 genes may have a different evolutional history than the rest of the second exon, including HVR_{I} and HVR_{II} [6,7]. Our findings are consistent with this interpretation, and a possible mechanism to account for this difference is suggested by DRB sequence analysis, as shown at the bottom of *Figure 1*. In the course of sequencing nearly 100 different DRB alleles from multiple species, several unique DRB6-like sequences were obtained, five of which are shown at the bottom of *Figure 1*, from *Macaca nemestrina, M. fascicularis*, and *Papio cynocephalus anubis* individuals. In each case, these genes were deleted in a specific intra-exon sequence extending from codon 60 to codon 80 [2]. These sequences likely represent DR pseudogenes which may represent the evolutionary remnant from an important genetic event, namely the segmental exchange of HVR_{III} among different DRB genes.

We propose that specific segmental interchange involving the HVR_{III} region has occurred among DR alleles, particularly in the primate DRB6 lineage. This is consistent with a recombinational hot-spot near class II HVR_{III}, as proposed earlier [7]. Similarly, a specific interlocus exon exchange has been hypothesized for the HLA-A locus [8]. Thus it is possible that segmental exchange is a general mechanism to maintain conserved motifs in diverse MHC lineages. The specific DRB6 HVR_{III} deletions observed presumably represent the vestigial donor sequences from such an event. This proposed genetic diversification mechanism is consistent with the observation that modern HVR_{III} segments are less diverse than the isogenic HVR_{I} and HVR_{II} segments, which presumably diversified by conventional mechanisms involving the gradual accumulation of mutations.

The known peptide binding functions of class II molecules establish structural constraints on the permitted extent of diversification for class II alleles, which presumably also limits the range of evolutionary variants which are observed. As suggested by others [9], such structural constraints are likely to encourage convergent evolutionary mechanisms, particularly within codons which correspond to peptide binding polymorphic sites (HVR_{II}, *Figure 1*). In addition, however, we suggest that the limited set of HVR_{III} sequence motifs is a successful adaptation to peptide binding and T cell recognition constraints, relatively resistant to additional diversification, which is conserved and maintained by a distinct genetic exchange mechanism.

Acknowledgments

The present study was supported in part by NIH grant RR00166 to the Washington Regional Primate Research Center, and by the Puget Sound Blood Center and Program.

References

1. Hughes AL, Nei M. Nucleotide substitution of major histocompatibility complex class II loci: Evidence for overdominant selection. *Proc Natl Acad Sci USA* 1989; 86: 958-62.
2. Gaur LK, Nepom GT. Ancestral major histocompatibility complex DRB genes beget conserved patterns of localized polymorphisms. *Proc Natl Acad Sci USA* 1997; 93 (in press).
3. Gaur LK, Snyder KE. Analysis of macaque MHC-DRB alleles by TCR-based oligotyping. *Ann Hum Biol* 1997 (in press).
4. Klein J. Origin of major histocompatibility complex polymorphism: the trans-species hypothesis. *Hum Immunol* 1987; 19: 155-62.
5. Figueroa F, Gunther E, Klein J. MHC polymorphism pre-dating speciation. *Nature* 1988; 335: 265-7.
6. Gyllensten U, Sundvall M, Ezcurra I, Erlich HA. Genetic diversity at class II DRB loci of the primate MHC. *J Immunol* 1991; 146: 4368-76.
7. Gyllensten UB, Sundvall M, Erlich HA. Allelic diversity is generated by intraexon sequence exchange at the DRB1 locus of primates. *Proc Natl Acad Sci USA* 1991; 88: 3686-90.
8. Hughes AL, Nei M. Ancient interlocus exon exchange in the history of the HLA-A locus. *Genetics* 1989; 122: 681-6.
9. Klein J, O'hUigin C. Class II B Mhc motifs in an evolutionary perspective. *Immunol Rev* 1995; 143: 89-111.
10. Marsh SG, Bodmer JG. HLA class II nucleotide sequences, 1995. *Tissue Antigens* 1995; 45: 258-80.

The influence of the MHC on survival of human isolates

A. Olivo, C. Alaez, H. Debaz, M. Moreno, M. Vázquez-Garciá, G. de La Rosa, C. Gorodezky

Department of Immunogenetics, INDRE SSA, Carpio 470, 1st floor, 11340 México DF, Mexico

The analysis of the MHC in Amerindian tribes is a very valuable tool to the understanding of many features of mankind. A very restricted MHC polymorphism is evident [1-3] and some studies suggest that certain class I variants present in Indians from Brazil and Ecuador have originated locally, suggesting that selective pressures have been important, possibly conferring advantage against infections [4]. Moreover, maintenance of polymorphic variants of HLA-*02 in different populations demonstrate that mutations can have a dramatic effect on antigen processing and presentation of different peptides derived from local pathogens [5]. Here we analyze one of the most interesting Indian groups in Mexico, reflecting a wonderful example of geographic, cultural and genetic isolation. The group is formed by 500 individuals inhabiting in the jungle of the State of Chiapas, located in the southeast of Mexico. They belong to the Mayance Family and their language is part of the Maya-Totonaco Group. The Lacandon Indians were never subdued by the Spaniards, because they escaped inside the jungle. They are highly endogamic and have very strict social and political organization. The prevalent diseases in them are malaria, tuberculosis, parasitic and intestinal infections, dengue and skin allergies. Among those caused by intermarriage, abortion, strabism, albinism and epilepsy are not uncommon [6]. The aim of this study was to analyze the molecular class II pattern of Lacandones in an attempt to look for their ancestral origins and migration patterns, as well as into the biological significance of their molecular profile. Selection mechanisms and the impact of the MHC on the epidemiology of the group is an important goal.

Methods

Population samples

DNA typing was done in 161 individuals belonging to 15 four generation families, of the 3 Lacandon communities: Metzabok, Nahá and Lacanjá. EDTA-blood was withdrawn from every individual and mixed with supplemented RPMI medium for the transfer to Mexico City. Mononuclear cells were isolated and kept at -196 °C.

DNA extraction, PCR amplification and oligonucleotide typing

DNA was obtained from the cells after treatment with proteinase K. Phenol/chloroform extraction was used for DNA isolation and isopropanol was used for precipitation. DNA amplification of the second exon of DRB1, B3, B4, DQA1 and DQB1 was done and the PCR products were dotted onto nylon membranes. The primers and probes used for hybridization, as well as the conditions were those recommended by the protocols of the 12 W. Detection was acomplished using a chemiluminiscent procedure. In some cases the PCR-SSP method was used to achieve a more accurate assignment of some DQA1 and DQB1 alleles [7]. Gene frequencies were determined by chromosome direct counting. Haplotypes were ensembled for each family member according to the segregation pattern. The incidence of homozygocity was obtained by direct counting from subjects that were less related; the Hardy-Weinberg test was applied for the analysis of each locus.

Results and discussion

Table I shows the allele frequencies of DRB1, DQA1 and DQB1 in the Lacandones. *Table II* lists their haplotype frequencies compared to other Amerindians. Their MHC pattern is restricted to only 13 haplotypes and it is interesting to point out that the results of the Hardy Weinberg test showed a good fit to the expected genotype distribution for each locus, indicating that although the allele variability is very limited, as expected in an inbred populaton, it is not accompanied by a deviation

Table I. Distribution of DRB1, DQA1 and DQB1 alleles among lacandones

Allele	No. Observed	Gene freq.	Allele	No. Observed	Gene freq.
DRB1			DQA1		
*0403	6	0.019	*0401	4	0.012
*0404	31	0.096	*0501	64	0.199
*0407	31	0.096	*3011	245	0.761
*0411	183	0.565	*03011/*0501#	7	0.022
*06	6	0.019			
*0801	4	0.012			
*1104	11	0.034	DQB1		
*1402	19	0.059	*0301	64	0.203
*1406	13	0.040	*0302	243	0.769
*1602	15	0.046	*0402	7	0.022

#This allele has a different pattern of hybridization. Probably a new variant. DRB1*01,*04,*0402,*0301;DQA1*0101/4 and DQB1*0201,*0501, are in < 0.6%. No. of individuals for DRB- 162; for DQA1- 161; and for DQB1- 158.

Table II. DRB1-DQA1-DQB1 haplotypes characteristic of lacandones compared to other amerindians

DRB1	DRB3/4/5	DQA1	DQB1	LAC N= 157	SERI[9] N= 101	XAV[1] N= 74	EAST[1] TOBA N= 135	MATAC[1] N= 49	TOBA[1] PILAGA N= 19	CAY[3] N= 100
*0404	*0101	*03011	*0302	7.9	0.5	13.5	10.4	20.4	5.3	4.0
*0403	*0101	*03011	*0302	1.3	0.0	0.0	0.0	0.0	0.0	0.5
*0407	*0101	*03011	*0302	9.6	44.6	14.9	11.9	0.0	10.5	27.0
*0411	*0101	*03011	*0302	55.4	0.0	0.0	11.9	14.3	15.8	3.0
*0411	*0101	*03011/*0501	*0302	1.9	0.0	0.0	0.0	0.0	0.0	0.0
*0411	*0101	*03011	*0402	0.6	0.0	0.0	0.0	0.0	0.0	0.0
*0404	*0101	*0301	*0402	0.3	0.0	0.0	0.0	0.0	0.0	0.0
*0802		*0401	*0402	0.0	36.6	45.9	40.0	2.0	21.1	13.0
*1402	*0101	*0501	*0301	5.4	13.9	51.4	20.7	44.9	15.8	18.0
*1402	*0301	*0501	*0301	0.3	0.0	-	-	-	-	-
*1406	*0101	*0501	*0301	2.8	0.0	0.0	41.5	30.6	42.1	0.0
*1406	*0301	*0501	*0301	1.3	0.0	-	-	-	-	-
*1602	*0201/2	*0501	*0301	4.5	0.0	51.4	3.0	0.0	0.0	9.0
*1104	*0201/3	*0501	*0301	3.5	0.0	0.0	3.7	0.0	0.0	0.0

The two haplotypes with DRB3*0301 have not been detected in other Amerindians.

in the frequency of homozygous individuals, suggesting strongly that the MHC itself is a unit of selection favouring heterozygocity. It has been claimed that this characteristic confers a selective advantage [5]. As an example, Amerindians have a very high frequency of DR4, but the distribution of the subtypes differs (*Table II*). DRB1*0411 is highly increased in Lacandones, moderate in Baris [2] but absent in North Amerindians [8] and in Mexican Seris (studied by us in this Workshop [9]). The prevalent DR4 alelle in Seris is *0407, while Lacandones have only 9.3%. Thus, even within Mexican Indians the class II profile is clearly distinct from one group to another. Eight Lacandones have Caucasian haplotypes (DRB1*0402, *03011,*01 and *0801), confirming that Indians accept sometimes visitors that intermix with their women. Unlike other Amerindians, Lacandones lack the DRB1*0802-DQA1*0401-DQB1*0402 haplotype. Their combinations are shown in *Table II*; the most frequent one is *0411-*03011-*0302.

Three individuals carry a new DR4 haplotype. DRB1*0411*DRB4*0101-DQA1*03011-DQB1-*0402, which is probably the result of a gene conversion event and a reminiscence of the *0802 haplotype. Seven people show *0411 with a peculiar DQA1 allele that hybridyzes with some *03011 and some *0501 probes. These two novel haplotypes, possibly reflect sequence exchanges within exon-2, between ancient and conserved domains, or with more recent variants. Their unique profile compared to other Amerindians, suggests either a different Asian ancestry or positive directional selection. The DR4 variants present in Lacandones probably confer selective advantage. For example, IDDM is absent in them, but the Mexican Mestizo IDDM patients carry *0405 [10], which does not exist in these Indians, although the frequency of DQB1-nonAsp and DQA1-Arg alleles is very high. Moreover, a strong influenza epidemics whipped out the group in 1946, and left about 50 people alive [6]. It is most likely that survivors were best adapted to fight a viral infection, they faced for the first time; probably DRB1*0411 carriers presented influenza peptides efficiently to Th1 cells and DRB1*0802 was lost either due to genetic drift or because this allele did not induce a good response against the virus. These two examples, one autoimmune disease and one infection, show how the mechanism of expression of certain illnesses may be explained through the immunogenetic features of the mysterious tribes of the world.

Acknowledgements

We are truly grateful to the Instituto Nacional Indigenista for their valuable help to access the Lacandones . To the members of the 3 Communities for their great cooperation. This work was partially supported by La Real Academia de Ciencias Exactas, Físicas y Naturales de España, by NIH Contract N01-A1-62-S23 and by Boheringer Mannheim Biochemica.

References

1. Cerna M, Falco M, Friedman H, Raymondi E, Maccagno A, Fernandez-Viña, Stastny P. Differences in class II alleles of isolated South American Indian populations from Brazil and Argentina. *Hum Immunol* 1993; *37:* 213-20.
2. Guédez BY. Layrisse Z, Domínguez E, Rodríguez-Larralde A, Scorza J. Molecular analysis of MHC class II alleles and haplotypes (DRB1, DQA1 and DQB1) in the Bari Amerindians. *Tissue Antigens* 1994; 44:125-8.
3. Titus-Trachtenberg, Rickards O, DeStefano GF, Erlich H. Analysis of HLA class II haplotypes in the Cayapa Indians of Ecuador: a novel DRB1 allele reveals evidence for convergent evolution and balancing selection at pos 86. *Am J Hum Genet* 1994,55:160-7.
4. Belich MP, Madrigal A, Hildebrand H, Zemmout J, Williams R, Luz R, Petzl-Erler ML, Parham P. Unusual HLA-B alleles in two tribes of Brazilian Indians. *Nature* 1992; *357*: 326-9.
5. Browning M Krausa P. Genetic diversity of HLA-A2: evolutionary and functional significance. *Immunol Today* 1996; 17:165-70.
6. Boremanse D. Los lacandones. In: Esponda Jimeno VM, ed. *La población indígena de Chiapas.* Gobierno del Edo de Chiapas, 1993: 271-81.
7. Olerup, O, Aldener A, Fogdell A. HLA-DQB1 and DQA1 typing by PCR amplification with sequence specific primers 8 PCR-SSP in 2 hours. *Tissue Antigens* 1993; 41:119-34.
8. Imanishi I, Akaza T, Kimura A, Gojobri T. Allele and haplotype frequencies for HLA and complement loci in various ethnic groups. In: Tsuji K, Aizawa M, Sasasuki T, eds. *HLA 1991. Proceedings of the 11th International Histocompatibility Workshop and Conference.* Oxford: Oxford University Press, 1992: 1065-220.
9. Debaz H, Alaez C, Olivo A, Pujol MJ, Duran C, Navarro JL, Juarez V, Gorodezky C.DNA profile of class II loci in Seris: a mexican Indian tribe. *12th Histocompatibility Workshop and Confrence, St Malo-Paris June 1996.* Sèvres : EDK, 1996 (abstr).
10. Gorodezky C, Olivo A, Debaz H, Rodriguez L, Altamirano N, Robles C.Los mecanismos moleculares de susceptibilidad y de protección dependientes del MHC en la diabetes tipo I en mexicanos. *Gaceta Médica* 1995; 131:395-404.

HLA DNA sequences from archaeological bone

M.P. Evison[1,2], D.M Smillie[2], A.T. Chamberlain[1]

1 Department of Archaeology and Prehistory, University of Sheffield, Sheffield S10 2TN, UK
2 Trent Centre, National Blood Service, Longley Lane, Sheffield S7 5JN, UK

Analysis of the HLA complex, when combined with DNA sexing methods, constitutes a unique tool for studying kinship and immunity in the archaeological record. Sequences recovered from mummified material have been assigned to class I and II HLA loci [1-4]. We analysed 92 teeth and bone specimens from archaeological skeletons recovered from excavations ranging in date from the Palaeolithic to the Medieval Period, using standard PCR based HLA-DPB1 typing and forensic DNA-sexing techniques.

Methods

Precautions were taken against contamination with intrusive DNA. Equipment was cleaned by soaking in 0.5 % sodium hypochlorite solution for 1 hr. Pre- and post-PCR activities were conducted in separate rooms and a laminar flow cabinet was used during the extraction step. Surfaces of bone or teeth were cleaned by washing with 0.05 % sodium hypochlorite solution or by abrasion with a grinding tip or drill bit, which was then discarded. Bone was ground to a fine powder in a coffee mill (Philips HR2811). Intact teeth were fractured longitudinally to expose the pulp cavity. We used a refinement of the silica method for DNA extraction [5]. Quantities of ~1.0 g of bone or ~0.1-0.7 g of tooth fragments were combined with 2.0 ml 0.5 M Na_2EDTA pH 8.0 and 25 µl proteinase K (20 mg / ml) in 4 ml Khan tubes and mixed on a rotary mixer for 48 hr at room temperature. Substrate residues were pelleted by centrifugation at 4,000 g for 5-15 min. Aliquots of 0.5 ml extract supernatant were bound to 20 µl silica suspension using 1.0 ml 4 M guanidine isothiocyanate by mixing for 2 hr in 1.5 ml Eppendorf tubes on a rotary mixer at room temperature. DNA/silica matrix was pelleted by microcentrifugation for 20 seconds at 13,000 g and washed twice in 1.5 ml 70 % ethanol and once in 1.5 ml acetone. The pellet was dried at 56 °C for 5 min. DNA was eluted from the silica into 115 µl sterile filtered distilled water by heating at 56 °C for 15 min, and vortexing every 5 min, to aid solution of the DNA. Silica was pelleted by centrifugation at 13,000 g for 2 min. Volumes of 105 µl DNA solution were taken off to avoid inadvertent removal of unwanted silicate. Samples were stored in 0.5 ml Eppendorf tubes at - 20°C.

All PCRs are of the sequence specific primer (SSP) type and were carried out using a Perkin-Elmer GeneAmp 9600 thermal cycler. PCR reaction mixtures and programs were optimised using modern DNA samples by D.S. Primer sequences are given in *Table I.*

Table I. Oligonucleotide primer sequences

5'CCC TGG GCT CTG TAA AGA ATA GTG3' (Amel-A)
5'ATC AGA GCT TAA ACT GGG AAG CTG3' (Amel-B)
5'GAG AGT GGC GCC TCC GCT CAT3' (DPB-AmpA)
5'GCC GGC CCA AAG CCC TCA CTC3' (DPB-AmpB)
5'ATG CTA AGT TAG CTT TAC AG3' (A)
5'ACA GTT TCA TGC CCA TCG TC3' (B)

The HLA-DPB1 primers (DPB-AmpA and -AmpB) amplify a 327 bp sequence of the polymorphic second exon [6]. The mtDNA analysis was included to provide a comparison of genomic and mtDNA survival. Primers A and B target a 121 bp segment of the non-coding region V [7]. The *Amel* primers (Amel-A and -B) target the X-Y homologous amelogenin gene [8]. The X homologue contains a 6 bp deletion. Products of 106 bp and 112 b.p are generated from the X and Y chromosomes, respectively. Blank controls were included in each extraction, purification and amplification phase to allow detection of contamination with intrusive DNA. Positive controls were included in extraction (50 µl

Table II. Table of results

	HLA-DPB1			Amel			mtDNA			Total		
	n	+	%	*n*	+	%	*n*	+	%	*n*	+	%
Forensic	89	41	46	119	97	82	89	73	82	297	211	71
Archaeological	92	34	37	92	9	10	92	43	47	276	86	31

Results of PCR analysis for HLA-DPB1, amelogenin (*Amel*) and mtDNA region V (mtDNA) in archaeological tooth and bone samples. Results from a separate study of forensic specimens are shown for comparison. Total number of samples (*n*), positive samples (+) , generating a PCR product of the appropriate size, and % of positive samples are given.

modern blood in 450 µl sterile filtered distilled water), purification (0.5 ml DNA solution at 10 ng / µl) and amplification (5 µl DNA solution at 10 ng / µl) steps. All specimens were extracted and amplified in duplicate.

Results

A degree of random contamination was experienced in extraction, purification and amplification blanks. Batches containing contaminated blanks were excluded from the study. A typical result is shown in *Figure 1.* Results are summarised in *Table II.* Results of a study of forensic specimens are shown for comparison. As expected, mtDNA PCR products predominated. HLA-DPB1 sequences were successfully amplified less than half as commonly. Only limited success was achieved with amplification of amelogenin sequences, despite the shorter length product. Reproducibility of results in duplicate samples was poor, but tended to be better for mtDNA. Consistency was also poor, with samples often amplifying for only one primer system, usually mtDNA region V. Results from UK archaeological specimens were generally poor, reflecting the poorer osteological structure (assessed macroscopically). Teeth tended to be a better substrate than bone. There was no correlation between the age of the material and the presence of amplifiable DNA.

Discussion

Ancient DNA results require scrupulous verification [9]. It should be possible to confirm the amelogenin sexing results by comparing them with the skeletal sex. All except two of the 39 amelogenin results were female, however, and sexing errors were exclusively "false females". We have observed false female results in previous experiments with forensic specimens (data not

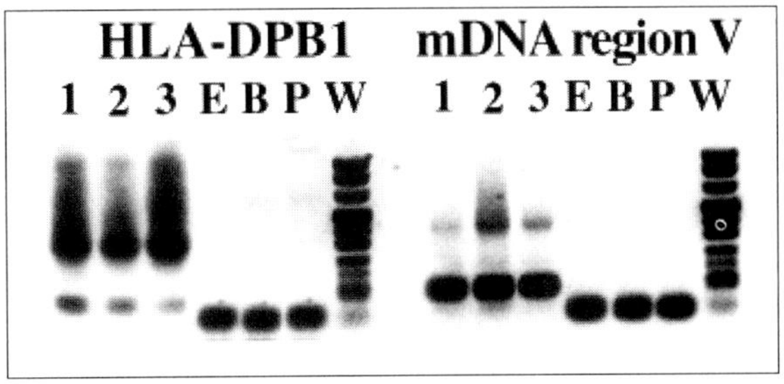

Figure 1. Photograph of 1.5 % agarose gel showing typical results for HLA-DPB1 and mtDNA region V analysis. Aliquots of 4 µl DNA solution were added to 1 µl X5 gel loading buffer (40 % sucrose, 0.1 % bromophenol blue, 50 mM Na_2EDTA, 50 mM Tris-HCl pH 7.6 and 5 % SDS) and run on a 1.5 % agarose gel (100 V., 20 min) containing 10 µl ethidium bromide (10 µg / ml). Single bands are generated by the amplification of 372 bp HLA-DPB1 sequences and 121 bp sequences of the mitochondrial non-coding region V. Samples 1-3: DNA extracted from archaeological bone, E: extraction blank, B: silicate binding (purification) blank, P: PCR blank, W: molecular weight marker (MWVIII).

shown) and attributed these to preferential amplification of the shorter (X-chromosome) product in degraded samples. Stone *et al.* [10] reported the recovery of sequences of the amelogenin gene from a sample of 20 archaeological skeletons. They avoided the problem of allelic drop-out by amplifying a 112 bp region of amelogenin occurring without deletion on both the X and Y chromosomes. They suggest that chance variation will influence whether the X or Y sequence tends to be amplified in males (in their comparison it again tends to be the X). Their attempts to apply the amelogenin sexing technique [8] we have used were not successful. Lack of robusticity in the amelogenin PCR system may explain why its shorter length product is amplified less frequently than the longer HLA-DPB1 product.

We doubt that the results can be explained by a fortuitous pattern of inhibition or contamination. Contamination might be expected to generate false males at least as frequently as false females and to effect each primer system similarly, especially if due to PCR carry over. False male results did not occur and there are distinct differences in the pattern of results obtained from the different primer systems. If the pattern of results is due to inhibition of amplification of a substantial background of contaminating DNA in a subset of the samples, more overall consistency in the results might be expected. Our archaeological DNA samples rarely inhibit amplification of modern DNA, further suggesting that this explanation is unlikely. It is possible that the apparent positive results are artefacts generated by *in vitro* recombination and "jumping PCR" occurring in degraded and fragmented samples, containing a minimal quantity of potentially contaminated DNA substrate. We are currently resolving the HLA-DPB1 alleles present in our sample by dot-blot hybridisation and direct sequencing. Putative HLA-DPB1 sequences were recovered at a rate which would make analysis of polymorphisms viable in phylogenetic studies of archaeological skeletal material.

Single copy nuclear DNA sequences are the most interesting and difficult target for ancient DNA analysis. The proportion of positive results obtained from archaeological material will be improved if teeth, which appear to be a better source than bone, are used, and if analysis is restricted to skeletons with good histological preservation. The silicate method of DNA extraction will remove inhibitors from most archaeological bone and tooth samples. Dedicated clean conditions, such as a clean room, are essential to reduce the likelihood of contamination. Cloning and sequencing of multiple PCR products will be necessary to establish the validity of HLA results from ordinary archaeological material. If possible, results should be verified via DNA independent controls. Skeletal sex and the ankylosing spondylitis pathology serve this purpose. We suggest that the extent of contamination and negative results should be reported, and that positive results should be reproduced in an independent HLA laboratory.

Acknowledgements

This study was supported by NERC and Trent Centre, National Blood Service, where the laboratory work was carried out. We thank Manthos Bessios, Birger Herzog, Nina Kyparissi-Apostolika, Maria Pappa and Beth Rega for access to archaeological material.

References

1. Lawlor DA, Dickel CD, Hauswirth WW, Parham P. Ancient HLA genes from 7,500-year-old archaeological remains. *Nature* 1991; 349: 785-8.
2. Hauswirth WW, Dickel CD, Rowold DJ, Hauswirth MA. Inter- and intrapopulation studies of ancient human remains. *Experientia* 1994; 50: 585-91.
3. Del Pozzo G, Guardiola A. Mummy DNA fragment identified. *Nature* 1989; 339: 431-2.
4. Woodward SR, King MJ, Chiu NM Kuchar MJ, Griggs CW. Amplification of ancient nuclear DNA from teeth and soft tissues. *PCR Methods and Applications* 1994; 3: 244-7.
5. Höss M, Pääbo S. DNA extraction from Pleistocene bones by a silica-based purification method. *Nucleic Acids Res* 1993; 21: 3913-4.
6. Kimura A, Sasazuki T. Eleventh International Histocompatibility Workshop reference protocol for the HLA DNA-typing technique. In: Tsuji K, Aizawa M, Sasazuki T, eds. *Proceedings of the Eleventh International Histocompatibility Workshop and Conference*. Oxford: Oxford University Press, 1992.
7. Wrischnik LA, Higuchi RG, Stoneking M, Erlich HA., Arnheim N, Wilson AC. Length mutations in human mitochondrial DNA - direct sequencing of enzymatically amplified DNA. *Nucleic Acids Res* 1987; 15: 529-42.
8. Sullivan KM, Mannucci A, Kimpton CP, Gill PA. Rapid and quantitative DNA sex test: flourescence-based PCR analysis of X-Y homologous gene amelogenin. *BioTechniques* 1993; 15: 636-41.
9. Richards MB, Sykes BC, Hedges REM. Authenticating DNA extracted from ancient skeletal remains. *J Archaeol Sci* 1995; 22: 291-9.
10. Stone AC, Milner GR, Pääbo S, Stoneking M. Sex determination of ancient human skeletons using DNA. *Am J Phys Anthropol* 1996; 99: 231-8.

HLA Diversity

MHC Regulation

Contents

• MHC Regulation

Structural diversity of the HLA-A regulatory complex

S. Köhler, J. Wehling, R. Blasczyk

Department of Internal Medicine, Division of Hematology and Oncology, Bloodbank, Virchow-Klinikum, Humboldt-Universität zu Berlin, Augustenburger Platz 1, 13353 Berlin, Germany

The transcriptional level of HLA class I genes is controlled by regulatory elements residing in the 5' flanking region. The sum of several cis-acting elements identified in the promoter region comprising kB enhancer elements, Interferon response sequence element (IRSE) and enhancer B, has become known as the MHC class I regulatory complex (CRC) [1]. A series of different transcription factors has been shown to bind to these elements [2,3], modulating the level of class I cell surface expression. HLA class I expression can be induced by a set of different cytokines [4], and suppressed by a number of viruses and oncogenes [5,6]. Locus or allele specific down-regulation of HLA class I glycoproteins has been found in several tumor cells. In some cases it has been demonstrated that the suppression was caused by altered binding of regulatory factors to class I enhancer sequences [7].

The CRC in the HLA-A gene is mapped to the region -216 to -92 bp upstream from the ATG start codon and has been shown to be locus specifically conserved (*Figure 1*) [8]. In this study we have sequenced the 5' flanking region of the majority of HLA-A alleles to define the structural basis for allele specific transcriptional regulation of HLA-A alleles. The sequence of a 450 bp fragment upstream from the ATG start codon was determined to identify allelic variations.

Materials and methods

A total of 32 HLA-A homozygous cell lines mostly from the 10th Histocompatibility Workshop and 95 PCR typed clinical samples were investigated, representing all serologic specificities and most of their subtypes. For template preparation, PCR amplification was performed haplotype specific using a generic 5' primer located in the 5' flanking region (5'AAG CTT ACT CTC TGG CAC CAA3', 21mer, Tm=62°C, matching nucleotides -501 - -521) and allele specific 3' primers in the 2nd or 3rd exon as described [9]. The resulting PCR products contained the first 521 bp of the 5' flanking region of a single allele.

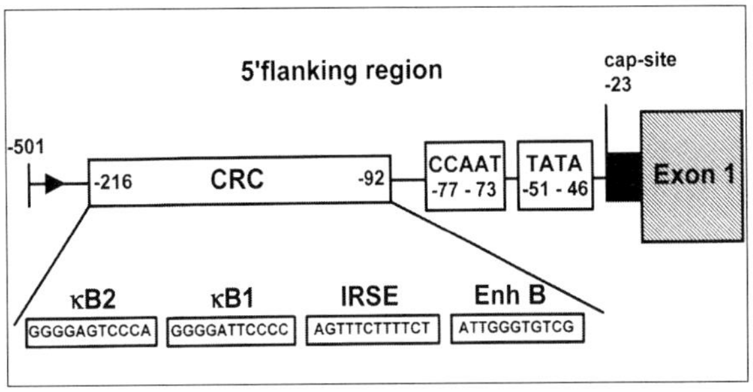

Figure 1. Schematic representation of the class I regulatory complex and the conserved cis-acting elements within the 5' flanking region. The 3' end of the generic 5' primer used for PCR amplification was located at position -501. CRC, class I regulatory complex; IRSE, Interferon response sequence element; Enh B, Enhancer B.

A 450 bp fragment upstream from the ATG start codon was sequenced in both directions using HLA-A gene specific nested sequencing primers in the 1st exon and the 5' flanking region. Sequencing reactions were performed as described elsewhere [9]. In brief, genomic DNA was amplified in a 100 µl volume, using 10 pmol biotinylated 3' or 5' primer. Single stranded templates were generated by magnetic beads technique (Dynal) and sequenced with Sequenase dye terminator chemistry. The sequences were analysed on an automatic DNA sequencer (Applied Biosystems 373A, software version 1.2.1).

Table I. Polymorhism of the HLA-A 5' flanking region within the first 450 bp

Position	6	44	53	54	65	103	141	154	163	198	208	225	247	273	296	297	303	308	331	342	360	374	407	413	415
Consensus	G	T	G	G	G	C	T	T	C	G	C	G	G	C	G	G	G	C	C	T	T	G	G	C	T
A*0101	-	-	-	T	-	-	A	C	-	-	-	-	-	-	-	-	C	-	-	C	-	-	-	T	A
A*0301	-	C	-	T	-	-	A	C	-	-	-	-	A	-	-	-	C	-	-	C	-	-	-	T	A
A*1101	C	-	C	T	T	-	A	C	-	-	-	-	-	-	-	A	C	-	-	C	-	-	-	T	A
A*3001/04	-	C	-	T	-	-	A	C	-	-	A	-	-	-	-	-	C	-	-	C	-	-	-	T	A
A*3002	-	C	-	T	-	-	A	C	-	-	A	-	-	-	-	-	C	-	-	-	-	-	-	T	A
A*2301	-	-	-	T	-	-	-	-	-	-	-	-	-	-	A	-	-	-	T	-	-	-	-	-	-
A*2402/05/07	-	-	-	T	-	-	-	-	-	-	-	-	-	-	A	-	-	-	T	-	-	-	-	-	-
A*0201-08/10/17	-	-	-	-	-	-	-	-	-	-	-	-	-	-	A	-	-	-	-	-	-	-	A	-	-
A*6801-02	-	-	-	-	-	-	-	-	-	-	-	-	-	-	-	-	-	-	-	-	A	-	A	-	-
A*6901	-	-	-	-	-	-	-	-	-	-	-	-	-	-	-	-	-	-	-	-	A	-	A	-	-
A*2501	-	-	-	-	-	-	-	-	-	-	-	A	-	-	-	-	-	-	-	-	-	-	A	-	-
A*2601	-	-	-	-	-	-	-	-	-	-	-	A	-	-	-	-	-	-	-	-	-	-	A	-	-
A*4301	-	-	-	-	-	-	-	-	-	-	-	A	-	-	-	-	-	-	-	-	-	-	A	-	-
A*3402	-	-	-	-	-	-	-	-	-	-	-	-	-	-	-	-	-	-	-	-	-	-	A	-	-
A*6601	-	-	-	-	-	-	-	-	-	-	-	-	-	-	-	-	-	-	-	-	-	-	A	-	-
A*6602-03	-	-	-	-	-	-	-	-	-	-	-	-	-	-	-	-	-	-	-	-	A	-	A	-	-
A*2902	-	-	-	-	-	-	-	-	G	-	-	-	-	-	-	-	-	A	-	-	-	-	-	-	-
A*3201	-	-	-	-	-	-	-	-	G	-	-	-	-	-	-	-	-	-	-	-	-	-	-	-	-
A*7401-03	-	-	-	-	-	-	-	-	G	-	-	-	-	-	-	-	-	-	-	-	-	-	-	-	-
A*3101	-	-	-	-	-	-	-	-	-	-	-	-	-	A	-	-	-	-	-	-	-	C	-	-	-
A*3301/03	-	-	-	-	-	-	-	-	-	-	-	-	-	A	-	-	-	-	-	-	-	C	-	-	-
A*8001	-	-	-	-	-	T	-	-	-	A	-	-	-	-	-	-	C	-	-	-	-	-	-	-	-

Results and discussion

Within the 450 bp fragment of the 5' flanking region 25 variable positions were identified yielding 14 different promoter sequences (*Table I*). The variations were group specific rather than allele specific. Exclusively within the A*30 and A*66 group divergent promoter sequences differing by a single nucleotide were observed between different allelic subtypes. These variations indicate most likely a different ancestral origin. A*6601 carried the same promoter as A*3402. The promoter sequences of A*6602 and 6603 were identical to that of the A28 group.

Within the 450 bp fragment of the 5' flanking region, 23 of the 25 variable positions were clustered around the cis-acting elements identified in the CRC. This diversity reflected the ancestral relationship of the HLA-A alleles rather than a functional relevance. The phylogenetic tree, constructed by the use of the neighbour-joining algorithm, separated the promoter sequences in six families corresponding to the ancestral HLA-A lineages with the exception, that the A28 group was closer related to A10 than to A2 (*Figure 2*). This finding is concordant with the similarity of the 5' coding sequences of the A10 and A28 groups which first diversify at the 3' part of the 2nd exon.

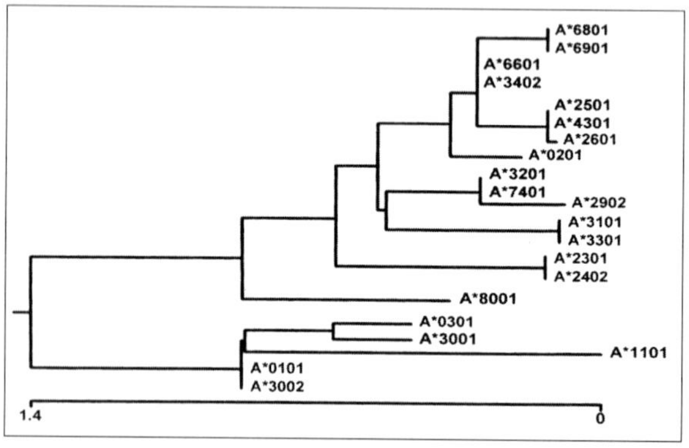

Figure 2. Phylogenetic tree of the 450 bp fragment of the HLA-A 5' flanking region using the neighbour-joining algorithm. The promoter sequences are divided in six families corresponding to the ancestral HLA-A lineages with the exception, that the A28 group is closer related to A10 than to A2.

```
                 -220        -210        -200        -190
Consensus ATGGATTGGGGAGTCCCAGCCTTGGGGATTCCCCAACTCCG
A*0201    -----------------------------------------
A*3001    -------[κB2]---A-------------[κB1]---------
A*3002    -------[   ]---A-------------[   ]---------
A*8001    -------------------------A---------------
```

Figure 3. Part of the class I regulatory complex showing the sequence of the kB enhancer elements. In A*8001 and the A*30 group the palindromes of kB1 and kB2, respectively, are interrupted. This probably indicates differing transcriptional regulation.

Two variable positions were located in the kB enhancer elements destroying their palindromic sequences (*Figure 3*). In the A*30 alleles a group specific point mutation interrupted the 3' palindrome of the kB2 element. In A*8001 the kB1 element was affected. Site-directed *in vitro* mutagenesis experiments have shown that nucleotide substitutions in the kB enhancer elements are able to reduce significantly reporter gene activity. Moreover, the kB1 element in A*8001 shows similarity to the sequence observed in HLA-C, for which no binding of nuclear factors could be observed [10]. This phenomenon has been made responsible for the low cell surface expression of HLA-C glycoproteins. These findings therefore provide a structural basis for a divergent transcriptional regulation of the HLA-A alleles.

Acknowledgments
This work was in part supported by a grant from the Wilhelm Sander-Stiftung.

References

1. David-Watine B, Israel A, Kourilsky P. The regulation and expression of MHC class I genes. *Immunol Today* 1990; 11: 286-92.
2. Ting JP, Baldwin AS. Regulation of MHC gene expression. *Curr Op Immunol* 1993; 5: 8-16.
3. Baldwin AS, Sharp PA. Two transcription factors, NF-kB and H2TF1, interact with a single regulatory sequence in the class I major histocompatibility complex promoter. *Proc Natl Acad Sci USA* 1988; 85: 723-7.
4. Hillman GG, Puri RK, Kukuruga MA, Pontes JE, Haas-GP. Growth and major histocompatibility antigen expression regulation by IL-4, interferon-gamma (IFN-gamma) and tumour necrosis factor-alpha (TNF-alpha) on human renal cell carcinoma. *Clin Exp Immunol* 1994; 96: 476-83.
5. Howcroft TK, Strebel K, Martin MA, Singer DS. Repression of MHC class I gene promoter activity by two-exon Tat of HIV. *Science* 1993; 260: 1320-2.
6. Lenardo M, Rustgi AK, Schivella AR, Bernards R. Suppression of MHC class I expression by N-myc through enhancer inactivation. *EMBO J* 1989; 8: 3351-5.
7. Blanchet O, Bourge JF, Zinszner H, Israel A, Kourilsky P, Dausset J, Degos L, Paul P. Altered binding of regulatory factors to HLA class I enhancer sequence in human tumor cell lines lacking class I antigen expression. *Proc Natl Acad Sci USA* 1992; 89: 3488-92.
8. Cereb N, Yang SY. The regulatory complex of HLA class I promoters exhibits locus- specific conservation with limited allelic variation. *J Immunol* 1994; 152: 3873-83.
9. Blasczyk R, Hahn U, Wehling J, Huhn D, and Salama A. Complete subtyping of the HLA-A locus by sequence-specific amplification followed by direct sequencing or single- strand conformation polymorphism analysis. *Tissue Antigens* 1995; 46: 86-95.
10. Park JH, Kim JD, Kim SJ. Nuclear protein binding patterns in the 5'-upstream regulatory elements of HLA class I genes. *Yonsei Med J* 1994; 35: 295-307.

Identification of a new regulatory element within the HLA-A promoter : regulation by the zinc finger protein ZFX

C. Gazin, M. L'Haridon, J.G. Xerri, L. Degos, P. Paul*

INSERM U93, Centre Hayem, Hôpital Saint-Louis, 1, avenue Claude Vellefaux, 75475 Paris Cedex 10, France
*Corresponding author

The human major histocompatibility complex (MHC) class I genes encode the heavy chain of the HLA-A, -B, and C membrane bound glycoproteins. The classical HLA class I genes (HLA-A, -B, -C) are often thought of as ubiquitously expressed antigens present on the surface of most cell types but, in fact their level of expression varies widely between tissues and stages of development [1, 2]. Expression is high in lymphoid cells but undetectable in neurones, mature sperm cells, acinar cells of the pancreas and trophoblast cells. Furthermore the level of MHC class I expression is often deregulated in tumour cells, during viral infections and auto-immune diseases [3, 4]. The expression of MHC class I genes can also be altered by various oncogenes (N-Myc, c-myc, c-fos) and viruses (HIV, HTLV1, Hepatitis, Cytomegalovirus, Adenovirus) and their transcription is modulated by IFN-α/β, IFN-γ, TNF, hormones and radiations. MHC class I gene expression is thus both tightly regulated and sensitive to various activation signals. Regulation of the human MHC class I promoter is controlled by a complex array of regulatory elements and factors. Among these regulatory elements are the enhancer A sequence which binds factors of the NF-kB family and is the target of TNF activation and an Interferon Responsive Element [5]. We have identified five additional upstream cis regulatory sequences within the HLA-A11 gene promoter which interact with nuclear factors to control the level of MHC class I transcription in human lymphoid cells [6]. To further characterise sites that indeed exert an effect on transcription levels, we identified nucleotide positions that are in contact with nuclear proteins by methylation interference and mutated those residues in reporter constructs allowing assessment of the HLA-A promoter activity.

Results

The -273/-205 positive regulatory element of the HLA-A11 promoter is essential to control transcription

The effect of sequences contained within the -335 to +2 promoter region of the HLA-A11 gene was assessed by introducing various portion of this region into a Chloramphenicol Acetyl Transferase (CAT) promoter-less reporter construct. CAT activity was assayed in EBV transformed cell lines transfected by these constructs. A positive regulatory element, distinct from the enhancer A sequence located in the -205/+2 construct, was characterised within the -335 to -206 region of the HLA-A11 promoter. The -335/+2 construct is 10 fold more active than the basal -90//+2 promoter construct which starts just upstream from the CAAT box and displays a 2.5 fold induction over the -205/+2 construct containing enhancer A. Mutation of protein binding sites characterised by methylation interference [6] within the -335 to +2 region allowed the identification of a regulatory element which is critical to maintain induction of transcription. Introduction of a BglII site at position -266 to -261 in the context of the 337/+2 construct resulted in a 20 fold reduction of promoter activity as compared to that of the 335/+2 construct (*Figure* 1). The integrity of this element is thus essential for the overall activity of transcription driven by the -337/+2 HLA-A promoter region.

The C-terminal Zinc fingers of the ZFX protein binds two sites within the HLA-A11 promoter

In order to further characterise the DNA-binding proteins that interact with this positive regulatory element we used a multimerised oligonucleotide spanning region

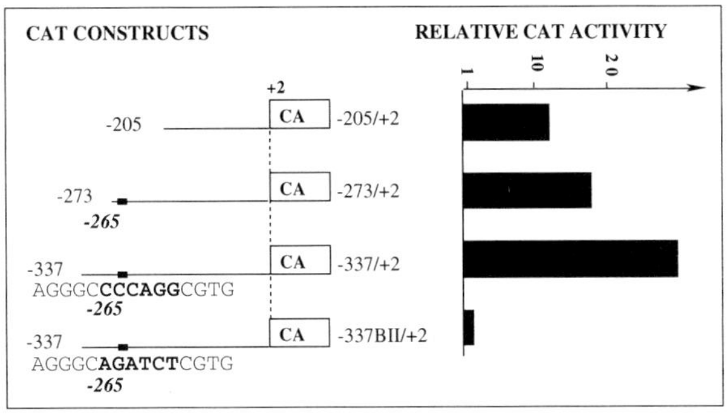

Figure 1. The -266 to -261 sequence is essential to the transcriptional activity of the HLA-A11 promoter. Functional analysis of transcriptional activity of HLA-A11 reporter constructs in a EBV transformed B cell line. Numbering is relative to the first nucleotide of exon1. Results are expressed as fold increase of CAT activity relative to the mutated -337/+2 HLA-A11 construct. Figure reproduced by permission of Oxford University Press [10].

-272 to -233 of the HLA-A11 promoter to screen a λgt11 cDNA expression library from Hela cells. We isolated a clone which displays strong specific binding to the -272/-233 site. A comparative analysis of the nucleic acid sequence of this clone shows a 100% identity with the C-terminal sequence of the ZFX gene [7]. The sequence contained in the cDNA insert starts in the middle of the ninth zinc finger of ZFX and thus retains 3 of the 13 zinc fingers found in ZFX which appear to be sufficient to bind the -272/-233 regulatory site. The DNA binding activity of the protein encoded by this cDNA was assayed by electrophoretic mobility shift assay of a fusion recombinant protein in a PGEX vector. The three C-terminal zinc fingers of the ZFX protein, produced as a GST fusion protein GST3ZF, specifically bind the -282/-250 labelled oligonucleotide (*Figure 2*). Methylation interference analysis of the interaction of the GST3ZF protein with DNA led us to define two sites centred at position -265 and -238 within the HLA-A11 promoter (8 , data not shown). Competition experiments using the two sites separated on different oligonucleotides -255/-224 and -282/-250 show that both sites abolish the binding of the three terminal zinc fingers to the radiolabelled -282/-250 site indicating that binding to each site occurs independently of the presence of the other site. The -282/-224 oligonucleotide mutated by introduction of a BglII site within the -266 to -261 positions did not interfere with binding while mutation of position -241 which was changed from A to T in the -255/-224 oligonucleotide clearly reduced the binding.

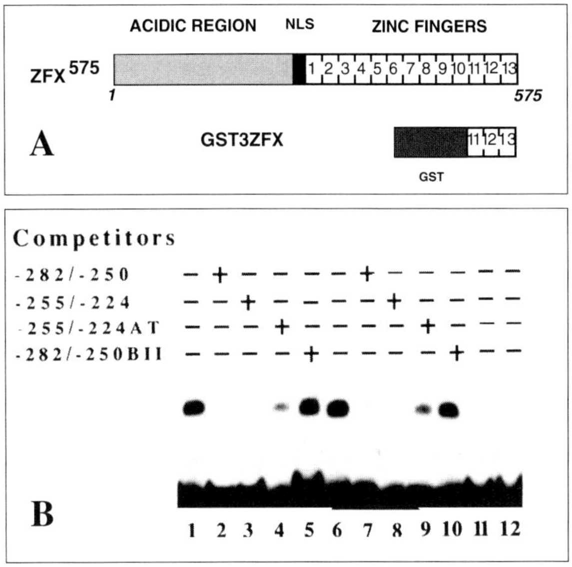

Figure 2. (A) Structure of the 575 amino acids isoform of the ZFX protein and position of the coding regions used to produce the three C terminal zinc fingers GST3ZFX fusion protein. (B) Electrophoretic mobility shift assay analysis of interaction of the purified GST3ZFX fusion protein (10ng) with the labelled HLA -A11 derived -282/-250 oligonucleotide sequence. Oligonucleotides used for competition were added in 1000 fold excess.

The ZFX protein is a positive regulator of the HLA-A11 promoter

A full length cDNA coding for the 575 Amino acids isoform of ZFX, ZFX^{575} was cloned in the eukaryotic expression vector PSG5. The effect of the $PSGZFX^{575}$ expression vector on HLA-A11 CAT reporter constructs was compared to that of the control vector PSG5 by co-transfection assays in various cell lines.

The PSG ZFX^{575} was found to stimulate the transcription of the -273/+2 promoter by a mean value of 20 fold in the murine Leydig cell line TM3 Its effect on the -205/+2 promoter CAT construct was a modest increase of 2 fold. Thus, in TM3, the main component of the transactivation was mediated through the -273/-205 region which was shown to contain binding sites for ZFX (*Figure 3*). The enhancement of the HLA-A promoter activity by ZFX was not detected in TM4, a murine Sertoli cell line nor in murine and human fibroblasts, EBV transformed B cell lines, or ATCC cell lines 293, T47D, HUT78 and thus appears to be quite specific of the TM3 cell type.

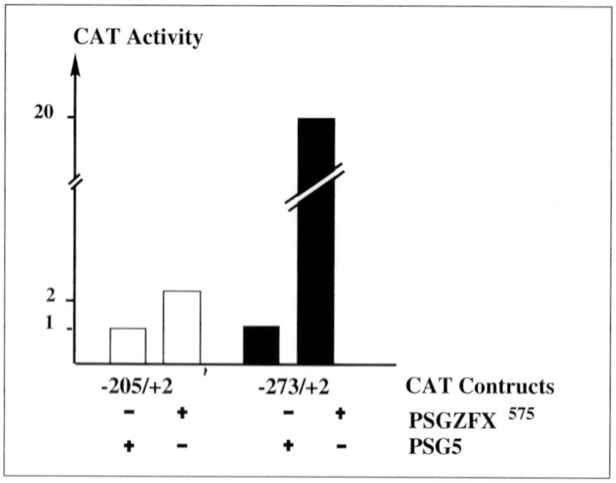

Figure 3. Transactivation of HLA-A11 promoter CAT constructs upon cotransfection with the ZFX 575 expression vector (PSGZFX575) in the TM3 leydig cell line. Control transfections are performed using the empty vector PSG5.

Discussion

We show that a critical regulatory region located in the -337 to -205 of the HLA-A11 promoter region activates transcription and that introduction of a mutation in the -266 to -261 sequence is sufficient to abolish this enhancer effect. An oligonucleotide encompassing this region was used to screen a λGT11 library and led to the identification of a partial cDNA encoding the C-terminal portion of the ZFX protein. The ZFX gene, located on the human X chromosome, is structurally similar to the ZFY gene. These genes encode highly homologous proteins containing an acidic N terminal region which activates transcription when fused to the GAL4 yeast DNA -binding domain, a nuclear localisation signal located in a short basic region and 13 zinc fingers encoded by a single exon (*Figure 2A*). Although these structural elements led to suspect the role of members of the ZFY family as transcription factors [9], we here demonstrate that this is indeed the case by defining a DNA binding site and a transcriptionnal effect of the ZFX protein. We show that the last three C-terminal zinc fingers of the ZFX protein bind to two regulatory sequences located in the -282/ -250 region of the HLA-A11 gene.

The second important aspect of this work is the fact that the 575 amino acids isoform of ZFX is able to activate transcription from an HLA-A promoter sequence through interaction with the DNA-binding site which binds the 3 C terminal zinc fingers motif. We previously described the 273/-250 region of the HLA-A11 promoter as a target for at least two transcription factors including the AP2 transcription factor which compete for their binding to overlapping sites [6]. The binding of ZFX to this same regulatory sites adds a higher level of complexity to the regulation trough this DNA element which integrity is crucial to maintain promoter activity. It is noteworthy that this transactivation level is specifically high in the Leydig cell line TM3 originating from mouse testis while it is not reproducibly observed in other cell type tested including the TM4 cell line originating from Sertoli cells of the testis. This cell type specific regulation suggests that the ZFX transcription factor may play a role in sex specific gene expression however the physiological significance of this observation remains to be established.

The ZFX binding site centred at position -265 is fairly well conserved among HLA-A, -G and E genes but is quite polymorphic when analysing sequences from the HLA-B and -C locus. This sequence is not found in a similar position of the murine MHC class I genes, however further experiments are needed to determine whether ZFX is likely to exert a locus specific regulation or whether its action is a general feature of HLA class I gene regulation. Similarly it would be interesting to evaluate the activity of other members of the ZFX family as well as other isoforms of the ZFX protein.

The identification of these co-operating or competing factors which assemble with the HLA-A11 promoter and the comprehension of their role in controlling cell specific class I transcription provides a new basis for the understanding of *in vitro* and *in vivo* physiological or pathological modulation of MHC class I transcription in human, including sexual differences observed in some of these phenomenons.

Acknowledgements

This work was supported by the Association Française contre les Myopathies (AFM) and by the Institut National de la Santé et de la Recherche Médicale (INSERM).

References

1. David-Watine B, Israël A, Kourilsky P. The regulation and expression of MHC class I genes. *Immunol Today* 1990; 11: 286-92.
2. Le Bouteiller P. HLA class I chromosomal region, genes, and products: facts and question. *Crit Rev Immunol* 1994; 14: 89-129.
3. Mc Fadden G, Kane K. How DNA viruses perturb MHC expression. *Adv Cancer Res* 1994, 63:117-209.
4. Garrido F, Cabrera T, Concha A, Glew S, Ruiz-Cabello F, Stern LP. Natural history of HLA expression during tumor development. *Immunol Today* 1993; 14:491-9.
5. Ting JPY, Baldwin AS. Regulation of MHC gene expression. *Curr Opin Immunol* 1993; 5: 8-16
6. Blanchet O, Gazin C, L'Haridon , Tatari Z, Degos L, Sigaux F, Paul P. Multiple nuclear factors bind to novel positive and negative regulatory elements upstream of the human major histocompatibility class I gene. *Int Immunol* 1994; 6: 1485-96.
7. Scheinder-Gädicke A, Beer-Romero P, Brown LG, Mardon G, Luoh SW, Page D. Putative transcription activator with alternative isoforms encoded by human ZFX gene. *Nature* 1989; 342: 708-11.
8. L'Haridon M, Paul P, Xerri JG, Dastot H, Dolliger C, Schmid M, de Angelis N, Grollet L, Sigaux F, Degos L, Gazin C. Transcriptional regulation of the MHC class I HLA-A11 promoter by the zinc finger protein ZFX. *Nucleic Acids Res* 1996; 24 (10): 1928-35.
9. Koopmann P, Ashworth A, Lovell-Badge R. The ZFY gene family in humans and mice. *Trends Genet* 1991; 7:132-6.
10. L'Haridon M, Paul P, Xerri JG, Dastot H, Dolliger C, Schmid M, de Angelis N, Grollet L, Sigaux F, Degos L, Gazin C. Transcriptional regulation of the MHC class I HLA-A11 promoter by the zinc finger protein ZFX. *Nucleic Acids Res* 1996; 24 (10): 1928-35.

Variation in HLA class I promoter sequences and differential regulation of HLA-A, -B, and -C alleles

J.L. Lee[1], D. Kim, P. Maye, N. Cereb, S.Y. Yang

1 Immunology Program, Sloan-Kettering Institute, New York, NY, USA
Laboratory of Biochemical Immunogenetics, Sloan-Kettering Institute, 1275 York Avenue, New York, NY 1002, USA

Transcriptional regulation of HLA class I genes is controlled by a series of cis-acting regulatory elements located [4] in the 5'-flanking upstream region and a variety of transcription factors that bind to them [1-3]. We have previously shown that HLA class I genes are highly polymorphic not only in the coding regions, but also in the upstream promoter where many cis-acting regulatory elements are located [4]. In that study, we showed that the κB1 site is conserved in all alleles of the HLA-A and -B genes examined, but not in the alleles of HLA-C gene. However, the κB2 site and its neighboring regions are conserved in a locus-specific manner [5]. These two tandemly arranged κB elements have been shown to play an important role in the transcription of class I genes [6]. Although HLA class I molecules are expressed in the majority of mature somatic cells, their cell surface expression is variable, tissue specific, and developmentally regulated. Cell surface expression of HLA-C gene products is relatively low. Locus-specific expression of HLA class I genes has been documented in a variety of tumor cells; many tumor cells showed a complete or selective loss of HLA-A or -B antigens [1-8]. In some cases, this is associated with the level of transcriptional factors that bind to the regulatory elements [9]. In this study, we measured the relative promoter strength for each of the locus-specific and allelic forms of HLA-A, -B, and -C promoters and examined κB-binding activities for each of the HLA class I loci.

Results and discussion

In a previous study, we identified 10 variant forms of the CRC region of HLA class I promoters, three HLA-A, three -B, and four HLA-C [5]. The upstream promoter region of these variants was amplified using locus-specific primers. Three allelic variants from the A locus represented by A2 (prototype), A26, and A30, three from the B locus represented by B7, B13 (prototype), and B37, and four from the C locus represented by Cw1 (prototype), Cw4, Cw7, and Cw17 we examined. Each of these PCR products was ligated into in a luciferase vector. Truncated CRC constructs from each locus (A2-120up, B7-120up, and Cw1-120up), and constructs which have only the CCAAT and TATA boxes of the upstream region of HLA class I (A2-TATA, B13-TATA, and Cw1-TATA) were also constructed in pGL2, the basic vector. These 10 allelic forms of the promoters in the luciferase expression vector each comprises a DNA fragment of 378 base pairs of the upstream region from each of the variants (*Figure 1*). The reporter gene assays were conducted using HLA-normal HeLa cells in transient transfection experiments. Of the 10 variants, the three HLA-A promoters showed the strongest luciferase activity, while the four HLA-C promoters showed the weakest, the HLA-B promoters showing an intermediate level. These results, represented by A2, B7, and Cw1 promoters, are shown in *Table I*. These promoter activities were correlated with the level of their transcripts in cells, as assessed by quantitative RT-PCR (data not shown). This result shows that the tandem-repeats of the κB motifs are involved in controlling the expression of the HLA-A and -B loci; compare the promoter strengths displayed by those of CRC-truncated promoter constructs (A2-120up and B7-120up). However, these CRC-truncated constructs derived from both HLA-A and -B alleles still maintain, though at reduced levels, luciferase activities. This suggests an important contribution of the enhancer B region which contains an inverted CCAAT box.

Our previous studies have shown that the two κB sites in the HLA-A2 bind two protein complexes, BI and BIII [6]. The BI complex contained the p50 homodimer and the BIII contained the p65 subunit of NF-κB. However, nei-

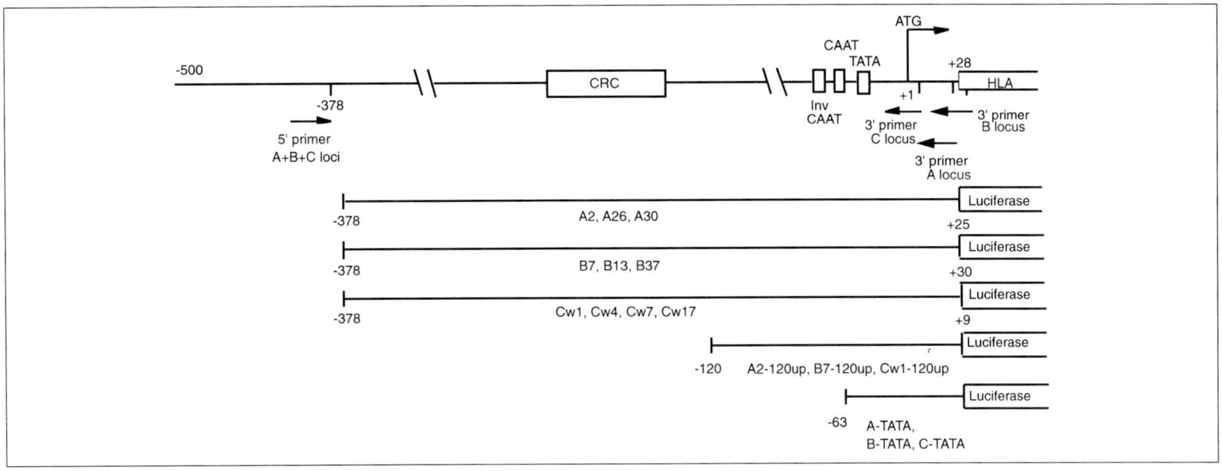

Figure 1. The upstream promoter region of HLA class I genes were amplified from A*0201, A*2601, A*3001, B*0702, B*1301, B*3701, Cw*0102, Cw*0401, Cw*0702, and Cw1701, using locus-specific primers. The amplified DNA fragment of 378 base pairs spans from -378 to +25 for A alleles, -378 to +30 for B alleles, and -378 to +9 for C alleles. All these PCR products were then ligated into Sma I-Hind III cut luciferase vector (pGL2. Basic; Promega, Madison, Wis). Truncated CRC constructs from each locus (A2-120up, B7-120up, and Cw1-120up), and constructs which having only the CCAAT and TATA boxes (A2-TATA, B13-TATA, and Cw1-TATA) were also constructed in the Sma I-Hind III site of pGL2, the basic vector. After cloning, the sequences of the constructs were confirmed using an automated sequencer (ABI 373). These reporter genes were tested in HeLa cells in transient transfection experiments. Cells were seeded into a 6-well culture plate the day before transfection at a density of 5 x 10^5 cells per well. After overnight incubation at 37°C, when cell density reached 60-70%, cells were transiently transfected using Lipofectin™ (Gibco BRL) according to the manufacture's protocol. Each transfection used 2.5 µg of luciferase reporter constructs and 0.25 µg of ß-galactosidase control vector, for normalization of transfection efficiencies. Following 48 hr incubation, cell lysates were assayed for luciferase and ß-galactosidase activity using a luciferase substrate (Promega) and Lumigal substrate (Lumigen), respectively, and read using a TopCounter (Packard Instrument.). The results in *Table I* are expressed in a relative value as a multiple of that obtained with the pGL2.Basic plasmid.

Table I. Promoter activities in luciferase reporter gene assay

Reporter construct	Relative Luciferase Activity			
	EXP #1	EXP #2	EXP #3	Mean ± S.D.
A2	286.71	218.89	138.89	214.86 ± 73.99
A2-120up	91.49	46.63	46.46	61.53 ± 25.95
A-TATA	12.23	7.94	7.50	9.23 ± 2.61
B7	174.56	162.23	112.44	149.74 ± 32.89
B7-120up	123.65	113.41	103.14	113.40 ± 10.25
B-TATA	15.05	10.04	8.86	11.32 ± 3.29
Cw1	46.23	50.31	11.81	36.12 ± 3.29
Cw1-120up	17.44	8.64	5.19	10.42 ± 6.31
C-TATA	1.55	1.34	1.78	1.56 ± 0.22
pGL2.Basic	1.00	1.00	1.00	1.00 ± 0.00

ther of them contained both the p50 and p65 subunits. Because the differential promoter activity of each locus may relate to the sequence variations in the κB sites, we examined protein binding capacity of those κB elements derived from prototypical A, B, and C promoters using nuclear extracts from unstimulated HeLa cells. Using electrophoretic gel mobility shift assays, we found no differences in binding capacity or patterns, between A- and B- loci. However, no binding was observed for the C-specific κB probe. Interestingly, although the κB2 motif of the B locus has some base substitutions, DNA binding was not affected by those variant sequences. This result is consistent with our previous observation that the κB1 site can bind both the BI and BIII complexes. It is possible that the relatively low promoter activity of HLA-B alleles compared to those of HLA-A, may be accounted for by the defect in the κB2 site. A recent report demonstrated that transactivating by, but not binding of, NF-κB is sensitive to seemingly minor sequence variations between canonical κB sites and the other κB-containing element [10].

The HLA-C-specific κB probe, which has a disruption in its palindromic κB1 sequence and substitutions in the κB2 site, showed no protein binding activity in low or high concentrations of potassium. HLA-C molecules are weakly expressed on the cells surface, at approximately 10% of the level of HLA-A or-B. It has been proposed that this low level of expression is caused by inefficient assembly and transport of the molecules [11] or by the HLA-C mRNA being unstable and rapidly degraded [12]. In this study, we have demonstrated that lower activity of the HLA-C promoter can be accounted for by the defect in the κB sites, especially the disrupted palindromic κB1 sequence.

In summary, we have shown that HLA-A alleles have the strongest promoters, and that HLA-C alleles have the weakest. These differential locus-specific promoter activities for HLA class I genes may result from the locus-specific sequence variations occurring in the κB sites. The weak expression of HLA-C alleles is apparently caused by the defect in their promoters, but other mechanisms at the post transcriptional level may also be involved.

References

1. Geragthy D. Structure of the HLA class I region and expression of its resident genes. *Curr Opin Genet Dev* 1993; 5 : 3.
2. Goust J. Major histocompatibility complex. *Immunol Series* 1993; 58 : 29.
3. Ting JY, Baldwin AS. Regulation of MHC gene expression. *Curr Opin Immunol* 1993; 5 : 8.
4. Cereb N, Yang SY. The regulatory complex of HLA class I promoters exhibits locus-specific conservation with limited allelic variation. *J Immunol* 1994; 152 : 3873.
5. Cereb N, Lee S, Maye P, Kong Y,Yang SY. Nonrandom allelic variation in the regulatory complex of HLA class I gènes. *Hum Immunol* 1994; 41 : 46-51.
6. Mansky P, Brown WM, Park JH, Yang SY. The secondary κB element, κB2, of the HLA-A class I regulatory complex is an essential part of the promoter. *J Immunol* 1994; 153 : 5082.
7. Momburg FZA, Harpprecht J, Moller P, Molgrnhauer G, Hammerling GJ. Selective loss of HLA-A or HLA-B antigen expression in colon carcinoma. *J Immunol* 1989; 142 : 352.
8. Peltenburg LTC, Schrier PI. Transcriptional suppression of HLA-B expression by c-Myc is mediated through the core promoter elements. *Immunogenetics* 1994; 40 : 54.
9. Blanchet O, Bourge J, Zinszner H, Israel A, Kourilsky P, Dausset J, Degos L, Paul P. Altered binding of regulatory factors to HLA class I enhancer sequence in human tumor cell lines lacking class I antigen expression. *Proc Natl Acad Sci USA* 1992; 89 : 3488.
10. Perkins ND, Schmid RM, Duckett CS, Leung K, Roce NR, Nabel GJ. Distinct combinations of NF-κB subunits determine the specificity of transcriptional activation. *Proc Natl Acad Sci USA* 1992; 89 : 1529.
11. Neefjes JJ, Pleogh HL. Allele and locus-specific differences in cell surface expression and the association of HLA class I heavy chain with β2-microglobulin: differential effects of inhibition of glycosylation on class I subunit association. *Eur J Immunol* 1988; 18 : 801.
12. McCutcheon JA, Smith KD, Lutz CT, Parham P. Low HLA-C expression at cell surface correlated with increased turnover of heavy chain mRNA. *J Exp Med* 1995; 181 : 2085.

Locus specific regulation of HLA class I gene expression

S.J.P. Gobin, V. Keijsers, A.M. Woltman, A. Peijnenburg, L. Wilson, P.J. Van den Elsen

Department of Immunohaematology and Blood Bank, Leiden University Hospital, PO Box 9600, 2300 RC Leiden, The Netherlands

The expression of HLA class I molecules is essential in the immune response as they present antigen-derived peptides to cytotoxic T-lymphocytes. In accordance with this key role in antigen presentation, the level of MHC class I expression is tightly controlled [1]. Regulation at the transcriptional level is mediated by several conserved *cis*-acting regulatory elements in the promoter region of MHC class I genes [1]. These include the enhancer A element, consisting of two κB-binding sites, and the flanking interferon stimulated response element (ISRE). Variation in the nucleotide sequence of these regulatory elements may explain the differential gene regulation of both the classical and non-classical HLA class I genes.

In this study, we assessed the capacity of the different regulatory elements of the promoter region of HLA-A, HLA-B, HLA-C, HLA-E, HLA-F and HLA-G to bind transcription factors of the NF-κB/Rel and interferon regulatory factor (IRF) families. This was related to the contribution of the various κB-binding sites and ISREs to transactivation, as evaluated by transient transfection studies of luciferase reporter constructs containing the various sites.

Binding properties and functioning of the κB-binding motifs in enhancer A

Electromobility shift assays using probes representing the enhancer A region of the different loci and nuclear extracts of B-cells, expressing HLA class I, revealed binding of several specific complexes. Proteins in these complexes could be identified as p50 and p65 in a so-called super-shift assay using specific antisera directed against these molecules.

The NF-κB-binding motifs κB1 and κB2 in HLA-A, κB1 in HLA-B, and κB1 in HLA-F were readily bound by protein complexes containing p50 and p65, whereas the two κB-binding motifs of HLA-G were only bound by p50 in gel shift assays (summarized in *Figure 1*). The κB-binding sites in HLA-C and HLA-E did not show any binding of specific complexes containing p50 or p65 (*Figure 1*). Whereas the κB1 site in HLA-A and HLA-B (GGGGATTCCCC) was readily bound by p50 and p65, the κB2 site of HLA-A (GGGGA<u>G</u>TCCCC), differing in one nucleotide from this concensus sequence, showed reduced binding of p50 and p65. Variation in two nucleotides from the concensus sequence in the κB1 site of HLA-F (G<u>A</u>G<u>A</u>ATTCCCC) had apparently no effect on the binding capacity of p50 and p65.

Enhancer A-containing reporter constructs were generated by cloning ds-oligonucleotides of the enhancer A sequence (κB1 and κB2) present in the various HLA genes linked to a 140 bp HLA-A2.1 promoter fragment and the luciferase gene in pGL3-Basic. In accordance with the results from the binding studies, enhancer A of HLA-A, containing two κB-binding concensus sequences, gave rise to a significant transcriptional activity in Tera-2 cells when co-transfected with p50 and p65, whereas transactivation of enhancer A of HLA-B (containing one concensus sequence) was relatively low (*Figure 1*). In contrast, none of the enhancer A of HLA-C, HLA-E, HLA-F or HLA-G gave rise to any significant NF-κB induced transactivation activity. In the case of HLA-G, this could be explained by a lack of transactivating activity by the p50 homodimer [2,3]. As concerns the enhancer A of HLA-F, lack of induced transactivation despite an apparent proper binding of NF-κB seems to be contradictory. However, it may be explained by binding specificities of p65 [3,4]. It is conceivable that p65 preferentially binds the anti-strand

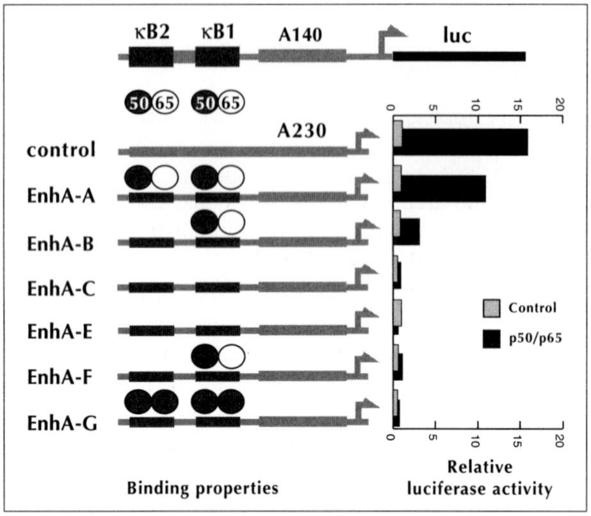

Figure 1. HLA class I gene regulation through enhancer A. Binding properties of the κB1 and κB2 sites in enhancer A (EnhA) of the various HLA class I loci as determined by electromobility shift assays. The relative contribution of enhancer A to transactivation was tested by transient co-transfection experiments in Tera-2 cells with luciferase reporter constructs containing the enhancer A region of the various HLA class I loci linked to the minimal promoter of HLA-A2.1, and RSV-driven expression vectors of p50 and p65. The β-galactosidase corrected luciferase values are expressed as the luciferase activity of the enhancer A-containing constructs divided by the luciferase activity value of pA140 and shown as mean of n=4.

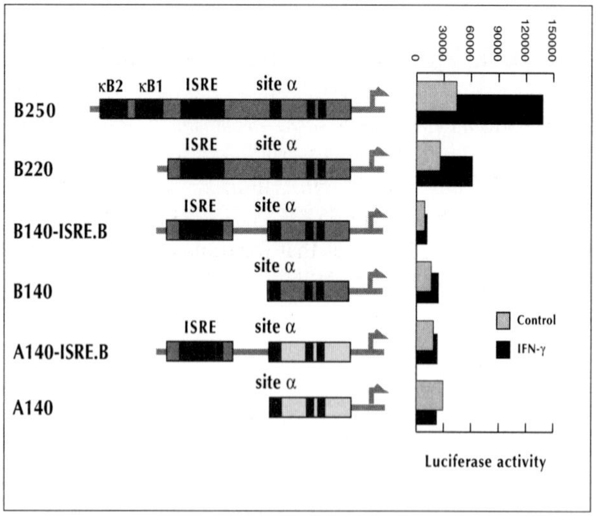

Figure 2. The 3'-flanking region of the ISRE is essential for IFN-γ-induced transactivation. The contribution of the different promoter sequences to IFN-γ-induced transactivtion was studied by transient transfection experiments in HeLa cells with luciferase reporter constructs, containing either PCR-generated HLA-B7 promoter fragments of different size or the ISRE of HLA-B linked to the minimal promoter of HLA-B7 or HLA-A2.1. The β-galactosidase corrected luciferase values are shown as mean of n=4.

of the 3' half-site in this κB motif, leading to binding of NF-κB in a reversed orientation which may not allow transactivation.

Binding properties and functioning of the ISRE and flanking sequence

Electromobility shift assays using probes representing the ISRE of the different loci and nuclear extracts from HeLa cells treated with IFN-γ, revealed binding of an IFN-γ induced complex to the ISRE of HLA-A, HLA-B/C and HLA-F (data not shown). This complex was most abundant after 2 hours of IFN-γ stimulation and still present at a reduced level after 18 hours. Further studies will be undertaken to assess the binding specificities of the ISREs of the other loci and the nature of the proteins in the ISRE-binding complexes. This complex is more likely to contain IRF-1 than other factors of the IRF family, such as ISGFγ and STAT1 since the ISGFγ/STAT1 complex can only bind this ISRE with weak affinity [5,6], but this remains to be confirmed by super-shift assays using specific antisera against these proteins.

Similar to the enhancer A-containing constructs, ISRE reporter constructs were generated by cloning ds-oligonucleotides of the ISRE sequence present in the different HLA loci linked to a 140 bp HLA-A2.1 promoter fragment and the luciferase gene in pGL3-Basic. Transient transfection experiments were performed in HeLa cells to assess the functional capacity of the different ISREs. Surprisingly, none of the cloned ISRE reporter constructs showed IFN-γ-induced transcriptional activity, whereas control constructs containing the 250 bp upstream promoter region of HLA-B7 or HLA-A2.1 were markedly induced (*Figure 2*; data not shown).

To find the possible cause of the lack of induced activity of the ISRE reporter constructs, other reporter constructs were generated. Transient transfection studies in HeLa demonstrated that the constructs with the ISRE of HLA-B linked to the 140 bp promoter fragment of either HLA-B7 or HLA-A2.1 (pB140-ISRE.B and pA140-ISRE.B, respectively) were not responsive to IFN-γ induction. However, pB220, which differs from pB140-ISRE.B only in the flanking sequence directly downstream from the ISRE, was induced by IFN-γ (*Figure 2*). This indicates that for transactivating activity mediated through the ISRE, the 3'-flanking sequence of the ISRE is required.

Conclusions

HLA class I gene expression is controlled by several conserved *cis*-acting regulatory elements of which the enhancer A and ISRE are best characterized. Locus specific variation of the nucleotide sequence within these elements allows differential regulation. In this study, it is shown that transactivation through the enhancer A is most important in HLA-A which contains two functional κB-binding motifs, and less marked through the enhancer A of HLA-B, which contains only one functional κB-binding site. The other HLA class I loci were not regulated by the enhancer A. Study on regulation through the ISREs of the different HLA loci, revealed that IFN-γ-induced transactivation was strongest for the ISRE in HLA-B/C and weak for the ISRE in HLA-A. Further, it was found that the 3'-flanking sequence is essential for functioning of the ISRE.

Acknowledgement

This research was supported by the Netherlands Organization for Research (NWO grant #901-09-200).

References

1. Le Bouteiller P. HLA class I chromosomal region, genes, and products: facts and questions. *Crit Rev Immunol* 1994 ; 14 : 89-129.
2. Kunsch C, Ruben SM, Rosen CA. Selection of optimal κB/Rel DNA-binding motifs: interaction of both subunits of NF-κB with DNA is required for trancriptional activation. *Mol Cell Biol* 1992 ; 12 : 4412-21.
3. Grilli M, Chiu JJ-S, Leonardo MJ. NF-kB and Rel: participants in a multiform transcriptional regulatory system. *Int Rev Cytol* 1993 ; 143 : 1-62.
4. Baeuerle PA, Henkel T. Function and activation of NF-κB in the immune system. *Annu Rev Immunol* 1994 ; 12 : 141-79.
5. Girdlestone J, Isamat M, Gewert D, Milstein C. Transcriptional regulation of HLA-A and -B: differential binding of members of the Rel and IRF families of transcription factors. *Proc Natl Acad Sci USA* 1993 ; 90 : 11568-72.
6. Bluyssen HAR, Muzaffar R, Vlieststra RJ, Van der Made ACJ, Leung S, Stark GR, Kerr IM, Trapman J, Levy DE. Combinatorial association and abundance of components of interferon-stimulated gene factor 3 dictate the selectivity of interferon responses. *Proc Natl Acad Sci USA* 1995 ; 92 : 5645-49.

HLA-C protein expression is regulated by regions 3′ to exon 3

J.A. McCutcheon

New York University, 345 E. 24th Street, New York, NY 10010, USA

HLA-C proteins have low cell surface expression compared with HLA-A and B molecules [1]. We demonstrated that HLA-C protein expression corresponds to mRNA levels; HLA-C mRNA levels are 2-10 fold lower than HLA-B mRNA levels [2]. Low HLA-C mRNA abundance results from a half life of approximately 30 minutes, compared with an HLA-B mRNA half life greater than 2 hours [2]. Finally, we found that low HLA-C protein expression corresponded to HLA-C sequences 3' to exon 3 [2].

Several gene families, including cytokines and proto-oncogenes, regulate protein expression by destabilizing mRNA (reviewed in [3]). The regulatory element is found in the 3' untranslated region (UTR). To determine if HLA genes contain mRNA destabilizing elements in their 3' UTR, I generated HLA-B/C chimeras exchanging the 3' UTR. In this report I present evidence suggesting that protein expression is regulated by at least two regions, one in the 3' UTR and another as yet unidentified, that act in *cis.*

Results and discussion

To determine the regulatory capabilities of HLA 3' UTRs, I generated chimeras containing either the entire coding sequence of HLA-B7 fused to the 3' UTR of HLA-Cw3 and the coding sequence of HLA-Cw3 fused to the 3' UTR of HLA-B7 (*Figure 1a*). These genes, along with parental HLA-B7 and Cw3 were transfected into 721.221, an Epstein Barr Virus transformed B lymphocyte cell line that contains no endogenous classical class I genes [4] as previously described [2]. Cell surface protein expression was determined by indirect flow cytometry using monoclonal antibodies (mAb) W6/32 and 4E (*Figure 1b*). The chimera formed from the coding sequence of HLA-B7 and the 3' UTR of HLA-Cw3 has cell surface protein expression similar to the parental HLA-B7 (*Figure 1b*, line 3), while the chimera formed from the coding region of HLA-Cw3 with the 3' UTR of HLA-B7 has double the cell surface expression of parental HLA-Cw3 (*Figure 1b*, line 4). These data show that by itself the 3' UTR of HLA-Cw3 gene has no regulatory effect, but removal of the 3' UTR permits increased protein expression. Because the cell surface expression of the chimeric Cw3/B7 (8) is lower than parental HLA-B7, this suggests that another region also controls regulation. Alone, this region can partially regulate protein expression. When combined in *cis* with the HLA-Cw3 3' UTR, complete protein regulation occurs. *Cis* acting regulatory elements that control constitutive gene expression have not been described. These data suggest that HLA-C genes are regulated by a novel mechanism.

References

1. Snary D, Barnstable CJ, Bodmer WF, Crumpton MJ. Molecular structure of human histocompatibility antigens: the HLA-C series. *Eur J Immunol* 1977; 8:580-5.
2. McCutcheon JA, Gumperz J, Smith KD, C.T. Lutz, Parham P. Low HLA-C expression at cell surfaces correlates with increased turnover of mRNA. *J Exp Med* 1995; 181:2085-95.
3. Hentze MW. Determinants and regulation of cytoplasmid mRNA stability in eukaryotic cells. *Biochem Biophys Acta* 1991; 1090:281-92.
4. Shimizu Y, DeMars R. Production of human cells expressing individual transferred HLA-A, -B, -C genes using an HLA-A,-B,-C null human cell line. *J Immunol* 1989;142:3320-8.

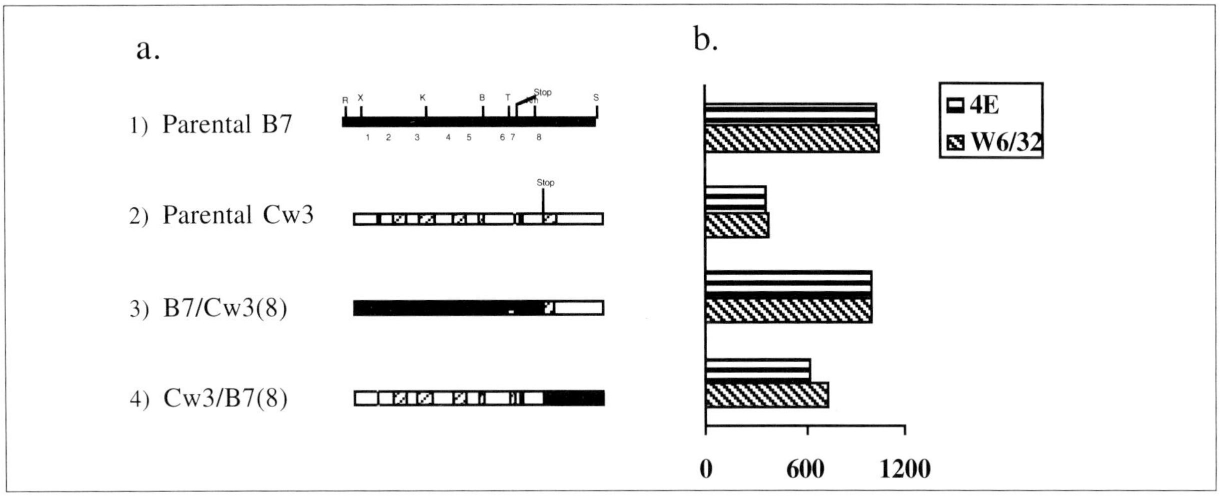

Figure 1. Effect of 3' UTR on HLA Protein Expression.
a. A schematic diagram of HLA-B7 and Cw3 parental and chimeric genes. HLA-B7 introns represented by gray boxes, exons are represented by black boxes, HLA-Cw3 introns are represented by white boxes and exons are represented by black boxes. Nomenclature: each chimera is named according to the source of the exons in parentheses, fusions between HLA-B7 and Cw3 are designated by a "/" . 1) Parental HLA-B7, 2) parental Cw3, 3) chimeric B7/Cw3(8), and 4) chimeric Cw3/B7(8). Exons are indicated by numbers below HLA-B7. Restriction enzymes are designated by the following: R=EcoRI, X=XbaI, K=KpnI, B=BsmI, T=Tth111I, Xm=XmnI, S=SalI. The translation stop site for both HLA-B7 and Cw3 has been noted.
b. Indirect flow cytometry using W6/32 and 4E. The x axis represents the change in mAb binding calculated by subtracting the mAb binding to untransfected 721.221 cells for each mAb. The y axis represents transfected cell line; the order is described above.
Methods : The chimeric B7/Cw3(8) was generated by digesting HLA-B7 KpnI to XmnI, Cw3 XmnI to SalI using standard restriction enzyme protocols. The chimeric Cw3/B7(8) was generated by digesting HLA-Cw3 KpnI to XmnI, B7 XmnI to SalI and pUC19 KpnI to SalI. The HLA-B7 and Cw3 pieces were separated on a 1% agarose gel, band isolated, and recovered using a Qiex kit (Qiagen) according to the manufacturer's instructions. All three fragments were ligated at room temperature for 4-8 hours, and the ligated plasmids transformed into H10B cells by electroporation according to the manufacturer's instructions. Positive colonies were confirmed by PvuII digestion. B7/Cw3(8) was subcloned into B7pHEBo KpnI to SalI, replacing the parental B7 gene between these restriction sites. Cw3/B7(8) was subcloned into Cw3pHEBo KpnI to SalI, replacing the parental Cw3 gene between these restriction sites. Restriction digestions, band isolations, ligations, and transformations were performed as previously described [2]. DNA for transfection was prepared using a Qiagen column (Qiagen) according to the manufacturer's instructions. Flow cytometry was performed on a Becton-Dickenson Facscan.

Promoter polymorphism of the HLA C locus

A. Volgger, Z. Yao, S. Scholz, E.D. Albert

Labor für Immungenetik, Kinderpoliklinik der LMU, Pettenkoferstrasse 8a, 80336 München, Germany

The expression of HLA C locus alleles on the cell surface is only about 10% of that of HLA A and B locus antigens [1]. Using the classical serological methods, the definition of HLA C alleles resulted in a high percentage of undetectable HLA C alleles. Using DNA typing procedures, practically all of these Cw blank alleles have been identified.

We have previously investigated the 5' untranslated regulatory region of the HLA B locus [2] and we could detect a series of nucleotide variations involving the enhancer B for HLA-B7 and B42 and in the rest of the cases substitutions outside of the known *cis*-acting elements. In this paper, we are reporting the results of the analysis of the first 350 bases upstream of the transcription initiation signal (ATG).

Materials and methods

Genomic DNA of lymphoblastoid cell lines (most of them Workshop cell lines) and homozygous and heterozygous panel individuals representing 13 HLA C locus specificities including two subtypes of Cw2, two subtypes of Cw3 and four subtypes of Cw7 have been investigated.

PCR amplification: based on the available HLA C locus sequencences [3], we constructed two primers for the amplification of the HLA C locus promoter region. The 5' sided primer (5'-GAGGCCTGGTGTAGGAGAAGAC-3') is located in the 5' untranslated region and the 3' sided primer (CTB) (5'-TCGTGGCGTCGCTGTCGAACCT-3') is placed in the intron 1 of the HLA C locus. The PCR amplification programme includes 30 cycles with denaturation at 96°C for 30 seconds, annealing at 57°C for one minute and extension at 72°C for one minute. Sequencing was performed using purified PCR products and a dideoxy-terminator cycle sequencing kit from Applied Biosystems (Foster City, California, USA). As described previously [3]. The amplification primers were also used as sequencing primers in the forward and reversed directions.

Results

Promoter sequences resulted in the identification of 18 polymorphic position and three positions at which insertions or deletions take place. The polymorphic positions are listed in *Table I.* As can be seen in *Table I*, there are 12 different promoter sequences, which means that some alleles as for example Cw6, Cw12 and Cw16 share the same promoter sequence at least in the first 350 bases upstream of the transcription initiation signal. The sequences of the promoters of the various alleles are usually fairly similar (*i.e.*, they differ only by one or two base exchanges). The most surprising feature of the HLA C promoter sequence polymorphism is the finding of a deletion for all Cw7 subtypes (from -163 to -165) and an instertion (-186 to -181) as well as a deletion (-42 to -35) for the allele Cw*1701. These deletions and insertions are the reasons for difficulties encountered in sequencing of heterozygous individuals with Cw7 or Cw17.

Discussion

The present investigation reveals a considerable polymorphism of the HLA C locus in the promoter region, of which the most outstanding feature is the presence of deletions and insertions for two alleles: Cw7 and Cw17. It has long been observed that the serological definition of Cw7 is very poorly reproducible and the question arises whether this might be due to the deletion in the

Table I.

	T -341	A -307	A -289	T -257	A -209, C-195, T -252, A - 243, C -237	T -241	G -202	T -162	A -151	A -89	G -48	G -21	C -20	G -7	Insert -186 -181	Del -42 -35	Del -163 -165	
Cw1	-	-	-	+	-	-	-	-	-	-	-	-	-	-	-	-	-	Cw1
Cw2	-	-	-	-	-	-	-	-	+	-	-	+	-	-	-	-	-	Cw2
Cw3	-	-	+	-	-	-	-	-	-	+	+	-	-	-	-	-	-	Cw3
Cw4	-	-	+	-	-	-	+	-	-	-	-	-	-	-	-	-	-	Cw4
Cw5	-	-	-	-	-	-	-	+	-	-	-	+	-	-	-	-	-	Cw5
Cw6	-	-	-	-	-	-	-	-	-	-	-	+	-	-	-	-	-	Cw6
Cw7	+	-	-	-	-	+	+	-	-	-	-	-	+	+	-	-	+	Cw7
Cw8	-	-	-	-	-	-	-	+	-	-	+	+	-	-	-	-	-	Cw8
Cw12	-	-	-	-	-	-	-	-	-	-	-	+	-	-	-	-	-	Cw12
Cw14	-	-	-	-	-	-	-	-	-	-	-	-	-	-	-	-	-	Cw14
Cw15	-	-	-	-	-	-	-	-	+	-	-	+	-	-	-	-	-	Cw15
Cw16	-	-	-	-	-	-	-	-	-	-	-	+	-	-	-	-	-	Cw16
Cw17	-	-	-	-	+	-	-	-	-	-	+	-	-	-	+	+	-	Cw17
	Cw7	Cw15	Cw3,4	Cw1, Cw8	Cw17	Cw7	Cw4, Cw7	Cw5,8	Cw15, Cw2	Cw3	Cw3, Cw17	Cw2,5, 6,8,12, 15,16	Cw7	Cw7	Cw17	Cw17	Cw7	

promoter, which reaches into the 3' end of the interferon response sequence. However, serological experience tells that Cw7 on HLA B7 haplotypes (almost always the subtype Cw*0702) is much better reproducible than Cw7 on the HLA B8 haplotype, which is almost always the subtype Cw*0701. Since all Cw7 subtypes have the same promoter sequence (at least up to position -355), it is more likely that the sequence variation observed in the transmembrane region [4] for the various Cw7 subtypes may be responsible for the above described serological observations.

The allele Cw17 is unusual, because it displays in the promoter sequence a relatively high number of substitutions, which do not occur in any other allele. This coincides with the exonic sequence, which is also somewhat apart from the other HLA C locus alleles.

References

1. Gussow D, Rein RS, Mejer I. Isolation, expression and the primary structure of HLA-Cw1 and HLA-Cw2 genes: evolutionary aspects. *Immunogenetics* 1987, 25:313-22.
2. Yang SY, Milford E, Hammerling U, Dupont B. Description of the reference panel of B-lymphoblastoid cell lines for factors of the HLA system: the B-cell line panel designed fro the 10th International Histocompatibility Workshop. In: Dupont B ed. *Immunobiology of HLA*. New York: Springer Verlag, 1989: 11-9.
3. Yao Z, Volgger A, Scholz S, Albert ED. Sequence polymorphism in the HLA-B promoter region. *Immunogenetics* 1995, 41:343-53.
4. Parham P, Lawlor DA, Lomen CE, Ennis PD. Diversity and diversification of HLA-A, B, C alleles. *J Immunol* 1989, 142:3937-50.
5. Bunce M, Welsh KI. Rapid DNA typing for HLA C using sequence-specific primers (PCR-SSP): Identification of serological and non-serologically defined HLA C alleles including several new alleles. *Tissue Antigens* 1994, 43:7-17.
6. Takiguchi M, Nishimura I, Hayashi H, Karaki S, Kariyone A, Kano K. The structure and expression of genes encoding serologically undetected HLA C locus antigens. *J Immunol* 1989, 143:1372-8.

Does HLA-Cw7 constitute a distinct family in the HLA-C locus ?

Z. Tatari[1], J.M. Cayuela[2], C. Fortier[1], C.J.T. Visser[1], C. Raffoux[1], D. Charron[1]

1 Laboratoire d'Immunologie et d'Histocompatibilité, Hôpital Saint-Louis and INSERM U.396, Paris, France
2 Laboratoire d'Hématologie moléculaire, Hôpital Saint-Louis, 1, avenue Claude Vellefaux, 75475 Paris Cedex 10, France

It has been reported that HLA-C molecules are expressed on the cell surface at levels much lower than either HLA-A or -B [1]. Different investigations suggested that levels of HLA-C mRNA in transfected cells were lower than those for other HLA class I loci [2]. However, other investigators found similar mRNA levels for HLA-B and -C in transfected B cell lines [3]. McCutcheon *et al.* [4] reported recently that the HLA-C mRNA is destabilized by a region 3' of exon3 and that its half-life is approximately 30 min while the HLA-B mRNA half-life is over 2 hours.

We investigated polymorphism of the HLA-C promotor region (-400bp to ATG). Direct sequencing was performed after a Nested-PCR and we classified the polymorphism observed in this region in 3 groups (*Table I*). We have observed that between all HLA-C promotor regions, HLA-Cw07 subtypes shared some characteristics which were specific for these alleles. Alignment and comparison of the Cw07 promotor with the promotor region of the other HLA-C alleles, HLA-B27 and H2-Ld in mice shows that the Cw07 promotor region has a distinct polymorphism more related to the HLA-B promotor region than to the other HLA-C alleles. These characteristics are summarized in *Table I*. A more interesting feature of this polymorphism is that at the NFκB site in the enhancer A region of Cw07 the critical nucleotides for protein binding are not disturbed by a mutation as is the case for the other alleles of the HLA-Cw promotor. In fact, the NFκB binding site is a perfect palindromic sequence (*Figure 1: a,b*). In the HLA-C promotor region (except Cw07), the semi palindrom 'a' has a nucleotide substitution (A instead G) which disturbs NFkB binding. The other semi palindrom 'b' is identical to the other HLA-C promotor and the difference observed with the HLA-B promotor region does not affect protein binding. Indeed, the Enhancer A region of Cw07 shared the polymorphism of both HLA-C and HLA-B (*Figure 1*).

Table I. Polymorphic positions which characterise the HLA-C promotor region

1- Polymorphic positions shared by promotor regions of all the HLA-Cw alleles comparing to HLA-B promotor region:

Positions:	- 213 T instead C
	- 157 C instead T

2- Polymorphic positions shared by promotor region of only some HLA-Cw :

- 375	T instead G	Cw14, Cw0402
- 342	C instead T	Cw0802
- 328	A instead T	Cw1601
- 310, -90	A instead G	Cw0302
- 51	G instead A	Cw0802, Cw0302

* Deletion of GAG (-357 to -359) for : Cw0602, Cw0402, Cw1601, Cw02, Cw01, Cw0501

3- Characteristic polymorphism of HLA-Cw07 compared with the other HLA-C promotor region :

Position	HLA-B27	HLA-C	HLA-Cw07
- 10	C	C	G
- 24	A	G	A
- 216	T	C	T
- 324	T	C	T
- 325	G	C	C
- 201	G	A	G

* Deletion of 3bp (-166 to -168)

```
-203                          -190
   GTT GAGGATTCTCC AC          HLA-Cw    Promotor
   GTT GGGGATTCCCC AC          HLA-B27
   GTT GGGGATTCTCC AC          HLA-Cw07
   GCT GGGGATTCCCC AC          H2-Ld
        o o o       o o
        ←           →
        a           b
        GGGRNNYYCC             Consensus
```

Figure 1. Enhancer A region. Corresponding sequences of protein-DNA interactions are shown by open circles. The arrows show the palindromic sequences (a and b).

Another characteristic of the Cw07 promotor region consists of a deletion of 3bp in position-168 to -166 following the Interferon Consensus Sequence (ICS). However, the ICS site is not disturbed (*Figure 2*).

```
-179                           -161
  GTTTCACTTCT TCTCCCAA          HLA-Cw     Promotor
  GTTTCACTTCT TCTCCCAA          HLA-B27
  GTTTCACTTCT . . . CCCAA       HLA-Cw07
  o      o   o    o
```

Figure 2. Interferon Consensus Sequence. Corresponding sequences of protein-DNA interactions are shown by open circles and the deletion is shown by (.).

Regarding the functional consequence of these polymorphisms, we have investigated the expression of Cw07 and compared its expression with the other HLA-Cw alleles. A northern blot, comparing the mRNA level of Cw07 with that of Cw0402, Cw0501, Cw0602 suggests that Cw07 is transcribed about two times more than the others. This result was supported by Quantitative- comparative/ PCR, where we compared the mRNA level of Cw07 relative to Cw05. This experiment shows that Cw07 is 2 or 3 times more transcribed than Cw05 (data not shown).

A previous study demonstrated [5] that in Gorilla gorilla (Gogo) a primate closely related to Homo sapiens and estimated to have diverged from a common ancestor 7-10 million years ago, there are two groups of Gogo-C sequences which are exceptionally divergent: Gogo C*01 and Gogo C*02. Comparison of the Gogo-C and HLA-C alleles reveals that the Gogo-C*02 group is more closely related to HLA-Cw07 than they are to Gogo-C*01. Moreover, Zemmour *et al.* [6] reported that Cw07 has a high degree of nucleotide substitution which distinguished them from the other alleles of HLA-C locus. Distinct restriction fragment length polymorphism patterns observed by Duceman *et al.* [7] suggested that HLA-Cw07 could be the product of a distinct but closely related locus. However, it has never been found that HLA haplotypes are expressing more than one HLA-C gene. The previous studies and the results obtained in our study about the polymorphism of the promotor region of HLA-Cw07 are in favor of the hypothesis that HLA-C locus possess two highly distinct families of alleles: Cw07 and the others. HLA-Cw07 may constitute an example of trans-species evolution of class I polymorphism described by Klein *et al.* [8].

References

1. Snary D, Barnstable CJ, Bodmer WF, Crumpton MJ. Molecular structure of human histocompatibility antigens : the HLA-C series. *Eur J Immunol* 1997 ; 8 : 580-5.
2. Shimizu Y, DeMars R. Production of human cells expressing individual transferred HLA-A, -B, -C genes using an HLA-A, -B, -C null human cell line. *J Immunol* 1989 ; 142 : 3320-8.
3. Tibensky D, Decary F, Delovitch TL. HLA-C genes are transcribed in HLA-C blank individuals. *Immunogenetics* 1988 ; 27 : 220-4.
4. McCutcheon J, Gumperz J, Smith KD, Lutz CT, Parham P. Low HLA-C expression at cell surfaces correlates with increased turnover of heavy chain mRNA. *J Exp Med* 1995 ; 181 : 2085-95.
5. Lawlor DA, Warren E, Taylor R, Parham P. Gorilla class I major histocompatibility complex alleles : Comparison to human and champanzee class I. *J Exp Med* 1991 ; 174 : 1491-509.
6. Zemmour J, Parham P. Distinctive polymorphism at the HLA-C locus : implications for the expression of HLA-C. *J Exp Med* 1992 ; 176 : 937-50.
7. Duceman EW, Ness D, Rendi R, Chorney MJ, Srivastava R, Greenspan DS, Pan J, Weissman SM, Grumet FC. HLA-JY 328 : mapping studies and expression of a polymorphic HLA class I gene. *Immunogenetics* 1986 ; 23 : 90.
8. Klein J. Origin of major histocompatibility complex polymorphism : the trans-species hypothesis. *Hum Immunol* 1987 ; 19 : 155.

IK: a new protein involved in the regulation of the MHC class II antigens expression

J. Vedrenne , D.J. Charron, P. Krief

INSERM U 396, Institut Biomédical des Cordeliers, 15, rue de l'École de Médecine, 75006 Paris, France

Major histocompatibility complex (MHC) class II antigens surface expression by the professional antigen presenting cells (APCs) is a pivotal aspect for a time adapted and a specific immune response. In our laboratory we have recently characterized a secreted factor (called IK) which inhibits the IFN-γ induced MHC class II antigens expression [1, 2]. Preliminary RT/PCR experiments *(Figure 1)* have led to the observation that the IK specific mRNA is less expressed in the MHC class II positive parental Raji cell line than in its MHC class II negative mutant RJ 2.2.5 [3]. These two cell lines provide the *in vitro* model used here to study the role of IK protein in the regulation of constitutive MHC class II expression.

Stable IK-transfection experiments of Raji cells were performed in order to express this protein in B cells which previously exhibit a wild type CIITA mRNA expression and a normal surface MHC class II level. RT/PCR analysis *(Figure 2A)* shows that 16 resistant transfected clones express the exogenous IK RT/PCR product. *Figure 2B* describes absence of specific HLA-DR RT/PCR product in these cells. In contrast, clones which have not integrated the exogenous IK mRNA still express the HLA-DR mRNA. The over-expression of IK protein in Raji cells may be related to a strong down-regulation of constitutive HLA-DR transcription inducing the lack of MHC class II antigens on the cell surface (data not shown). Class II transactivator (CIITA) is essential for both the IFN-γ induced and the constitutive MHC class II expression [4, 5]. This observation led us

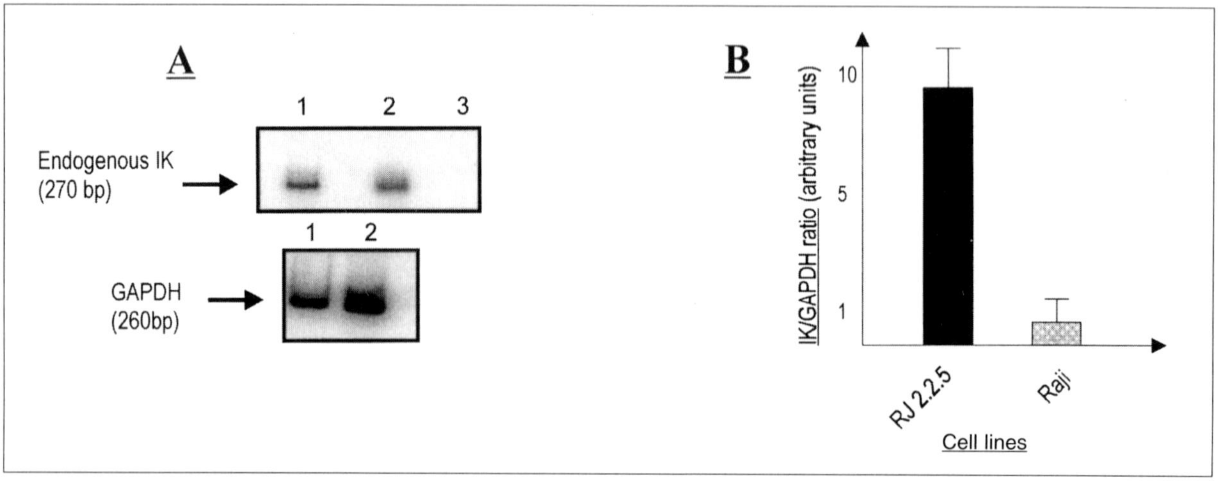

Figure 1. (A) High sensitive RT/PCR analysis of IK mRNA allows the detection of an endogenous IK-specific amplification product (270 bp) in RJ 2.2.5 (lane 1) but also in Raji cells (lane 2). Lane 3: negative control of PCR amplification carried out without cDNA. (B) In comparison with the intensity of the GAPDH amplification product we show that endogenous IK mRNA is more highly expressed in RJ 2.2.5 cells than in Raji cell line.

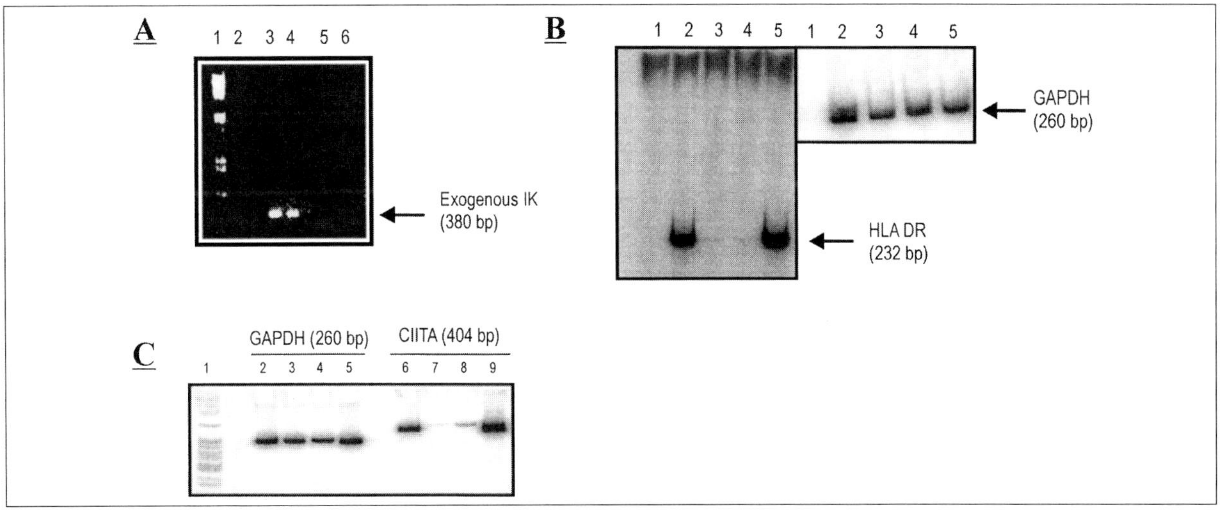

Figure 2. (A) Ethidium bromide revelation of IK-specific RT/PCR products (380 bp) shows the presence of exogenous IK mRNA in stably IK-transfected Raji cells (lanes 3 and 4). This signal is logically not detected in Raji/pHyg cells (lanes 5 and 6). Lane 2: negative control of PCR amplification carried out without cDNA. (B) High sensitive RT/PCR analysis of HLA-DR mRNA. As previously described, Raji cells (lane 2) are positive for HLA-DR mRNA expression and RJ 2.2.5 (lane 3) negative. Moreover, the HLA-DR specific RT/PCR signal (232 bp) is totally reduced in Raji/pCDM8-IK clones (lane 4) in contrast with the result observed in Raji/pHyg cells (lane 5). Lane 1: negative control of PCR amplification carried out without cDNA. (C) High sensitive RT/PCR analysis shows as previously described the lack of CIITA transcript expression in RJ 2.2.5 (lane 7) in contrast with the expression observed in Raji cell line (lane 6). Lane 8 shows the inhibitory effect of IK over-expression on CIITA transcript level in Raji/pCDM8-IK cells (lane 8). No effect is detected in Raji-pHyg-transfected clones (lane 9).

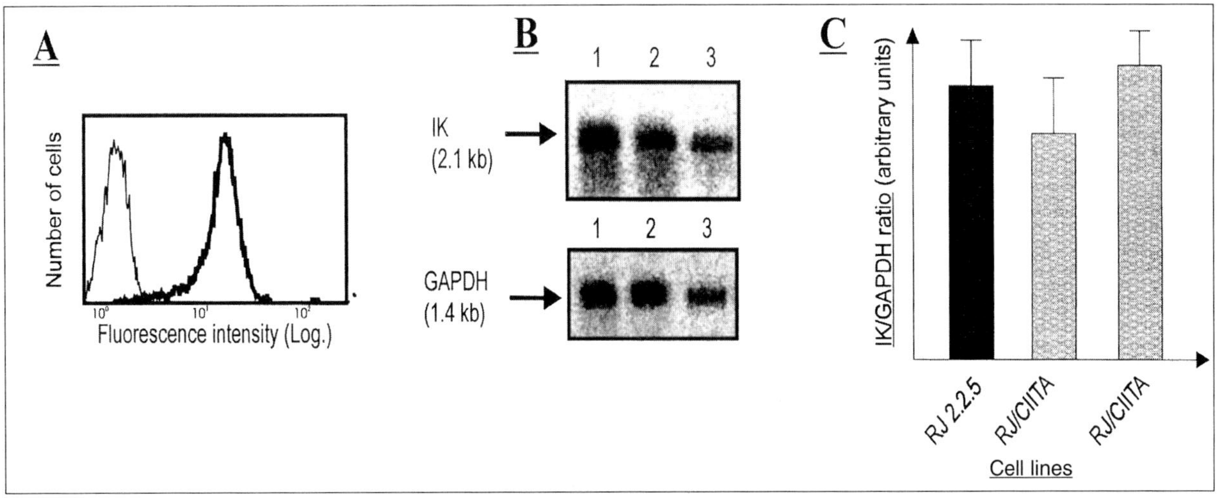

Figure 3. (A) Flow cytometric analysis of HLA-DR surface expression on CIITA-transfected RJ 2.2.5 cells shows the recovery of a positive HLA-DR phenotype. (B and C) Northern blot assay on mRNA extracted from CIITA-transfected RJ 2.2.5 cells and GAPDH-relative quantification show the absence of modulation in IK transcript level between RJ 2.2.5 cells (lane 1) and two CIITA-transfected RJ 2.2.5 clones (lanes 2 and 3).

to assess the CIITA mRNA level by RT/PCR analysis after stable IK-transfection. This experiment described a strong decrease in CIITA mRNA expression in the exogenous IK-positive clones *(Figure 2C)*.
The cytoplasmic localization of the IK protein suggests an indirect inhibition of CIITA transcription due to the sequestration in the cytoplasm of one or more CIITA positive transcriptional factors. These protein/protein interactions demonstrate the importance of proteins levels (IK, CIITA, not identified IK-ligand) in the regulation of MHC class II expression. Differences in HLA-DR phenotype may be driven by these proteins ratios. For example Raji cells may express IK protein below the threshold level which induces CIITA transcriptional inhibition. Moreover, over-expression of IK protein could indirectly maintains a low CIITA expression level responsible of a latent HLA-DR transcription repression state.
To acknowledge the mechanism by which IK influences the constitutive MHC class II expression we have analyzed modulations of IK mRNA level in CIITA-transfected RJ 2.2.5 cells. Restoration of CIITA expression is confirmed by the high HLA-DR surface expression observed in 28 resistant clones *(Figure 3A)*. Northern blot analysis shows no detectable modulation of endogenous IK transcription in these transfected cells *(Figure 3 B, C)*. The regulation of IK mRNA expression is not driven by CIITA. These results suggest that IK acts upstream of CIITA in the MHC class II regulatory pathway.
Characterization of potent intracellular IK-ligand(s) will be of great interest in the understanding of IK-mediated regulation of MHC class II expression.

References

1. Krief P, Boucheix C, Billard C, Mishal Z, Van Agthoven A, Fiers W, Azzarone B. Modulation of expression of class II histocompatibility antigens by secretion of a cellular inhibitor in K562 leukemic cells. *Eur J Immunol* 1987; 17: 1021-5.
2. Krief P, Augery-Bourget Y, Plaisance S, Merck MF, Assier E, Tanchou V, Billard M, Boucheix C, Jasmin C, Azzarone B. A new cytokine (IK) down regulating HLA class II: monoclonal antibodies, cloning, and chromosome localization. *Oncogene* 1994; 9: 3449-56.
3. Accolla RS. Human B cell variants immunoselected against a single Ia antigen subset have lost expression of several Ia antigen subsets. *J Exp Med* 1983; 157: 1053-8.
4. Steimle V, Otten LA, Zufferey M, Mach B. Complementation cloning of an MHC class II transactivator mutated in hereditary MHC class II deficiency (or bare lymphocyte syndrome). *Cell* 1993; 75: 135-46.
5. Steimle V, Siegrist CA, Mottet A, Lisowska-Grospierre B, Mach B. Regulation of MHC class II expression by interferon-gamma mediated by the transactivator gene CIITA. *Science* 1994; 265: 106-9.

Allele-specific transcriptional control of HLA-DQB1 is cell-type dependent

J.S. Beaty, G.T. Nepom

Virginia Mason Research Center, Seattle, Washington 98101, USA and Department of Immunology, University of Washington School of Medicine, Seattle, Washington 98195, USA

Expression of HLA-DQB1 is regulated largely at the transcriptional level by a set of DNA sequence elements, including the W, X1, X2 and Y boxes shared by all HLA class II genes (reviewed in [1] and [2]). Expression of HLA-DR, DQ and DP genes is often coordinate [3], but isotype-specific transcriptional control elements exist, as well [4]. In the region immediately 5' of the X1 element, alleles of the DQB1 locus contain sequences of two distinct types, differing by the presence or absence of the specific dinucleotide, TG. We have shown that equivalent fragments of the 5' regions of two alleles which differ at this site, DQB1*0301 and *0302, drive expression of the chloramphenicol acetyltransferase (CAT) reporter gene with different efficiencies in transient transfections of human B lymphoblastoid cells (B-LCL) [5]. This polymorphism affects regulation of transcription through two mechanisms: by changing the spacing between the W and X1 boxes and by changing the pattern of regulatory protein binding near the X1 element [6]. The increased W-X1 spacing in DQB1*0302 due to the presence of the TG dinucleotide at positions -180/-179 is the dominant effect and it correlates with reduced expression compared to that of the *0301 allele. A similar optimal spacing restriction occurs between the W-X1 elements of the DRA gene [7]. The presence of TG in *0302 is also associated with the binding of a nuclear protein that is missing from the array of DNA binding proteins interacting with the *0301 allele. Although this factor appears to be a strong positive effector of transcription, the effect of its binding to the *0302 regulatory region is superseded by the transcriptional down-regulating effect of the increased W-X1 spacing. Recently, the gene encoding this DQB1*0302-binding protein was cloned and sequenced in our laboratory; the protein has been identified as the zinc finger transcription factor,YY1 [8]. YY1 participates in the transcriptional control of a broad range of genes and can function as either a repressor or activator of transcription, depending on the structural context of the YY1 binding site in these regulatory regions [9]. Transcription of HLA-DRA is enhanced by the binding of YY1 to a site in the first exon of that gene; elements with significant sequence similarity are located downstream of the transcriptional start sites in DRB, DPA and B, and DQA, but interestingly, not in DQB [10].

The functional significance of such transcriptional regulatory sequence polymorphism has been confirmed by results of steady-state DQB1 mRNA analysis. Quantitative RT-PCR of the allele-specific mRNAs derived from endogenous DQB1*0301 and *0302 in heterozygous primary skin fibroblasts showed that interferon-γ (IFN-γ) induced transcription of *0301 occurs earlier and at higher levels than does *0302 expression [6]. The level of *0301 mRNA is about seven-fold higher than *0302 mRNA levels after 24 h. induction, for example [6]. To determine if the allele-specific difference in DQB1 mRNA levels observed in these cells was reflected by an earlier and higher level appearance of DQ3.1 protein on the cell surface, cells from the same experiment were harvested and treated with DQ3.1- and 3.2-specific antibodies and analyzed by flow cytometry. Over the course of IFN-γ treatment, the DQ3.1 level at the cell surface steadily increased, while that of DQ3.2 increased only slightly (*Figure 1*). In other words, the relative cell surface levels of DQ proteins in these DQB1-heterozygous cells exactly paralleled the relative levels of the *0301 and *0302 specific mRNA species which encoded them.

The appearance of DQ protein at the cell surface in these experiments lagged behind the appearance of DQB1-

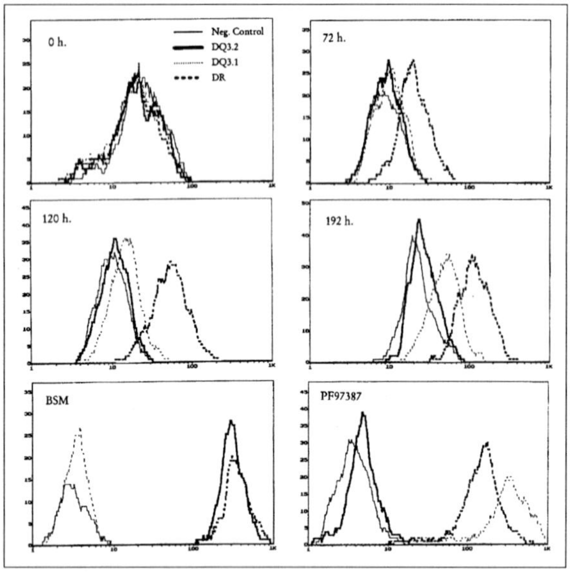

Figure 1. Cell surface expression of DQ proteins following induction. Flow cytometry of IFN-γ treated DQB1-heterozygous primary skin fibroblasts, stained with the following 1° antibodies: anti-IG2 (NN4, negative control), anti-DQ3.2 (200.1), anti-DQ3.1 (159.1) and anti-DR (L243). The 2° antibody was FITC-conjugated goat anti-mouse IgG. BSM and PF97387 are B-LCL which are DQB1*0302/*0302 and DQB1*0301/*0301, respectively.

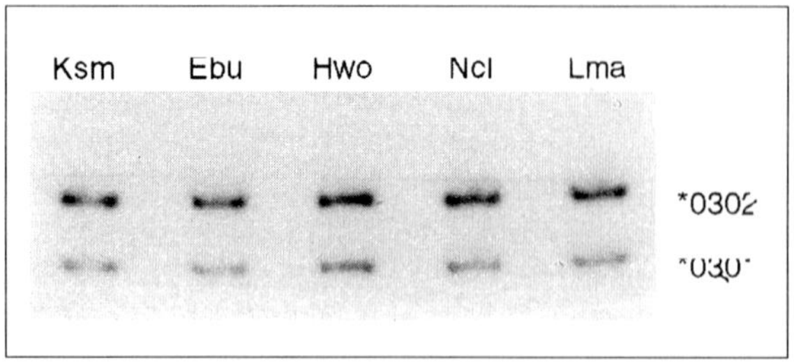

Figure 2. Comparison of DQB1 expression in primary skin fibroblasts and adherent PBL obtained from the same DQB1-heterozygous individual. Gel electrophoresis of HpaII-treated RT-PCR products which were generated from fibroblasts treated with IFN-γ for 120 h. and adherent PBL is described in [6]. BSM and PF97387 are B-LCL which are DQB1*0302/*0302 and DQB1*0301/*0301, respectively.

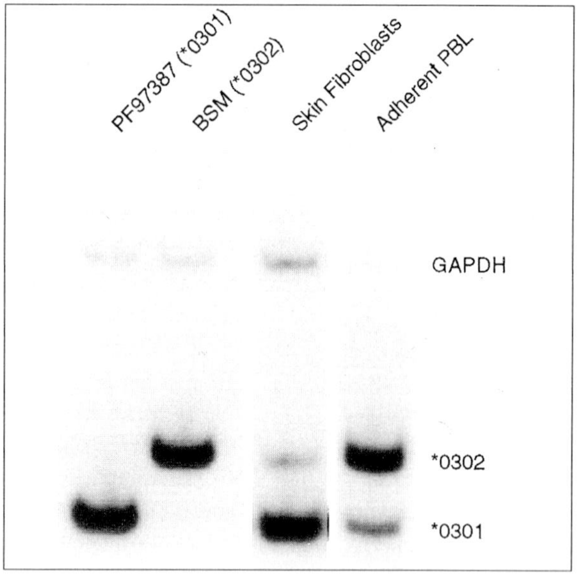

Figure 3. Steady-state levels of DQB1*0301 and *0302 mRNAs in heterozygous EBV-transformed B-LCL. Gel electrophoresis of HpaII-treated RT-PCR products [6].

specific mRNA within the IFN-γ treated primary fibroblasts by approximately 72 hours. Expression of DQ genes also lagged significantly behind that of DR, which appeared on the cell surface less than 48 hours after IFN-γ induction. Enhanced induction of DQB1 occured when primary skin fibroblasts were treated with IFN-γ plus GM-CSF compared to IFN-γ alone, although the ratio of DQB1*0302 to *0301 mRNAs was unaffected (not shown). No synergy was observed when cells were treated with IFN-γ and IL-4 together.

These differential levels of DQ allelic expression were detected using the inducible fibroblasts, but not with B-LCL, which constitutively express HLA-DQ. Both DQ3.2 and DQ3.1 molecules are expressed at high levels on B-LCL and no consistent differences in allelic expression were apparent by FACS analysis of cell surface staining. To investigate the transcriptional expression in B-LCL and in other lymphoid cell populations, we compared the fibroblast transcript patterns derived by RT-PCR with similar studies of autologous and HLA-matched peripheral blood lymphocytes (PBL) and B-LCL.

Quantitative RT-PCR of the allele-specific mRNAs from heterozygous DQB1*0301/*0302 donors were performed on primary skin fibroblasts and on adherent PBL (*Figure 2*). As summarized in *Table I*, relative patterns of expression were highly tissue-specific. In each case, the DQB1*0302 and *0301 transcripts were different from each other, with the hierarchy reversed between the cell types. DQB1*0301 was consistently 4.5 to 7-fold higher in induced fibroblasts; DQB1*0302 was consistently about 5-fold higher in adherent PBL. DQB1 genes were fully induced in these PBL; mRNA levels and the relative amounts of transcript from each allele were unaffected by treatment with IFN-γ.

Table I. Relative expression of HLA-DQB1*0301 and *0302 is tissue-specific

DQB1 Heterozygous Tissue Donor	Cell Type	Relative Expression Levels of Endogenous DQB1 Alleles
RuFo	1° Skin Fibroblast	0301>0302
	Adherent PBL	0302>0301
PaBr	1° Skin Fibroblast	0301>0302
	Adherent PBL	0302>0301
GlSc	1° Skin Fibroblast	0301>0302
	Adherent PBL	ND

DQB1 allele-specific expression was determined by quantitative RT-PCR [6]. Primary skin fibroblasts were treated with 250 U IFN-γ per ml.

Figure 3 shows the results of similar experiments using five different DQB1 heterozygous Epstein Barr virus-transformed B-LCL. In each cell line, while the *0302 and *0301 mRNA levels were also different from each other, the hierarchy was reversed from that observed in primary skin fibroblasts. Depending on the cell line, DQB1*0302 was present at levels which were from 3- to 5-fold higher than those of *0301.

The cell-type dependence of DQB1 allele-specific transcriptional control described here is most likely due to qualitative and/or quantitative differences in the nuclear proteins which are required for normal expression of the gene. It is possible, for example, that YY1, which may be responsible for most of the allele-specific expression differences in DQB1, is differentially expressed in various cell types. Tissue-specific variation in expression of particular HLA alleles may contribute to specificity of immune regulation and, possibly, autoimmunity by influencing the threshold of site-specific immune activation.

Acknowledgments

This work was supported by grant DK41801 from the National Institutes of Health.

References

1. Glimcher LH, Kara CJ. Sequences and factors: a guide to MHC class II transcription. *Annu Rev Immunol* 1992 ; 10 : 13-49.
2. Mach B, Steimle V, Martinez-Soria E, Reith W. Regulation of MHC class II genes: lessons from a disease. *Annu Rev Immunol* 1996 ; 14 : 301-31.
3. Benoist C, Mathis D. Regulation of major histocompatibility complex class-II genes: X, Y and other letters of the alphabet. *Annu Rev Immunol* 1990 ; 8 : 681-715.
4. Ono SJ, Song Z. Mapping of the interaction site of the defective transcription factor in the class II major histocompatibility complex mutant cell line clone-13 to the divergent X2-box. *J Biol Chem* 1995 ; 270 : 6396-402.
5. Andersen LC, Beaty JS, Nettles JW, Seyfried CE, Nepom GT, Nepom BS. Allelic polymorphism in transcriptional regulatory regions of HLA-DQB genes. *J Exp Med* 1991 ; 173 : 181-92.
6. Beaty JS, West KA, Nepom GT. Functional effects of a natural polymorphism in the transcriptional regulatory sequence of HLA-DQB1. *Mol Cell Biol* 1995 ; 15 : 4771-82.
7. Vilen BJ, Penta JF, Ting JPY. Structural constraints within a trimeric transcriptional regulatory region: Constitutive and interferon-gamma inducible expression of the HLA-DRA gene. *J Biol Chem* 1992 ; 267 : 23728-34.
8. Sukiennicki T, Beaty JS, Nepom GT. *In preparation* 1996.
9. Shi Y, Seto E, Chang LS, Shenk T. Transcriptional repression by YY1, a human GLI-Kruppel-related protein, and relief of repression by adenovirus E1A protein. *Cell* 1991 ; 67 : 377-88.
10. Hehlgans T, Strominger JL. Activation of transcription by binding of NF-E1 (YY1) to a newly identified element in the first exon of the human DRα gene. *J Immunol* 1995 ; 154 : 5181-7.

Molecular basis for differences in the transcriptional activities of HLA-DRB genes in different haplotypes

X. Qiu, D.P. Singal

Department of Pathology, McMaster University Hamilton, Ontario, L8N 3Z5 Canada

The HLA class II (DR,DQ,DP) molecules of the human major histocompatibility complex, which are expressed on the surface of immunocompetent cells such as B lymphocytes, activated T cells and macrophages, present foreign antigenic peptides to peripheral helper T lymphocytes for initiating specific immune responses and to immature thymic T cells for education. These antigens therefore play a crucial role in regulation of immune response and in generation of T cell repertoire in the thymus. Since the expression of class II antigens on antigen presenting cells affects the extent of T cell activation and immune response, the level of cell-surface expression of these molecules determines the quality of immune response. For example, differences in level of expression of DRB1 and DRB3 genes restrict and activate distinct CD4+ T lymphocytes.

The expression of HLA class II genes is transcriptionally regulated by a complex interaction between the *cis*-acting elements and the *trans*-acting factors. The cis-acting elements consist of DNA sequences primarily localized to the proximal promoter region and contain a series of conserved sequence motifs, including from 3' to 5' direction the TATA, CCAAT, Y, X2, X1 and W boxes. We and others have reported polymorphisms in the conserved consensus motifs in promoter regions of DRB genes [1]. The polymorphisms in some of the conserved motifs affected DNA-protein interactions in the gel mobility shift assay and the promoter strength in the CAT assay [2-7]. In the present study, we utilized normal and mutated promoter elements and examined the effect of polymorphisms in the X1 and Y box motifs on the transcriptional activity of DRB1 promoters. In addition, we examined the effect of these polymorphisms in binding *trans*-regulatory proteins.

Materials and methods

Genomic DNA from homozygous B lymphoblastoid cell lines, belonging to the DR1 and DR51, DR52 and DR8, and DR53 haplotype groups, obtained from the Tenth International Histocompatibility Workshop, were separately amplified for promoter regions of DRB genes by PCR [1]. The PCR-amplified DNA was ligated into Bluescript KS^- vector and competent cells (DHα) were transformed. DNA isolated from multiple clones in each case was separately sequenced. The promoter alleles were assigned to DRB1 genes in different haplotypes on the basis of similarities in the transcript and signal peptide region sequences [3,4]. Site-directed point mutations were introduced at position -183 in the X1 box and at position -150 in the Y box of DRB1 promoter in different haplotype groups by PCR [5].

For construction of plasmids, 243 bp (-223 to +20) DRB1 promoter fragments were subcloned in the pCAT basic plasmid to generate plasmids containing promoters of DRB1 genes from different haplotype groups as well as those with site-directed point mutations in the X1 and Y box motifs. The construction integrity of various normal and mutant DRB1 promoter-CAT constructs was confirmed by sequence analyses. Plasmid pCH110 containing the simian virus 40 early promoter encoding β-galactosidase was used as control for transfection efficiency. Raji cells were transfected with plasmid constructs by the DEAE-dextran method, incubated for 48h, harvested and lysed by repetitive freeze-thaw cycles. CAT activity was normalized with values of β-galactosidase assay and relative strengths of different promoter constructs were calculated.

The gel mobility shift assays with nuclear proteins from a homozygous B lymphoblastoid cell line (BM14) and double-stranded oligonucleotides containing polymorphic nucleotides in the X1 box (position -183) and the Y box (position -150) were performed as described previously [2,5]. Competition experiments were performed with unlabeled double-stranded oligonucleotides.

Results and discussion

The nucleotide sequences of DRB1 promoters in different DR haplotype (DR1 and DR51, DR52 and DR8, and DR53) groups showed polymorphisms in various consensus motifs (X1 = -183, Y = -150, CCAAT = -125, and TATA = -88) and in spacers (-166, -137, -121, -99, and -98) between these boxes (*Figure 1*). In the DR1, DR51 haplotype group the CCAAT box is mutated to CCAAC sequence and the Y box carries an inverted CCAAT motif. In contrast, the CCAAT box is unmutated in the DR52, DR8 and DR53 haplotype groups and the Y box has a nucleotide substitution resulting in an imperfect inverted CCAAT sequence.

The relative CAT activities of different pDRB1 CAT plasmids showed that the activity of DRB1 promoters in the DR1, DR51 haplotype group is about four- to five-fold higher ($p<0.0005$) than that of DRB1 promoters in DR52 and DR8, and DR53 groups (*Figure 1*).

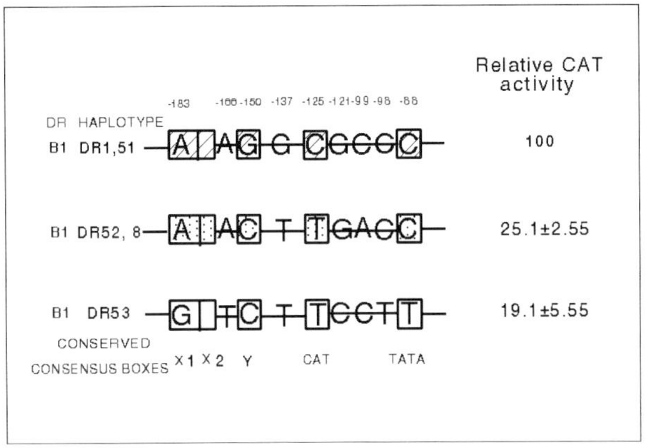

Figure 1. Nucleotide polymorphisms and relative CAT activities of upstream promoter regions of DRB1 genes in the DR1 and DR51, DR52 and DR8, and DR53 haplotype groups.

To elucidate the functional role of polymorphisms in the X1 box at position -183 and in the Y box at position -150, we mutated these boxes in DRB1 promoters in various DR haplotype groups. The transcriptional activities of these mutated promoters were compared with those of parental elements in the respective DR haplotype group (*Figure 2*). It is evident that in the DR1,DR51 group, substitution of nucleotide A by G at position -183 in the X1 box and of nucleotide G by C at position -150 in the Y box significantly reduced the CAT activity. In the DR53 group, substitution of nucleotide G by A at position -183 in the X1 box caused slight but non-significant increase in the promoter strength. In contrast, substitution of nucleotide C by G at position -150 in the Y box, and of nucleotide G by A in the X1 box and C by G in the Y box significantly increased the CAT activity. Similarly, substitution of nucleotide C by G at position -150 in the Y box of DRB1 promoters in the DR52 group significantly enhanced the promoter strength. These results show that polymorphisms in both the X1 and Y box motifs affect the transcriptional activities of DRB1 promoters. In addition, the present data suggest that the Y box with an inverted CCAAT sequence enhances the promoter strength, whereas the Y box with an imperfect inverted CCAAT motif has an inhibitory effect on the transcriptional activity of DRB1 promoters.

We then carried out gel mobility shift assays with polymorphic X and Y box oligonucleotides (XB1.1, XB1.2, YB1.1 and YB1.2) and nuclear proteins from a B cell line. The results with polymorphic X box-specific oligonucleotides showed that polymorphism at position -183 affected protein-DNA interactions (data not

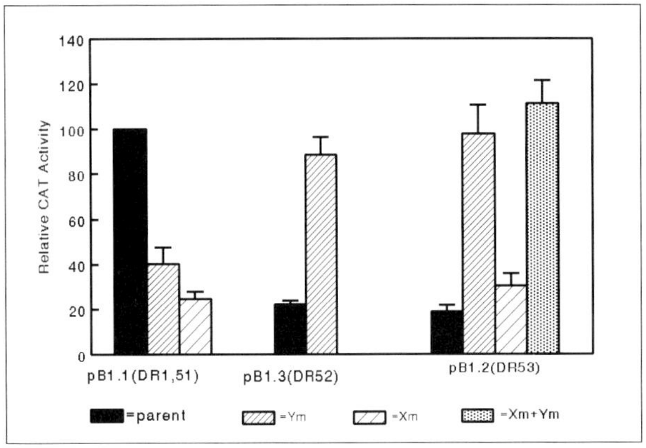

Figure 2. Relative activities of CAT reporter plasmids containing normal (parent) DRB1 promoters from the DR1 and DR51 (pB1.1), DR53 (pB1.2), and DR52 (pB1.3) haplotype groups, and the mutated (Ym, Xm and Xm+Ym) DRB1 promoter fragments.

shown). The protein-DNA complex showed specificity in that it was inhibited only by the relevant oligonucleotide. Similarly, when oligonucleotide YB1.2 containing imperfect inverted CCAAT sequence was used as a probe, the protein-DNA complex was competed efficiently only with YB1.2. In contrast, when Y box oligonucleotide (YB1.1) containing an inverted CCAAT motif was used as a probe, the protein-DNA complex was competed equally by both YB1.1 and YB1.2 oligonucleotides. These results suggest that the *trans*-regulatory nuclear proteins have higher affinity for YB1.2 than for YB1.1.

We now extend our earlier studies on DRB1 promoters in the DR1 and DR51, and DR53 haplotype groups to the DR52 and DR8 group and show that the substitution of a single nucleotide in both the X1 and Y box motifs play a dominant role on the promoter strength in the transfection experiments [5]. In addition, the present data demonstrate that polymorphisms in the X and Y box elements result in variations in binding nuclear proteins in the gel mobility shift assay. The results in the present study on the dominant role of the X-box region on the transcriptional activity of DRB1 promoters are in agreement with those published earlier [5-7]. The present data further demonstrate that nucleotide polymorphism at position -150 in the Y box also plays a dominant role on the level of expression of DRB1 genes, as suggested by us earlier [5]. In addition, the results in the present study extend earlier data in that the binding affinities of Y box-binding nuclear proteins (NF-Y and NF-YB) have inverse relationships to the promoter strength [5,6]. For example, NF-YB which binds to the Y box with an imperfect inverted CCAAT sequence has inverse relationship to the promoter strength. Furthermore, the present results demonstrate that the Y box with an inverted CCAAT sequence enhances the promoter strength, whereas the Y box with an imperfect inverted CCAAT motif has an inhibitory effect on the transcriptional activity of DRB promoters.

References

1. Singal DP, Qiu X, D'Souza M, Sood SK. Polymorphism in the upstream regulatory regions of HLA-DRB genes. *Immunogenetics* 1993 ; 37 : 143-7.
2. Singal DP, D'Souza M, Sood SK, Qiu X. Sequence-specific interactions of the nuclear proteins with polymorphic upstream regulatory regions of HLA-DRB genes. *Transplant Proc* 1993 ; 25 : 180-2.
3. Singal DP, Qiu X. Polymorphism in the upstream regulatory region and level of expression of HLA-DRB genes. *Mol Immunol* 1994 ; 31 : 1117-20.
4. Qiu X, Singal DP. Allelic polymorphism in the upstream regulatory region of HLA-DRB genes : functional role of conserved consensus motifs. *Transplant Proc* 1995 ; 27 : 682-3.
5. Singal DP, Qiu X. Polymorphism in both X and Y box motifs controls level of expression of HLA-DRB1 genes. *Immunogenetics* 1996 ; 43 : 50-6.
6. Emery P, Mach B, Reith W. The different level of expression of HLA-DRB1 and -DRB3 genes is controlled by conserved isotypic differences in promoter sequence. *Hum Immunol* 1993 ; 38 : 137-47.
7. Louis P, Vincent R, Cavadore P, Clot J, Eliaou JE. Differential transcriptional activities of HLA-DR genes in the various haplotypes. *J Immunol* 1994 ; 153 : 5059-67.

Constitutive and inducible expression of HLA class II genes in normal cells is under the control of the AIR-1-encoded CIITA *trans*-activator

G. Rigaud[1,4], A. De Lerma Barbaro[2], S. Sartoris[1], G. Tosi[2], R.S. Accolla[2,3]*

1 Institute of Immunology and Infectious Diseases, University of Verona, Italy
2 Advanced Biotechnology Center, Largo Rosanna Benzi, 10, 16132 Genova, Italy
3 Chair of General Pathology and Immunology, Medical School, Varese, Italy
4 Present address : Unité d'Immunogénétique, INSERM U276, Institut Pasteur, Paris, France
* Corresponding author

The MHC-restricted recognition of antigen by T cells is the final result of a developmentally regulated process taking place mostly in the thymus where T cells learn to recognize self antigens presented by MHC class II molecules particularly expressed on thymic epithelial cells (TEC) [1]. It is generally believed that during the maturation process, T cells expressing TCR with high affinity for self MHC-antigen are negatively selected and die [2]. As a consequence, only the T cells with low affinity TCRs are allowed to leave the thymus and to colonize the periphery. Thus the expression of MHC class II molecules is fundamental for modelling the T cell repertoire, for the acquisition of tolerance, and for recognition of antigen.

The expression of MHC class II antigens is a highly regulated, developmentally controlled process. On differentiated cells, class II antigens are expressed only on few cell types, mainly confined to, or in strong contact with, the immune system as it is the case of B cells, macrophages and TEC [3]. Moreover the mode of expression of class II genes is distinct in the various cell types. B cells express class II genes constitutively, whereas macrophages and TEC express them after induction with a variety of stimuli, among which the cytokine IFN-γ is certainly one of prominent biological relevance. The expression of class II molecules is mainly controlled at transcriptional level. Crucials *cis* acting elements involved in the transcriptional control of class II genes map within a limited sequence of 300 bp of the class II promoter immediately 5' to the transcription start site [4] One of the most important loci controlling class II gene expression is the AIR-1 locus [5]. This locus encodes a transcriptional activator, CIITA [6], which exerts its action on the class II promoter region by modifying the relative binding of DNA-interacting proteins at distinct sites [7], although itself is probably not a DNA binding protein. CIITA is usually not expressed in class II-negative cells. Thus, it appeared to us of importance to analyze the molecular mechanisms by which class II genes are induced in human thymic epithelial cells at very early stages of *in vitro* primary cultures, particularly in regard to the expression of CIITA and to the possible modifications of the crucial 300 bp class II promoter region in uninduced and IFN-γ induced TEC. These situations were compared to those found in B cells.

Material and methods

MHC class II cell surface phenotyping of TEC and B cells by means of monoclonal antibodies, RNA analysis, and *in vivo* genomic footprinting after DNase I digestion have been extensively described in recent publications [7,8].

Results and discussion

In vitro cultured TEC do not express cell surface class II antigens (*Figure 1B, histogram c*). However, after IFN-γ treatment they express class II DR molecules in an homogeneous fashion (*Figure 1B, histogram d*), and at levels approaching those of the B cell line Raji (*Figure 1A, histogram b*). This induction takes place also for the other class II molecular subsets, DQ and DP and correlates with de novo accumulation of class II mRNA (data not shown).

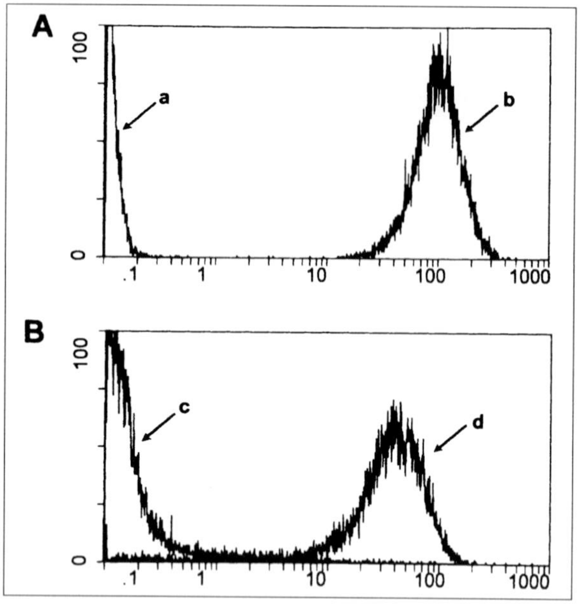

Figure 1. Flow cytofluorometric analysis of thymic epithelial cells (panel B) after staining with a mAb specific for DR antigens, followed by the rabbit anti-mouse FITC, before (c) and after (d) incubation with IFN-γ. As a control (panel A), the histograms of Raji cells stained with (b) or without (a) the anti-DR mAb are depicted. Values are expressed as log of fluorescence intensity in the abscissa, and number of cells in the ordinate.

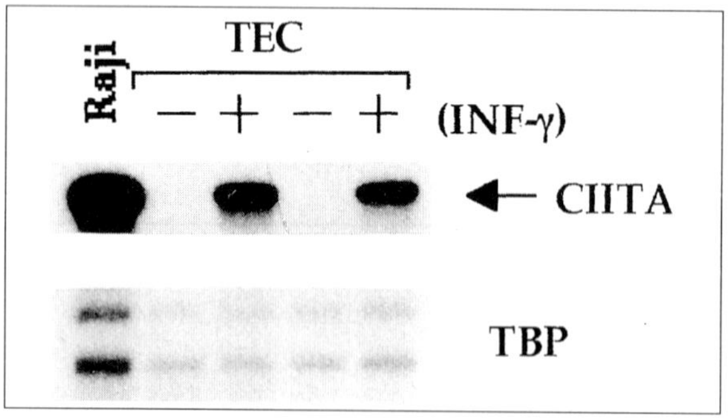

Figure 2. Expression of CIITA specific mRNA. RNase protection assay of CIITA in TEC incubated with (+) or without (-) IFN-γ. Raji mRNA was used as positive control. The TBP probe was used as reference. In this case two primary cultures of TEC obtained from distinct donors were analyzed.

Because of the central role played by the AIR-1 locus product on the transcriptional control of class II genes, we subsequently analyzed whether CIITA transcripts were present in TEC before and after IFN-γ induction. *Figure 2* shows that CIITA specific message was not detectable in uninduced TEC but was clearly present in IFN-γ induced TEC. Thus, IFN-γ activation of MHC class II genes in TEC is associated with *de novo* accumulation of CIITA mRNA. The induction of CIITA after cytokine treatment was a common finding in many cell lines expressing inducible class II genes, particularly tumor cell lines derived from both sarcomas and adenocarcinomas (data not shown).

It was therefore important to assess, by *in vivo* genomic footprinting, whether the IFN-γ mediated induction of class II genes could result in a modification of the class II promoter occupancy *in vivo* and, if so, how this modification could compare to the one observed in class II constitutive B cells. As it can be seen in *Figure 3*, changes in the DRA promoter occupancy of IFN-γ treated TEC were observed on multiple sites and on distinct regulatory elements.

On the upper strand (*Figure 3*), strong protections to the DNase I digestion were observed between uninduced and induced TEC on the O, Y, X2 and V boxes (open rectangles), whereas the X1 box showed only slight protection. The protection observed on the O box was accompanied by a nuclease hyper-reactivity (arrow) immediately downstream of the protected area (open rectangle). On the W/S box, no significant changes between uninduced and induced TEC were observed.

Comparison between TEC and B cells, revealed interesting features. The footprint patterns observed in IFN-γ induced TEC and in Raji B cells at the X1, X2, Y and O boxes were almost superimposable. Particularly in the X2 and in the Y boxes, the unprotected sites in uninduced TEC which were protected in induced TEC, were also protected in B cells (see open rectangle).

On the other hand the footprint pattern in the region within and around the W/S box in B cells was not superimposable to the one observed in TEC induced or not induced. In B cells this region was caracterized by a more intense hyper-reactivity even at sites which were clearly protected in TEC (see asterisks).

Important differences between B cells and TEC could be also observed within and around the negative regulatory V element [9]. In B cells this element included a

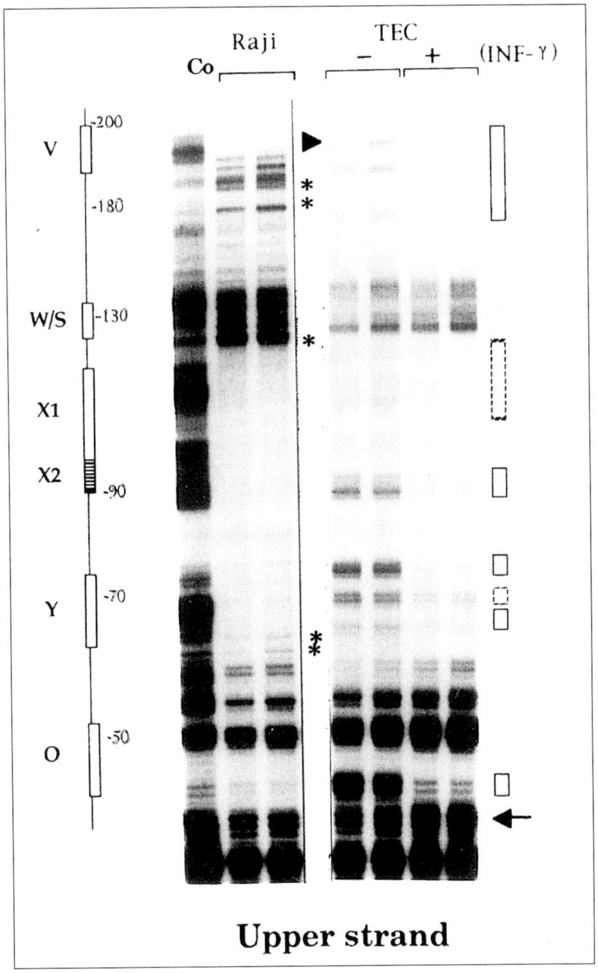

Figure 3. DNase I *in vivo* footprint analysis of the MHC class II DRA gene promoter in uninduced and IFN-γ induced TEC. (A) Upper strand ; For each cell type analyzed, two DNase I concentrations are shown. Cell derivation is indicated on the top of each lane. Conserved regulatory elements and positions relative to the start site are indicated on the left side of the figure. Arrows indicate DNase I hyper-reactivity in IFN-γ induced TEC. Arrowheads point to unprotected sites present in TEC and absent in Raji cells, whereas asterisks indicate hyper-reactive sites present in B cells and absent in TEC. Protections are indicated by open rectangles. Hatched rectangles indicate partial protections in IFN-γ treated TEC with respect to untreated cells. Control (Co) was obtained by DNase I digestion of nacked DNA.

protected and an unprotected area. Immediately downstream the V box one hyper-reactive and one unprotected site, were found (see asterisks). In contrast, in IFN-γ induced TEC, the V box showed a strong protection extending 3' to the hyper-reactive sites observed in B cells. It must be noted that in uninduced TEC, one relevant unprotected site was seen within the V box (full arrowhead). This site was protected in B cells.

The results presented in this report are important in several aspects. First of all we demonstrate that IFN-γ induction of class II genes in TEC is accompanied by *de novo* expression of CIITA , the transcriptional *trans*-activator which plays a key role in the control of the constitutive class II expression in B cells. Second, we provide evidence that, upon cytokine treatment, the class II promoter undergoes a dramatic conformational change, as a result, most likely, of the binding of distinct *trans*-acting factors.

Third, although strong similarities were found between IFN-γ induced TEC and B cells, cell type specific differences were also observed at several sites of the promoter between TEC cells, either induced or uninduced, and B cells. Many of these differences, were found in and around the W/S and the V boxes. Taken together these results indicate that tissue specific factors, interacting with the class II promoter region, exist and may contribute to the distinct mode of class II gene expression observed in the various cell types.

The necessary corollary is that different conformations of the class II promoter, dictated by the interaction with qualitatively and/or quantitatively different factors, may produce similar effects on gene transcription, provided that crucial factors, such as CIITA, stabilizing protein-DNA interaction at given sites, are present.

Acknowledgements

The Authors wish to thank Drs D. Ramarli and AP Riviera for help in preparing TEC cultures, and Miss T. Cestari and Miss M. Nicolis for technical support.

This work was supported by the following grants to R.S.A.: ISS First National Project Tuberculosis; ISS IX Project AIDS; MURST 40% Immunoregulation; PNR National Research Project Neurobiologic Systems.

References

1. Boyd RL, Tukey CL, Godfrey DI, Izon DJ, Wilson TJ, Davidson NJ, Bean AGD, Ladyman HM, Ritter MA, Hugo P. The thymic microenvironement. *Immunol Today* 1993 ; 14 : 445-59.
2. Von Boehmer H. Developmental biology of T cells in T cell receptor transgenic mice. *Annu Rev Immunol* 1990 ; 8 : 531-56.
3. Accolla RS, Dellabona P, Scarpellino L, Carra G, Sartoris S. A family of trans-acting factors with distinct regulatory functions control expression of MHC class II genes. *Immunol Res* 1990 ; 9 : 20-33.
4. Benoist C, Mathis D. Regulation of major histocompatibility complex class-II genes : X, Y, and other letters of the alphabet. *Annu Rev Immunol* 1990 ; 8 : 681-715.
5. Accolla RS, Jotterand-Bellomo M, Scarpellino L, Maffei A, Carra G, Guardiola J. aIr-1, a newly found locus on mouse chromosome 16 encoding a trans-acting activator factor for MHC class II gene expression. *J Exp Med* 1986 ; 164 : 369-74.
6. Steimle V, Otten LA, Zufferey M, Mach B. Complementation cloning of an MHC class II transactivator mutated in hereditary MHC class II deficiency (or Bare Lymphocyte Syndrome). *Cell* 1993 ; 75 : 135-46.
7. Rigaud G, Paiola F, Accolla RS. *In vivo* modification of major histocompatibility complex class II DRA promoter occupancy mediated by the AIR-1 trans-activator. *Eur J Immunol* 1994 ; 24 : 2415-20.
8. Rigaud G, De Lerma Barbaro A, Nicolis M, Cestari T, Ramarli D, Riviera AP, Accolla RS. Induction of CIITA and modification of *in vivo* HLA-DR promoter occupancy in normal thymic epithelial cells trated with IFN-γ. *J Immunol* 1996 ; 156 : 4254-8.
9. Wright KL, Ting JPY. *In vivo* analysis of the HLA-DR gene promoter : cell-specific interaction at the octamer site and up-regulation of X box binding by interferon γ. *Proc Natl Acad Sci USA* 1992 ; 89 : 7601-5.

Symposium communications

HLA Diversity

HLA typing and sequencing

Function of HLA

Transplantation biology and medicine

HLA and Diseases

HLA typing and sequencing

Technical advances in HLA typing

Contents

Effect of low ionic strength for keeping single stranded DNA and application to MHC allele typing and matching

E. Maruya, H. Saji, S. Yokoyama

Department of Research Kyoto Red Cross Blood Center, 644 Sanjusangendo mawarimachi, Higashiya Maku, Kyoto 605, Japan

We developed a simple and efficient procedure to control the formation of single stranded DNA (ssDNA) and then applied it to classical and non classical HLA allele typing, and DNA crossmatching (X'm) for unrelated bone marrow transplantation. The low ionic strength (LIS) conditions inhibited the duplex formation of ssDNA. By changing ionic strength, the ratio of ssDNA / double stranded DNA (dsDNA) was controlled easily after heat denaturation. We utilized the LIS effect to SSCP (single stranded conformation polymorphism) [1], DCP (DNA conformation polymorphism), which was based upon consolidating two conformation polymorphisms, SSCP and heteroduplex formation (HDF), in a gel, and pretreatment for hybridization of PCR-MPH (microtiter plate hybridization; a kind of reverse SSO using microtiter plate) [2]. These methods are referred to as PCR-LIS-SSCP, PCR-LIS-DCP and PCR-LIS-MPH.

Materials

The classical and non-classical HLA allele typing

Genomic DNAs were obtained from 100 healthy Japanese. These samples had been typed for *DRB1*, *DQB1* and *DPB1* by PCR-RFLP [3] and *A* alleles by PCR-SSOP [4]. The DNAs of the Terasaki DNA Exchange Program and the 10th International Histocompatibility Workshop cell line panels were used as reference for *class II* and *TAP* [5] allele typing, respectively. Group specific, locus and group specific, and exon specific primers were used for *class II*, *class I* and *TAP* amplifications, respectively.

DNA crossmatching

Genomic DNAs were obtained from 60 pairs of Japanese related and unrelated bone marrow transplantations. These DNAs were typed *DRB1*, *DQA1*, *DQB1*, and *DPB1* by PCR-RFLP [3] and *A* and *B* alleles by PCR-SSOP [4] and PCR-LIS-SSCP. Generic primers were used for amplification of *DRB*, *DQB* and *DPB* region. The *class I* exons 2 and 3 were amplified with exon specific primers which are able to co-amplify *A*, *B*, *C* and other *class I* loci.

Methods

LIS-SSCP

One microliter of PCR product was added to 20µl of LIS solution (10% saccharose, 0.01% bromophenol blue, and 0.01% xylene cyanol FF). The mixture was incubated for 2 mins at 97 °C and 4-10µl of the mixture was applied to 8 - 15% polyacrylamide gel (acrylamide: bisacrylamide = 49 : 1) on a minigel electrophoresis apparatus with a constant temperature control system (AE-6410, Atto). Electrophoresis was carried out in 45mM Tris-borate (pH8.0) / 1mM EDTA at an optimal running temperature and 15mA for 2 hours. DNAs in the gel were detected by silver staining (Daiichi Pure Chemicals, Tokyo, Japan). To evaluate the optimal conditions of gel concentration and running temperatures for electrophoresis, we performed the electrophoresis in 10 or 12.5% polyacrylamide gel at 22 °C at first and then modified the condition to 8 , 15 or 20%, and 32 or 4 °C

LIS-DCP

To form the optimal ratio of ssDNA and dsDNA (homo- and hetero-duplex), 3µl (for *DRB*, *DPB* and *class I exon 2*) or 7 µl (for *DQB* and *class I exon 3*) of amplified products (donor, recipient and mixture which was mixed with equal volumes of donor/recipient products) were added 7µl of LIS solution in each three tube. These mixtures were incubated for 1 min at 95 °C and then 1 min at 55 °C, followed by incubation for 10 mins at room temperature. Two-four μl portions of the mixtures were applied to the 10% polyacrylamide gel and electrophoresis was carried out as described above, at 22 °C for 80 mins. DNA banding profiles were observed after silver staining.

LIS-MPH

Fifty μl of *DRB* generic amplified product was added 150 μl of LIS solution. The mixture was incubated for 10 mins at 95 °C and added to each well of the 'DRB generic typing plate'. The usual protocol was used for other procedures.

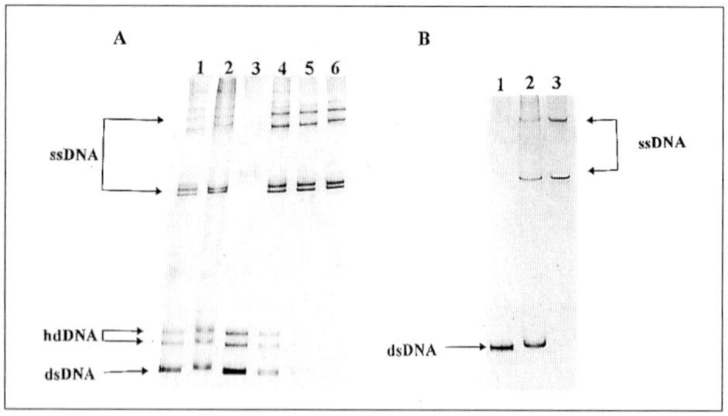

Figure 1. The effect of low ionic strength for keeping ssDNA after heat denaturation.
(A) Lane 1: heat denatured DNA, lane 2: heat denatured with formamide (DNA solution: formamide=1:7), lane 3: untreated DNA, lane 4: heat denatured with LIS (DNA solution: LIS=1:1), lane 5: heat denatured with LIS (1:5), lane 6: heat denatured with LIS (1:10). The amplified product was *HLA-DRB1*1501/1602*. (B) Lane 1: untreated DNA, lane 2: heat denatured with formamide (1:7), lane 3: heat denatured with LIS (1:20). The amplified product was HLA-*DRB1*1501* and applied in equivalent volume to each lane. Electrophoresis was carried out in 10% gel at 22 °C, 80 mins.

Results and discussion

The effect of low ionic strength for keeping ssDNA after heat denaturation

Figure 1 A and *B* show the effect of low ionic strength. Equivalent amounts of amplified product were resolved in each lane. The dsDNA bands decreased with increasing volume of added LIS solution into amplified products. Therefore, the ratio of ssDNA / dsDNA formation after heat-denaturation was controllable by changing ionic strength of DNA solution. In B, lanes 1 (untreated) and 2 (formamide) show the dsDNA bands, but disappeared in lane 3 (LIS). Therefore, LIS was more efficient for ssDNA formation than formamide.

Classical HLA allele typing

HLA-class II allele typing

A total of 72 alleles {DR1 (*DRB1*0101~3*), DR2 (*DRB1*1501~3, 1505, 1601~2*), DR3 (*DRB1*0301*), DR4 (*DRB1*0401~8, 0410, 0411*), DR5 (*DRB1*1101~4, 1201, 1202*), DR6 (*DRB1*1301~5, 1401~3, 1405, 1406*), DR8 (*DRB1*0801~4, 0806*), DQ5 (*DQB1*0501~3*), DQ6 (*DQB1*0601~0604, 0609*), DQ2 (*DQB1*0201*), DQ3 (*DQB1*0301~3*) DQ4 (*DQB1*0401, 0402*), *DPB1*0101, 0201, 0202, 0301, 0401, 0402, 0501, 601, 0901, 1001, 1101, 1401, 1701, 1901, 2101, 2701, 4701*} could be typed using a combination of LIS-SSCP with group-specific amplification. *Figure 2* shows several examples of LIS-SSCP profiles.

HLA-class I allele typing

We applied this method to the allele typing of *A2*, *A26* and *B61* which were polymorphic in Japanese. Ten *A2* (*A*0201~0208, 0210* and *0211*), 5 *A26* (*A*2601~5*) and 3 *B61* (*B*4002, 4003* and *4006*) alleles could be typed using a combination of this method with the nested PCR, locus and group specific amplification. *Figures 3-4* show the LIS-SSCP profiles of *A2 and B61* alleles.

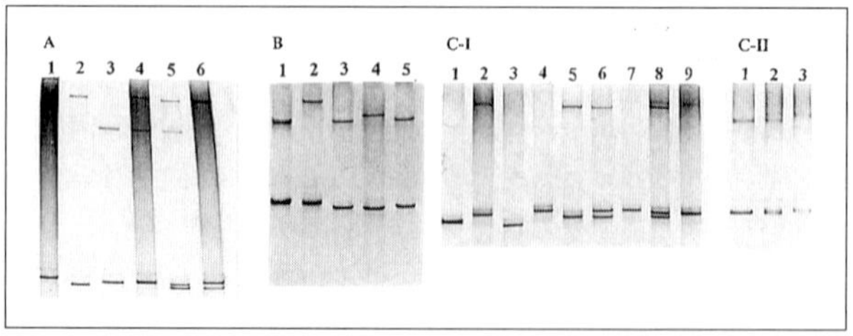

Figure 2. PCR-LIS-SSCP analysis of *HLA-class II (DR1, DR2, and DR8/12).*
(A) Lane 1: *DRB1*0101*, lane 2: *DRB1*0102*, lane 3: *DRB1*0103*, lane 4: *DRB1*0103/0101*.
(B) Lane 1: *DRB1*1501*, lane 2: *DRB1*1502*, lane 3: *DRB1*1602*, lane 4: *DRB1*1601*.
(C-I) Lane 1: *DRB1*0804*, lane 2: *DRB1*0801*, lane 3: *DRB1*0802*, lane 4: *DRB1*0803*, lane 5: *DRB1*0806*, lane 6: *DRB1*0806/0803*, lane 7: *DRB1*0803*, lane 8: *DRB1*0801/0806*, lane 9: *DRB1*0801*.
(C-II) lane 1: DRB1**1201*, lane 2: DRB1**1201/1202*, lane 3: DRB1**1202*. Electrophoresis was carried out in 12.5% gel at 22 °C in A and B, at 4 °C in C-I, at 32 °C in C-II.

Non-classical HLA allele typing

Three of four *TAP1* alleles (*0101*, *0201*, *0301* and *0401*), and all four *TAP2* alleles (*0101*, *0102*, *0103* and *0201*) were identified using a combination of LIS-SSCP

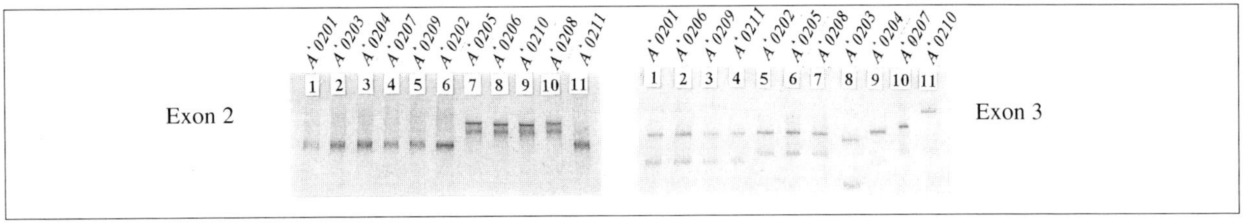

Figure 3. PCR-LIS-SSCP analysis of *HLA-class I* (*A2*).
Eleven alleles in this group (A*0201 ~ 0211) were examined.

(A) Six profiles of the amplified exon 2

Profiles	Lanes	Alleles
I	1-5	*A*0201=0203=0204=0207=0209*
II	6	*A*0202*
III	7	*A*0205*
IV	8-9	*A*0206=0210*
V	10	*A*0208*
VI	11	*A*0211*

(B) Six profiles of the amplified exon 3

Profiles	Lanes	Alleles
I	1-4	*A*0201=0206=0209=0211*
II	5-7	*A*0202=0205=0208*
III	8	*A*0203*
IV	9	*A*0204*
V	10	*A*0207*
VI	11	*A*0210*

=: identical sequences in the amplified region. The sequences of A*0201 and A*0209 are identical in exons 2 and 3. Therefore, these alleles could not be distinguished.

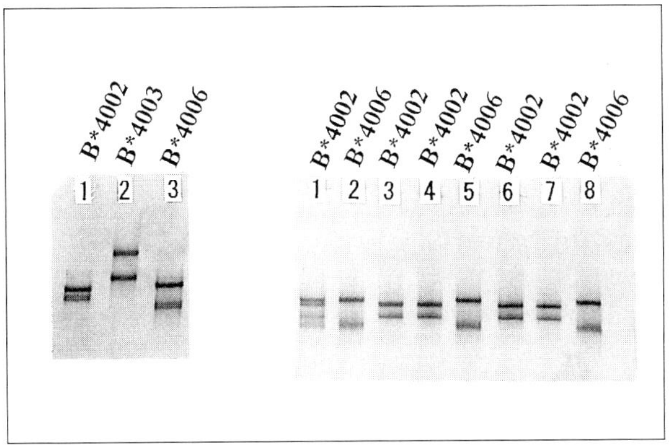

Figure 4. PCR-LIS-SSCP analysis of *HLA-class I* (B61). Three alleles in this group (*B*4002, 4003, 4006*) were examined, exon 3 amplified.

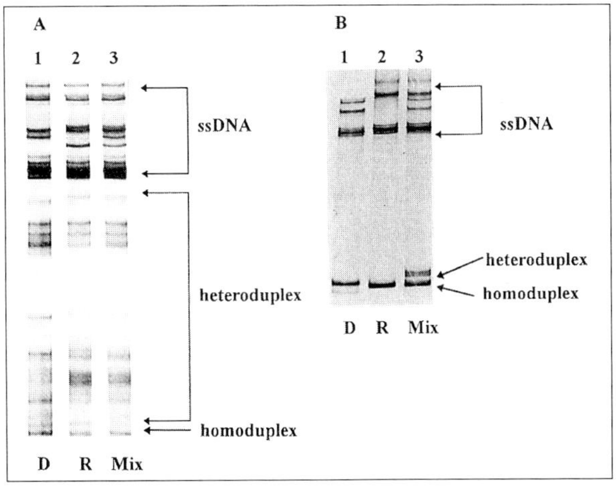

Figure 5. DNA X'm by PCR-DCP.
(A) This is the result of *DRB* X'm in an incompatible pair. Lane 1: donor, lane 2: recipient, lane 3: mixture of donor and recipient. The profiles of three lanes were different. (B) This is the result of *DPB* X'm in an incompatible pair. Lane 1: donor, lane 2: recipient, lane 3: mixture of both. A newly formed heteroduplex could be detected in lane 3.

with the exon specific amplifications. The allele frequencies of *TAP1* were similar in the Japanese and the Caucasian population [6], although those of *TAP2* were different (*Table I*). Moreover we found a new sequence variation at codon 577 (ATG→GTG: Met→Val). This variation was found in 12.4% of healthy Japanese (allele frequency: 6.6%), exhibited a strong linkage disequilibrium with *DRB1**0803-DQB1*0601* and leaded to a new *TAP2* allele, *TAP2**Bky2* (allele frequency: 5.1%).

Table I. Determination and allele frequencies of *TAPs*

		Japanese	Caucasian	Codons					
		AF(%)	AF(%)	379	565	577	651	665	687
	0101	32.2	40.0	Val	Ala	Met	Arg	Thr	Stop
	0103	9.3	not tested	Val	Ala	Met	Cys	Thr	Stop
	0201	27.7	23.8	Val	Ala	Met	Arg	Ala	Gln
TAP2	*Bky2*[##]	5.1	not tested	Val	Ala	Val	Arg	Ala	Gln
	C[#]	9.9	6.0	Ile	Ala	Met	Arg	Thr	Stop
	D[#]	0.0	4.5	Ile	Thr	Met	Arg	Thr	Stop
	0102	7.0	0.7	Val	Thr	Met	Arg	Thr	Stop
	Hky1[##]	1.9	0.0	Ile	Ala	Met	Arg	Ala	Gln
	Unknown	6.9	9.9						
		AF(%)	AF(%)	333	637				
	0101	86.3	83.0	Ile	Asp				
TAP1	*0201*	12.7	11.5	Val	Gly				
	0301	0.9	2.2	Val	Asp				

AF: Allele frequency
#: taken from Powis *et al.*
##: designated in this study

DRB1 allele

		I	C
DRB X'm	I	15	2*
	C	0	43

R: 0.918

DQB1 allele

		I	C
DQB X'm	I	12	1#
	C	0	47

R: 0.951

DPB1 allele

		I	C
DPB X'm	I	23	1$
	C	0	36

R: 0.966

HLA-class I A, B allele

		I	C
class I X'm	I	14	8
	C	3&	35

R: 0.596

Table II. The association between *HLA-class I, II* allele matching
and DNA crossmatching
*: One case was *DRB1*04* allele typing error. Another was *DRB5* deficiency
#: *DQB1*03* allele typing error, 0302 versus 0303.
$: *DPB1* allele typing error was caused by DNA contamination.
&: *A*0201* and *A*0206* were indistinguishable.
I: incompatible, C: compatible

DNA crossmatching [7]

DRB, DQB, DPB, class I exons 2 and *3* X'm were performed with 60 pairs of related and unrelated bone marrow transplantations by LIS-DCP. It was based on matching electrophoretic mobility of SSCP and HDF in amplified regions. Figure 5 shows examples of DNA X'm results. The predictability of matching with allele type was observed in *class II* but not in *class I* (*Table II*). By DNA X'm, we could detect 3 cases of allele typing errors in *class II* and a *DRB5* deficient case. This method could be used not only for locus but also 'region' matching. In *class I* X'm, it was difficult to detect the difference between *A*0201 and A*0206* and to evaluate the predictability of *class I* X since *C* locus alleles were not typed in all pairs.

HLA-DRB1 generic typing by PCR-LIS-MPH

DRB1 "generic typing" was performed by LIS-MPH on over 1,000 samples. Spending volume of amplified DNA was reduced and color development on positive probes improved.

Conclusion

The ratio of ssDNA / dsDNA formation after heat denaturation could be controlled by changing the ionic strength of the DNA solution. We utilized the LIS effect to SSCP, DCP and pretreatment for hybridization of PCR-MPH. The application of LIS effect to allele typing and crossmatching technique is simple, rapid and cost effective.

References

1. Orita, M, Iwahana H, Kanazawa H, Hayashi K, Sekiya T. Detection of polymorphisms of human DNA by gel electrophoresis as single-strand conformation polymorphisms. *Proc Natl Acad Sci USA* 1989; 86: 2766-70.
2. Kawai, S, Maekawajiri S, Tokunaga K, Juji T, Yamane A. A simple method of HLA-DRB typing using enzymatically amplified DNA and immobilized probes on microtiter plate. *Hum Immunol* 1994; 41: 121-6.
3. Uryu, N, Maeda M, Ota M, Tsuji K, Inoko H. A simple rapid method for HLA-DRB and-DQB typing by digestion of PCR-amplified DNA with allele specific restriction endonucleases. *Tissue Antigens* 1990; 35**:** 20-31.
4. Kimura A, Date Y, Sasazuki T. DNA typing of the HLA-A gene. *Transplantation Now* 1994; 7 (suppl): 10-22.
5. Powis SH, Tonks S, Mockridge I *et al.* Alleles and haplotypes of the MHC-encoded ABC transporters *TAP1* and *TAP2*. *Immunogenetics* 1993; 37: 373-80.
6. Powis SH, Cooper MD, Trowsdale J, Zhu ZB, Volanakis JE. Major histocompatibility haplotypes associated with immunoglobulin-A deficiency and common variable immunodeficiency: analysis of the peptide transporter genes *TAP1* and *TAP2*. *Tissue Antigens* 1994; 43: 261-5.
7. Clay TM, Bidwell JL, Howard MR, Bradley BA. PCR-fingerprinting for selection of HLA matched unrelated marrow donors. *Lancet* 1991; 337: 1049-52.

PCR-SSO hybridization in microplate method using single-stranded DNA dissociated by alkaline-magnetic beads

K. Kobayashi[1], Y. Hata[1], M. Iwasaki[1], M. Atoh[1], H. Suzuki[2], S. Sekiguchi[1]

1 Department of Laboratory Medicine
2 Department of Blood Transfusion, National Defense Medical College, 3-2 Namiki, Tokorozawa, Saitama 359, Japan

More recently, the following molecular typing methods based on polymerase chain reaction (PCR) have been developed: sequence-specific oligonucleotide (SSO) [1], reverse dot-blot hybridization [2], restriction fragment length polymorphism (RFLP) [3], sequence-specific primer (SSP) [4], and single-strand conformation polymorphism (SSCP) [5]. The conventional PCR-SSO typings are performed in batch mode, so that the procedures are taken too long and are unsuitable for small numbers of sample. We have developed a novel PCR oligotyping method using oligonucleotide probes and biotinylated single-stranded PCR products attached avidin that immobilized in microplate by a high gauss magnet. This method are some advantages that it is suitable for small numbers of sample, the assay time is short, and some HLA class II loci are able to react in same microplate simultaneously.

Materials and methods

All samples used in the present examinations had been typed by PCR-RFLP, PCR-SSO or PCR-SSP. DNA was extracted by a rapid isolation method using guanidine thiocyanate method.

The principle of our method is shown in *Figure 1*. The exon 2 of the HLA-DRB1 or DRB genes was amplified by PCR using biotinylated downstream primer (DRBAMP-B or DRBAMP-4) and unlabeled upstream primer (DRBAMP-A). The downstream primers were biotinylated to immobilize the PCR products. Genomic DNA (500 ng) was amplified in a total volume of 100 µl containing 10 mM Tris-HCl (pH 8.3), 50 mM KCl, 1.5 mM $MgCl_2$, 200 µM dNTP, 0.5 µM each of primer and 2 units of Taq DNA polymerase. The PCR profile consisted of initial denaturation by heating to 96°C for 2 min followed by 30 cycles at 96°C for 1 min, 60°C annealing for 1 min, and 72°C elongation for 1 min. A final elongation step of 5 min at 72°C was added.

The oligoprobes used in this study were based on the 11th and 12th International Histocompatibility Workshops. Digoxigenin-11-ddUTP was attached to the probes by incubating for 15 min at 37°C each sequence-specific oligonucleotide (SSO) probe (100 pmol) with 50 units of terminal transferase in 1x tailing buffer (200 mM potassium cacodylate, 25 mM Tris-HCl (pH 6.6), 0.25 mg/ml bovine serum albumin) containing 5 mM $CoCl_2$, and 40 nmol digoxigenin-11-ddUTP.

The PCR products (80 µl) were bound with 40 µl of avidin coated beads (10 µg/µl, Dynal Japan, Tokyo, Japan)

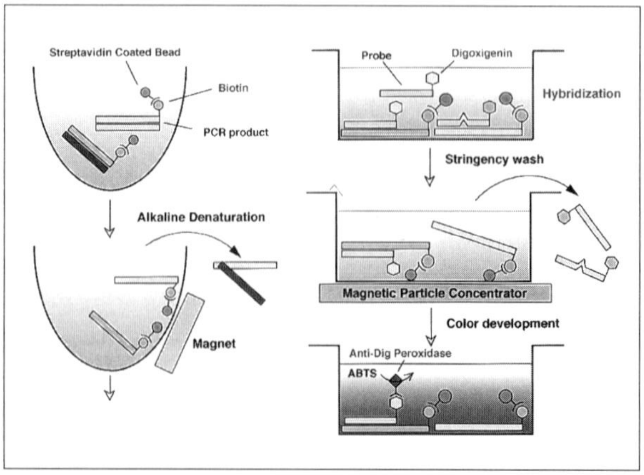

Figure 1. Principle of the magnetic SSO method.
The PCR product was attached with streptavidin coated Dynabeads. The DNA was denatued with NaOH and collected only antisense DNA by attaching a magnet. The antisense DNA and digoxigenin labeled probe were hybridized in micrplate well. After washing with TMAC, the hybridized DNA was detected by using anti-digoxigenin-peroxidase and a chrogenic substrate.

in a microtubes and incubated for 15 min. The avidin binded DNA sample was denatured for 10 min by adding 16 µl of 0.4 M NaOH. The single-stranded avidin-biotin-DNA complex was captured by Dynal Magnetic Particle Concentrator (MPC)-E-1 (Dynal Japan), and then the complex was washed with 0.1 M NaOH and with hybridization buffer [5x SSC, 0.5% blocking reagent , 0.1% sodium N-lauroylsarosinate, 0.02% SDS]. The DNA was resuspended with 1.3 ml of hybridization buffer. The 50 µl of the single stranded avidin-biotin-DNA in hybridization buffer and 0.36 pmol oligonucleotide probes were loaded to each microplate well, and then incubated for 30 min at 54°C to allow hybridization. The hybridized DNA was immobilized on the bottom of the wells by attaching MPC-96 magnet (Dynal Japan) and the plate was washed twice with 2x SSPE, 0.1% SDS at room temperature and once with 3 M tetramethylammonium chloride solution for 30 min at 59°C. Finally, the tray was rinsed with 2x SSC at room temperature. After the stringency wash was completed, the plate was rinsed with washing buffer (0.1 M maleic acid, 0.15 M NaCl, 0.3% Tween 20, pH 7.5) and with buffer 2 (1% blocking reagent, 0.1 M maleic acid, 0.15 M NaCl, pH 7.5).
Binding of the digoxigenin-labeled probe was detected by anti-digoxigenin-conjugated enzyme followed by color development. Anti-digoxigenin-peroxidase (15 µU/100 µl) diluted with buffer 2 were added to the plate. The plate was incubated for 15 min and was rinsed twice with washing buffer and with ABTS substrate buffer (Boehringer Mannheim, Tokyo, Japan). Finally, 0.05% ABTS substrate was added to each well, the tray was incubated in the dark for 60 min. After the color development was completed, the results were scored by visual inspection.

Results

The biotinylated strand was recovered by attaching a high gauss magnet and the unlabeled strand was removed by wash with NaOH. Five microgram of beads per 1 µl of PCR sample was suitable to detect the hybridization by visual inspection. The denatured antisense DNA was hybridized with digoxigenin labeled probe on the well. The probes applied in this experiment were similar to those used in the 11th and 12th International Workshops. The concentrations of probe and PCR product were examined with positive and negative DNA samples for the specific alleles recognized by these probes. From these preliminary tests, the best concentrations of probe and DNA at which it give a strong signal with the known positives and no cross-hybridization with known negatives was selected. The sensitivity and no cross-reactivity were shown as same as the conventional method when examined at 0.36 pmol of probe and 3 µl of PCR sample per well. After stringency washes, the specific-binded DNA was detected with anti-digoxigenin-peroxidase conjugate and ABTS substrate. In all eliminative procedure, the DNA was immobilized by attaching a magnet under the microtiter plate. In this enzymatic detection method, positive reactions are in the wells with green color, making it easy to determine positive and negative reactions by visual inspection after 1 hour and the color is stable for a few days. An alternative substrate for alkaline phosphatase, p-nitrophenylphosphate (pNPP), produced a yellow, but the color development was very slow (3 hours or longer). The color was developed in all wells in next day.
The results of testing PCR-amplified DNA from selected members of our reference cell panel typed with 23 DRB generic probes and 18 DR4 allelic probes are shown in *Table I* and *Figure 2*. This microplate hybridization method and chemiluminecent filter dot-blot procedure showed correspondence in this experiment.

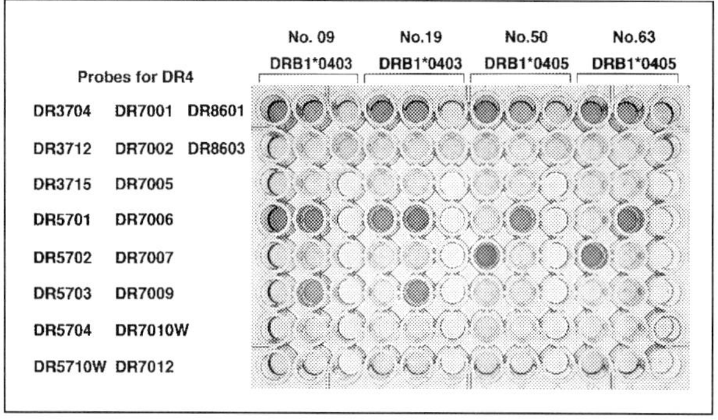

Figure 2. HLA-DR4 allele typing using the magnetic SSO method.
This shows a example of the DR4 allele typing using this magnetic SSO method. This typing results showes good reactivities and specificities. In this enzymatic detection method, positive reactions are in the wells with green color, making it easy to determine positive and negative reactions by visual inspection after 1 hour.

Table I. DRB1 generic typing using the magnetic SSO method

	Oligonucleotide Probes		Tested DRB Alleles			
No.	Name	Specificities	DRB1*0406 DRB1*0406 DRB4*0101 DRB4*0101	DRB1*0101 DRB1*0802	DRB1*1302 DRB1*1405 DRB3*0202 DRB3*0301	DRB1*1302 DRB1*1501 DRB3*0301 DRB5*0101
1	DRB1001	DRB1*01	-	+	-	-
2	DRB1003	DRB1*03+DRB1*11 +DRB1*13+DRB1*14 (except DRB1*1404)	-	-	+	+
3	DRB1004	DRB1*04+DRB1*1410	+	-	-	-
4	DRB1005	DRB1*08+DRB1*12+ DRB1*1404+DRB1*1411 +DRB1*1105	-	+	-	-
5	DRB1006	DRB1*07	-	-	-	-
6	DRB1007N	DRB1*09	-	-	-	-
7	DRB1008	DRB1*10	-	-	-	-
8	DRB1009N	DRB5	-	-	-	+
9	DRB1010	DRB3*0101	-	-	-	-
10	DRB1011	DRB3*0201+DRB3*0202 +DRB3*0301	-	-	+	+
11	DRB2801	DRB1*01	-	+	-	-
12	DRB2802	DRB1*12	-	-	-	-
13	DRB2803	DRB1*07	-	-	-	-
14	DRB2804	DRB1*09	-	-	-	-
15	DRB2805N	DRB5*0101	-	-	-	+
16	DRB2810	DRB4*0101+DRB4*0102	+	-	-	-
17	DRB3707	DRB1*09+DRB5 (except DRB5*0101)	-	-	-	-
18	DRB3709	DRB5*0101	-	-	-	+
19	DRB5703	DRB1*11	-	-	-	-
20	DRB7011	DRB1*02	±	-	-	+
21	DRB8601		-	+	+	+
22	DRB8602	DRB1*12+DRB1*0102* +DRB5*02	-	-	-	-
23	DRB8603		+	-	+	+

Discussion

In the conventional dot-blot hybridization method, the following specific materials are required: dot blotter, oven or crosslinker, plastic bag sealer, nylon membranes, x-ray film and so on. Our method, however, does not require any of these specific materials, although high gauss magnet, incubator and/or waterbath are necessary to apply this method. Most reagents are on the market but some buffers. This method does not need radioisotope such as ^{32}P to detect hybridizations. And so this method can be performed in any laboratory. No special training is necessary and the method is feasible for laboratories with little experience in molecular techniques.

Our method is used only (-) strand DNA isolated by alkaline-magnet capturing, so that the false reactions are decreased and the signals are intensified compared to the denatured DNA containing (+) and (-) strands. To validate the accuracy of the procedure, we have compared it to conventional dot-blot hybridization. The results obtained with both methods were identical.

The microplate method described by Kostyu *et al.* [7] and Lazaro *et al.* [8] required denaturation in wells, and then oligonucleotide probes were added in these wells. Since our method does not need the denaturation of DNA in the well of the microplate, the digoxigenin labeled probes can be stored in the well of the plate for long period in a freezer. Consequently, by this method, DNA typing can be immediately performed.

A principal advantage of this method is the points that is easily performed in small numbers of sample and in short assay time. This typing assay can be completed within 3 hours after PCR amplification. As the another advantage, this method is able to perform DRB1 and DQB1 genotyping or generic and allele typing on the same microplate simultaneously.

References

1. Saiki RK, Bugawan TL, Horn GT, Mullis KB, Erlich HA. Analysis of enzymatically amplified γ-globin and HLA-DQα DNA with allele-specific oligonucleotide probes. *Nature* 1986; 324:163-6.
2. Saiki RK, Walsh PS, Levenson CH, Erlich HA. Generic analysis of amplified DNA with immobilized sequence-specific oligonucleotide probes. *Proc Natl Acad Sci USA* 1989; 86:6230-4.
3. Ota M, Seki T, Nomura N, Sugimura K, Mizuki N, Fukushima H, Tsuji K, Inoko H. Modified PCR-RFLP method for HLA-DPB1 and DQA1 genotyping. *Tissue Antigens* 1991; 38:60-71.
4. Olerup O, Zetterquist H. HLA-DR typing by PCR amplification with sequence-specific primers (PCR-SSP) in 2 hours: an alternative to serological DR typing in clinical practice including donor-recipient matching in cadaveric transplantation. *Tissue Antigens* 1992; 39:225-35.
5. Kimura A, Hoshino S, Yoshida M, Harada H, Sasazuki T. HLA 1991, vol. 1. New York: Oxford University Press, 1992.
6. Kimura A, Sasazuki T. HLA 1991, vol. 1. NewYork: Oxford University Press, 1992.
7. Kostyu DD, Pfohl J, Ward FE, Lee J, Murray Al, Amos DB. Rapid HLA-DR oligotyping by an enzyme-linked immunosorbent assay performed in microtiter trays. *Hum Immunol* 1993; 38:148-58.
8. Lazaro AM, Fernandez-Vina MA, Liu Z, Stastny P. Enzyme-linked DNA oligotyping - A practical method for clinical HLA-DNA typing. *Hum Immunol* 1993; 36:243-8.

DNA typing of the HLA-A gene and its clinical applications

A. Kimura[1]*, Y. Date[1], S. Yasunaga[2], T. Sasazuki[2]

1. Department of Tissue Physiology, Division of Adult Diseases, Medical Research Institute, Tokyo Medical and Dental University, Kandasurugadai 2-3-10, Chiyoda-ku, Tokyo 101, Japan
2. Department of Genetics, Medical Institute of Bioregulation, Kyushu University, Fukuoka 812, Japan
* Corresponding author

Precise genotyping of HLA genes is important to investigate the biological role of HLA molecules in controlling the susceptibility to autoimmune diseases and the recognition of allogeneic cells. One of the methods allowing for the precise HLA genotyping is the PCR-SSOP-based DNA typing system which has been established for the HLA class II genes [1]. We have applied the PCR-SSOP method in developing the DNA typing system for HLA-A gene [1]. In our system, a DNA region of the HLA-A gene, from exon 1 to exon 3, was amplified by the PCR and its polymorphisms in exon 2 and exon 3 were examined by hybridization with 91 types of SSOPs [2] to distinguish HLA-A alleles except for two combinations of HLA-A2 alleles, A*0201 vs A*0209 and A*0207 vs A*0215N, which have identical exon 2 and exon 3 sequences and are different in exon 4 sequence. We then analyzed exon 4 in these HLA-A2 alleles by using a group-specific PCR and hybridization with 5 types of SSOPs [2], finally allowing to define all HLA-A alleles at the DNA level. We report here the clinical applications of our HLA-A DNA typing method.

Results and discussion

HLA genotypes were determined in a large panel of healthy unrelated Japanese individuals, and the genotyping results showed that there were considerable heterogeneities of HLA-A2, A11, A24, and A26 in the Japanese population [2]. In addition, 4 new HLA-A alleles, A*2407, A*2408, A*2605, and A*2606, were suggested from the hybridization patterns and were confirmed for the presence by subsequent sequencing analysis [2].
One of the clinical applications of the HLA-A DNA typing is to investigate the disease-associated HLA-A alleles at the DNA level. We have previously reported that the susceptibility to Graves' disease (GD) and Hashimoto's thyroiditis (HT), both are autoimmune thyroid diseases, was associated with HLA-A2 in the Japanese population [3, 4], while different HLA class II alleles were associated with the diseases; DPB1*0501 with GD [3] and DRB4*01 with HT [4]. Because GD and HT were often found in the same multiplex families, it has been speculated that there is a common HLA-linked genetic factor in GD and HT, and the common genetic factor might be in strong linkage diseqilibrium with HLA-A2 [5]. We then examined the HLA-A gene in 87 patients with GD and 100 patients with HT and compared the frequencies of HLA-A2 alleles, DPB1*0501, and DRB4*01 in the patients with those in 493 healthy controls. All patients and controls were genetically unrelated. As shown in *Table I*, significant positive associations with HLA-A2 alleles were found in both GD and HT, confirming the association of HLA-A2 and autoimmune thyroid diseases. However, the associated HLA-A2 alleles were different in GD and HT; HLA-A*0206 in GD and HLA-A*0207 in HT. These observations suggested that the common genetic factor to GD and HT was not in the HLA-A locus. Because the binding motifs were different in HLA-A2 subtypes [6], it

Table I. Association of HLA alleles with autoimmune thyroid diseases

HLA allele	% controls	Graves' disease % patients		Hashimoto's disease % patients	
	(n=493)	(n=87)	RR#1	(n=100)	RR#1
A*0201	20.2	27.6		23.0	
A*0206	15.4	32.2	2.8	16.0	
A*0207	7.2	13.8		17.0	2.4
A*0210	1.3	1.1		1.0	
DPB*0501	60.2	86.2	4.1	62.0	
DRB4*01	64.5	64.4		83.0	2.7

#1 Relative risk. Only those with statistical significance (pc<0.05) are shown.

was postulated that self-antigens which may be presented by HLA-A2 molecules, if any, might be different in GD and HT.

Another clinical application of the HLA-A DNA typing is to examine the correlation between HLA-A match and prognosis of recipients or graft outcome in transplantation, especially in the bone marrow transplantation (BMT). A total of 239 serologically A, B, DR-identical unrelated BMT pairs was analyzed for HLA-A match at the DNA level. Matches in DRB1, DQA1, DQB1, DPA1, and DPB1 loci also were analyzed by the PCR-SSOP method [7] in these BMT pairs. It was found that 25.1% of BMT pairs had at least one HLA-A subtype mismatch in the graft versus host direction, while the mismatches also were found in 18.8, 10.9, 17.2, 49.8, and 64.4% of BMT pairs in DRB1, DQA1, DQB1, DPA1, and DPB1 loci, respectively. High frequencies of mismatches at the DP loci may be due to that the BMT pairs were selected by serological identity of HLA-A, B, and DR specificities and that there is no tight linkage disequilibria between alleles in DRB1 locus and those in DP loci. It was noted that only 19.2% of BMT pairs had no mismatch in the analyzed loci. To examine for the significance of HLA-A match in the clinical prognosis of BMT recipients, we have analyzed the 1 year survival rate and the frequency of graft versus host disease (GVHD) more than grade II in DRB1, DQA1, and DQB1-identical BMT recipients *(Table II)*. Although the number of BMT cases in each category was small, lower 1 year survival rate and higher frequency of severe GVHD were observed in HLA-A mismatched cases *(Table II)*, suggesting that the HLA-A mismatch also affect the clinical prognosis of unrelated BMT. Because similar effect of HLA-A subtype mismatch on the graft survival was also observed in kidney transplantation [8], it was strongly suggested that HLA-A matching at the DNA level would be needed for better clinical prognosis in transplantation.

Conclusion

We have extensively analyzed the polymorphisms in the HLA-A gene by developing a PCR-SSOP-based typing method. Our typing method allowed us to distinguish all HLA-A alleles including several new alleles at the DNA level. The typing method was applied to investigate the association of HLA-A2 and autoimmune thyroid diseases, demonstrating that defferent HLA-A2 alleles were associated with GD and HT. It also was applied to examine the HLA match in unrelated BMT, suggesting that the mismatch at the HLA-A locus also affect the clinical prognosis of serologically A, B, DR-identical and DRB1, DQA1, DPB1-identical BMT.

Table II. Correlation between HLA mismatch and clinical prognosis of recipients in serologically A, B, DR-identical and DRB1, DQA1, DQB1-identical unrelated BMT

HLA mismatch#1	n#2	1 year survival rate#3	frequency of GVHD#4
none	46(45)	69.6%	31.1%
A	16(15)	43.8	46.7
DPB1	30(29)	63.3	34.5
A+DPB1	10	20.0	50.0
DPA1	7	71.4	28.6
A+DPA1	6	16.7	66.7
DPA1+DPB1	50	60.0	36.0
A+DPA1+DPB1	13	46.2	38.5

#1 Mismatch in GVH direction.
#2 Number of recipients who were categolized in each group. Some patients were died within a few days after BMT before developing GVHD and were not included in the analysis of GVHD. Numbers of the patients analyzed for GVHD were in parentheses.
#3 Combined 1 year survival rates in A-mismatched cases (n=45) and A-matched cases (n=133) were 35.6% and 64.7%, respectively. The difference was statistically significant, $p<0.01$.
#4 Occurrence of GVHD more than grade II. Combined frequencies of severe GVHD in A-mismatched (n=40) and A-matched cases (n=131) were 43.9% and 33.6%, respectively. The difference was not significant.

Acknowledgments
We thank Drs T. Juji, T. Akaza, K. Tokunaga, and research committee of unrelated BMT in Japan for their contributions in the analysis of correlation between HLA match and prognosis in unrelated BMT. This work was supported in part by research grants from the Ministry of Health and Welfare, Japan.

References

1. Kimura A, Sasazuki T. Eleventh International Histocompatibility Workshop reference protocol for the HLA DNA-typing technique. In: Tsuji K, Aizawa M, Sasazuki T, eds. *HLA 1991* vol 1. Oxford: Oxford University Press, 1992: 397-419.
2. Date Y, Kimura A, Kato H, Sasazuki T. DNA typing of the HLA-A gene: population study and identific-

ation of four new alleles in Japanese. *Tissue Antigens* 1996: 47: 93-101.
3. Dong RP, Kimura A, Ohkubo R, Shinagawa H, Tamai H, Nishimura Y, Sasazuki T. HLA-A and DPB1 loci confer susceptibility to Graves' disease. *Hum Immunol* 1992: 35: 165-72.
4. Wan XL, Kimura A, Dong RP, Honda K, Tamai H, Sasazuki T. HLA-A and DRB4 genes in controlling the susceptibility to Hashimoto's thyroiditis. *Hum Immunol* 1995: 42: 131-6.
5. Sasazuki T, Kimura A, Dong RP, Sudo T, Honda K, Shinagawa H, Kuma K, Morita T, Matsubayashi S, Tamai H. Immunogenetics of Hashimoto's thyroiditis. In : Nagataki S, Mori T, Torizuka K eds. *80 years of Hashimoto Disease*. Tokyo: Elsevier, 1993: 13-8.
6. Sudo T, Kamikawaji N, Kimura A, Date Y, Savoie CJ, Nakashima H, Furuichi E, Kuhara S, Sasazuki T. Difference in MHC-class I self peptide repertoires among HLA-A2 subtypes. *J Immunol* 1995: 155: 4749-56.
7. Kimura A, Dong RP, Harada H, Sasazuki T. DNA typing of HLA class II genes in B-lymphoblastoid cell lines homozygous for HLA. *Tissue Antigens* 1992: 40: 5-12.
8. Shintaku S, Kimura A, Fukuda Y, Date Y, Tashiro H, Hoshino S, Furukawa M, Sasazuki T, Dohi K. Polymerase chain reaction-based HLA-A genotyping and its application to matching in kidney transplantation. *Transplant Proc* 1995: 27: 682-9.

A high resolution molecular typing method for simultaneous identification of HLA class I alleles

R. Arguello[1], H. Avakian[1], J.M. Goldman[1,2], J.A. Madrigal[1,2,3]

1 Anthony Nolan Research Institute, The Royal Free Hospital, Pond Street, Hampstead, London NW3 2QG, UK
2 Department of Hematology, Royal Postgraduate Medical School, London UK
3 Department of Hematology, Royal Free Hospital School of Medicine, London UK

Improvements in DNA based typing methods [1] for detection of the HLA polymorphism have enabled more accurate HLA typing for transplant donors and patients. Current typing methods include sequence-specific primer amplification (SSP) [2, 3], hybridization with sequence specific oligonucleotide probes (SSO) [4, 5], heteroduplex analysis [6, 8], single strand conformation polymorphism (SSCP) [9,10] and direct nucleotide sequencing [10, 11]. Due to the extensive sequence homology between the A, B and Cw loci [12] and between class I classical and non-classical genes and pseudogenes [13], each of these methods requires large numbers of specific reagents for high resolution typing. Although direct sequencing can be used for high resolution analysis of the class I alleles [10, 11], prior typing and group specific amplification is required in order to avoid ambiguous results from certain heterozygous combinations.

We have developed a novel high resolution DNA based typing method for HLA class I alleles. This is based on locus specific amplification of exons 2 and 3 of HLA-A, B and Cw loci followed by the separation of the allelic products which allows the isolation of individual allelic segments. The separated allelic segments from each locus are isolated, blotted onto membranes and hybridized with 40 oligonucleotide probes. The HLA class I alleles are identified by their unique hybridisation patterns with these universal probes.

Locus specific amplification

Polymorphism of exons 2 and 3 of class I genes account for over 95% of the allelic variations, these were amplified using locus specific primers [14], only 3 amplification reactions per sample were required. The 3' primer used for amplification was biotinylated at the 5' end, thus the anti-sense strands of the amplified product possess biotin.

Separation of the allelic products

This has been achieved by a novel technique that relies on formation of duplexes with a reference DNA strand and the electrophoretic separation of the duplexes. The technique, Complementary Strand Analysis (CSA) has wider applications, it can be used for obtaining DNA for direct sequencing or it can be employed as a diagnostic method.

PCR products are icubated with magnetic beads coated with streptavidin and the PCR reaction components are

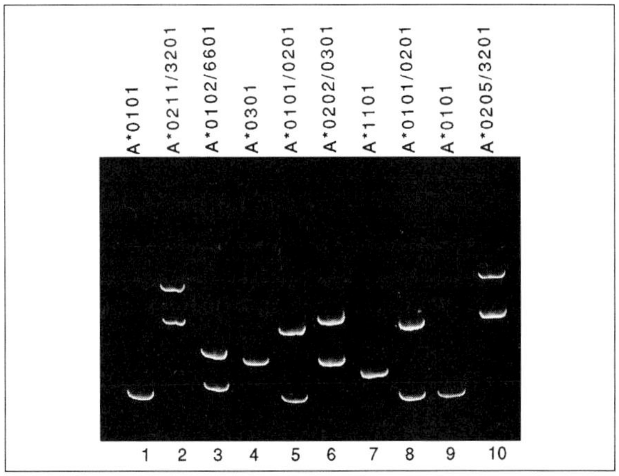

Figure 1. Complementary Strand Analysis of some HLA-A alleles. DNA from IHW cell lines were processed as described in the text. Homozygous samples yield one band and heterozygous samples two bands.

washed away. The beads are then treated with 0.15 M NaOH at 37 °C to dissociate and remove the non-biotinylated sense strand. The anti-sense strand is detached from the beads by heating at 95 °C. Reference strands for each locus are prepared with the same PCR primers except the 5' primer is biotinylated. We have selected A*0101, B*4402 and Cw*0701 as the alleles for reference strands for A, B and Cw loci respectively, these alleles are amplified from DNA prepared from homozygous cell lines. The relevant reference strand (A,B,Cw) is added to the anti-sense single strand preparations of the sample DNA, denatured at 95 °C allowed to anneal, the resulting duplexes are resolved in PAGE *(Figure 1)*. During initial testing DNA from different homozygous cell lines were mixed and then analysed successfully by CSA (results not shown). In practice we prepare combined gel cassettes with PAG and low melting point agarose and the migrating DNA bands are visualised and isolated from the agarose phase. The purified A, B and Cw locus products are blotted on nylon membrane, one dot per allele from each locus, on the same membrane. Each membrane carries DNA from 15 samples (2 dots per locus, 6 dots per sample) and a control track *(Figure 2)*.

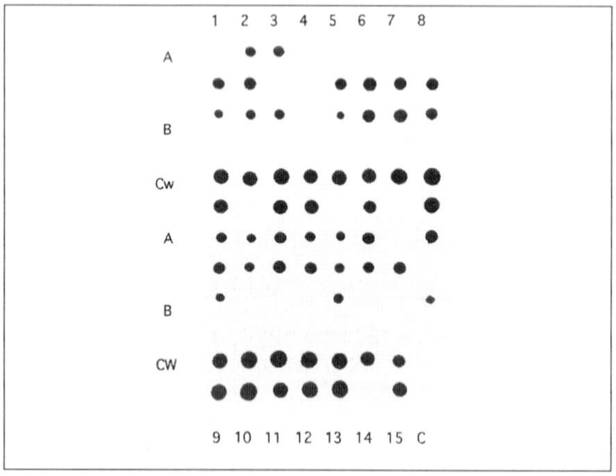

Figure 2. URSTO hybridisation pattern of HLA-A B and Cw alleles with prob 37.
DNA from 15 IHW cell lines were processed by CSA and the isolated bands were blotted on nylon memebrane. The membrane was hybrised with probe 37, developed and autoradiographed as described.

Hybridization with 40 universal probes

Most class I alleles lack unique base substitutions for identification purposes; instead within the exon sequences of each allele there are a number of conserved sequence motifs which reflect the evolutionary development of that allele [15, 16]. Comparison of HLA-A, B, Cw allelic sequences reveals a patchwork pattern of motifs in which a given allele comprises a unique combination of these sequence motifs. We have performed a detailed analysis of the recurring motifs in exons 2 and 3 of class I alleles and established that alleles can be identified by the specific combination of these motifs. Based on the DNA sequences of 221 reported alleles there are a large number of these recurring motifs, however a minimum set of 40 selected motifs can be used to identify the majority of the recognized alleles *(Table II)*. On the basis of this analysis we generated 201 motif combinations which were employed for typing of class I alleles regardless of the locus specificity. We have synthesised 40 oligonucleotides based on the sense sequences of these motifs *(Table I)*, these are designated Universal Recombinant Site Targeting Oligonucleotides (URSTO), the HLA alleles are identified by their unique hybridisation pattern (6-16 probes per allele) according to the predicted motif combinations *(Table II)*.

In a routine run the membranes with allelic samples are hybridized with the probes at the same temperature, the washing and stringency conditions are also uniform for all probes. We have used digoxigenin as the ligand for these probes and reactivity is visualised by chemiluminescence and autoradiography. Normally we prepare 20 membranes for a complete HLA-A, B and Cw typing.

Typing of HLA class I alleles

We have for HLA-A, B and Cw, 63 cell lines which expressed 81 different class I alleles *(Table III)*. These cell lines were selected to include allele combinations in which more than one base sequence motif was present for the same sequence range. In this way it was possible to test the probes that were targeted at different substitutions at a given location which could possibly have cross hybridized and produced false signals. The separation of the allelic products, in all heterozygous combinations which we have tested was achieved by CSA method described above. The advantage of this step is that

Table I. Nucleotide sequences and the sites of URSTO probes for the HLA class I genes

ID	Sequence	Location	ID	Sequence	Location
2	GGC CCG GCC GCG GGG AGC	113 - 130	23	ACC AGT TCG CCT ACG ACG	413 - 430
3	CTC ACA GAT TGA CCG AGT	282 - 299	24	ATT GGG ACC GGA ACA CAC	248 - 265
4	CGG ATC GCG CTC CGC TAC	307 - 324	25	TAC CTG GAG GGC ACG TGC	557 -574
5	TAC CTG GAG GGC CTG TGC	547 - 564	26	TGT ATG GCT GCG ACG TGG	365 - 382
6	CAG AGG ATG TAT GGC TGC	358 - 375	28	GCC CAG TCA CAG ACT GAC	277 - 292
7	ACA CCC TCC AGA GGA TGT	350 - 367	29	ACC GAG TGG ACC TGG GGA	293 - 310
8	CAG AGG ATG TTT GGC TGC	358 - 375	30	CGG AAC CTG CGC GGC TAC	307 - 324
9	CGA CGT GGG GCC GGA CGG	375 - 392	31	ATT TCT ACA CCT CCG TGT	92 - 109
10	CTC ACA TCA TCC AGA GGA	347 - 364	32	GCC CGT GTG GCG GAG CAG	520 - 537
11	TGT ATG GCT GCG ACC TGG	365 - 382	33	GAT CTC CAA GAC CAA CAC	267 - 284
12	CCA GCA GGA CGC TTA CGA	411 - 428	34	TGA CCA GTC CGC CTA CGA	411 - 428
13	GTG CGT GGA CGG GCT CCG	561 - 578	35	AAC ACA CAG ATC TAC AAG	259 - 276
14	GCG GAC ACG GCG GCT CAG	478 - 495	36	CGC GGG CGC CGT GGG TGG	212 - 229
15	GGA GCA GTG GAG AGC CTA	531 - 548	37	AGA TAC CTG GAG AAC GGG	580 - 597
16	GGA GCA GTT GAG AGC CTA	531 - 548	40	TCT CAC ACC CTC CAG	346 - 360
17	GTG CGT GGA GTG GCT CCG	561 - 578	41	ACC AAC ACA CAG ACT GAC C	277 - 295
18	GGA GCA GCT GAG AGC CTA	531 - 548	42	GGC GGA GCA GCG GAG A	528 - 543
19	AGG GGC CGG AGT ATT GGG	236 - 253	43	CAG GAC GCC TAC GAC GGC	415 - 432
20	GGC CCG ACG GGC GCC TCC	382 - 400	44	GAG GAC CTG CGC TCC TGG	454 - 471
22	TCC GCG GGC ATA ACC AGT	401 - 418	45	GAA GGA GAC GCT GCA GCG	597 - 614

Table II. URSTO hybridisation patterns of some class I alleles

	Probe ID number
A*0201	2 6 16 17 25 26 29 37 45
A*0202	2 6 7 15 17 25 26 29 37 40 45
A*0203	2 6 15 17 25 26 29 37 45
A*0204	2 16 17 25 26 29 37 45
A*0205	2 6 7 15 17 25 26 29 31 37 40 45
A*0206	2 6 16 17 25 26 29 31 37 45
A*0207	2 16 17 25 29 37 45
A*0210	2 8 16 17 25 29 31 37 45
A*0211	2 3 6 16 17 25 26 29 37 45
A*0212	2 6 17 25 26 29 37 45
A*0213	2 6 17 25 26 29 37 45
A*0214	2 6 7 16 17 25 26 29 31 37 40 45
A*0215N	2 16 17 25 29 37 45
A*2402	2 4 13 19 25 37 40 45
A*2403	2 4 17 19 25 37 40 45
A*2404	2 13 19 25 37 40 45
B*3501	2 5 6 10 11 17 18 19 20 24 30 32 34 37 45
B*3502	2 5 6 10 11 17 18 19 22 24 30 32 37 45
B*3503	2 5 6 10 11 17 18 19 20 23 24 30 32 37 45
B*3504	2 5 6 10 11 17 18 19 20 22 24 30 32 37 45
B*3505	2 5 17 18 19 20 24 30 32 34 37 40 45
B*3506	2 5 6 10 11 17 18 19 20 22 23 24 30 32 37 45
B*3507	5 6 10 11 17 18 19 20 24 30 32 34 37 45
B*3508	2 5 6 10 11 17 19 20 24 30 32 34 37 42 45
B*3509	2 5 6 10 11 17 18 19 20 22 24 30 32 37 44 45

	Probe ID number
B*3512	2 5 9 10 17 18 19 22 24 30 32 37 45
B*3513	2 5 6 10 11 17 18 19 20 23 30 32 37 45
B*3701	2 9 17 19 23 25 32 33 37 45
B*3801	2 4 7 9 17 22 23 24 25 31 32 37 40 45
B*3802	2 7 9 17 22 23 24 25 31 32 37 40 45
B*39011	2 7 9 17 22 23 24 25 30 31 32 37 41 45
B*39013	2 7 9 17 22 23 24 25 30 31 32 37 40 41 45
B*39021	2 7 9 17 22 23 25 30 31 32 33 37 40 41 45
B*39022	2 7 9 17 19 22 23 25 30 31 32 33 37 40 41 45
B*4402	2 5 9 10 19 32 33 37 43 45
B*44031	2 5 9 10 18 19 32 33 37 43 45
B*44032	2 5 6 9 10 18 19 26 32 33 37 43 45
B*4404	2 9 10 19 25 32 33 37 42 43 4
B*4405	2 5 9 10 19 32 33 37 45
B*4406	2 4 5 9 10 19 24 32 37 43 4
Cw*0602	11 14 15 17 19 20 25 34 37 40 44 45
Cw*0701	6 7 11 17 18 19 20 25 30 34 36 37 40 44 45
Cw*0702	7 17 18 19 20 25 30 34 36 37 40 44 45
Cw*0703	7 17 18 19 20 30 34 36 37 40 44 45
Cw*0704	6 11 17 19 20 23 25 30 37 44
Cw*1201	7 14 15 17 19 20 25 30 37 40 44 45
Cw*12021	7 14 15 17 19 20 25 30 34 36 37 40 44 45
Cw*12022	7 14 15 17 19 20 25 30 34 36 37 40 44 45
Cw*1203	11 14 15 17 19 20 25 30 34 36 37 40 44 45
Cw*1701	6 11 14 17 18 19 20 23 36 44 45

The probe numbers correspond to ID numbers in *Table I.*

Table III. HLA class I alleles tested

HLA-A (n=33)
A*0101, A*0102, A*0201, A*0202, A*0203, A*0204, A*0205, A*0206, A*0207, A*0208, A*0209, A*0210, A*0211, A*0212, A*0213, A*0216, A*0217, A*0301, A*1101, A*2301, A*2402, A*2403, A*2501, A*2601, A*2902, A*3001, A*3002, A*3101, A*3201, A*3301, A*6601, A*6602, A*6802

HLA-B (n=30)
B*0702, B*0801, B*1302, B*1402, B*1501, B*1502, B*1520, B*1801, B*3501, B*3701, B*3801, B*4001, B*4002, B*4101, B*4201, B*4402, B*4403, B*4601, B*4701, B*4801, B*4901, B*5001, B*5101, B*5201, B*5301, B*5502, B*5701, B*5801, B*5802, B*6701.

HLA-Cw (n=18)
Cw*0102, Cw*0202, Cw*0302, Cw*0303, Cw*0304, Cw*0401, Cw*0501, Cw*0602, Cw*0701, Cw*0702, Cw*0704, Cw*0802, Cw*1202, Cw*1203, Cw*1402, Cw*1502, Cw*1601, Cw*170

Numbers of different heterozygous combinations tested were: HLA-A 19; HLA-B 14 and HLA-Cw 11.

individual allelic sequences can be identified unambiguously with the URSTO probes.

The results indicate that in all cases the alleles could be identified by their unique hybridization patterns. The class I alleles that were tested included 33 A, 30 B and 18 Cw alleles and 44 different heterozygous combinations. The specificity of the probes were tested rigorously since there are several common sequences in all three loci that differ by one nucleotide only. These differences were found to be sufficient to prevent cross hybridization and all alleles tested in this study were identified unambiguously by these probes. In addition, during repeated tests individual alleles produced hybridisation patterns which were identical and agreed with the predicted probe combinations.

The combination of the two techniques described here has enabled the unambiguous and high resolution typing of HLA class I alleles in 63 cell lines. The resolution obtained was at the allelic level and comparable to DNA sequencing techniques. In addition, since the probes are based on common inter-locus sequences, the same set can be used to type HLA-A, B and Cw loci simultaneously on the same membrane. The same probes have the potential to identify new alleles without the need to modify the published probe sequences. In addition the selection of the target motifs for these probes ensures that for a coherent pattern no two probes for the same sequence location can hybridize with the product from a single allele. This approach offers a unique high resolution typing method for most routine and research applications.

References

1. Bidwell J L. Applications of the polymerase chain reaction to HLA class II typing. *Vox Sang* 1992; 63:81-9.
2. Krausa P, Brywka III M, Savage D, Hui KM, Bunce M, Ngai JLF, Teo DLT, Ong YW, Barouch D, Allsop CEM, Hill AVS, McMichael AJ, Bodmer JG, Browning MJ. Genetic polymorphism within HLA-A*02: significant allelic variation revealed in different populations. *Tissue Antigens* 1995; 45:223-31.
3. Krausa P, Bodmer JG, Browning MJ. Defining the common subtypes of HLA A9, A10, A28 and A19 by use of ARMS/PCR. *Tissue Antigens* 1993; 42:91-9.
4. Allen M, Liu L, Gyllensten U. A comprehensive polymerase chain reaction-oligonucleotide typing system for HLA class I A locus. *Hum Immunol* 1994; 40:25-32.
5. Gao X, Jakobsen IB, Serjeantson SW. Characterization of the HLA-A polymorphism by locus-specific polymerase chain reaction amplification and oligonucleotide hydridization. *Hum Immunol* 1994: 41:267-79.
6. Clay TMC, Bidwell JL, Howard MR, Bradley BA. PCR-fingerprinting for selection of HLA matched unrelated marrow donors. *Lancet* 1991; 337:1049-52.
7. Tong JY, Hammad A, Rudert WA, Trucco M, Hsia S. Heteroduplexes for HLA DQB1 identity of family members and kidney donor-recipient pairs. *Transplantation* 1994; 57:741-5.
8. Sorrentino R, Cascino I, Tosi R. Subgrouping of DR4 alleles by DNA heteroduplex analysis. *Hum Immunol* 1992; 33:18-23.
9. Hoshino S, Kimura A, Fukuda Y, Dohi K, Sasazuki T. Polymerase chain reaction-single-strand conformation polymorphism analysis of polymorphism in DPA1 and DPB1 genes: A simple, economical, and rapid method for histocompatibility testing. *Hum Immunol* 1992; 33:98-107.
10. Blasczyk R, Hahn U, Wehling J, Huhn D, Salama A. Complete subtyping of the HLA-A locus by sequence-specific amplification followed by direct sequencing or single-strand conformation polymorphism analysis. *Tissue Antigens* 1995; 46:86-95.
11. Petersdorf EW, Hansen JA. A comprehensive approach for typing the alleles of the HLA-B locus by automated sequencing. *Tissue Antigens* 1995; 46:73-85.
12. Arnett KL, Parham P. HLA class I nucleotide sequences, 1995. *Tissue Antigens* 1995; 45:217-57.
13. Garaghty DE, Koller BH, Hansen JA, Orr HT. Examination of four HLA class I pseudogenes. Common events in the evolution of HLA genes and pseudogenes. *J Immunol* 1992; 149:19-34.
14. Cereb N, Maye P, Lee S, Kong Y, Yang, SY. Locus-specific amplification of HLA class I genes from genomic DNA. *Tissue Antigens* 1995; 45:1-11.
15. Madrigal JA, Belich M, Hildebrand W, Benjamin R, Little AM, Zemmour J, Ennis P, Ward F, Petzl-Erler M, du Toit E, Parham P. Distinctive HLA-A, B antigens of black populations formed by interallelic conversion. *J Immunol* 1992: 149: 3411-5.
16. Parham P, Adams E, Arnett KL. The Origins of HLA-A, B, C Polymorphism. *Immunol Rev* 1995; 143:141-80.

Typing of HLA-B alleles by single-tube nested PCR-SSP

H. Bellot, K. Böttcher, J. Hein, H. Kirchner, G. Bein

Institute of Immunology and Transfusion Medicine, University of Lübeck, Medical School, Ratzeburger Allee 160, 23538 Lübeck, Germany

HLA class I typing at the DNA level is confronted with the extensive sharing of sequence elements both within a single locus and among other members of the HLA class I multigene family [1]. As one single sequence element can appear in different alleles there is frequently a lack of allele-specific sequence motifs. Thus the differentiation of distinct alleles, especially in heterozygous individuals, requires a method that recognizes a specific combination of sequence elements on one single chromosome, *i. e.* in *cis* localisation.

We previously described a procedure for low resolution DNA typing by a two-step PCR amplification with nested sequence-specific primers (nPCR-SSP) which allows identification of all homozygous and heterozygous combinations within the HLA-B5 cross-reactive group [2]. However, for reasons of practical handling, extension of this approach is not suitable for clinical purpose. We thus developed a one-tube nested PCR assay [3-5] where one PCR reaction defines the presence or absence of a serologically defined specifity, *e.g.* HLA-B*51. This procedure minimizes the risk of pipetting mistakes and cross-contamination between the two amplification rounds and simplifies interpretation of the typing results.

Material and methods

Reference DNA samples and DNA extraction

EBV-transformed B-lymphoblastoid cell lines of the 10th International Histocompatibility Workshop served as amplification and specificity controls: BM92 (B51), RML (B51), AMAI (B53), and E4181324 (B52). genomic DNA was isolated essentially according to the salting-out procedure [6].

PCR primers

Primers were designed using a recent compilation of the WHO-recognized HLA class I sequences [7] and referring to the primers published by J. Hein [2] *(Table I)*. All primers were provided by a commercial supplier (TIB Molbiol, Berlin, Germany).

PCR amplification and visualization of amplification products

PCR reactions were carried out either in thin-walled tubes or in MicroAmp™ Reaction Tubes in a total reaction volume of 20 µl. Each reaction mix consisted of: 50 ng genomic DNA, 2 µl of 10x Taq buffer (Perkin Elmer), dNTPs (4 pmol), the outer primers (2 pmol each), the inner primers (5 pmol each), the internal control primers HGH I and HGH III (1.5 pmol each), and 0.5 U Taq polymerase (Perkin Elmer). AmpliWax™ beads (Perkin Elmer) were used to perform the hot start technique [8]. After an initial denaturation step at 96°C for 2 min, the samples were subjected to 15 cycles of 96°C for 10 sec, 70°C for 30 sec, and 72°C for 30 sec. This was followed by 10 cycles of 96°C for 10 sec, 63°C for 30 sec, and 72°C for 30 sec, then 10 cycles where the annealing temperature was dropped to 52°C for 30 sec to increase the amount of the amplified product. The reactions were completed by a final extension step at 72°C for 5 min. 10µl aliquots of the reaction products were subjected to gel electrophoresis on

Table I.

Primer	Nucleotide number	Sequence (5'-3'-orientation)	$Tm_{(2+4)}$ in °C
63 N	168 - 189	GCC GGA GTA TTG GGA CCG GAA C	72°C
163 L	559 - 578	CGG AGC CAC TCC ACG CAC AG	68°C
81 A	226 - 241	GAG AAC CTG CGG ATC G	52°C
114 N	412 - 428	TCG TAG GCG TAC TGG TT	52°C
HGH I	5556 - 5580	CAG TGC CTT CCC AAC CAT TCC CTT A	76°C
HGH III	6609 - 6633	CCT TGT CCA TGT CCT TCC TGA AGC A	76°C

standard 2% agarose gels. After ethidium bromide staining the results were examined under UV transillumination and documented by photography.

Results and discussion

The one-tube nested PCR is based on the principle that primers with a high Tm can anneal to the template DNA at a high annealing temperature whereas shorter primers with a lower Tm will not be able to anneal until the temperature is dropped to a certain level. This allows during the first amplification step to generate a PCR product that will only be primed by the outer, longer primers if the annealing temperature is kept at a high level.

To prevent the outer primers from competing for the amplification with the inner primers during the second amplification step their concentration in the reaction mix has to be limited. We therefore investigated different concentrations of the outer primers at a given concentration of the inner primers as well as a number of cycling protocols to obtain maximum specificity and efficiency of the PCR during the different amplification steps. Only at the reaction conditions described above were we able to detect the product of the first amplification step as well as that of the second. Under all other cycling-conditions either the detected signal was too weak, or the specificity of the PCR was poor.

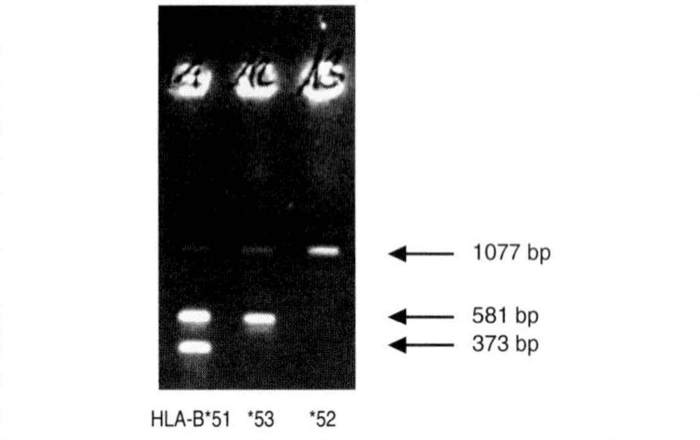

Figure 1. The electrophoresis shows a typing result by the HLA-B*51 single-tube assay. In the first lane there is a DNA (RML) to which all four primers match completely: the product of the first amplification step is located at 581 bp, the product of the second amplification step at 373 bp. The second lane shows a DNA (AMAI) with a single mismatch for one inner primer, only the product of the first amplification step can be seen. The DNA in the third lane (E4181324) has a mismatch for one of the outer primers, only the signal of the internal control, a 1077 bp fragment of the human growth hormone gene, is detectable.

Once the PCR conditions were established we were able to detect the product of the outer primer pair as well as of the inner primer pair only if all four primers completely matched the template DNA. If there was a single mismatch for the inner primers only the product of the first amplification step was detectable. A mismatch for the outer primers led to no signal at all except for that of the internal control *(figure 1)*.

HLA-B typing by this technique offers an excellent degree of resolution since the location of four sequence motifs on one chromosome is detected in a single assay. It therefore provides more distinct information than one-step PCR-SSP or PCR-SSO typing. Its extension might allow a complete and easy to handle low resolution typing of the HLA-B locus if equal PCR parameters can be applied for the other serologically defined specificities.

References

1. Geraghty DE, Koller BH, Hansen JA, Orr HT. The HLA class I family includes at least six genes and twelve pseudogenes and gene fragments. *J Immunol* 1992; 149: 1934-46.
2. Hein J, Böttcher K, Grundmann R, Kirchner H, Bein G. Low resolution DNA typing of the HLA-B5 cross-reactive group by nested PCR-SSP. *Tissue Antigens* 1995; 45: 27-35.
3. Erlich HA, Gelfland D, Sninsky JJ. Recent advances in the polymerase chain reaction. *Science* 1991; 252: 1643-51.
4. Pecharatana S, Pickett MA, Watt PJ, Ward ME. Genotyping ocular strains of *Chlamydia trachomatis* by single-tube nested PCR. *PCR Methods Appl* 1993; 3: 200-4.
5. Wilson SM, McNerney R, Nye PM, Godfrey-Fausset PD, Stoker NG, Voller A. Progress toward a simplified polymerase chain reaction and its application to diagnosis of tuberculosis. *J Clin Microbiol* 1993; 31: 776-81.
6. Miller SA, Dykes DD, Polesky HF. A simple salting out procedure for extracting DNA from human nucleated cells. *Nucleic Acids Res* 1988; 16: 12-5.
7. Fernandez-Vina M. HLA-B nucleotide sequences. *Internet ASHI homepage* (last updated on March), 1996.
8. D'Aquila RT, Bechtel LJ, Videler JA, Eron JJ, Gorczyca P, Kaplan JC. Maximizing sensitivity and specificity of PCR by preamplification heating. *Nucleic Acids Res* 1991; 19: 37-49.

A nested PCR-RFLP method for high-resolution typing of HLA-B locus alleles

S. Mitsunaga[1], A. Ogawa[1], K. Tokunaga[1,2], T. Akaza[1], K. Tadokoro[1], T. Juji[1]

1 Department of Research, Japanese Red Cross Central Blood Center, 4-1-31 Hiroo, Shibuya-ku, Tokyo 150, Japan
2 Department of Human Genetics, University of Tokyo, 7-3-1 Hongo, Bunkyo-ku, Tokyo 113, Japan

PCR-RFLP methods are useful for high resolution HLA typing of a relatively small number of samples. However, use of this method has been limited to HLA class II typing until now. Only exon 2 is highly polymorphic in HLA class II genes, and locus specific amplification of the exon is relatively easy. On the other hand, both exon 2 and exon 3 are highly polymorphic in HLA class I genes, and locus specific amplification of each exon is very difficult, as there are no locus specific nucleotide sequences at the boundary regions of exon 2 and exon 3. It is theoretically possible to analyze the region containing exon 2, intron 2 and exon 3 using a PCR-RFLP method instead of separately analyzing both exons. However, data on the intron 2 nucleotide sequence of most HLA-B alleles are not available.

We adopted a nested PCR system for locus specific amplification of exon 2 and exon 3 of HLA-B gene. The first PCR achieves HLA-B locus specific amplification of the region containing exon 2, intron 2 and exon3. Then, exon 2 and exon 3 are specifically amplified separately by the second PCR using the diluted first PCR product as template. The primer pairs for the second PCR are exon specific but not locus specific. However, locus specificity is guaranteed by the first PCR.

The first PCR amplification of genomic DNA using outer primers was performed for 30 cycles (96 °C for 30 seconds and 74 °C for 1 minute) followed by a final extension step at 72 °C for 5 minutes. The primers described by Cereb *et al.* [1], 5BIn1-57 and 3BIn3-37, were used for the HLA-B locus specific first PCR. After the first PCR, exon 2 and exon 3 were amplified separately using nested primer pairs. A group specific amplification system was used for the second PCR to simplify the following RFLP analysis. Namely, two primer sets, ex21/N4 and ex23/N4, were used for exon 2 amplification, and three primer sets, BF-E31/Bga, BF-E31/Bac and BF-E31/Bct, were used for exon 3 amplification. In the second PCR, 2 μl of 1/1000 diluted first PCR product was used as template and amplified for 25 cycles (96 °C for 30 seconds, 54 °C for 1 minute and 72 °C for 30 seconds). After amplification, products were denatured at 96 °C for 2 minutes and gradually reannealed by decreasing the temperature to 70 °C at a rate of 1°C per 5 minutes to avoid heteroduplex formation [2]. Both the first and second PCRs were carried out in a 100 μl volume using the same reaction mixture except for primers: 50 mM Tris-HCl pH8.8, 10 mM $(NH_4)_2SO_4$, 1.5 mM $MgCl_2$, 250 mM each of dNTP, 2.5 units of Taq polymerase, and 50 pmol of each primer. The reaction mixture and PCR conditions which were reported by Cereb *et al.* [1] were also used for the first PCR. The specificity of the group specific PCR amplification was confirmed by amplification of serologically typed samples. Only expected samples from serological typing data were amplified (data not shown). Nucleotide sequences of each primer are as follows:

ex21, 5'-GGTATTTC(TC)ACACC(TG)CCG-3'
ex23, 5'-GGTATTTC(TC)ACACCGCCA-3'
N4, 5'-TCGCTCTGGTTGTAGTAG-3'
BF-E31, 5'-GGG(CT)CA(GA)GGTCTCACA-3'
Bga, 5'-GCCACTCCACGCACTC-3'
Bac, 5'-GCCACTCCACGCACGT-3'
Bct, 5'-GCCACTCCACGCACAG-3'.

The Bct primer has mismatches at nucleotide positions 571 and 572 compared with some alleles. However, we confirmed this primer could be used to amplify B*4403 and B*5103 which possessed mismatches at these positions.

A total of 143 HLA-B alleles [3] were analyzed by computer for expected PCR-RFLP patterns using various endonucleases. The number of alleles which were predicted to be amplified with the primer pair ex21/N4 and

Table I. Numbers of different PCR-RFLP patterns predicted by computer analysis

Group (total number)	Restriction enzymes		No. of RFLP patterns	Total RFLP patterns for each exon
exon 2-ex21 (47)*1	AvaII, BsrI, Cac8I, DdeI, DpnII, HaeIII, MnlI, NciI, SspI	(9)	21	
exon 2-ex23 (96)*1	BanII, BsmAI, BsoFI, BsrDI, BsrI, DpnII, MboII, MnlI, Sau96I, SspI	(10)	33	54 (exon 2)
exon 3-Bga (31)*1	AluI, BglII, BstNI, DdeI, FokI, KpnI, MspA1I, NlaIII	(8)	19	
exon 3-Bac (32)*1	AluI, BslI, BsrI, NlaIII, RsaI	(5)	14	
exon 3-Bct (80)*1	BsaHI, BslI, Bsp1286I, BsrI, Cac8I, DdeI, FokI, HphI, RsaI, SacII	(10)	40*2	73 (exon 3)
total: 143 alleles				total: 122 PCR-RFLP patterns (exon 2 + exon 3)

*1 Number of alleles included.
*2 B*1526N can be distinguished from B*1527 by XcmI digestion.
*2 B*3505 can be distinguished from B*3517 by MaeII digestion.

ex23/N4 were 47 and 96, respectively. Results of computer analysis on the recognition sites of various endonucleases predicted that 47 HLA-B alleles of the ex21/N4 group would be resolved into 21 PCR-RFLP patterns using nine restriction endonucleases, and 96 HLA-B alleles of the ex23/N4 group would be resolved into 33 PCR-RFLP patterns using ten restriction endonucleases *(Table I)*. As for exon 3, 31, 32 and 80 alleles were predicted to be amplified with the primer pairs BF-E31/Bga, BF-E31/Bac and BF-E31/Bct, respectively. Similarly, results of computer analysis predicted that 31 alleles of the BF-E31/Bga group, 32 alleles of the BF-E31/Bac group and 80 alleles of the BF-E31/Bct group would be resolved into 19, 14 and 40 PCR-RFLP patterns, using 8, 5 and 10 restriction endonucleases, respectively. The total number of predicted PCR-RFLP patterns for exon 2 was 54, and 73 for exon 3. Moreover, 122 PCR-RFLP patterns were predicted to be obtained by the combination of exon 2 and exon 3 patterns. All of the 143 HLA-B alleles except for the following could be distinguished using the present PCR-RFLP method: B*1501 = 1512 = 1514 = 1519, B*1502 = 1521, B*1509 = 1510, B*1511 = 1515 = 1528, B*1526N = 1527, B*2703 = 27052 = 2710, B*3501 = 3503 = 3506 = 3511, B*3505 = 3517, B*3510 = 3513, B*39011 = 39013 = 3905, B*40011 = 40012, B*5101 = 5102 = 5103 and B*5501 = 5502. Among these alleles, B*1526N can be distinguished from B*1527 by XcmI digestion, and B*3505 can be distinguished from B*3517 by MaeII digestion.

We analyzed 32 samples which were distributed at the International Cell Exchange held by Terasaki laboratory (UCLA), using present PCR-RFLP method. We identified

27 HLA-B alleles in these samples. Only the results obtained with one sample contradicted the consensus results of other laboratories due to partial digestion with one restriction enzyme. We also used this method for the analysis of post-transfusion graft-versus-host disease (PT-GVHD) [4]. In almost all cases of PT-GVHD, no information is available on the HLA types of patient and donors. However, we could identify HLA-B alleles and HLA-A, -DRB1, -DQB1 and -DPB1 successfully using PCR-RFLP methods described here and elsewhere (2). Various PCR-based HLA-B typing methods have been reported. The PCR-SSOP method is one of the most reliable method and is used widely for HLA class I typing, including HLA-B, and HLA class II typing. However, it is not practical to use this method for typing of a relatively small number of samples due to the requirement of a large number of probes. A nested PCR-RFLP method described here is a reliable and suitable method for high resolution typing of a relatively small number of samples.

References

1. Cereb N, Maye P, Lee S, Kong Y, Yang SY. Locus-specific amplification of HLA class I genes from genomic DNA: locus-specific sequences in the first and third introns of HLA-A, -B, and -C alleles. *Tissue Antigens* 1995: 45: 1-11.
2. Mitsunaga S, Oguchi T, Tokunaga K, Akaza T, Tadokoro K, Juji T. High-resolution HLA-DQB1 typing by combination of group-specific amplification and RFLP. *Hum Immunol* 1995: 42: 307-14.
3. Marsh SGE. Nomenclature for factors of the HLA system, update January 1996. *Tissue Antigens* 1996: 47: 262-3.
4. Nishimura M, Uchida S, Mitsunaga S, Tokunaga K, Tadokoro K, Juji T. Evidence of involvement of cytotoxic antibodies directed against patient's HLA class II produced by transfused donor-derived B cells in post-transfusion graft-versus-host disease. *Br J Haematol* 1996: 92: 1011-3.

Optimization of high resolution DNA typing of HLA-A and -B alleles

A.M. Lazaro, M.A. Fernandez-Vina, C.J. Nulf, V.M. Fish, J.E. McGarry, C.Y. Marcos, P. Stastny

Department of Internal Medicine, University of Texas, Southwestern Medical Center, 5323 Harry Hines boulevard, Dallas TX 75235, USA

HLA class I genes comprise 3 classical genes encoding the major histocompatibility antigens HLA-A, -B and -C and 3 non-classical genes -E, -F, and -G, and the pseudogenes -H, -J, -K, and -L. The HLA-complex presents the largest allelic polymorphism of the entire human genome. Many of the polymorphic sequences are shared not only by alleles of a given locus, but are also present in other classical and non-clasical class I genes. HLA-B is the most polymorphic locus of the class I genes. The regions with the highest sequence variability are localized in exons 2 and 3, which encode the peptide-binding α1 and α2 domains of the class I molecules. Due to the large number of class I loci, PCR–SSOP typing requires the development of locus-specific and/or group-specific primer sets. Previously, we reported a comprehensive procedure for high resolution DNA typing of HLA-B locus alleles [1]. We have now simplified, improved, and expanded this procedure. PCR conditions were improved by using a buffer containing 15 mM ammonium sulphate, 10mM beta-mercaptoethanol and 10% dimethyl sulfoxide (DMSO). The addition of these two co-solvents as an aid for PCR amplification has been previous described [2].

All amplifications were carried out under identical conditions in a thermal cycler (Gene Amp PCR System 9600, Perkin Elmer Corporation, Norwalk, CT). Amplified DNA was immobilized on nylon membranes by dot-blotting.

Figure 1 shows the DNA-amplification strategy used. HLA-A locus typing was performed with the primers RAP1007 (AGGATCCAGACGCCGAGGATGGCCG) and DB337 (CAGGATCCCTCCTTCCCGTTCTC-CAGGT) described by Bugawan *et al.* [3]. The amplified fragment of 990 bp spans from the first exon to the end of exon 3 of locus A, including the intervening introns. A set of 93 SSOP 19 nucleotide-long were locally designed ([4] and unpublished) to analyze all polymorphic segments of exons 2 and 3. Genotypes were assigned according to the corresponding hybridization patterns of currently recognized alleles.

HLA-B typing included two PCR-SSOP steps. The first involved an initial screening by PCR-SSOP hybridization of polymorphisms in codons 45-46 to classify the samples into one of the four groups of alleles: B7-8 (includes B7-8-14-16-27-42-48-55-56-59-67-70-73-81-82), B12-40 (includes B12-21-40-41-47-B*3519), B5-35 (includes B5-18-35-37-53-58-78-B*1522-B*4406), B15-57 (includes B15-13-57). B-locus specific amplification was obtained with the primers 5'Bin (spanning nucleotides 36 to 57 of first intron; GGGAGGAGCGAGGG-GACC(GC)CAG) and 3'Bin (spanning nucleotides 37 to 59 of 3rd intron GGAGATGGGGAAGGCTCCCCACT) described by Cereb *et al.* [2]. In addition to the analysis of codons 45-46, these PCR products were also tested for the polymorphisms of the first segment of exon-2 (which is not amplified with the group-specific primers) that distinguish subtypes of B14, B39 and B35.

The second step involved group–specific amplification (GSA). The 5' primers spanning the polymorphisms of codons 45-46, previously described by us [1] were combined with the B-locus 3' intron primer (3Bin). Four different sets of probe of about 50 SSOP each were used to analyze all the polymorphic sites of exon 2 and exon 3. Alleles were assigned on the basis of their hybridization patterns. There are currently 145 HLA-B alleles ([5] and S. Marsh, 1996 update). The resolution achieved by the GSA-SSOP typing method here described is quite high, since it allows identification of 143 distinguishable patterns that correspond to 141 alleles and to 2 pairs of alleles. The couples B*1512/1519 and B*0705/0706 differ from each other in exons 4 and 5 respectively which could not be analyzed with the primers used. The sharing of sequences between alleles did not interfere with the assignment of the majority of genotypes, since it was possible distinguish 10278 genotypes of 10296 genotypic combinations (considering 143 alleles). Only 18 genotypes (9 pairs) were ambiguous.

In this study we performed high resolution typing of HLA-A (n=400) and -B (n=1509) alleles of a panel comprising samples from Caucasoid, African-American, Hispanic and Oriental subjects as well as from individuals from North American and South American Indian tribes. Eighty-five cell lines of the Tenth International Histocompatibility Workshop (10th IHWS) were used as controls.

The results showed a good correlation of DNA typing with serology in the majority of the broad HLA-B specificities. However, some serological splits such as B51, B52, B56, B62, B63 had a poor correlation with r values between 0.50 and 0.85 or very poorly correlation as B65, B75 and B64 with $r < 0.50$. Two novel alleles found in the course of this work (B*3519 and A*0219) were serological blanks. Certain serological antigens may be represented by several subtypes at similar frequency in the same ethnic group. Therefore, the chances of finding identity for DNA-defined variants based on serologic typing of B-locus alleles could be low even among pairs from the same ethnic group. Matching for HLA-B locus by serological typing has an impact in allograft survival in kidney transplantation [6, 7]. It is not known whether matching for DNA-defined alleles improves graft survival or if the mismatch subtypes are involved in rejection in bone marrow transplantation. However other studies [8] have shown that minor mismatches between B-locus alleles can be distinguished by T lymphocytes.

In the course of this study, we could identify 97 HLA-B locus alleles and found 25 novel hybridization patterns. These were consistent with new alleles sequenced by other investigators [9] and our group [10, 11]. The novel alleles differ from their postulated progenitors by few residue subtitutions. Those substitutions may affect the structure of the peptide binding specificity pockets and could also affect T cell recognition.

In summary, we developed and optimized a batch-mode procedure for high resolution DNA-typing of HLA-A

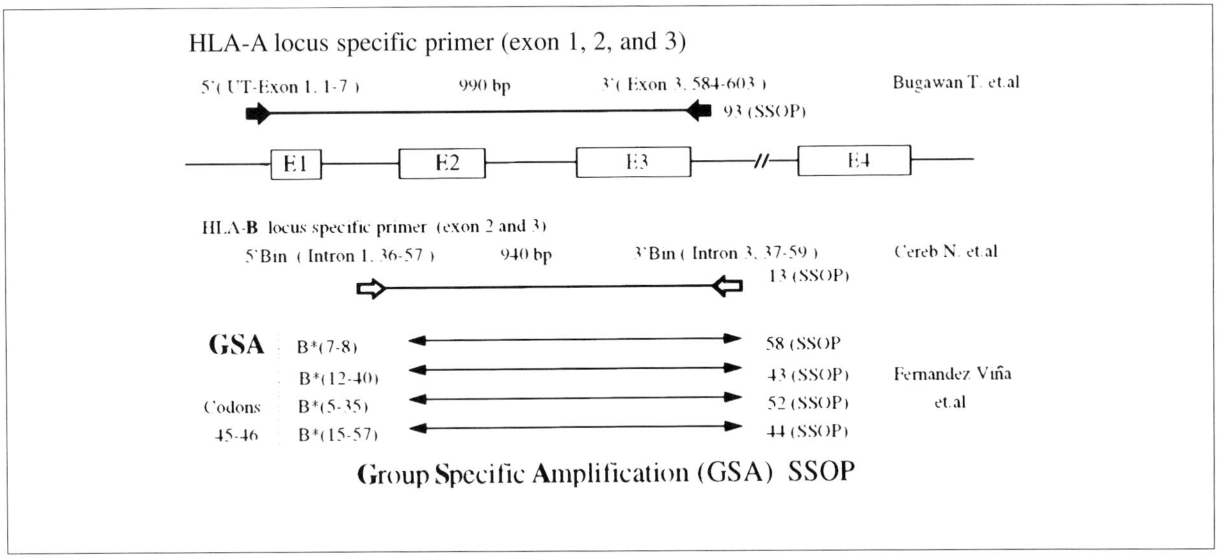

Figure 1. DNA amplification strategy selected for molecular typing of HLA-A and B loci. Genomic DNA was amplified by PCR with locus- and group-specific primers (GSA). The amplified HLA-A fragment spans from exon-1 to the end of exon-3. HLA-B typing involved two types of amplifications. HLA-B locus amplification included a segment extending from intron-1 to intron-3. Four B-locus group-specific amplifications (GSA) were obtained with primers spanning the polymorphism of codons 45-46 combined with the monomorphic B-locus 3'primer 3'Bin. The numbers preceding (SSOP) correspond to those used to hybridize the different amplifications performed.

and -B loci which allows to distinguish 99.82 percent of all the possible genotypes.This methodology can be applied to the typing of large numbers of donors for registries of unrelated bone marrow transplants.

References

1. Fernandez Vina MA, Lazaro AM, Sun Y, Miller S, Forero L, Stastny P. Population Diversity of B-locus alleles observed by high-resolution DNA typing. *Tissue Antigens* 1995: 45:153-68.
2. Cereb N, Maye P, Lee S, Kong Y, Yang SY. Locus-specific amplification of HLA class I genes from genomic DNA: locus-specific sequences in the first and third introns of HLA-A, -B and -C. *Tissue Antigens* 1995: 45:1-11.
3. Bugawan TL, Apple R, Erlich HA. A method for typing polymorphism at the HLA-A locus using PCR amplification and immobilized oligonucleotide probes. *Tissue Antigens* 1994: 44:137-47.
4. Fernandez-Vina MA, Falco M, Sun Y, Stastny P. DNA typing for HLA class I alleles: I. Subsets of HLA-A2 and of A28. *Hum Immunol* 1992: 33:163-73.
5. Marsh SGE. Nomenclature for factors of the HLA system, update January 1995. *Tissue Antigens* 1995: 45:220-2.
6. Opelz G. Importance of HLA antigen splits for kidney transplant matching. *Lancet* 1988: 2:61-6.
7. Takemoto S, Terasaki PI, Cecka JM, Cho YW, Gjertson DW. Survival of nationally shared, HLA-matched kidney transplants from cadaveric donors. The UNOS Scientific Renal Transplant Registry (see comments). *N Engl J Med* 1992: 327:834-9.
8. Fleischhauer K, Kernan NA, O'Reilly RJ, Dupont B, Yang SY. Bone marrow allograft rejection by T lymphocytes recognizing a single amino acid difference in HLA-B44. *N Engl J Med* 1990: 323:1818-22.
9. Arnett KL, P P. HLA Class I nucleotide sequences, 1995. *Tissue Antigens* 1995: 46:217-57.
10. Marcos CY, Fernandez-Vina MA, Lazaro AM, Raimondi EH, S. Novel HLA-B35 subtypes from native Americans. Putative gene conversion events with donor sequences of alleles common in native Americans (B*4002 or B*4801). 1997 (in press).
11. Garber TL, Butler LM, Trachtenberg EA, *et al.* HLA-B alleles of the Cayapa of Ecuador. New B39 and B15 alleles. *Immunogenetics* 1995: 42:19-27.

Rapid subtyping for HLA B27 by denaturing gradient gel electrophoresis (DGGE)

R. Tamouza[1], F. Marzais[1], R. Krishnamoorthy[2], C. Besmond[2], C. Raffoux[1], D. Charron[1]

1 Laboratoire d'Imunologie et d'Histocompatibilité, Hôpital Saint-Louis and INSERM U396, 1, avenue Claude Vellefaux, 75010 Paris, France
2 INSERM U120, Hôpital Robert Debré, Paris, France

The extreme polymorphism of both class I and II genes results in the most highly variable system of functional alleles presently known. However, molecular typing of HLA class I genes and in particular of the HLA B locus has been delayed due to structural characteristics of the locus namely that the polymorphic sites, distributed in 2 exons, are concentrated on short area of both exons. Among the functional implications of the MHC class I, several associations have been described between a disease and a specific allele or group of alleles. In this context, ankylosing spondylitis (AS) was found to be strongly associated with the HLA class I specificity B27 [1] and has become a classical example in HLA and disease studies. At the molecular level, HLA B27 represent a group of nine closely related alleles that differ in a restricted number of nucleotides substitution, clustered in the 3' and 5' parts of exons 2 and 3 respectively. A molecular typing was reported using PCR-SSOP for the different subtypes of HLA B27 [2]. In contrast to this investigation using multiples targetted probes, we choose a global approach which could not only discriminate between the differents subtypes but also identify a potentially unknown mutant in the region studied. The denaturing gradient gel electrophoresis (DGGE) method [3], allows the resolution of DNA fragments differing by a single nucleotide substitution. The method is based on the electrophoretic mobility of a double strand DNA molecule through linearly increasing concentrations of a denaturing agent. During the migration, a position will be reached where the concentration of denaturing agent equals the melting temperature (Tm) of the DNA fragment lowest melting domain, causing denaturation and consequent retardation of its electrophoretic mobility.

In this study, we describe a DNA subtyping system based on the allelic polymorphism within the HLA-B27 group involving allele specific amplification in combination with denaturing gradient gel electrophoresis of PCR products for exons 2 and 3. This approach is able to discriminate 8 alleles. The subtyping was completed by RFLP for the identification of B*2707.

Materials and methods

Subjects

Thirty homozygous and heterozygous HLA B27 positive cell lines of known B27 subtypes were use.

PCR amplification

Specific amplification of B27

Three PCR amplifications necessary for the complete subtyping of HLA B27 indicated as A, B and C, were performed in the same conditions. A fourth locus B exon 2 PCR, D, is systematically carried out to differenciate between B27 homo and heterozygotes alleles. Primers sequences, specificities, locations, orientations, and reaction conditions are given in *Table I.*

Subtyping procedure

Artificial heteroduplexing

A heteroduplexing step is performed by the artificial mixing of the PCR product to be analysed and a known and common B27 subtype PCR product.

DGGE analysis

The gel apparatus for the DGGE analysis was as described previously [3]. The conditions used for the PCR products of exon 2 and 3 are in brief the following.

One third of the amplifications mix was electrophoresed through a 6% polyacrylamide gel with linearly increasing gradient from 40% to 80% for the two PCR products of exons 2 and 3.

Table I. A. Sequences, directions and positions of primers used for amplification of HLA B27 and HLA B related alleles. B. PCR conditions and specificity

A

Primer	Sequence 5'-->3'	Direction	Position
E40s*	GCCGCGAGTCCGAGAGA	sense	aa 40-45
Spe B	CCACGTCGCAGCCATACATA	antisense	aa 97-104
E91As*	GGGTCTCACACCCTCCAGAAT	sense	aa 91-97
3BIn3-37**	GGAGGCCATCCCCGGCGACCTAT	antisense	Int3: 37-59
E91Bs*	GGGTCTCACACCCTCCAGAGC	sense	aa 91-97
E181as*	GCGCTGCAGCGTCTCCTT	antisense	aa 175-181
5BIn1-57**	GGGAGGAGCGAGGGGACCG	sense	Int1: 36-57
E90as*	GGCCTCGCTCTGGTTGTA	antisense	aa 85-90

B

PCR	Pair	T°C	MgCl2	bp	Specificity
A	E40s/Spe B	63°C	1.0	436	Exon2 + Intron2/B27
B	E91As/3BIn3-37	-	-	335	Exon3/B27
C	E91Bs/E181as	-	-	273	Exon3/B2707+B alleles
D	5BIn1-57/E90as	-	-	362	Exon2/B alleles

* and **: primers previously described [2,5].

The melting behaviour of both amplified fragments was simulated by computer analysis using the MELT87 program [4].

Strategy

After the B27 specificity determination, the two specific PCR product of exons 2 and 3 were subjected to a DGGE run. This step could resolved 8 out of the 9 subtypes. At the same time, the third PCR product was digested by a B2707 specific enzyme, BsrI (Biolabs Beverly MA).

Results

For analysis of the polymorphisms by DGGE, DNA segments containing the variable regions of exons 2 and 3 could be amplified specifically with exception for B*2707. The two regions studied were assimilated to two distinct fragments, respectively A and B.

Fragment A (Fg A), 436 bp in length, contain a second half of exon 2, intron 2 and the beginning of the third exon. Fragment B (Fg B), 335 bp, consist of the entire exon 3 and a part of the third intron.

Fg A

B* 2701, 02, 03, and 08 shows a distinct and clear different pattern, while B*2705, 09 and B*2704, 06 which exhibit the same sequence in this region shows the same pattern.

Fg B

The analysis of this fragment, served to discriminate between B*2704 and 06, and between B*2705 and 09. All the polymorphic areas were located in the low Tm domain of the two fragments.

For the determination of B*2707 which cannot be amplified by the specific B27 primers, the third PCR amplication of B locus exon 3 (C) was digested by BsrI which is in this case allele specific.

To clarify B27 homozygosity or heterozygosity, we amplify systematically exon 2 of locus B (D) and digest with a B27 specific enzyme StyI (Biolabs Beverly MA). This is essential to interpret an abnormal profile encountered in heteroduplexes analysis.

Discussion

Starting from the fact that the HLA B27 specificity is one of the diagnosis elements for ankylosing spondylitis, we investigated the most suitable approach of DNA subtyping in routine use. Several techniques based on the global study of the target DNA fragment are developed at the present time. We have choosen a proven technology with well defined mathematical rationale: DGGE is caracterised by a computer algorithm to simulate the melting behaviour of the choosed fragments. Furthermore, in the HLA B27 subtyping, even without using GC clamps, the variable regions of the two exons lie in the low melting domains. Hence, every sequence difference results in a mobility difference and could be resolved. Also, if the homoduplexes show a different but close migration, we take advantage of the resolving power of heteroduplexes analysis. In addition, the fact that all the amplification reactions, and the electrophoresis can be realized under the same conditions and at the same time in one day's work for the two exons, represent an important advantage in terms of time.

Finaly, DGGE is very well suited for the identification and charaterization of yet undefined alleles due to its intrinsic ability to analyse DNA polymorphism without knowledge of the nucleotide sequence.

All these features make DGGE well suited for the tissue typing clinical laboratory. Overall, this technology offers a simple, rapid and reliable alternative to the existing methods for subtyping HLA alleles. With its capacity to score new alleles efficiently in population studies, the DGGE is a valid intermediate between targetted screening and untargetted nucleotide sequencing.

References

1. Schlosstein L, Terasaki PJ, Bluestone R, Pearson CM. High association of HLA antigen W27 with ankylosing spondylitis. *N Engl J Med* 1973; 288: 704.
2. Lopez-Larrea C, Sujirachato K, Mehra NK, Chiewsilp P, Isarangkura D, Kanga U, Dominguez O, Coto E, Pena M, Setien F, Gonzalez-Roces S. HLA-B27 subtypes in Asian patients with ankylosing spondylitis. Evidence for new associations. *Tissue Antigens* 1995; 45:169-76.
3. Myers RM, Maniatis T, Lerman LS. Detection and localisation of single base changes by denaturing gradient gel electrophoresis. In Wu R, ed. *Methods in Enzymology*, vol.155. New York: Academic Press, 1987: 501-27.
4. Lerman LS, Silverstein K. Computational simulation of DNA melting and its application to denaturing gradient gel electrophoresis. In Wu R, ed. *Methods in Enzymology*, vol.155. New York: Academic Press, 1987: 482-501.
5. Cereb N, Maye P, Lee S, Kong Y, Yang SY. Locus-specific amplification of HLA class I genes from genomic DNA: locus-specific sequences in the first and third introns of HLA-A, -B, and -C alleles. *Tissue Antigens* 1995; 45: 1-11.

HLA-DQB1 and -DPB1 allele typing by PCR-PHFA method

S. Moriyama[1], K. Tokunaga[1,2], S. Mitsunaga[1], K. Tadokoro[1], T. Oka[3], S. Maekawajiri[3], A. Yamane[3], T. Juji[1]

1 Department of Research, Japanese Red Cross Central Blood Center, 4-1-31, Hiroo, Shibuya-ku, Tokyo 150, Japan
2 Department of Human Genetics, University of Tokyo, Tokyo, Japan
3 Institute for Biotechnology Research, Wakunaga Pharm. Co., Hiroshima, Japan

Recently, a number of methods such as PCR-sequence-specific oligonucleotide probes (SSO), PCR-sequence-specific primer (SSP), PCR-single-strand conformation polymorphism (SSCP), and PCR-restriction fragment length polymorphism (RFLP) have been introduced for HLA typing in accordance with the increasing requirements for HLA typing in various medical fields. We have developed a reliable high resolution typing method, PCR-preferential homoduplex formation assay (PHFA) [1], for HLA-DQB1 and DPB1 alleles and applied it to our population samples.

Materials and methods

DNA preparation
Genomic DNAs were prepared from peripheral blood leukocytes of unrelated Japanese according to a previously described simple procedure [2].

PCR amplification
PCR-PHFA was applied for the polymorphic second exon of class II genes. The DQB1 gene was amplified by PCR using two primer pairs, QB1P55 [2] /DQBAMP-C (5'-CCCGCGGTACGCCACCTC-3') and QB1P55/DQBAMP-D (5'-TCGTGCGGAGCTCC AACTG-3'), which correspond to DQ5 and DQ6 groups, and DQ2, DQ3 and DQ4 groups, respectively. The DPB1 gene was also amplified, using DPBAMP-A/DPBAMP-B [1]. Amplification was carried out in 100μl of reaction mixture for 35 cycles in a thermal cycler, using a step program (denaturation at 95 °C for 30 seconds, annealing at 60 °C for the DQB1 gene and at 55 °C for the DPB1 gene for 30 seconds, and finally extension at 72 °C for 30 seconds).

Principle of PCR-PHFA
The principle of this method is based on preferential homoduplex formation during hybridization between double (DNP and biotin)-labeled standard and unlabeled sample DNA. Labeled and unlabeled PCR products are mixed and heat-denatured. When the sequence of the sample DNAs is identical to that of the labeled standard, mutually strand exchange occurs. As a result, the amount of double labeled ds (double-stranded) DNAs decreases due to dilution with the unlabeled sample DNAs. On the other hand, when there are differences between the two sequences, most of double-labeled dsDNA recovered. Double-labeled dsDNA was detected using a format similar to that of ELISA with a microtiter plate coated with streptavidin and anti-DNP antibody conjugated alkaline phosphatase.

Preparation of standard DNA
Genomic DNAs from homozygous individuals were used to prepare standard DNAs. Some control DNAs were prepared from heterozygous individuals by cloning. These control DNAs were amplified with double (DNP and biotin)-labeled primers and the products of the amplification were used as standard DNAs.

Preferential homoduplex formation
Preferential homoduplex formation was performed in 30μl reaction mixture containing 20μl of diluted standard DNA solution (0.5μl of double-labeled standard DNA, 9μl of 10xSSC, 3μl of DMSO, 7.5μl of distilled water) and 10μl of unlabeled sample PCR product. For homoduplex formation, temperature of mixture was slowly cooled down to 70°C from 98°C at a rate of 1°C per 10 min in a thermal cycler.

Detection of double-labeled molecules
After homoduplex formation, the reaction mixture was transferred to a streptavidin-coated microtiter plate with 100μl of solution I containing anti-DNP antibody conjugated alkaline phosphatase [1]. After incubation for 30

Table I. DQB1 allele typing for DQ2,3,4 groups by PCR-PHFA

Unlabeled DNA (Sample)	*Index* [1)] Labeled Standard DNA *0201	*0301	*0302 [2)]	*0303	*0401	*0402	Assigned by PCR-PHFA	Assigned by PCR-RFLP
A	88	90	[3]	29	79	80	0302	0302
B	87	[4]	77	63	90	86	0301	0301
C	91	[8]	75	61	[4]	10	0301 /0401	0301 /0401
D	[4]	76	89	88	10	[4]	0201 /0402	0201 /0402
E	87	55	20	[2]	135	93	0303	0303
F	80	[6]	16	[2]	80	75	0301 /0303	0301 /0303
G	92	87	[3]	20	88	80	0302	0302

The intensity of the resulting yellow color development was measured at 405nm.

1) Results were presented as *index* values calculated from a net absorbance .

$\textit{Index} = 100 \times A_{405}$ **sample /** A_{405} **DDW**

2) The data in boxes represent positive signals.

Table II. DPB1 allele typing by PCR-PHFA

Unlabeled DNA (Sample)	*Index* [1)] Labeled Standard DNA *0201 [2)]	*0202	*0301[5)]	*0401	*0402	*0501	*0901	*1301	Assigned by PCR-PHFA	Assigned by PCR-RFLP
A	[8]	54	77	64	37	[10]	91	96	0201 /0501	0201 /0501
B	[13]	47	62	60	[15]	73	68	93	0201 /0402	0201 /0402
C[4)]	88	77	[12]	70	89	[11]	44	88	0301 /0501	0301 /0501
D	22	[6]	84	50	[5]	80	85	99	0202 /0402	0202 /0402
E	42	69	91	64	[17]	[16]	93	101	0402 /0501	0402 /0501
F	81	66	95	19	62	[19]	87	95	0401 /0501	0401 /0501
G[3)]	92	86	100	79	85	100	81	[20]	1301	1301
H	71	[19]	100	70	89	[15]	94	103	0202 /0501	0202 /0501
I[3)]	94	102	73	105	105	106	[9]	101	0901	0901

The intensity of the resulting yellow color development was measured at 405nm

1) Results were presented as *index* values calculated from net absorbance at 405nm.

$\textit{Index} = 100 \times A_{405}$ **sample /** A_{405} **DDW**

2) The data in boxes represent positive signals.

3) When only one allele was detected using 8 standard DNAs, another PCR-PHFA was performed using 5 additional standard DNAs to detect rare alleles.

4) DPB1*0301 was distinguished from DPB1*1401 using restriction enzyme Rsa I.

min at room temperature, the plate was washed three times with 350µl of solution I and incubated with 100µl of substrate solution (p-nitrophenyl phosphate disodium salt, Sigma). After incubation at room temperature for 30 min, absorbance was measured using an ELISA reader [3].

PCR-RFLP analysis

To discriminate DQB1*0602 from DQB1*0603, and DPB1*0301 from DPB1*1401, PCR-RFLP method was performed using the restriction enzyme *Rsa* I.

Results and discussion

Most of the DQB1 and DPB1 alleles examined in the present study could be distinguished from each other. Even a one base substitution in the DQB1 gene (*e.g.* DQB1*0302 vs. DQB1*03032) or in the DPB1 gene (*e.g.* DPB1*02012 vs. DPB1*0402) could be clearly detected. Although DQB1*0602 and DQB1*0603, DPB1*0301 and DPB1*1401 were not able to be clearly distinguished using the PCR-PHFA method, those alleles were easily typed using the PCR-RFLP method with one restriction enzyme. In the present study, one hundred healthy Japanese were typed for DQB1 alleles, and 376 Japanese samples were typed for DPB1 alleles using this typing system. The results for both loci agreed well with those obtained using the PCR-RFLP method.

This method is suitable for routine typing, because of simple operation and flexibility for both small and large numbers of samples.

References

1. Oka T, Matsunaga H, Tokunaga K, Mitsunaga S, Juji T, Yamane A. A simple method for detecting single base substitutions and its application to HLA-DPB1 typing. *Nucleic Acids Res* 1994; 22: 1541-7.
2. Mitsunaga S, Oguchi T, Tokunaga K, Akaza T, Tadokoro K, Juji T. High-resolution typing by combination of group-specific amplification and restriction fragment length polymorphism. *Hum Immunol* 1995; 42: 307-14.
3. Kawai S, Maekawajiri S, Tokunaga K, Juji T, Yamane A. A simple method of HLA-DRB typing using enzymatically amplified DNA and immobilized probes on microtiter plate. *Hum Immunol* 1994; 41: 121-6.

A comparative study of HLA-DRB typing by PCR/SSOP versus transcription-mediated amplification (TMA) and probe hybridization protection analysis (HPA)

A.G. Smith, K. Matsubara, A. Marashi, L.A. Guthrie, L. Regen, E. Mickelson, J.A. Hansen

Fred Hutchinson Cancer Research Center, 1124 Columbia Street, E612, Seattle, WA 98104, USA

DNA typing methods have proven far superior to traditional methods for analysis of HLA class II DR genetic traits. The forward dot blot PCR/SSOP method of HLA-DRB typing has been found to be highly accurate for both medium and large scale (50 to 250 samples per week) testing [1,2]. However, this process is labor intensive and poorly suited to large scale automation [3]. In order to evaluate alternative HLA-DNA typing methods, we have used the system of transcription mediated amplification (TMA) [4,5] with probe hybridization protection analysis (HPA) [6] in a microtiter plate format developed by the Chugai Pharmaceutical Co (Tokyo, Japan), to perform intermediate level DRB typing for 502 individual samples. The Chugai typing kit included DNA preparation reagents, an amplification mix with TMA enzymes supplied in lyophilized aliquots, vacuum sealed 96 well microtiter plates containing lyophilized probes with reagents for 4 sample typings per plate, and the hybridization and detection reagents. Plate incubations at 60°C were performed in a microplate shaker incubator (Tomy Tech, Palo Alto, CA) and the chemiluminescent probe signals were detected with a luminometer (Anthos Biotec, Salzburg, Austria) which transmitted the data to a Chugai computer analysis program to print the probe hybridization values and the deduced DRB typing. Up to 24 DNA samples were prepared and typed by TMA/HPA in 11 hours, whereas PCR/SSOP typing of up to 40 samples took approximately 72 hours. 252 samples from patients and family members submitted to our Clinical Immunogenetics Laboratory were prospectively tested concurrently with a locally developed intermediate level DRB PCR/SSOP assay [2] in a double blind fashion. In addition, 250 retrospective samples of archived frozen cells or DNA from clinical and research panels, previously typed by allele level DRB1 PCR/SSOP, were chosen to include 66 distinct DRB1 alleles representing Caucasian, American Black, Asian, and native American ethnic groups.

When the TMA/HPA and PCR/SSOP results of the prospective clinical samples were compared, five samples were found to have discrepant typing. Four of the discordant results occurred in the first two TMA/HPA assays with false negative identification of DRB1*01 (n=3) and DRB1*03 (n=1). The microtiter plate cooling method was modified after these first assays so that, subsequently, plates were carefully nested in a water/ice slurry. Repeat TMA/HPA analysis of the four samples with methodology related problems was concordant with PCR/SSOP. Only one other prospective clinical sample was discordant: DRB1*1001, 0301/0305 (PCR/SSOP) versus DRB1*1001, "X" (TMA/HPA). The same ambiguous HPA pattern was seen in 3 separate tests with the same sample. This sample was ultimately typed as concordant with PCR/SSOP using both the original DNA sample diluted 1:3 and an independent DNA preparation, giving HPA reactions consistent with DRB1*1001, 0301/0305. The problem encountered in TMA/HPA typing this sample was apparently related to the quality of the original sample DNA. *Figure 1* gives the frequency distribution of the DRB1 specificities assigned among the 252 clinical samples by PCR/SSOP versus TMA/HPA after repeat typing of the four samples from the problematic assays, so that only the single false negative TMA/HPA DRB1*03 assignment is noted as discrepant.

The 250 retrospective samples included two unique alleles of DRB1*12, three alleles each of DRB1*01 and

*03, six of DRB1*02, eight alleles each of DRB1*08 and *13, eleven alleles each of DRB1*04, *11, and *14, and DRB1*0701, *0901 and *1001. Particular effort was made to test multiple heterozygous combinations for alleles characteristic of racial and ethnic groups not represented in the Japanese population. For example, DRB1*0302 (n=18), found primarily in American Blacks, and DRB1*1305 (n=17), common in the Jewish population, were each tested in ten different heterozygous combinations; and DRB1*0411 (n=7), found in native Americans, was tested in seven different combinations. Evaluated at the intermediate typing level, TMA/HPA testing of the 250 retrospective samples detected all of the DRB1 alleles present with the exception of false negative identification of DRB1*1402 and *1406 alleles (n=2) in the presence of DRB1*0301, due to the absence of an HPA probe for the LLEQR sequence at codons 67-71 in those DR14 alleles. The highly polymorphic nature of the DR13 and DR14 alleles makes it very difficult to identify all DR6 alleles in the presence of DR3 or DR11 with a limited probe panel by either PCR/SSOP or TMA/HPA. Any sample typed by intermediate level DRB typing as homozygous for DRB*03, *11, *13, or *14 should be analyzed by high resolution analysis to confirm homozygosity. At the high resolution level, the patterns of 12 HPA probes specific for polymorphisms at codons 37, 47, 57, 60, and 67 to 71 were used to evaluate specificity and sensitivity among the 250 retrospective samples. At this level, TMA/HPA identified seven samples as discordant with the previous PCR/SSOP typing. Repeat DR52-associated DRB1 allele level PCR/SSOP with the current panel of probes and allele specific primers [7] determined that TMA/HPA analysis was correct in six samples, all of which involved the identification of sequences at codons 67 to 71 in samples heterozygous for two DR52-associated DRB1 alleles. One sample that typed by PCR/SSOP as DRB1*0405,0807 showed a consistent cross-reaction with the HPA probe for codon 57 D (aspartic acid).

In summary, we have found the TMA/HPA DRB typing system to provide rapid, reliable and accurate clinical typing results. DNA amplification problems were less frequent in TMA/HPA (2%) compared to PCR/SSOP (4.4%). Final TMA/HPA typing of clinical samples was concordant for all 462 DRB specificities identified by medium resolution PCR/SSOP. Among the 250 retrospective samples, a single HPA probe for codon 57 aspartic acid consistently cross-reacted with the codon 57 valine sequence of the DRB1*0807 allele. HPA probes were more specific than local PCR/SSOP, however, in the detection of sequences from codons 67 to 71 among samples heterozygous for two alleles of DRB1*08, 11, 12, or 13.

The current TMA/HPA methodology could be improved by the use of a molded plastic cold block to provide more consistent and secure microtiter plate cooling than the current water/ice slurry. Nevertheless, this methodology, based in a microtiter plate format but without the usual plate washing steps of the traditional ELISA format, has superior potential for microplate handling and reagent distribution with a robotics system and a work surface incorporating microplate heating and cooling units.

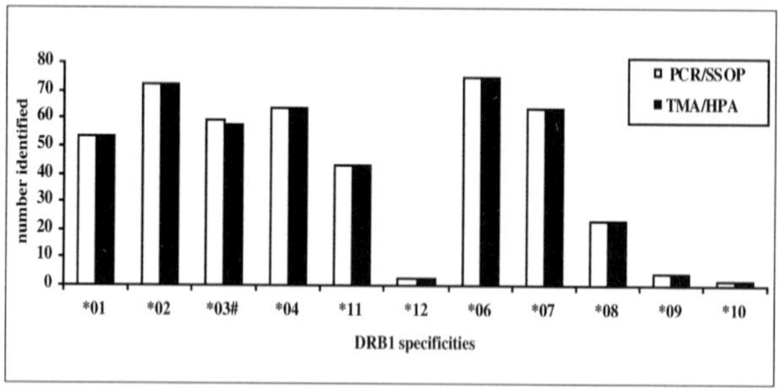

Figure 1. Distribution of HLA-DRB1 specificities assigned by TMA/HPA versus PCR/SSOP among 252 prospectively typed clinical samples.
One sample typed by PCR/SSOP as DRB1*1001, 0301/0305 and by TMA/HPA as DRB1*1001, X, with another DR allele detected but not identified. One of 462 (0.998%) DRB assignments were discordant, after repeat typing of 4 samples in 2 early TMA/HPA assays

References

1. Ng J, Hurley CK, Carter C, Baxter-Lowe LA, Bing D, Chopek M, Hegland J, Lee TD, Si TC, Tse L, KuKuruga D, Mason JM, Monos D, Noreen H, Rosner G, Schmeckpeper B, Dupont B, Hartzman RJ. Large-scale DRB and DQB1 oligonucleotide typing for the NMDP registry: progress report from year 2. *Tissue Antigens* 1996; 47: 21-6.

2. Mickelson E, Smith A, McKinney S, Anderson G, Hansen JA. A comparative study of HLA-DRB1 typing by standard serology and hybridization of non-radioactive sequence-specific oligonucleotide probes to PCR-amplified DNA. *Tissue Antigens* 1993; 41: 86-93.
3. Baxter-Lowe LA, Asu U, Dinauer D, Majewski D, Glumm R, Gorski J. HLA class II oligotyping: summary of a 4-year experience. In: *HLA 1991, Proceedings of the Eleventh International Histocompatibility Workshop and Conference*, vol. 1. New York: Oxford University Press, 1992: 515-8.
4. United States Patent Number 5,399,491. Inventors: Dacian DL, Fultz TJ. Assignee: Gen-Probe Inc, San Diego, CA. Date of Patent: March 21, 1995.
5. Jonas V, Alden MJ, Curry JI, Damisango K, Knott CA, Lankford R, Wolfe JM, Moore DF. Detection and identification of *Mycobacterium tuberculosis* directly from sputum sediments by amplification of rRNA. *J Clin Microbiol* 1993; 31: 2410.
6. Matsubara K, Koide Y, Kobayashi A, Kaida R, Takeda S, Matsuda E, Matsuoka Y, Yoshida TO. A rapid and sensitive method for HLA-DRB1 typing by Acridinium-ester-labeled DNA probes. *Hum Immunol* 1992; 35: 132-9.
7. Smith AG, Nelson JL, Donadi E, Mickelson EM, Regen L, Guthrie LA, Hansen JA. Six new DRB1 alleles reflect the variety of mechanisms which generate polymorphism in the MHC. *Tissue Antigens* 1996; 48: 118-26.

Successful strategy for the large scale development of HLA-human monoclonal antibodies

A. Mulder, M.J. Kardol, J.G.S. Niterink, J.H. Parlevliet, M. Marrari, J. Tanke, J.W. Bruning, R.J. Duquesnoy[1], I. Doxiadis, F.H.J. Claas

Leiden University Hospital, Leiden, SVM-Foundation, Bilthoven, The Netherlands
University of Pittsburgh, Medical Center, W1550 Biomedical Science Tower, Pittsburgh, PA 15261, USA

Serological typing methods rely heavily on the availability of allosera, derived from multiparous women. To circumvent the problems of supply of these reagents, we embarked upon the development of human monoclonal HLA-antibodies (HuMAbs), to supplement, and eventually replace the classical allosera for tissue typing. We have focussed our efforts towards the development of HLA-class I specific HuMAbs. [1, 2] For this work, the B-lymphocytes from donors, who had developed alloantibodies upon sensitization were immortalized by sequential Epstein Barr virus tranformation and fusion to generate hybridomas, and the ensuing HuMAbs were characterized in complement dependent cytotoxicity asssays against panels of HLA-typed PBLs. This contribution summarizes the result of our strategy for the development of human monoclonal antibodies developed in our laboratory.

Materials and methods

Cell immortalization

Peripheral blood lymphocytes for immortalization are taken 10-20 weeks post partum from multiparous women. Two methods are followed for Epstein Barr Virus transformation. PBL are treated with L-leucyl-leucyl-O-methyl Ester, to inactivate suppressive cells, washed and incubated for 3hr at 37° C in the EBV containing supernatant of marmoset cell line B95-8. Freshly transformed cells are *(a)* plated out in 96 wells plates in media containing cyclosporin A or *(b)* supplemented with a mouse anti CD40 antibody, rIL-6 and cyclosporin A and plated out in 96 well plates previously loaded with irradiated CDw32 transfected L-fibroblasts. Antibody productive EBV cell lines are expanded and electrofused with either the mouse myeloma Ag8.653, or the heteromyeloma SHM-D33 and cultured in the presence of HAT and ouabain and hybridoma growth factor.

Antibody specificity determination

We use a semi automated cytotoxicity method for screening supernatants for the presence of HLA antibodies, against small informative cell panels. Large scale screening of final antibody products is performed in the NIH microcytotoxicity, against panels of serologically HLA-typed PBLs.

Results and discussion

In a comparison of the two culture methods for freshly EBV transformed B-lymphocytes of a single individual we found a seven fold increase in the number of Ab productive EBV cell lines when using the CD40 system [3]. Cessation of antibody production, which is a common problem of EBV cell lines, was circumvented by establishing hybridomas using electrofusion.

HuMAbs generated were tested in cytotoxicity assays and the results are summarized in *Table I.* Monoclonal antibodies fall roughly in three categories. (a) HuMAbs reactive with single alleles. (b) HuMAbs reactive with a determinant shared by two alleles (c) broadly specific HuMAbs reactive with determinants shared by a combination of alleles. Comparison of amino acid sequences of class I molecules revealed the epitopes responsible for binding of some of the broadly specific HuMAbs (Manuscript in preparation). Even for a HuMAb reactive with a large array of alleles, *e.g.* OK 4F9, the epitope can be pinpointed to a single amino acid 74(D) with

Table I. Specificities of Human monoclonal antibiodies

HuMAb	isotype	reactivity by cytotoxicity	n	tp	fn	fp	tn	r
OK2F3	IgM	A3	4199	1186	2	31	4198	.98
VN2F1	IgM	B17	151	8	0	0	143	1.0
GK31F12	IgM	B13	263	10	0	2	251	.86
BRO11F6	IgG	A11	183	17	3	6	172	.91
HDG8D9	IgG	B51	184	7	7	4	166	.88
M13E12	IgM	B12	175	45	0	0	130	1.0
FVS8B4	IgM	B37	226	3	5	2	216	.94
DK1G8	IgG1	A29	151	10	0	1	140	.98
BVK5C4	IgM	A9	151	31	0	0	120	1.0
BVK5B10	IgM	B8	105	13	0	1	91	.98
SN607D8	IgG	A2 / A28	151	93	0		57	.99
SN66E3	IgM	A2/A28	151	93	0	1	57	.99
Ha5C2	IgM	A2+A28 (not A*0203)	88	57	4	1	26	.89
SN230G6	IgG	A2/B17	107	60	0	0	47	1.0
AE 9D9	IgM	B8/B14	151	29	1	1	120	.97
NIE44B8	IgM	A25/A26	129	5	2	1	121	.95
Ha2C10	IgM	B60/B48	180	20	0	0	160	1.0
OK2H12	IgM	A3/A11/A32/A1	261	171	3	5	83	.93
OK3C8	IgM	A3/A11/A32	260	114	8	16	122	.82
OK5A3	IgM	A3/A11/A24/A36/weak A1	261	187	4	6	64	.89
OK4F9	IgM	A1/A3/A11/A34/A66/A29/A30/A31/A33	262	184	5	0	72	.95
OK8F12	IgG	B72/B71/B62/B46/B35/B51	262	70	39	5	148	.67
FVS4G4	IgM	B37/B35/B17/B62/B51/B52/B53/B14/B72/B18/B38	273	161	5	0	107	.96
OK3F10	IgM	B15/B35/B70/B21/B17/B46/B56/B52	261	99	14	8	140	.83
OK6H10	IgM	B15/B35/B56/B21/B72	261	89	6	6	160	.90
IND2D12	IgM	B15/B56/B17/B35/B21/B75	151	69	3	3	76	.92
VD1F11	IgM	B15/B35/B17/B21/B60/B46/B55/B56/B51/B52/B72	151	99	3	1	48	.95
HDG2G7	IgG	A19(notA30)/B63/B57/A25/B49	182	39	5	7	145	.87
HDG4B1	IgG	B57/B63/A32/A25	151	15	0	6	130	.92

tp : true positive.
fn : false negative.
fp : false positive.
r : correlation coefficient.

a critical contribution from residues GTLRG at positions 79-83. These broadly reactive HuMAbs aid in the definition of public epitopes [4] that were previously recognized by sera with high panel reactivity.

Although our methodology efficiently produces HLA-HuMAbs of HLA-typing quality, a complete set of monoclonals has not yet been produced. Since this methodology is dependent on the immunization status of the cell donor, rare specificities are still elusive. *In vitro* (re)immunization of human PBLs, which we have successfully employed for the development of some monoclonals [1, 2] should alleviate this problem.

We are in the process of testing these monoclonals against cell lines that are being disseminated in the framework of this workshop. Although generally in good agreement with the specificities outlined here the number of cell lines tested is too low to make definite conclusions.

Since the majority of HuMAbs, besides being cytotoxic, are also binding their ligands in FACS assays, alternative usage for our HuMAbs emerge : *e.g.* the studies of allele specific down regulation of HLA molecules in cervical tumors.

References

1. Mulder A, Kardol M, Blom J, Jolley WB, Melief CJM, Bruning JW. Characterization of two human monoclonal antibodies reactive with HLA-B12 and HLA-B60, respectively, raised by *in vitro* secondary immunization of peripheral blood lymphocytes. *Hum Immunol* 1993; 36:186-92.
2. Mulder A, Kardol M, Blom J, Jolley WB, Melief CJM, Bruning H. A human monoclonal antibody, produced following *in vitro* immunization, recognizing and epitope shared by HLA-A2 subtypes and HLA-A28. *Tissue Antigens* 1993; 42:27-34.
3. Peyron E, Nicolas JF, Reano A, Roche P, Thivolet J, Haftek M, Schmitt D, Peronne C, Banchereau J, Rousset F. Human monoclonal autoantibodies specific for the bullous pemphigoid antigen 1 (BPAg1). *J Immunol* 1994; 153:1333-9.
4. Duquesnoy R, White LT, Fierst JW, Vanek MV, Banner BF, Iwaki Y, Starzl, TE. Multiscreen serum analysis of highly sensitized renal dialysis patients for antibodies toward public and private class I HLA determinants. *Transplantation* 1990; 50: 427-37.

Ligation based typing (LBT) of HLA-DQA1 alleles by detecting polymorphic sites in exon 2

M. Petrasek, I. Faé, W.R. Mayr, G.F. Fischer

Department of Blood Group Serology, University of Vienna, Waehringer Guertel 18-20, A-1090 Vienna, Austria

Tissue typing which is based on the detection of polymorphic sequences in amplified DNA by oligonucleotide probes is commonly referred to as PCR-SSO [1, 2] typing. While the classical SSO typing relies on differential hybridisation [3], we have recently developed an alternative method which makes use of the discriminatory capacity of a heat stable ligase [4]. We call the technique ligation based typing (LBT) [5]. Briefly, a pair of oligonucleotide probes hybridises to PCR amplified DNA in fluid phase. In case of perfect match the probes become ligated, otherwise they stay separated. Biotinylation of one oligonucleotide and hapten labelling of the other allows immobilisation on an avidin coated plate and the detection of the ligated product by an ELISA [6].

Application to HLA-DRB and DQB1, HLA-B27 and HPA-1 to HPA-5 typing has been described in detail elsewhere [5, 7, 8]. Here we want to describe an HLA-DQA1 typing system which is based on the detection of polymorphic sites in exon 2 of the DQA1 gene.

Primers (DQA1AMP-A and DQA1AMP-B, *Table I*) specific for exon 2 of the DQA1 gene are used for PCR. If necessary, *i.e.* if the first typing indicates the presence of an HLA-DQA1*01 allele, a second PCR with DQA1*01 specific primers (DQA1AMP-A and DQA1AMP-B55, *Table I*) is performed. The latter primer pair leads to amplification only in HLA-DQA1*01 positive individuals; the specificity of the HLA-DQA1*01 specific primer combination was confirmed by amplification of a panel of 50 typed [9] individuals when only amplification products of DNA samples of HLA-DQA1*01 positive individuals could be detected after electrophoresis in agarose gels stained with ethidium bromide.

The probes (purchased from Genset, Paris, France) are listed in *Table II*. In a first step the specificities DQA1*01, *0201, *03, *0401, *05, and *0601 were discriminated with six probe pairs *(Table II)*. DQA1*01 positive individuals were further amplified with the DQA1*01 specific primers and typed using four different probe pairs (see *Table II*). Since these probes detect only polymorphic sites in exon 2 the discrimination of HLA-DQA1*0101 and *0104 cannot be achieved.

Using this probe panel all heterozygous combinations can be determined unambiguously with the exception of the HLA-DQA1*0103/0401 genotype which cannot be discriminated from HLA-DQA1*0103/0601.

The optimal concentration of probes was determined in titration experiments, where PCR amplified DNA from typed individuals was used. The signal to noise ratio in these experiments ranged from 16 to 24. Thus, discrimination between positive and negative was clear cut.

HLA-DQA1 alleles of 355 healthy unrelated blood donors were typed using the ligation based technique. Individuals showing only one allele were assumed to be homozygous. The distribution of alleles is listed in *Table III*. While these frequencies do not significantly differ from the ones obtained with RFLP analyses [9] the resolution is higher. The rarest allele observed in our study was HLA-DQA1*0601 which appeared in two chromosomes only. It belongs most probably to an HLA-DRB1*08-DQB1*03 haplotype. Analysis of the Hardy-Weinberg equilibrium gave sufficient fit ($p>0.4$). The HLA-DQA1 database may serve for comparison in disease association - and anthropological studies.

As already observed in the DR/DQ LBT typing system a major advantage of LBT as compared to classical SSO typing is the simple designing and use of the probes. While for hybridisation the exact incubation and washing conditions have to be established for each

Table I. PCR-primers used in this study

Name	Sequence (5'/3')
DQA1AMP-A	ATG GTG TAA ACT TGT ACC AGT
DQA1AMP-B	TTG GTA GCA GCG GTA GAG TTG
DQA1AMP-B55	CCC TGC GGG TCA AAA CCT CC

Table II. Sequences and specificities of probes used for DQA1 specific amplified alleles

probes	alleles detected	Sequence (5'/3')
QA561GUS QA562GDS	01	GGC CTG AGT TCA GCA AAT TTG GAG GTT TTG ACC CGC AGG GTG CA
QA471AUS QA472ADS	0201	GAG AGG AAG GAG ACT GTC TGG A AGT TGC CTC TGT TCC ACA GAC TTA
QA562GUS QA563ADS	03	GCC TCT GTT CCG CAG ATT TAG AAG ATT TGA CCC GCA ATT TGC ACT GAC
QA691AUS QA692CDS	0401 0601	TTG CAC TGA CAA ACA TCG CTG TGA CAA AAC ACA ACT TGA ACA TCC TGA TTA AAC
QA752GUS QA753TDS	05	CGC TGT CCT AAA ACA TAA CTT GAA CAG TCT GAT TAA ACG CTC CAA CTC TAC C
QA251TUS QA252TDS	0103 0201 0601	see below TCA CCC ATG AAT TTG ATG GAG AiG AG

Sequences and specificities of probes used for DQA1*01 specific amplified alleles

probes	alleles detected	Sequence (5'/3')
QA251TUS QA252ADS	0101/04 0102	TTA CGG TCC CTC TGG CCA GT ACA CCC ATG AAT TTG ATG GAG AiG AG
QA333GUS QA341CDS	0102 0103	CAC CCA TGA ATT TGA TGG AGA TGA G CAG TTC TAC GTG GAC CTG GAG
QA333GUS QA341GDS	0101/04	see above GAG TTC TAC GTG GAC CTG GAG
QA411AUS QA412ADS	0103	AGT TCT ACG TGG ACC TGG AGA AGA AGG AGA CTG CCT GGC GG

Table III. Distribution of HLA-DQA1 alleles in the Austrian population

DQA1*	Allele frequency
0101/04	0,1648
0102	0,2014
0103	0,0817
02	0,1268
03	0,1211
04	0,0254
05	0,2760
06	0,0028

probe, the only requirement for probes in LBT is that their melting temperatures are above 68°C. The automation of the procedure is easily accomplished, since there is no necessity of incubation and washing of membranes. It is notable that identical ligation as well as ELISA conditions are used in all applications of LBT developed so far. This strongly indicates that LBT can be easily expanded to several allelic systems, and thus is a versatile tool in genotyping.

References

1. Saiki RK, Bugawan TL, Horn GT, Mullis KB, Erlich HA. Analysis of enzymatically amplified beta-globin and HLA-DQ alpha DNA with allele-specific oligonucleotide probes. *Nature* 1986; 324:163-66.
2. Saiki RK, Walsh PS, Levenson CH, Erlich HA. Genetic analysis of amplified DNA with immobilized sequence-specific oligonucleotide probes. *Proc Natl Acad Sci USA* 1989; 86:6230-4.
3. Conner JC, Reyes AA, Morin C, Itakura K, Teplitz RL, Wallace RB. Detection of sickle cell ßS-globin allele by hybridization with synthetic oligonucleotides. *Proc Natl Acad Sci USA* 1983; 80:278-82.
4. Barany F. Genetic disease detection and DNA amplification using cloned thermostable ligase. *Proc Natl Acad Sci USA* 1991; 88:189-93.
5. Fischer GF, Faé I, Petrasek M, Moser S. A combination of two distinct in vitro amplification procedures for DNA typing of HLA-DRB and -DQB1 alleles. *Vox Sang* 1995; 69:328-35.
6. Nickerson DA, Kaiser R, Lappin S, Stewart J, Hood L, Landegren U. Automated DNA diagnostics using an ELISA-based oligonucleotide ligation assay. *Proc Natl Acad Sci USA* 1990; 87:8923-7.
7. Fischer GF, Faé I, Moser S, Petrasek M, Bäßler HMS, Menzel GR, Mayr WR. Ligation based HLA-B*27 typing. *Tissue Antigens* 1996; 48: 148-52.
8. Legler TJ, Köhler M, Ohto H, Panzer S, Mayr WR, Fischer GF. Genotyping for the human platelet antigen systems HPA-1, HPA-2, HPA-3, HPA-4 and HPA-5 by multiplex PCR and ligation based typing. *Transfusion* 1996; 36: 426-31.
9. Fischer GF, Faé I, Pickl WF. Distribution of polymorphic HLA-DR and -DQ alleles as determined by restriction fragment length polymorphism analysis in an Austrian population. *Vox Sang* 1992; 62:236-41.

Molecular DNA crossmatching of HLA-DR subtypes by temperature gradient gel electrophoresis (TGGE)

M. Uhrberg [1], J. Enczmann [1], M. Giphart [2], H. Grosse-Wilde [3], J. McCluskey[1], P. Wernet [1]

1 Bone Marrow Donor Center (with Stem Cell Bank and Transplantation Immunology), Boulevard 14.80, Heinrich-Heine University, Moorenstrasse 5 , 40001 Düsseldorf, Germany
2 Academisch Ziekenhuis Leiden, The Netherlands
3 Institut für Immunologie, Universitätsklinikum Essen, Germany
4 Red Cross BTS, Adelaide, Australia

The TGGE (temperature gradient gel electrophoresis) molecular crossmatching approach enables the rapid and safe definition of HLA-DR identity by mixing the PCR products of UD-BMT (unrelated donor bone marrow transplantation) pairs. Subtypic differences in the genes of the DRB1, 3, 4, and 5 locus in different UD-BMT settings with multiple donors were safely detected performing a simple electrophoresis run of the PCR samples in a thermal gradient. The study presented here provides an objective evaluation of the potential of the TGGE technique to improve currently used UD-BMT selection strategies. Of the 106 UD-BMT pairs which were crossmatched by TGGE, 9 pairs were found to be mismatched by TGGE. In all of these cases, allelic differences were independently found by HLA-DR subtyping, thereby confirming the TGGE results. Furthermore, in a comparative TGGE study, which was performed in two different laboratories (Düsseldorf and Leiden) no differences in the TGGE results of both laboratories could be found, demonstrating that HLA-DR crossmatching by TGGE is a robust and reproducible technique.

Materials and methods

PCR amplification

PCR primers complementary to conserved regions of intron 1/exon 2 and exon 2 of the DRB1, DRB3, DRB4, and DRB5 genes were used for amplification of genomic DNA as described [1]. Cycle profile: 30s at 94°C; 30s at 55°C; heat to 72°C in 30s; 30s at 72°C ; 35 cycles. The amplification products were verified on 2% agarose gels.

Sample preparation

To generate the crossmatch sample, the PCR products of potential donor and recipient were mixed prior to TGGE. Six µl of each PCR product were mixed with an equal amount of a denaturation buffer, containing 8M urea and 0,4M MOPS and applied to a denaturation/renaturation cycle consisting of a 10 min. incubation at 98°C and subsequent cooling to 25°C.

TGGE

TGGE is a denaturing gradient PAGE system, in which a linear temperature gradient is superimposed parallel to the electric field on a horizontal polyacrylamide gel. TGGE was performed with a commercially available instrument (Diagen TGGE-System, Diagen, 4010 Hilden, Germany) as described by Rosenbaum *et al.* [2]. The instrument consists of a horizontal gel electrophoresis system equipped with a thermoplate and two thermostats. Up to 27 samples could be applied on a 5% polyacrylamide gel and were electrophoresed for 165 min. Subsequently, the banding patterns were detected by a rapid silver staining protocol as described [1]. The optimal temperature gradient for the separation of HLA-DR exon 2 fragments was defined as described [3]: 40°C for the water bath at the non-denaturing side were the samples are applied and 65°C for the water bath at the denaturing side.

HLA typing

HLA-DR subtyping was performed in Essen (32 pairs) by high resolution SSP typing and in Adelaide (72 pairs) by high resolution SSO typing.

Results and discussion

A total of 106 UD-BMT pairs was analysed by TGGE. Of the 106 UD-BMT pairs which were crossmatched by TGGE, 9 pairs (8,5%) were found to be mismatched by TGGE and 97 pairs (91,5%) were matched. All of these pairs were independently HLA-DR subtyped. The results of the comparison between the TGGE crossmatching and the HLA-DR subtyping which was performed in Essen (32 pairs) and Adelaide (74 pairs) is shown in *Table I.*

Table I. Comparison between TGGE crossmatching and HLA-DR subtyping results

	HLA-DR subtype	
	identical	non-identical
TGGE match	96	1
TGGE mismatch	0	9

All the TGGE-mismatched pairs had also a subtype difference at the HLA-DR locus. This is shown in *Table II.* In five cases a difference was found at the DRB1 locus. Also in five cases a subtype difference was detectable at the DRB3 locus. On the other hand, all the TGGE-matched pairs except one (which was TGGE-identical and SSO-typed as DRB1*0101 vs DRB1*0103) were also identical on the subtype level. The overall concordance between TGGE crossmatching and the HLA-DR subtyping was more than 99%. Seventy-two out of the 106 pairs were tested in two different laboratories by TGGE (Leiden and Düsseldorf). Independently, in all cases the same crossmatch results were generated.

Table II. HLA-DR subtype of all TGGE-mismatched samples

BMT pairs	DRB1*	DRB1*	DRB3*	DRB4*	DRB5*
R1	1501	**1407**[1]	n. t.[2]	null	0101
D1	1501	**1408**	n. t.	null	0101
R2	1501	**1201**	**0202**	null	0101
D2	1501	**1202**	**0301**	null	0101
R3	**0804**	**1101**	0202	null	null
D3	**0801**	**1104**	0202	null	null
R4	1301	1501	**0101**	null	0101
D4	1301	1501	**0202**	null	0101
R5	0407	1301	**0101**	n. t.	null
D5	0407	1301	**0202**	n. t.	null
R6	0301	**1101**	n. t.	null	null
D6	0301	**1108**	n. t.	null	null
R7	0301	**1104**	n. t.	null	null
D7	0301	**1101**	n. t.	null	null
R8	1201	1501	**0201**	null	0101
D8	1201	1501	**0202**	null	0101
R9	0103	1301	**0201**	null	null
D9	0103	1301	**0101**	null	null

1: mismatched alleles are written in bold; 2: not determined.

One important result for the donor selection process is, that all of the TGGE-mismatched pairs were actually also HLA-DR-subtype mismatched. This means that there is no risk of negatively selecting an identical donor due to a false mismatched TGGE result.

It was previously shown that TGGE is capable of safely detecting single base pair mutations in the homozygous and heterozygous state in different diseases [4,5]. Here, it is shown, that the TGGE technique is also ideally suited for the safe detection of subtypic differences in the complex HLA-DR system. The combination of TGGE crossmatching and direct sequencing [6] was previously found to result in the rapid and safe selection of unrelated bone marrow donors [1], leading to the detection of all allelic differences at the HLA-DR locus. The present analysis of more than 100 different UD-BMT pairs by TGGE confirms the previous experience, that TGGE crossmatching is a highly valuable method for the unrelated donor selection process in BMT. The comparative analysis of more than 70 UD-BMT pairs by TGGE in Leiden and Düsseldorf shows, that the technique could be performed without any standardisation problems in different laboratories resulting in the same high matching quality.

References

1. Uhrberg M, Enczmann J, Wernet P. Rapid DNA crossmatch analysis of HLA class II genotypic polymorphisms by temperature gradient gel electrophoresis in unrelated bone marrow donor selection. *Eur J Immunogenet* 1994; 21:313-24.
2. Rosenbaum V, Riesner, D. Temperature-gradient gel elctrophoresis. Thermodynamic analysis of nucleic acids and proteins in purified form and in cellular extracts. *Biophys Chem* 1987; 26:235.
3. Uhrberg M, Hinney A, Enczmann J, Wernet P. Analysis of the HLA-DR gene locus by temperature gradient gel electrophoresis and its application for the rapid selection of unrelated bone marrow donors. *Electrophoresis* 1994; 15:1044-50.
4. Hernández A, Uhrberg M, Enczmann J, Wernet P. Rapid screening of point mutations in the protein C gene by multiperpendicular temperature gradient gel electrophoresis. *Genet Anal* 1994; 11:102-5.
5. Wenzel M, Enczmann J, Uhrberg M, Schuch B, Ebert T, Schmitz-Draeger B, Ackermann R, Wernet P. Two novel mutations of the von Hippel-Lindau (VHL) tumor suppressor gene in renal carcinoma. *Hum Mol Genet* 1997, in press.
6. Knipper AJ, Hinney A, Schuch B, Enczmann J, Uhrberg M, Wernet P. Selection of unrelated bone marrow donors by PCR-SSP typing and subsequent non-radioactive sequence-based typing for HLA DRB1/3/4/5, DQB1, and DPB1 alleles. *Tissue Antigens* 1994; 44:275-4.

Sequencing Based HLA Typing

Contents

A novel approach for the computer analysis and allele assignment of complex HLA class I sequences

L. Johnston-Dow, M. Conrad, M. Kronick

Applied Biosystems Division of Perkin Elmer, 850 Lincoln Centre Drive, Foster City, 944404 CA, USA

SBT of class II HLA genes is rapidly finding acceptance in routine use for high resolution allele assignment in HLA typing labs. In general, the strategies described all depend on the analysis of a single informative exon in the class II gene which contains all the information necessary to provide a correct allele assignment. However, the allele assignments for the HLA class I genes requires a different approach for the data analysis since the informative regions span at least two and in some cases three exons. In most class I SBT strategies the region to be sequenced requires anywhere from two to six separate sequencing reactions that must then be analyzed with respect to each other, the class I gene architecture and a database of known allele sequences. Depending on sequencing strategy, these independent sequence segments may or may not overlap thus complicating the analysis process. We have developed an approach that combines both he prior knowledge of the region sequenced with the immediate data to yield a clear and unambiguous method for the data analysis of sequences resulting from these related yet discontinuous genomic regions.

Materials and methods

Class I sequence data was obtained by using the method as described in the 12th IHWS sequencing based typing (SBT) Handbook and in of Johnston-Dow *et al.* [2]. Genomic DNA from 12th International Histocompatibility Workshop cell lines was used for PCR templates and was obtained from the ECACC. Briefly, a locus specific PCR amplification of a 2 kb span of the genomic region of HLA A from exons 1 through 5 is performed. The sequence of the polymorphic exons 2 and 3 can then be obtained by the use of sequencing primers in the flanking introns as shown in *Figure 1*. This amplification results in a single PCR product which serves as the template for all the sequencing reactions. Sequencing is performed as previously described [2] using AmpliTaqFS (Perkin Elmer) in a cycle sequencing protocol with fluorescently-labeled primers. The dye-labeled sequencing primers have been previously described and anneal to sites which flank the 5' and 3' intron-exon borders of exons 2 and 3, respectively as shown in *Figure 1*. Sequence is thus determined for each of exons 2 and 3 in both the 5' and 3' orientation. Electrophoresis and data capture were performed as recommended by Applied Biosystems for the ABI Automated DNA Sequencer. Primary data analysis was performed using factura HLA and sequence navigator (Perkin Elmer). In addition, SeqApp [3] was used for sequence comparisons and motif analysis. Sequence library analysis was performed using allele [1].

Results and discussion

The data analysis scheme is outlined in *Figure 1*. Briefly, factura HLA (Perkin Elmer) was used to screen each sequence against an exon-specific consensus sequence to eliminate any intron region from subsequent consideration. In addition, the relative peak heights at each position were determined and IUB (International Union of Biology) ambiguity codes assigned to mixed-base or heterozygous positions. The resultant sequences were assembled into a project using sequence navigator (Perkin Elmer) and a pre-existing locus-specific template. The template included a consensus sequence for the gene of interest from exons 1 through 4 in a sequence navigator multiple sequence alignment layout, as is shown in *Figure 2*. The sequences were then assembled into a project that contains the exon sequences as determined from exons 2 through 3 or 4. This assemblage is then aligned to the gene consensus for inspection and editing in sequence navigator. A view of the resultant project is shown in *Figure 2*.

The ability to view, manipulate and compare multiple sequences is critical for HLA class I SBT. The complex nature of the data includes 75 potential polymorphic positions in the combined exons 2 and 3 as calculated from a

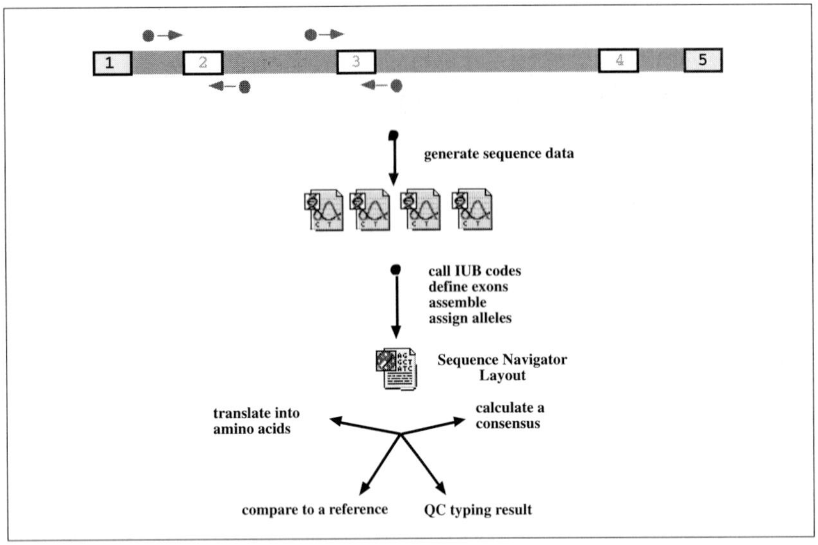

Figure 1. The above figure is a schematic diagram for the steps involved in the SBT of HLA class I genes and resultant analysis of the subsequent data.

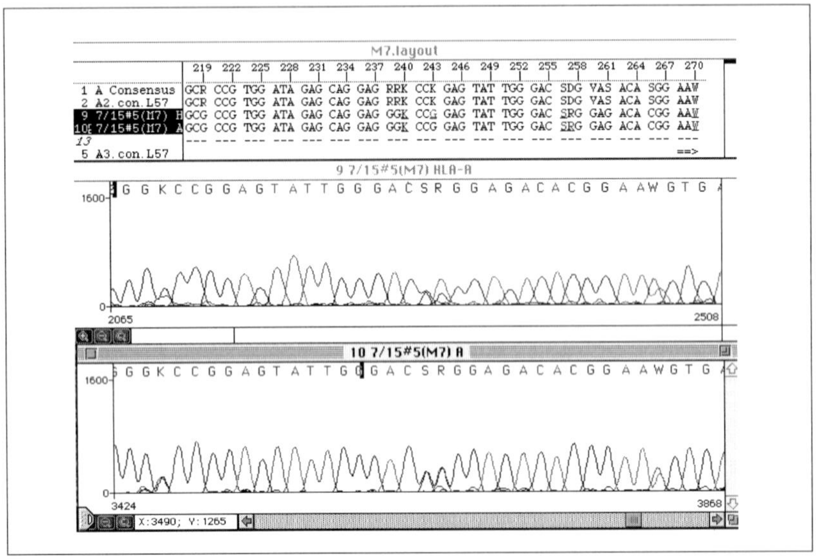

Figure 2. The above figure shows a screen capture of an HLA A SBT project file for the 12th IHWS cell M7. Electropherograms of the aligned data, in both orientations and to a HLA A consensus, are displayed as groups of codons for ease of analysis and translation into peptide sequence. Reference sequences can be easily imported for additional comparison and quality control.

58 allele database. The large number of polymorphic positions and their potential interactions to produce anomalous sequence motifs make the inspection of primary sequence data from both orientations critical. In addition, the ability to compare test electropherograms of heterozygous combinations to a database of known heterozygous and homozygous data can be quite helpful in the consideration of this type of SBT data.

Acknowledgments

We would like to thank Peter Parham for his encouragement, helpful discussions and contribution of class I sequence data and Erik Rozmuller for the gift of allele and the information regarding the ambiguous combinations.

References

1. Rozmuller E, Tilanus M. *Hum Immunol* 1993; 37:207.
2. Johnston-Dow L, Versluis L, Chadwick R, Parham P, Tilanus M, Kronick M. A general approach for the sequencing based typing of the HLA-A. *Hum Immunol* 1995; 44(1):160.
3. SeqApp v1.9a169, Don Gilbert (SeqApp@Bio.Indiana.Edu) 1992.

Sequencing based typing for DQA : a simple method for routine DQA typing

V. Schaeffer, D. Charron

Hôpital Saint-Louis, 1, avenue Claude Vellefaux, 75010 Paris, France
Laboratoire d'histocompatibilité and INSERM U396, Institut des Cordeliers, 15, rue de l'École de Médecine, 75006 Paris, France

The genes of the HLA class II region constitute one of the most polymorphic genetic systems in humans. HLA class II allelic diversity is commonly defined using PCR-SSO [1, 2] or PCR-RFLP [3, 4] techniques. These methods are time consuming and cumbersome. Other methods, such as sequencing based typing (SBT), have been developed to overcome the increasing number of probes used for the PCR-SSO method, to discover new alleles and to resolve typing problems. Previously, a radioactive SBT method was developed for DRB, DQB, and DPB [5] and a non radioactive method for DPB [6, 7] and DRB.
We report here on a high resolution SBT method for DQA and a comparison of generic and specific SBT methods.

Materials and methods

DNA samples

DNA from twenty three cell lines from the 10th Workshop and thirty four bone marrow donors were typed using this SBT method and a generic DQA amplification method. DNA from fifteen 10th Workshop cell lines, twenty four local panel and fourteen bone marrow transplantation patients were amplified with group or allele specific primers for DQA1*01,DQA1*02/03 and DQA1*04/06. The positive amplifications were sequenced.

Sequencing method

Generic amplification

The DQA alleles were amplified with two primers "DQA-forward" (5' TGT AAA ACG ACG GCC AGT ATG GTG TAA ACT TGT ACC AGT 3') and "DQA-reverse" (5' CAG GAA ACA GCT ATG ACC TTG GTA GCA GCG GTA GAG TTG 3'), which were chosen in the 5' generic region and 3' generic region of the exon 2 of DQA1 respectively . The 5' primer has the -21M13 recognition sequence and the 3' primer has the M13 reverse recognition sequence at the 5' end. The PCR (25 µl total volume) is composed of 1x PCR buffer, 400 µM total dNTPs, 200 nM each primer, 45 mM $MgCl_2$, 0.625 units ampliTaq and 2 ng/µl DNA. The amplification was done on a Perkin Elmer 9600 thermocycler, with one cycle at 96°C for 5 min, followed by 35 cycles at 96°C for 30 seconds, 55°C for 30 seconds, 72°C for 30 seconds, and finally one cycle at 72°C for 5 min. The PCR product is about 228 bp.

*Specific DQA1*01, DQA1*02/03 and DQA1*04/06 amplification*

A second method was developed to overcome the effect of the deletion of three nucleotides in the alleles DQA1*0201, 0401, 05 and 06. This direct sequencing method was done with specific amplifications. The common 5' primer "DQA - forward" was used in association with one of the following specific 3' primers, which also contain a M13 reverse tail at the 5' end : "DQA*01 - reverse" (5' CAG GAA ACA GCT ATG ACC GAT GTT CAA GTT GTG TTT TGC 3') and "DQA*04/06 - reverse" (5' CAG GAA ACA GCT ATG ACC GAT GTT CAA GTT GTG TTT TGT 3') to sequence the DQA1*01 and DQA1*04/06 alleles respectively. The specific 5' primer "DQA*02/03 - forward" (5' TGT AAA ACG ACG GCC AGT GCT GAC CAT GTT GCC TCT TAC 3') was used in association with the generic 3' primer "DQA - reverse" to sequence the DQA1*02 and DQA1*03 alleles.
First, the samples were screened by a low resolution method such as PCR-SSP and the DQA alleles present identified. For DQA1*01 and DQA1*04/06, the PCR mix (23.5 µl total volume) was composed of 1.06x PCR buffer, 425 µM total dNTPs, 213 nM of each primer, 8.5 mM $MgCl_2$, 0.625 units ampliTaq polymerase and 1.5 ng/µl DNA. The PCR mix (23.5 µl total volume) for DQA1*02/03 was composed of 1x PCR buffer, 400 µM total dNTPs, 200 nM of each primer, 16 mM $MgCl_2$, 0.625 units ampliTaq and 2 ng/µl DNA. The cycling program for DQA1*01 was one cycle at 96°C for 5 min, 30 cycles at 96°C for 30 seconds, 59°C for 20 seconds, 72°C for 30 seconds and finally one cycle at 72°C for 5 min. The amplification of DQA1*02/03 was done with

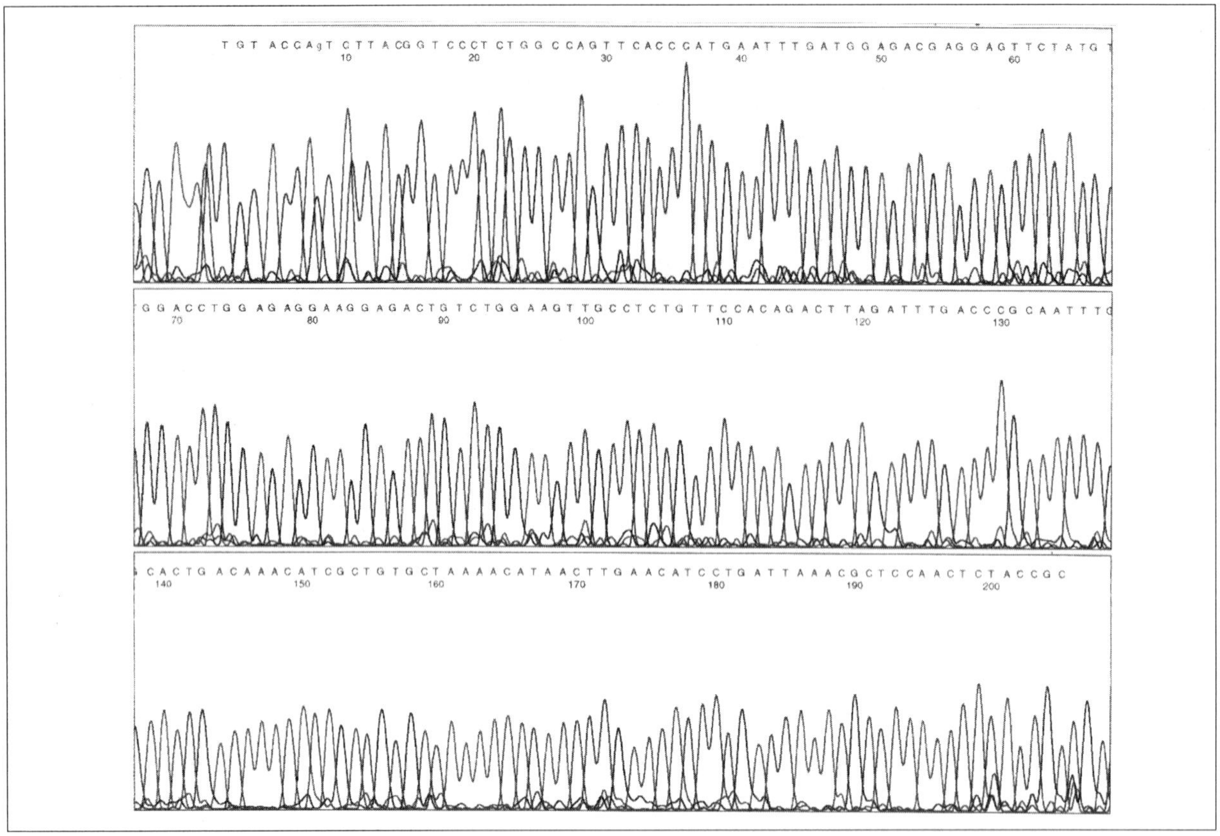

Figure 1. Sequence of a specific DQA1*02/03 amplification of a DNA typed DQA1*0201/0601 by oligotyping.

one cycle at 96°C during 5 min, followed by 30 cycles with 96°C for 30 secondes, 60°C for 30 seconds, 72°C for 30 seconds, and finally one cycle at 72°C for 5 min. The amplification of DQA1*04/06 was done with one cycle at 96°C for 5 min, followed by 30 cycles at 96°C for 30 seconds, 62°C for 15 seconds, 72°C for 30 seconds and finally one cycle at 72°C for 5 min.

Sequencing reactions

After the control and the verification of the intensity of the PCR product on a 1% agarose gel, the PCR product was diluted 1/10 with distilled water. The sequencing reaction was performed with dye-primer sequencing kits : -21M13 ready reaction kit and M13 reverse ready reaction kit with Taq FS (Applied Biosystems). The cycle sequencing was performed on the Perkin Elmer 9600 thermocycler. The cycling program contains 15 cycles with three steps of 96°C for 20 seconds, 59°C for 30 seconds and 72°C for 30 seconds, followed by another 15 cycles which included two steps of 96°C for 20 seconds and 72°C for 30 seconds. After precipitation with ethanol, the reactions were loaded onto a 377 DNA sequencer (Applied Biosystems).

Sequence analysis and interpretation

To facilitate the DQA typing by SBT method, software (Factura and Sequence Navigator) has been developed by Applied Biosystems (Applied Biosystems, division of Perkin Elmer, Foster City, USA). Factura was used to interpret the sequence data and assign heterozygosity codes (NC-IUB codes) to the heterozygous positions. Subsequently the alleles were identified by reference to a library of HLA DQA sequences (subdivided into one library for deleted alleles and one for non-deleted alleles) included in the software. Sequence Navigator was used to study the alignment of sequences obtained in the forward and reverse directions and to inspect the quality of the sequence data.

Results

A comparison between the two sequencing techniques, generic or several specific amplifications, showed that the former was more difficult to interpret. This difficulty come from the fact that for certain alleles (DQA1*0201, DQA1*0401, DQA1*0501.1, DQA1*0501.2, DQA1*0502, DQA1*0503 and DQA1*0601), there is a deletion of three nucleotides at positions 166, 167 and 168 of the DQA sequence. For the specific amplifications, the primers were chosen to amplify groups of alleles with the deletion (DQA1*04/06) or without the deletion (DQA1*01) (except for DQA1*02 and 03).

Figure 1 shows the electrophoregram of the specific DQA1*02/03 amplification of a cell typed DQA1*0201/0601 by oligotyping. The low background and clearly distinguishable peaks can be seen.

The software enables quick and precise typing of the cells. But, its use was limited in the case of generic amplification of cells which were heterozygous for the deletion. For the specific amplification, this problem disappears, except in the case of a cell typed DQA1*02/DQA1*03, which is only represented in about 2% of our reference panel.

The sequencing method with generic and specific amplications were set up with our panel of cells, which included most of the DQA alleles : DQA1*0101, DQA1*0102, DQA1*0103, DQA1*0201, DQA1*0301, DQA1*0302, DQA1*0401, DQA1*05, DQA1*0601. The typing of the cell lines, done with generic and specific amplification, was in full accordance with the reference DQA typing. The results obtained with the local panel was also identical to the oligotyping.

Discussion and conclusions

The techniques using specific or generic amplification gave some ambiguities. In exon 2 of DQA, the only difference between DQA1*0101 and DQA1*0104 is located at the beginning (position 5), upstream of the 5' primer used for the PCR. Concerning the alleles DQA1*0301.1 and DQA1*0302, the difference is also located at the beginning of the exon 2, at position 28. These ambiguities came from the choice of the 5' primer(s) and 3' primer(s), used for the PCR. This amplification problem was identical for generic and specific amplification. Unfortunatly, for the present, we have not completed establishing the method for specific sequencing of DQA1*05. The recommended sequencing method for HLA-DQA is the technique with specific amplification. Although the steps of the PCR are not identical for the different specific amplifications, the sequencing program is identical and the different amplifications can be included on the one sequencing gel. With this method, the DQA alleles can be easily typed. There is no problem of interpretation with the software except in the case of a DQA1*02/DQA1*03 heterozygote, which represent only 2% of our reference french population. Moreover, new alleles can be discovered. The specific SBT method is sensitive, reproductible and is a high resolution typing technique. The typing can be obtained in one and a half days. Typing interpretation is greatly facilitated by the use of the software Factura.

Acknowledgements

We thank Leslie Johnson-Dow and Mel Kronick from Applied Biosystems, Foster City, for the HLA software for DQA and J. Williamson and F. Christiansen for their help in writing this manuscript.

References

1. Angelini G, Bugawan TL, Delfino L, Erlich HA, Ferrara GB. HLA-DP typing by DNA amplification and hybridization with specific oligonucleotides. *Hum Immunol* 1989; 26: 169.
2. Peponnet C, Schaeffer V, Lepage V, Chatelain F, Rodde I, Alsayed J, Boucher P, Hermans P, Montplaisir N, Charron D. Comparison of two HLA-DRB high resolution microtiter plate reverse hybridization typing methods: advantage of a codon-86 valine or glycine PCR segregation. *Tissue Antigens* 1995; 45: 129-38.
3. Uryu N, Maeda M, Ota M, Tsuji K, Inoko H. A simple method for HLA-DRB and -DQB typing by digestion of PCR amplified DNA with allele specific restriction endonucleases. *Tissue Antigens* 1990; 35 : 20-31.
4. Maeda M, Uryu N, Muryama M, Ishii H, Ota M, Tsuji K, Inoko H. A simple and rapid method for HLA-DP genotyping by digestion of PCR-amplified DNA with allele specific restriction endonucleases. *Hum Immunol* 1990; 27: 111.
5. Santamaria P, Boyce-Jacino MT, Linstrom AL, Barbosa JJ, Faras AJ, Rich SS. HLA class II "Typing" : direct sequencing of the *DRB*, *DQB* and *DQA* genes. *Hum Immunol* 1992; 33: 69-81.
6. Verluis LF, Rozemuller EH, Tonks S, Marsh SGE, Bouwens AGM, Bodmer JG, Tilanus MGJ. High-resolution HLA-DPB typing based upon computerized analysis of data obtains by fluorescent sequencing of the amplified polymorphic exon 2. *Hum Immunol* 1993; 38: 277-83.
7. Rozemuller EH, Chadwick B, Charron D, Baxter-Lowe LA, Eliaou JF, Johnston-Dow L, Tilanus MGJ. Sequenase sequence profiles used for HLA-DPB1 sequencing based typing. *Tissue Antigens* 1996; 47: 72-9.

A concept for HLA class I typing using cycle-sequencing and fluorescent-labelled sequencing primers exemplified by the HLA-A locus

L. Norgaard, L. Fugger, B.K Jakobsen, A. Svejgaard

Tissue Typing Laboratory, Department of Clinical Immunology, Section 7631, National University Hospital (Rigshospitalet), 20 Tagensvej, 2200 Copenhagen, Denmark

During the last few years the number of different alleles recognised in the HLA class I and II loci has increased considerably. A fast and accurate method for HLA typing meeting this high degree of polymorphism holds relevance for a number of areas including transplantation biology, studies of disease susceptibilities, population genetics as well as an attempt to elucidate the evolutionary mechanisms underlying the polymorphism itself.

Sequencing-based typing (SBT) methods offer the highest resolution possible, as the assignment of alleles is obtained by determining the underlying sequences of the amplified alleles. A number of protocols considering class I, as well as class II loci, have already been published [1-5]. These protocols all vary in the use of different strategies, including a DNA versus mRNA/cDNA based approach, generic versus group-specific amplification, and different kinds of sequencing chemistries.

Here we describe a mRNA based protocol for typing HLA-A locus alleles using cycle-sequencing with AmpliTaq® DNA Polymerase, FS and fluorescent-labelled sequencing primers. Using this method we investigated more than 50 different clinical samples and cell lines from the International Histocompatibility Workshop Cell Panel, the latter obtained from ECACC (European Collection of Animal Cell Cultures). Our results were in good accordance with the serological profiles obtained in our own laboratory and the DNA-based assignment given by the ECACC, respectively.

The concept

Figure 1 outlines the strategy used in the present protocol. In short, our protocol is based on the following.

mRNA/cDNA as starting material

In this way a PCR product without intervening introns is obtained. This gives a more effective utilisation of the

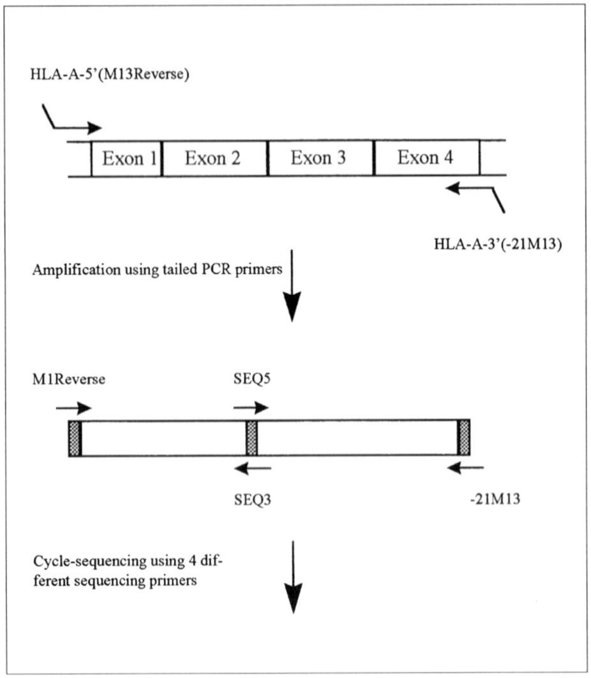

Figure 1. Outline of the strategy used in the present protocol. As cDNA constitute the template in the PCR reaction, a product without intervening introns is obtained. The HLA-A-5' and HLA-A-3' PCR primers used for A-locus-specific amplification incorporate the recognition sites for the M13Reverse and -21M13 sequencing primers, respectively. This creates a protocol, in which the same PCR product serves as template in all the subsequent cycle-sequencing reactions using AmpliTaq® DNA Polymerase, FS and fluorescent-labelled sequencing primers. A reliable sequence throughout the amplified region can be obtained with the M13Reverse and -21M13 sequencing primers alone. The sequence of both strands can be obtained by including the two internal sequencing primers, SEQ5 and SEQ3, annealing to the middle of the amplified product.

subsequent sequencing reactions, especially in class I loci, where more than one exon has to be considered in order to obtain a sufficient level of resolution.

Only one locus-specific PCR reaction
This reaction amplifies an 824 bp. product covering exons 1-3 and most of exon 4. The inclusion of exon 4 creates a protocol able to discriminate between closely related alleles differing in this exon only, *e.g.* A*0201/*0209 and A*31011/*31012; however, our protocol is not able to discriminate A*0207 from the newly recognised A*0215N allele, as the single nucleotide difference between these alleles resides outside the region amplified in this protocol. Moreover, considering a relatively large part of the gene gives a more reliable assignment of alleles as more polymorphic positions are included in the analysis.

Tailed primers for PCR amplification
The addition of the recognition sites for the M13 Reverse and -21M13 sequencing primers to the 5'end of the HLA-A-5' and HLA-A-3' PCR primers respectively, creates a PCR product that can be sequenced with these well-characterised and often used sequencing primers. In this way a time-consuming and expensive process of primer-design and -optimisation can be avoided. Moreover, as noted by others [5], the use of tailed primers for amplification will facilitate the integration of two or more loci into the same SBT protocol. However, the use of tailed primers significantly increases the requirement for a fully optimised PCR reaction, as primer/dimers and other kinds of oligomerization products are targets for the M13Reverse and -21M13 primers in the subsequent sequencing reactions.

Fluorescent-labelled sequencing primers
The sequences produced with this chemistry, in contrast to those produced with fluorescent-labelled terminators, are characterised by a low background and, most important, relatively even peak heights throughout the electropherogram, as shown in *Figure 2*. For this reason the identification of heterozygous positions becomes reproducible and highly reliable; an advantage when determining the differences between closely related alleles. However, this chemistry is also characterised by the presence of false stops, which, depending of their position might affect the assignment of alleles. This problem was, however, easily resolved by sequencing the opposite strand with one of the two internal primers, SEQ5 and SEQ3, designed for all three class I loci and thus usable in a protocol integrating these loci.

Direct cycle-sequencing with AmpliTaq® DNA Polymerase, FS
This enzyme combines the relative ease of performing cycle-sequencing with a quality of data previously obtained only with the much more laborious T7 Sequenase® chemistry. Moreover, the use of the FS enzyme circumvent the requirement for time-consuming purification of the PCR product, as a simple dilution in water constitutes the only step necessary prior to sequencing.

Automatic sequencing
The use of automated sequencing creates a protocol easily extended with different kinds of software for handling and automatic assignment of alleles. This opportunity was, however, not used in the present work.

Results

The more than 50 cell lines and clinical samples investigated during this study, represented 33 of the 59 different alleles recognised from this locus [6], thus indicating the ability of the PCR reaction to amplify all alleles of the A-locus. The reliability of the sequencing reactions are documented by the ability of the protocol to discriminate between closely related alleles, differing in only a few, or even at single, positions throughout the gene, as shown in *Figure 2*.

Discussion

The number of different alleles now recognised in each loci of the HLA system and the potential impact of previously undetected differences between these in some situations, *e.g.* bone marrow transplantation [7], constitute a major challenge in HLA typing. The ability of SBT protocols to discriminate between closely related alleles with only a limited number of primers and reactions make these a powerful approach in this situation. However, for routine use, these protocols still need to be improved in several ways, *e.g.* in regard to the time and labour involved.

The present protocol was established with two purposes. First of all, we wanted to take advantage of the time-savings offered by the enzyme AmpliTaq® DNA Polymerase, FS. The possibility to use direct cycle-sequencing constitutes a major progress in regard to the

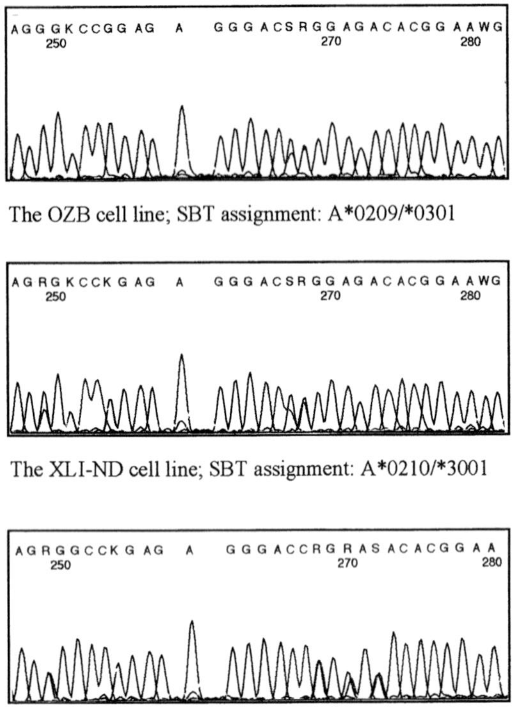

The OZB cell line; SBT assignment: A*0209/*0301

The XLI-ND cell line; SBT assignment: A*0210/*3001

The CRB cell line; SBT assignment: A*3002/*6602

Figure 2. Sequencing electropherograms, obtained with the M13Reverse sequencing primer, from three different cell lines, all heterozygous in the A-locus. From above: OZB (IHW No.:9216), XLI-ND (IHW No.: 9220), and CRB (IHW NO.: 9234). The IUB codes for mixed base positions were added manually. The electropherograms display the low background and the even peak heights produced by the AmpliTaq FS enzyme and fluorescent-labelled primers; characteristics making the identification of heterozygous positions very reliable.

demand for purification of the PCR product prior to sequencing, compared to protocols using either T7 Sequenase® [4,5] or other kinds of cycle-sequencing [2]. As shown here, this was done without compromising the quality of data. Secondly, we wanted to create a protocol easily extended to cover all loci of class I. This was accomplished by restricting the locus-specificity to the PCR reaction alone. As the cDNA synthesis and all of the sequencing reactions are designed for use in B- and C-loci as well, the addition of one or more PCR reactions specific for each of these loci will create a method integrating all three loci of class I into the same SBT protocol.

Acknowledgements

This work was supported by the Danish Cancer Society. We thank Professor Soren Buus, University of Copenhagen, for his gift of a number of cell lines, Dr Mel N. Kronick, Perkin Elmer Corp., for valuable advice during this work, and Ms. Gitte Kolander for skilful technical assistance.

References

1. Santamaria P, Lindstrom AL, Boyce-Jacino MT *et al.* HLA class I sequence-based typing. *Hum Immunol* 1993; 37: 39-50.
2. Petersdorf EW, Hansen JA. A comprehensive approach for typing the alleles of the HLA-B locus by automated sequencing. *Tissue Antigens* 1995; 46: 73-85.
3. Rozemuller EH, Bouwens AGM, Van Oort E *et al.* Sequencing-based typing reveals new insight in HLA-DPA1 polymorphism. *Tissue Antigens* 1995; 45: 57-62.
4. Blasczyk R, Hahn U, Wehling J, Huhn D, Salama A. Complete subtyping of the HLA-A locus by sequence-specific amplification followed by direct sequencing or single single-strand conformation polymorphism analysis. *Tissue Antigens* 1995; 46: 86-95.
5. McGinnis MD, Conrad MP, Bouwens AGM, Tilanus MGJ, Kronick MN. Automated, solid-phase sequencing of DRB region using T7 sequencing chemistry and dye-labelled primers. *Tissue Antigens* 1995; 46: 173-9.
6. Arnett KL, Parham P. HLA class I nucleotide sequences, 1995. *Tissue Antigens* 1995; 45: 217-57.
7. Fleischhauer K, Kernan NA, O'Reilly RJ, Dupont B, Yang SY. Bone marrow- allograft rejection by T lymphocytes recognizing a single amino acid difference in HLA-B44. *N Engl J Med* 1990; 323: 1818-22.

Improved direct sequencing system for accurate detection of heterozygosity in HLA-A, B and C loci

M.P. Bettinotti, Y. Mitsuishi, M. Lau, P.I. Terasaki

UCLA Tissue Typing Laboratory, 950 Veteran Avenue, Los Angeles, CA 90095, USA

The need for accurate typing of HLA class I molecules in the tissue typing laboratory has been firmly established. The most direct approach is to obtain the DNA sequence of the alleles present. Cloning and sequencing the whole gene from cDNA [1] is however too expensive and time consuming for clinical purposes. An alternative is the direct sequencing of PCR products [2, 3] encompassing exons 2 and 3, which are sufficient for the discrimination of most alleles.

We designed a method for direct sequencing of PCR products obtained from genomic DNA that can be used for the typing of HLA-A, B and C loci.

Strategy

The template to be sequenced is the product of a nested PCR amplification and contains a mixture of both alleles present in each locus.

A PCR fragment that includes exons 2 and 3 is amplified from genomic DNA using three different pairs of primers, one pair specific for each locus: HLA-A, B and C. The 5' primer lies on the 5' untranslated region and the 3' primer on the third intron.

The PCR products obtained are used as template for a second round of amplifications with two sets of primers flanking exons 2 and 3 respectively. The 5' primers include the T7 promoter sequence and the right hand primers the -21M13 sequence. The PCR products are thus tailed with the T7 and -21M13 sequences.

Sequencing with the T7 primer provides the sense sequence and with -21M13 the antisense sequence.

The direct and reverse sequences obtained for each locus are compared with a consensus sequence of exon 2 or exon 3 of HLA class I genes. The heterozygous positions are determined. The two possible sequences are compared to the aligned known sequences for the loci A, B and C. The two most probable alleles are assigned.

Materials and methods

First PCR amplification

A PCR fragment, extending from the 5'untranslated region to the third intron, is amplified from genomic DNA. For locus A the primers are 5'UT-A and 3'I3-A (1107 bp product); for locus B, 5'UT-B and 3'I3-B-1+2 (1088 bp product) and for locus C, 5'UT-C and 3'I3-BC-1+2 (1114 bp product) *(Table I)*.

The final reaction mix (20 µl) contains 0.2 units of Ampli Taq DNA Polymerase (Perkin-Elmer, Branchburg, NJ, USA) and 15 pmol of each primer in a 50 mM KCl, 1.5 mM $MgCl_2$, 25 mM Tris.HCl pH 8.9, 1% glycerol and 200 µM of each dNTP solution. A hot start PCR with separation of primers is done in order to avoid primer-dimer amplification. The temperature profile for the Perkin-Elmer Thermal Cycler model 480 is: one cycle of 4 min at 96 °C and 35 cycles of 1 min at 96 °C, 1 min at 63 °C and 2 min at 72 °C.

Secondary PCR amplification

After a 1 in 300 dilution in water, the PCR products are used as template for a second round of amplifications. The primers flanking the second exon are 5'EX2-t and 3'EX2-m and produce a 291 bp long fragment. In the case of exon 3, the left-hand primer, 5' EX3-t, is common to the three loci and the right-hand primers are: 3'I3-A-m for locus A (396 bp product), 3'I3-B-m for locus B (365 bp product) and 3'I3-BC-m for locus C (342 bp product) *(Table I)*.

The concentrations of all reagents are the same as in the first PCR except for the absence of glycerol. The thermal program consists of 5 cycles of 1 min at 96 °C, 1min at 57 °C and 1 min at 72 °C and 28 cycles of 1 min at 96 °C, 1 min at 65 °C and 1 min at 72 °C.

Table I. Primers for primary and secondary PCR amplification

Primer	Sequence	Position	
5'UT-A	5'TTCTCCCCAGACGCCGAGGATGGCC3'	5'UT- EX1	-19 to -1 1-6
5'UT-B	5'ACCCACCCGGACTCAGAATCTCCT3'	5'UT	-35 to -12
5'UT-C	5'GAGAAGCCAATCAGCGTCTCCGCA3'	5'UT	-83 to -60
3'I3-A	5'TGTTGGTCCCAATTGTCTCCCCTC3'	intr3	94-71
3'I3-B-1	5'GGAGGCCATCCCCGGCGACCTAT3'	intr3	64-36
3'I3-B-2	5'GGAGGCCATCCCCGGCGATCTAT3'	intr3	64-36
3'I3-BC-1	5'GGAGATGGGGAAGGCTCCCCACT3'	intr3	34-12
3'I3-BC-2	5'GGAGATGGGGAAGGCTCCCCATT3'	intr3	34-12
5'EX2-t	5'TACGACTCACTATAGGGCACTCCATGAGGTATTTC3'	EX2	6-22
3'EX2-m	5'GTAAAACGACGGCCAGTTCTGGTTGTAGTAGC3'	EX2	261-247
5'EX3-t	5'TACGACTCACTATAGGGGGCCAGGGTCTCACA3'	intr2 EX3	273-278 1-9
3'I3A-m	5'GTAAAACGACGGCCAGTCAATTGTCTCCCCTC3'	intr3	85-71
3'I3-B-m	5'GTAAAACGACGGCCAGTCCCCGGCGACCTAT3'	intr3	49-36
3'I3-BC-m	5'GTAAAACGACGGCCAGTGGAAGGCTCCCCACT3'	intr3	26-12

5'UT: 5' untranslated region; EX: exon; intr: intron

Sequencing

After purification using a QIA quick PCR Purification Kit (QIAGEN, Chatsworth, CA, USA), the PCR products are submitted to automated fluorescent sequencing in an Applied Biosystems Automated Sequencer model 373 A. The sequencing reactions are carried out using the standard protocol recommended for the ABI/Perkin-Elmer Dye Primer Cycle Sequencing Core Kit with Amplitaq DNA polymerase FS (Applied Biosystems / Perkin-Elmer, Foster City, CA, USA).

Data analysis

The direct and reverse sequences obtained for each locus are compared with a consensus sequence of exon 2 or exon 3 of HLA class I genes using the Sequence Navigator program.

Discussion and conclusion

The advantages of the method are:

1. The sample is genomic DNA, which is easy to obtain and very stable. By contrast, to obtain cDNA large quantities of fresh cells or the establishments of cell lines are necessary.
2. The nested PCR amplification provides a very clean and abundant template for sequencing.
3. Cycle sequencing allows the use of the PCR product directly as template without need of preparation of a single stranded template.
4. Dye-primer chemistry provides homogeneous electrophoregram peaks and therefore clear discernment of heterozygous position.
5. Commercial dye-fluorescent primers are less expensive than custom primers and provide robust sequencing reactions.

The method still needs adjustments:

1. Incorporation of new primers into the first PCR reaction to cover HLA-B alleles that are being missed (HLA-B27, 39, 61).
2. Replacement of the 5' secondary amplification primers with sequences 20 to 50 bp further into the introns in order to obtain the whole clear exonic sequence. This is important because some polymorphic regions essential for allele assignment are close to the end of the exons.
3. Sequencing of other exons to discern some alleles with characteristic polymorphic positions outside of exons 2 and 3.

References

1. Ennis PD, Zemmour J, Salter RD, Parham P. Rapid cloning of HLA-A, B cDNA by using polymerase chain reaction: Frequency and nature of errors produced in amplification. *Proc Natl Acad Sci USA* 1990; 87: 2833-2837.
2. Santamaria P, Lindstrom AL, Boyce-Jacino MT *et al.* HLA class I sequence-based typing. *Hum Immunol* 1993; 37: 39-50.
3. Petersdorf E W and Hansen J A. A comprehensive approach for typing the alleles of the HLA-B locus by automated sequencing. *Tissue Antigens* 1995; 46: 73-85

Subtyping of HLA-A2 by reversed dot blot and sequencing based typing: a comparative study

S. Scheltinga[1], T. Van den Berg[1], L. Versluis[1], O. Avinens[2], J.F. Eliaou[2], L. Johnston-Dow[3], M. Tilanus[1]

1 University Hospital Utrecht, Department of Pathology, PO Box 85500, 3508 GA Utrecht, The Netherlands
2 Centre Hospitalier et Universitaire de Montpellier, 34295 Montpellier Cedex, France
3 Perkin Elmer, Applied Biosystems Division, 850 Lincoln Centre Drive, Foster City 94404, CA, USA

The HLA-A2 allele has the highest frequency (~40%) in various human populations. HLA-A2 along with A28 (A68 and A69) comprise a single related group. Many monospecific reagents exist for the A2 group and one for A28. However, it is difficult to discriminate between A68 and A69. Molecular methods are required for high resolution typing, which include the identification of all A2 subtypes. We compared HLA-A2 subtyping by Reversed Dot Blot and sequencing based typing. Reversed Dot Blot subtyping was developed to discriminate between A*0201 to A*0210 and Sequencing Based Typing was developed for high resolution HLA-A typing.

Material and methods

We investigated a cell panel of 22 DNA samples representing most A2 subtypes. Samples from the ECACC and our laboratory are studied and listed in *Table I*. DNA is isolated by the 'salting-out' method [1].

Reversed Dot Blot

HLA-A2 positive samples were identified by serological methods. Subsequently, exons 2 and 3 are amplified which results in a 600 bp PCR product. PCR amplifications were carried out in 50 µl volumes containing 5 µl 10 X PCR buffer I (Perkin Elmer), 0.8 mM $MgCl_2$ (Perkin Elmer), 1 U Taq DNA Polymerase-FS (Perkin Elmer), 5 µl DMSO (concentrated), 125 nmol of each dNTP and 2 % DIGdUTP, 25 µmol of each amplification primer (shown in *Table I*) and 1 µg of target DNA. Thermalcycling was performed in a Perkin Elmer 9600 with the following temperature profile: 5' 95 °C, 35 cycli of 30" 92 °C, 1' 66 °C, 1' 72 °C and finally 1' 72 °C [2]. The probes used are listed in *Table II*. The names of the probes include both a letter and a number, which stand respectively for the kind of amino acid and the number of the codon. For example, F9 codes for phenylanaline at codon number 9. The probes are spotted on a nylon membrane, dried, then hybridized with the HLA-A PCR product. Each sample required a single nylon membrane with probes. When the PCR product binds a probe it is visualized by a light sensitive reaction on a film. The negative control contains all the necessary reagents with exception of the probe. The reaction pattern on the blot gives an identification of the HLA-A2 subtype.

Sequencing Based Typing

The protocol for amplification and sequencing is described by Johnston-Dow *et al.* elsewhere in this volume. Briefly, exons 1 to 5 of HLA-A are amplified by PCR and serve as a template for all sequence reactions. Amplification primers are listed in *Table III*. Amplification is HLA-A generic and results in a 2 kb PCR product. Exons 2 and 3 are sequenced with AmpliTaq DNA polymerase-FS (Perkin Elmer) and fluorescently labelled primers (also listed in *Table II*). Analysis is performed with HLA software [3], which compare the sequencing results with a sequence library and allows the comparison of the data.

Results

The typing results of Reversed Dot Blot compared with Sequencing Based Typing are shown in *Table III*. Also the data from the literature is listed. An example of typical sequence data is shown in *Figure 1*.

Reversed Dot Blot could not identify 5 of the in total 20 DNA samples. This is shown in *Table III* with 'no result'.

In 14 DNA samples Sequencing Based Typing and Reversed Dot Blot gave comparable typing results, which also agreed with the data from the literature.

As well as in Reversed Dot Blot as in Sequencing Based

Table I. Typing results of Reversed Dot Blot compared with Sequencing Based Typing

sample name	IHW number	previously assigned	Reversed Dot Blot	Sequencing Based Typing
273 Lyon		A2	0202	0202/0301
60 Lyon		A2/3	0201 or 0209 or 0211 or 0217	0201/0301 or 0209/0301
278 Lyon		A2/24	no result	0201/2402 or 0209/2402
352 A Lyon		A2/2	0202/0210	0201/0205 or 0209/0205 or 0202/0206
306 A Lyon		A2/28	0201 or 0209 or 0211 or 0217	0201/6802 or 0209/6802
BSM	9032	A*0201	0201 or 0209 or 0211 or 0217	0201 or 0209
HAG	9297	A*0201	0201 or 0209 or 0211 or 0217	0201 or 0209
KOSE	9056	A2	0201 or 0209 or 0211 or 0217	0201 or 0209
LUY	9070	A*0201	0201 or 0209 or 0211 or 0217	0201 or 0209
Delprado			0202	0202/2402
M7	9215	A*0202/0301	0202	0202/0301
LV8		A*0203	0203	0203/0301
CLA	9209	A*0206/2402	0206	0206/2402
KNE	9214	A*0207	0207	0101/0207 or 0101/0215N
KLO	9213	A*0101/0208	no result	0101/0208
OZB	9216	A*0209/0301	0201 or 0209 or 0211 or 0217	0210 or 0209/0301
XLI-ND	9220	A*0210	0210	0210/3001
AMALA	9064	A*0217	no result	0217
AMAL	9010	A28	no result	6802
MGAR	9032	A*2601	no result	2601

Table II. Amplification primers and probes for Reversed Dot Blot

	name	sequence	orientation/ exon
Amplification primers	PA1	5' CTC GTC CCC AGG CTC TCA CTC C 3	forward exon 2
	PA6	5' GGA GTG GCT CCG CAG ATA C 3'	reversed exon 3
probes	F9	5' GGT ATT TCT TCA CAT CCG T 3'	exon 2
	Y9	5' GGT ATT TCT ACA CCT CCG T 3'	exon 3
	R43	5' GCG AGC CGG AGG ATG GAG 3'	exon 2
	Q43	5' GCG AGC CAG AGG ATG GAG 3'	exon 2
	K66	5' GAC ACG GAA AGT GAA GGC C 3'	exon 2
	F73	5' CCA CTC ACA GAT TGA CCG 3'	exon 2
	C99	5' CGC AGC CAC ACA TCC TCT G 3'	exon 3
	F99	5' GAG GAT GTT TGG CTG CGA C 3'	exon 3
	Q99	5' ACC CTC CCA GAT GAT GTT TGG 3'	exon 3
	Y99	5' GAG GAT GTA TGG CTG CGA C 3'	exon 3
	T149	5' AGT GGG AGA CGG CCC ATG A 3'	exon 3
	W156	5' CGG AGC AGT GGA GAG CCT 3'	exon 3
	Q156	5' CGG AGG AGC AGA GAG CCT 3'	exon 3
	F162	5' TAC CTG GAG GGG CGA TGC 3'	exon 3

Table III. Amplification and sequence primers for Sequencing Based Typing

	name	sequence	orientation
Amplification primers	A5.4	5' CGC CGA GGA TGG CCG TC 3'	forward exon 1
	A3.2 (c/t)	5' GGA GAA CC/TA GGC CAG CAA TGA TGC CC 3'	reversed exon 5
Sequence primers	A5.9 (a/g)	5' cagga-TCG GGC A/GGG TCT CAG CC 3'	forward exon 2
	B3.6	5' cagga-CAC TCA CCG GCC TCG CTC TGG 3'	reversed exon 2
	A5.10 (c/t)	5' cagga-GGG CTC GGG GGA CT/CG GG 3'	forward exon 3
	A3.4	5' cagga-GAG GCG CCC CGT GGC 3'	reversed exon 3

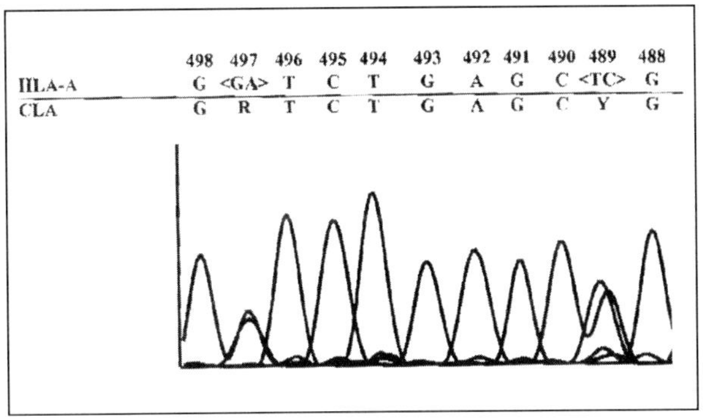

Figure 1. An electropherogram of CLA obtained with sequence primer A3.4 (exon 3 reversed). CLA is a heterozygous sample, because of the presence of double peaks. The typing result of CLA is A*0206/2402.

Typing we encountered ambiguities. The Reversed Dot Blot detects 7 of the known A2 subtypes. No discrimination was possible between A*0201 and A*0209 where exon 4 is required for a final HLA-A2 typing. Sequencing Based Typing also requires exon 4 for discrimination between A*0201 and A*0209. Exon 4 sequence information is also necessary to resolve the ambiguous combination A*0207 and A*0215N, which is found in the sample KNE. In Reversed Dot Blot A*0211 and A*0217 can not be detected, because both belong to the high numbered A2 subtypes. The heterozygous sample 352 A Lyon resulted in the ambiguous combination A*0201/0205 and A*0202/0206. GSAPs (group specific amplification primers) are necessary to resolve this ambiguity.
In the samples 306 A Lyon and AMAL, Reversed Dot Blot could not detect the members of the A28 group, in those cases A68. Sequencing Based Typing could type all alleles of the A2 group.

Conclusions

In situations where the probe did not hybridize with a PCR product the DNA sample was not a member of the A2 group.
For the samples that gave a hybridization pattern, comparable results were seen by Reversed Dot Blot and Sequencing Based Typing. In addition, they were concordant with typing results reported for these samples in the literature. In either system it was not possible to discriminate between A*0201 and A*0209, because of the difference located in exon 4. This is also found for the allele combination A*0207 and A*0215N, which also requires exon 4 sequence information.
The combination A*0207 or A*0215N is not found in Reversed Dot Blot. The system was designed for A*0201 to A*0210 and there is no probe for A*0215N yet.
Reversed Dot Blot is useful in typing the A2 subtypes for A*0201 to A*0210. The higher numbers are inconvenient, because new probes have to be developed.
In Sequencing Based Typing we only encounter one ambiguity: A*0201/0205 and A*0202/0206. In Reversed Dot Blot we expect a lot of ambiguities especially in heterozygous samples. Different heterozygous samples should give the same reaction patterns on the blot.
Reversed Dot Blot cannot type for the members of the A28 group (A68 and A69) and other alleles, whereas Sequencing Based Typing gives typing of all HLA-A alleles.
Reversed Dot Blot is applicable for A2 subtypes and Sequencing Based Typing gives a direct high resolution typing of the A2 group.

Acknowledgements
We thank Applied Biosystems Division of Perkin Elmer, Foster City, CA, for their financial support and M. Kronick and group for their advise.
This study was performed with the contribution of the travel grant obtained by MWO (MW-MWO-INSERM).

References

1. Kimura A, Sasazuki T. Eleventh International Histocompatibility Workshop reference protocol for the HLA DNA-typing technique. In: Tsuji K, Aizawa M, Sasazuki T, eds. *HLA 1991*, vol. 1. *Proceedings of the Eleventh International Histocompatibility Workshop and Conference*. Oxford: Oxford University Press; 1992: 397-419.
2. Eliaou JF, Palmade F, Avinens O, Edouard E, Ballaguer P, Nicolas JC, Clot J. Generic HLA-DRB1 gene oligotyping by a nonradioactive Reverse Dot Blot methodology. *Hum Immunol* 1992; 35: 215-22.
3. Rozemuller EH, Chadwick B, Charron D, Baxter-Loxe LA, Eliaou JF, Johnston-Dow L, Tilanus MGJ. Sequenase sequence profiles used for HLA-DPBI sequencing based typing. *Tissue Antigens* 1996; 47 (1): 72-9.

Nucleotide sequencing analysis of HLA-C alleles

I. Faé, M. Petrasek, E. Broer, W.R. Mayr, G.F. Fischer

Department of Blood Group Serology, University of Vienna, Waehringer Guertel 18-20, A-1090 Vienna, Austria

HLA-C molecules can be detected on the surface of most types of human nucleated cells. There is evidence that they are involved in peptide presentation to cytotoxic T-lymphocytes as well as in the interaction with natural killer cells [1, 2]. Compared with HLA-A and HLA-B molecules their level of expression, however, is considerably lower, be it because of intrinsic properties of the HLA-C heavy chain or because of different regulatory events at the transcriptional level [3, 4].

At present, 35 HLA-C alleles have obtained an official designation [5]. The eight specificities Cw1 to Cw8 comprise a total of 20 alleles. The other alleles, although expressed [6], have not been shown to elicit alloantibody production, therefore, they are typed as C blank. In the Austrian population the gene frequency of C blank encoding alleles can be estimated as up to 25%.

To assess further the significance of the HLA-C polymorphism on immune response, it seems essential to characterise HLA-C alleles at the nucleotide level. For that we have worked out a cDNA based sequencing protocol. RNA isolation from 10^5 - 10^6 peripheral blood lymphocytes has been performed with magnetic beads (Dynabeads mRNA Direct™ Kit, Dynal, Oslo, Norway). cDNA was generated using primer CPRIM *(Table I)* and MuLV reverse transcriptase (Boehringer Mannheim, Mannheim, Germany). CPRIM is complementary to an mRNA stretch of exon 4 common to all HLA-C alleles described. Aligning of HLA-class I sequences shows that at the 3' end of the primer HLA-C alleles have an additional triplet when compared to HLA-A and HLA-B alleles implicating high locus specificity of the primer. The precipitated cDNA was used as template in four separate PCR reactions using the primer pairs M13ClassIAMP and C874REV, M13C432REV and ClassIAMP, M13C874REV and ClassIAMP, and M13C441AMP and C874REV *(Table I)*. "M13" in the name of a primer indicates that it has been tailed with the M13 universal primer sequence, "AMP" that it is derived from the sense and "REV" that is derived from the non-sense strand. The number after a "C" indicates the position of the primer's 3' end in the cDNA sequence. The 5' amplification primer ClassIAMP is from the 5' untranslated region immediately after the initiation codon. The amplification products allow sequencing of a region of HLA-C alleles that comprises exons 1 to 3 and a large part of exon 4.

The PCR products were directly sequenced using a cyle sequencing protocol including labelled primers on a robotic workstation (Catalyst 800). Electrophoresis of sequenced material was performed on a fluorescent sequencing device (373A DNA sequencer; all reagents and machines from ABI, Foster City, CA). Since one PCR primer in each reaction contained an M13 universal primer tail, only one labelled primer could be used for all sequencing reactions.

Seventy-seven individuals were subjected to HLA-C specific sequence analysis. All had been previously typed by serology. After having established a correlation between serology and sequencing based typing in individuals showing two HLA-Cw specificities (n=20) they have been selected for the (putative) presence of HLA-C blank alleles. Either they were completely HLA-C blank (n=13) when typed with a panel of HLA-C specific sera or they displayed one (n=44) HLA-C specificity.

With the exception of one allele all sequences obtained were identical to known HLA-C sequences or, in heterozygous individuals, were compatible with combinations of them. This indicates that the cDNA generation was specific for the HLA-C locus and no HLA-A or HLA-B specific sequences were amplified. The exception occured during the sequencing analysis of alleles encoding the HLA-Cw5 specificity in six individuals. We observed, consistently, at position 576 a "C" instead of a "G" which was expected according to the published sequence. The question whether we have observed a novel allele or if there exists an error in the database has

Table I. Primers used for cDNA generation and sequencing of HLA-C alleles

Name	Sequence (5 → 3')
CPRIM	GCT AGG ACA
M13ClassIAMP	TGT AAA ACG ACG GCC AGT CTC AGA ATC TCC CCA GAC GCC G
M13C441A	TGT AAA ACG ACG GCC AGT GCC TAC GAC GGC AAG GAT TAC
M13C874REV	TGT AAA ACG ACG GCC AGT CTC AGG GTG AGG GGC TC
M13C432REV	TGT AAA ACG ACG GCC AGT TTC AGG GCG ATG TAA TCC TTG
C874REV	CTC AGG GTG AGG GGC TC
ClassIAMP	CTC AGA ATC TCC CCA GAC GCC G

Table II. HLA-C blank encoding alleles observed

Allele	n
0102	2
0803	1
1202	1
1203	14
1402	7
1502	14
1505	2
1601	9
1602	1
1701	7

to be addressed in retypings of the reference cells.

Apart from this one nucleotide discrepancy we did not observe any novel sequences in our typings and the unambigous assigning of HLA-C alleles was possible.

Discrepancies between serological typing and sequencing based typing were observed only in two individuals, where an HLA-C*0803 and an HLA-C*0102 allele could not be detected. Otherwise there was perfect correlation between serology and molecular typing. Fourty four of the individuals tested displayed only one HLA-C specificity. In twelve of them only one HLA-C allele could be detected using sequencing based typing. The others were heterozygous and possessed an allele encoding an HLA-C blank specificity. *Table II* compiles the distribution of alleles encoding HLA-C blanks in our sample. The reason for the discrepancy between molecular typing and serology regarding the HLA-C*0102 and HLA-C*0803 alleles could be a trivial typing error. However, the typings have been repeated and gave consistent results. Furthermore we observed in a family study that both, the molecularly defined HLA-C*0102 and *0803 alleles segregate but cannot be detected by serology in two generations. Six other individuals carrying the HLA-C*0102 allele possessed the HLA-Cw1 specificity. Thus future studies will have to address the possibility that a mutation outside the part of the HLA-C alleles which has been sequenced by now could give rise to a non-expressed molecule. The other alleles listed in *Table II* indicate that polymorphism among HLA-C blank alleles exists in the Austrian population. A larger database will be necessary to establish their exact gene frequencies, however.

Serological typing of the products of the HLA-C locus has been notoriously difficult and therefore the function of this molecule is less well characterised than that of HLA-A or HLA-B molecules. Sequencing based typing is a practicable means of characterisation of the HLA-C polymorphism and application in routine typing will help to assess the functional role of HLA-C.

References

1. Towsend A, Bodmer H. Antigen recognition by class I-restricted T lymphocytes. *Annu Rev Immunol* 1989; 7: 601-24.
2. Colonna M, Borsellino G, Falco M, Ferrara GB, Strominger JL. HLA-C is the inhibitory ligand that determines dominant resistance to lysis by NK1- and NK2 - specific natural killer cells. *Proc Natl Acad Sci USA* 1993; 90: 12000-4.
3. Zemmour J, Parham P. Distinctive polymorphism at the HLA-C locus: implication for the expression of HLA-C. *J Exp Med* 1992; 176: 937-50.
4. McCutcheon JA, Gumperz J, Smith KD, Lutz CT, Parham P. Low HLA-C expression at cell surfaces correlates with increased turnover of heavy chain mRNA. *J Exp Med* 1995; 181: 2085-95.
5. Bodmer JG, Marsh SGE, ALbert ED, Bodmer WF, Bontrop RE, Charron D, Dupont B, Erlich HA, Mach B, Mayr WR, Parham P, Sasazuki T, Schreuder G, Strominger JL, Svejgaard A, Terasaki PI. Nomenclature for factors of the HLA system, 1995. *Tissue Antigens* 1995; 46: 1-18.
6. Hajek-Rosenmayr A, Jungl L, Stammler M, Kirnbauer M. HLA-C 'blank' alleles express class I gene products. Biochemical analysis analysis of four different HLA-C 'blank' polypeptides. *Immunogenetics* 1989; 30: 399-404.

Sequence based typing (SBT) of HLA-C alleles in 214 Caucasians using the automated DNA sequencer ALF

B.C. Schlesinger, B. Laumbacher, R. Wank

Institut für Immunologie, Universität München, Goethestrasse 31, 80336 München, Germany

Due to decreased surface expression serological typing of HLA-C antigens is more difficult than typing of HLA-A and -B antigens. At present 34 different alleles have been characterised mostly by sequencing [1], but only 8 antigens can be recognised serologically. To our knowledge, the allele frequencies for HLA-C have not been studied at a population level up to now. In this study we used direct sequencing of PCR products to determine HLA-C allele distribution in a panel of 214 healthy Caucasian individuals.

Material and methods

Subject panel and template preparation

Peripheral blood lymphocytes (PBL) from healthy unrelated Caucasian individuals were isolated by Ficoll gradient centrifugation. Total RNA was prepared from 5 x 10^6 freshly isolated cells or after anti-CD3 stimulation using the Micro RNA isolation kit (Stratagene, La Jolla, CA92037, USA). RNA was transcribed into cDNA by RAV-2 reverse transcriptase (Amersham, Braunschweig, Germany) and subjected to PCR amplification. Serological HLA class I antigen typing was performed according to the NIH method [2] with minor modifications for automated reading [3] using workshop reagents, our own monoclonal antibodies, and reagents obtained by exchange.

Amplification and sequencing primers

The sequence, length, and localisation of the primers are shown in *Table I*. The primer for reverse transcription is specific for class I alleles. The PCR primer pair amplified a 1018 bp fragment of HLA-C alleles spanning the 5'end of exon 2 up to the 3' untranslated region (PCR-protocol: 1. 94°C - 2 min - 1 cycle; 2. (94°C - 30 seconds, 65°C - 30 seconds, 72°C - 1 min) - 35 cycles; 3. 72°C - 2 min - 1 cycle). The sequencing primers were hybridised to conserved regions of HLA alleles. Following amplification PCR products were sequenced directly after strand separation with Streptavidin coated Dynabeads M-280 (Dynal, Hamburg, Germany).

Sequence based typing (SBT)

Sequencing was performed using Fluoreprime or Indodicarbocyanine (Cy5) labelled primer *(Table I)* and the Pharmacia Autoread-Kit according to the manufacturers protocol. Gels were run on an automated DNA Sequencer ALF or ALF Express (Pharmacia, Freiburg, Germany). Both strands of every PCR product were sequenced.

Results

HLA-Cw alleles and their correlation with serological specificities

In our random panel of 214 Caucasian individuals we found only one encoding allele, HLA-Cw*0102, Cw*0401, Cw*0501, and Cw*0602, respectively, coding for the serologically characterised HLA antigens Cw1, Cw4, Cw5 and Cw6 *(Figure 1)*. Cw*02021 and Cw*02022 encoded the Cw2 antigen, with the later being found in 96.6% of the cases. Cw*0304 with 57.69%, Cw*0303 with 39.74%, and Cw*0302 with 2.5% encoded the Cw3 antigen. Cw*0701 with 49.54%, Cw*0702 with 39.44%, and Cw*0704 with 11.00% were found to encode for the Cw7 antigen. The Cw*0802 allele, which is mainly found in Caucasians, encoded all Cw8 antigens with one exception where Cw8 was encoded by Cw*0803. This allele has been described previously in South American Indians of the Kaingang tribe [4]. HLA-C alleles that have not been characterised serologically (Cw blank) were present at 11.9% in our panel *(Figure 1)*. The alleles Cw*1202, Cw*1402, Cw*1403, Cw*1501/02, Cw*1505, and Cw*1701 occurred in frequencies below 1%. Cw*1601 was found in 2.57% and Cw*1203 in 5.61% of our panel.

Table I. Sequence, length, and localisation of the primers used for template preparation and sequencing

usage	Name	Orientation	Sequence	Length	Localisation+
reverse transcription	HLA-RT	antisense	5' TTGAGACAGAGATGGAGACA 3'	19mer	3'UT (236 - 256) from stop-codon
PCR	HLA-Ex1-2	sense	5' B*-AGACCTGGGCCTGCTCCCACTCC 3'	23mer	Exon1 / Exon2 (62 - 84)
	HLA-ALC	antisense	5' GGGAATTGCTGCATCTCAGTCCCACACAGGC 3'	31mer	3'UT (8 - 32) from stop-codon
sequencing	F-B1	antisense	5' F#-CCTCGCTCTGGTTGTAGTAGC 3'	21mer	Exon2 (320 - 340)
	F-G1	antisense	5' F#-GCTGCAGCGTCTCCTTCCCGTTCT 3'	24mer	Exon3 (590 - 613)
	F-K1	sense	5' F#-GTGGGCTACGTGGACGACAC 3'	20mer	Exon2 (145 -164)
	F-C1	sense	5' F#-GCCTACGACGGCAAGGATTAC 3'	21mer	Exon3 (421 - 441)

+ Nucleotide positions are counted from the start-codon (A = 1) unless indicated otherwise. *B-biotinylated, #F-Fluoreprime/Cy5 labelled.

Table II. Correlation between serological typing of HLA-C antigens and sequence based typing

	Serological typing		
Antigen	False positive	False negative	r
Cw1	5,88 %	-	0,968
Cw2	4,34 %	8,30 %	0,933
Cw3	1,69 %	3,33 %	0,970
Cw4	9,30 %	2,50 %	0,932
Cw5	16,66 %	16,66 %	0,821
Cw6	25,92 %	28,57 %	0,705
Cw7	23,61 %	32,92 %	0,664
Cw8	8,33 %	26,66 %	0,813

Table III. Association between HLA-C alleles and HLA-B antigens

HLA-C allele	HLA-B antigen	Fisher's exact p
Cw*0303	B62	$1,19 \times 10^{-6}$
Cw*0304	B40	$6,29 \times 10^{-12}$
Cw*0304	B62	$1,85 \times 10^{-8}$
Cw*0701	B8	$5,40 \times 10^{-17}$
Cw*0702	B7	$4,25 \times 10^{-18}$
Cw*0704	B44	$9,17 \times 10^{-4}$
Cw*1203	B38	$6,86 \times 10^{-7}$

We found a strong correlation between serological typing and sequence based typing for Cw1, Cw2, Cw3, and Cw4 antigens with r > 0,9 and false positive or false negative results below 10% *(Table II)*. For Cw5, Cw6, Cw7, and Cw8 false positive or false negative results were obtained in over 10% of the cases reaching up to 32.92% false negative results in the Cw7 group *(Table II)*.

Linkage disequilibria between HLA-B antigens and HLA-C alleles

In this study we could confirm linkage disequilibria between Cw*02022/B27, Cw*0401/B35, Cw*0501/B44, Cw*0802/B14, Cw*1202/B52, Cw*1402/B51, and Cw*1601/B44 as previously described [5].

For HLA-C antigen groups with more than one encoding allele we found allele specific associations with HLA-B antigens (see *Table III* for p values): Cw*0303 was associated with B62, while for Cw*0304 the association with B40 was stronger than with B62. Cw*0701 was associated with B8, Cw*0702 with B7 and Cw*0704 weakly associated with B44. Cw*1203 was associated with B38 and not with B52 as described for Cw*1202.

Discussion

In our panel, 11.9% of the HLA-C alleles encode molecules for which no antisera are available. Sequence based typing of HLA-C alleles allows not only detection of Cw blank alleles but also the exclusion or detection of

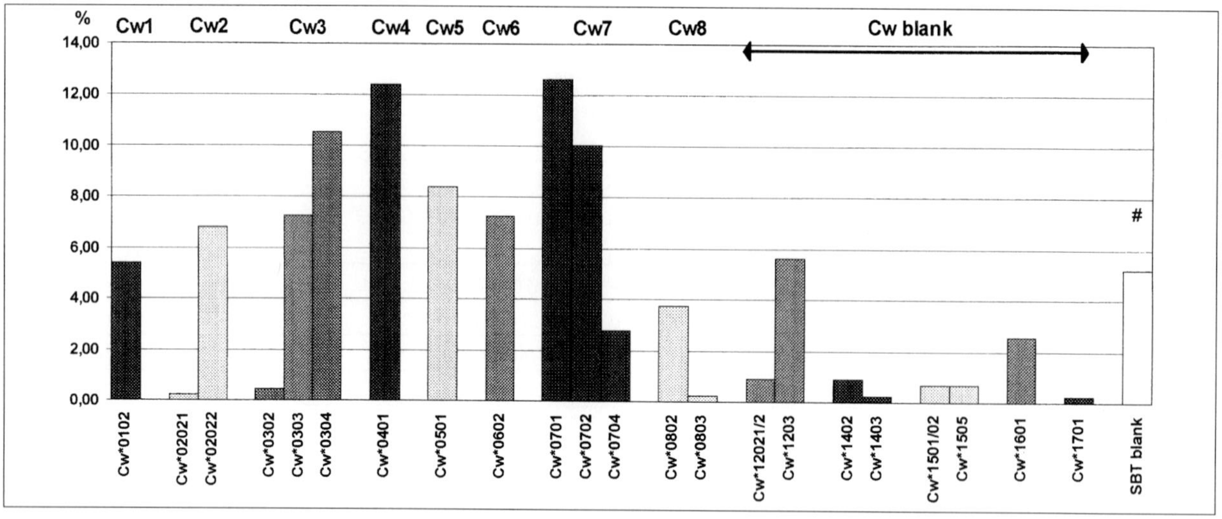

Figure 1. Frequencies of HLA-C alleles in a normal Caucasian population (n = 214).
SBT blank alleles are calculated from the percentage of individuals with only one allele typed by SBT minus the percentage of expected homozygous individuals.

alleles that are incorrectly characterized by antibodies. We could identify at least one HLA-C allele in every individuals of our population. Heterozygosity was assertained in 81%. The number of individuals with only one HLA-C allele was 10.4% higher than the expected number of homozygotes. Despite the improved accuracy of SBT versus serological typing we cannot exclude the presence of so far undetected alleles, at a rate of 5.2% in our population, that we are not able to amplify with our primer set.

HLA-B antigens were mostly associated with one HLA-C subgroup allele. The observed association of both HLA-Cw*0303 and Cw*0304 with B62 may separate into a more specific association with one of the alleles encoding HLA-B62.

References

1. Arnett KL, Parham P. HLA class I nucleotide sequences. *Tissue Antigens* 1995; 45: 217-57.
2. Terasaki PI, Mc Clelland JD. Microdroplet assay of human serum cytotoxins. *Nature* 1964; 204: 998.
3. Wimmer A, Graf A, Wank R. Automated measurement of cell destruction. *Infusionstherapie* 1992; 19: 130-3.
4. Belich MP, Madrigal JA, Hildebrand WH, Zemmour J, Williams RC, Luz R, Petzl-Erler ML, Parham P. Unusual HLA-B alleles in two tribes of Brazilian Indians. *Nature* 1992; 357: 326-9.
5. Baur MP, Danilovs JA. Reference tables for two and three locus haplotype frequencies of HLA-A, B, C, DR, Bf, and GLO. In: Terasaki PL, ed. *Histocompatibility testing 1980*. Los Angeles: UCLA Tissue Typing Laboratory, 1980: 994-1210.

Automated DNA sequencing : a fast and accurate method for high resolution HLA class II typing

M. Bielefeld[2], E. Van den Berg-Loonen[1], C. Voorter[1], P. Savelkoul[1], L. Björkesten[2]

1 Laboratory for Tissue Typing, Maastricht, The Netherlands
2 Pharmacia Biotech AB, Bjorkgatam 30, S-7518 Uppsala, Sweden

Sequencing is becoming an acknowledged method for high resolution HLA typing. It solves several problems which are system dependent in other methods like low resolution, The setting up of large quantities of PCR* reactions and changing the primer sets.
Here we want to describe an easy and economical way to perform sequence based typing. Typing is performed with data derived from sequencing within exon II. The system is based on a concept originally published by Spurkland *et al.* [1]. As most of the data were produced within the DRB1 system, we shall use this example for a detailed description. The DQB primers are in the process of being evaluated and work similarly. For SBT of the DPB locus, we have applied the system described in the Technical Handbook of the 12th International Workshop and Conference [2].

Methodology

Amplification and sequencing primers

The 5' primers are located in the group specific region between codons 5 and 15. The 3' primer which is biotinylated for solid phase sequencing and the sequencing primer are generic and situated at codon 88 - 94 and codon 14 - 19 respectively *(Figure 1)*.

Amplification

For the amplification, two slightly different approaches were used.
1. One amplification with a mixture of all group specific 5' primers and the generic 3' primers is performed. Both alleles are amplified together in the same reaction. This method is easy and economical, however since not all possible combinations have been tested up to now, preferential amplification of one allele could occur in certain heterozygous combinations.

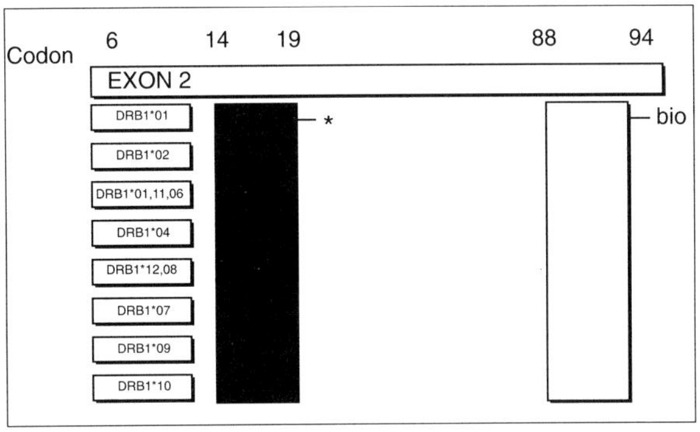

Figure 1. Amplification and sequencing scheme for the DRB 1 locus.

2. Separate PCR reaction with each 5' group specific primer and the 3' generic primer are performed. The two positive reactions are mixed before sequencing. This involves more PCR reactions in the beginning, but gives higher security as preferential amplification can be excluded. More data should however be evaluated to give preference to either method.

Sequence reactions

The subsequent sequencing is performed using the heterozygous PCR sample. Solid phase sequencing with the AutoLoad™ system [3] has shown to be the most accurate and convenient method.
Electrophoresis and sequence determination: the automated sequencers ALF™ and ALF*express*™ with their software dedicated for heterozygote detection proved to be a perfect platform to facilitate data generation and analysis. The possibility to work with raw data at all times allows an interactive control of the sequence data, increasing the confidence in the typing result. Runs were performed under standard conditions using denaturing acrylamide gels and a constant running temperature of 55° C. The average running time was 220 minutes.

* PCR (polymerase chain reaction) is covered by US patents 4,683,195 and 4,683,202

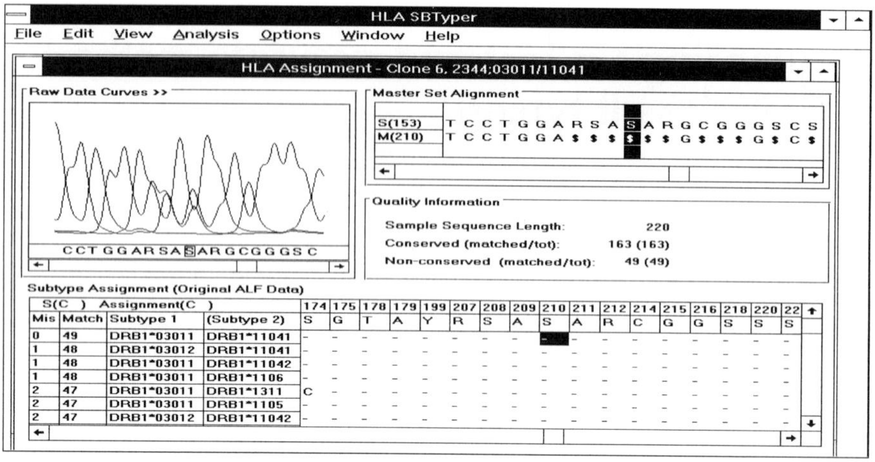

Figure 2.
Result of an automated HLA typing with HLA SB*Typer.*

Automated HLA typing with HLA SB*Typer*™

The automated analysis with this software is based on the comparison with a data base containing all known alleles of the respective loci. Typing is performed in two steps which are automatically performed. First the test sample is aligned to the data base sequence. Then the combinations of the non-conserved positions for all possible pairs of alleles are compared with those of the sample sequence. The best fits are displayed as result. In addition information on the quality of the sequence and typing data is given. The result can easily be re-investigated if necessary using the direct link to the ALF raw data curves *(Figure 2).*

Resolving multiple assignments

With the result from one sequencing reaction about 75% of all heterozygous combinations can be resolved immediately (this value can vary depending on the population). In order to analyse the remaining cases, 2 methods can be chosen.

Group specific amplification

When the sequence of the heterozygous sample gives more than one possible allele combination the single alleles can be separately amplified, when they are derived from different groups. By subsequent sequencing an unambiguous typing result will be obtained.

Codon 86 primers

The DRB1 genes can be split into 2 groups based on codon 86 - one containing TG the other GT at this position. The use of 3' amplification primers specific for one or the other form has proven to be a powerful method to split allele pairs that amplify with the same primer (DRB1*11/*13 for example).

All cases analysed in our studies could be typed unambiguously by performing one more PCR reaction and subsequent sequencing as described [4,5].

More than 500 different samples have been analysed using the methods described. They were compared with typing results derived from SSP and for a number of cases also serology. No contradictory results have been observed. In all cases where SSP could not give a clear answer (difficult combination or new allele), the typing could be performed to the allele level with SBT.

Reference

1. Spurkland A, Knutsen I, Markussen G, Vartdal F, Egeland T, Thorsby E. HLA matching unrelated bone marrow transplant pairs: HLA-DRB1 and DQB1 genes using magnetic beads as solid support. *Tissue Antigens* 1993; 41: 155 - 64.
2. Technical Handbook, Twelfth International Histocompatibility Workshop and conference. Utrecht: AZU-printing office and Paris HLA et Médecine, 1996.
3. Lagerkvist A, Steward J, Landegren LFM, Landegren U. Manifold sequencing: efficient processing of large sets of sequence reactions. *Proc Natl Acad Sci USA* 1994; 91: 2245 -9.
4. Voorter CEM, Rozemuller EH, de Bruyn-Geraerts D, Van der Zwaan AW, Tilanus MGJ, van den Berg-Loonen EM. Comparison of DRB sequence based typing using different strategies. 1997, in press.
5. De Bruyn-Geraerts D, Voorter CEM, Lie J, van den Berg-Loonen EM. High resolution DRB1 typing by sequencing based typing in 77 DR4 positive rheumatoid arthritis patients. *Abstract book, 12th International Histocompatibility Conference.* New York: Elsevier, 1996.

Symposium communications

HLA Diversity

HLA typing and sequencing

Function of HLA

Transplantation biology and medicine

HLA and Diseases

Function of HLA

Assembly and traffic of MHC molecules. Antigen processing and presentation

Contents

The function of HLA-DM during peptide loading onto MHC class II molecules

H. Kropshofer, G. Moldenhauer, G.J. Hämmerling, A.B. Vogt

German Cancer Research Center, Department of Molecular Immunology, Im Neuenheimer Feld 280, D-69120 Heidelberg, Germany

Shortly after biosynthesis MHC class II molecules bind to the invariant chain (Ii) which prevents premature loading with peptides [1]. Owing to an Ii targeting signal class II:Ii complexes are sorted to endocytic compartments where Ii is degraded [2]. The residual Ii fragment by which Ii has bound to the class II αβ dimers, is designated CLIP (class II-associated Ii peptide) [3]. Antigenic peptide loading onto αβ dimers requires the release of CLIP, since it occupies the peptide binding groove [4]. At endosomal pH, CLIP can dissociate by itself to a certain extent, as shown for several class II alleles [5]. Analysis of mutant antigen presenting cell lines mainly expressing αβ:CLIP complexes at the cell surface, led to the identification of a key player involved in peptide loading [6]: the non-classical MHC class II molecule HLA-DM (DM).

In vitro studies have shown that DM facilitates peptide loading directly, as it accelerates CLIP release from DR molecules [7]. Moreover, several reports implied that DM may function in substoichiometric amounts and, therefore, may act as a catalyst of loading [8]. Consistent with this view, DM was found to bind only weakly to DR molecules *ex vivo* [9].

However, so far there is no evidence for the catalytic nature of DM, likewise, little is known about its substrate specificity and about further roles of DM during loading of αβ dimers beyond the stage of CLIP release.

Results and discussion

DM is a catalyst of loading

To analyze the role of DM as a catalyst, we purified DM from human spleen cells and a putative substrate, DR1:CLIP complexes, from the DM-negative mutant T2 transfected with DR1. Using a ratio DR1:DM of 40:1 in an *in vitro* peptide binding assay based on high-performance size exclusion chromatography (HPSEC), DM reduced the half-maximal time of binding to DR1 of *influenza* virus hemagglutinin-derived HA peptide from 300 to 25 min at pH 5.0.

To determine the rate of DM-catalyzed exchange of CLIP for HA peptide according to the model of Michaelis and Menten, we measured the amount of DR1:HA complexes formed during the initial linear phase of loading using different DR1:CLIP concentrations. We could deduce a turnover-number of 4±1 DR1:CLIP complexes per minute per DM molecule, reminiscent of low-capacity enzymes, such as lysozyme or protein-disulphide isomerase. Thus, at endosomal pH substoichiometric amounts of DM appear to be powerful enough to catalyze quantitative loading of αβ dimers in 1-2 hours, the time loading takes *in vivo*.

DM does not acts as a peptide receptor

We treated purified DM with 0.1% TFA and separated potential low-molecular-weight ligands by ultrafiltration, essentially as described for the acid elution of classical class II moleules [10]. Analysis by mass spectrometry did not yield any signals in the mass range m/z = 1000-4000. Lack of binding at pH 5.0 or 7.0 was also observed in a HPSEC assay: neither CLIP nor several other peptides known to bind promiscuously to DR molecules failed to bind stably to DM, irrespective of the incubation time. We conclude, that DM does not serve as a "sink" for CLIP or as a peptide shuttle.

DM:DR interaction is peptide-dependent

In order to visualize putative DM:DR complexes that are expected to have only low affinity, recombinant DM generated in insect cells was covalently immobilized on a sensor chip and DR1:CLIP complexes were passed over this DM surface at pH 5.0. Plasmon resonance measurements allowed us to detect a dose-dependent interaction of DR1:CLIP with DM in real time.

Importantly, DR1:peptide complexes isolated from the DM-positive lymphoblastoid cell line WT-100 revealed to interact less well with DM compared to DR1:CLIP complexes. These data suggest that DM cannot efficiently associate with αβ dimers once they are loaded with stably binding non-CLIP peptides.

DM stabilizes "empty" DR molecules in a chaperon-like manner

Again, we chose DR1:CLIP complexes as a starting material, because CLIP has been shown to dissociate very rapidly in our experimental setup at low pH, thereby generating "empty" DR1 molecules. Such class II molecules with an unoccupied binding groove tend to become functionally inactivated, as verified in our case: the number of DR1 molecules available for subsequent binding of HA peptide decreased with increasing preincubation time. However, when DR1:CLIP was preincubated together with DM, functional inactivation of DR1 could be prevented in a dose-dependent manner. Furthermore, a 15-min incubation revealed that HA peptide bound in the presence of DM with an 80-fold higher apparent affinity than in the absence of DM *(Figure 1)*.

These findings emphasize that DM acts beyond the stage of CLIP release: it is able to stabilize empty DR molecules by forming DR:DM complexes at the same time enhancing the entry of new peptides into the binding groove. Thus, DM functions as a molecular chaperon that keeps the peptide binding groove accessible for loading.

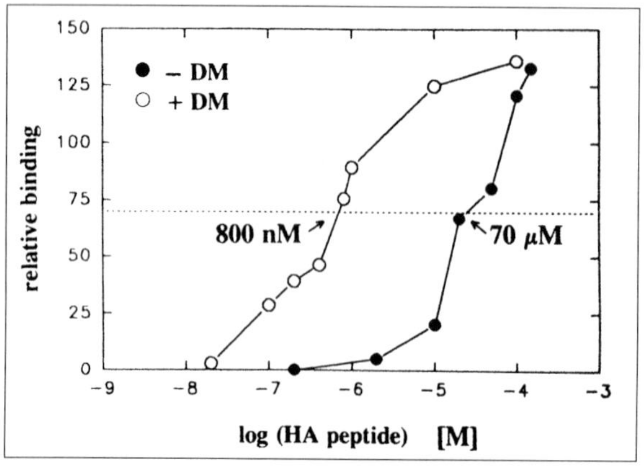

Figure 1. DM enhances the apparent affinity of high-stability peptides.

DM functions as a peptide editor

Up to now it was unclear whether DM is able to remove peptides other than CLIP and, if it does, how this would be accomplished mechanistically. Therefore we added DM to DR:peptide complexes purified from various lymphoblastoid cell lines and could identify a sizeable fraction of non-CLIP self-peptides being susceptible to DM-mediated removal.

The structural basis for the DM-sensitivity was elucidated by a novel highly sensitive mass spectrometry binding assay: mimicking the situation *in vivo,* mixtures of peptides, distinguishable by their unique masses, were offered to purified DR:CLIP with and without DM, the so formed complexes isolated by ultrafiltration, bound peptides acid-eluted and analyzed by mass spectrometry. We found that only those peptides resist DM removal that display an intrinsically high kinetic stability, but not necessarily those with a high steady state affinity. Consequently, DM removed peptides that contained at least one suboptimal anchor residue or that were shorter than 11 residues *(Figure 2)*, providing a rationale for the minimal length requirements of DR-associated peptides *in vivo*.

Together, DM can function as a versatile editor that selects for high-stability class II:peptide complexes by a kinetic proofreading mechnism.

Kinetic proofreading model

The low pH of lysosomal or prelysosomal loading compartments favors binding of DM to DR αβ dimers. However, it seems to be the peptide occupying the DR binding groove that determines the half-life of the DR:DM complex *(Figure 3):* low-stability peptides, such as CLIP, are released by DM which remains bound to the αβ dimer. Conversely, high-stability pepties cause rapid dissociation of DM from DR. In mechanistic terms, binding of DM is likely to induce a sort of "open" state of the binding groove, whereupon a peptide bound with low stability will be released. In contrast, peptides with the appropriate number and spacing of anchor side-chains and sufficient length will resist the DM-induced "opening" of the groove and will remain bound, whereupon DM dissociates and starts a new round of editing. This type of kinetic proofreading by DM skews the class II-associated peptide repertoire towards a population of stably binding peptides. Moreover, it minimizes the number of αβ dimers that may lose unstably bound peptides and be subsequently degraded due to disassembly en route to or at the cell surface.

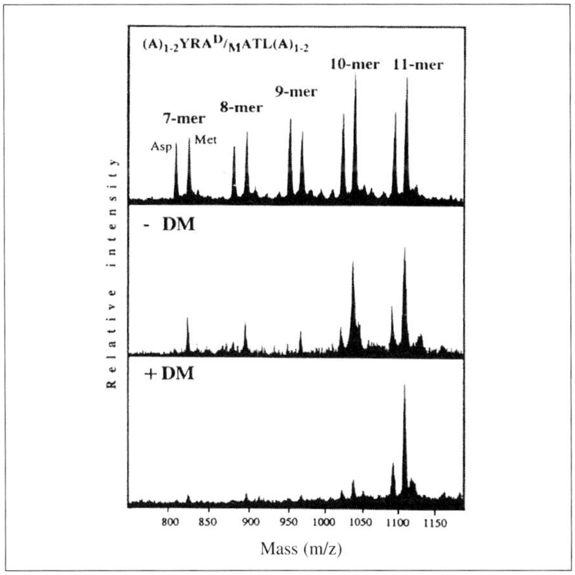

Figure 2. DM acts as a peptide editor.

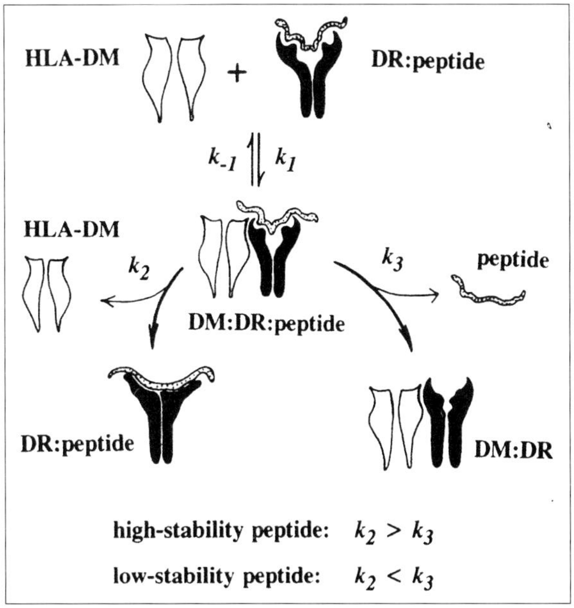

Figure 3. The kinetic proofreading model.

References

1. Roche PA, Marks MS, Cresswell P. Formation of a nine-subunit complex by HLA class II glycoproteins and the invariant chain. *Nature* 1991; 354: 392-4.
2. Bakke O, Dobberstein B. MHC class II-associated invariant chain contains a sorting signal for endosomal compartments. *Cell* 1990; 63: 707-15.
3. Riberdy JM, Newcomb JR, Surman MJ, Barbosa JA, Cresswell P. HLA-DR molecules from an antigen processing mutant cell line are associated with invariant chain peptides. *Nature* 1992; 360: 474-7.
4. Ghosh P, Amaya M, Mellins E, Wiley DC. The structure of HLA-DR3 complexed with CLIP, an intermediate in peptide loading. *Nature* 1995; 387: 457-62.
5. Kropshofer H, Vogt AB, Stern LJ, Hämmerling GJ. Self-release of CLIP in peptide loading of HLA-DR molecules. *Science* 1995 ; 270 : 1357-9.
6. Kelly AP, Monaco JJ, Cho S, Trowsdale J. A new human HLA class II-related locus. *Nature* 1991; 353: 571-3.
7. Sloan VS, Cameron P, Porter G, Gammon M, Amaya M, Mellins E, Zaller DM. Mediation by HLA-DM of dissociation of peptides from HLA-DR. *Nature* 1995; 375: 802-6.
8. Denzin LK, Cresswell P. HLA-DM induces CLIP dissociation from MHC class II αβ dimers and facilitates peptide loading. *Cell* 1995 ; 82 : 155-65.
9. Sanderson F, Thomas C, Neefjes J, Trowsdale J. Association between HLA-DM and HLA-DR *in vivo*. *Immunity* 1996; 4: 87-96.
10. Vogt AB, Kropshofer H, Kalbacher H, Kalbus M, Rammensee HG, Coligan JE, Martin R. Ligand motifs of HLA-DRB5*0101 and DRB1*1501 molecules delineated from self-peptides. *J Immunol* 1994; 153: 1665-73.

A lymphoblastoid cell line lacking the LMP2 proteasome subunit

H. Teisserenc[1], M. Belich[3], C. Lafaurie[2], E. Mickelson[4], J. Trowsdale[3], D. Charron[1]

1 INSERM U396 and 2 U93, Centre Hayem, Hôpital Saint-Louis, 1, avenue Claude Vellefaux, 75010 Paris, France
3 Imperial Cancer Research Fund, London, UK
4 Fred Hutchinson Cancer Research, Seattle, USA

MHC class I molecules display peptides derived from endogenous proteins to cytotoxic T lymphocytes. These peptides are transported from the cytosol into the lumen of the endoplasmic reticulum, by a heterodimeric peptide transporter (TAP), where they bind class I molecules. The TAP transporter is encoded by two genes, *TAP1* and *TAP2*, located in the class II region of the MHC. The TAP genes are closely associated with loci for two proteasome components, *LMP2* and *LMP7* [1-3] The proteasome is a non lysosomal protease that is involved in ubiquitin dependent and independent intracellular protein degradation. The functions of the proteasome may be regulated by the subunit composition. Several lines of evidence, including that from *LMP2* and *LMP7* knock-out mice and from mutant human B lymphoblastoid cells lines [4-7], are consistent with a role for the proteasome containing LMP subunits in antigen processing. However, these studies also show that the LMP subunits are not essential for antigen processing since in their absence other, constitutive proteins are incorporated into the proteasome [8-10]. Proteasomes containing either the LMP subunits or their replacements (MB1 and delta) appear to function in antigen processing although with some subtle variations in performance [10]. The current report describes the case of an individual who lacks the LMP2 subunit.

Results

In an exercise to find new *LMP2* and *LMP7* polymorphisms, coding regions of these genes were studied by RT-PCR and SSCP on 60 B-lymphoblastoid cell lines taken both from our laboratory and from the Xth workshop.

Two alternatively LMP2 spliced transcripts
LMP2 cDNA amplification revealed the presence of two products. One was at the expected size and corresponds to the *LMP2* cDNA sequence previously reported. The second is shorter and lacks the 132 bp corresponding to the entire exon 3, without disruption of the open reading frame. These two transcripts were present in all B-LCL studied.

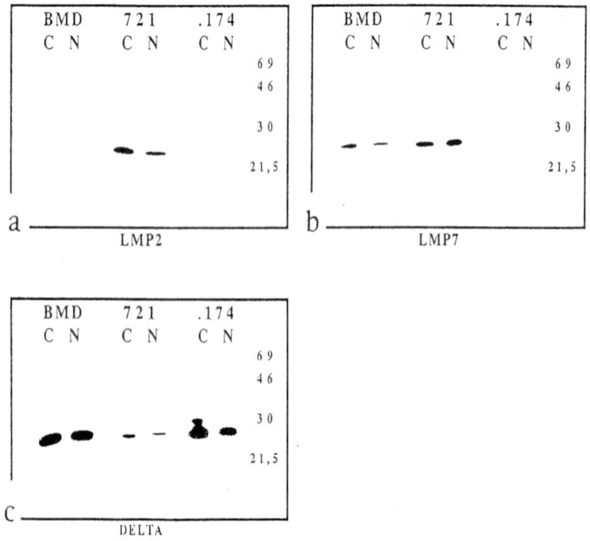

Figure 1. Analysis of LMP2, LMP7 and Delta protein expression in the cytoplasm and nuclei of the BMD LMP2 mutant B-cell line. 721 and .174 were used as controls. Cytoplasmic and nuclear lysates are indicated by "C" and "N" respectively. LMP2, LMP7 and Delta antisea were used at concentrations of 1:1000. 40mg of total cytoplasmic or nuclear lysates were loaded per lane/per cell. Western blots were probed with the following antisera: (a) anti-LMP2, (b) anti-LMP7 and (c) anti-Delta.

A B-LCL lacking the LMP2 subunit

In the BMD B-LCL, *LMP2* cDNA amplification gave only the shorter transcript even though the exon 3 is present at the genomic level. A similar result was obtained using the PBLs from which the BMD cell line was derived. In order to identify the mechanism leading to the preferential expression of the shorter transcript we analyzed *LMP2* intron sequences in BMD. A homozygous single bp substitution in the acceptor splice site of exon 3 was found. Since disruption of exon 3 does not alter the open reading frame, we next studied expression of the LMP2 subunit in BMD. As shown in figures 1a and 1b, Western-Blot analysis using antisera against carboxyterminal peptides from LMP2 and LMP7 did not detect any LMP2 protein in BMD. Moreover, Delta, the proteasome component highly homologous to LMP2, is upregulated in BMD as it is in the LMP deficient cell line 721.174 *(Figure 1c).*

Consequences of the LMP2 defect in the BMD individual

Since *LMP2* or *LMP7* knockout mice present some anomalies (decreased CD8+ population and reduced levels of MHC-class I cell surface expression respectively), we investigated these parameters in the cells from individual from which BMD was derived. As shown in *Figure 2*, HLA class I molecule expression was slightly decreased (78% vs 95% in PBL controls) with a more marked reduction of the mean of fluorescence. Contrary to the *LMP2* knockout mice, no significant variation of the CD8+hi population was detected in PBLs from BMD, whereas the CD8+lo population was increased. Strikingly, the NK population was highly increased in BMD. 46% of the PBLs of this individual were CD16+CD56+ cells (*Figure 3* shows the CD56+ cells in BMD compared to a PBL control).

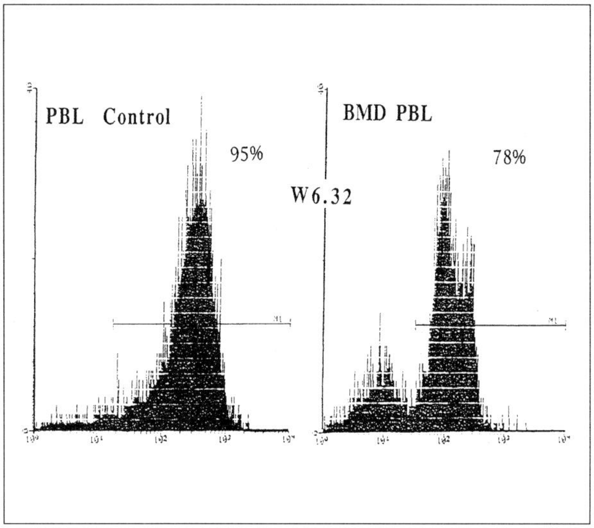

Figure 2. Cell surface expression of MHC class I molecules. PBLs from BMD and control were analyzed by FACS using the W6/32 Ab.

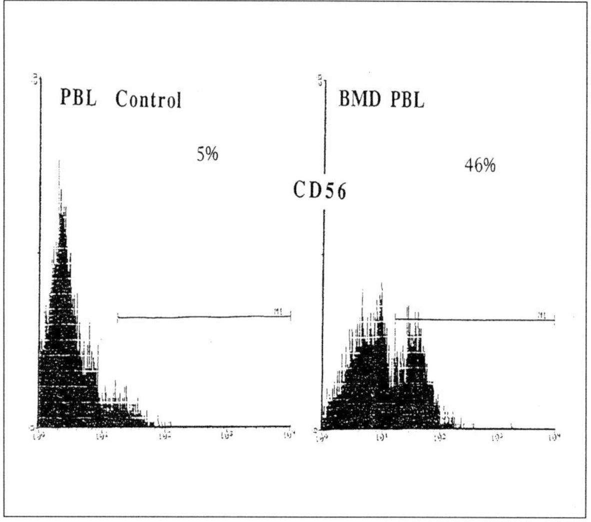

Figure 3. PBLs from BMD have increased levels of NK cells. PBLs from BMD and control individual were stained for CD56-expressing cells. Cells were gated for lymphocytes. The numbers indicate the percentage of positive cells.

Discussion

This report describes for the first time the case of an individual who lacks one of the two proteasome subunits encoded within the MHC. BMD is a "healthy" bone marow donor who has never suffered from recurrent infections or autoimmune diseases. The *LMP2* defect in BMD causes the upregulation of Delta subunit expression. This may explain the slight effect on HLA class I expression, by Delta, the constitutive counterpart of LMP2 allowing sufficient peptides to be generated for association with HLA molecules. The high number of

NK found in BMD suggests that LMP2 replacement is only partially efficient in terms of antigen presentation. Indeed, the number or the nature of peptides that bind to HLA class I molecules could be unsuitable for normal immune surveillance *via* CD8+ T cells and the NK cell expression may be perturbed, or may be upregulated, to fulfil this role. In order to validate this hypothesis, functional assays are underway.

References

1. Monaco JJ, McDevitt HO. H-2 linked low molecular weight polypeptide antigens assemble into an unusual macromolecular complex. *Nature* 1984; 309: 797-9.
2. Glynne R, Powis SH, Beck S, Kelly A, Kerr LA, Trowsdale J. A proteasome-related gene between the two ABC transporter loci in the class II region of the human MHC. *Nature* 1991; 353: 357-60.
3. Kelly A, Powis SH, Glynne R, Radley E, Beck S, Trowsdale J. Second proteasome related gene in human MHC class II region. *Nature* 1991; 353: 667-8.
4. Fehling HJ, Swat W, Laplace C, Kühn R, Rajewsky K, Müller U von Bohmer H. MHC class I expression in mice lacking the proteasome subunit LMP7. *Science* 1994; 265: 1234-7.
5. Van Kaer L, Ashton-Rickardt PG, Eichelberger M, Gaczynska M, Nagshima K, Rock KL, Goldberg AL, Doherty PC, Tonegawa S. Altered peptidase and viral-specific T cell response in LMP2 mutant mice. *Immunity* 1994; 1: 533-41.
6. Cerundolo V, Kelly A, Elliott T, Trowsdale J, Townsend A. Genes encoded in the major histocompatibility complex affecting the generation of peptides for TAP transport. *Eur J Immunol* 1995; 25: 554-62.
7. Kuckelkorn U, Frentzel S, Kraft R, Kostka S, Groettrup M, Kloetzel PM. Incorporation of major histocompatibility complex-encoded subunits LMP2 and LMP7 changes the quality of the 20S proteasome polypeptide processing products independent of interferon-g. *Eur J Immunol* 1995; 25: 2605-11.
8. Arnold D, Driscoll J, Androlewicz M, Hughes E, Cresswell P, Spies T. Proteasome subunits encoded in the MHC are not generally required for the processing of peptides bound by MHC class I molecules. *Nature* 1992; 360: 171-4.
9. Momburg F, Ortiz-Navarette V, Neefjes J, Goulmy E, Van de Walt Y, Spits H, Powis SJ, Butcher GW, Howard JC, Walden P, Hämmerling GJ. Proteasome subunits encoded by the major histocompatibility complex are not essential for antigen presentation. *Nature* 1992; 360: 174-7.
10. Belich M, Glynne RJ, Senger G, Sheer D, Trowsdale J. Proteasome components with reciprocal expression to that of the MHC-encoded LMP proteins. *Curr Biol* 1994; 4: 769-76.

Presentation of T cell epitope by Antennapedia homeodomain

M.P. Schutze-Redelmeier[1], H. Gournier[1], F. Garcia-Pons[1], M. Moussa[1], A.H. Joliot [2], M. Volovitch[2], A. Prochiantz[2], F.A. Lemonnier[1]

1 Département SIDA-Rétrovirus, Unité d'Immunité Cellulaire Antivirale, Institut Pasteur, 28, rue du Dr Roux, 75724 Paris Cedex 15, France
2 CNRS URA 1414, École Normale Supérieure, 46, rue d'Ulm, 75230 Paris Cedex 5, France

Induction of $CD8^+$ cytolytic T lymphocytes (CTL) and recognition of target cells are primarily dependent on cell surface expression of MHC class I molecules loaded with antigenic peptides. As a rule, these peptides are produced in the cytosol, mainly by proteasomes, translocated in the endoplasmic reticulum (ER) by TAP peptide-pumps and loaded on nascent MHC class I molecules. Better knowledge of the early steps of antigen processing might result in the design of more efficient vaccine vectors. Studying *in vitro* neuronal differentiation, we observed that the antennapedia homeodomain (AntpHD, a 61 aminoacid peptide structured in 3 α helices) translocates spontaneously across cell plasma membranes [1]. Translocation being energy independent, non saturable and observed with many types of cells, we investigated the immunological potential of AntpHD fusion peptides [2].
As a model system, we tested fusion peptides in which a T cell epitope (pCw3, position 170-179 of the second domain of the HLA-Cw3 molecule), bounded by processing permissive nucleoprotein (NP) influenza derived sequences, was linked to the AntpHD C-terminus. C myc-tag sequences were also included to follow the intracellular fate of the fusion peptides (*Figure 1A*). This epitope is presented by $H\text{-}2K^d$ mouse class I molecules and recognized by a CTL clone (CAS 20) isolated in the laboratory.
Cytosolic penetration is illustrated in *Figure 1B*, following incubation of fibroblastic cells with recombinant proteins for 2 h. Penetration was similarly observed at 4°C confirming the energy independence of the process. Internalization of radiolabeled AntpHD fusion peptides was not reduced by a 1000x molar excess of unlabeled material substantiating the fact that penetration is not saturable (not shown).
AntpHD-pCw3 treated cells were next tested as targets in a 4 h cytolytic assay. Testing P815 ($H\text{-}2^d$) target cells, specific $H\text{-}2K^d$ restricted lysis was observed, down to 0.1 µg/ml (10^{-8} M) of fusion peptide and 5 h incubation (*Figure 2A*).

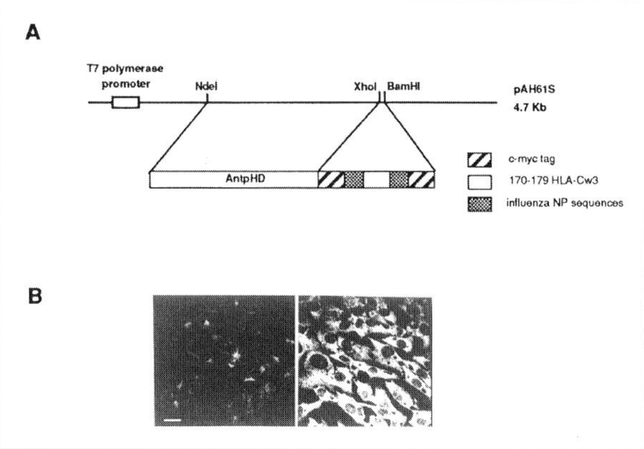

Figure 1. A. Representation of the AntpHD-pCw3 fusion peptide: sequences of c-myc tag (EQKLISEEDL), 170-179 pCw3 (RYLKNGKETL), NP amino (CAEIDL) and carboxy (LRTED) terminus.
B. Confocal analysis of fibroblastic cells incubated 2 h at 37°C (right panel) or not (left) with 1 µg/ml of purified AntpHD-pCw3 fusion peptide.

Inhibition by brefeldin A but not chloroquine suggested that fusion peptides were processed in the cytosol and that the Cw3 epitope was TAP translocated in the ER and loaded on $H\text{-}2K^d$ molecules (*Figure 2B*).
We then tested whether AntpHD-pCw3 fusion peptides could prime CTL responses *in vivo*. Injection of fusion peptides alone was unsuccessful. Similar failure was observed coinjecting them with alum, saponin or incomplete Freund adjuvant. However, mixing them with sodium dodecyl sulphate, we regularly induced CTL responses which were documented following *in vitro* restimulation by synthetic pCw3 peptides (*Figure 3*). Under such conditions, injection of equimolar amounts of synthetic pCw3 peptides failed to prime the CTL response. Similar induction was obtained with another construction containing an $H\text{-}2K^d$ restricted NP influenza (147-156) derived epitope. Whether such a

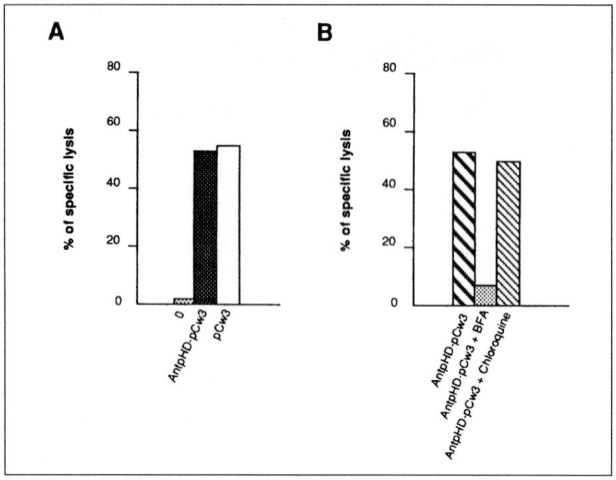

Figure 2. Recognition of P815 cells preincubated overnight with AntpHD-pCw3 fusion peptides.
A. Chromium (^{51}Cr)-labeled P815 cells preincubated with 1 µM of AntpHD-pCw3 fusion peptides were tested using CAS 20 CTL at a 3:1 effector to target (E/T) ratio in a 4 h cytolytic assay. Control experiments were performed with unsensitized P815 cells, and cells pulsed with 1 µM of pCw3 synthetic peptides. Specificity was further documented testing different AntpHD fusion peptides (not shown).
B. P815 target cells incubated overnight with 1 µM of AntpHD-pCw3 fusion peptides in the presence or absence of Brefeldin A (BFA, 0.5 µg/ml) or chloroquine (Chlor. 10 µM) were tested as in 2A. Control experiments (not shown) pulsing these cells with 1 µM of pCw3 synthetic peptides established that their antigen presentation capacity was unaltered.

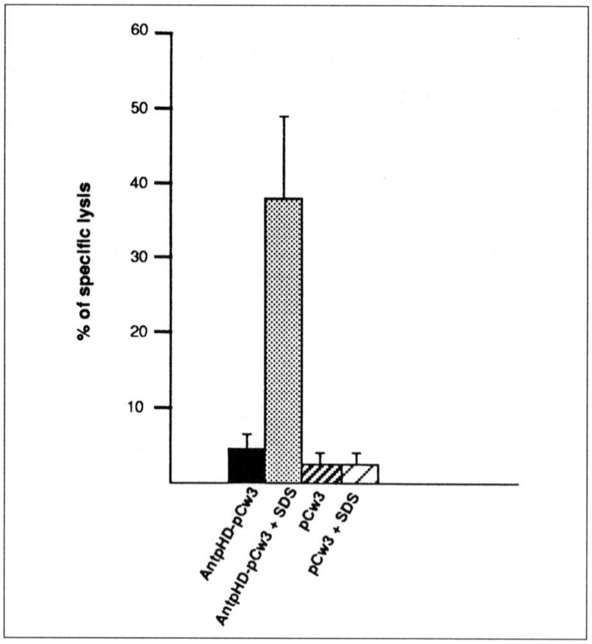

Figure 3. CTL response of DBA/2 mice to AntpHD-pCw3 fusion peptides.
Mice were immunized i.p. on day 0 and 7 with AntpHD-pCw3 (50 µg) fusion or pCw3 (5µg) synthetic peptides, alone or with 500 µg of Sodium Dodecyl Sulphate (SDS). Spleen cells were restimulated *in vitro* (7 days post last immunization) for 5 days with 10 µM of pCw3 synthetic peptide and tested at a 60:1 E/T ratio against P815 HLA-Cw3 transfected cells.

strategy will be of general interest remains however to be established, since it has so far not been possible to significantly protect C57Bl/6 mice against Lewis lung carcinoma cells, by injecting them with AntpHD fused to mutated connexin peptides (L. Eisenbach, personal communication). Nevertheless, AntpHD fusion peptides provide us with a direct access to the MHC class I associated antigen processing pathway. Constructing AntpHD fusion peptides deprived of lysine residue we observed that they sensitized cells to lysis, implying that processing of antigens does not entirely rely on ubiquitination (M.P. Schutze-Redelmeier, unpublished data). Finally, since the 16 amino acid-long third helix of AntpHD is sufficient for internalization [3], fusion peptides containing several CTL epitopes (up to 94 aminoacids) could be prepared.

Acknowledgements
This work was supported by grants from the Fondation pour la Recherche Médicale (SIDACTION, A. Prochiantz, M. Volovitch), the Pasteur-Weizmann Joint Research Program, the Association pour le Développement de la Recherche sur le Cancer and from the Institut Pasteur.

References

1. Perez F, Joliot A, Bloch-Gallego E, Zahaoui A, Triller A, Prochiantz A. Antennapedia as a signal for the cellular internalization and nuclear addressing of a small exogenous peptide. *J Cell Sci* 1992; 101: 717-22.
2. Schutze-Redelmeier MP, Gournier H, Garcia-Pons F, Moussa M, Joliot AH, Volovitch M, Prochiantz A, Lemonnier FA. Introduction of exogenous antigens into the MHC class I processing and presentation pathway by Drosophila Antennapedia homeodomain primes cytotoxic T cells *in vivo*. *J Immunol* 1996; 157: 650-5.
3. Derossi D, Joliot A, Chassaing G, and Prochiantz A. The third helix of the Antennapedia homeodomain translocates through biological membranes. *J Biol Chem* 1994; 269: 10444-50.

A strategy for prediction of peptide binding affinities for the human transporter associated with antigen processing

S. Daniel[1], J. Hammer[2], F. Gallazzi[2], F. Sinigaglia[2], S. Caillat-Zucman[1], P.M. van Endert[1]

1 INSERM U25, Hôpital Necker, 161, rue de Sèvres, 75743 Paris Cedex 15, France
2 Roche Milano Richerche, 58 Via Olgettina, 20132 Milan, Italy

Identification of peptide epitopes presented by HLA class I proteins to cytotoxic CD8+ T cells has been greatly facilitated by a growing inventory of "peptide binding motifs" which allow a limited prediction of peptides binding to individual HLA class I alleles based on the residues in specific anchor positions [1]. However, the power of these predictions is not only limited by little understood inhibitory effects on HLA binding of residues in non-anchor positions, but also suffers from the fact that only a minority of high affinity peptides are antigenic, *i.e.* found to be efficiently presented by cells expressing the protein they are derived from [2]. The latter phenomenon is presumably due to selective intracellular processing of protein antigens entailing inefficient generation of many potential epitopes to HLA class I molecules. Next to selective cleavage of proteins by the cytosolic proteasome complex, selective translocation of antigenic peptides into the ER by the TAP complex may be a prime cause for selective intracellular antigen processing for HLA class I proteins [3].
Investigation of the effects of an allelic polymorphism in the rat TAP2 protein has provided convincing evidence that the selectivity of the TAP complex *can* have profound effects on the nature of epitopes presented by HLA class I proteins. In this example, inefficient transport of peptide substrates with C-terminal basic residues leads to delayed assembly of a rat class I allele using such C-terminals as "anchors" with peptides frequently carrying unusual (*i.e.* other than basic) residues at the C-terminus [4]. In the case of the functionally monomorphic human TAP complex, formal proof for an epitope selection by the transporter has not yet been reported. Peptide transport assays involving ER-restricted glycosylation of peptide substrates with different C-terminals did not provide evidence for selective peptide translocation [5]. However, the employed assay measures end point accumulation of glycosylated substrates in the ER and is likely to possess low sensitivity. Using a sensitive alternative technique measuring direct binding of peptides to TAP complexes [6], we have been able to establish a peptide binding motif for the human TAP complex that is based mainly on favorable and unfavorable effects on TAP affinity of the residues in the N- and C-terminal positions of short peptides [7].
We have now undertaken a systematic analysis of the effects of substitutions in 9-mer peptides on TAP binding affinity. The results of this analysis allow us to predict TAP binding affinities of 9-mer peptides with satisfactory precision, thereby enabling us to probe large numbers of natural HLA class I ligands or peptides with known HLA class I binding affinities for their transporter affinity and to establish the role of the human TAP complex in epitope selection.

Effects of substitutions in a 9-mer poly-Ala peptide on TAP affinity

We synthesized a library of 171 peptides comprising substitutions of each position in the sequence Ala-Ala-Ala-Ser-Ala-Ala-Ala-Ala-Tyr by 19 natural amino acids (except cysteine for reasons of synthesis). We chose a starting sequence including Tyr at position 9 (P9) to confer medium to high affinity, and Ser at P4 to increase solubility. Peptides were synthesized on a multiple peptide synthesizer and routinely possessed at least 70% and in most cases more than 80% purity, as assessed by HPLC analysis. Peptide binding affinities for the human TAP complex were measured as described [6]. Briefly, Sf9 insect cell microsomes over-expressing human TAP1/2 complexes were incubated at 4°C with 25 pMol of iodinated reporter peptide R-9-L (Arg-Arg-Tyr-Asn-

Table I.

Residue	*P1*	*P2*	*P3*	*P4*	*P5*	*P6*	*P7*	*P8*	*P9*
Ala	1	1	1	1.3	1	1	1	1	78
Gly	11.2	11.9	16.6	2.3	4.2	0.64	18.9	0.3	600
Ser	6.6	0.76	0.56	1	1.4	2.2	2.3	0.3	3000
Leu	12.8	0.41	0.58	1.0	0.4	1.4	0.63	0.86	24.3
Tyr	20.8	0.76	0.08	0.42	0.45	3.0	0.23	1.2	1
Arg	1.8	0.52	0.5	0.3	0.78	0.46	1.0	1.3	7.5
Asp	104	21.4	15.4	0.69	1.7	1.4	6.8	1	828
Pro	72.2	160	0.8	0.45	0.4	1.3	0.2	0.78	52.2

Ala-Ser-Thr-Glu-Leu) and an increasing molar excess of unlabeled competitor peptides. Microsomes were immediately centrifuged, washed once and reporter peptide bound to TAP complexes was counted. As a correlate of peptide affinity for TAP, normalized molar excess of competitor required for 50% inhibition of binding of reporter peptide (IC50) was determined.
IC50s for selected substitutions in the poly-Ala peptide normalized with reference to the IC50 of unsubstituted competitor peptide are shown in the *Table I*.
Several conclusions can be drawn from the shown data: firstly, strong favorable as well as unfavorable effects on binding affinity are observed. Secondly, major effects are restricted to substitutions in specific positions, namely P1, P2, P3 and P9, while replacements in other positions (for example P4) have little effect. Thus, binding affinity depends mainly on the residues in the C- and N-terminal positions. Finally, most amino acids have different effects depending on their position. For example, aromatic hydrophobic residues increase affinity in P2, P3 and P9 while being deleterious in P1. Pro has strong or moderate unfavorable effects in P1 and P2 or in P9 , but affects affinity not at all when present in P3. Acidic residues reduce binding affinity when present in any of the important positions, while only Arg is favorable for binding in any position.

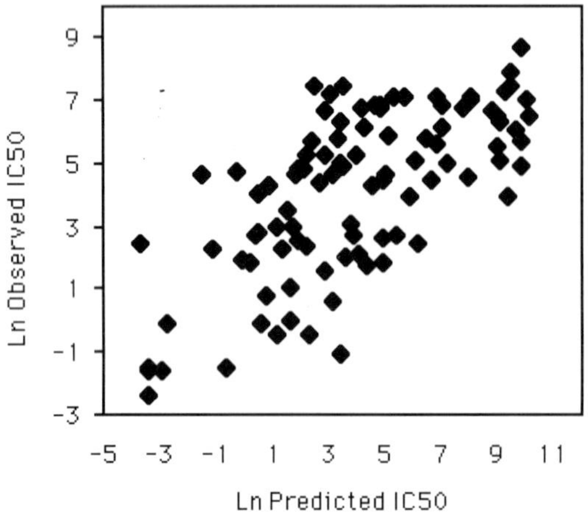

Figure 1. Observed and predicted IC50s for 100 random sequence peptides.

Prediction of TAP binding affinities of random peptides

To find out whether these effects can be observed in any 9-mer peptide, we transformed the observed IC50s to logarithms to generate a matrix allowing prediction of binding affinity (*i.e.* IC50) of 9-mer peptides based on addition of logarithmic values for the amino acids in each position. We then tested performance of matrix-based IC50 predictions by measuring TAP binding of 100 peptides with computer-generated random sequences. A comparison of predicted and observed IC50s is shown in the *Figure 1*.
Predicted IC50 values correlated significantly with observed values. At an overall correlation of r=0.7 between observed and predicted affinities, predictive performance was slightly better for high affinity peptides (Aroc=0.90) than for medium (Aroc=0.85) or low affinity (Aroc=0.84) peptides. Thus, for the large majority of 9-mer peptides with highly variable sequences, binding affinity could be predicted based on the effects of amino acid substitutions observed in the poly-Ala peptide. These effects therefore appear to be largely independent of sequence context.
Using the described strategy and a parallel neural net approach with a higher performance (N. Petrovsky, V. Brusiç and P.M.van Endert, unpublished), we have now

started to analyze TAP affinities of large numbers of data base-retrieved peptides binding to various HLA class I alleles or eluted from them. The results of this analysis are in accordance with direct measurements of TAP affinities of 80 natural ligands of various HLA class I alleles (unpublished) and provide overwhelming evidence that the extent of coordination between the ligand preferences of HLA class I molecules and the TAP complex varies strongly according to the class I alleles. Most or all peptides binding to some alleles, such as B27, Cw07 or A31 possess high transporter affinities, while other class I alleles (A2, B40, B7) bind peptide ligands with moderate to low affinities. Further analysis will show whether naturally processed (*i.e.* HLA protein-eluted) peptides display higher TAP affinities than control peptides with comparable binding affinities for the respective HLA class I alleles.

References

1. Rammensee HG, Friede T, Stefanoviç S. MHC ligands and peptide binding motifs: first listing. *Immunogenetics* 1995; 41: 178-228.
2. Sette A, Vitiello A, *et al.* The relationship between class I binding affinity and immunogenicity of potential cytotoxic T cell epitopes. *J Immunol* 1994; 153: 5586-92.
3. Germain RN. MHC-dependent antigen processing and peptide presentation: providing ligands for T lymphocyte activation. *Cell* 1994; 76: 287-99.
4. Powis SJ, Young LL, *et al.* The rat *cim* effect: TAP allele-dependent changes in a MHC class I anchor motif and evidence against C-terminal trimming of peptides in the *ER. Immunity* 1996; 4: 159-66.
5. Momburg F, Roelse J, Howard JC, Butcher GW, Hämmerling GJ, Neefjes JJ. Selectivity of MHC-encoded peptide transporters from human, mouse and rat. *Nature* 1994; 367: 648-51.
6. Van Endert PM, Tampé R, Meyer TH, Tisch R, Bach JF, McDevitt HO. A sequential model for peptide binding and transport by the transporters associated with antigen processing. *Immunity* 1994; 1: 491-500.
7. Van Endert PM, Riganelli D, Greco G, Fleischhauer K, Sidney J, Sette A, Bach JF. The peptide-binding motif for the human transporter associated with antigen processing. *J Exp Med* 1995; 182: 1883-95.

Substrate specificity of TAP peptide transporters

F. Momburg, J.O. Koopmann, E.A. Armandola, M. Post, G.J. Hämmerling

German Cancer Research Center, Department of Molecular Immunology, Im Neuenheimer Feld 280, D-69120, Heidelberg, Germany

MHC class I molecules are mostly loaded with antigenic peptides originating from proteins expressed in the cytoplasm. The peptide fragments are likely to be generated by the proteasome, a large, barrel-shaped complex of cytosolic proteases with multiple cleavage specificities. In order to associate with the peptide binding groove of class I molecules, the peptides need to be translocated across the membrane of the endoplasmic reticulum (ER). This function is carried out by the transporter associated with antigen processing (TAP) (reviewed in [1]).

TAP belongs to an evolutionary conserved family of ATP-binding cassette (ABC) transporters that specifically translocate through membranes a variety of substrates possessing a wide range of chemical properties and masses. In TAP molecules, the common four-domain structure of ABC transporters is organized in two noncovalently associated subunits, TAP1 and TAP2, each consisting of a hydrophobic domain predicted to span the ER membrane 6-10 times, and a hydrophilic domain extending into the cytoplasm. The C-terminal cytoplasmic domain contains the nucleotide binding site. Usually, the presence of both TAP subunits is required for class I loading and subsequent antigen presentation suggesting that the peptide transporter functions as a heterodimer. The *Tap1* and *Tap2* genes have been mapped to the class II region of the MHC and are inducible by interferon-γ (reviewed in [1]).

Radio-iodinated peptides containing an NXT glycosylation signal are accessible to the peptide transporter when incubated with cells that are permeabilized at the plasma membrane with streptolysin O. Using this in vitro translocation assay we have previously shown that TAP-mediated peptide translocation into the ER is dependent on the hydrolysis of ATP [2].

To analyze the influence of the peptide sequence we used various series of glycosylatable model peptides that were substituted either at the C-terminal residue, at internal positions, or at the N-terminal residue. Translocation of these peptides was studied with cells expressing rat, mouse or human TAP1/2. In the rat, allelic forms of TAP2 exist that fall into two functional groups (TAP2-A and TAP2-B) characterized by differential loading of class I molecules with antigenic peptides (reviewed in [1]). We and others have shown that rat transporters of the A and B type differ in their specificity for synthetic peptide substrates [3, 4]. Rat (r) TAP1/2^{u} and other rTAP1/2-B transporters preferentially translocate peptides containing hydrophobic C-terminal residues, while rTAP1/2^{a} and other rTAP1/2-A transporters also translocate peptides with polar or charged C-terminal amino acids. The specificity of mouse TAP is similar to the restricted transport pattern of rTAP1/2^{u}, and the nonselective phenotype of rTAP1/2^{a} is shared by human TAP [3]. An influence on the efficiency of translocation, but no species- or allele-specific differences, were found when substitutions at other positions within the peptide sequence were analyzed [5]. In contrast to the functionally relevant polymorphism of rat TAP2, the rather limited sequence polymorphism described for allelic variants of human or mouse TAP subunits does not significantly alter peptide transport specifities.

To analyze which of the 25 polymorphic residues determine the different transport patterns of rTAP2^{a} and rTAP2^{u} (703 a.a.), hybrid molecules were constructed [6]. By using 5 restriction sites shared between TAP2^{a} and rat TAP2^{u} cDNAs, 14 rTAP2$^{a/u}$ hybrids were generated in which a single swap segment or combinations of the resulting segments (I through VI) were exchanged in a criss-cross fashion. The chimeric rTAP2 molecules were co-expressed with rTAP1 in TAP-deficient T2 cells and tested for their transport specificities with peptides varied at the C-terminal residue (RYWANATRSX or TVDNKTRYX). The polymorphic residues 374 and 380 contained in segment V were found to control the transport of small, polar and charged C-terminal residues. Introduction of segment V^a into the u environment converted the selective peptide transport of rat $TAP1/2^u$ into a nonselective. The residues 217/218 present in segment II additionally influenced the transport of basic C-terminal residues. Introduction of II^a into $TAP2^u$ molecule strongly enhanced transport of peptides with C-terminal Arg or His while in the inverse hybrid, the acceptance of basic C-terminal residues was reduced. A contribution of polymorphic TAP2 residues in fragments III and VI was noted, but appeared to be minor [6].

In accord with these findings, a single point mutation in hTAP2 (374 A→D) significantly reduced the transport of RYWANATRSX peptides with small and polar C-terminal residues in comparison with wild-type hTAP2 [7]. Based on computer-assisted predictions of the location of membrane-spanning segments in TAP2 it can be assumed that the two pairs of residues identified as being important for TAP specificity are located in cytoplasmic loops close to the membrane [6].

To assess the relative contribution of TAP1 and TAP2 subunits to transport specificity, TAP subunits of rat, mouse (m), or human (h) origin were co-expressed in T2 cells, or in Sf9 insect cells after infection with recombinant baculoviruses. The transport specificity with regard to C-terminal peptide residues was found to be mainly influenced by TAP2, but TAP1 can also contribute, *e.g.*, the interspecies hybrid mTAP1/hTAP2 showed a restricted transport pattern in contrast to the permissive hTAP1/2 transporter [7]. Crosslinking studies with photoactivatable peptides have clearly demonstrated that both the TAP1 and the TAP2 half-transporters are involved in the binding site for peptide. Interestingly, the region of TAP1 that was labelled with photoconjugates encompassed the residues corresponding to #374/#380 on the TAP2 chain [8].

Class I molecules are usually loaded with peptides of 8-11 amino acids, but as an exception to this rule, a few class I molecules, *e.g.* HLA-B27, have been reported to bind much longer peptides. To address the question of length selection by TAP we studied the transport of peptides with the tyrosine residue for radio-iodination at one end and the glycosylation signal at the other [9]. Because loss of one of the tagged extremities will render the peptide undetectable in the translocation/ glycosylation assay, this approach circumvents the problem that long peptides can undergo partial degradation by proteases associated with permeabilized cells (or microsomes) while remaining ligands for TAP. Three sets of individual peptides or partially randomized peptide libraries ranging between 6 and 40 residues were employed. For three different transporters, $rTAP2^a$, $rTAP2^u$ and hTAP, the most efficient was observed for peptides with 8–12 amino acids. 6-mers and longer peptides of up to 40 amino acids were also translocated, albeit less efficiently. For two of the three sets of length variants analyzed, $rTAP1/2^a$ showed a less stringent length selection than $rTAP1/2^u$ and hTAP. We carefully controlled that the superior transport of the 10-mer of the TNKT..Y series was not due to faster degradation or less efficient glycosylation of shorter or longer length variants.

Additionally, microsomes derived from $T2.rTAP1/2^a$ cells were used to monitor peptide binding at 4°C in the absence of ATP [10]. A high binding affinity for the radiolabelled 10-mer (K_D = 580 nM) was found followed by the TNKT..Y 14-mer with 1300 nM, while other length variants were clearly inferior [9]. Thus, TAP binds and translocates preferentially peptides with a length suitable for binding to MHC class I molecules, but peptides that are considerably longer may also be substrates. About 10^5 peptide binding sites per cell equivalent of $T2.rTAP1/2^a$ microsomes were determined providing an estimate for the number of TAP complexes in the ER membrane.

Using TAP-containing microsomes in a modified transport assay, we have recently begun to analyze the kinetics of TAP-mediated peptide translocation. V_{max} and K_m values were determined for a variety of iodinated peptides including glycosylatable peptides and natural class I-binding peptides. In agreement with the affinity constants obtained in the above mentioned binding assay, K_m values for transport ranged between 0.4 and 20 μM. Remarkably, some of the class I binding peptides, *e.g.* the B27 peptide RRYQKSTEL, the D^d peptide KGPDKGNEY, or the K^d peptide TYQRTRALV, were among the most efficiently transported peptides, as indicated by V_{max} values > 10 pmol/min x µg microsomal protein. Furthermore, we have analyzed the kinetic values for the co-substrate ATP, as well as for GTP, CTP and UTP which might also serve as substrates. ATP was with K_m = 200 µM the best substrate, followed by CTP (310 µM), GTP (890 µM) and UTP (2970 µM). Since GTP is present in the cytosol at high concentrations similar to ATP (~1 mM), *in vivo* this nucleotide may be utilized by TAP to some extent in addition to ATP.

References

1. Heemels MT, Ploegh H. Generation, translocation, and presentation of MHC class I-restricted peptides. *Annu Rev Biochem* 1995; 64: 463-91.
2. Neefjes JJ, Momburg F, Hämmerling GJ. Selective and ATP-dependent translocation of peptides by the MHC-encoded transporter. *Science* 1993; 26 : 769-71.
3. Momburg F, Roelse J, Howard JC, Butcher GW, Hämmerling GJ, Neefjes JJ. Selectivity of MHC-encoded peptide transporters from human, mouse and rat. *Nature* 1994; 367: 648-51.
4 Heemels MT, Schumacher TNM, Wonigeit K, Ploegh HL. Peptide translocation by variants of the transporter associated with antigen processing. *Science* 1993; 262: 2059-63.
5. Neefjes JJ, Gottfried E, Roelse J, Grommé M, Obst R, Hämmerling GJ, Momburg F. Analysis of the fine specificity of rat, mouse and human TAP peptide transporters. *Eur J Immunol* 1995; 25: 1133-6.
6. Momburg F, Armandola EA, Post M, Hämmerling GJ. Residues in TAP2 peptide transporters controlling substrate specificity. *J Immunol* 1996; 156: 1756-63.
7. Armandola EA, Momburg F, Nijenhuis M, Bulbuc N, Früh K, Hämmerling GJ. A point mutation in the human transporter associated with antigen processing (TAP2) alters the peptide transport specificity. *Eur J Immunol* 1996; 26: 1748-55.
8. Nijenhuis M, Schmitt S, Armandola EA, Obst R, Brunner J, Hämmerling GJ. Identification of a contact region for peptide on the TAP1 chain of the transporter associated with antigen processing. *J Immunol* 1996; 156: 2186-95.
9. Koopmann J-O, Post M, Neefjes JJ, Hämmerling GJ, Momburg F. Translocation of long peptides by transporters associated with antigen processing (TAP). *Eur J Immunol* 1996; 26: 1720-8.
9. Van Endert PM, Tampé R, Meyer TH, Tisch R, Bach JF, McDevitt HO. A sequential model for peptide binding and transport by the transporters associated with antigen processing. *Immunity* 1994; 1: 491-500.

HLA class II superdimers are expressed by B lymphocytes and monocytes

C. Roucard, M.L. Ericson, F. Garban, N.A. Mooney, D.J. Charron

INSERM U396, 15, rue de l'École de Médecine, 75006 Paris, France

The surprising finding made by Brown *et al.* that HLA class II molecules of the DR isotype can self-associate as parallel double-dimers in crystals [1] may have important implications for the understanding of T cell antigen recognition. Activation of the CD4+ helper T cells is a key-event in the cellular immune response. It can be imagined that a double-dimer, or superdimer, of αβ class II molecules could crosslink two T cell receptor molecules. The increased avidity of the interaction would be likely to translate into an enhanced activation signal in the T cell and perhaps also in the antigen-presenting cell (APC) [2]. The CD4 costimulatory molecule on the T cell membrane interacts both with the T cell receptor and with the class II molecule on the APC. Since CD4 appears to have a bivalent mode of binding to the class II molecule it could further stabilize such multi-protein aggregates by cross-linkage [2]. A hypothetical formation of large, symmetrical lattices of aggregated molecules is also compatible with available structural data [3].

Recently [4], a 120 kDa form of MHC class II molecules was detected on murine splenocytes. It was suggested that the 120 kDa species represented class II superdimers and that these may be involved in low affinity T cell interactions. We have provided evidence in a previous study for $(\alpha\beta)_2$ superdimers on cord blood B cells [5] and we here present evidence for $(\alpha\beta)_2$ superdimers on B cells and monocytes from adult peripheral blood and on the human lymphoblastoid B cell line Raji.

Results

We have studied the HLA-DR molecules expressed on different types of APC (freshly isolated B cells and monocytes from human peripheral blood and immortalized Raji B cells) by use of monoclonal antibodies (mAbs) recognizing different structural determinants of DR molecules. By labelling cell surface molecules with a ^{35}S sulphur reagent, followed by immunoprecipitation of the DR molecules with the D1.12 mAb, we identified a new HLA class II 120 kDa species. The 120 kDa form was present on both monocytes and B cells indicating that it was not cell type specific (data not shown). This molecule, that we believe represents a superdimer $(\alpha\beta)_2$, is stable in SDS at room temperature indicating that it is stably loaded with peptide antigens [6]. The $(\alpha\beta)_2$ dissociates into 60 kDa αβ complexes at 50°C and into monomers at 100°C proving that the 120 kDa form does not result from an association of αβ complexes with other cellular proteins. The D1.12 mAb recognizes an epitope of the DRα chain located near the peptide binding site [7]. According to the crystallographic structure this epitope is exposed on the surface of the superdimer and should indeed be available for antibody-binding.

By *in vivo* labelling of the cells and subsequent immunoprecipitation with D1.12, we obtained a similar electrophoretic migration pattern *(figure 1)*. When using the 2.06 mAb however the result was different: mature and SDS-resistant αβ dimers (50-60 kDa) were observed as well as immature and SDS-unstable αβIi complexes migrating as separate monomers. No 120 kDa molecules could be precipitated with the 2.06 mAb (data not shown). The antigenic determinant of this mAb is believed to be located on a monomorphic portion of the DRβ [8], and we hypothesize that the binding site for 2.06 is not available for antibody-binding in the $(\alpha\beta)_2$ structure. In conclusion, these two mAbs permitted us to distinguish two different conformations of SDS-stable HLA-DR molecules.

In a pulse-chase experiment with Raji cells, the superdimers were first detected after 1h of chase concomitant

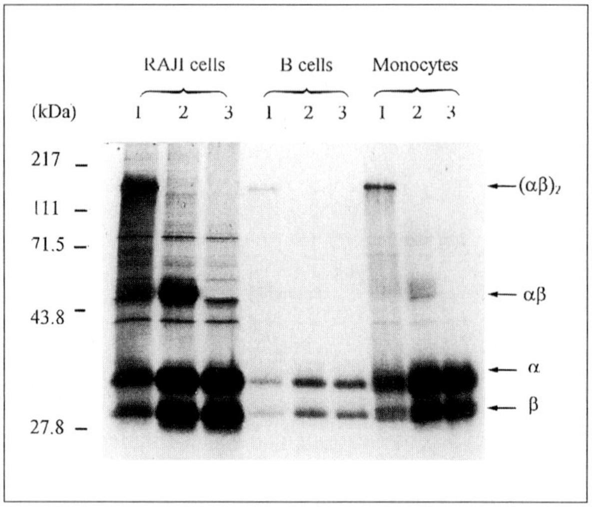

Figure 1. Raji cells, B cells and monocytes express superdimers. B cells, monocytes (freshly purified from peripheral blood) and Raji cells were pulse-labelled with [^{35}S] methionine and [^{35}S] cysteine for 30 minutes and chased for 4h at 37°C. HLA-DR molecules were immunoprecipitated with D1.12 mAb. Each sample was divided in three aliquots and incubated in reducing SDS sample buffer for 30 minutes at 20°C (lane 1) or at 50°C (lane 2), or boiled for 5 minutes (lane 3), and loaded on a 10% SDS-polyacrylamide gel. After electrophoresis, the gel was dried and autoradiographed.

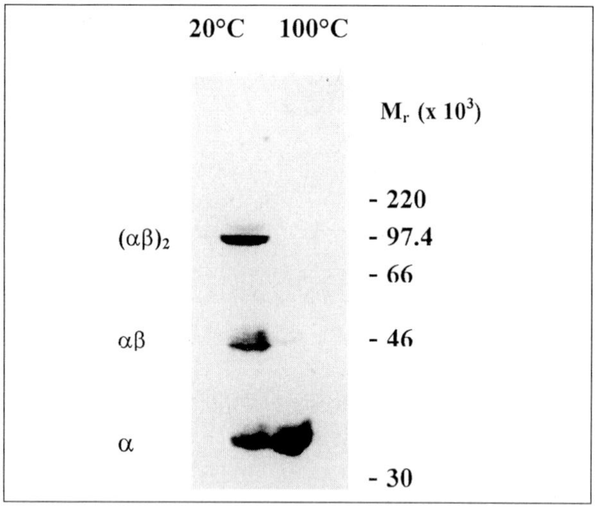

Figure 2. Western-blot analysis of Raji B cell HLA-DR molecules. Raji cells were lysed in a 0,1% Triton X-100 lysis buffer on ice for 30 min. Lysates were cleared of debris by a 10,000 x *g* centrifugation at 4°C. Samples were incubated in reducing SDS-sample buffer at 20°C for 30 min or boiled for 10 min, and loaded on a 10% SDS-polyacrylamide gel. Proteins were transferred to a nitrocellulose membrane and HLA-DRα chains were revealed with the DA6.147 mAb and by electrochemiluminescence. HLA class II dimers (αβ), superdimers $(\alpha\beta)_2$ and the α-chains are denoted.

with the appearance of the p22 proteolytic fragment of the invariant chain Ii (data not shown). Degradation of the Ii chain precedes peptide-loading and migration to the cell surface. This indicates that $(\alpha\beta)_2$ are formed intracellularly before cell surface expression and interaction with TCR on CD4+ T cells. They are probably formed in a post-Golgi compartment as indicated by the glycosylation pattern and resistance to endoglycosidase H digestion [9].

A general objection that can be raised to the immunoprecipitation procedure is that an aberrant electrophoretic behaviour of precipitated protein (due to non-dissociated antibody) can not be formally excluded. We addressed this problem by using a different approach to detect MHC superdimers in a human EBV-transformed B cell line, Raji. Cells were lysed in 0.1% Triton X-100 on ice and cellular debris were eliminated by centrifugation. Lysates were incubated 30 minutes at room temperature in a reducing SDS-sample buffer or boiled for 10 minutes and then subjected to SDS-polyacrylamide gel electrophoresis. Electrophoretically separated proteins were transferred to a nitrocellulose membrane by Western-blotting and we then used the DA6.147 mAb to detect the human class II DRα chain. Stably peptide-loaded MHC class II molecules that are refractory to denaturation by SDS at room temperature and therefore migrate as 50-60 kDa αβ dimers [6] can be seen in *Figure 2* (20°C). However, a higher molecular weight species of 100-120 kDa is also readily detectable. The molecular weight corresponds to the superdimer previously observed. When boiled, both forms dissociate into free α- and β- chains.

Conclusion

We have identified a dimer of MHC class II heterodimers or "superdimers" on human antigen presenting cells from adult peripheral blood. We propose that the superdimers form intracellularly in a post-Golgi compartment before being transported to cell surface. The superdimers may play an important role during the interaction between the HLA class II molecules and the TCR, leading to cellular activation. The presence of superdimers (that could interact with two CD4 molecules) and the capability of CD4 to form oligomers or tetramers [3] may theoretically permit the formation of a lattice composed of multiple complexes of CD4/MHC class II molecule/TCR. This lattice would result in a cross-linking of the TCR essential for the T cell activation and may also be of importance for intracellular signals in the APC. An obvious question that remains to be answered is whether the $(\alpha\beta)_2$ superdimers present two different or two identical peptides. It seems reasonable to assume that the superdimer has to present two identical peptides in order to elicit a strong T cell response.

During infection, B cells and monocytes presumably accumulate large amounts of antigens internalized *via* antigen receptors (surface immunoglobulins and Fc receptors). These antigens will be degraded and concentrated in the MIIC (MHC class II compartment) [10] where they will bind to class II molecules. The probability, under these circumstances, of having two identical peptides on the two αβ subunits in a superdimer will perhaps be sufficient to elicit an immune response *via* the HLA class II superdimers.

References

1. Brown JH, Jardetzky TS, Gorga JC, Stern LJ, Urban RG, Strominger JL, Wiley DC. Three-dimensional structure of the human class II histocompatibility antigen HLA-DR1. *Nature* 1993; 364: 33-9.
2. Germain RN. Seeing double. *Curr Biol* 1993; 3: 586-9.
3. Sakihama T, Smolyar A, Reinherz EL. Molecular recognition of antigen involves lattice formation between CD4, MHC class II and TCR. *Immunol Today* 1995; 16: 581-7.
4. Schafer PH, Pierce SK. Evidence for dimers of MHC class II molecules in B lymphocytes and their role in low affinity T cell responses. *Immunity* 1994; 1: 699-707.
5. Garban F, Ericson M, Roucard C, Rabian-Herzog C, Teisserenc H, Sauvanet E, Charron D, Mooney N. Detection of empty HLA class II molecules on cord blood B cells. *Blood* 1996; 87: 3970-6.
6. Sadegh-Nasseri S, Germain RN. A role for peptide in determining MHC class II structure. *Nature* 1991; 353: 167-70.
7. Fu XT, Karr RW. HLA-DRα chain residues located on the outer loops are involved in nonpolymorphic and polymorphic antibody-binding epitopes. *Hum Immunol* 1994; 39: 253-60.
8. Charron DJ, McDevitt HO. Analysis of HLA-D region-associated molecules with monoclonal antibody. *Proc Natl Acad Sci USA* 1979; 76: 6567-71.
9. Roucard C, Garban F, Mooney NA, Charron DJ, Ericson ML. Conformation of human leucocyte antigen class II molecules, evidence for superdimers and empty molecules on human antigen presenting cells. *J Biol Chem* 1996; 273: 12993-4000.
10. Peters PJ, Neefjes JJ, Oorschot V, Ploegh HL, Geuze HJ. Segregation of MHC class II molecules from MHC class I molecules in the Golgi complex for transport to lysosomal compartments. *Nature* 1991; 349: 669-76.

In vivo single particle imaging reveals the formation of cell surface HLA-DR dimer of dimers

K.M. Wilson, I.E.G. Morrison, R.J. Cherry, N. Fernandez

Department of Biological and Chemical Sciences, Central Campus, University of Essex, Wivenhoe Park, Colchester CO4 3SQ, Essex, UK

The factors controlling the organization of MHC immunoreceptors at the cell surface of living antigen presenting cells have not yet been fully elucidated. It is likely that class II are displayed in 'functional domains' comprising more than one pair of heterodimers. The molecules must therefore have the capacity to 'redistribute' under the influence of constraints imposed by the cytoskeleton and the modulatory activity exerted upon receptor-density by, for example cytokines. Fully assembled MHC class II molecules consist of single alpha and beta heterodimers bound to a short peptide. This complex is anchored to the cell surface *via* the transmembrane domain of both the alpha and beta chains of the class II dimers. Because of the lipid environment and the fluidity of the membrane the molecules can potentially undergo mobility (lateral diffusion) and clustering (*ie.*, dimerization of heterodimers). At the cell surface the peptide/class II structure becomes a ligand for reactive T cells to form a tetrameric structure. It follows that class II receptor recruitment in an optimal conformation must be critical for T cell activation.

We have been interested in setting up a system that would allow us to study the behaviour (mobility and receptor clustering) of MHC at the cell-surface on single living cells and eventually relate this to the function of class II mediated responses. For this purpose, a molecular probe and a single particle imaging system for living cells based on a cooled slow-scan coupled charged device (CCD) digital camera was developed. The main property of the system is that it allows nanometer-scale resolution of receptors on single cells under culture conditions and thus, in essence, permits the study of receptors in their native configuration. The system obviates the use of biochemical extraction procedures such as the use of non-ionic or zwitterionic detergents that disrupt the cell membrane and hence affect protein-protein interactions.

The molecular probe we have produced consists of R-phycoerythrin (PE), a small size, high yield fluorescent protein isolated from cyanobacteria and eukaryotic algae which can be coupled to intact IgG or Fab fragments of a monoclonal antibody [1]. We have succeeded in coupling PE in a 1:1 molar ratio to Fab fragments derived from a monoclonal-antibody specific for HLA-DR monomorphic epitopes without affecting the specificity of the antibody for its target epitope. Coupling Fab fragments to PE reduces the overall size of the probe compared to IgG and obviates crosslinking by the presence of intact IgG which may otherwise occur. The probe is then used to bind cells expressing the specific antigen reactive with the monoclonal antibody. During the imaging analysis the cells are kept under culture conditions and subjected to analysis under the microscope in a technique called single particle imaging. This technique can be used for both mobility analysis [2] and clustering analysis to determine, for example receptor self-associations [3].

In order to calibrate the imaging detection system and obtain a measure of the intensity of single PE-Fab particles, an aliquot of PE-Fab was loaded onto a microculture poly-L-lysine slide, without cells, and then imaged using the CCD camera. A representative example of this type of image is shown in *Figure 1A*. As expected the image shows a constellation of spots of similar size and intensity. The particles appear as diffraction limited spots covering a number of pixels; their approximate positions are identified by a simple image analysis algorithm and then quantified by least-squares fitting the pixels in this immediate area with a 2-dimensional Gaussian function. This fit procedure gives values for the spot widths, which can be used for artefact rejection (only spots near to the diffraction limited width are accepted, and spots with large deviations in the width or high residual variance values are rejected) and

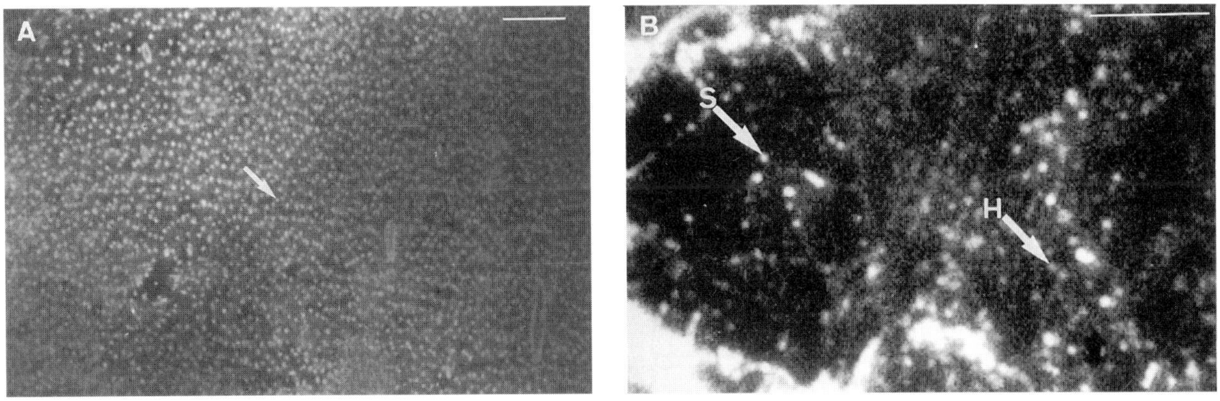

Figure 1. Single particle imaging of: (A) PE-Fab particles (arrowed) bound to a control poly-L-lysine coated microscope slide and (B) PE-Fab bound to HLA-DR molecules on a fibroblast cell co-transfected with HLA-DR α and β chains and the invariant chain. HLA-DR heterodimers (H) can be distinguished from HLA-DR dimers of dimers (S) by comparision of the relative fluorescent intensities. The scale bar represents 10 μm.

spot intensity above local background [3]. This allows the intensity distribution of single PE-Fab particles to be obtained. *Figure 2A* shows that the peak fluorecence intensity of a single PE-Fab particle was approximately 25 counts above local background. In principle, PE particles should have uniform intensity; the observed distribution width is probably caused by a combination of detector non-uniformity and focal imperfections (both considerably small) and photon-counting effects -*i.e.* a measure of the probability of emitted photons entering the detection optics of the system.

We then used the PE-Fab probe to determine the aggregation state of cell surface HLA-DR molecules. For these experiments, we utilised a transfected fibroblast cell line kindly supplied to us by professor R. Lechler. The cell line designated M1DR1/Ii has large, approximately flat areas that facilitate optical imaging and real-time analysis. The untransfected M1DR1/Ii fibroblast is devoid of detectable HLA class II expression. This phenotype was reversed by co-transfection of exogenous HLA-DR A and HLA-DR B genes and the invariant chain gene. Upon transfection M1DR1/Ii synthesize fully assembled HLA class II heterodimers at the cell surface [4]. *Figure 1B* shows a typical example of the images obtained for PE-Fab bound to M1DR1/Ii cells maintained at 22 °C. The image shows significant differences from that shown in *Figure 1A*. The fluorescent spots in *Figure 1B* show a large variation in intensity and a significant number of fluorescent patches which may correspond to large clusters. All the fluorescent spots in the images from these experiments were analysed in an identical manner to those for control poly-L-lysine slides and the total spot intensity distribution for PE-Fab bound to M1DR1/Ii cells at 22°C obtained. *Figure 2B-C* shows that the peak fluorescence intensity of PE-Fab bound to cells at 22°C was approximately 30 counts above local background. This peak intensity corresponds well to that found for PE-Fab bound to control poly-L-lysine slides and therefore represents the PE-Fab bound to single HLA-DR heterodimers. However, a significant secondary fluorescence intensity peak at approximately 60-70 counts above background was also present. This indicates the presence of a sizeable number of HLA-DR clusters at 22°C.

In order to test whether the state of aggregation of HLA-DR molecules at the cell surface is temperature-dependent we then used the PE-Fab HLA-DR probe to bind cells maintained at 37°C. These images were analysed in an identical manner to those for control poly-L-lysine slides and the total spot intensity distribution for PE-Fab bound to M1DR1/Ii cells at 37 °C obtained. *Figure 2D-E* shows that the peak fluorescence intensity of PE-Fab bound to cells at 37°C was approximately 25 counts above local background. This peak corresponds to PE-Fab bound to single HLA-DR heterodimers. However, a small secondary fluorescence intensity peak at approximately 60-70 counts above background was also present. This indicates the presence of a small proportion of HLA-DR clusters at 37 °C.

These data were further analysed by computer software which can deconvolve the distributions into 1, 2, and 3 particle components as previously described [3]. This

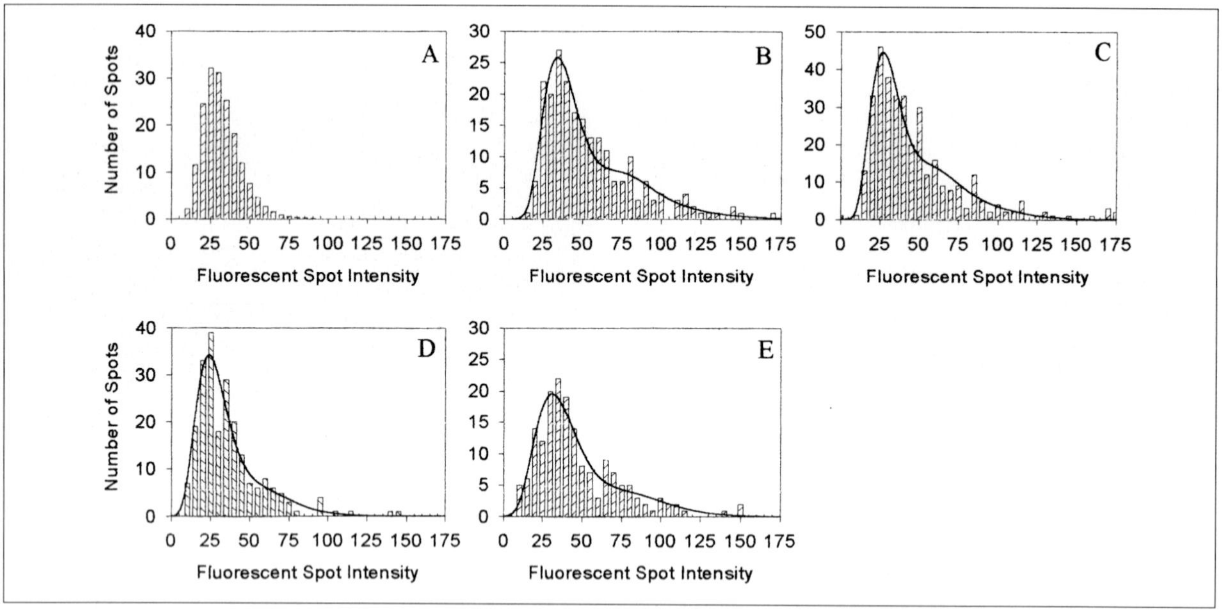

Figure 2. Fluorescence intensity distribution histograms obtained from images of: (A) PE-Fab bound to control poly-L-lysine coated sldes, (B-C) PE- Fab bound to HLA-DR molecules on fibroblast cells at 22 °C and (D-E) PE-Fab bound to HLA-DR molecules on fibroblast cells at 37 °C. The solid lines show the the 1-particle with 2-particle and 3-particle deconvolution, best fitted using the poly lysine slide distribution as the single particle function. This analysis allows the relative proportions of single HLA-DR heterodimers (1-particle contribution) and HLA-DR dimers of dimers (2-particle contribution) to be calculated.

enables the proportions of single HLA-DR heterodimers, dimers of heterodimers (dimer of dimers) and larger clusters to be calculated as shown in *Table I.* Approximately 25% of the total cell surface pool of HLA-DR molecules (spots) are configured as dimer of dimers at 22°C. However, at 37°C, the proportion of dimer of dimers falls to approximately 15% of the total HLA-DR detectable spots. These data suggest the existence of a temperature dependent equilibrium between individual heterodimers and dimers of dimers. However, more experiments are necessary to ascertain this issue.

The factors controlling the formation of dimers of dimers of MHC class II are at present unknown. In our experiments the HLA-DR dimer of dimers are unlikely to be formed as a result of the binding of the HLA-DR molecules with the fluorescent probe since Fab fragment was used, thus minimising the possibility of cross-linking. The existence of dimerised structures have been also postulated by Karjalainen (Basel) for the T cell receptor. In his model two TCR combining sites in the superdimer could be readily superimposed on the structure of dimerised peptide/ MHC class II molecules [5]. Our data support the notion that class II form dimer of dimers to enhance the stability of the reaction with the TCR molecules on responding T cells.

Table I. Percentage of cell surface HLA-DR single heterodimers, dimers of dimers and larger clusters at 22 °C and 37 °C

Cell Number	Temp. (°C)	No of spots	Percentage HLA-DR Heterodimers	Percentage HLA-DR Superdimers	Percentage larger clusters
Cell #1	22	220	71 ±4	25 ±3	3 ±3
Cell #2	22	340	70 ±4	25 ±3	4 ±3
Cell #3	22	270	64 ±4	30 ±3	6 ±3
Cell #4	22	143	95 ±2	5 ±4	2 ±3
Cell #5	37	161	82 ±5	18 ±3	0 ±3
Cell #6	37	217	85 ±15	15 ±3	0 ±3

An obvious question is whether the formation of HLA-DR dimer of dimers [6] preceeds the ligation of the T cell receptor and the accessory molecule CD4. It is possible that dimer of dimers assemble as such after insertion into the cell membrane since its fluidity would facilitate the mobility and physical redistribution of the class II molecules withing the lipid bilayer. This process could, however, be slowed or even abolished by restrictions imposed by cytoskeletal restraints. It is also possible that some dimer of dimers can be formed in intracellular compartments (*eg.*, endoplasmic reticulum) or in the endosomes of an antigen presenting cell. A potential binding site for pairs of class II is the β_2 domain of HLA-DR, which is the binding site for the CD4 accessory molecule.

The physiological role of cell-surface dimer of dimers has not yet been documented. Such structures could increase in number on engagement of TCR and CD4. Data to support the notion that transmission of signals *via* HLA class II requires dimerisation and cross-linking has also been reported [7]. It is possible to envisage that a rapid increase in serially engaged class II dimer of dimers may result in a rapid crosslinking of T cell receptors on T cells, generating an amplified signalling in both the APC and responding T cell [8]. Thus, HLA class II dimer of dimers may have a role as an efficient mechanism for (a) amplifying TCR signal transduction and signal delivery and in turn (b) upregulating co-accessory receptor-ligand pairs required for antigen presentation.

In conclusion, we have developed an *in vivo* non-invasive single particle imaging approach that allows one to determine the state of aggregation of HLA-DR molecules in ther native configuration. The system is well suited for detailed molecular interactions at the cell surface of antigen presenting cells using similar molecular probes to the PE-Fab DR-specific probe used in this study.

Acknowledgements

This work was supported by BBSRC and the University of Essex Research Promotion Fund.

References

1. Smith PR, Wilson KM, Morrison IEG, Cherry RJ, Fernandez N. Imaging of individual cell surface mhc antigens using fluorescent particles. In: Fernandez N, Butcher G, eds. *MHC biochemistry and genetics*. Oxford: Oxford University Press, 1997 (in press).
2. Wilson KM, Morrison IEG, Smith PR, Fernandez N, Cherry R J. Single particle tracking of cell surface HLA-DR molecules using R-phycoerythrin labeled monoclonal antibodies and fluorescent digital imaging. *J Cell Sci* 1996; 109: 2101-9.
3. Morrison IEG, Anderson CM, Georgiou GN, Stevenson GVW, Cherry RJ. Analysis of receptor clustering on cell surfaces by imaging fluorescent particles. *Biophys J* 1994; 67: 1280-90.
4. Dodi A, Brett S, Nordeng T, Sidhu S, Batchelor RJ, Lombardi G, Bakke O, Lechler RI. The invariant chain inhibits presentation of endogenous antigens by a human fibroblasts cell line. *Eur J Immunol* 1994; 24: 1632-9.
5. Karjalainen K. TCR superdimer formation-prelude to T cell activation. *Basel: Institute for Immunology, Annual Report*, 1995: 38.
6. Roucard C, Garban F, Mooney NA, Charron DJ, Ericson ML. *J Biol Chem* 1996; 271: 13993-4000.
7. Brickghannam C, Mooney N, Charron D. Signal transduction in B lymphocytes. *Hum Immunol* 1991; 30: 202-7.
8. Germain RN. MHC dependent antigen and peptide presentation: providing ligands for T lymphocyte activation. *Cell* 1994; 76: 287-99.

Intracellular pathway of MHC class II molecules in human dendritic cells

C. Saudrais, D. Spehner[1], H. de la Salle[1], A. Bohbot[3], J.P. Cazenave[2], B. Goud, D. Hanau[1], J. Salamero

UMR 144 CNRS, Institut Curie, Laboratoire compartimentation et dynamique cellulaire, 75005 Paris, France
1 CJF INSERM 94-03, Laboratoire d'Histocompatibilité, and
2 INSERM U311, Etablissement de Transfusion Sanguine, 10, rue Spielmann, 67065 Strasbourg, France
3 Service d'Onco-Hématologie, Hôpital de Hautepierre, 67200 Strasbourg, France

Dendritic cells (DCs) are among the most potent antigen presenting cells [1]. They present exogenous antigenic peptides complexed with major histocompatibility class II (MHC-II) molecules to CD4+ T cells. α and β chains of the MHC-II molecules are cotranslationaly translocated into the endoplasmic reticulum were they associate with a third polypeptide, known as the invariant chain (Ii). After transport through the Golgi apparatus, αβIi complexes are directed toward the endocytic pathway. Following Ii degradation, free αβ dimers eventually bind antigenic peptides derived from exogenous proteins. The efficiency of DCs in MHC-II restricted antigen presentation, and the importance of MHC-II molecules transport led us to analyze the intracellular pathway of MHC-II molecules in human DCs.

It is now widely accepted that a combination of granulocyte/macrophage colony stimulating factor (GM-CSF) and interleukin 4 (IL4) provides the best conditions for the generation of cells with the characteristic phenotype and function of naive DCs from human monocytes [2]. As a starting material, we used highly purified human blood monocytes [3].

Biosynthesis and intracellular transport of αβIi complexes

Most studies concerning intracellular transport of MHC-II molecules have been performed in B cells [4]. We compared the fate of these molecules in a pulse chase experiment in BEBV, freshly isolated blood monocytes and DCs. Using a rabbit antiserum directed against the luminal domain of Ii, p33, p35 and p41 isoforms of Ii were detected in all cell types. The oligomerization of Ii isoforms with MHC-II molecules, as well as rapid degradation of Ii were also similar. On the other hand, the ratio of p41 versus p33 dramaticaly differs between BEBV (10%) or monocytes (14%), and naive dendritic cells where it reaches 50%.

Cell surface biotinylation over the time course of a pulse chase experiment was used to measure plasma membrane arrival of proteins. We verified that very small quantities of αβIi were transported to the cell surface in both fresh monocytes and BEBV [5]. In contrast, we showed here that a significant amount of newly synthesized αβIi complexes were rapidly and transiently expressed at the cell surface of DCs. Indeed, they reached the cell surface as rapidly as MHC-class I molecules, suggesting their direct transport from the trans golgi network to the plasma membrane of DCs. We also observed that all mature Ii isoforms reached the plasma membrane as αβIi complexes.

A new intracellular pathway for generation of αβ-peptide complexes

We then investigated the behaviour of the αβIi complexes transiently expressed at the plasma membrane of DCs. As a first indication, electron microscopy experiment coupled to immunogold detection showed that cell surface αβIi complexes were rapidly internalized into coated pits. They were detected in late endosomal or lysosomal structures enriched in MHC-II molecules after further internalisation.

We next asked whether these internalized αβIi complexes could be converted into free αβ dimers. DCs were surface biotinylated at chosen times of a pulse chase experiment (see *Figure 1A*). Lysates were first immunoprecipitated with L243 mAb which recognizes essentially αβ dimers (HLA-DR) free of Ii chains. All immunoprecipitations were analyzed by SDS-polyacrylamide gel electrophoresis and quantified by phosphorimager. We estimated that almost all αβ dimers were

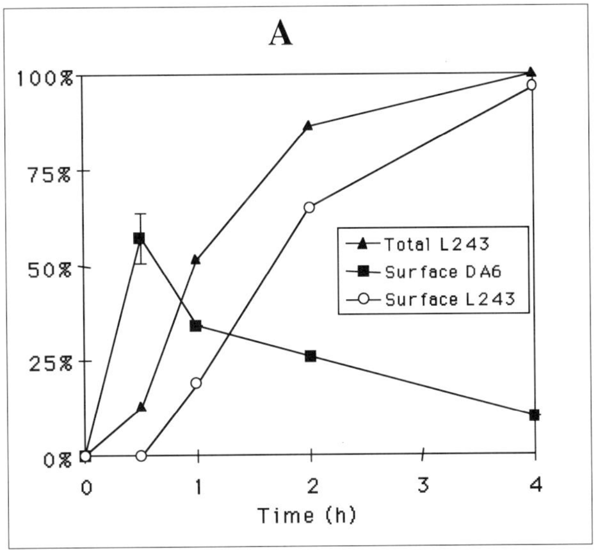

Figure 1A.

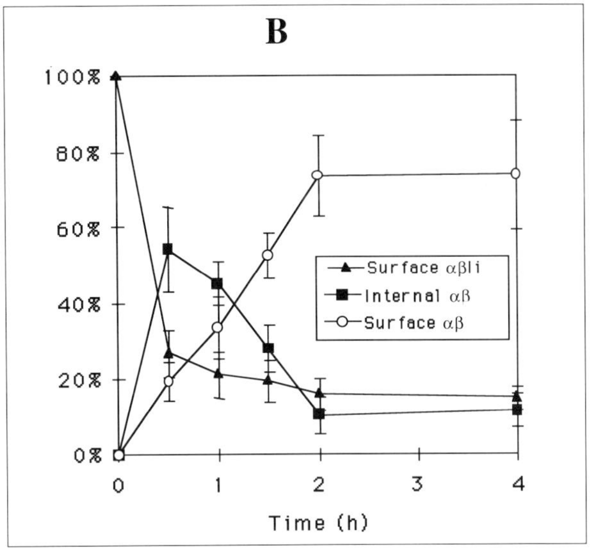

Figure 1B.

detected at the cell surface 4 hours after a short pulse labeling of human DCs (open circles in *Figure 1A*) . In a similar experiment, cell lysates preadsorbed with L243 were submitted to immunoprecipitation with the DA6.147 mAb (anti-DRα) allowing the recovery of residual DR molecules mainly present as precursor αβIi forms. We calculate that at least 55% (± 13%) of the αβ dimers expressed at the plasma membrane 4 hours after their synthesis had first trafficked *via* the cell surface of DCs and were rapidly reinternalized as αβIi precursor form (filled squares in *Figure 1A*).

We confirmed that αβIi complexes transiently expressed at the plasma membrane can be converted into αβ dimers. Radiolabeled DCs were incubated 30 minutes at 37°C in order to allow the transport of αβIi complexes toward the plasma membrane. Previous experiments showed that at this time point no αβ dimers were detected at the plasma membrane. Cells were surface-biotinylated (time 0 in *Figure 1B*) and re-incubated at 37°C for different periods of time. By using specificity of the L243 mAb, we were able to directly follow the conversion of cell surface biotinylated αβIi complexes (filled triangles in *Figure 1B*) into biotinylated αβ dimers (filled squares in *Figure 1B*). These dimers were detected as soon as 15 minutes after the biotinylation. A large proportion of the dimers were SDS-stable [6], betraying association with peptides.

Using a cleavable biotin and a membrane impermeant reducing agent (2-mercaptoethanesulfonic acid) we were able to follow the return of these biotinylated dimers to the cell surface. At least 80% of cell surface biotinylated αβIi complexes were internalized and converted into αβ dimers which were transported back to the plasma membrane within 2 hours (open circles in *Figure 1B*).

Discussion

We here describe an alternative intracellular transport of MHC-II molecules which allows a large proportion of these molecules to travel through the entire endocytotic pathway of DCs. The blocking of transport from early to late endosomal compartments by microtubule depolymerisation did not seem to affect the conversion of surface biotinylated αβIi complexes into SDS-stable dimers. Our experiments suggest that in human DCs Ii degradation and binding of peptides to MHC-II molecules may occur in different compartments all along the endocytic pathway. This could reinforce the suspected "sentinel" role of DCs in the whole body [1] by helping these cells to identify and activate more trace clones of antigen-reactive T cells.

High expression of the p41 form of Ii enhances MHC-II restricted antigen presentation [7]. Whether the p41 form of Ii which is highly expressed in DCs when compared to other antigen presenting cells plays a specific role in the intracellular transport of MHC-II molecules in naive DCs remains to be evaluated.

References

1. Steinman RM. The dendritic cell system and its role in immunogenicity (review). *Annu Rev Immunol* 1991; 9: 271-96.
2. Sallusto F, Lanzavecchia A. Efficient presentation of soluble antigen by cultured human dendritic cells is maintained by granulocyte/macrophage colony-stimulating factor plus interleukin 4 and downregulated by tumor necrosis factor α. *J Exp Med* 1994; 179: 1109-18.
3. Faradji A, Bohbot A, Schmitt-Goguel M, Siffert JC, Dumont S, Wiesel ML, Piemont Y, Eischen A, Bergerat JP, Bartholeyns J, Poindron P, Witz JP, Oberling F. Large scale isolation of human blood monocytes by continuous flow centrifugation leukapheresis and counterflow centrifugation elutriation for adoptive cellular immunotherapy in cancer patients. *J Immunol Methods* 1994 ; 174 : 297-309.
4. Cresswell P. Assembly, transport, and function of MHC class II molecules. *Ann Rev Immunol* 1994; 12: 259-93.
5. Roche PA, Teletski CL, Stang E, Bakke O, Long EO. Cell surface HLA-DR-invariant chain complexes are targeted to endosomes by rapid internalization. *Proc Nate Acad Sci USA* 1993; 90: 8581-5.
6. Germain RN, Hendrix LH. MHC class II structure, occupancy and surface expression determined by post-endoplasmic reticulum antigen binding. *Nature* 1991; 353: 134-9.
7. Peterson M, Miller J. Antigen presentation enhanced by the alternatively spliced invariant chain product p41. *Nature* 1992; 357: 596-8.

Invariant chain determines MHC class II molecules transport into and out of lysosomes

V. Brachet, G. Raposo, I. Mellman[1], S. Amigorena

Institut Curie, Section de Recherche, 12, rue Lhomond, 75005 Paris, France
1 Yale University, Department of Cell Biology, New Haven, CT 06510, USA

Understanding the molecular basis of antigen processing requires characterization of intracellular compartments in which immunogenic peptides are generated and loaded onto class II molecules. Rapidly after their synthesis in the ER, MHC αβ dimers associate with a third polypeptide, the invariant (Ii) chain, which plays a central role in class II biosynthesis and function [1]. Ii is involved in the proper folding and the transport of class II molecules to the endocytic pathway. Ii also regulates peptide binding ; only upon Ii degradation in endosomes αβ dimers efficiently bind antigenic peptides. However, Ii degradation alone is not sufficient for peptide binding. A peculiar monomorphic MHC class II molecule, HLA-DM in humans and H2-M in mice, is also required for peptide loading [2]. In the past year, something of a breakthrough occurred with the identification of specialized compartments that host antigen processing and/or peptide loading, designated MIIC and CIIV [3,4]. However, it is becoming increasingly clear that these compartments are themselves heterogeneous and not always distinct from conventional endosomes and lysosomes.

To question the relationship between conventional and specialized endocytic compartments, we analyzed the effect of leupeptin, an inhibitor of lysosomal proteases which interferes with Ii degradation [5], on the intracellular distributions of class II molecules. In murine A20 B lymphoma cells, MHC class II molecules are principally found in specialized endocytic class II vesicles (CIIV) related to endosomes, but lacking lysosomal markers. In the presence of leupeptin, a 10 kDa Ii-fragment remained associated to αβ dimers and retained class II molecules intracellularly [5,6]. Under these conditions, the Ii-p10 αβ complexes were found in lysosomal compartments, which morphologically resembled to MIIC (they were multivesicular, contained class II, H2-M and lysosomal markers). Moreover, MHC class II molecules in these lysosomal compartments were not destined for degradation, since upon removal of leupeptin, Ii-p10 was degraded and peptide-loaded αβ dimers were transported to the cell surface.

Therefore, the rate of Ii degradation determines the transport of class II molecules through the endocytic pathway : when Ii is degraded slowly (due, for example, to the presence of leupeptin) class II molecules are found in lysosomal compartments. Differences in the intracellular localization of class II molecules in various cells could therefore be due to distinct efficiencies of endosomal degradation of Ii in particular cell types. Our results also question the nature of the late endocytic compartments were class II molecules are found. Is leupeptin inducing the formation of MIIC in cells which normally only have CIIV, or are class II molecules simply transported to conventional lysosomes under certain conditions ?

References

1. Cresswell P. Assembly, transport, and function of MHC class II molecules. *Ann Rev Immunol* 1994 ; 12: 259-93.
2. Roche PA. HLA-DM: an *in vivo* facilitator of MHC class II peptide loading. *Immunity* 1995 ; 3 : 259-62.
3. Peters PJ, Neefjes JJ, Oorschot V, Ploegh HL, Geuze HJ. Segregation of MHC class II molecules from MHC class I molecules in the Golgi complex for transport to lysosomal compartments. *Nature* 1991 ; 349 : 669-76.
4. Amigorena S, Drake JR, Webster P, Mellman I. Transient accumulation of new class II molecules in a novel endocytic compartment in B lymphocytes. *Nature* 1994 ; 369 : 113-20.
5. Neefjes JJ, Ploegh HL. Inhibition of endosomal proteolytic activity by leupeptin blocks surface expression of MHC class II molecules and their conversion to SDS resistant alpha beta heterodimers in endosomes. *EMBO J* 1992 ; 11 : 411-6.
6. Amigorena S, Webster P, Drake JR, Newcomb J, Cresswell P, Mellman I. Invariant chain cleavage and peptide loading in major histocompatibility complex class II vesicles. *J Exp Med* 1995 ; 181 : 1729-41.

Function of HLA

HLA and peptides in Physiology and Diseases

Contents

Distinct effects of altered allopeptide analogs on a human self-restricted T cell clone

A.I. Colovai, Z. Liu, P.E. Harris, J. Kinne, S. Tugulea, J. Molajoni, R. Cortesini, N. Suciu-Foca

College of Physicians and Surgeons of Columbia University, Department of Pathology, 630 West 168th Street, 14-401, New York, NY 10032, USA

Direct evidence has been provided for two distinct, but not mutually exclusive, mechanisms of allorecognition [1]. In the direct pathway, T cells recognize intact allo-MHC complexes displayed on the surface of donor cells. This type of recognition prevails in early post-transplantation, before the departure of donor dendritic cells from the graft, and engages a highly heterogeneous population of T cells. In contrast, the indirect pathway of allorecognition involves a limited repertoire of T cells which recognize donor MHC antigens in the form of peptides processed and presented by self MHC proteins, in a manner similar to the recognition of nominal antigens. Increasing evidence indicates that indirect recognition may be crucial for initiating and perpetuating the rejection of an allograft by providing help for alloantibody production, delayed-type hypersensitivity and T cell cytotoxicity against the graft [2,3]. Hence, specific suppression of indirect recognition may have a profound effect on the graft outcome.

Previous studies have shown that in both the animal and human systems, an allo-MHC molecule usually comprises a single dominant immunogenic peptide, which is recognized in the context of one self MHC restriction element [4,5]. Moreover, the repertoire of T cells involved in the recognition of donor HLA-derived allopeptides is biased to a limited set of TCR VB genes [6]. For these reasons, selective immune interventions aimed at suppressing indirect recognition can be envisioned. One of the most promising approaches in this direction resides in the use of analogs of the immunogenic allopeptides, which can modulate the response of specific T cells in a beneficial manner [7]. To determine whether single residue substitutions in the MHC and/or TCR contact area result in the generation of TCR agonists and antagonists, we have engineered analogs of the dominant determinant of the HLA-DR1 molecule which is recognized by HLA-DRB1*1101 positive responders. One of these peptide analogs carries the binding motif of the heat-shock protein.

The present study reports on the structure of peptide analogs which either enhance or suppress the response of alloreactive T cells. These investigations demonstrate that allopeptide reactivity can be inhibited by induction of high zone tolerance or by use of TCR antagonists.

Materials and methods

Peptides

Peptide DR1/22-35 (ERVRLLERCIYNQE) and its analogs were obtained from Chiron Mimotopes (San Diego, CA). The purity of each peptide was higher than 95% as indicated by HPLC and mass spectrometry.

Cells

A human alloreactive Th cell clone (ZL #1), which recognizes the dominant immunogenic peptide of the DRB1*0101 molecule (peptide DR1/22-35), was generated by *in vitro* immunization of PBMCs from a healthy volunteer carrying the DRB1*1101/1201 genotype, as previously described [5]. The proliferative response of ZL #1 T cell clone was restricted by DRB1*1101 protein and was measured by [^{3}H]TdR incorporation in 3-day blastogenesis assays. Because high numbers of T cells were required for blocking and competition assays, ZL #1 T cell clone was transformed by infection with Herpes virus Saimiri, as previously described [8]. The reactivity of the transformed clone (HVS-ZL #1) was studied by measuring the amount of IFN-g secreted by the T cells upon 24 hrs of stimulation.

Binding assays

The binding affinity of the different peptides for soluble DR11 protein was measured in a competition ELISA assay. Briefly, the biotinylated peptide corresponding to residues 22-35 from DRB1*0101 protein (1µM) was incubated with recombinant DRB1*1101 protein (rDR11) (0.1µM) and various concentrations (0.1-100µM) of the peptide analog, for 48 hr at room temperature. The biotinylated rDR11 peptide complexes were quantitated by using the avidin-peroxidase detection system (Pierce Co., Rockford, IL) in ELISA plates pre-coated with anti-HLA-DR mAb L243. The concentration of the peptide analog required to displace 50% of the biotinylated peptide (IC50) was calculated.

ELISA for quantitation of IFN-γ

HVS-ZL #1 T cell clone (2x104 cells/well) was stimulated for 24 hr with self APCs (5x104 cells/well) pre-pulsed with peptide DR1/22-35 and individual peptide analogs. One hundred µl of culture supernatants were transferred to ELISA plates pre-coated with anti-human IFN-g mAb (Pharmingen, San Diego, CA). Quantitative ELISA for measuring the amount of IFN-γ produced by T cells was performed according to the protocol provided by Pharmingen.

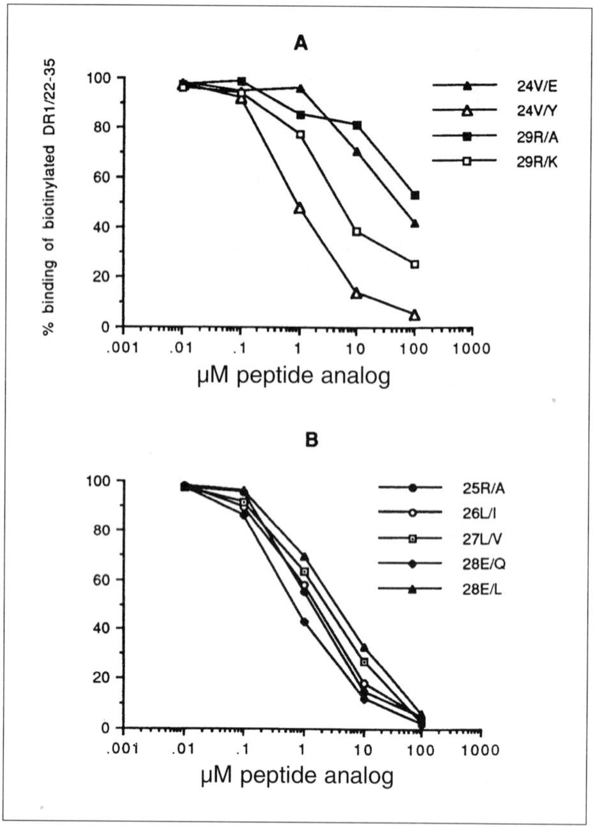

Figure 1. Inhibition of DR1/22-35 peptide binding to soluble DR11 protein by peptide analogs. Binding of biotinylated DR1/22-35 (1µM) to soluble DR11 protein (0.1µM) in the presence of various concentrations of peptide analogs was measured in a competition ELISA assay. Analogs carrying single amino acid substitutions at MHC anchor positions, 24V and 29R (panel A), and at TCR contacts 25R, 26L, 27L and 28E (panel B), were tested for their ability to inhibit the binding of the wild-type peptide.

Results and discussion

MHC binding affinity of peptide analogs

Because T cells only recognize peptides which bind to the MHC molecule above a certain threshold (60-200 complexes/cell) and because peptide antigenicity is often (but not always) proportional to the affinity of binding [9], the various analogs were tested in a competition assay for their ability to block the binding of the wild-type peptide to soluble DRB1*1101 protein *(Figure 1)*.

Two peptides with non-conserved substitutions at potential MHC contact residues, 24V/E and 29R/A, showed a low binding affinity for DR11 protein (IC50>50µM), *i.e.* failed to block the binding of the wild-type peptide. In contrast, homologous substitutions at the same positions, 24V/Y and 29R/K, generated analogs which bound relatively well to DR11 (IC50=0.9µM for 24V/Y peptide, and IC50=4µM for 29R/K peptide) *(Figure 1A)*. These findings indicate that position 24 and 29 serve as anchors for the binding of peptide 22-35 to DR11 protein. It is, therefore, likely that positions 25 through 28 comprise TCR rather than MHC contact residues.

Indeed, both homologous (26L/I and 27L/V) and non-homologous (25R/A, 28E/L and 28E/Q) substitutions at these positions had no significant effect on binding of peptide DR1/22-35 to DR11 molecule, suggesting that residues at positions 25 through 28 project outside the MHC binding groove *(Figure 1B)*.

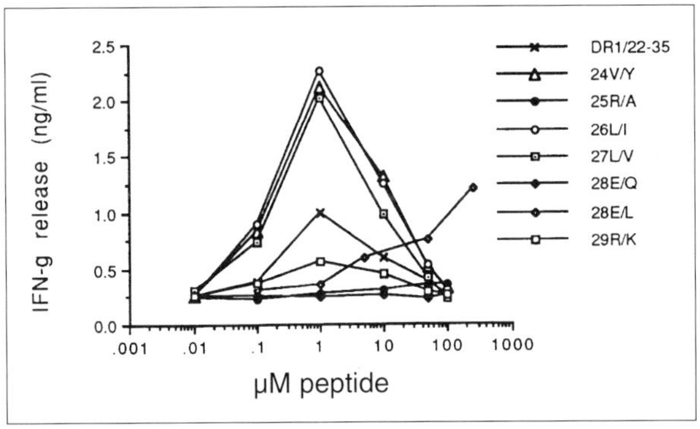

Figure 2. Effect of peptide DR1/22-35 and its analogs on HVS-ZL #1 T cell clone. The stimulatory activity of peptide DR1/22-35 and indicated analogs was assessed by measuring the amount of IFN-γ secreted by HVS-ZL #1 T cell clone in the presence of autologous APCs and various concentrations of the test peptide. The amount of IFN-γ released in 100µl culture supernatant was quantitated by ELISA.

Stimulatory capacity of peptide analogs

The capacity of the analogs which bound to the DR11 molecule to stimulate the function of HVS-ZL #1 T cell clone was determined by quantitation of IFN-g production. Each peptide was tested at concentrations of 0.01-100µM and the effect was compared to that of the wild-type peptide *(Figure 2)*.

As expected, the stimulatory activity of analogs 24V/Y and 29R/K, carrying substitutions at MHC anchor positions, varied in parallel with their binding affinity for DR11 protein. In contrast, the substitutions introduced at positions 25 through 28, which did not affect the binding capacity, resulted in significant changes in the stimulatory activity of the analogs compared to the wild-type peptide. Thus, two peptide analogs, 25R/A and 28E/Q, failed to elicit IFN-γ production, while analogs 26L/I and 27L/V induced stronger stimulation than the wild-type peptide. This demonstrates that positions 25-28 are involved in the interaction of peptide DR1/22-35 with the TCR.

All stimulatory peptides, except for analog 28E/L, induced high-zone tolerance, suppressing clonal proliferation at concentrations higher than 10µM. Chronic stimulation of alloreactive T cells with such analogs of enhanced immunogenicity may result in clonal exhaustion and deletion [10]. Analog 28E/L, however, augmented IFN-γ production at concentrations which were tolerogenic for the other peptides. This analog contains the heat-shock protein binding motif (aliphatic amino acids at positions i, i+2, and i+4, corresponding to 24V, 26L, and 28L in the sequence of peptide 28E/L). Peptides carrying this motif were previously shown to act as effective blockers of alloreactive cytotoxic T cells [10]. The fact that peptide 28E/L was stimulatory to HVS-ZL #1 T clone suggests that peptide binding to the heat shock proteins does not prevent the function of alloreactive T helper cells.

Inhibitory activity of peptide analogs

To determine whether non-immunogenic peptide analogs can be used for inhibition of T cell function, peptides 25R/A and 28E/Q were tested for their ability to block the response of ZL #1 T cell clone to the wild-type peptide. At concentrations higher than 5µM, both of these peptides inhibited the function of TCL-ZL by 50-95% *(Figure 3)*. Inhibition was dose-dependent, suggesting that it was caused by MHC blockade. However, both of these peptides also behave as TCR antagonists (Colovai *et al.*, in preparation).

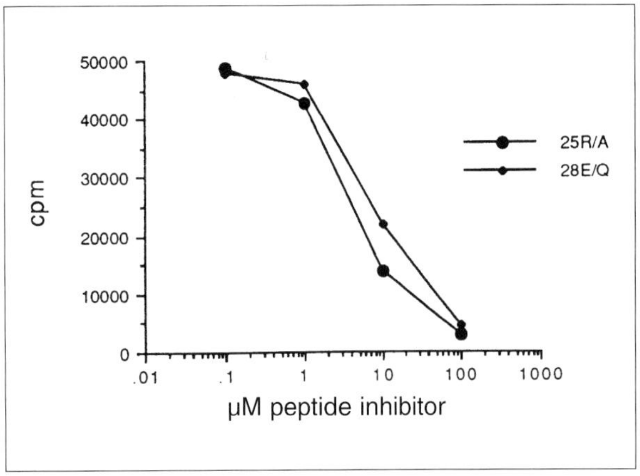

Figure 3. Inhibitory activity of analogs 25R/A and 28E/Q. The capacity of non-stimulatory analogs 25R/A and 28E/Q to inhibit the response of ZL #1 T cell clone induced by peptide DR1/22-35 (wild-type) was measured in a 3-day blastogenesis assay. ZL #1 T cells (20,000 cells/well) were incubated with irradiated autologous APCs (50,000 cells/well), the wild-type peptide (1µM) and individual analogs at indicated concentrations. After 48 hrs, cells were labeled with 3H[TdR] and harvested 18 hrs later.

Conclusions

Recent studies suggest that the use of peptide agonists and antagonists opens new perspectives to selective immunotherapy of autoimmune diseases [7]. The present study shows for the first time that structural variants of dominant alloepitopes may act as potent suppressors of the indirect allorecognition pathway. The finding that non-conservative substitutions in the TCR contact area generate inhibitory peptides suggests a viable option to achieve specific immunosuppression. This is particularly important for prevention and/or treatment of chronic rejection which cannot be reversed by any of the currently available therapies. Further studies of amino acid substitutions which can render dominant allopeptides tolerogenic are required for understanding the mechanisms of TCR antagonism.

References

1. Sherman LA, Chattopadhyan S. The molecular basis of allorecognition. *Annu Rev Immunol* 1993 ; 11 : 385-402.
2. Suciu-Foca N, Reed E, Marboe C, Xi YP, Sun YK, Ho E, Rose EA, Reemtsma K, King DW. Role of anti-HLA antibodies in heart transplantation. *Transplantation* 1991 ; 51 : 716-24.
3. Lee RS, Grusby MJ, Glimcher LH, Winn HJ, Auchincloss JR H. Indirect recognition by helper cells can induce donor-specific cytotoxic T lymphocytes *in vivo*. *J Exp Med* 1994 ; 179 : 865-72.
4. Benichou G, Takizawa PA, Olson CA, McMillian M, Sercarz EE. Donor major histocompatibility complex (MHC) peptides are presented by recipient MHC molecules during graft rejection. *J Exp Med* 1992 ; 175 : 305-8.
5. Liu Z, Harris PE, Colovai AI, Reed EF, Maffei A, Suciu-Foca N. Indirect recognition of donor MHC class II antigens in human transplantation. *Clin Immunol Immunopathol* 1996 ; 78: 228-35.
6. Liu Z, Sun YK, Xi YP, Hong B, Harris PE, Reed EF, Suciu-Foca N. Limited usage of TCR VB genes by allopeptide specific T cells. *J Immunol* 1993 ; 150 : 3180-6.
7. Jameson SC, Bevan MJ. T cell receptor antagonists and partial agonists. *Immunity* 1995 ; 2 : 1-11.
8. Grassmann R, Fleckenstein B, Desrosiers RC. Viral transformation of human T lymphocytes. *Adv Cancer Res* 1994 ; 63 : 211-44.
9. Sette A, Vitiello A, Reherman B, Fowler P, Nayersina R, Kast Wm, Melief CJ, Oseroff C, Yuan L, Ruppert J, *et al.* The relationship between class I binding affinity and immunogenicity of potential cytotoxic T cell epitopes. *J Immunol* 1994 ; 153 : 5586-92.
10. Nobner E, Goldberg JE, Naftzger C, Lyu SC, Clayberger C, Krensky AM. HLA-derived peptides which inhibit T cell function bind to members of the heat-shock protein 70 family. *J Exp Med* 1996 ; 183 : 339-48.

Naturally processed HLA-DR bound peptides from fibroblast cell lines as facultative antigen-presenting cells

H. Kalbacher[2], J. Gamper[1], T. Halder[2], G.A. Müller[3], H.E. Meyer[4], C.A. Müller[1]

1 Section of Transplantation Immunology, Medical Hospital, University of Tübingen, 72076 Tübingen, Germany
2 Medical and Natural Sciences Research Center, University of Tübingen, 72074 Tübingen, Germany
3 Department of Nephrology, University Center of Internal Medicine, 35075 Göttingen, Germany
4 Institute for Physiological Chemistry, University of Bochum, 44780 Bochum, Germany

Major histocompatibility complex (MHC) class II molecules are highly polymorphic membrane glycoproteins involved in the binding of peptides from foreign and self antigens. MHC class II molecules bound peptides have been shown to vary in length (12-35 amino acid residues), and to carry allele specific anchor positions [1-4]. Current understanding of the molecular constraints of these antigenic peptides have been mostly obtained from human EBV-transformed B cell lines which are professional antigen presenting cells (APC) which constitutively express HLA class II molecules to stimulate $CD4^+$ T cell subpopulations. In tissues, however, T cell responses against foreign-, self- or allo-antigens may be influenced by the presentation of peptide/MHC complexes on organ specific cells [5]. Beside professional APC like B cells and monocytes, fibroblasts and epithelial cells are known to exert facultative HLA class II antigen-presenting capacity after stimulation with IFNγ [6]. For an analysis of differences in the peptide pattern bound to HLA-class II molecules of professional and facultative APC, we used two human, SV-40-immortalized, renal fibroblast cell lines derived from a normal kidney biopsy and from a kidney with renal interstitial fibrosis. Both cell lines were analyzed for HLA-DR bound peptides after stimulation with IFNγ, and these peptides were compared with naturally processed peptides bound to similar HLA class II alleles from EBV-transformed B cell lines.

Materials and methods

Cell lines

HLA-DR molecules were purified from two heterozygous renal fibroblast cell lines which were grown from primary fibroblast cultures of a normal kidney biopsy (TK 173: DRB1*0701/DRB1*1303), and of a kidney with interstitial fibrosis (TK 188: DRB1*0101 /DRB1*0801) after transfection with a transforming plasmid containing the SV40 large T antigen. The constitutively HLA class II negative fibroblast cell lines were stimulated with IFNg (1000 U/ml) for 72 hours to induce the expression of HLA-DR molecules. The cell lines were maintained *in vitro* at 37 °C, 10 % CO_2, in Dulbecco's MEM 1640 supplemented with 10% heat-inactivated fetal calf serum (FCS) and antibiotics.

Immunofluorescence staining for FACS analysis

Immunophenotyping of the renal fibroblast cell lines was performed according to standard procedures. Cells were washed with PBS supplemented with 0,8% BSA and 0.1% sodium azide after blocking unspecific binding via the Fc receptor with polyglobin for 10 minutes and labeled for 30 minutes on ice with the monoclonal antibodies L243 (anti HLA-DR), TÜ22 (anti HLA-DQ), and B7/21 (anti HLA-DP). Cells were then again washed twice, and treated with a subclass-specific secondary antibody conjugated with fluorescein isothiocyanate (FITC). Stained cells were resuspended in PBS, and analyzed by a FACScan flow cytometer (Becton Dickinson) for their expression of HLA molecules.

Isolation of HLA-DR molecules and endogenous peptides

Cells were lysed in 2 % NP40 and the resulting homogenate was submitted to immunoaffinity chromatography with the monoclonal antibody L243 (anti HLA-DR), immobilized to sepharose. After washing with 100 mM phosphate buffer supplemented with 0,1 % Zwittergent-12, pH 8.0, two thirds of the column-bound HLA-DR molecules were used to elute the peptides by acid extraction [2]. One third of the column was used to

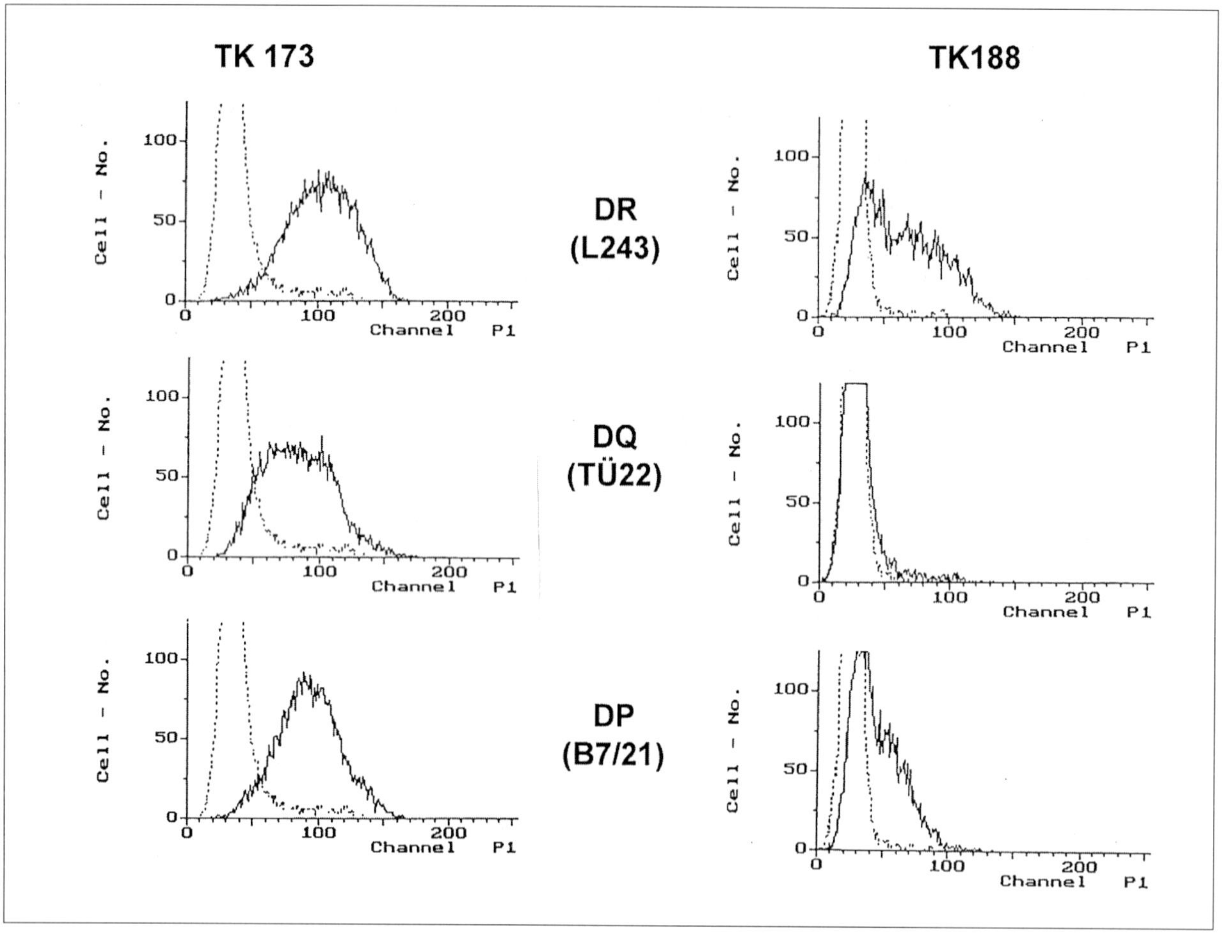

Figure 1. Induction of HLA class II molecules on the renal fibroblasts cell lines TK 173 and TK 188 after stimulation with IFNγ.

isolate the intact HLA-DR molecules by elution at pH 11.0 (100 mM phosphate buffer, 0,1 % Zwittergent-12) [7,8]. These MHC molecules were checked for quality and quantity by SDS-PAGE and used for binding experiments.

Peptide separation

The peptide pools were separated by micro bore reversed phase HPLC on a Vydac protein C_4 column (125 x 2,0 mm) using an acetonitrile gradient. The peaks were collected and stored at -80°C until subsequent analysis [7].

Sequence analysis

Matrix-assisted laser desorption ionisation (MALDI, Finnigan MAT) served to determine the masses and the homogeneity of the collected peaks. Homogenous peaks were directly submitted to an automated Edman microsequencer (ABI 477A).

Results and discussion

For an analysis of differences in dominant peptide patterns bound to HLA class II molecules of professional and facultative APC, fibroblast cell lines derived from a normal (TK173) as well as from a fibrotic kidney (TK188) were investigated for HLA-DR bound peptides after stimulation with IFNγ. The resulting self peptides were compared with naturally processed HLA-DR bound peptides from similar HLA-DR alleles of EBV-transformed

Table I. Naturally processed peptides from the renal fibroblast cell line TK173 (HLA-DRB1*1303 / DRB1*0701)

Time [min]	Sequence	Source protein [human]	Residues	MW [found / theor.]
19.6	FSHDYKGSTSHHLVS	Apolipoprotein B-100	1942-1956	1716.3 / 1701.8
29.8	NPGGYVAYSKAATVTGKL	Transferrin receptor	215-232	1803.2 / 1797.1
41.4	KPQYFEFMKV...	unknown	-	1855.3

Table II. Naturally processed peptides from the renal fibroblast cell line TK188 (HLA-DRB1*0101 / DRB1*0801)

Time [min]	Sequence	Source protein [human]	Residues	MW [found / theor.]
20.0	WPKYFEMVMVFGN	unknown	-	1650.9 / 1648.0
23.3	RPAGDRTFQKWAAVVVPSGEE	HLA-B13	234-254	2304.1 / 2300.6
23.3	RPAGDRTFQKWAAVVVPSGEEQ	HLA-B13	234-255	2431.8 / 2428.7
26.2	DVGVYRAVTPQGRPDA	HLA-DQ6	43-58	1697.9 / 1700.9
44.8	LPKPPKPVSKMRMAT	Invariant chain	80-94	1699.3 / 1680.0
49.0	LPKPPKPVSKMRMATPLLMQALPM	Invariant chain	80-103	2684.2 / 2676.5
49.0	QNQFVQMILNSLINK...	CD36	150-16x	-

human B-cell lines. Induction of HLA class II antigens on the renal fibroblast cell lines TK173 and TK188 is shown in *Figure 1.* Both cell lines were found to strongly express HLA class II molecules after stimulation with IFNγ, although TK188 seemed to be less inducible in its expression for surface HLA-DR and -DP molecules and almost completely lacked induction of HLA-DQ antigens indicating differences in HLA class II expression. SDS-PAGE of immunoaffinity purified HLA-DR molecules showed the typical bands at 60 kD (α/ß dimer), α chain (34 kD) and the ß chain (29 kD) suggesting that the DR-molecules were intact and capable of presenting self peptides.

Naturally processed peptides were acid-extracted from immunoaffinity-purified HLA-DR molecules, ranging from 15-24 amino acid residues in length, and further characterized by mass spectrometry and Edman microsequencing. Seven major peptides from endogenous proteins were found associated with HLA-DR molecules of TK173, three with those of TK188 *(Tables I* and *II).*

Self proteins contributed to the large majority of bound peptides and were derived from membrane proteins (predominantly from MHC class I and II, the invariant chain, and the transferrin receptor) and from an exogenous source (bovine apolipoprotein B-100, which is abundant in serum supplemented culture media). Some of the sequences could not be defined as peptides from known proteins. Corresponding synthetic peptides bound to the purified HLA-DR1 and HLA-DR7 molecules in a high-performance size-exclusion chromatography (HPSEC)-binding assay [6] (data not shown). Although the renal fibroblasts did not differ from professional APC in most of the HLA-DR associated peptides such as those derived from other HLA-molecules, they were found to carry also some newly identified endogenous peptides complexed to HLA-DR like the CD36 peptide and the unknown sequences which might be characteristic for renal fibroblasts. To ensure the hypothesis of presentation of tissue-specific self peptides further HLA class II-associated self peptides from non classical APC have to be identified. For melanoma cells at least one tissue-specific self peptide has been described [7].

References

1. Chicz RM, Urban RG, Gorga JC, Vignali AA, Lane WS, Strominger J. Specificity and promiscuity among naturally processed peptides bound to HLA-DR-alleles. *J Exp Med* 1993;178: 27-47.

2. Rammensee HG, Friede T, Stevanovic S. MHC ligands and peptide motifs: first listing. *Immunogenetics* 1995; 41: 178-228.
3. Stern LJ, Brown JH, Jardeztky TS, Gorga JC, Urban RG, Strominger JL, Wiley DC. Crystal structure of the human class II MHC protein HLA-DR1 complexed with an influenza virus peptide. *Nature* 1994; 368: 215-21.
4. Kropshofer H, Max H, Müller CA, Hesse F, Stevanovic S, Jung G, Kalbacher H. Self-peptide released from class II HLA-DR1 exhibits a hydrophobic two residue contact motif. *J Exp Med* 1992; 175: 1799-803.
5. Freed JH, Marrack P. Tissue-specific expression of self peptides bound by major histocompatibility complex class II molecules. *In* Sette A, ed. *Naturally Processed Peptides, vol. 57, Chem Immunol.* Basel : Karger, 1993 : 88-112.
6. Steimle V, Siegrist CA, Mottet A, Liskowksa-Grospierre B, Bach B. Regulation of MHC class II expression by interferon gamma mediated by the transactivator gene CIITA. *Science* 1994, 265: 106-9.
7. Halder T, Pawelec G, Kirkin AF, Zeuthen J, Meyer HE, Kalbacher H. A peptide from the known class I restricted melanoma-specific tumor antigen GP100 is presented by HLA-DR in the melanoma cell line FM3. In : Charron D, ed. *Genetic diversity of HLA. Functional and medical implication,* vol. II. Sèvres : EDK, 1997.
8. Max H, Halder T, Kalbus M, Gnau V, Jung G, Kalbacher H. A 16mer peptide of the human autoantigen calreticulin is a most prominant HLA-DR4Dw4-associated self-peptide. *Hum Immunol* 1994 ; 41 : 39-45.

Specificity of naturally processed peptides from HLA-DQA1*0501-DQB1*0301 : influence of the DQα chain?

I. Daher-Khalil, F. Boisgérault, J.P. Feugeas, V. Tieng, A. Toubert, D. Charron

Laboratoire d'immunogénétique Humaine, INSERM U396, Institut Biomédical des Cordeliers 15, rue de l'École de Médecine, 75006 Paris, France

Recently, the nature of peptide binding motifs and structural interaction has been well studied with respect to multiple HLA-DR allotypes [1], much less is known concerning peptide binding motifs for HLA-DQ molecules [2, 3]. In HLA-DR molecules, while structural diversity is limited to the polymorphic β chain, which contributes all the critical functional residues to influence variability in peptide binding interaction, HLA-DQ contains both polymorphic α and β chains that could independently influence specific peptide interaction. Moreover, as some DQαβ dimers are associated with a variety of autoimmune diseases, sequence information from self peptides bound to DQαβ dimers sharing b chain and linked to autoimmune diseases, will allow a better understanding of the molecular mechanisms of these diseases and of the influence of the DQα chain in peptide binding. To evaluate such questions, self peptides bound to purified HLA-DQ7, (DQA1*0501-DQB1*0301) and (DQA1*0301-DQB1*0301), negatively associated to IDDM [4], were eluted and characterized and their binding to a variety of HLA-DQαβ dimers tested.

Results and discussion

Self peptides bound to immunoaffinity purified HLA-DQ7 molecules (DQA1*0501-DQB*0301) and (DQA*0301-DQB1*0301) expressed on EBV-transformed B-LCL Sweig and Jhaf respectively, were isolated and characterized. The bound peptides were released by acid elution and separated by HPLC [5]. The specific predominant peaks of HLA- DQA1*0501-DQB*0301 were sequenced by Edman microsequencing. Twelve complete sequences were obtained, which derived from 5 proteins including MHC associated molecules (A29, the most abundant peptide sequenced, and DRα) and other integral membrane proteins *(Table I)*. Peptides derived from the majority of these proteins have been previously isolated from several HLA-DR and some HLA-DQ molecules [1, 2]. As expected, peptides varied in length from 9 to 22 amino acids and contained nested sets with ragged N- and/or C-terminal ends. The sequencing of the predominant peaks of HLA DQA*0301-DQB1*0301 is in process.

Peptide binding

The ability of the transferrin receptor derived self peptide, termed N16G, to bind with HLA-DQA1*0501 DQB1*0301 molecule on B-LCL Sweig was examined *(Table II)*. This peptide was synthetized and biotinylated at the N-terminus for direct binding. Binding was performed on paraformaldehyde-fixed cells as previously described [6]. Briefly, after incubation of biotinylated N16G peptide with fixed B-LCL, cells were then lysed and the lysate was transfered to wells coated with DQ or DR specific mAb. The capture of DQ or DR /peptide complex on the plates were detected by Streptavidin-POD. Binding data described in *Table II* shows that N16G peptide was not only able to bind to DQA1*0501-DQB1*0301 dimer but also to DRB1*1101 molecule on Sweig BLCL. Moreovere, the verification of the specificity of these binding interaction using cell lines expressing different DQ and DR molecules *(Table II)* indicates that while N16G peptide was a promiscous DR peptide, it preferentially bound to DQA1*0501-DQB1*0301 and DQA1*0502-DQB1*0301.

Influence of DQα chain in peptide binding

To examine the effect of DQα polymorphism on N16G peptide binding, cell lines Sweig, Amala, Jhaf and Luy, which express the same DQβ chain (DQB1*0301), but

Table I. Naturally processed peptides bound to HLA-DQA1*0501-DQB1*0301

Source protein	Residue	Category	peptide sequence	Length	RT
transferrin receptor	217-230	membrane	NPGGYVAYSKAATVTVTG	16	65
INF-induced protein	89-103		VGDVTGAQAYASTAK	15	23
HLA-DRα	76-98	membrane	SFEAQGALANIAVDKA	16	35
	77-98	membrane	FEAQGALANIAVDKA	15	43
	78-98	membrane	EAQGALANIAVDKA	14	35
HLA-A29	168-177	membrane	QRKWEAARVA	10	25
	169-178	membrane	RKWEAARVAE	10	25
	170-180	membrane	KWEAARVAEQL	11	34
	170-181	membrane	KWEAARVAEQLR	12	34
	171-185	membrane	WEAARVAEQLRAYLE	15	35
	171-179	membrane	WEAARVAEQ	9	25
CLIP	98-119	membrane	PKPPKPVSKMRMATPLLMQESQ	22	46
			KPPKPVSKMRMATPLLMQESQ	21	47

Residues describing the peptide binding motif are shown in either bold or underlined.

Table II. Binding of peptide N16G to different DQ and DR alleles expressed on B-LCL

B-LCL	Sweig	Amala	Jhaf	Luy	Bm14	HID	DBB	Cox	Spoo10
DQA1*0	501	502	301	601	301	301	201	501	102
DQB1*0	301	301	301	301	302	303	303	201	502
N16G	++	++	-	-	-	-	-	-	-
DRB1*0	1101	1401	407	803	401	901	702	301	1101
N16G	+	-	+	-	-	++	++	-	+

DQ or DR from $1x10^6$ cells were assayed with 50 mM biotinylated N16G. Anti-DQmAb L2 and anti-DR mAb L243 were used as capturing mAb. ++ > 0,7; + < 0,7; - < 0,1 U OD 492nm.

have different DQα chains, were used *(Table II)*. Peptide N16G binding was detected with DQA1*0501-DQB1*0301 and DQA1*0502-DQB1*0301 dimers. No binding was seen to DQA1*0301-DQB1*0301 and DQA1*0601-DQB1*0301 dimers. These results are in agreement with those described by Kwok *et al.* [6] which demonstrated that peptide specifically binding to DQA1*0301-DQB1*0301 does not bind to DQA1*0501-DQB1*0301. The two DQ dimers, which bind N16G, differ by only one amino acid, the residue 59 with Arg instead of Pro in the DQA1*0501 chain. Modeling of HLA-DQ molecules according to the known structure of HLA-DR1 [7] reveals that residue 59 is located outside the different binding pockets. Therefore, this difference should not prevent N16G binding.

DQA1*0501-DQB1*0301, which bind N16G, and DQA1*0301-DQB1*0301 and DQA1*0601-DQB1*0301 dimers, which do not, differ by residues located in pocket 1 and 9 of the DQ molecules. For example, in the pocket 1, DQA1*0501-DQB1*0301 has an aliphatic Leu and a large amide Gln at α chain position 51 and 53 respectively, while DQA1*0301-DQB1*0301 has aromatic Phe and a positively charged Arg residues. These two residues at site 51 and 53 might be expected to restrict the size and the charge of permitted residues in peptide bound in DQA1*0501-DQB1*0301 compared to DQA1*0301-DQB1*0301. Differences in pocket 1 and 9 likely account for our findings that these molecules have distinct specificity for the N16G peptide. Based on our results and data previously described by Kwok *et al.* [6, 8] describing the peptide binding motif for DQA1*0301-DQB1*0302, DQA1*0301-DQB1*0301 and DQA1*0301-DQB1*0303, peptide binding motif for DQA*0501-DQB1*0301 could be proposed to be :

	1 4 7 9		1 4 7 9
either	GxxAxSxxA	or	YxxxAxVxxI
	V A S		F G L T
	A V Q		

References

1. Chicz RM, Urban RG, Gorga JC, Vignali DAA, Lane WS, Strominger JL. Specificity and promiscuity among naturally processed peptides bound to HLA-DR alleles. *J Exp Med* 1993; 178 : 27-47.
2. Falk K, Rötzschke O, Stevanovic S, Jung G, Rammensee HG. Pool sequencing of natural HLA-DR, DQ and DP ligands reveals detailed peptide motifs, constraints of processing and general rules. *Immunogenetics* 1994; 39 : 230-42.
3. Chicz RM, Lane WS, Robinson RA, Trucco M, Strominger JL, Gorga JC. Self-peptides bound to the type 1 diabetes associated class II MHC molecules HLA-DQ1 and HLA-DQ8. Int Immunol 1994; 6 : 1639-49.
4. Khalil I, Deschamps I, Lepage V, Degos L, Hors J. Dose effect of cis and trans encoded HLA-DQab heterodimers in IDDM susceptibility. *Diabetes* 1992; 41:378-84.
5. Boisgérault F, Khalil I, Tieng V, Connan F, Tabary T, Cohen JMH, Choppin J, Charron D, Toubert A. Definition of the HLA-A29 peptide ligand motif allows prediction of potential T-cell epitopes from the retinal soluble antigen, a candidate autoantigen in birdshot retinopathy. *Proc Natl Acad Sci USA* 1996; 93 : 3466-70.
6. Kwok WW, Nepom GT, Raymond FC. HLA-DQ polymorphisms are highly selective for peptide binding interaction. *J Immunol* 1995; 155 : 2468-76.
7. Stern LJ, Brown JH, Jardetzky TS, Gorga JC, Urban RG, Strominger JL, Wiley DC. Crystal structure of the human class II MHC protein HLA-DR1 complexed with an inflenza virus peptide. *Nature* 1994; 368 : 215.
8. Kwok WW, Domeier ME, Raymond FC, Byers P, Nepom GT. Allele-specific motifs characterize HLA-DQ interactions with a diabetes-associated peptide derived from glutamic acid decarboxylase *J Immunol* 1996;156 : 2171-7.

Interactions of peptide side chains with structurally complementary pockets in DQ molecules are critical for allele-specific peptide binding and T cell reactivity

W.W. Kwok, D. Koelle, G.T. Nepom

Virginia Mason Research Center,
1000 Seneca Street, Seattle, WA 98101, USA

The DQB1*0302 allele is associated with an increased risk of susceptibility to insulin dependent diabetes mellitus (IDDM) in the Caucasian population [1]. We analyzed two structurally similar alleles DQB1*0301 and DQB1*0303, in order to identify molecular parameters characteristic of the disease-associated DQB1*0302 allele. The DQ polypeptide encoded by the DQB1*0302 allele differs from DQB1*0303 only at codon 57, and differs from DQB1*0301 at four positions in the first extracellular domain, *i.e.*, codons 13, 26, 45 and 57. We have investigated how these polymorphisms influence peptide binding and T cell reactivity involved in antigen-specific DQ-restricted immune recognition.

X-ray crystallographic studies of the MHC/peptide complex have shown that peptides are bound to MHC in an extended conformation utilizing four major binding

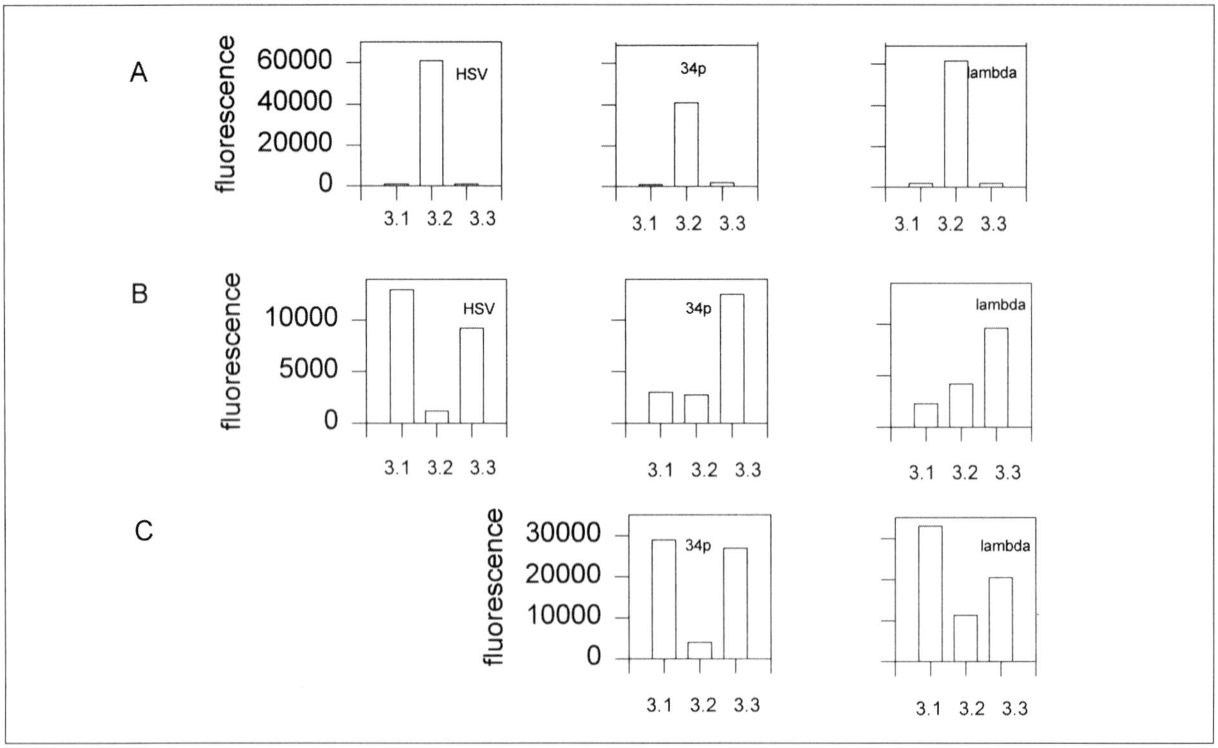

Figure 1. Binding of biotinylated peptides to different B-LCL expressing different DQ alleles as described [4]. (1A) Binding of HSV-2 433-445, 34p and R12-24. (1B) Binding of biotinylated peptide with Ala substitution at position n+8. (1C) Binding of biotinylated peptide with Ala substitution at position n+3 and n+8.

Table I. DQ-binding peptides used in this study

	A. native peptides	B. Ala (n+8)	C. Ala (n+3, n+8)
HSV-2 433-445	DMTPADALDDFDL	DMTPADALDAFDL (10A)	-
34P	IARFKMFPEVK	IARFKMFPAVK (9A)	IARAKMFPAVK (4A, 9A)
λR12-24	LEDARRLKAIYEK	LEDARRLKAIYAK (12A)	LEDARRAKAIYAK (7A, 12A)

pockets, *i.e.*, pockets 1, 4, 6 and 9 within the DR molecule [2, 3]. Though such studies have not yet been extended to DQ molecules, the extensive similarity in DR and DQ amino acid sequences suggests that peptides likely also bind in an extended conformation to DQ molecules using homologous binding pockets. Polymorphism of residues of both DQα and DQβ chains can contribute to the different environments of each binding pocket in different alleles [4]. However, each of the DQB1*03 alleles which were described in these studies pair with the identical DQA1*0301 allele. Therefore, peptide bindings in these studies show allelic specificity depending solely on the polymorphism of the DQB1 chain.

In a series of previous experiments, we have identified 3 peptides that bind avidly to DQ3.2, but not to DQ3.1 and DQ3.3 *(Figure 1A)* [4-6]. These peptides are the glutamate decarboxylase peptide (GAD) 253-263 (or 34p), λ-repressor peptide 12-24 (λR 12-24) and the HSV-2 VP16 peptide 433-445 (HSV-2). Comparison of amino acid sequences of the three DQ3.2 binding peptides showed the presence of a negatively charged residue near the carboxyl terminal end of the peptide *(Table IA)*.

Molecular modeling of the DQ molecules based on the DR1 crystal structures suggested that codon 13 and 26 are located within the proximity of pocket 4, while codon 57 is located within the proximity of pocket 9 (codon 45 is not associated with the peptide-interaction pockets). For pocket 9, DQ3.1 and DQ3.3 have an Asp at codon 57, while DQ3.2 has an Ala. This codon 57 polymorphism is similarly present in many DR, DQ and murine I-A alleles. An Asp at this position may form a salt bridge with a conserved Arg residue which is present in codon 76, 79 and 80 of DRα, DQα and I-Aα respectively. The presence of this salt bridge should influence both the size and charge environment of pocket 9. In the absence of the Asp at codon 57, the Arg in the α chain may be favored to interact with other negatively charged residues contributed by the bound peptide. To test this hypothesis, substitution of the negatively charge residues on each of the 3 peptides to an Ala were carried out *(Table IB)*.

Figure 1B shows that these Ala substituted peptides lost binding to DQB1*0302, and gained binding affinity for DQB1*0303. The HSV-2,10A peptide could also bind to DQB1*0301. For DQ3.1, pocket 4 has Ala and Tyr (codon 13 and 26 respectively). For DQ3.2, pocket 4 has Gly and Leu. As Ala is larger than Gly, and Tyr is larger than Leu, pocket 4 in DQ3.1 may be constrained to accommodate a residue with a small side chain. This model fits well with the HSV-2-10A peptide, in which position n+3 also has an Ala and the peptide can bind to DQ3.1. To further test this hypothesis, the n+3 position residue for both the λR 12-24-12A peptide and the 34p9A peptide was modified to an Ala *(Table IC)*.

These modified peptides were examined for the ability to bind to DQ3.1. In contrast to the unmodified peptides, these substituted peptides with Ala at position n+3 and n+8 bound better to DQ3.1 and DQ3.3 compared with DQ3.2 *(Figure 1C)*. Binding experiments with peptides in which only the n+3 residue was modified to an Ala show that these peptides are incapable of binding to the DQ3.1 molecules (data not shown). All these data support the concept that polymorphisms of pocket 9 allows for the selective binding of peptides to either DQ3.2 or DQ3.3, where a negatively charged side chain at position 9 is favored for binding to DQ3.2 and a noncharged residue is favor for binding to DQ3.3. In additional to the polymorphisms of pocket 9, polymorphisms of pocket 4 also influence the selective binding of peptide to either DQ3.2 and DQ3.1, where a noncharged residue at position 9 and a small residue at position 4 are favored for binding to DQ3.1 compared with DQ3.2.

A DQ3.2 T cell clone that recognizes the HSV-2 VP16 peptide was tested for its ability to recognize the modi-

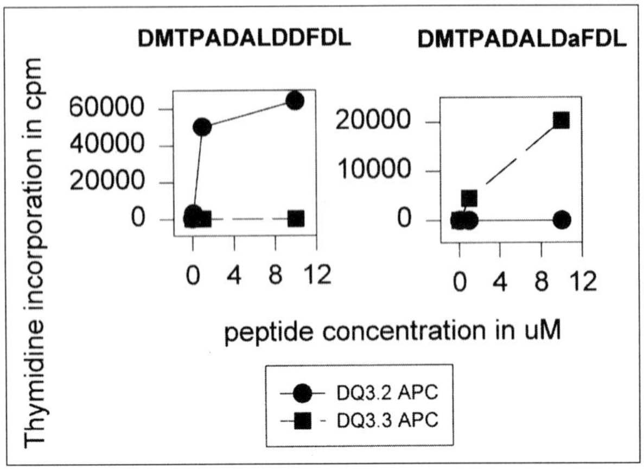

Figure 2. Modulation of T cell recognition by HSV 433-445 analogs.

fied peptides. This clone did not recognize the 433-445, 10A peptide presented by DQ3.2, nor did it recognize the wild type 433-445 peptide presented by a DQ3.3 APC *(Figure 2)*. However, this T cell clone recognized the 433-445, 10A peptide presented by a DQ3.3 APC *(Figure 2)*. These experiments show that codon 57 region of the DQB1 chain is an important immunodominant region for T cell recognition through a peptide-dependent mechanism, where negatively charged residue at codon 57 is favored to interact with an small non-charged residue on position 9 of the peptide and a non-charged residue at codon 57 is favored to interact with a negatively charged residue on position 9 of the peptide. In both cases, the resulting MHC-peptide complex is sufficient for comparable T cell recognition.

References

1. Nepom GT, Erlich H. MHC class II molecules and autoimmunity. *Ann Rev Immunol* 1991 ; 9 : 493-525.
2. Stern LJ, Brown JH, Jardetzky TS, Gorga JC, Urban RG, Strominger JL, Wiley DC. Crystal structure of the human class II MHC protein HLA-DR1 complexed with an influenza virus peptide. *Nature* 1994; 368 : 215-21.
3. Ghosh P, Amaya M, Mellins E, Wiley DC. The structure of an intermediate in class II MHC maturation: CLIP bound to HLA-DR3. *Nature* 1995 ; 378 : 457-62.
4. Kwok WW, Nepom GT, Raymond FC. HLA-DQ polymorphisms are highly selective for peptide binding interactions. *J Immunol* 1995 ; 155 : 2468-76.
5. Kwok WW, Domeier ME, Raymond FC, Byers P, Nepom GT. Allele-specific motifs characterize HLA-DQ interactions with a diabetes-associated peptide derived from glutamic acid decarboxylase. *J Immunol* 1996 ; 156 : 2171-7.
6. Kwok WW, Domeier ME, Johnson ML, Nepom GT, Koelle DM. HLA-DQB1 codon 57 is critical for peptide binding and recognition. *J Exp Med* 1996 ; 183 : 1253-8.

Motif for HLA-DQ2 (α1*0501, β1*0201) : anchors at P1, P4, P6, P7 and P9

F. Vartdal[1], B.H. Johansen[1], T. Friede[2], C.J. Thorpe[3], S. Stevanovič[2], J.A. Eriksen[4], K. Sletten[5], H.G. Rammensee[2], E. Thorsby[1], L.M. Sollid[1]

1 Institute of Transplantation Immunology, Rikshospitalet, N0027 Oslo, Norway
2 Departement of Immunology, Deutsches Krebsforschungszentrum, Heidelberg, Germany
3 Departement of Crystallography, Birkbeck College, London, England
4 Departement for Medicinal and Organic Chemistry, Norsk Hydro Research Centre, Porsgrunn, Norway
5 Departement of Biochemistry, University of Oslo, Oslo, Norway

To define the peptide binding motif of HLA-DQ2 [*i.e.* DQ(α1*0501 β1*0201)], we have sequenced individual peptides and a pool of peptides eluted from affinity-purified DQ2 molecules. Identification of the peptide binding motif of this molecule is interesting, as this molecule is associated to celiac disease and to insulin dependent diabetes mellitus.

Materials and methods

Peptides were eluted from DQ affinity-purified from DQ2-homozygous EBV-transformed B cell lines. The low molecular weight material (< 10 kD) of the eluate was separated on reverse-phase HPLC. The individual peaks and a pool of the remaining non-peak material were collected and subsequently sequenced by automated Edman degradation in a pulsed-liquid protein sequencer. The sequences of the indvidual peptides were compared with sequences of proteins in the Swissprot databank. Analysis of peptide binding to DQ2 was performed as described previously [1]. Models of peptide/DQ2 complexes of DQ2 with the peptides used in this study were constructed from the crystallographic structure of HLA-DR1 binding the HA peptide using the homology modeling tools incorporated into the QUANTA/CHARMm molecular modeling package (Molecular Stimulation/Biosym, San Diego, USA).

Results and discussion

Variants of eight different peptides with a length of 9-19 amino acids were identified; among them the class II-associated invariant chain peptides (CLIP) and peptides that stem from HLA class I α, HLA-DQα1*0501, Ig κ and CD20 molecules and from two non-identified sources.

Binding studies of synthetic variants of eluted peptides showed that HLA class I α 46-60 bound with a high binding affinity (IC50 =130 nM), while the remaining peptides displayed lower binding affinities. Since the HLA class I α 46-60 peptide has a high binding affinity, we performed biochemical binding analyses of synthetic truncated and serially single Lys- or Ala- substituted variants of this peptide. This showed that that HLA class I α 52-60 is the core peptide binding to DQ2, and that substitutions of Ile52, Glu55, Pro57, Glu58 and Trp60 with Lys lead to a profound reduction (>32-fold) in binding affinity. This indicates that the DQ2 binding motif has anchors at positions P1, P4, P6, P7 and P9. This is consistent with a previous study on binding of synthetic variants of another DQ2-binding ligand (Ova 267-276Y), where we have shown that P4 (aliphatic or negatively charged residues), P7 (negatively charged residues) and P9 (bulky hydrophobic residues) are included in the DQ2 binding motif [2]. The present study further elucidates the DQ2 binding motif. The results demonstrate that P1 and P6 are also anchors and that bulky hydrophobic residues are well accepted at P1, while Pro or negatively charged residues are preferred at P6.

The pool sequencing essentially corroborated the binding data, by showing a peak of bulky hydrophobic residues corresponding to P1, of Val, Leu and Glu corresponding to P4, of Glu and Asp corresponding to P6/P7 and a weak peak of Tyr at positions reflecting P9. Computer modelling of the DQ2/HLA class I α-peptide demonstrated that the side chains of Ile52 (P1) and Trp60 (P9) fit into two large pockets at both ends of the class II binding trench, while the side chains of Glu55, Pro57 and Glu58 are well accomodated in the P4, P6 and P7 pockets, respectively.

Conclusion

The present and our previous study [2] together suggest that the peptide binding motif of DQ2 is:
P1: bulky hydrophobic residues ;
P4: aliphatic or negatively charged residues ;
P6: Pro or negatively charged residues ;
P7: negatively charged residues ;
P9: bulky hydrophobic residues.

References

1. Johansen BH, Buus S, Vartdal F, Viken H, Eriksen JA, Thorsby E, Sollid LM. Binding of peptides to HLA-DQ molecules: peptide binding properties of the disease associated HLA-DQ(α1*0501, β1*0201) molecule. *Int Immunol* 1994; 6: 453-61.
2. Johansen BH, Vartdal F, Eriksen JA, Thorsby E, Sollid LM. Identification of a putative motif for binding of peptides to HLA-DQ2. *Int Immunol* 1996, 8: 177-82.

An allo-specific peptide derived from HLA-A2 is presented by HLA-DQ7

J.P. Feugeas [1,2], S. Lemaire[2], I. Khalil[1], G. Haentjens[2], A. Toubert[1], C. Derappe[2], D. Néel[2], M. Aubery[2], D. Charron[1]

1 INSERM U396, 15, rue de l'École de Médecine, 75006 Paris, France
2 INSERM U180, 45, rue des Saints-Pères, 75006 Paris, France

Recognition of peptide fragments presented by class II HLA molecules to T cell receptor (TCR) is a central event in the development of immune response. The determination of structural motif and origin of peptides capable of binding to the different HLA alleles is of a considerable interest for a better understanding of HLA-disease associations. Here we analysed peptides eluted from HLA-DR11 and -DQ7 molecules.

Method

HLA molecules and peptides were purified from the homozygous Epstein-Barr virus-transformed B cells JVM(HLA-A2-DRB1*1102-DQA1*0501-DQB1*0301) as described [1] using immunoaffinity columns with the mAbs L2 (anti-DQ) and D1.12 (anti-DR). Selected fractions were analysed by electrospray ionisation-mass spectrometry and sequenced by pulsed liquid automated Edman degradation. Other fractions were analysed by pool sequencing.

Potential peptide binding motifs
(Tables I and II)

Sequences of peptides eluted form HLA-DR11 (DRB1*1102, abbreviated 1102) and pool sequencing suggested the following motif: Pro or other hydrophobic amino-acid at position i, Ile at i + 3 and Lys i + 7. The motif described for DRB1*1104 [2] is Pro at position i and Lys at position i + 7 without Ile at position i + 3. The presence of Arg β71 in the pocket 4 of HLA-DRβ*1104 instead of Glu β71 for 1102 may account for that difference. The motif described for DRB1*1101 [1] is (W,Y,F) at position i, (M,L,V,I) at i + 3, (R, K) at i + 5 and (R,K) at i + 7. Differences with 1102 can be explained by the fact that amino-acids β86 (in pocket 1), β71 (in pockets 4 and 7), β67 (in pocket 7) are not the same for 1102 and 1101 alleles (amino-acids in the pocket 9 are identical).

For peptides eluted from HLA-DQ7 the most significant signal was Ala or Gly in the middle of the peptide as also described by Falk *et al.* [3] and Kwok [4]. Pool sequencing showed that other frequent amino-acids were Pro at position 2 and aromatic/hydrophobic amino-acids at position 4, 7 and 9.

Source of peptides *(Tables I and II)*

Three peptides eluted from HLA-DR11 (-DRB1*1102) appeared to derive from known proteins. One peptide matched 100% to macrophage inflammatory protein (MIP-1α). The same peptide was found by Harris *et al.* [2] eluted from an other HLA-DR11 (DRB1*1104) molecule. The presentaion of the same self peptide by two different cell lines underlines that a few proteins are major peptide donors for several different class II molecules.

Source proteins of three peptides eluted from HLA-DQ7 (-DQA1*0501-DQB1*0301) were identified. Unexpectedly, one peptide was identical to a part of the NMDA-glutamate receptor which is a membrane receptor of nerve cells. EBV transformed cells may express this receptor or a homologous unknown protein. An other peptide eluted from HLA-DQ7 was a polymorphic part of the HLA-A2 heavy chain called peptide A2.56-69. Peptides derived from polymorphic part of class I molecules have also been identified bound to several HLA-DR and -DQ allotypes [5] although it was not yet described for HLA-DQ7. We suggest that the presentation of those allo-specific peptides is not a coincidence and may play a role in discrimination between self and non-self. Further functional studies are necessary to explore that hypothesis. However in 1987 Krensky *et al.* (10th international workshop) have already used a synthetic A2.56-69 pep-

Table I. Peptides eluted from HLA-DR11 (-DRB1*1102)

Source protein	Peptides													
MIP-1		K	P	G	V	**I**	F	L	T	**K**	R	S	R	
Adenylate cyclase		V	A	G	V	**I**	G	A	K	**K**	P	Q	Y	D
ATP synthase	H	P	K	I	T	**I**	E	R	K	**K**	Q	F	V	
unknown		F	P	Q	E	**I**	V	E	V	**K**	Y	T	A	G

Table II. Peptides eluted from HLA-DQ7 (-DQA1*0501-DQB1*0301)

Source protein	Peptides														
glutamate receptor	R	R	I	I	P	R	**G**	E	A	R	L	P	S		
unknown	X	P	D	H	A	S	**A**	P	P	Y	S	S			
HLA-A2	G	P	E	Y	W	D	**G**	E	T	R	K	V	K	A	H
RNA polymerase	I	P	K	P	E	D	**A**	P	E	S	F	R	L	L	V
unknown	X	P	V	Q	M	Q	**A**	R	P	V	X	T	K	Q	F

tide to modulate lysis by HLA-A2-specific cytotoxic T lymphocytes. These authors have shown that this peptide could sensitize HLA-A69-DR5-DQ7 target cells to HLA-A2 specific CTL. They suggested that A2.56-69 peptide was presented by HLA-A69 (closely related to HLA-A2) to the HLA-A2 specific CTL. According to our results the A2.56-69 peptide could also be presented by class II HLA molecules providing help for cytolysis of the target cells. Indeed it is now known that «indirect» recognition of allo-peptides by helper cells can induce cytotoxic T lymphocytes both *in vitro* and *in vivo* [6].

References

1. Newcomb JR, Cresswell P. Characterization of endogenous peptides bound to purified HLA-DR molecules and their absence from invariant chain-associated αβ dimers. *J Immunol* 1993 ; 150 : 499-507.
2. Harris PE, Maffei A, Liu Z, Colovai I, Reed EF, Inghirami G, Suciu-Foca N. Naturally processed cytokine-derived peptide bound to HLA-class-II molecules. *J Immunol* 1993 ; 151 : 5975-83.
3. Falk K, Rötzschke O, Stevanovic S, Jung G, Rammensee HG. Pool sequencing of natural HLA-DR, DQ, and DP ligands reveals detailed peptide motifs, constraints of processing, and general rules. *Immunogenetics* 1994 ; 39 : 230-42.
4. Kwok WW, Domeier ME, Raymond FC, Byers P, Nepom GT. Allele-specific motifs characterize HLA-DQ interactions with a diabetes-associated peptide derived from glutamic acid decarboxylase. *J Immunol* 1996 ; 156 : 2171-7.
5. Chicz RM, Lane WS, Robinson RA, Trucco M, Strominger JL, Gorga JC. Self-peptides bound to the type I diabetes associated class II MHC molecules HLA-DQ1 and HLA-DQ8. *Int Immunol* 1994 ; 6 : 1639-49.
6. Lee RS, Grusby MJ, Glimcher LH, Winn HJ, Auchincloss H. Indirect recognition by helper cells can induce donor-specific cytotoxic T lymphocytes *in vivo*. *J Exp Med* 1994 ; 179 : 865-72.

A highly efficient, universal and unbiased approach to address MHC specificity. Quantitation by peptide libraries and improved prediction of binding

A. Stryhn[1], L. Østergaard Pedersen[1], T. Romme[1], C. Bisgaard Holm[2], A. Holm[2], S. Buus[1]

1 Department of Experimental Immunology, Institute of Medical Microbiology and Immunology, University of Copenhagen, Blegdamsvej 3, 2200 Copenhagen, Denmark
2 Research Center for Medical Biotechnology, Chemistry Department, Royal Veterinary and Agricultural University, Copenhagen, Denmark

Considerable interest has focused on understanding how MHC specificity is generated and characterizing the specificity of MHC molecules with the ultimate goal being to predict peptide binding [1]. Two fundamentally different, but complementary, approaches are currently used to determine the peptide binding specificity of MHC [2]. One approach consists of sequencing the peptides already bound to MHC molecules of a given allotype [3], whereas the other approach consists of examining which peptides will bind to the MHC [4, 5], comparing binding *versus* non-binding peptides to establish the specificity involved [6]. Both approaches have advantages and disadvantages [2]. The latter approach - the direct binding method [4, 5] - allows the one to identify and quantitate both positively and negatively interacting residues, whereas the sequencing method only allows the identification of the most dominant of the positively interacting residues. We have used the direct binding method and generated a highly efficient, universal and unbiased approach to address MHC specificity through a strategy whereby all possible peptides of a particular size are distributed into "positional scanning combinatorial peptide libraries" (PSCPL, [7]).

Methods

MHC class I molecules were purified, and peptides synthesized, as previously described [5]. For each MHC molecule, an indicator peptide was radioiodinated. Complexes between purified MHC molecules and labelled indicator peptide were quantitated by high-flux spun column gel filtration [8]. The concentration of test peptide (or library) needed to obtain 50% inhibition of the binding of the indicator peptide - the IC_{50} - was determined. The lower: the IC_{50} - the better: the binding of the test peptide. The assay requires that the MHC class I in question can be purified and that a high affinity binding indicator peptide has been identified. These requirements can be met for all MHC molecules, in particular, indicator peptides can readily identified once the peptide elution motif has been established [3].

Results and discussion

The Influenza virus haemagglutinin octamer peptide, $Ha_{255-262}$ (FESTGNLI), has been identified as a minimal epitope in H-2^k mice restricted by the MHC class I molecule, K^k [9]. To investigate the specificity of K^k, each amino acid of the FESTGNLI peptide was, one by one, replaced with any of the other natural occurring amino acids (except cysteine; a total of 8 x 18 = 144 analogs) and each analog was tested for its ability to bind to K^k. The effect of the substitution was expressed as IC_{50}(FESTGNLI) divided with IC_{50}(analog) *(Figure 1A)*. The majority of the single substitutions had a moderate effect upon binding K^k as 127 out of 144 (88%) replacements led to less than a 10-fold decrease in binding. The deleterious substitutions were entirely concentrated in positions 2, which preferred E, and 8, which preferred I.

Strikingly, all naturally occurring L-amino acid appeared more or less acceptable in all the non-primary anchor positions (in particular for positions 3, 4, and 6). This result led to the idea that any amino acid could be introduced at these positions and consequently that soluble peptide libraries generated by introducing mixtures of amino acids during synthesis could bind to class I molecules. Pilot experiments demonstrated that a random 8-mer peptide library (XXXXXXXX or X_8) contained sufficient peptide binders to be detected in the K^k inhibition of binding assay (data not shown). Subsequently, all possible peptides of a given size and composition under consideration were represented by a systematic set of sub-libraries. In each sub-library, one amino acid in one position is kept constant whereas the remaining positions contain mixtures of amino acids (see *Table I*, a design termed "positional scanning combinatorial peptide libraries" (PSCPL, [7]). A complete eight-mer PSCPL was synthesized. Each PSCPL sub-library was tested for its ability to bind to class I molecules. To express the data, the IC_{50} of the PSCPL sub-library was related to the binding of the random X_8 library by calculating a "relative binding factor", RB, as $IC_{50}(X_8)$ divided with IC_{50}(PSCPL sub-library). The RB indicates whether a given amino acid in a particular position increases (RB> 1) or decreases (RB< 1) binding compared to an "average amino acid" in that position.

Comparing the binding matrices of the three MHC class I molecules demonstrated that the PSCPL detected a MHC dependent specificity *(Figure 1B-D)*. The most distinctive specificities corresponded to the known primary anchor residues. Notably, they were all correctly identified. The C-terminal residue was the most critical for all three class I molecules (I for K^k, L for K^b and V for HLA-A*0204). The second most important residues was in position 2 (E for K^k and L for HLA-A*0204) or position 5 (F for K^b). Characteristically, the primary anchor positions, in particular the C-terminal primary anchor, were exceptionally choosy in the sense that hardly any other amino acid was acceptable here. This fits well with the accepted definition of a primary anchor position as a position where one amino acid is strongly preferred and the majority of the remaining amino acids are disfavoured.

The RB values could be tabulated as partially exemplified in *Table II*. For each MHC class I molecule, this matrix considers 160 possible binding events. The PSCPL identified amino acids, which could increase or decrease binding (primary and secondary anchors for RB > 2, upper 95% confidence limit; disfavored residues for RB < 0.5, lower 95% confidence limit) in every position. About 10% of the possible residues were secondary anchor residues and about 40% of the possible residues were disfavouring. The frequent occurrence of disfavoured amino acids demonstrates that negating the binding potential of primary and secondary anchor residues plays an important role in shaping the specificity of MHC class I. The matrixes generated were also used to predict binding. A panel of peptides with "locked primary anchors" (like in [10]) was synthesized. For each of these peptides binding was predicted as well as determined experimentally. A highly significant correlation was found with the PSCPL

Table I. Design of peptide libraries

Position 1	Position 2	....	Position 8
AXXXXXXX (AX_7)	XAXXXXXX (XAX_6)	....	XXXXXXXA (X_7A)
CXXXXXXX (CX_7)	XCXXXXXX (XCX_6)	....	XXXXXXXC (X_7C)
DXXXXXXX (DX_7)	XDXXXXXX (XDX_6)	....	XXXXXXXD (X_7D)
...	....	....	....
YXXXXXXX (YX_7)	XYXXXXXX (XYX_6)	....	XXXXXXXY (X_7Y)

Table II. Example of the tabulation of the relative binding factors (RB) *in casu* for K^k. The table gives the relative binding factor (RB) of each natural amino acid corresponding to each position of a 8-mer. The RB is calculated as $IC_{50}(X_8)$ divided with IC_{50}(PSCPL sublibrary)

Aa	Position								Aa
	1	2	3	4	5	6	7	8	
A	0.57	0.60	0.78	1.09	**2.46**	0.86	1.17	*0.19*	A
C	1.03	*0.32*	*0.12*	*0.45*	*0.08*	*0.15*	*0.42*	*0.01*	C
D	1.72	1.70	*0.39*	0.55	*0.46*	*0.26*	*0.41*	*0.001*	D
E	0.73	**9.73**	*0.39*	1.09	*0.12*	*0.18*	0.64	*0.001*	E
F	1.72	*0.37*	**2.28**	1.30	1.24	0.71	**2.01**	1.14	etc

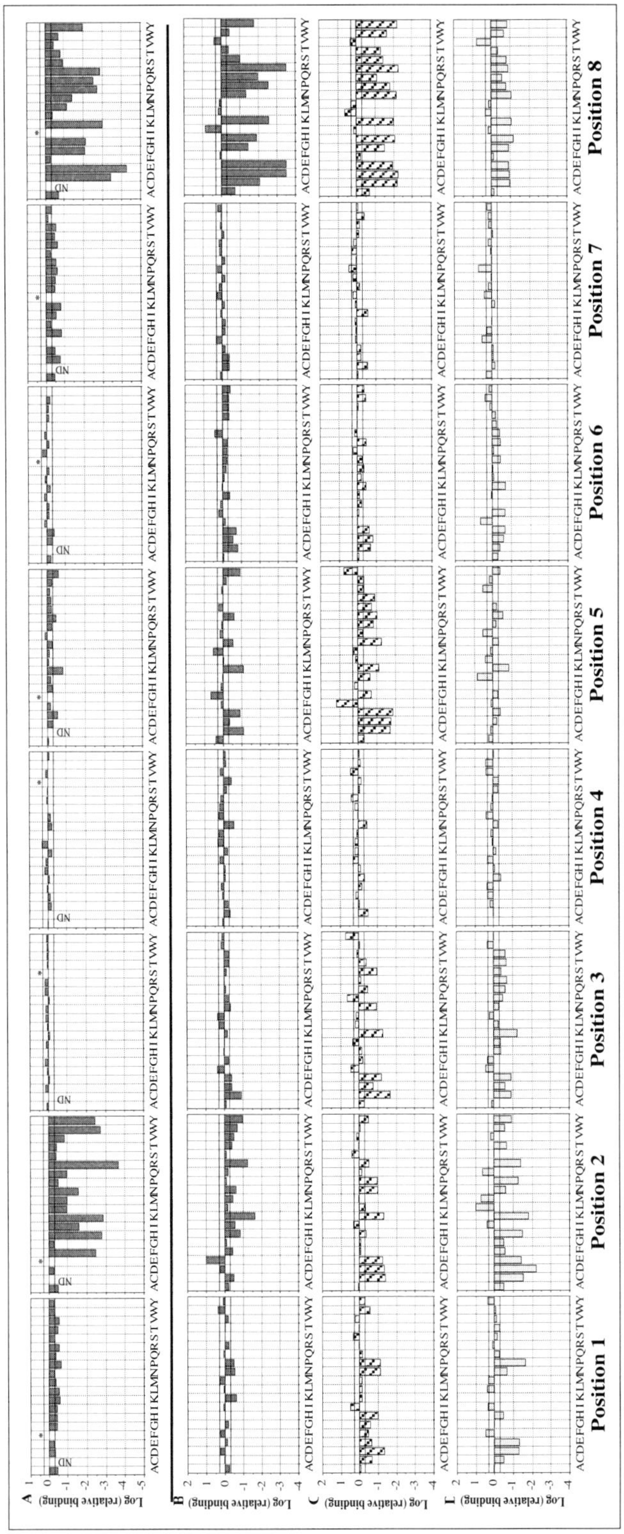

Figure 1. The specificity of three MHC class I molecules determined analog scanning and by positional scanning combinatorial peptide libraries (PSCPL).
A: FESTGNLI analogs, K^k;
B: PSCPL, K^k;
C: PSCPL, K^b;
D: PSCPL, HLA-A*0204.
Increasing concentrations of analog or PSCPL sub-libraries were added to MHC binding reactions to determine the IC_{50} of the various sub-libraries. For (A) binding is expressed as "relative binding", which is calculated as IC_{50} of the analog divided with the IC_{50} of the native FESTGNLI peptide. For (B-D) binding is expressed as "relative binding" (RB), which is calculated as IC_{50} of the PSCPL sub-library divided with the IC_{50} of the random X_8 library. The theoretical maximum value for the PSCPL RB is 10, whereas the minimum value is zero. Shown is the logarithm of the relative binding for each of the substituted analogs, position by position. Indicated are the upper 95% significance level, which was 2, and the lower 95% significance level, which was 0.5. Note, that the graphs for K^k binding in *Figures 1A* and *1B-D* are not readily comparable since *Figure 1A* normalizes binding to FESTGNLI whereas *Figure 1B-D* normalizes binding to X_8.

matrix being better at predicting than a matrix extracted from the analog data in *Figure 1A*.

One major accomplishment of the PSCPL approach is the unbiased and quantitative description of all functionally important residues. It is universal since many different MHC molecules can be addressed with the same set of PSCPL sub-libraries, and assays to test PSCPL binding can be developed for any MHC molecule. Conveniently, PSCPL significantly reduces the experimental set-up and the subsequent data handling. It also leads to improved peptide binding predictions, which might be important for the development of rational immune therapy in the future.

Postscriptum

This workshop and conference celebrated significant progress in HLA-typing, and the importance of typing was frequently stressed. The time is now ripe to shift the attention to the biology of HLA, that is the specificity of HLA molecules. Information on the specificity of HLA molecules may have many practical and clinical applications. By way of example, transplantation matching, selection of optimal parasite subunits for vaccine development, and the identification of MHC associated auto-immune epitopes could all be improved. The development of specific immunotherapy (*e.g.* raising anti-virus or anti-tumor responses) could be tailored to a given patient. A detailed mapping of the many MHC specificities would be a very large task, indeed. More than 200 HLA class I haplotypes have been entered into the international histocompatibility workshops listings of the human MHC class I allotypes and these numbers are still growing. An international concerted action would be needed and the IHCW could be instrumental in generating consensus and disseminating information.

References

1. Rammensee HG, Friede T, Stevanonic S. MHC ligands and peptide motifs : first listing. *Immunogen etics* 1995; 41:178.
2. Buus S, Pedersen LØ, Stryhn A. The analysis of peptide binding to MHC and of MHC specificity. In Claassen E, Zegers N, eds. *Immunological recognition of peptides in medicine and biology*. New York : CRC Press, 1995: 61.
3. Falk K, Rötzschke O, Stevanovic S, Jung G, Rammensee HG. Allele-specific motifs revealed by sequencing of self-peptides eluted from MHC molecules. *Nature* 1991 ; 351:290.
4. Babbitt BP, Allen PM, Matsueda G, Haber E, Unanue ER. Binding of immunogenic peptides to Ia histocompatibility molecules. *Nature* 1985 ; 317:359.
5. Olsen AC, Pedersen LØ, Hansen AS, Nissen MH, Olsen M, Hansen PR, Holm A, Buus S. A quantitative assay to measure the interaction between immunogenic peptides and MHC class I molecules. *Eur J Immunol* 1994 ; 24:385.
6. Sette A, Buus S, Apella E, Smith JA, Chesnut RW, Miles C, Colon SM, Grey HM. Prediction of major histocompatibility complex binding regions of protein antigens by sequence pattern analysis. *Proc Natl Acad Sci USA* 1989 ; 86:3296.
7. Pinilla, Appel JR, Blanc P, Houghten RA. Rapid identification of high affinity peptide ligands using positional scanning synthetic peptide combinatorial libraries. *Biotechniques* 1992 ; 13:901.
8. Buus S, Stryhn A, Winther K, Kirkby N, Pedersen LØ. Receptor-ligand interactions measured by an improved spun column chromatography technique. A high efficiency and high throughput size separation method. *Biochim Biophys Acta* 1995; 1243:453.
9. Gould KG, Scotney H, Brownlee GG. Characterization of two distinct major histocompatibility complex class I Kk -restricted T-cell epitopes within the influenza A/PR/8/34 virus hemagglutinin. *J Virol* 1991 ; 65:5401.
10. Rupert J, Sidney J, Celis E, Kubo R, Sette A. Prominent role of secondary anchor residues in peptide binding to HLA-A2.1 molecules. *Cell* 1993 ; 74:929.

The differentially disease-associated HLA-B*2704 and B*2706 subtypes differ in their binding of peptides with C-terminal tyrosine residues

J.R. Lamas, B. Galocha, J.A. Villadangos, J.P. Albar[1], J.A. López de Castro

Centro de Biología Molecular Severo Ochoa (CSIC-UAM), Universidad Autónoma de Madrid, Facultad de Ciencias, and Immunology and Oncology Department, Pharmacia-CSIC, Centro Nacional de Biotecnología, Cantoblanco, 28049 Madrid, Spain

B*2704 and B*2706 are two closely related HLA-B27 subtypes, which are essentially restricted to Asian populations. B*2704 differs from the most common B*2705 subtype by two amino acid changes in the peptide binding site: Asp>Ser77, implying loss of an acidic residue in the C/F pocket, and Val>Glu152, implying replacement of an acidic residue for an aliphatic one. B*2706 differs from B*2704 by two additional changes: His>Asp114 and Asp>Tyr116, implying gain and loss of acidic residues, respectively. In addition, both subtypes differ from B*2705 by a conservative change (Ala>Gly211) in the a3 domain, which is unlikely to be relevant for peptide binding [1]. B*2704, but not B*2706, is associated to ankylosing spondylitis in an Asian population [2]. In this study, the peptide binding specificity of the B*2704 and B*2706 subtypes, and of mutants mimicking their polymorphism, was comparatively analyzed using peptides naturally presented by the disease-associated B*2705 and B*2702 subtypes. The goal was to establish the functional differences that underline the differential association of B*2704 and B*2706 to spondyloarthropathy. A quantitative assay [3], based on the stabilization of HLA-B27 expression on the TAP-deficient RMA-S cells by exogenously added peptide, was used to assess binding.

Results and discussion

Binding of some peptides naturally presented by B*2705 (05.Pi) or B*2702 (02.Pi) to B*2704 and B*2706 is shown in Table I. Peptides with basic C-terminal residues bound to B*2704 with intermediate affinity, and yet more poorly to B*2706. The B*2704 subtype bound very efficiently peptides with C-terminal aliphatic or aromatic residues, suggesting that it can present many of the peptides naturally presented by B*2702 and B*2705. The B*2706 subtype also bound efficiently peptides with C-terminal Leu and Phe but,

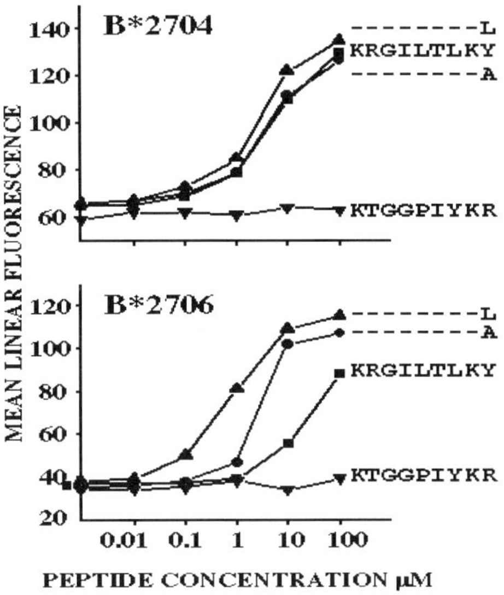

Figure 1. Binding of 02.P6 (KRGILTLKY) and its synthetic analogs with Leu9 or Ala9 to B*2704 and B*2706. Synthetic peptides were incubated at various concentrations with HLA-B27+-RMA-S cells at 26°C, and HLA-B27 fluorescence was measured at a given time after transfer to 37°C [3]. The HLA-A68-bound peptide KTGGPIYKR was used as negative control. The 02.P6 peptide bound better to B*2704 than to B*2706 (see also *Table I*). Changing the C-terminal Tyr to Leu or Ala had no effect with B*2704, but significantly improved binding to B*2706.

Table I. Peptide binding to HLAB27 subtypes[a]

PEPTIDE	SEQUENCE	B*2705	B*2704	B*2706
05.P2	R**R**IKEIVK**K**	0.8	10	100
05.P6	G**R**IDKPIL**K**	2	20	70
05.P5	R**R**SKEITV**R**	2	10	30
05.P8	K**R**FEGLTQ**R**	2	20	40
05.P10	R**R**ISGVDR**Y**	3	5	40
02.P6	K**R**GILTLK**Y**	4	2	40
02.P2	G**R**LTKHTK**F**	4	4	4
02.P3	R**R**FVNVVPT**F**	2	2	1
05.P1	R**R**YQKSTE**L**	1	1	0.5

[a]Binding to each HLA-B27 variant is expressed as the µM EC50 value, that is the concentration of peptide required to obtain half the maximum HLA-B27-associated fluorescence on RMA-S transfectants of the peptide that binds best (i.e. the one with the lowest EC50) among the 05.P or the 02.P sets. Peptides with EC50≤5µM were considered to bind with high affinity, as these were the values obtained for most of the B*2705- and B*2702-bound peptides with B*2705 and B*2702, respectively. EC50 values >5µM and <50µM and EC50≥50µM indicate intermediate and low affinity, respectively.

unlike B*2704, peptides with C-terminal Tyr bound worse. The lower suitability of C-terminal Tyr was directly demonstrated with peptide analogs in which this residue was changed to either Leu or Ala . One example is shown in *Figure 1*. Whereas these changes had little effect on binding to B*2704, they improved binding to B*2706. C-terminal Tyr was also unsuitable for B*2709 [4], which is the only other subtype reported to be not associated to ankylosing spondylitis [5]. In contrast, besides B*2704, the disease-associated B*2705 and B*2702 subtypes bind peptides with C-terminal Tyr and present them *in vivo* [6]. Thus, efficient presentation of peptides with C-terminal Tyr is a feature that distinguishes between disease-associated and non-associated subtypes, and may be relevant for the association of HLA-B27 to spondyloarthropathy.

Introduction of an acidic residue at either position 114 or 152 greatly decreased binding of many peptides. Removal of single acidic charges in the C/F pocket (S77, Y116) improved binding of peptides with C-terminal Leu or Phe, but did not impaired binding of those with C-terminal basic residues *(Table II)*. Thus, removal of more than one acidic charge in the C/F pocket is required to abrogate the specificity of HLA-B27 for peptides with C-terminal Arg or Lys. The efficient binding of peptides with aliphatic or aromatic C-terminal residues to B*2704 implies that the S77 change compensates for the negative effects of the E152 one. Similarly, the equally efficient binding of peptides to both the Y116 and D114Y116 mutants revealed that the Y116 change compensates for the disrupting effect of D114. Finally, a comparison of the binding properties of B*2706 with the mutants mimicking the changes in this subtype indicates that the high suitability of this subtype for nonpolar residues and its low suitability for polar ones, including Tyr, requires that the acidic charges at both positions 77 and 116 are removed. Thus, the peptide specificity of B*2706, which may be the basis of its low association to spondyloarthropathy, results from the joint effect of its four changes relative to B*2705, and is not explained by the separate binding properties of B*2704 and D114Y116 mutant.

Table II . Peptide binding to HLA-B27 mutants mimicking B*2704 and B*2706 subtypes[a]

PEPTIDE	SEQUENCE	S77	E152	D114	Y116	D114Y116
05.P2	R**R**IKEIVK**K**	0.5	6	60	0.1	0.1
05.P6	G**R**IDKPIL**K**	1	20	5	1	0.3
05.P5	R**R**SKEITV**R**	1	20	40	3	3
05.P8	K**R**FEGLTQ**R**	0.6	>100	90	2	2
05.P10	R**R**ISGVDR**Y**	0.8	>100	40	5	4
02.P6	K**R**GILTLK**Y**	0.3	30	10	5	2
02.P2	G**R**LTKHTK**F**	0.9	5	8	1	0.4
02.P3	R**R**FVNVVPT**F**	0.5	3	4	0.4	0.5
05.P1	R**R**YQKSTE**L**	1	5	20	0.1	0.2

[a]See footnote to *Table I.*

Acknowledgments

This work was supported by grant SAF 94-0891 from the Plan Nacional de I+D. We acknowledge the Fundación Ramón Areces for an institutional grant to the CBMSO.

References

1. Rudwaleit M, Bowness P, Wordsworth P. The nucleotide sequence of HLA-B*2704 reveals a new amino acid substitution in exon 4 which is also present in

HLA-B*2706. *Immunogenetics* 1996; 43:160-2.

2. López-Larrea C, Sujirachato K, Mehra NK, Chiewsilp P, Isarangkura D, Kanga U, Dominguez O, Coto E, Peña M, Setien F, Gonzalez-Roces S. HLA-B27 subtypes in Asian patients with ankylosing spondylitis. Evidence for new associations. *Tissue Antigens* 1995; 45:169-76.
3. Villadangos JA, Galocha B, Garcia F, Albar JP, Lopez de Castro JA. Modulation of peptide binding by HLA-B27 polymorphism in pockets A and B, and peptide specificity of B*2703. *Eur J Immunol* 1995; 25:2370-7.
4. Fiorillo MT, Greco G, Sorrentino R. The Asp116-His116 substitution in a novel HLA-B27 subtype influences the acceptance of the peptide C-terminal anchor. *Immunogenetics* 1995; 41:38-9.
5. D'Amato M, Fiorillo MT, Carcassi C, Mathieu A, Zuccarelli A, Bitti PP, Tosi R, Sorrentino R. Relevance of residue 116 of HLA-B27 in determining susceptibility to ankylosing spondylitis. *Eur J Immunol* 1995; 25:3199-201.
6. Rötzschke O, Falk K, Stevanovic S, Gnau V, Jung G, Rammensee HG. Dominant aromatic/aliphatic C-terminal anchor in HLA-B*2702 and B*2705 peptide motifs. *Immunogenetics* 1994 ; 39:74-7.

Analysis of endogenous peptides eluted from HLA-B*2705 and B*2703 subtypes

A. Toubert, F. Boisgérault, V. Tieng, N. Dulphy, M.C. Stolzenberg, I. Khalil, D. Charron

Laboratoire d'Immunogénétique Humaine, INSERM U. 396, Institut Biomédical des Cordeliers and Hôpital Saint-Louis, 1, avenue Claude Vellefaux, 75475 Paris Cedex 10, France

HLA-B27 has been one of the most studied HLA class I allele because of its association to spondylarthropathies (SA). Its 3-dimensional structure has been solved as well as the peptide binding motif of its major subtype B*2705 [1]. HLA-B27 has been subdivided into at least 9 subtypes, B*2701 to B*2709, differing from B*2705 by 1 to 5 aminoacids in the peptide binding groove. They also differ in frequency and in their ethnic distribution. Frequent subtypes, such as B*2705 or B*2702 among Caucasians and B*2704 in Orientals are certainly associated with SA while other subtypes, B*2703 in West Africa [2], B*2706 in the Thai population [3] and B*2709 in Sardinia [4] could be less strongly associated. B*2703 is unique among B27 subtypes and even among HLA class I molecules since it differs from B*2705 by a single aminocid at position 59, His instead of Tyr. This Tyr residue is conserved among HLA class I molecules and participates in the hydrogen bounds stabilizing the N-termini of peptides. Functional and peptide binding studies indicate that the B*2703 peptides could include a subset of the whole B*2705 associated peptides [5, 6]. In view of the possible preferential association between B*2705 and SA compared to B*2703, it would be of interest to investigate the endogenous peptides bound by these 2 subtypes. From previous studies [7] and considering the position of the substitution in pocket A, it could be expected that sequences from individual HPLC fractions instead of pool sequencing would be needed to observe differences between these variants.

Material and methods

Peptide elution and HPLC fractionation were carried out as in [8] from 3.10^9 to 10^{10} cells in each experiment. C1R-B*2705 and B*2703 [7] transfectants were used. N-terminal Edman's sequencing was performed on the major HPLC fractions. Synthetic peptides (Neosystem, Strasbourg, France) were tested in a stabilization assay of empty class I molecules expressed at the surface of T2-B*2705 or B*2703 cell lines [5, 9]. The results were expressed in relative fluorescence index (RFI) as the ratio of mean fluorecence intensities obtained with peptide-treated cells (100μM overnight) to that of cells incubated without peptide.

Results and discussion

The analysis of pool sequencing data from C1R-B*2705 and B*2703 eluted peptides showed differences in agreement with previous studies [5, 8] : basic residues (Arg, Lys, His) were preferred at the first position (P1) of B*2703 peptides, the requirement for Arg at P2 was clear for both subtypes but stronger for B*2703 than for B*2705 while aromatic residues (Tyr, Phe) or aliphatic residues (Ile, Leu, Val) were equally represented at P3. At the C-terminus, aromatic residues (Tyr or Phe) were overrepresented in both alleles. Individual sequences yielding a match in protein databases are presented in *Table I.* Some peptides are common to both subtypes, such as the histone H3.3 or the proteasome C5 peptides. Several peptides have been already reported in previous studies (histone H3.3, rat ribosomal L36, proteasome C5) indicating that dominant endogenous peptides are repeatedly presented by the same HLA allele in different cell types or culture conditions.

The stabilization of empty class I molecules expressed at the surface of TAP-deficient cells T2-B*2705 and B*2703 in presence of synthetic peptides was chosen to assess the allelic specificity of peptide binding *(Table I)*. Viral peptides known to bind both alleles (HIV-1 gp120 314-322) or preferentially B*2705 (influenza A virus

Table I. Peptide sequences and *in vitro* binding to T2-B*2705 and B*2703 (see *Material and methods*). Results are expressed as relative fluorescence index (RFI): - = RFI<1.5; + = RFI 1.5 to 2.5; + + = RFI 2.5 to 4

PEPTIDE SEQUENCE	ORIGIN	BINDING T2-B*2705	T2-B*2703
HIV-1 gp120 GRAFVTIGK	viral	+ +	+ +
Influenza A nucleoprotein SRYWAIRTR	viral	+	-
Histone H3.3 RRYQKSTEL	C1R-B*2705 C1R-B*2703	+	+
Proteasome C5 RRFMPYYVY	C1R-B*2705 C1R-B*2703	+ +	+ +
Rat ribosomal L36 GRLTKHTKF	C1R-B*2705	+	-
HLA class I RRYLENGKETL	C1R-B*2705	+	-
Initiation factor eIF-2 KRFEKHWRL	C1R-B*2703	+	+

nucleoprotein 383-391) were used as controls. As expected, endogenous peptides found in both subtypes (H3.3, proteasome C5) bound both alleles *in vitro*. The initiation factor eIF-2 peptide derived from B*2703 bound also equally well to both subtypes. At the opposite, two endogenous peptides eluted from B*2705 (ribosomal L36, HLA class I) bound specifically to B*2705 and were totally negative on B*2703. Rat ribosomal L36 peptide is a poor B*2703 binder probably because of the nature of the P1 residue (Gly) which is unfavorable for this allele. Conversely, the class I derived peptide carries Arg at P1 which is a residue of choice for B*2703. In that case, it could be argued that the length of the peptide (11-mer) could contribute to its decreased binding affinity to B*2703. Therefore, in the case of B*2705 and B*2703, differences in binding affinity and in the selection of endogenous peptides could involve additional parameters than the nature of the P1 residue alone such as the peptide length or interactions among residues in the peptide.

In conclusion, we show here that a single difference in one residue in pocket A outside peptide anchors binding pockets could have profound effects on the nature of the endogenous peptides bound. This could have important consequences in the selection of T cell repertoire in the thymus, induction of tolerance and susceptibility to autoimmunity.

Acknowledgements

*We wish to thank Dr. J. Lopez de Castro for providing us the C1R-B*2705 and B*2703, Dr. P. Cresswell the T2-B*2705 and Dr. J. Frelinger the T2-B*2703 cell lines. This work was supported in part by a grant from the Association de Recherche sur la Polyarthrite (ARP).*

References

1. Jardetzky TS, Lane WS, Robinson RA, Madden DR, Wiley DC. Identification of self peptides bound to purified HLA-B27. *Nature* 1991; 353: 326-9.
2. Hill AV, Allsopp CE, Kwiatkowski D, Anstey NM, Greenwood BM, McMichael AJ. HLA class I typing by PCR: HLA-B27 and an African B27 subtype. *Lancet* 1991; 337: 640-2.

3. Lopez-Larrea C, Sujirachato K, Mehra NK, Chiwsilp P, Isarangkura D, Kanga U, Domingez O, Coto E, Pena M, Setién F, Gonzalez-Roces S. HLA-B27 subtypes in Asian patients with ankylosing spondylitis. *Tissue Antigens* 1995; 45: 169-76.
4. D'Amato M, Fiorillo MT, Carcassi C, Mathieu A, Zucarelli A, Bitti PP, Tosi R, Sorrentino R. Relevance of residue 116 of HLA-B27 in determining susceptibility to ankylosing spondilytis. *Eur J Immunol* 1995; 25: 3199-201.
5. Colbert RA, Rowland-Jones S, McMichael AJ, Frelinger JA. Differences in peptide presentation between B27 subtypes: the importance of the P1 side chain in maintaining high affinity peptide binding to B*2703. *Immunity* 1994; 1: 121-30.
6. Villadangos JA, Galocha B, Garcia F, Albar JP, Lopez de Castro JA. Modulation of peptide binding by HLA-B27 polymorphism in pockets A and B, and peptide specificity of B*2703. *Eur J Immunol* 1995; 25: 2370-7.
7. Rojo S, Garcia F, Villadangos JA, Lopez de Castro JA. Changes in the repertoire of peptides bound to HLA-B27 subtypes and to site-specific mutants inside and outside pocket B. *J Exp Med* 1993; 177: 613-20.
8. Boisgérault F, Khalil I, Tieng V, Connan F, Tabary T, Cohen JMH, Choppin J, Charron D, Toubert A. Definition of the HLA-A29 peptide ligand motif allows prediction of potential T-cell epitopes from the retinal soluble antigen, a candidate autoantigen in birdshot retinopathy. *Proc Natl Acad Sci USA* 1996; 93: 3466-70.
9. Stuber G, Leder GH, Storkus WJ, Lotze MT, Modrow S, Szekely L, Wolf H, Klein E, Kärre K, Klein G. Identification of wild-type and mutant p53 peptides binding to HLA-A2 assessed by a peptide loading-deficient cell line assay and a novel major histocompatibility complex class I peptide binding assay. *Eur J Immunol* 1994; 24: 765-8.

Identification of HLA-A2 binding peptides from cytomegalovirus and its recognition by cytotoxic T lymphocytes

A. Solache, A.K. Ruprai, J. Grundy[1], A. Madrigal

Anthony Nolan Research Institute and
1 Department of Immunology, the Royal Free Hospital, Pond Street, Hampstead, London NW3 2QG, UK

Infection due to cytomegalovirus (CMV) represents a significant complication in BMT. However, after allogeneic BMT, the recovery of $CD8^+$ cytotoxic T lymphocytes (CTL) responses to CMV is correlated with an improved outcome from CMV disease [1,2]. On the other hand, while infection by CMV is a common occurrence in healthy individuals, it remains largely asymptomatic, with the virus persisting in a latent state for many years if not for life. In the peripheral blood of such normal asymptomatic CMV seropositive individuals, CTL's specific for CMV are present at a relatively high frequency [3].

The size of human CMV genome (235 kbp) allows for a large potential coding capacity, and thus there are obvious difficulties in determining whether individual viral proteins are immunodominant with respect to the CTL response. It has been suggested that virion coat proteins introduced exogenously as parts of the virus particle are processed and presented by class I HLA molecules. One of the key structural proteins is the lower matrix 65 kDa phosphoprotein (pp65) that has been shown to be a predominant viral antigen recognised by CMV-specific CTL's after infection [4]. However, the specific viral epitopes recognised by cytotoxic T cells have not yet been characterised.

Class I molecules of the MHC present antigens in the form of short peptides to CTL. Several murine as well as human cell lines with defects in the class I mediated antigen processing pathway have recently been of particular importance in the elucidation of intracellular events associated with antigen presentation. The T2 cell line [5,6], derived from the Epstein-Barr virus transformed B lymphoblastoid cell line *.174* has a large deletion in the MHC class II region including the TAP1 and TAP2 genes which encode the transporters proteins. These cell lines are unable to present endogenously synthesised peptides. However, the addition of appropriate peptides induces assembly of the class I molecules from the constituent subunits [6]. The T2 cell line expresses HLA-A2 and HLA-B5 molecules, but only HLA-A2 molecules are present at a low density, on the cell surface of the T2 cell line. Using this T2 cell line, we have analysed the binding of several pp65-CMV peptides to HLA-A2 molecules.

Results

We have used the amino acid sequence of the CMV pp65 protein to design peptides sharing consensus motifs that matched the published consensus sequence for HLA-A2-binding peptides. The dominant anchor residues for HLA-A2 have been shown to be leucine, valine, isoleucine or methionine at position 2 and valine, leucine, isoleucine or alanine at position 9 or 10. Consequently, 17 CMV pp65 peptides were synthesised with this anchor motif in mind. Nonamer peptides from the influenza A matrix M1 protein and nucleoprotein that have been described as having high binding affinity for the HLA-A2 molecule [7] were also synthesised for use as positive controls in the T2 binding assay. The HLA-B27 binding peptide (residues 383-392), from influenza nucleoprotein was used as a negative control *(Table I)*.

Using the T2 assay, we have found that some CMV pp65 peptides are able to stabilise the HLA-A2 molecules on the surface of the T2 cells to different degrees *(Figure 1)*. While the positive control, a HLA-A2-binding influenza matrix 58-66 peptide AE41, resulted in a 6 fold increase in cell surface HLA-A2 stabilisation (fluorescence intensity), the negative control HLA-B27 binding peptide AE43 showed not increase. The remaining CMV peptides designed with the HLA-A2 binding motif showed increased fluorescence ranging from

Table I. CMV and control peptides used in T2 binding assay. Anchor residues are underlined

CMV-PP65 PEPTIDES

		I2 - V9			**L2 - L9**		
AE42	NLVPMVATV	AF83	VIGDQYVK V	AF91	VLPHETRL L		
AE44	VLGPISGH V	AF84	KISHIMLD V	AF92	ALFFFDID L		
AE45	MLNIPSIN V	AF85	RIFAELEG V	AF93	GLSISGNL L		
AE46	TLESFCED V						
AE48	RLLQTGIH V	**L2 - I9**		**I2 - L9**			
AE47	LLQTGIHVR V	AF86	VLCPKNM II	AF89	SIYVYALPL		
AE49	ILARNLVPM V	AF87	NLLMNGQQ I	AF90	DIYRIFAE L		

CONTROL PEPTIDES

AE41	GILGFVFTL V	(HLA-A*0201)
AE43	SRYWAIRTR	(HLA-B27)

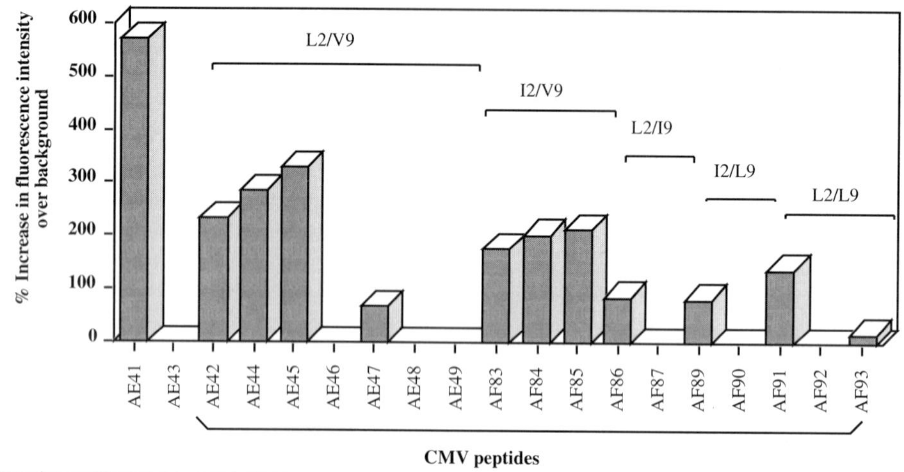

Figure 1. The T2 assay was done as described elsewhere [8]. Briefly, 5x 10^5 T2 cell aliquots were incubated overnight with 100 µM of synthetic peptide at 37 °C. A control aliquot of T2 cells to which no peptide was added was set up in parallel. Cell surface HLA molecules were then detected by indirect immunofluorescence. The HLA class I specific antibody W6/32, was used as the primary staining step and binding was detected using FITC-conjugated sheep-anti-mouse IgG as the secondary antibody. The level of class I stabilisation was then determined using flow cytometric analysis.

1.5 to 3.5 fold compared with control no peptide. In particular peptides AE42, AE44 and AE45 bearing anchor residues leucine and valine at positions 2 and 9 respectively showed good HLA class I stabilisation. These peptides also have in their sequences several hydrophobic residues like is the case of the peptide AE42 valine and alanine in positions 6 and 7.

In contrast, peptides AE46, AE47, AE48 and AE49 showed no stabilisation, although they possessed the same anchor residues. However, these peptides contain at least one charged residue in secondary positions which may explain their poor binding. Interestingly, the peptide AE46, does not stabilise the HLA -A2 molecule although it has an aromatic residue (phenylalanine) in position 5 which has been shown to be associated with preferential binding [9]. However, its lack of affinity can be explained by the presence of two negatively charged residues (glutamic acid) in positions 3 and 7. Since it is known that a negatively charged residue at position 3 is common in non-binding peptides [10]. The same observation that hydrophobic and aromatic residues in secondary positions are relevant for preferential binding and that negatively or positively charged residues are associated with poor binding or non binding can be also applied to the rest of our pp65-CMV peptides bearing different anchor motifs (I2-L9, L2-I9, L2-L9 or I2-V9). Our observations confirm previous studies where the importance of the binding motif and secondary residues was outlined [9,10].

Discussion

Using the T2 binding assay, a number of nonamer sequences from pp65 that stabilise the HLA-A2 molecules present in the T2 cell lines have been identified. However, although such peptides stabilise HLA-A2 molecules, one might find the problem that CTL's stimulated *in vitro* with peptides may not always recognise endogenously processed antigens. Similarly, even if these peptides bind to the HLA-A2 molecule, they may not be recognised by CMV-specific CTL's. Therefore, the CTL response to these peptides is being analysed in order to determine: (a) if they are able to generate specific CTLs that can recognise CMV infected targets and (b) if they can be recognised by CMV or pp65 specific CTLs. In addition, pp65 peptides designed with consensus binding motifs for other HLA class I alleles will be investigated using the described systems.

The identification of the CMV antigenic peptide will aid the generation of recombinant vaccines that could be used to immunise patients against CMV infection. And the development of CTL's could be helpful to investigate the potential for selective reconstitution of CMV-specific immunity in bone marrow transplant recipients by the adoptive transfer of CMV-specific T cell clones generated from the respective bone marrow donor. Thus the identification of specific CTL target antigens may be useful in the design of methods to increase CMV-specific immunity in BMT recipients.

References

1. Reusser P, Riddell SR, Meyers, JD, Greenberg PD. Cytotoxic T- lymphocyte response to cytomegalovirus after human allogeneic bone marrow transplantation: pattern of recovery and correlation with infection and disease. *Blood* 1991; 78 : 1373 - 80.
2. Quinnan Jr GV, Kirmani N, Rook AH, Manischewitz, JF, Jackson L, Moreschi G, Santos GW, Saral R, Burns WH. Cytotoxic T cells in cytomegalovirus infection: HLA-restricted T-lymphocyte and nonT-lymphocyte cytotoxic response correlate with recovery from cytomegalovirus infection in bone marrow transplant recipients. *N Engl J Med* 1982; 307 : 6-13.
3. Borysiewicz LK, Graham S, Hickling JK. Human cytomegalovirus-specific cytotoxic T cells: their precursor frequency and stage specificity. *Eur J Immunol* 1988; 18 : 269-75.
4. Riddell SR, Rabin M, Geballe AP, Britt WT, Greenberg PD. Class I MHC-restricted CTL recognition of cells infected with human cytomegalovirus does not require endogenous viral envelope expression. *J Immunol* 1991; 146 : 2795-804.
5. DeMars R, Rudersorf R, Chang C, Petersen J, Strandtmann J, Korn N, Sidwell B, Orr HT. Mutations that impair a postranscriptional step in expression of HLA-A and -B antigens. *Proc Natl Acad Sci USA* 1985; 82 : 81-3.
6. Cerundulo V, Alexander J, Anderson K, Lambi C, Cresswell P, McMichael A, Gotch F, Townsend A. Presentation of viral antigen controlled by a gene in the major histocompatibility complex. *Nature* 1990; 345 : 449-52.
7. Morrison J, Elvin J, Latron F, Gotch F, Moots R, Strominger JL, McMichael A. Identification of the nonamer peptide from influenza A matrix protein and the role of pockets of HLA-A2 in its recognition by cytotoxic lymphocytes. *Eur J Immunol* 1992; 22:903-7.
8. Elvin J, Cerundulo V, Elliot T, Townsend A. A quantitative assay of peptide-dependent class I assembly. *Eur J Immunol* 1991; 21:2025-31.
9. Drijfhout JW, Brandt RMP, D'Amaro J, Kast WM, Melief CJM. Detailed motifs for peptide binding to HLA-A*0201 derived from large random sets of peptides using a cellular binding assay. *Hum Immunol* 1995; 43: 1-12.
10. Ruppert J, Sidney J, Celis E, Kubo RT, Grey HM, Sette A. Prominent role of secondary anchor residues in peptide binding to HLA-A2.1 molecules. *Cell* 1993; 74: 929-37.

Unusual expression of the LINE-1 retrotransposon in autoimmune disease-prone mice: possible presentation by an MHC class I molecule

K. Benihoud[1], C. Chischportich[1], P. Bobé[1, 2], N. Kiger[1]

1 Inserm U267, 14, avenue Paul-Vaillant-Couturier, 94807 Villejuif Cedex, France
2 Université Paris XI, Orsay, France

During aging, MRL/Mp-lpr/lpr (MRL/lpr) mice develop a syndrome similar to human SLE and rheumatoid arthritis [1], both pathologies in which the events triggering the autoimmune response are unknown. These mice express the autosomal recessive *lpr* mutation, recently characterized as an *ETn* retrotransposon insertion into the *fas* gene [2] which is responsible for a defect in the apoptotic process leading to the proliferation of a large number of CD4⁻ CD8⁻ lymphocytes in the lymph nodes (LN). However, introduction of this gene into other genetic backgrounds has only produced lymphoproliferation associated with mild disease and therefore cannot account for the entire autoimmune syndrome of MRL/lpr mice. These autoimmune disease-prone mice, which are of the H-2^k haplotype, are issued from the following series of backcrosses adapted from Murphy [1]:

AKR/J (H-2^k)	F1-F5	F1	F1	F1-F3			MRL/l (F40) (H-2^k)
X →	X →	X →	X →	X →	F1-F11 →	F12:	
C57BL/6J (H-2^b)	C57BL/6J (H-2^b)	C3H/Di (H-2^k)	AKR/J (H-2^k)	LG/J (H-2^d)			MRL/n(F32) (H-2^k)

An unexpected reactivity to MHC-specific antibodies

Surprisingly, lymphoid and peritoneal cells from some old MRL/lpr mice exhibited, in addition to the expected anti-H-2^k reactivity, an unexpected reactivity towards polyclonal and monoclonal antibodies [3] recognizing an epitope of a polypeptide encompassing the variable amino-acid residues 61-70 of the Aβ^d chain; this epitope is defined as the major determinant of the serologic alloantigenicity [4]. Therefore, the MHC of several mice presenting these unexpected specificities were genotyped by RFLP analysis, using a number of MHC class I and II probes and restriction enzymes known to discriminate between the k and d haplotypes, and it was concluded that these mice were of the H-2^k haplotype [5]. However, these results did not rule out the possibility of short stretches of H-2^d DNA, inherited from the LG strain and "converted" into H-2^k genes, which could not be detected by RFLP analysis.

Molecular cloning of the sequences encoding the unexpected specificities

To distinguish between this hypothesis and the possibility of translation, in this particular strain, of a molecule exhibiting antigenic mimicry with an allogeneic class II chain, a λgt11 expression library was constructed from splenic and LN cells and screened with polyclonal and monoclonal antibodies directed against the Aβ^d determinant. We isolated 30 cDNA clones sharing high sequence homology (>80%) with the 3' end (open reading frame (ORF) 2 encoding a reverse transcriptase) of a LINE-1 (L1) element *(Figure 1)*, a highly repeated endogenous retroviral-like sequence propagated through the mammalian genome *via* retrotransposition [6]. The full-length genomic sequence (6800 bp) of L1 is bordered by short direct repeats, it presents two ORF, and terminates in a 3' polyA$^+$-rich tail. Most elements are truncated to varying degrees at the 5' end, with a fixed 3' end, including a polyA$^+$ tail; heterogeneously sized L1 RNA can be transcribed from both strands giving rise to a majority of defective cDNA copies, which may nevertheless be integrated into host sequences [7]. In some cases, full-length polyadenylated L1 sense-strand transcripts have been detected in murine and human lymphoma cell lines or teratocarcinoma cells as well as in blastocysts.

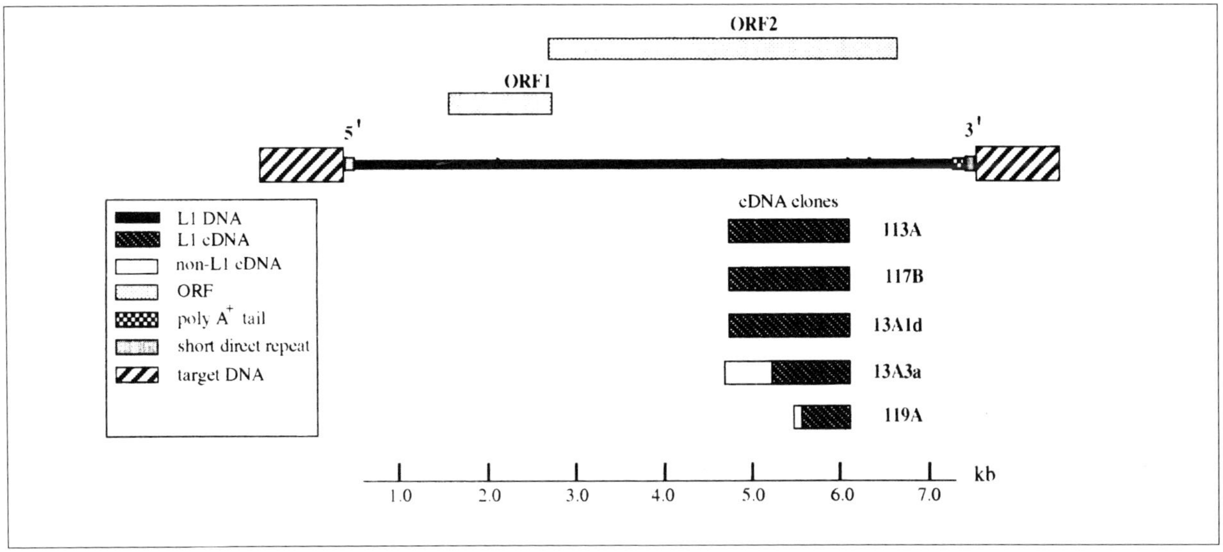

Figure 1. Diagram comparing 5 of the cDNA clones that were isolated to the known LINE-1 element.

Expression of L1 sequences in MRL/lpr mice

Using a cDNA probe that detects transcripts from both strands, we previously observed an overexpression of total L1 RNA in the spleen of the MRL/lpr mouse used for the construction of cDNA library in comparison to its ancestor strains [6]. In order to detect only the sense-strand (susceptible to being translated) transcription of L1 sequences in MRL/lpr, we undertook a systematic study in different lymphoid (spleen, LN, thymus) and non-lymphoid (liver, heart, brain, intestine, lung) organs using antisense RNA probes. The results showed that full-length (7 kb) sense-strand polyA$^+$ RNA are transcribed in all MRL/lpr organs (including liver, spleen, LN, thymus) not only in old but also in newborn mice. *Figure 2* illustrates the sense-strand transcription in the thymus of a newborn mouse and that in the murine teratocarcinoma cell line F9, used as a positive control, and shows that both heterogeneously sized and full-length transcripts are present at birth. Nevertheless, radioimmunoassays have shown that the L1/Aβ^d cross-reactive mAb only recognizes lymphoid cells from old MRL/lpr mice. We immunoprecipitated the molecules recognized by the anti-Aβ^d 34-5-3 mAb : after metabolic labeling of spleen and LN cells with ^{35}S methionine. As expected, this antibody coprecipitated class II α and β chains in the d haplotype (not shown). In contrast to other H-2^k

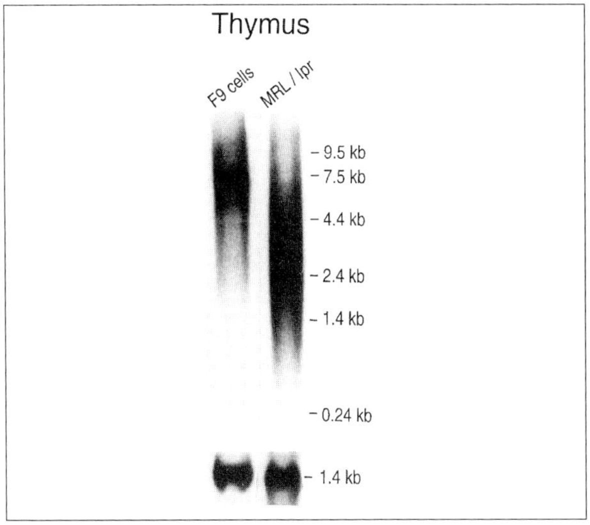

Figure 2. Expression of LINE-1 (top) and GAPDH (bottom) polyA+ RNA in newborn thymus, and F9 cells. Hybridization of the coding-strand RNA-specific riboprobe recognizing the 5' end of the Northern-blotted retrotransposon (L1). The blots were dehybridized and then rehybridized with the control GAPDH riboprobe.

strains, two molecules, 45 and 12 kDa, were coprecipitated from MRL/lpr spleen and LN lysates. Under reducing conditions, MRL/lpr lysates were highly contaminated by unassociated light and heavy immunoglobulin chains; under the non-reducing conditions used in the experiment reported in *Figure 3*, these contaminants were less important in the spleen and disappeared from LN (organ poor in B lymphocytes) lysates in which only the 45- and 12- kDa molecules were found. These molecules migrated exactly like class I molecules coprecipitated by the anti-(H-2KD)^k 3-83 mAb or by an anti-β2-microglobulin (β2m) antiserum (not shown). Furthermore, these two bands can be eliminated by preclearing MRL/lpr lysates with the anti-β2m antiserum coupled to protein-A-sepharose prior to immunoprecipitation with mAb 34-5-3 (not shown). These findings suggest that a peptide derived from the L1 reverse transcriptase is presented at the cell surface in association with a class I molecule in the MRL strain.

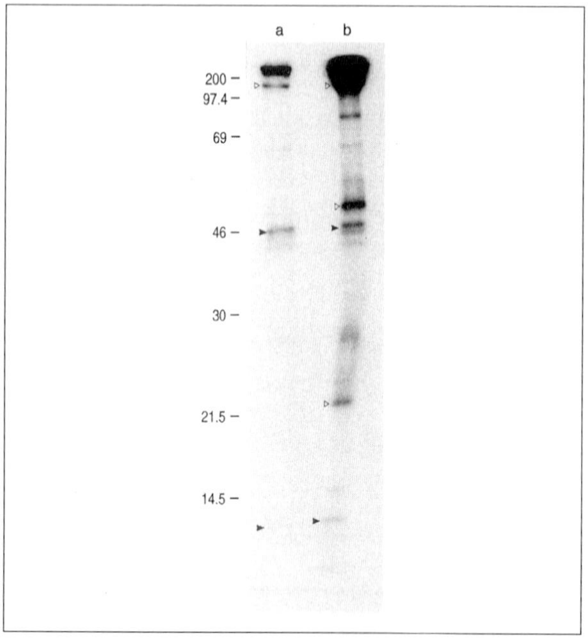

Figure 3. Analysis on 12% SDS-PAGE under non-reducing conditions of the proteins immunoprecipitated by mAb 34-5-3 from MRL/lpr LN (a) and splenic (b) lysates. White arrowheads: contaminating free and associated heavy and light immunoglobulin chains, black arrowheads: the immunoprecipitated molecules. On the left are the molecular masses (kDa).

There is increasing evidence of an association between autoimmune manifestations and retroviruses [8]. Systemic autoimmune diseases are characterized by defects in immune tolerance to self antigens which could include products of endogenous retroviral sequences and retrotransposons. Triggering by an infectious virus antigenically similar to the endogenous retroviral protein could elicit such an autoimmune response. This possibility is illustrated by studies demonstrating a loss of tolerance to an endogenous viral protein in a transgenic mouse after virus infection [9]. Therefore, the expression of a full-length L1 transcript encoding a reverse transcriptase highly similar to a viral protein and the possible transport of its peptidic product to the cell membrane by a class I molecule could be a possible mechanism at work in disease induction.

References

1. Murphy ED. Lymphoproliferation (lpr) and other single-locus models for murine lupus. In : ME Gerswin, B Merchant, eds. *Immunologic Defects in Laboratory Animals*. New York : Plenum Publishing Co, 1981: 143-73.
2. Nagata S, Golstein P. The Fas death factor. *Science* 1995; 267: 1449-56.
3. Bobé P, Gachelin G, Kiger N. Spontaneous autocytotoxicity against an unexpected H-2d haplotype in MRL/lpr (H-2k) autoimmune disease-prone mice. *Immunogenetics* 1987; 25: 251-7.
4. Buerstedde JM, Pease LR, Bell MP, Nilson AE, Buerstedde G, Murphy D, McKean DJ. Identification of an immunodominant region on the I-Aβ chain using site-directed mutagenesis and DNA-mediated gene transfer. *J Exp Med* 1988; 167: 473-87.
5. Delarbre C, Bobé P, Kiger N, Kourilsky P, Gachelin G. Further serological and RFLP analysis of the MRL-+/+ and MRL-lpr/lpr mice. *J Immunogenet* 1988; 15: 307-19.
6. Bobé P, Benihoud K, Kiger N. Allogenic MHC class II determinant(s) in MRL/lpr autoimmune-prone mice. *J Immunol* 1993; 151: 2813-9.
7. Singer MF, Krek V, McMillan JP, Swergold GD. LINE-1: a human transposable element. *Gene* 1993; 135: 183-8.
8. Krieg AM, Gourley MF, Perl A. Endogenous retroviruses: potential etiologic agents in autoimmunity. *FASEB* J 1992; 6: 2537-44.
9. Zinkernagel RM, Cooper S, Chambers J, Lazzarini RA, Hengartner H, Arnheiter H. Virus-induced autoantibody response to a transgenic viral antigen. *Nature* 1990; 345: 68-71.

HLA-peptide interactions: theoretical and experimental approaches

D. Monos [1], A. Soulika [1], E. Argyris [1], J. Gorga [2], L. Stern [3], V. Magafa [4], P. Cordopatis [4], I. Androulakis [5], C. Floudas [5]

1 Department of Pediatrics, University of Pennsylvania, Children's Hospital of Philadelphia, 1208B Abramson Research Building, 34th and Civic Center Boulevard, Philadelphia, PA 19104, USA
2 Department of Pediatrics, Childrens Hospital of Pittsburgh and University of Pittsburgh-School of Medicine, 6115 Rangos Research Center, 3705 Fifth Avenue, Pittsburgh, PA 15213, USA
3 Department of Chemistry, Massachusetts Institute of Technology, 77 Massacusetts Avenue,Cambridge, MA 02139, USA
4 Laboratory of Pharmacognosy and Chemistry of Natural Products, Department of Pharmacy, University of Patras, Patras 26500, Greece
5 Department of Chemical Engineering, Princeton University, Princeton, NJ 08544-5263, USA

A number of methods have been developed that investigate the HLA/peptide interactions and involve cocrystallization of HLA protein with a single peptide, biochemical isolation and characterization of naturally HLA-associated peptides and a variation of a binding assay that involves employment of random phage-peptide libraries. These methods have provided useful insights and has become apparent that almost every residue on a particular peptide influences the interaction with either the HLA or the T cell receptor molecule. The already made progress has adequately established that the complex interacts in a specific manner, its complexity, however, is such that invites alternative approaches for studying these molecular interactions.
The approach taken in this study consists of a combined theoretical and experimental study. The basic idea is to examine whether the results provided by the predictive power of the theoretical studies concerning HLA/peptide interactions, are in accord with actual experimental data obtained by employing binding assays. For this purpose the potential energy of the interaction between each individual aminoacid with pocket 1 of DR1, was compared to the binding affinity of the haemagglutinin (306-318) peptide analog, carrying that particular aminoacid at position 308, as it was interacting with DR1.

Methods

The modeling and global optimization studies were performed as described in 1-3. Human DR1 from the lymphoblastoid cell line LG2 and insect DR1 from culture supernatans of Sf9 cells were purified as previously described [4]. Radiolabeling and peptide binding was performed as previously described [5].

Results

Modeling and global optimization of interacting peptides

The modeling and optimization studies of the interactions between the HLA-DR1 protein and an influenza virus peptide are based on a novel decomposition approach. This decomposition approach consists of the following stages.

Stage 1

This first stage consists of a decomposition of the interactions between the HLA-DR1 protein and an influenza virus peptide into the interactions of the five pockets of the HLA-DR1 protein, identified explicitly in the crystallographic studies described by Stern [6], with each of the naturally occuring aminoacids. This decomposition allows us to focus first on the interactions of each pocket with each naturally occuring aminoacid and has as key objective the study of the binding affinity of each aminoacid separately.

Stage 2

In this stage, pocket 1 of the HLA-DR1 protein is represented by a number of residues. The work by Stern [6] provides information on the constituent aminoacids of each pocket of the HLA-DR1 protein.

Stage 3

For pocket 1 interacting with each naturally occuring aminoacids, a mathematical model was constructed that represents all the energetic atom-to-atom interactions. These interactions are classified as (1) intra-interactions

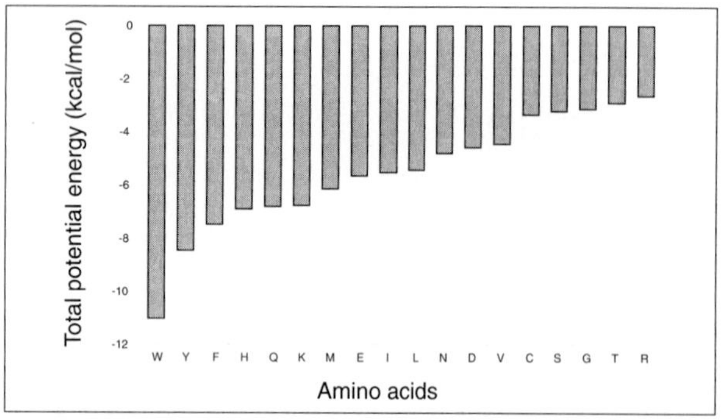

Figure 1. Calculated total potential energy for every single amino acid indicated in the horizontal axis as it interacts with pocket 1 of DR1.

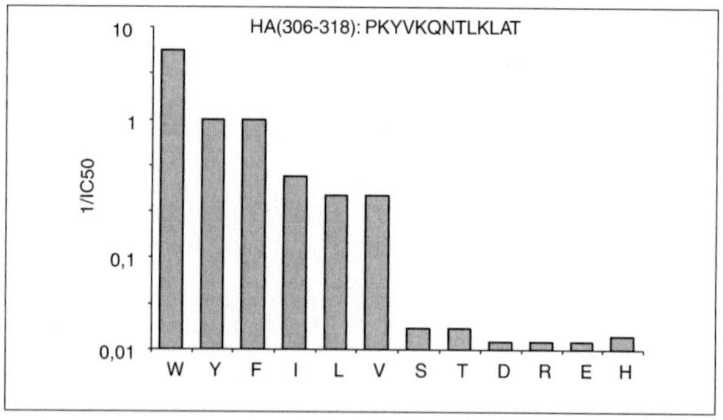

Figure 2. Binding of HA(306-318) and its analogs to DR1: Y(308)-HA (306-318) has been susbstituted with every single amino acid indicated in the horizontal axis. 1/IC50 reflects relative binding.

between the atoms of the residues that define a pocket of the HLA-DR1 protein and the atoms of the considered naturally occuring aminoacid, and (2) inter-interactions between the atoms of the considered naturally occuring aminoacid. These interactions consist of electrostatic, nonbonded, hydrogen-bonds, torsional, and cystine loop-closing components.

Stage 4

Having a mathematical model which accounts for all the interactions of a given pocket and a given naturally occuring aminoacid, in this stage we formulated the global optimization problem which minimizes the total potential emergy subject to lower and upper bounds on the degrees of freedom.

Stage 5

In this stage, an energetic-based criterion that allows for the comparison of the binding between a given pocket and each naturally occuring aminoacid was introduced. This measure, which is denoted as DE, corresponds to the difference of (1) the global minimum total potential energy that is obtained in stage 4 and which is indicated as $\varepsilon_{HLA+BPi}$, and (2) the global minimum potential energy of the considered naturally occuring aminoacid when it is very far away from the pocket and which is denoted as ε^0_{BPi}. This criterion represents a measure of the binding affinity of each aminoacid to a given pocket, in the sense that it quantifies the tendency of an aminoacid to bind with a pocket of the HLA-DR1 molecule. The aminoacid that exhibits the least DE corresponds to the one with the best possible binding to that pocket of the HLA-DR1 protein.

Stage 6

In this stage, we repeat stages 3-5 for each naturally occuring aminoacid and hence create a rank ordered list for the binding of each aminoacids to a given pocket.

Our preliminary modeling and global optimization studies of the interactions of the HLA-DR1 protein with the influenza virus peptide, have focused on pocket 1 of the HLA-DR1 molecule and consist of stages 1-5 of the aforementioned decomposition approach. The total potential energy that accounts for the intra and inter types of interactions does not include any solvation contributions, and the results in the form of rank-ordered list are as shown in *Figure 1*.

Binding assays of influenza HA peptide (306-318) analogs to HLA-DR1

The objective of this series of binding assays was to provide the experimental basis that would evaluate the modeling and global optimization studies, as applied on the DR1/HA(306-318) complex. Since the HA(306-318) peptide residue that interacts with P1 is Y(308) a number of analog peptides were synthesized that substituted the Y(308) residue with 11 different aminoacids. The relative binding affinity of each HA (306-318) substituted peptide to the baculovirus expressed DR1 molecule was evaluated by competition binding assays. Immunoaffinity purified soluble DR1 molecules from culture medium of Sf9 insect cells were incubated with ^{125}I-labelled Y(308)-HA(306-318) peptide and a competitive analog peptide X(308)-HA(306-318), where X is one of the 11 aminoacids tested, at concentration 0.2, 2, 20 and 200 μM. After 20 hours of incubation at 37°C the DR/peptide complex was analyzed by native polyacrylamide gel electrophoresis (PAGE). The degree of competition between the labelled natural HA peptide and its analog for DR1 was evaluated by scanning the band that corresponded to the dimer DR on an imaging film. Relative binding values were derived from the reciprocal of 50% inhibitory concentration (IC50) of each peptide. *Figure 2* illustrates the relative binding of the individual analog peptides.

Three groups of binding affinities were basically observed. The first group included analog peptides with W, Y and F. These peptides bound with the highest affinity to DR1. The second group included the analog peptides with I, L and V and characterized by an intermediate level of affinity for DR1. Analogs with Q, K, M, N, G and A at 308-HA(306-318) were not synthesized.

These results are in agreement with studies that have identified the peptide motif of DR1 by sequencing analysis of eluted peptides or by employing phage peptide libraries [7]. According to these motifs, the prefered anchor residues for P1 are Y, F, W, V, L, M and I. Furthermore, studies on the binding of HA(308) peptide analogs to DR1 have been previously reported [8]. The affinity of single substituted HA (308) peptides was evaluated for F,K,S and D. The reported results are in direct agreement with the results in *Figure 2*.

Additional studies have evaluated the effect of single amino acid substitutions at the anchor residue Y to the binding of the YRSMAAAAA peptide to DR1 [9]. Even though the employed peptide in this study is very different from HA(306-318) and the source of DR1 is human BLCL, the relative binding affinities of the analog peptides were identical to the relative binding affinities of our study (*Figure 1*). These data suggest that irrespectively of the differences in the overall sequence the anchor residue p1(p1 being the residue that interacts with P1 of the HLA) is critical for binding and that the contribution of the other residues, for the two different peptides, should be comparable and comprise only a small fraction of the total energy required for their binding affinity. These conclusions are in accord with previous reports addressing not only the issue of pocket specificity [9] but also issues related to the thermodynamics of this interaction [10].

Discussion

The global optimization studies provided a rank ordered list where the three amino acids W,Y and F have had the lowest potential energies for binding to P1 of DR1 (*Figure 1*). This is in absolute agreement with the binding studies, where analog peptides of HA (306-318) with W,Y or F at position 308 provided the best affinities for DR1 (*Figure 2*). Furthermore the aminoacids I, L and V as they interacted with P1 of DR1 were characterized by potential energies that corresponded to 9th, 10th and 13th position, on the list respectively. When analog peptides with these aminoacids were tested in binding assays they resulted in intermediate level of affinities for DR1. The DE value of -4,441 kcal/mol for the binding of V, reflects an approximate increase of 60%, as compared to Tryptophane's potential energy that is -11.023 kcal/mol. Provided that an increase of 32% (W-F) in potential energy reflects a group of strong binders, an increase of up to 60% could very well reflect a group of intermediate level binders.

The characteristic increase of DE 1.12 kcal/mol that separates V (-4,441 kcal/mol) from C (-3.32 kcal/mol) may signal interactions of aminoacid and P1 with potential energies that reflect the third group of low affinity analogs in the binding assay system. This group includes the HA(306-318) analogs with S, T, D, E, R and H at 308. Characteristically the algorithm provided potential energies for S, T and R that are indeed at the bottom of the list, with DE of -3.221, -2.905 and -2.601 kcal/mol respectively. Aminoacids H, E and D however appear on the list as 4th, 8th and 12th respectively, deviating significantly from what would have been expected based on the binding affinities of the respective analogs. It is noteworthy that these three aminoacids are charged molecules which are highly hydrophilic and therefore unlikely to fit comfortably in the hydrophobic environment of P1 pocket. Yet the algorithm seems not to account succesfully for this fact.

Finally there is a number of aminoacids including Q, K, M, N, C, G and A for which no analogs were synthesized. For these aminoacids we can not comment directly. However it is already known that peptides with M at p1 are intermediate level binders [8], while peptides with A at p1 result in loss of peptide binding [9]. The potential energy of -6.150 kcal/mol for M and -2.969 kcal/mol for A, rate these amino acids as 7th and 17th respectively and are consistent with the reported binding studies. Indirect data therefore support the results obtained with the global optimization algorithm.

It should be mentioned that no direct relationship has yet been established between actual levels of potential energies and values of affinities of the corresponding analogs for the DR1 molecule. The comparisons made among DE values of interactions and affinities of the analogs are only relative to each other. Provided we establish a satisfactory relationship between the two approaches we will then investigate whether an exact quantitative relationship exist between the two methods.

References

1. Maranas CD, Floudas CA. A deterministic global optimization approach for molecular structure determination. *J Chem Phys* 1994; 100: 1247-61.
2. Androulakis IP, Maranas CD, Floudas CA. aBB : a global optimization method for general constrained nonconvex problems. *J Global Optimization* 1995; 7: 337-63.
3. Maranas CD, Androulakis IP, Floudas CA. A deterministic global optimization approach for the protein folding problem. In : Pardalos PM, Shallaway, Xue, eds. *DIMACS Series in Discrete Mathematics and Computer Science* 1996; 133-50.
4. Gorga JC, Horejsi V, Johnson DR, Raghupathy R, Strominger JL. Purification and characterization of class II histocompatibility antigens from a homozygous human B cell line. *J Biol Chem* 1987; 262: 16087-94.
5. Scheirle A, Takacs B, Kremer L, Marin F, Sinigaglia F. Peptide binding to soluble HLA-DR4 molecules produced by insect cells. *J Immunol* 1992; 149 : 1994-9.
6. Stern LJ, Brow JH, Jardetzky TS, Gorga JC, Urban RG, Strominger JL, Wiley DC. Crystal structure of the human class II MHC protein HLA-DR1 complexed with an influenza virus peptide. *Nature* 1994; 368 : 215-21.
7. Rammensee HG, Friede T, Stevanovic S. MHC ligands and peptide motifs:first listing. *Immunogenetics* 1995; 41: 178-228.
8. Jardetzky TS, GorgaJC, Bush R, Rothbard J, Strominger JL, Wile DC. Peptide binding to HLA-DR1: a peptide with most residues substituted to alanine retains MHC binding. *EMBO J* 1990; 9: 1797-803.
9. Hammer J, Belunis C, Bolin D, Papadopoulos J, Walsky R, Higelin J, Danho W, Sinigaglia F, Nagy ZA. High-affinity binding of short peptides to major histocompatibility complex class II molecules by anchor combinations. *Proc Natl Acad Sci USA* 1994; 91 : 4456-60.
10. Hill CM, Liu A, Marshall NW, Mayer J, Jorgensen B, Yuan B, Cubbon RM, Nichols EA, Wicker LS, Rothbard JB. Exploration of requirements for peptide binding to HLA DRB1*0401. *J Immunol* 1994; 152: 2890.

Function of HLA

Signal transduction. NK receptors and function

Contents

• Signal transduction. NK receptors and function

Engagement of HLA class I induces tyrosine phosphorylation of cytoskeletal proteins in human EBV-transformed B cells

W. Di Berardino, V. Imbert[1], J.F. Peyron[1], O. Munoz, J.L. Cousin

Unité de Recherche sur les Interactions Cellulaires en Immunologie et Immunopathologie, INSERM U343, Hôpital de l'Archet, route Saint-Antoine de Ginestière, BP 79, 06202 Nice Cedex 03, France
1 Laboratoire d'Immunologie Cellulaire et Moléculaire, INSERM U364, Faculté de Médecine Pasteur, 06107 Nice Cedex 02, France

In addition to their well-established role in antigen-specific presentation, the MHC molecules can function as signal transduction components. Cross-linking HLA class I molecules can activate the phosphoinositide pathway with subsequent mobilization of free-Ca^{2+} from internal stores [1]. HLA class I antigens also play a role in cell adhesion that requires the integrity of the cytoskeleton [2]. It has been shown that during cell adhesion, the cytoskeleton is reorganized and several proteins are phosphorylated. Among them, the focal adhesion-associated protein $pp125^{FAK}$ plays a central role. This protein is associated with the cytoskeletal protein paxillin [3], that link actin filament bundles to the plasma membrane at sites of cell adhesion [4]. Paxillin and $pp125^{FAK}$ become coordinately phosphorylated on tyrosine in response to various stimuli [5]. Recently, talin, another focal adhesion protein, has also been shown to interact with $pp125^{FAK}$ [6]. Talin can associate to vinculin (116 kD) that have a binding site for paxillin [3]. All these proteins are potential substrates for $pp125^{FAK}$. *In vitro* binding experiment using the $pp59^{fyn}$ SH2 domain indicate that this PTK binds to the major site of autophosphorylation of $pp125^{FAK}$ [7]. We demonstrate that engagement of the HLA-class I molecules enhances the kinase activity of $pp125^{FAK}$ and $pp59^{fyn}$ and induces tyrosine phosphorylation of the cytoskeleton-associated proteins paxillin, talin and vinculin. These events are observed only with anti-HLA class I B9.12.1 mAb promoting B cell homotypic aggregation [2].

Results and discussion

Tyrosine phosphorylations induced by anti-class I mAbs

Previous studies have shown that changes in the phosphorylation of several proteins regulate their structure and function during cell adhesion *in vivo*. These events are also associated with major rearrangements of the actin cytoskeleton (reviewed in [8]). Therefore we investigated the effects of B9.12.1 on tyrosine phosphorylation of cytoskeleton-associated proteins. Cells were treated with anti-HLA-class I or irrelevant mAb and lysed in RIPA buffer. Tyrosine-phosphorylated proteins were immunoprecipitated with anti-phosphotyrosine, separated by SDS-PAGE and transferred to Immobilon membrane. Samples were assayed for paxillin, talin and vinculin by immunoblot using appropriate monoclonal antibodies. As shown in *Figure 1*, B9.12.1 mAb strongly stimulated tyrosine phosphorylation of talin (225 kDa), vinculin (116 kD) and paxillin (68 kD).

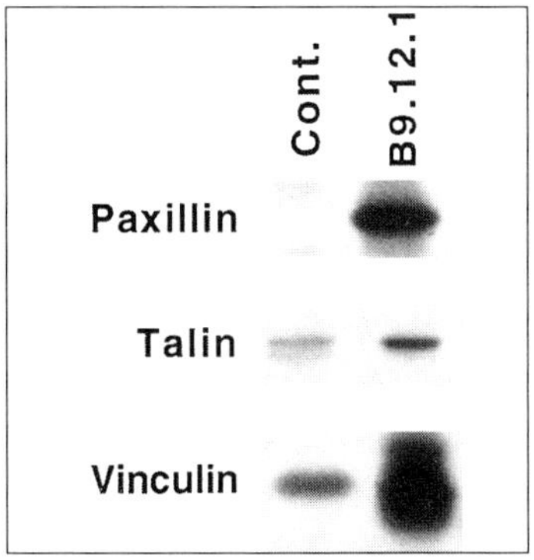

Figure 1. Induction of paxillin, talin and vinculin tyrosine phosphorylation by HLA class I. SKW6.4 cells were treated for 10 min at 37°C with the mAbs, washed and lysed in RIPA buffer. Tyrosine phosphorylation of paxillin, talin and vinculin were analyzed by immunoprecipitation with an anti-phosphotyrosine mAb (UBI, 5 mg/assay) and immunoblotting with anti-paxillin (Transduction laboratories, 1: 250), anti-talin (Sigma, 1: 200) or anti-vinculin (Sigma, 1: 400).

p125^{FAK} phosphorylation in HLA class I-treated cells

Recently, the coordinate tyrosine phosphorylation of pp125^{FAK} and paxillin has been observed in many systems. Consequently, we examined whether HLA class I mAbs trigger tyrosine phosphorylation of pp125^{FAK} in B lymphocytes. Lysates from cells stimulated for 5 min with anti-HLA class I mAbs were immunoprecipitated with either anti-p125^{FAK} or isotype-matched control mAb. Immunoprecipitates were incubated with [γ-^{32}P]ATP *(Figure 2)*. Clearly, B9.12.1 mAb induced a marked incorporation of [^{32}P] in pp125^{FAK} component. Another band of 60 kDa is also observed in anti-p125^{FAK} immunoprecipitates from B9.12.1-treated cells suggesting that a src kinase coprecipitated with pp125^{FAK}.

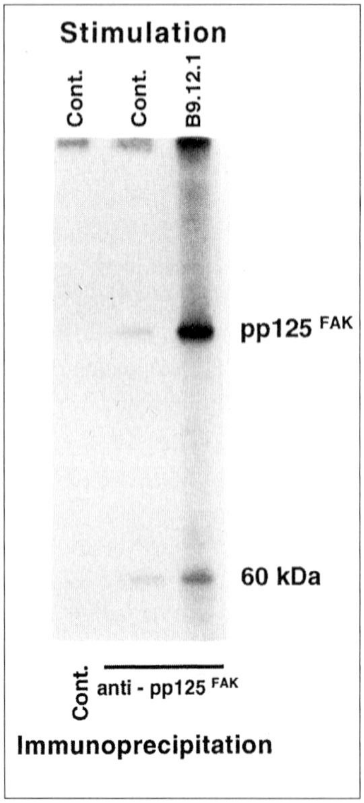

Figure 2. Stimulation of pp125^{FAK} tyrosine kinase activity. Cells were stimulated with the mAbs for 5 min and lysed in RIPA buffer. After preclearing with protein A immunoadsorbant, lysates were immunoprecipitated with anti-p125^{FAK} (UBI, 5 mg/assay) or control mAb. Immunocomplexes were incubated with [γ-^{32}P]ATP for 20 min. Phosphorylated proteins were separated by SDS-PAGE and revealed by autoradiography.

Stimulation of pp59^{fyn} protein tyrosine kinase activity

Recently, pp59^{fyn} has been involved in pp125^{FAK} and paxillin phosphorylation [10]. Analysis of pp59^{fyn} activity was performed on immunoprecipitates from cells untreated or stimulated for 5 min with anti-class I mAbs. As shown in *Figure 3*, engagement of HLA-class I molecules with B9.12.1 mAb activates the protein tyrosine kinase pp59^{fyn}.

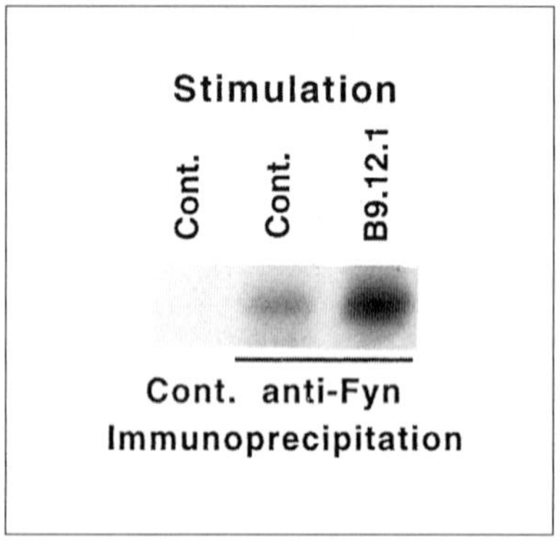

Figure 3. Activation of pp59^{fyn} tyrosine kinase activity by the HLA class I mAb B9.12.1. Cells were treated for 5 min at 37°C with the mAbs, washed and lysed in lysis buffer. pp59^{fyn} was precipitated using a specific antiserum (UBI, 1: 100). Kinase assay was performed in the presence of [γ-^{32}P]ATP. Samples were separated by SDS/PAGE and phosphoproteins visualized by autoradiography.

Conclusion

We demonstrated that engagement of HLA class I antigens in EBV-transformed B lymphocytes induces a rapid activation of protein tyrosine kinases pp125^{FAK} and pp59^{fyn} and the phosphorylation of the cytoskeletal components paxillin, talin and vinculin [9] that correlated with homotypic aggregation. This suggests that tyrosine phosphorylations of cytoskeletal protein bring about cytoskeletal rearrangement leading to activation or surface expression of an adhesion molecule.

References

1. Geppert TD, Davi, LS, Gur H, MC, W, Lipsky P E. Accessory cell signals involved in T cell activation. *Immunol Rev* 1990; 117: 5-66.
2. Ødum N, Ledbetter J A, Martin P, Geraghty D, Tsu T, Hansen J A, Gladstone P. Homotypic aggregation of human cell lines by HLA-class II, -class Ia and HLA-G-specific monoclonal antibodies. *Eur J Immunol* 1991; 21: 2121-31.
3. Turner CE., Miller JT. Primary sequence of paxillin contains putative SH2 and SH3 domain binding motifs and multiple LIM domains: identification of a vinculin and $pp125^{FAK}$-binding region. *J Cell Sci* 1994; 107: 1583-91.
4. Burridge K, Fath K, Kelly T, Nuckolls G, Turner C. Focal adhesions: transmembrane junctions between the extracellular matrix and the cytoskeleton. *Annu Rev Cell Biol* 1988; 4: 487-525.
5. Burridge K, Turner CE, Roher L H. Tyrosine phosphorylation of paxillin and $pp125^{FAK}$ accompanies cell adhesion to extracellular matrix: a role in cytoskeletal assembly. *J Cell Biol* 1992; 119: 893-903.
6. Chen HC, Appeddu PA, Parsons JT, Hildebrand JD, Schaller MD, Guan JL. Interaction of focal adhesion kinase with cytoskeletal protein talin. *J Biol Chem* 1995; 270: 16995-9.
7. Cobb BS, Schaller MD, Leu TH, Parsons J T. Stable association of pp60src and $pp59^{fyn}$ with the focal adhesion-associated protein tyrosine kinase, $pp125^{FAK}$. *Mol Cell Biol* 1994; 14: 147-55.
8. Luna EJ, Hitt AL. Cytoskeleton-plasma membrane interactions. *Science* 1992; 258: 955-64.
9. Groech ME, Otto JJ. Purification and characterization of a 85 kDa talin-binding fragment of vinculin. *Cell Motil Cytoskeleton* 1990; 15: 41-50.
10. Thomas SM, Soriano P, Imamoto A. Specific and redundant roles of src and fyn in organizing the cytoskeleton. *Nature* 1995; 376: 267-71.

The role of HLA class I molecules in endothelial cell activation

H. Bian, P.E. Harris, E.F. Reed

Department of Pathology, College of Physicians and Surgeons, Columbia University, 630 West 168th street, New York 10032, USA

Accelerated graft vasculopathy, a type of chronic rejection, is responsible for the majority of late graft failures. This condition is characterized by a diffuse, concentric, intimal occulsive lesion which leads to gradual fibrosis of the transplanted organ [1]. The mechanism of chronic rejection is poorly understood, but it is suspected that the associated vascular changes are a result of anti-HLA antibody-mediated injury to the endothelium [2-4].

In this study, we have explored the hypothesis that anti-HLA antibodies initiate chronic rejection by binding to EC and transducing signals which result in alterations in EC function. Our studies demonstrate that anti-HLA antibody ligation to HLA class I molecules expressed by EC transduces activation and proliferation signals which contribute to the development of graft atherosclerosis.

Materials and methods

Antibodies

The following monoclonal (mAb) and polyclonal antibodies were used : W6/32, a murine mAb that binds to a monomorphic epitope on HLA class I antigens; BB7.2, a murine mAb specific for HLA-A2, A69; Hu-009 (IgM),a human mAb specific for HLA-A2; goat anti-mouse IgG used to cross-link the mouse mAb; mouse IgG mAb and human IgM mAb isotype controls.

Endothelial cells

EC-pSV1 is a stable human SV40-transfected endothelial cell line [5]. The HLA class I phenotype of this cell line is HLA-A2, A3, B51, B27. EC-pSV1 was grown at 37 °C, 5% CO_2, in endothelial cell growth medium (EGM) containing 10ng/ml hEGF, 3 mg/ml Bovine Brain extract, 5% FCS. Assays were performed on EC monolayers that were 80-90% confluent.

Phosphotyrosine immunoblotting

Tyrosine phosphorylation was measured by immunoblotting endothelial cell lysates with the anti-phosphotyrosine mAb PY20. EC (1.4 x 10^6) were incubated for 16 hours in EGM medium without supplements and stimulated for various times with (10 ug/ml) of anti-HLA mAbs, isotype control antibodies and/or crosslinking antibodies at 37 °C. The samples were lysed directly in SDS sample buffer, boiled for 5 min and centrifuged for 10 min at 14,000 x g. The supernatant was electrophoresed on 5-20% gradient SDS-PAGE, blotted on a PVDF membrane and blocked. The immunoblot was incubated with biotinylated PY20 for 1 hour, washed and incubated with avidin-alkaline phosphatase for 1 hour at room temperature. The blot was washed, developed and analysed.

Analysis of inositol phosphates

EC-pSV1 cells were incubated for 16 hours in EGM medium without supplements followed by a 10 min incubation with 10 mM LiCl. Cells were treated with anti-HLA antibodies or control antibodies for the indicated times at 37 °C. The release of (1,4,5)$InsP_3$ was measured using a commercially available Inositol 1,4,5 triphosphate RIA assay kit (Amersham International).

Endothelial cell proliferation assay

EC-pSV1 cells were seeded in 96-well flat bottom plates at 5000 cells /well in EGM. After 18 hours of incubation, EGM was removed and replaced with EGM without supplements. On day 3, anti-MHC class I mAbs or isotype control mAb were added to the cultures. [^{3}H]TdR incorporation was determined after 24, 48, and 72 hours.

Table I. Stimulation of EC-pSV1 proliferation by anti-HLA class I mAbs

Time	Antibody		
(Hours)	IgG Isotype Control	W6/32	BB7.2
24	605*	671	118
48	572	3048	2225
72	320	1913	2401

* [^{3}H]TdR incorporation was determined and the data expressed as the mean cpm of triplicate determinations.

Results and discussion

To determine whether ligation of HLA class I molecules on the surface of EC with anti-HLA antibodies stimulates tyrosine phosphorylation of intracellular proteins we performed Western blot analysis. EC-pSV1 cells were treated with the anti-HLA class I mAb W6/32 alone or in conjunction with a secondary cross-linking antibody for various periods of time. Treatment of EC with W6/32 resulted in an increase in tyrosine phosphorylation of cellular proteins at approximate molecular masses ranging from of 35 kDa and 45 kDa. This response was seen with the primary antibody alone, yet was enhanced upon cross-linking with the secondary antibody. Tyrosine phosphorylation of intracelluar proteins was not observed when EC were treated with isotype matched control antibodies.

Similar patterns of tyrosine phosphorylation were observed when EC were treated with the murine anti-HLA-A2 mAb (BB7.2) and the human anti-HLA-A2 mAb (Hu-009). After 10 min. of antibody ligation, increased tyrosine-phosphorylation of proteins between 35 and 45 kDa was observed. No increase in tyrosine phosphorylation of intracellular proteins was observed after incubation with the isotype control antibodies. These studies show that anti-HLA antibody ligation to HLA class I molecules on the surface of the endothelial cell results in tyrosine phosphorylation of specific intracellular proteins.

To determine if anti-HLA class I antibodies stimulate the release of calcium from intracellular stores of EC, we measured the production of Inositol (1,4,5)-triphosphate [(1,4,5)InsP$_3$] following antibody ligation. Treatment of EC-pSV1 with W6/32 resulted in the generation of 3.0 and 3.8 pm/10^6 cells of (1,4,5)InsP$_3$ at 3 and 7 minutes, respectively. (1,4,5)InsP$_3$ release was unaffected by reacting the cells with isotype control antibodies. These data suggest that HLA class I engagement by specific antibodies triggers the activation of phospholipase C and subsequent hydrolysis of phosphatidylinositol, and generation of (1,4,5)InsP$_3$ and Ca^{+2} flux.

The capacity of mAb to class I MHC antigens to induce endothelial cell proliferation was next examined. EC-pSV1 failed to proliferate in the presence of soluble isotype control antibody. In contrast, EC-pSV1 proliferated when cultured with W6/32 or BB7.2 for 24 and 48 hours. These results demonstrate that ligation of anti-HLA antibodies to HLA antigens expressed by EC induces cellular proliferation *(Table I)*.

We conclude that anti-HLA antibodies are able to initiate signaling events in EC, including increased tyrosine phosphorylation of intracellular proteins and inositol phosphate generation which culminate in cell proliferation. We propose that these events contribute to the development of accelerated graft vasculopathy.

References

1. Azuma H, Tilney NL. Chronic graft rejection. *Curr Op Immunol* 1994; 6: 770-6.
2. Suciu-Foca N, Reed E, D'Agati VD, Ho E, Cohen DJ, Benvenisty AI, McCabe R, Brensilver JM, King DW, Hardy MA. Soluble HLA-antigens, anti-HLA antibodies and anti-Idiotypic antibodies in the circulation of renal transplant recipients. *Transplantation* 1991; 51: 593-601.
3. Suciu-Foca N. , Reed E, Marboe C, Xi YP, Sun YK, Ho E, Rose E, Reemstma K, King DW. Role of anti-HLA antibodies in heart transplantation. *Transplantation* 1991; 51: 716-24.
4. Reed, EF, Hong B, Ho E, Harris PE, Weinberger J, Suciu-Foca N. Monitoring of soluble HLA alloantigens and anti-HLA antibodies identifies heart allograft recipients at risk of transplant associated coronary artery disease. *Transplantation* 1996; 61: 566-72.
5. Lassalle P, LaGrou C, Delneste Y, Sanceau J, Coll J, Torpier G, Wietzerbin J, Stehelin D, Tonnel AB, Capron A. Human endothelial cells transfected by SV40 T antigens: characterization and potential use as a source of normal endothelial factors.*Eur J Immunol* 1992; 22: 425-31.

CD1a mediated signalling on human thymocytes

N. Mooney, S. Laban, M.T. Zilber, D. Charron, C. Gelin

INSERM U396, 15, rue de l'École de Médecine, 75006 Paris, France

Bacterial superantigens (SAg) are a family of proteins which are potent activators of T cells [1]. Some aspects of the model involving a trimolecular complex between MHC-class II, TcR and SAg, are not explained by current data [2] and it has been suggested that MHC non-classical molecules can also present the bacterial enterotoxins. In an attempt to identify such proteins, we have studied the response of human thymocytes to the toxins SEA and TSST-1. Our data demonstrate the involvement of the CD1a molecule in this response.

Results and discussion

A significant proliferation of CD2+ class II- thymocytes could be induced by the SAg SEA or TSST-1, indicating that the SEA (or TSST-1) induced signalling on thymocytes can be MHC-class II independent. An MHC- class II independent cell-to-cell contact can be sufficient for induction of thymocyte proliferation by bacterial SAg as described for human T cell clones. To identify the molecules involved in thymic activation by SEA or TSST-1, the effects of mAbs directed against various thymic surface molecules was tested. The most intriguing result was the clear inhibition observed after the addition of a CD1a mAb (70% inhibition). By contrast, mAbs directed against the CD1b and c molecules did not influence this activation. These results demonstrated that the CD1a molecule is involved in bacterial SAg activation of thymocytes and the ability of CD1a molecules to transmit signals was therefore examined. Firstly, an intracellular calcium flux was induced after stimulation *via* the CD1a molecule and costimulation of CD1a and CD3 resulted in a partial inhibition of the CD3 mediated flux. Secondly, we have examined the effects of CD1a binding on tyrosine phosphorylation using immunoblotting *(Figure 1)*. A CD1a mAb induced a rapid tyrosine phosphorylation of some substrates phosphorylated *via* CD3. The addition of the toxins SEA or TTST-1 to thymocytes lysates did not induced any detectable protein tyrosine phosphorylation. Interestingly, although prestimulation of thymocytes with SEA or TSST-1 had no effect on the phosphorylation pattern induced *via* CD3, such a treatment inhibited the CD1a mediated phosphorylation.

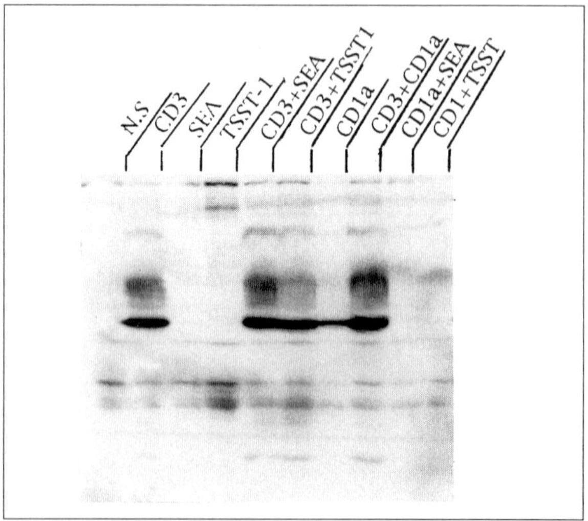

Figure 1. Tyrosine phosphorylation induced *via* CD1a is inhibited by prestimulation with SEA or TSST-1. Thymocytes were cultured in microfuge tubes. At time = -10 min, 10 mg/ml of CD3 , and/or CD1a mAbs were added to the medium. Cells were then lysed and subjected to SDS-PAGE. Following transfer, the filters were incubated with anti-phosphotyrosine mAb. Prestimulation with SEA or TSST-1 (1,5mg/ml) was performed during 20 min before addition of CD3 or CD1a mAbs.

These data represent the first demonstration of a role for the CD1a molecule in the response of human thymocytes to bacterial SAg and show that the signal transduction initiated *via* CD1a might be instrumental in this activation. The peculiar function of the CD1a molecule in the SAg activation as compared to the role of the CD1b and c molecules may reflect the differences in the cytoplasmic tails of these three molecules. The CD1 system has recently been identified as a novel family of Ag presenting molecules separate from those encoded by the MHC [3]. The results described indicate that the CD1a molecule participates in the SAg presentation although it is not yet clear whether this arises *via* direct binding of the SAg or by interaction with the SAg binding molecule.

References

1. Marrack P, Kappler J. The staphylococcal enterotoxins and their relatives. *Science* 1990; 248: 705-11.
2. Yagi J, Uchiyama T, Janeway CA. Stimulator cell type influences the response of T cells to staphylococcal enterotoxins. *J Immunol* 1994; 152: 1154-62.
3. Blumberg RS, Gerdes D, Chott A, Porcelli S, Balk S. Structure and function of the CD1 family of MHC like cell surface proteins. *Immunol Rev* 1995; 147: 5-29.

Structural analysis of the signalling apparatus of the HLA class II molecule

T. Rich, S. Laban, D. Charron , N. Mooney

Laboratoire d'Immunogénétique Humaine, INSERM U396, Institut Biomédical des Cordeliers, 15, rue de l'école de Médécine, 75006 Paris, France

We report here the preliminary results of a mutation study undertaken to examine signal transduction mediated via ligation of the class II histocompatibility antigen. Several lines of evidence indicate that signal pathways may be activated following class II ligation of APC's [1, 2]. The antibody mediated cross-linking of class II expressed by primary human B cells has been shown to result in an increase in intracellular calcium whereas PKC mobilization and activation was observed following class II cross-linking on a human lymphoblastoid B cell line. Similar cross-linking studies in murine cell lines resulted in cAMP elevation and PKC translocation [3]. This PKC activation event was distinct to that seen in human cells as a translocation to the nucleus rather than to the membrane was observed.Therefore different signalling pathways may be active in human and mouse cells prompting us to further investigate signal transduction mediated by human class II antigens.

Several reports have indicated that the cytoplasmic tails of the Ia class II alpha and beta chains are required for efficient plasma membrane expression and signal transduction [4-7]. Clearly any fluctuation in plasma membrane expression of class II or its altered trafficking will alter the efficacy of signal transduction and possibly result in the expression of different class II peptide complexes. We have generated cell cultures expressing mutant class II dimers to evaluate the contribution of the cytoplasmic and transmembrane domains of the human DR class II antigen to signal transduction. Data presented here reports the differing intracellular fate of these mutants.

Results and discussion

Premature termination codons were introduced into cDNAs of the DRα and DRβ chain to generate constructs which lacked 10 amino acids of the alpha chain cytoplasmic domain ($\alpha\Delta10$) and 4, 10 and 12 amino acids of the beta chain cytoplasmic domain ($\beta\Delta4$, $\beta\Delta10$, $\beta\Delta12$). In addition the cytoplasmic tail residues βGly 254 and βHis 255 were substituted with Ala residues (GH mutant). This replacement was to test the findings of a previous report suggesting a role for these residues in murine signal transduction [4].

Transient transfection of the human kidney epithelial cell line 293-EBNAI (Invitrogen) was performed using the Lipofectamine reagent (Gibco-BRL). Cultures expressing mutant and wildtype (WT) alpha and beta chains were established either with or without the simultaneous transfection of invariant chain (li). 48-72 hours post-transfection the expression of class II dimers was assessed using immunofluorescence microscopy (Axiophot fluorescence microscope, Zeiss, Germany) of permeabilised cells with a fluorescein conjugated antibody specific for an epitope expressed on a luminal portion of the folded α chain (L243). Confocal microscopy of these cells was also performed using the fluorescein conjugated L243 antibody. The nucleus was identified using a DNA co-stain (*Figure 1*).

Fluorescence microscopy of DRWT dimers expressed without invariant chain revealed reticular staining, staining that could represent the Golgi apparatus and some vesicular staining. Co-transfection with li resulted in an elevation of class II staining of vesicular structures. This was particularly apparent by confocal microscopy. A 'wild type' pattern of staining was seen in cells expressing αGH +/- li. Cells expressing $\alpha\Delta10/\beta\Delta12$-li also showed a similar pattern of staining to that seen with DRWT-li. However, co-transfection of li resulted in a very heavy perinuclear staining of class II. This may represent a retention of the class II dimers at the endoplasmic reticulum (ER). Transfections performed with single truncated chains paired with a WT partner indicate that residues in both chains influence intracellular routing of the dimer as single chain truncations could result in vesicular staining. *Table I* summarises the data obtained from these transfections.

Table I. Transfections prepared using the 293 EBNA cell line. 48-72 hours post-transfection class II expression was evaluated using normal fluorescence microscopy and confocal microscopy using the fluorescein conjugated antibody, L243. The first three columns indicate the DR class II mutant constructs transfected with or without li chain. +/- indicates degree of class II staining. FM indicates data acquired using only the Axiophot fluorescence microscope. Other data was collected using confocal microscopy also

alpha chain	beta chain	invariant chain	vesicular staining	intracellular retention
α WT	β WT	no	+/-	+
α Δ10	β WT	no	+/-	+
α WT	β WT	yes	+++	-
α Δ10	β WT	yes	+++	-
α Δ10	β Δ12	no	-	+
α Δ10	β Δ12	yes	-	+++
α WT	β Δ12	yes	++ (FM)	+/- (FM)
α Δ10	β Δ4	yes	+/-(FM)	+ (FM)
α WT	β GH	yes	+++	-

Clearly deletion of portions of the cytoplasmic tail of the alpha or beta chain of the class II antigen is influencing its subcellular localisation. Co-expression with li chain results in an increased staining with the L243 antibody. This probably relects the stabilisation of the folded epitope recognised by L243. The chaperone properties of li have been described in detail elsewhere [8,9]. A second ER resident protein, calnexin, has also been shown to play a role in stabilization of free class II chains and partially assembled αβli complexes [10]. It has been suggested that the step wise addition of αβ dimers to the trimeric li chain scaffold results in the eventual masking of an N-terminal ER retention signal in the li chain and subsequent egress of the αβli complex. However, this has not been firmly established. Here we provide evidence that residues contributed by both the α and β chain are responsible for masking the li ER retention signal. Loss of these residues results in heavy perinuclear expression as a result of ER retention. Clearly we must be very cautious in the interpretation of any subsequent signalling data obtained using these mutants bearing in mind their differing intracellular trafficking fates.

Panel A.

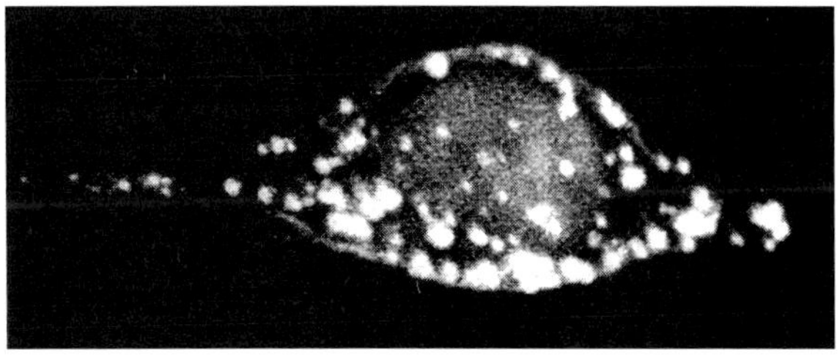

Panel B.

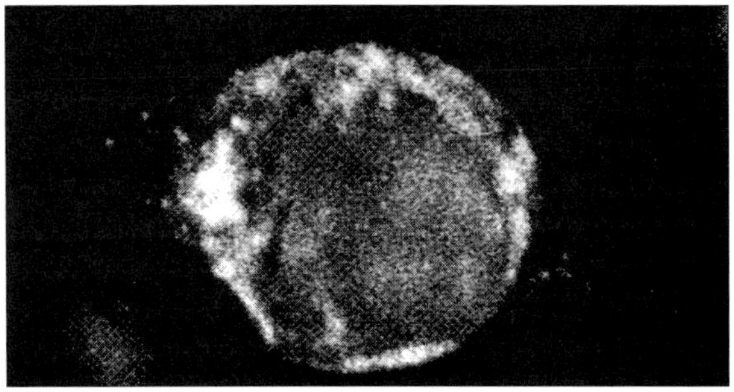

Figure 1. Confocal microscopy performed using permeabilised transient cultures. Class II was stained using the fluorescein conjugated L243 antibody. The upper panel (A) shows vesicular staining of DRWT+li. The lower panel (B) shows the heavy perinuclear staining seen in cells transfected with the αΔ10βΔ12+li constructs.

Acknowledgments
This work was supported by grants from INSERM, ANRS and LNFCC.

References

1. Mooney NA, Grillot-Courvalin C, Hivroz C, Ju L, Charron D. Early biochemical events after MHC class II-mediated signaling on human B-lymphocytes. *J Immunol* 1990: 145: 2070-6.
2. Brick-Ghannam C, Huang FL, Temime N, Charron D. Protein kinase C (PKC) activation via human leucocyte antigen class II molecules. *J Biol Chem* 1991: 266: 24169-75.
3. Cambier JC, Newell MK, Justement LB, McGuire JC, Leach KL, Chen ZZ. Ia binding ligands and cAMP stimulate nuclear translocation of PKC in B lymphocytes. *Nature* 1987: 327:629-32.

4. Harton, JA, Van Hagen AE, Bishop GA. The cytoplasmic and transmembrane domains of MHC class II β chains deliver distinct signals required for MHC class II-mediated B cell activation. *Immunity* 1996: 3: 349-358.
5. Chervonsky AV, Gordon L, Sant AJ. A segment of the MHC class II β chain plays a critical role in targeting class II molecules to the endocytic pathway. *Int Immunol* 1994:6:973-982.
6. Smiley ST, Rudensky AY, GlimcherLH, Grusby MJ. Truncation of the class II β chain cytoplasmic domain influences the level of class II/invariant chain-derived peptide complexes. *Proc Natl Acad Sci USA* 1996: 93: 241-244.
7. Nabavi N, Ghogawala Z, Myer A, Griffith IJ, Wade WF, Chen ZZ, McKean DJ, Glimcher LH. Antigen presentation abrogated in cells expressing truncated Ia molecules. *J Immunol* 1989: 142: 1444-1447.
8. Wolf PR, Ploegh HL. How MHC class II molecules acquire peptide cargo *Annu Rev Cell Dev Biol* 1995: 11: 267-306.
9. Xu X, Song W, Cho H, Qiu Y, Pierce SK. Intracellular transport of invariant chain-MHC class II complexes to the peptide-loading compartment. *J Immunol* 1995: 155: 2984-2992.
10. Arunachalam B, Cresswell P. Molecular requirements for the interaction of class II major histocompatibility complex molecules and invariant chain with calnexin. *J Biol chem* 1995: 270: 2784-2790.

T cell MHC class II molecules down-regulate CD4+ T cell responses following LAG-3 binding

F. Triebel, B. Huard

Laboratoire d'Immunologie Cellulaire, INSERM U333, Institut Gustave-Roussy, 39, rue Camille Desmoulins, 94805 Villejuif, France

Compared to the extensively studied CD4 or CD8 molecules, little is known about the function of the third MHC ligand, *i.e.* LAG-3 (lymphocyte activation gene-3), expressed on activated T and NK lymphocytes [1]. *In vivo*, it is selectively expressed in inflammatory lymphoid tissues, such as tonsils or lymph nodes [2]. LAG-3 is closely related to CD4 at the gene and protein level [1] and we have identified a specific LAG-3/HLA class II interaction in a cellular adhesion assay [3]. LAG-3 is therefore a second ligand for MHC class II molecules. The consequence of this interaction in the antigenic response of T cell clones has been investigated with LAG-3 exerting a negative regulatory role on antigen-dependent stimulation [4].

We constructed the fusion protein LAG-3Ig, a soluble molecule comprising the extracellular Ig domains of LAG-3 joined to human IgG1. This molecule is known to compete for CD4/MHC class II interaction in intercellular adhesion (rosette formation between CD4-transfected COS cells and MHC class II$^+$ B cells), but do not compete in CD4/MHC class II-dependent T cell cytotoxicity assay [5]. These results suggest that co-engagement of the TcR with CD4 alters the CD4/MHC class II molecular interaction to become insensitive to LAG-3Ig competition [5].

Here, we report the direct binding of LAG-3Ig to class II molecules on the cell surface. LAG-3Ig, in contrast to CD4Ig or CD8Ig, has a very good binding avidity for class II molecules. Saturation in terms of mean fluorescence intensity with LAG-3Ig plus GAH is usually obtained at 30μg/ml with 3×10^6/ml Daudi B cells. LAG-3Ig stained all class II$^+$ cells tested including B cells, activated T and NK cells, as well as xenogenic MHC class II molecules expressed on murine B cells or monkey PHA blasts. This binding was blocked by the 17B4 LAG-3-specific mAb.

Inhibition of CD4+ T cell clone antigen-specific proliferation and cytokine secretion was obtained when LAG-3Ig crosslinked MHC class II molecules expressed on the effector T cells. This effect was also found with anti-CD3 mab, PHA plus PMA or low dose IL-2 driven stimulation in the absence of APC. Inhibition was observed only when a cross linking reagent (GAH) was added as a second step, leading to T cell MHC class II molecule agregation and rapid induction of cell death as assessed by propidium iodide incorporation at 6 hrs. It is concluded that LAG-3 may represent a physiological ligand activating this MHC class II negative regulatory pathway. These results highlight the importance of T-T cell interactions in the control of T cell-mediated immune responses. Overall, the LAG-3 protein and its counter-receptors (MHC class II molecules) are both activation antigens in vivo whose interaction may result in the down-regulation of the ongoing T cell response [6].

References

1. Triebel F, Jitsukawa S, Baixeras E, Roman-Roman S, Genevee C, Viegas-Pequignot E, Hercend T. LAG-3, a novel lymphocyte activation gene closely related to CD4. *J Exp Med* 1990; 171: 1393-8.
2. Huard B, Gaulard P, Faure F, Hercend T, Triebel F. Cellular expression and tissue distribution of the human LAG-3-encoded protein, a MHC class II ligand. *Immunogenetics* 1994; 39: 213-7.
3. Baixeras E, Huard B, Miossec C, Jitsukawa S, M Martin, Hercend T, Auffray C, Triebel F, D Piatier-Tonneau D. Characterization of the lymphocyte activation gene 3-encoded protein. A new ligand for human leukocyte antigen class II antigens. *J Exp Med* 1992; 176: 327-32.
4. Huard B, Tournier M, Hercend T, Triebel F, Faure F. Lymphocyte-activation gene 3/major histocompatibility complex class II interaction modulates the antigenic response of CD4+ T lymphocytes. *Eur J Immunol* 1994; 24: 3216-22.
5. Huard B, Prigent P, Tournier M, Bruniquel D, Triebel F. CD4/major histocompatibility complex class II interaction analyzed with CD4- and lymphocyte activation gene-3 (LAG-3)-Ig fusion proteins. *Eur J Immunol* 1995; 25: 2718-21.
6. Huard B, Prigent P, Pages F, Bruniquel D, Borie N, Triebel F. T cell MHC class II molecules downregulate CD4+ T cell responses following LAG-3 binding. *Eur J Immunol* 1996; 26: 1180-6.

Mechanisms of HLA class II mediated death of splenic B cells

J.P. Truman, C. Choqueux, D. Charron, N. Mooney

INSERM U396, Immunogénétique Moléculaire, 15, rue de l'École de Médecine, 75006 Paris, France

Programmed cell death (PCD) is an active process where the cell commits suicide as a response to a particular condition. This may be due to depravation of cytokines, certain metabolic inhibitors, or being killed by cytotoxic T cells or natural killer cells. PCD or apoptosis differs from necrosis, or passive cell death, in that it generally exhibits the following phenomena: a shrinkage of the cell, condensation of the chromatin, fragmentation of the genomic DNA into ~180 base pair fragments, and the fragmentation of the cell including nucleus into small, membrane-enclosed particles [1]. These particles are rapidly engulfed *in vivo* by the surrounding cells, leaving no trace of the cell. This mode of death is therefore particularly useful as it does not liberate any potentially dangerous proteases from the cell's interior, in marked contrast to death by necrosis.

Until recently, MHC class II mediated signal transduction was considered only in terms of cellular activation [2, 3]. Recently, it has been observed that MHC class II mediated signalling could induce the apoptosis of resting mouse splenocytes, and we have described that HLA class II signalling could induce programmed cell death (PCD) in activated splenic B cells and B cell lines [4, 5].

Fas (also called APO-1 or CD95) is a member of the tumour necrosis (TNF) receptor family, which when trimerised by it's physiological ligand (a member of the TNF family), named Fas ligand (FasL), induces PCD [6]. It has a role in graft rejection, immunological privilege and also in cytotoxicity. However, on non-activated cells, Fas trimerisation generally has no effect. This could be a safeguard against the induction of PCD of 'bystander' cells, that is, cells that are not directly involved in the immune response. Activation of T or B cells restores the death inducing qualities of Fas, which suggests that these cells are now 'ready to die' using the Fas mechanism [7]. Indeed, it has been shown that T cells die by a process known as activation-induced cell death, or AICD, that uses Fas/FasL interactions [6]. HLA class II signalling also potentiates the death-inducing properties of Fas. This is not a consequence of cellular activation, as HLA class II cross-linking increases Fas-mediated death in many B cell lines [8]. As these cells can be considered as activated, it becomes clear that HLA class II signalling 'prepares' the B cell to die *via* a Fas-induced pathway.

Splenic B cells activated *via* HLA class II signalling, either through the use of monoclonal antibodies (mAb) or via superantigens, die after a period of time in excess of three days. The use of agonistic anti-Fas mAbs (clone CH-11) also induces more cell death after HLA class II stimulation. To try to account for this increased sensitivity to Fas-mediated cell death, we looked for FasL induction in splenic B cells. FasL mRNA was detected after 4 hours of HLA class II cross-linking either by mAb (L227 XL) or superantigens (toxic shock syndrome toxin-1, TSST-1) in splenic B cells. By using mAb specifically against FasL, increasing levels of FasL protein were observed. Furthermore, the use of antagonistic Fas antibodies or of anti-FasL antibodies blocked HLA class II mediated death in these cells, probably by inhibiting efficient trimerisation of Fas. Therefore, this can be considered an indirect pathway of HLA class II-mediated PCD, since HLA class II signals only set in motion a series of events in which apoptosis is a consequence of the activated state of the B cell *(Figure 1)*.

It is interesting to note here that FasL has not been detected previously in B cells induced to die following cross-linking of their membrane immunoglobulins [6]. We have also failed to detect any FasL in splenic B lymphocytes stimulated through the surface immunoglobulins using anti-μ antibodies, although an efficient increase in the sensitivity of the cells to Fas ligation was observed.

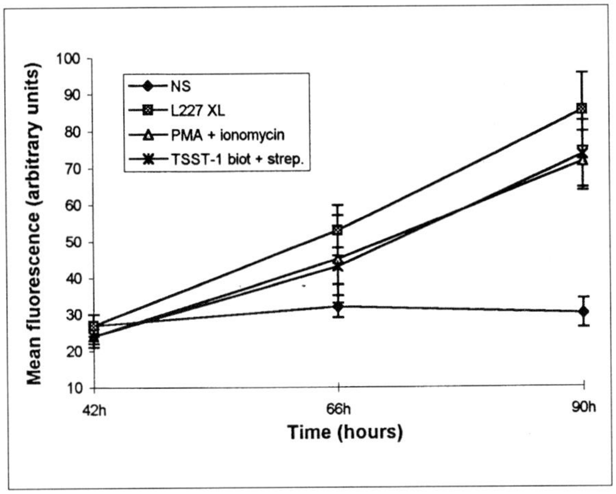

Figure 1. FasL surface expression on splenic B cells after treatment. Note that the level of fluorescence remains constant up to 42hours after treatment, so earlier time points are not shown.

It has been known for some time that MHC class II ligation induces a rapid calcium flux, increased transcription and activation of several protein kinase C (PKC) isoforms, and the activation of several protein tyrosine kinases (PTKs) [3, 9]. These events have been associated with cellular activation. We have observed that HLA class II mediated PCD in activated B cells required phosphatase activity and the participation of the cytoskeleton [5]. It was of interest to study whether the events leading to PCD also affected cellular activation, or vice-versa.

By blocking the transcription and/or the translation of genes, we were able to inhibit HLA class II mediated cellular activation. This lead to an increase in PCD of the resting splenic B cells, which we then tried to inhibit using other inhibitors known for their effects on signal transduction. The results suggested that PTKs, intracellular calcium, and PKC were important for the activation of non-activated B cells, while the cytoskeleton, phosphatases (PP1A and PP2A), PKC and the influx of extracellular calcium were important for HLA class II mediated PCD [10]. The requirements for PTK, intracellular calcium for activation and phosphatases, cytoskeleton and extracellular calcium were independent of each other, suggesting that two separate pathways are initiated following the cross-linking of HLA class II. This pathway of PCD induction can be considered as a direct pathway, as HLA class II signalling directly cause PCD.

Further evidence for a role of extracellular calcium in PCD induction came with the finding that cord blood B cells, which do not generate a calcium flux after HLA class II ligation, do not die but can still undergo cellular activation. The increase of intracellular calcium using a calcium ionophore (ionomycin) induced PCD in cord blood B cells if the HLA class II molecules were subsequently cross-linked.

The role of PKC in both cellular activation and PCD is intriguing. The PKC family of serine/threonine kinases contains many different isoforms, which appear to have differing roles in the cell. The simple answer to this dual role would be to suggest that some isoforms of PKC are involved in PCD, while others are involved in cellular activation.

FasL induction, along with CD40-ligand induction (also a member of the TNF family) both require an intracellular calcium flux. It is possible that the induction of an intracellular calcium flux by ionomycin in the cord blood B cells allows the induction of FasL. Other findings have suggested that the nuclease involved in DNA fragmentation is also calcium-dependent. The induction of the calcium flux may allow activation of the nuclease in response to HLA class II signalling. This finding suggests that cord blood B cells may die if HLA class II is cross-linked at the same time that a calcium flux is induced through another receptor.

These results also imply that many of the secondary messengers observed after cellular activation may be signals for cell death. Concurrent cell death and cell activation signalling would allow the possibility of cell death when cellular activation can not proceed. This could act as a safeguard against aberrant or inappropriate activation of the cell. We propose that the two distinct mechanisms of HLA class II-mediated death have different physiological roles. In the first instance, the resting B cell is activated by the T cell after antigen presentation. Once activated, the B cell has a limited time of survival (3-5 days) before it dies by apoptosis. Should a T cell encounter the activated B cell and recognise the peptide presented to it, the B cell dies more rapidly, instead of gaining yet another activation signal. The production of FasL by the B cell also raises the possibility of B cell cytotoxicity.

To summarise, we have identified two major mechanisms of induction of PCD after HLA class II signalling, an indirect pathway which involves Fas and FasL which occurs when non-activated B cells are activated *via* HLA class II, and a direct pathway which is induced in activated B cells.

References

1. Duvall E, Wyllie AH. Death and the cell. *Immunol Today* 1986; 7: 115-9.
2. Mooney NA, Grillot-Courvalin C, Hivroz C, Ju LY, Charron D. Early biochemical events after MHC class II-mediated signaling on human B lymphocytes. *J Immunol* 1990; 145: 2070-6.
3. Scholl PR, Geha RS. MHC class II signaling in B-cell activation. *Immunol Today* 1994; 15: 418-22.
4. Newell MK, VanderWall J, Beard KS, Freed JH. Ligation of major histocompatibility complex class II molecules mediates apoptotic cell death in resting B lymphocytes. *Proc Natl Acad Sci USA* 1993; 90: 10459-63.
5. Truman JP, Ericson ML, Choqueux-Séébold CJM, Charron DJ, Mooney NA. Lymphocyte programmed cell death is mediated *via* HLA class II DR. *Int Immunol* 1994; 6: 887-96.
6. Nagata S, Golstein P. The Fas death factor. *Science* 1995; 267: 1449-55.
7. Daniel PT, Krammer PH. Activation induces sensitivity toward APO-1 (CD95)-mediated apoptosis in human B cells. *J Immunol* 1994; 152: 5624-32.
8. Yoshino T, Cao L, Nishiuchi R, Yamadori I, Kondo E, Teramoto N, Hayashi K, Takahashi K, Kamikawaji N, Akagi T. Ligation of HLA class II molecules promotes sensitivity to CD95 (Fas antigen, APO-1)-mediated apoptosis. *Eur J Immunol* 1995; 25: 2190-4.
9. Brick-Ghannam C, Ericson ML, Schelle I, Charron D. Differential regulation of mRNAs encoding protein kinase C isoenzymes in activated human B cells. *Hum Immunol* 1994; 41: 216-24.
10. Truman JP, Choqueux C, Charron D, Mooney N. HLA class II molecule signal transduction leads to either apoptosis or activation *via* two different pathways. *Cell Immunol* 1996; 172: 149-57.

Similarities and differences between HLA class II signalling in foetal versus adult B lymphocytes

F. Garban, J.P. Truman, J. Lord, J. Plumas, M.C. Jacob, J.J. Sotto, D. Charron, N. Mooney

INSERM U396 , Institut des Cordeliers, 15, rue de l'École de médecine, 75006 Paris France
University of Birmingham Medical School, Birmingham, UK

Cord blood B lymphocytes may be considered 'naive' since in the majority of cases they have not been exposed to exogenous antigen. Previous studies of foetal B cells from cord blood have reported a phenotype similar to that of a mature B cell. Their capacity to generate antibody forming cells in response to activated T cells or mitogens is reduced in comparison with peripheral adult B cells. Immunoglobulin production is also lower than in adult B cells [1]. A previous study has reported similarities between cord blood B cells and B lymphocytes from patients with chronic lymphocytic leukemia (B-CLL) [2].

HLA class II molecules are transmembrane glycoproteins associated in heterodimers composed of a 34 kD α chain and a 28 kD β chain. Our recent studies have revealed HLA class II molecules associated in dimers of dimers or 'superdimers' on both foetal and adult antigen presenting cells [3,4]. Crosslinking of HLA class II molecules leads to the generation of second messengers, including an intracellular calcium flux (Ca^{++}_i), activation of tyrosine kinases, activation of phospholipase C (PLC), generation of diacylglycerol (DAG) [5,6], and activation of protein kinase C (PKC) [7,8]. This study compares the generation of second messengers and the functional consequences of HLA class II signalling on adult foetal B lymphocytes. Preliminary studies on B cells from patients with B-CLL or mantle zone lymphomas are also described.

Second messenger study

The generation of an intracellular calcium flux (Ca^{++}_i) via HLA class II was studied by flow cytometry on cells loaded with the calcium binding fluorochrome indo-1. Intracellular levels were unchanged in foetal B lymphocytes after stimulation via either HLA class II or CD 19 *(Figure 1)*. However calcium mobilization occured after cross linking of surface immunoglobulins although the level of the intracellular calcium flux was considerably lower on cord blood than observed with adult B lymphocytes *(Figure 1)*. On the contrary resting adult B splenocytes (small dense cells on Percoll gradient fractionation), generated an intracellular calcium flux after cross linking of HLA class II molecules or after stimulation with the anti-CD19 antibody. Surprisingly, no Ca^{++}_i was observed in adult lymphocytes from B chronic lymphocytic leukemia *(Figure 1)* or mantle zone lymphoma after signalling *via* HLA class II molecules. Similarly to cord blood B cells, stimulation via surface IgM could generate an Ca^{++}_i.

Although a defect has been observed with regard to Ca^{++}_i after stimulation via HLA class II molecules, the capacity to transmit signals is preserved with regard to the activation of tyrosine kinase (s) and PKC activation *Table I*. In cord blood and in adult B cells a 53 kD substrate could be detected by immunoblotting with an anti-phosphotyrosine antibody. We then examined activation of the serine/threonine kinase PKC by confocal microscopy using isoform specific antibodies directed against the PKC family: (1) after stimulation *via* HLA class II three PKC isoforms were activated, α βII and δ (2) a translocation towards the membrane has been observed for the three PKC isoforms, (3) a translocation towards the nucleus could be also detected for PKC βII.

Functional aspects: rapid aggregation and proliferation

Aggregation of B cells is one of the first steps mediated by HLA class II DR molecule signaling and is mediated by adhesion molecules including ICAM- 1 and LFA-1. Despite expression of these molecules on cord blood B

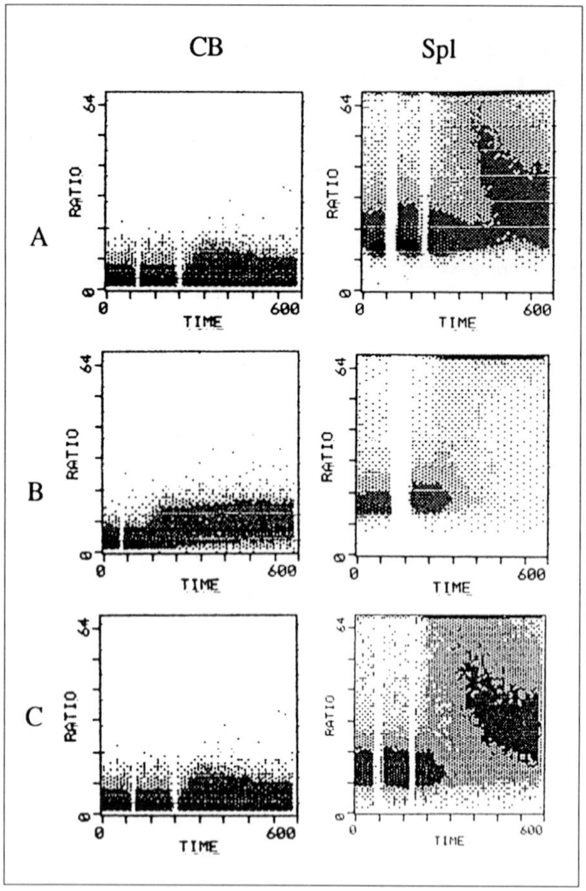

Figure 1. Figure 1 shows the intracellular calcium levels in cord blood B lymphocytes (CB) versus adult B splenocytes (Spl). A: stimulation *via* CD19 results in a significant intracellular calcium flux in Spl, although a minor flux was observed in CB this was not significant. B: signal transduction *via* surface IgM results in a small but prolonged and significant intracellular calcium flux in CB and a marked calcium flux in adult B splenocytes. C: HLA class II DR molecule signaling induces a calcium flux in adult B splenocytes but a calcium flux was not observed in CB B lymphocytes. It should be noted that the base level of intracellular calcium is lower in foetal compared with adult B lymphocytes.

lymphocytes, rapid aggregation of these cells was not observed in contrast to the rapid aggregation of adult B lymphocytes. However late aggregation of cord blood B cells was observed (after 24 hours of stimulation) albeit to a lesser degree than that observed in HLA class II stimulated adult B splenocytes (data not shown).

Table I. Provides a summary of the second messengers (calcium mobilization, tyrosine kinases, Protein kinase C) and the dainstream consequences involved in HLA class II signalling throughout B lymphocyte ontogeny

	Calcium mobilization	Tyrosine kinases	Protein kinase C	Early aggregation	Cell proliferation
Cord blood B cells	0	+	+	0	+
Resting splenocytes	++	+	+	++	+
Mantle cell lymphomas	0	+	Not done	0	+
B-CLL lymphocytes	0	+	Not done	0	+

Cell proliferation was studied by examining the distribution of isolated nuclei in the different phases of the cell cycle (G1 , S, G2 and M). Cord blood B cells were cultured for 24 hours with or without monoclonal anti-DR antibody. A significant proportion of cord blood B cells progress into the G2/M phases >10% (data not shown) by HLA class II stimulation thereby confirming that HLA class II mediated signalling mediates proliferation of cord blood B cells.

Discussion

This work reports the differences between resting adult B lymphocytes and cord blood B cells concerning their response to HLA class II signalling. A crucial feature is the lack of Ca^{++}_i after cross linking of HLA class II molecules on foetal B cells. The trivial explanation concerning the lower cell surface expression of HLA class II antigens on cord blood B cells [4] is unlikely since the same defect could be observed in lymphocytes from B cells of chronic lymphocytic leukemia or mantle zone lymphoma which express an extremely high level of HLA class II. Furthermore cord blood B cells are clearly capable of HLA class II mediated signalling since tyrosine kinase activation, PKC activation and proliferation were observed despite the deficient Ca^{++}_i and the lack of rapid aggregation. These data lead us to suggest that cord blood B cells are 'hyporesponsive' rather than immature since their characteristics with regard to HLA class II signalling could be observed in adult cells in a particular stage of differenciation such as B-CLL lymphocytes. The importance of HLA class II signaling is underlined by it's conservation throughout B lymphocyte ontogeny.

References

1. Splawsky JB, Jelinek DF, Lipsky PE. Delineation of the functional capacity of human neonatal lymphocytes. *J Clin Invest* 1991; 87: 545-53.
2. Schroeder HW Dighiero G. The pathogenesis of chronic lymphocytic leukemia: analysis of the antibody repertoire. *Immunol Today* 1994; 15: 288-94.
3. Roucard C, Garban F, Mooney NA, Charron DJ, Ericson ML. Conformation of HLA class II molecules: evidence for superdimers and empty molecules on human antigen presenting cells. *J Biol Chem* 1996; 273: 12993-4000.
4. Garban F, Ericson M, Roucard C, Rabian-Herzog C, Teisserenc H, Sauvanet E, Charron D, Mooney N. Detection of empty HLA class II molecules on cord blood B cells. *Blood* 1996; 87: 3970-6.
5. Mooney N, Grillot Courvalin C, Hivroz C, Ju LY, Charron D. Early biochemichal events after MHC class II mediated signalling on human B lymphocytes. *J Immunol* 1990; 145: 2070-6.
6. Lane PJ, McConnel FM, Shieven GL, Clark EA, Ledbetter JA. The role of class II molecules in human B cell activation association with phosphatidyl inositol turnover protein tyrosine phosphorylation and proliferation. *J Immunol* 1990; 144: 3684-92.
7. Cambier JC, Newell MK, Justement LB, McGuire JC, Leach KL, Chen ZZ. Ia bindings ligands and cAMP stimulate nuclear translocation of PKC in B lymphocytes. *Nature* 1987; 327: 629-32.
8. Brick Ghannam C, Huang FL, Temine N, Charron D. Protein kinase C activation via human leukocyte antigen class II molecules, a novel regulation of PKC activity 1991 *J Biol Chem* 1991; 35: 24169-75.

A novel member of the p58/p70 family of inhibitory receptors, which is characterized by three Ig-like domains and is expressed as a 140 kDa disulphide-linked dimer, is specific for HLA-A alleles

D. Pende, R. Biassoni, C. Cantoni, S. Verdiani, M. Falco, C. Di Donato, L. Accame, C. Bottino, A. Moretta, L. Moretta

Istituto Scientifico Tumori and Centro Biotecnologie Avanzate, Largo Rosanna Benzi 10, 16132 Genova, Italy

So far, different types of inhibitory NK receptors specific for distinct groups of HLA-C (p58 molecules) or HLA-B (p70/NKB1 molecules) alleles have been identified [1, 2]. Thus, p58.1 (reactive with EB6 mAb) recognized a group of HLA-C alleles (HLA-Cw2, -Cw4, -Cw5 and -Cw6) characterized by the amino acid residues N77/K80. p58.2 (reactive with GL183 mAb) recognized HLA-Cw1, Cw3, Cw7 and Cw8 alleles characterized by S77/N80. p70/NKB1 (reactive with Z27 mAb) recognized a group of HLA-B alleles belonging to the Bw4 supertypic specificity (*e.g.* HLA-B2705, -B51, -B58 and -B44). Cloning of these receptors revealed new members of the immunoglobulin (Ig) superfamily characterized by two (p58) or three (p70/NKB1) Ig-like domains in their extracellular portions and by a long cytoplasmic tail associated with a non polar transmembrane [3, 5].

In the present study we identified a novel surface molecule expressed by a subset of human NK cells which functions as receptor specific for defined HLA-A alleles [6]. For mouse immunization we selected the GL183-EB6-Z27- NK cell clone DP7, which displayed specificity only for HLA-A3 molecules, when tested against a large panel of different HLA class I cell transfectants. The hybridoma supernatants were first screened for their ability to reconstitute lysis of CIR-A3 by the immunizing DP7 clone. Q66 mAb (IgM) exerted this functional effect and selectively reacted with the immunizing DP7 clone and other NK clones displaying HLA-A3 specificity. Analysis of the cell distribution of the surface molecules recognized by Q66 mAb revealed that, in fresh PBL, $Q66^+$ cells represent a subset of $CD16^+$ NK cells, while among $CD3^+$ cells are few. *Figure 1* shows a double fluorescence analysis of a cultured polyclonal NK population. The subset of $Q66^+$ cells is distinguishable from that of $p58^+$ cells (as revealed by staining with a mixture of EB6 and GL183 mAbs) or $p70/NKB1^+$ cells (as stained by Z27 mAb). In modulation experiments we could demonstrate that, in clones $Q66^+EB6^+$, the two molecules, Q66 and p58.1, are not physically associated at the surface.

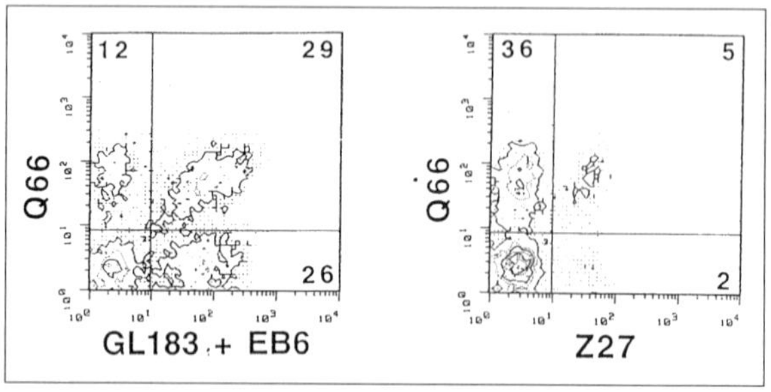

Figure 1. Two colour-cytofluorimetric analysis of the distribution of Q66 mAb-reactive molecules compared with the other NK receptors in a cultured $CD3^-56^+16^+$ bulk population.

Among NK clones which did not recognize HLA-C or HLA-B alleles (and did not express p58 or p70 molecules), we selected $Q66^+$ clones which were analyzed for their cytolytic activity against four B-EBV cell lines expressing an informative HLA-class I haplotype. As shown in *Figure 2*, it's evident that two cell lines (HOM2 and WT100BIS) were resistant to lysis by $Q66^+$ clones while the other two (SP0010 and A51) were efficiently lysed. According to the HLA haplotype of the four

B-EBV target cell lines it is possible to conclude that neither HLA-C nor HLA-B are involved in the protective effect. Indeeed, the two protected cell lines expressed Cw1 or Cw6, belonging to the two different groups of NK-defined HLA-C specificities; moreover they expressed HLA-B27 or -B35, belonging to the Bw4 or Bw6 supertypic specificities. The analysis of the expressed HLA-A alleles, suggested that HLA-A3 and HLA-A11 conferred protection. The target cell lines that were susceptible to lysis expressed HLA-C and HLA-B alleles belonging to the same groups of the protected targets, but lacked HLA-A3 or HLA-A11 (they were both homozygous for HLA-A2). The HLA-A3 specificity of Q66 clones was confirmed also by the use of C1R transfected with different HLA-A and -B alleles. p70⁻p58⁻Q66⁻ clones, tested in comparison, did not show any HLA-A3 specificity. Moreover, the addition of Q66 mAb to the cytolytic assay could restore lysis of HLA-A3 protected targets by Q66$^+$ NK cell clones. These data support the notion that Q66 mAb-defined molecules represent inhibitory NK receptors specific for HLA-A3 and -A11 alleles. In addition, the receptors for Bw4 and those for HLA-A3 were functionally independent as shown by the analysis of Z27$^+$Q66$^+$ clones. Thus, when tested against target cells coexpressing HLA-Bw4 and HLA-A3 alleles (*e.g.* HOM2) lysis was achieved only by mAb-mediated masking of both receptors; Q66 mAb could restore lysis only when tested against C1R-A3, but not against C1R-B27 which requires Z27 mAb.

Q66$^+$, but not Q66$^-$ NK cell clones expressed mRNA coding for a novel 3Ig domain protein homologous to the HLA-C (p58) and HLA-B (p70) receptors. The corresponding cDNA, named cl 1.1, was used to generate transient and stable transfectants in COS7 and NIH3T3 cell lines, respectively. Both types of transfectants were specifically stained by Q66 mAb *(Figure 3)*. Since the cytoplasmic tail of Q66-reactive molecules was at least 11 aminoacid longer than the other p58/p70 molecules, we could generate an antiserum specific for the C-terminus of Q66-reactive molecules, termed PGP3. Western blot analysis using PGP3 on total cell lysates revealed, only in Q66+ NK cells and cl 1.1 transfected NIH3T3 cell line, molecules displaying a MW of 140 kD, under non reducing conditions, which resolved , under reducing conditions, in a 70 kD band. Thus, differently from the other p58/p70 receptors, Q66-reactive molecules appear to be expressed as disulphide linked dimers and were thus termed p140. The comparative analysis of the aminoacid sequences of p58, p70 and p140 molecules revealed the existence of two cysteins proximal to the transmembrane region, only in the amino acid sequence of p140 molecules.

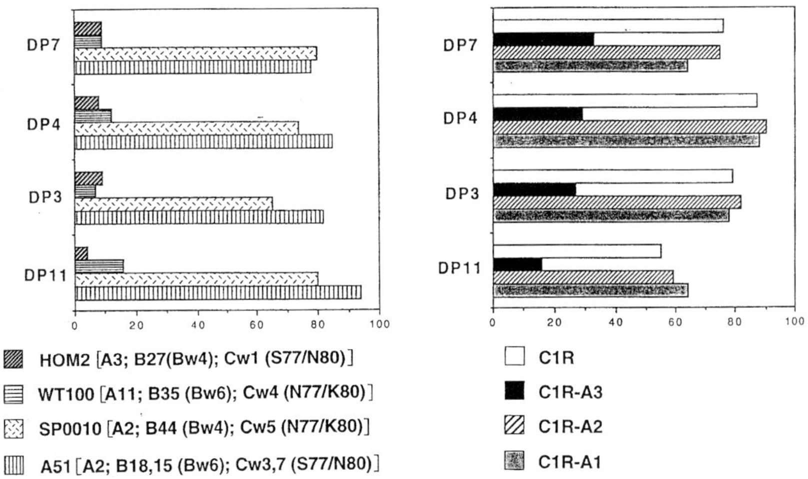

Figure 2. HLA-A3 and -A11 expression on target cells confers protection from lysis by Q66$^+$ clones. Four representative EB6$^-$, GL183$^-$, Z27$^-$, Q66$^+$ clones were assessed for cytolytic activity against the indicated target cells. Data are expressed as a % specific lysis.

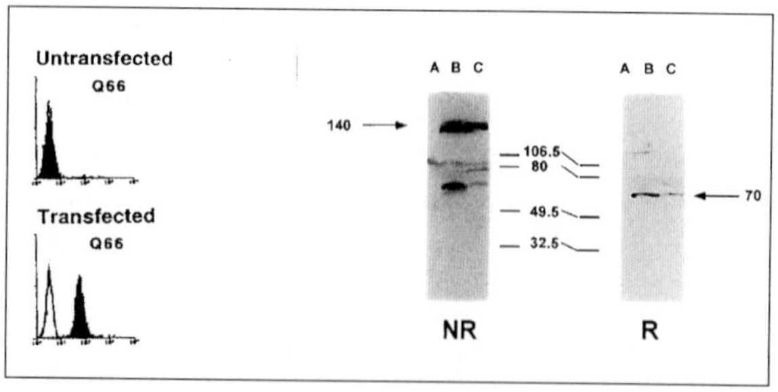

Figure 3. Cell surface expression (left panel) and western blot analysis (right panel) of Q66 mAb-reactive proteins in cl. 1.1 transfected NIH-3T3 cells.
Left: solid histograms represents cells stained with Q66 mAb and empty histograms are cells with cIg.
Right: western blot analysis under non reducing (NR) and reducing (R) conditions of untransfected (A) and cl. 1.1 transfected (B) NIH-3T3 cells compared with a Q66+ NK cell population (C).

References

1. Moretta A, Bottino C, Vitale M, Pende D, Biassoni R, Mingari M.C, Moretta L. Receptors for HLA-class I-molecules in human natural killer cells. *Ann Rev Immunol* 1996; 14: 619-48.
2. Lanier LL, Phillips JH. Molecular and cell biology of inhibitory MHC class I receptors on NK cells and T cells. *Immunol Today* 1996; 17: 86-100.
3. Wagtmann N, Biassoni R, Cantoni C, Verdiani S, Malnati MS, Vitale M, Bottino C, Moretta L, Moretta A, Long EO. Molecular clones of the p58 NK cell receptor reveal immunoglobulin related molecules with diversity in both the extra- and intra-cellular domains. *Immunity* 1995; 2: 439-49.
4. D'Andrea A, Chang C, Franz-Bacon K, McClanahan T, Phillips JH, Lanier LL. Molecular cloning of NKB1. A natural killer cell receptor for HLA-B allotypes. *J Immunol* 1995; 155: 2306-10.
5. Colonna M, Samaridis J. Cloning of immunoglobulin-superfamily members associated with HLA-C and HLA-B recognition by human natural killer cells. *Science* 1995; 268: 405-08.
6. Pende D, Biassoni R, Cantoni C, Verdiani S, Falco M, Di Donato C, Accame L, Bottino C, Moretta A, Moretta L. The natural killer cell receptor specific for the p58/p70 family of inhibitory receptors which is characterized by three Ig-like domains and is expressed as a 140 kD disulphide-linked dimer. *J Exp Med* 1997; 184: in press.

Does BY55 monoclonal antibody identify a novel NK receptor?

V. Schiavon, S. Agrawal, L. Boumsell, A. Bensussan

INSERM U448, Faculté de médecine de Créteil, 8, rue du Général Sarrail, 94010 Créteil Cedex, France

Natural killer (NK) cells are T-cell receptor (TCR) negative circulating large granular lymphocytes which are able to lyse tumor or virally infected cells [1]. The characteristic surface markers expressed by these cells are CD16, CD56, CD11b and CD122. Recently, several molecules including NKB1 [2] , p58 molecules [3], and CD94 [4], have been reported as being NK cell receptors. It has been established that the ligand of these molecules are MHC-Cl I molecules which protect targets cells from NK-mediated lysis. In our laboratory, we have developed a monoclonal antibody (mAb) called BY55 to further characterize circulating cells with cytotoxic activity [5]. BY55 mAb was obtained by repeated Balb/c mice immunization with YT2C2, a human cell line which possesses NK cell functional characteristics. BY55 mAb reacts with a new 80-kDa protein structure expressed exclusively by the immunizing cell line, YT2C2 (and its related parental cell lines) and by a subset of circulating lymphocytes.

BY55 mAb characterizes a unique lymphocyte subset

The representative two-color immunofluorescence stainings of PBL (peripheral blood lymphocytes) from a normal individual *(Figure 1)* show that BY55 mAb reacts neither with B lymphocytes nor with CD4+ lymphocytes, whereas it labels most of the CD3- cells. Among BY55+ lymphocytes, 60% are CD3-, 20%

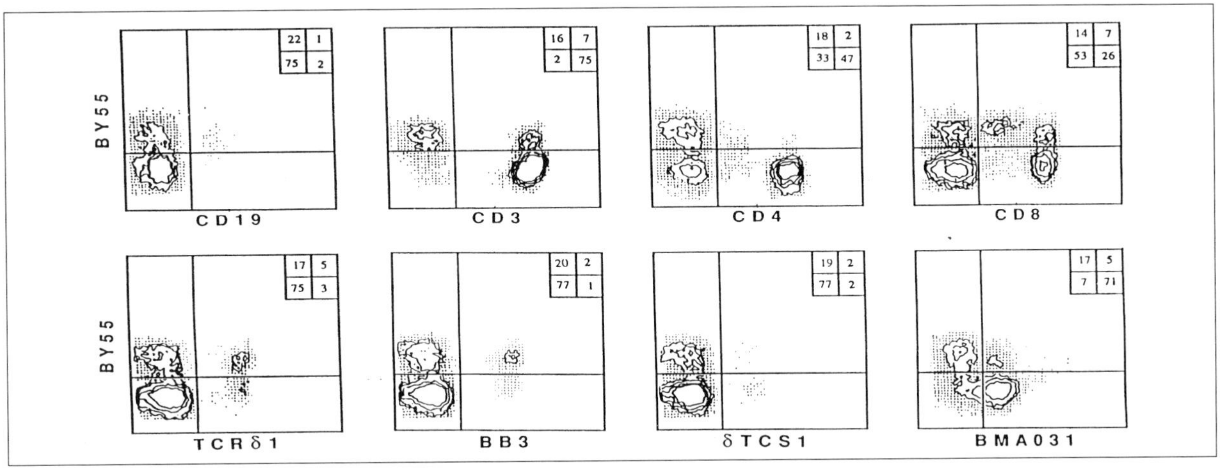

Figure 1. Two-color immunofluorescence analysis of BY55 expression in peripheral blood lymphocytes. Cells from a representative donor were first labeled with CD19, CD3, CD4, CD8, TCRδ1 (TCRγδ), BB3 (Vδ2) , δTCS1 (Vδ1) or BMA031 (TCRαβ) mAb coupled with FITC in combination with BY55 mAb. After washing, cells were incubated with a PE anti-mouse IgM. Samples were then analysed by flow cytometry. Division in quadrants was established on the basis of one-color immunofluorescence analysis of samples for each individual experiment. Numbers in the top right corner of two-dimensional contour plots indicate the percent of cells included within each quadrant.

Table I. Two-color immunofluorescence analysis of BY55 expression with other NK cells characteristic surface markers. Cells from a representative donor were first labeled with FITC-conjugated CD16 and CD57 or with unconjugated CD56, CD94 (Kp43) and p58 (EB6 and GL183) mAb. After washing, unconjugated mAb labeled cells were incubated with a FITC-labeled anti-mouse IgG+M. After futher washing and the eventually remaining anti-mouse IgG+M was saturated by an excess of mouse Ig and then cells were incubated with PE- conjugated BY55 mAb. Samples were then analysed by flow cytometry. Results are the percentages of a representative experiment

Percentage of PBL Coexpressing CD16, CD56, CD57, CD94, EB6 or GL183 Molecule with BY55 mAb reactive Antigen

	CD16-	CD16+	CD56-	CD56+	CD57-	CD57+
BY55+	7.5	5.6	8.5	9.3	8.8	7.2
BY55-	84.6	2.3	76.5	5.7	80.2	3.7

	CD94-	CD94+	EB6-	EB6+	GL183-	GL183+
BY55+	11.5	6.7	17.6	2.1	13.6	4.6
BY55-	75.3	6.4	78.9	0.5	80.3	1.5

CD3+TCRαβ+ and 20% are CD3+TCRγδ+. Further, within BY55+ TCRγδ+ cells, an equal proportion reacted with BB3 (Vδ1) or δTCS1 (Vδ2) mAb. Also, it should be noted that BY55 mAb stains not only CD3- cells but also $CD8^{dim}$ and also a subpopulation $CD8^{bright}$ cells. Thus, BY55 mAb characterizes a cellular subset clearly different from all other well known T cell subsets.

The cell subset defined by BY55 mAb is different from those defined by other NK cell-associated markers

PBL from a normal individual were double-stained with BY55 mAb and other NK cell surface markers. The results shown in *Table I* clearly indicate that the subset defined by BY55 mAb does not exactly overlap with any of the subsets defined by: CD16, CD56, CD57 or by the recently described NK receptors, CD94 and the two p58 molecules (identified by EB6 and GL183 mAbs). BY55 mAb labels two-third of CD16+, CD56+ and CD57+ cells, one-half of CD94+ cells and most of p58+ cells.

BY55 mAb characterizes functional NK cells

As most of the CD3- lymphocytes were stained by BY55 mAb, we looked at whether NK activity was exhibited by BY55+ cells. Thus, PBL were labeled with BY55 mAb and sorted into BY55+ and BY55- cells using a FACS. The results from a representative experiment are shown in *Figure 2*.

Whole PBL and BY55 mAb labeled PBL of this donor exhibit strong NK activity against the NK sensitive cell

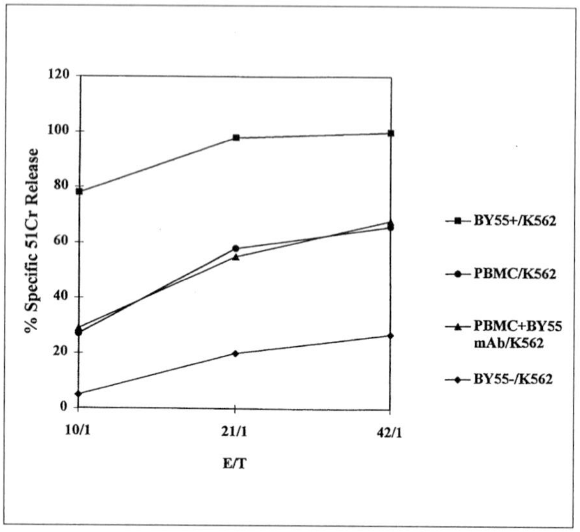

Figure 2. Determination of the NK activity mediated by FACS sorted BY55+ and BY55- PBL. Freshly isolated PBL were labeled with BY55 mAb for indirect immunofluorescence. These treated cells were either used directly as effector cells (triangles), or sorted into BY55+ (squares) and BY55- (diamonds) effector cells. Untreated PBL were also tested as effector cells (circles) against K562 target cells.

Table II. Human NK receptors EB6, HP-3E4, GL183, dx9 and 5.133 belong to the immunoglobulin superfamily (Ig-SF). Their intracellular tail possess either two or three Ig-SF domains and their ligands have been shown to be MHC Cl-I molecules which protect the target cell from NK lysis

Human NK Inhibitory Receptors and MHC Class I Ligands				
Receptor				**Ligand**
cDNA	Structure	mAb	mw	MHC Cl I ligands
NKAT1	Two Ig-SF domains	EB6, HP-3E4	55	HLA-Cw4, -CW5, -Cw6
NKAT2	Two Ig-SF domains	GL183	58	HLA-Cw1, -Cw3, -Cw7, -Cw8
NKT5	Two Ig-SF domains	GL183	50	--
NKAT3	Three Ig-SF domains	dx9, 5.133	70	HLA-B5101, -B5801, -B2705
NKAT4	Three Ig-SF domains	5.133	70	HLA-A0301

line, K562. The BY55+ cell population is greatly enriched in cells mediating NK activity, whereas the BY55- cell population is almost deprived of NK function. It is also to be noted that BY55 mAb does not modify NK activity (*Figure 2*).

At the cDNA level, the molecule recognized by BY55 mAb is different from all the other described NK cell receptors.

Recently, the gene of the molecule recognizes by BY55 mAb has been cloned in the COS system (Gordon Freeman personal communication). The analysis of the cDNA sequence clearly indicates that this is a new molecule which belongs neither to the C-type lectin nor to the immunoglobulin superfamilies. Thus, this molecule is different from the other NK receptors recently cloned (*Table II*), such as the p58 and the p70 molecules which possess extracellular immunoglobulin superfamily domains [6]. Moreover, unlike other NK receptors, the BY55 molecule is not a transmembrane molecule but a PIG-linked one.

Presently, the function of the BY55 molecule is unknown but in view of the new molecular data, we propose investigating the possible immunoregulatory function of this molecule. Indeed, we have recently shown that this molecule disappears from the cell surface of peripheral blood mononuclear cells as early as four hours after *in vitro* culture with BY55 mAb (data not shown). The next step of this study will be to determine whether this molecule activates or inhibits the cytolytic activity of NK cells. In conclusion, we have described a new PIG-linked protein expressed on functional circulating NK cells. Thus, this molecule may represent a new type of NK receptor.

References

1. Trincheri G. Biology of NK cells. *Annu Rev Immunol* 1989; 47: 187-276.
2. Litwin V, Gumperz J, Parham P, Philipps JH, Lanier LL. NKB1: a natural killer cell receptor involved in the recognition of polymorphic HLA-B molecules. *J Exp Med* 1994; 180: 537-43.
3. Bottino C, Vitale M, Olcese L, Sivori S, Morelli L, Augugliaro R, Ciccone E, Moretta L, Moretta A. The human natural killer cell receptor for major histocompatibility complex class I molecules. Surface modulation of p58 molecules and their linkage to CD3z chain, FceRIg chain and p56lck kinase. *Eur J Immunol* 1994; 24: 2527-34.
4. Moretta A, Vitale M, Olcese L, Sivori S, Bottino C, Morelli L, Augugliaro R, Babaresi M, Pende D, Ciccione L, Lopez-Bottet M, Moretta L. Human natural killer cell receptor for HLA-B alleles. *J Exp Med* 1994; 180: 545-55.
5. Maiza H, Leca G, Mansur IG, Schiavon V, Boumsell L, Bensussan A. A novel 80-kDa cell surface structure identifies human circulating lymphocytes with natural killer activity. *J Exp Med* 1993; 178: 1121-6.
6. Colonna M. Natural killer cell receptors specific for MHC class I molecules. *Curr Op Immunol* 1996; 8: 101-7.

The HLA-C-specific "activatory" or "inhibitory" natural killer cell receptors display highly homologous extracellular domains but differ in their transmembrane and intracytoplasmic portions

R. Biassoni[1], C. Cantoni[1], M. Falco[1], S. Verdiani[1], C. Bottino[1], M. Vitale[2], R. Conte[1], A. Poggi[1], A. Moretta[2,4], L. Moretta[1,3]

1 Istituto Nazionale per la Ricerca sul Cancro, Centro Biotecnologie Avanzate, Largo Rossana Benzi 10, 16132 Genova, Italy
2 Istituto di Istologia ed Embriologia Generale, Università di Genova, Italy
3 Istituto di Patologia Generale, Università di Genova, Italy
4 Dipartimento di Scienze Biomediche e Biotecnologie, Università di Brescia, Italy.

Natural killer cells (NK) express clonally distributed receptors able to recognize different groups of HLA class I alleles. In particular, receptors specific for two groups of HLA-C alleles have been characterized, displaying 58 kDa as molecular weight [1, 2]. p58.1, recognized by EB6 mAb, is specific for HLA-Cw4 and related alleles (-Cw2, -Cw5, -Cw6), while p58.2, stained by GL183 mAb, is specific for HLA-Cw3 and related alleles (-Cw1, -Cw7, -Cw8) [1, 2]. Interaction between NK receptor and its ligand leads to the inhibition of the NK-mediated target cell lysis. Recently, additional 50 kDa molecular forms of EB6 or GL183-mAb reactive receptors (p50) have been identified, able to trigger rather than to inhibit NK cell functions [3]. These receptors share the same HLA-C specificity as the corresponding inhibitory ones. Importantly, single NK cells do not coexpress p58 and p50 receptors with an identical HLA-C specificity. Genes encoding for inhibitory p58 NK receptors have been isolated; they encode for type I surface proteins belonging to the Immunoglobulin (Ig) superfamily [4].

In this study we isolated genes encoding for the novel activatory p50 forms of NK receptors. To this end a large panel of NK cell clones with known phenotype and function was analyzed by PCR. We utilized specific pairs of primers deduced from DNA sequences of inhibitory p58 receptors. Full-length cDNAs encoding for p50 EB6-reactive (EB6ActI) and for p50 GL183-reactive (183ActI) molecules were amplified from activatory EB6+ and GL183+ NK cell clones respectively [5]. Comparative analysis of p58 inhibitory versus p50 activatory amino acid sequences revealed that p50 are highly homologous to p58 in their extracellular regions formed by two Ig-like domains. However at least 11 amino acid residues in the extracellular domains were unique of EB6- or GL183-reactive molecules independently from the inhibitory or activatory function. In contrast, major differences exist in their transmembrane and cytoplasmic portions. Inhibitory p58 receptors display a 76-84 amino acid cytoplasmic tail, containing two immunoreceptor tyrosine-based inhibitory motifs (ITIM), spaced by 26 amino acids [5, 6]. On ther other hand activatory p50 molecules are characterized by a shorter 39 aminoacid tail, which does not contain any ITIM motif [5]. In addition, while p58 have a non polar transmembrane portion, p50 contain the charged amino acid Lys, which could be responsible for the association with accessory molecule(s) potentially involved in the signal transduction *(Figure 1)*.

EB6ActI and 183ActI cDNAs were transiently transfected in COS cell line, indicating that EB6ActI encoded a protein stained by EB6 but not GL183 mAb, while the contrary was true for 183ActI (data not shown). As shown in *Figure 2*, Jurkat cells stably transfected with EB6ActI (activatory p50.1) or EB6cl.42 (inhibitory p58.1) cDNAs were both brightly stained by EB6 but not by GL183 mAb. Moreover,

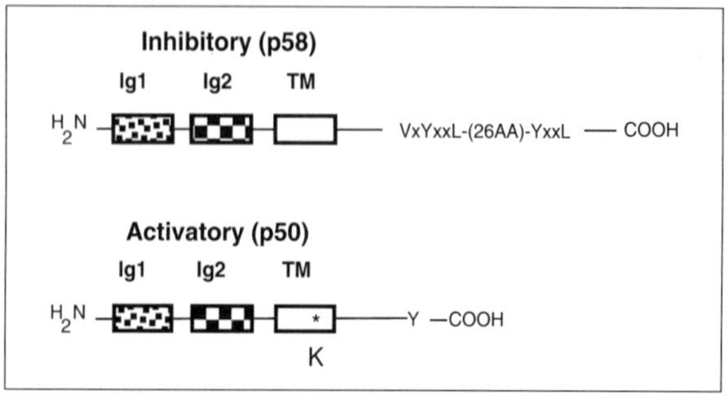

Figure 1. Schematic representation of p58/p50 NK receptors.

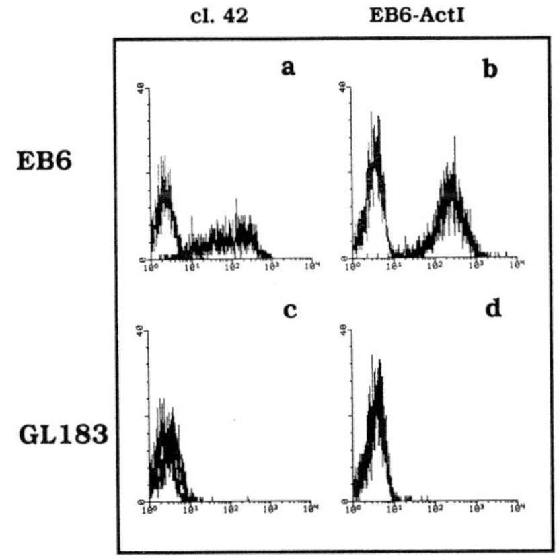

Figure 2. Jurkat cells transfected with RSV.5gpt/cl42 (inhibitory EB6) or RSV.5gpt/EB6-ActI (activatory EB6) were analyzed for cell surface expression of p58/p50 molecules by using EB6 (a, b) or GL183 (c, d) mAb.

EB6 mAb immunoprecipitated 50 kDa molecules from EB6ActI cell transfectants and 58 kDa molecules from EB6cl42 transfectants *(Figure 3)*. In addition, N-glycanase digestion of EB6 molecules immunoprecipitated from EB6ActI and EB6cl.42 Jurkat transfectants resulted in molecules of 36 and 42 kDa, respectively, in agreement with previous data on NK cell clones (data not shown).

In conclusion these data indicate that the HLA-C specific NK receptors mediating either cell triggering or inhibition display a sequence homology in their extracellular domains, but not in their transmembrane or cytoplasmic portions. Therefore, receptors with identical specificity and mAb reactivity may transduce signals of opposite sign due to structural differences in the portions involved in signal transduction.

Acknowledgements

S.V. C.C. and M.F. are recipients of an A.I.R.C., I.S.S. and postdoctoral fellowships, respectively. Partially supported by C.N.R. and A.I.R.C. grants to R.B, A.M. and L.M.

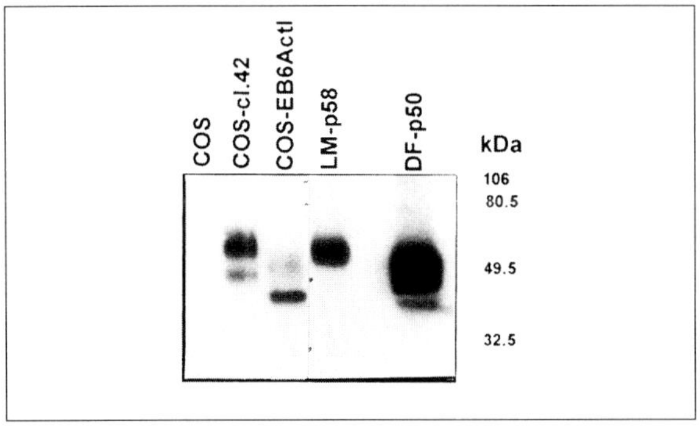

Figure 3. Immunoprecipitation of p58/p50 molecules from COS 7 cell transfectants. EB6+ polyclonal NK cell populations expressing inhibitory p58.1 (LM-p58) or activatory p50.1 (DF-p50) NK receptors and COS 7 cells untrasfected or transfected with RSV.5gpt/cl.42 and RSV.5gpt/EB6-ActI were lysed in 1% NP40 lysis buffer and immunoprecipitated with EB6 mAb coupled with CNBr-Sepharose. Samples were size-fractionated in a 8.5% SDS-PAGE and analyzed by Western-blot with 125I-EB6 mAb. On the right vertical side of the figure the position of molecular weight standard is reported.

References

1. Moretta A, Bottino C, Vitale M, Pende D, Biassoni R, Mingari MC, Moretta L. Receptors for HLA class I molecules in human natural killer cells. *Annu Rev Immunol* 1996; 14: 619-48.
2. Moretta A, Bottino C, Pende D, Tripodi G, Tambussi G, Viale O, Orengo A M, Barbaresi M, Merli A, Ciccone E, Moretta L. Identification of four subsets of human CD3-CD16+ NK cells by the expression of clonally distributed functional surface molecules. Correlation between subset assignment of NK clones and ability to mediate specific alloantigen recognition. *J Exp Med* 1990; 172: 1589-98.
3. Moretta, A, Sivori S, Vitale M, Pende D, Morelli M, Augugliaro R, Bottino C, Moretta L. Existence of both inhibitory (p58) and activatory (p50) receptors for HLA-C molecules in human natural killer cells. *J Exp Med* 1995; 182: 875-84.
4. Wagtmann N, Biassoni R, Cantoni C, Verdiani S, Malnati MS, Vitale M, Bottino C, Moretta L, Moretta A, Long EO. Molecular clones of the p58 NK cell receptor reveal immunoglobulin related molecules with diversity in both the extra- and intracellular domains. *Immunity* 1995; 2: 439-49.
5. Biassoni R, Cantoni C, Falco M, Verdiani S, Bottino C, Vitale M, Conte R, Poggi A, Moretta A, Moretta L. The HLA-C-specific "activatory" or "inhibitory" natural killer cell receptors display highly homologous extracellular domains but differ in their transmembrane and intracytoplasmic portions. *J Exp Med* 1996; 183: 645-50.
6. Olcese L, Lang P, Vély F, Cambiaggi A, Marguet D, Bléry M, Hippen KL, Biassoni R, Moretta A, Moretta L, Cambier JC, Vivier E. Human and mouse natural killer cell inhibitory receptors recruit the PTP1C and PTP1D protein tyrosine phosphatases. *J Immunol* 1996; 156: 5431-9.

Recognition of threonine 80 on HLA-B27 subtypes by NK clones

I. Luque[1], D. Galiani[1], R. Gonzalez[1], F. García[2] , J.A. Lopez de Castro[2], J. Peña[1], R. Solana[1]

1 Departamento de Inmunologia, Facultad de Medicina, Hospital Reina Sofia, Universidad de Cordoba, 14004 Cordoba, Spain
2 Centro de Biologia Molecular Severo Ochoa, Consejo Superior de Investigaciones Cientificas. Universidad Autonoma de Madrid, Cantoblanco 28049 Madrid, Spain

Recognition of MHC class I molecules on target cells by natural killer (NK) cells inhibits NK cell mediated lysis. Three different NK specificities have been defined according to their capacity to recognize Class I polymorphic motifs [1,2]. This effect is mediated by different NK inhibitory receptors, [1,2], namely, NK1,NK2 and NK3 which are inhibited by HLA-C alleles with Lys80, HLA-C alleles with Ser77 [3] and by HLA-Bw4 alleles with Ile80 [4] respectively.
In an attempt to further analyze how NK cells recognize HLA-B27, we have studied the effect induced by the different HLA-B27 subtypes and some HLA-B*2705 mutants on the lytic capacity of some NK clones.

Materials and methods

NK clones were obtained as previously described [5]. The HLA class I deficient EBV-transformed B lymphoblastoid cell line C1R was used as target without and transfected with the HLA-B*0702,HLA-B*2701, B*2702, B*2703, B*2704, B*2705 and B*2706 genes and with HLA-B*2705 site-directed mutated at positions 74 (Y74), 80 (I80) 81 (A81) and double mutated at positions 77 and 80 (N77I80) [6]. NK cytotoxicity was measured by the standard ^{51}Cr release assay [5].
The selection of NK clones were done by screening for their ability to lyse the B cell line C1R and its variants transfected with HLA-B*0702 and HLA-B*2705 genes. Five NK clones were selected based in their capacity to specifically be inhibited by HLA-B*2705 but not HLA-B*0702 gene transfection (*Table I*). These five NK clones were used to analyze their cytotoxic capacity against target cells transfected with HLA B27 subtypes and mutants. The clone RJ141, which was not inhibited by HLA gene transfection, was used as control.

Results and discussion

The results shown in *Table II* indicate that whereas B*2701, B*2703, B*2704 and B*2706 induced strong protection to lysis by these particular NK clones, HLA-B*2702 was unable to induce protection.
HLA-B27 subtypes are particularly polymorphic at the aminoacids defining the HLA-Bw4 epitope [6]. A feature which differentiates B*2702 from all other subtypes, is the presence of Ile at position 80 in B*2702, whereas the remaining HLA-B27 subtypes analyzed have Thr in this position. Thus our results suggested that Thr80 of HLA-B27 is of particular relevance in the induction of resistance to lysis by these NK clones.
To confirm the role of Thr80 in HLA-B27 recognition by NK cells, C1R cells transfected with the B*2705 gene specifically mutated in positions 74, 80 and 81 to mimic the changes in the B*2702 at single positions, were used as target cells. The cytotoxicity of these clones was subsequently analyzed against these transfectants. The results in *Table II*, show that the protection conferred by B*2705 to lysis was reverted when Thr80 was changed to Ile80, whereas mutations at positions 74 (D → Y) or 81 (R → A) did not affect B*2705 induced protection to lysis.
Our results demonstrate the critical role played by Thr80 on HLA-B*2705 on recognition by a group of NK clones, adding to previous studies that underline the importance of residue 80 for NK recognition. Thus, it has been shown that cytotoxicity of a subset of NK clones expressing the NKB1 receptor was inhibited by the Bw4 epitope (residues 77-83) in HLA-B27, B58 and B51 [7]. However the recognition pattern of these clones was not affected by the different sequences of the Bw4 molecules in residue 77-81 (*i.e.* D77T80L81 in B*2705 or N77I80A81 in B*5101 and B*5801), and therefore

Table I. Lysis of C1R and HLA transfectants by NK clones from a single donor (HLA- B27/-B18)

Number of clones	NK Lysis C1R	C1R-B*0702	C1R-B*2705
45	+	- [(1)]	-
6	+	-	+
5	+	+	-
1	+	+	+
11	-	nt	nt

[(1)] When cytotoxicity against an HLA class I transfectant was diminished by 50% or more compared with untransfected C1R cells.

Table II. Lysis of C1R transfected with B27 subtypes and B*2705 mutants by specific B*2705 specific clones

Target C1R Transfected with	NK clones RJ18	RJ48	RJ76	RJ19	RJ43	RJ141 (1)
None	+	+	+	+	+	+
B*2701	-	-	-	-	-	+
B*2702	+	+	+	+	+	+
B*2703	-	-	-	-	-	+
B*2704	-	-	-	-	-	+
B*2706	-	-	-	-	-	+
B*2705 wildtype	-	-	-	-	-	+
B*2705-Y74	-	-	-	-	-	+
B*2705-I80	+	+	+	+	+	+
B*2705-A81	-	-	-	-	-	+
B*2705-N77/I80	-	-	+/-	+/-	+/-	+

(1) control clone

were not significantly affected by Thr80/Ile80 polymorphism. Furthermore, NK3 clones have been defined by recognition of Ile80 in HLA-Bw4 (4), NK1 clones by recognition of Lys80 in HLA-Cw4 allele and NK2 by recognition of Ser77 in HLA-Cw3 allele [3].

The fact that residue 80 is involved in the structure of pocket E and F of the peptide binding groove [8], suggests that the peptides bound to MHC molecules could participate in the specificity of NK recognition. Although other results analyzing the effect of single mutations in NK recognition and in particular the results of Malnati *et al.* [9], further support this possibility, the issue still remains controversial as the murine NK inhibitory receptor Ly-49A recognize MHC molecules independently of the type of bound peptide [10]. Two additional NK clones obtained from a different donor were also selected by their capacity to lyse C1R transfected with B*2702 but not C1R transfected with B*2705 and screened using I80 and N77/I80 mutants transfected C1R line, confirming that NK resistance induced by B*2705 was reverted by T→ I mutation in position 80.

This work was supported by grants CICYT1001/92 and FIS95/1169 (J.P.), FIS1541/94 (R. S.) and SAF94/0891 and an institutional grant of the Foundation Ramon Areces to the CBMSO (J.A.L-C.). rIL-2 was generously provided by Hoffmann-La Roche, Nutley, NJ.

References

1. Solana R, Peña J. MHC antigens and NK cells, 1st ed. Austin, TX: R.G. Landes Company, 1994.
2. López-Botet M, Moretta L, Strominger J. NK-cell receptors and recognition of MHC class I molecules. *Immunol Today* 1995; 17: 212.
3. Biassoni R, Falco M, Cambiaggi A, Costa P, Verdiani S, Pende D, Conte R, Donato C, Parham P, an Moretta L. Amino acid substitution can influence the natural killer (NK)-mediated recognition of HLA-C molecules. Role of serine-77 and lysine-80 in the target cell protection from lysis mediated by "group 2" or "group 1" NK clones. *J Exp Med* 1995; 182: 605.

4. Cella M, Longo A, Ferrara GB, Strominger JL, Colonna M. NK3-specific natural killer cells are selectively inhibited by Bw4-positive HLA alleles with isoleucine 80. *J Exp Med* 1994; 180: 1235.
5. Luque I, Solana R, Galiani MD, González R, García F, López de Castro JA, Peña J. Threonine 80 on HLA-B27 confers protection to lysis by a group of NK clones. *Eur J Immunol* 1996; 26: 1974.
6. Lopez de Castro JA. Structural polymorphism and function of HLA-B27. *Curr Op Rheumatol* 1990; 7: 270.
7. Gumperz JE, Litwin V, Philips JH, Lanier LL, Parham P. The Bw4 public epitope of HLA-B molecules confers reactivity with natural killer cells clones that express NKB1, a putative HLA receptor. *J Exp Med* 1995; 181: 1133.
8. Madden DR, Gorga JC, Strominger JL, Wiley CD. The structure of HLA-B27 revels nonamer self peptides bound in an extended conformation. *Nature* 1991; 353: 321.
9. Malnati MS, Peruzzi M, Parker KC, Biddison WE, Ciccone E, Moretta A, Long EO. Peptide specificity in the recognition of MHC class I by natural killer cell clones. *Science* 1995; 267: 1016.
10. Correa I, Raulet DH. Binding of diverse peptides to MHC class I molecules inhibits target cell lysis by activated natural killer cells. *Immunity* 1995; 2: 61.

Downregulation of $\gamma\delta$ T cell recognition by receptors for HLA class I molecules

H. Nakajima, H. Tomiyama, Y. Ikeda Moore, M. Takiguchi

Department of Tumor Biology, Institute of Medical Science, University of Tokyo, 461 Shirokanedai, 108 Tokyo, Japan

It is well known that natural killer (NK) cells have receptors for major histocompatibility complex (MHC) class I molecules that negatively regulate the cytotoxicity with respect to the target cells of NK cells. Several genes encoding the murine and human NK cell inhibitory receptors have been cloned, and recent studies have shown that some $\alpha\beta$ T cells also carry these receptors which inhibit the recognition of T cells [1]. In humans $\gamma\delta$ T cells are a minor fraction of all T cells, but they have a unique role in immune systems to recognize antigens in a different way of $\alpha\beta$ T cells. It is shown that some $\gamma\delta$ T cells also express the receptors [2].Here we show that some $\gamma\delta$ T cell clones were also negatively downregulated by receptors for HLA class I molecules [3]. There was a diversity of reactions against polymorphic HLA class I molecules, implying the existence of heterogeneous populations of receptors.

After stimulations of PBL from HIV-1 patients with HIV-1 peptides, CTL clones were generated by a limiting dilutions. CTL clones having non specific killing activity were selected for this study and eight $\gamma\delta$ T cell clones out of these CTL clones were used in this study. To investigate the effect of HLA class I expression on target cells, we tested these $\gamma\delta$ T cell clones for the ability to lyse a panel of C1R transfectants expressing HLA-A, -B, -C molecules. Relative percentage value of specific lysis of C1R transfectants for C1R cells were shown in *Table I*. Recognition of seven $\gamma\delta$ T cell clones were downregulated by the expression of polymorphic HLA class I molecules. The HLA class I molecules which inhibited the cytolysis by these CTL clones were different in each $\gamma\delta$ T cell clones. These results suggest that the inhibitory effect on cytolysis by these $\gamma\delta$ CTL clones is mediated by heterogenous populations of receptors for HLA class I molecules. HLA-B*0702 showed strong inhibitory effects, which were observed in six of eight clones. In contrast, the expression of tested 10 HLA class I molecules failed to inhibit the cytolysis of one $\gamma\delta$ T cell clone carrying both CD8 and CD56 (T-HIV-B35-14-320). By flowcytometric analysis with anti-p58, anti-CD94, and anti-NKB1 mAbs, seven of eight clones did not carry known receptors for HLA class I molecules. No clones expressed NK cell related surface molecule CD16 (FcIIIγ receptors).

Moreover, we investigated whether the cytolysis of C1R transfectants is restored in the presence of mAb specific for HLA class I molecules. The cytolysis of C1R-B*0702 cells by two $\gamma\delta$ T cell clones (T-HIV-B35-14-10 and T-HIV-B35-SF2-24-20) was tested using W6/32 anti-HLA class I mAb, SFR8-B6 anti-Bw6 mAb, and MB40.2 anti-HLA-B7 mAb. The cytolysis by both CTL clones were restored in the presence of W6/32 mAb at a dose-dependent fashion. On the other hand, SFR8-B6 and MB40.2 mAbs failed to restore the cytolysis of C1R-B*0702, which is stained strongly with the two mAbs. Scince SFR8-B6 recognizes residues 77-83, which provide Bw6 epitopes, the results suggest that the binding site of the receptors of these $\gamma\delta$ T cell clones is different from that of known NK receptors. Moreover, these clones recognize a site different from a MB40.2 binding site.

We tested the effect of mAb specific for CD3 or $\gamma\delta$ TCR on cytolysis by T-HIV-B35-SF2-24-20 clone in order to clarify the role of $\gamma\delta$ TCR on antigen recognition. The cytolysis of C1R cells by T-HIV-B35-SF2-24-20 clone was inhibited by both mAbs, indicating that $\gamma\delta$ TCR recognizes antigens on C1R cells and acts as a stimulatory receptor. On the other hand, these mAbs failed to restore the cytolysis of C1R-B*0702 cells by this clone, suggesting that $\gamma\delta$ TCR does not act as an inhibitory receptor.

Table I. The expression of class I molecules inhibits the lysis of C1R cells

	C1R	.A*0201	.A*2401	.A*3302	.B*0702	.B*3501	.B*3901	.B*5101	.B*5201	.B*4001	.Cw*0702	K562
T-HIV-B35-14-10	100	49	60	62	16	78	47	88	80	50	57	2
T-HIV-B35-14-206	100	92	28	36	3	29	34	48	43	19	104	2
T-HIV-B35-14-210	100	131	169	66	9	38	77	58	64	22	94	0
T-HIV-B35-14-212	100	106	57	19	1	7	42	12	31	7	64	0
T-HIV-B35-14-320	100	106	133	131	84	125	103	124	127	116	89	9
T-HIV-B35-SF2-24-20	100	124	107	140	37	141	104	217	140	60	135	6
T-HIV-B35-SF2-24-34	100	111	52	47	1	30	34	49	49	18	75	0
YY-D3-1	100	-	69	-	70	132	-	19	21	-	-	-

- No Data   <20%   <50%

Relative percentage values (RPV) of specific lysis of C1R transfectants for C1R cells is presented.
RPV=% specific lysis of C1R transfectant / % specific lysis of C1R cells x100.

Only one out of eight γδ T cell clones, YY-D3-1, expressed NKB1 receptors which recognize residues 77-80 of the HLA-Bw4 structural motif. To investigate the effect of NKB1 molecules on γδ T cell, we tested this clone for the ability to lyse five C1R transfectants expressing HLA-Bw4 or HLA-Bw6 molecules *(Table I).* Expression of HLA-B*5101 and -B*5201 molecules carrying Bw4 motif well inhibited the lysis of YY-D3-1 clone. The lysis against C1R-B*5101 and -5201 were restored by the blocking of NKB1 molecules on YY-D3-1 clone with DX9 mAb. On the other hand, expression of HLA-A*2402 molecules having the Bw4 epitope did not effectively prevent the cytolysis of C1R transfectants by YY-D3-1 clone. Moreover the cytolytic activity of this CTL clone against C1R-A*2402 did not upregulate in the presence of DX9 mAb. These results indicate that NKB1 receptors on γδ CTL clone actually recognized HLA-B*5101 and -B*5202 but not -A*2402 carrying the Bw4 epitope. Scince Bw4 positive HLA-B binding peptides is different from HLA-A*2402 bind peptides, it is suspected this receptor recognize a peptide bound to HLA-Bw4 molecules. Our recent study showed that position 8 of nonamer peptides influenced the binding of Tü109 anti-Bw4 mAb[4]], implying that NKB1 molecules recognize a comformational structure formed by Bw4 motif and position 8 of binding peptides.

In this study we demonstrated the exsistence of the heterogenic inhibitory receptors for HLA class I molecules on γδ T cell. Heterogeneity of these receptors may correspond to the polymorphism of MHC class I molecules and MHC class I binding peptides. Scince most Ag-specific γδ T cells show no MHC restriction, the recognition of γδ T cell may be negatively regulated by the expression of MHC class I molecules on target cells. γδ T cells have a crucial role on eliminating tumor cells as well as virus- and bacteria-infected cells lacking MHC class I molecules through antigen recognition *via* γδ TCR. The immune recognition might be cooperatively regulated by both receptors of CTL.

References

1. Phillips JH, Gumperz JE, Parham P, Lanier LL. Superantigen-dependent, cell-mediated cytotoxicity inhibited by MHC class I receptors on T lymphocytes. *Science* 1995;268:403-5.
2. Ferrini S, Cambiaggi A, Meazza R, Sforzini S, Marciano S, Mingari MC, Moretta L. T cell clones expressing the natural killer cell-related p58 receptor molecule display heterogeneity in phenotypic properties and p58 function. *Eur J Immunol* 1994;24:2294-8.
3. Nakajima H, Tomiyama H, Takiguchi M. Inhibition of γδ T cell recognition by receptors for MHC class I molecules. *J Immunol* 1995;155:4139-42.
4. Takamiya Y, Sakaguchi T, Miwa K, Takiguchi M. Role of HLA-B*5101 binding nonamer peptides in formation of the HLA-Bw4 public epitope. *Int Immunol* 1997 (in press).

Fas lytic activity mediated by human cord blood lymphocytes

Z. Brahmi, A. Montel, G. Hommel-Berrey

Department of Medicine and Microbiology-Immunology, IU School of Medicine, 702 Barnhill Drive, Indianapolis, IN, USA

As of this study, more than 200 bone marrow transplants have been performed using cord blood as the source of stem cells. We and others have recently shown that freshly isolated umbilical cord blood cells (UCBC) failed to lyse NK tumor targets by the traditional exocytosis mechanism involving perforin and the granzymes, but that they regain their lytic potential after 18 hour treatment with IL-2, IL-12 or IL-15. The reason for this hyperesponsiveness is not completely understood, although we have demonstrated that soluble HLA may be responsible, at least in part, for this lack of activity [1]. To date, however, no study has investigated whether or not fresh UCBC can mediate tumor lysis via the newly described Fas lytic pathway. This pathway is triggered when the FAS ligand (FasL), present on the effector cells (EC) engages the Fas antigen, present on the target cells (TC). The interaction results in the generation of apoptotic death signals that lead to the demise of the TC involving DNA degradation into small oligonucleotide fragments, membrane blebbing and chromatin condensation. The Fas lytic pathway was first described in a rat CTL hybridoma clones and in peritoneal exudate lymphocytes from mice [2]. Subsequently, Arase *et al.* [3] have shown that murine NK cells constitutively express FasL mRNA and our laboratory has demonstrated that upon stimulation with PMA and ionophore (PIO), human NK cells increase FasL mRNA levels [4]. More recently, Eischen *et al.* demonstrated that human NK clones have high levels of FasL mRNA and they can use the Fas lytic pathway when stimulated with immobilized anti-Fc receptor antibody [5].

In the current study, we wanted to determine whether fresh, unstimulated and stimulated UCBC can lyse Fas+ tumor TC *via* the Fas lytic pathway.

Materials and methods

Umbilical cord blood cells

UCBC were obtained from the umbilical cord of full term newborn children. Lymphocytes were isolated by Ficoll-Hypaque [6].

^{51}Cr-release assays

Standard ^{51}Cr-release assays were performed as previously described [6]. As TC, we used Fas+ cell lines (BL41-B95, an EBV^{+} derivative of the Burkitt lymphoma cell line BL-41 (a gift of Dr Elliott Kief) and Jurkat F+; and Fas- TC (K562, gpt 2, a transfectant derived from BL-41 and Fas-Jurkat, a generous gift of Dr P.H. Krammer (German Cancer Research Center, Heidelberg, Germany).

Reverse transcription chain reaction (RT-PCR)

Total RNA was isolated from 0.5 x 10^6 cells using Tri-reagent (Molecular Research Center, Inc., OH) and reverse transcribed as instructed by the manufacturer for the first strand cDNA synthesis kit (Boehringer Mannheim, Indianapolis, IN) and using an oligo-p(dt)$_{15}$ as primer. Five microliters from each 20 µl RT reaction were used to amplify a 503 bp fragment of Fas with FasL specific primers. In addition, 5 µl from each reaction were used to amplify a 213 bp fragment of histone 3.3 (internal standard). Ten µl of PCR product were electrophoresed in a 1.4% agarose gel, transferred to a nylon membrane and probed with FasL (or H 3.3) PCR products labeled with ^{32}P-dCTP and ^{32}P-dATP using the Megaprime DNA labeling Kit (Amersham). After washing, the membranes were exposed to film.

Results and discussion

First, we wanted to determine whether freshly collected, unstimulated UCBC or UCBC stimulated with PIO could lyse a Fas+ TC in a standard 4 hour ^{52}Cr-release assay. Neither Fas+ TC nor Fas- TC were lysed (data not shown).

Next, we wanted to determine whether or not by incubating UBCB in medium alone or in medium supplement with IL-2 we could boost Fas-mediated lytic function. As we previously reported, NK lytic activity mediated by UCBC incubated with IL-2 for 18 hours was high, but with medium alone the activity was low (*Table I*). UCBC had essentially no lytic activity against either gpt 2 (Fas-) or BL41B95 (Fas+) TC in 4 hour ^{51}Cr-release assays, even after treatment with PIO. We obtained essentially the same results when UCBC were kept up to 5 days in culture.

Table I. Cord blood cells (UCBC) were kept in culture for up to 5 days in medium alone or in medium supplemented with IL-2; UCBC were then tested for lytic activity in 4 hr ^{51}Cr-release assays in the presence or absence of PMA and ionophore (PIO)

EC	Target cells			Incubation
	K562(F-)	GPT2(F-)	BL41B95(F+)	Time
UCBC in medium	10.5+7.17	3.5+1.32	1.0	3 days
"+PIO	12.1+6.08	1.25+.25	2.25.+.75	3 days
"IL2	44.7+19.8	23.7+8.5	10.0+3.87	3 days
"+IL2+PIO	28.7+14.4	6.2+2.3	7.0+3.67	3 days
UCBC in medium	14.6+7.80	6.0+2.51	1.0	5 days
" + PIO	6.33+3.52	1.3+.33	2.7+1.2	5 days
" + IL2	51.3+8.81	39.3+4.0	20.7+8.7	5 days
"+IL2+PIO	29.7+13.1	14+7.5	23+7.5	5 days

In the experiments described above, UCBC were not pretreated with PIO, but rather PIO was added at the beginning of the 4 hour ^{51}Cr-release assays. Next, we theorized that by pretreating UCBC with PIO for 2 hours, this will allow the FasL to be expressed on the surface of UCBC. We therefore pretreated UCBC with PIO for 2 hours, then tested the cells against Jurkat Fas+ and Jurkat Fas-TC in 18 hour ^{51}Cr-release assays. Jurkat Fas+ have been shown to be exquisitely sensitive to lysis by the FasL. In addition, to distinguish between granule-mediated and Fas-mediated lysis, we added EGTA to the medium to chelate calcium and thus inhibited the granule-mediated lysis (*Table II*).

To ensure that the lytic activity observed against the Fas+ TC in the presence of EGTA was mediated by the Fas lytic pathway, we added a monoclonal antibody

Table II. Unstimulated and cord blood cells pre-stimulated with PMA/ ionophore for 2 hours were tested against Fas+ and Fas-TC in 18 hr ^{51}Cr-release assays. Fresh NK cells and YT, an NK-like cell line that expresses the Fas ligand constitutively, were used as controls

EC	Target cells		
	Jurkat F+	Jurkat F+/EGTA	Jurkat/F-
UCBC	25.2+2.13	13.7+2.2	14.8+2.7
UCBC +PIO	18.8+2.5	24.5+2.9	3.8+1.3
NK	13+1.1	5.5+.6	9.0+1.0
NK + PIO	12.5+7.5	19.1+3.0	2.2+1.3
YT	31	15	31
YT+ PIO	35	18	19

(M3, a generous gift of Dr David Lynch, Immunex) that blocks the Fas pathway [7] . As a control, we used a non Fas blocking antibody (M33). M3 inhibited lysis of Jurkat Fas+ in the presence of EGTA by about 70 percent, whereas M33 did not (it actually increased it slightly, *Table III*).

Table III. UCBC unstimulated or pre-stimulated with PIO for 2 hours were tested against Jurk F+ and Jurk F- in 18 Hr ^{51}Cr-release assays with or without EGTA. A Fas blocking monoclonal Ab (M3) and a non-blocking one (M33) were also used. YT-INDY, an NK-like cell line expressing the FasL constitutively was used as a control

	Jurkat F+	Jurkat F+/EGTA	Jurkat/F-
UCBC	10.6+3.1	-1.66+0.7	2.6+11.0
UCBC +PIO	26.2+5.2	19.8+3.6	15.7+2.3
UCBC +PIO+M3	7.6		
UCBC +PIO+M33	26.5		
YT	35.8	22.6	7.9
YT+PIO	48.1	30.8	5.1
YT+M3	16.7	3.3	
YT+M33	27.5	26.1	

Finally, when we extracted RNA from UCBC and reverse transcribed it by RT-PCR, we showed that unstimulated UCBC did have the message for the Fas ligand and treatment with PIO did increase the message level substantially (*Figure 1*).

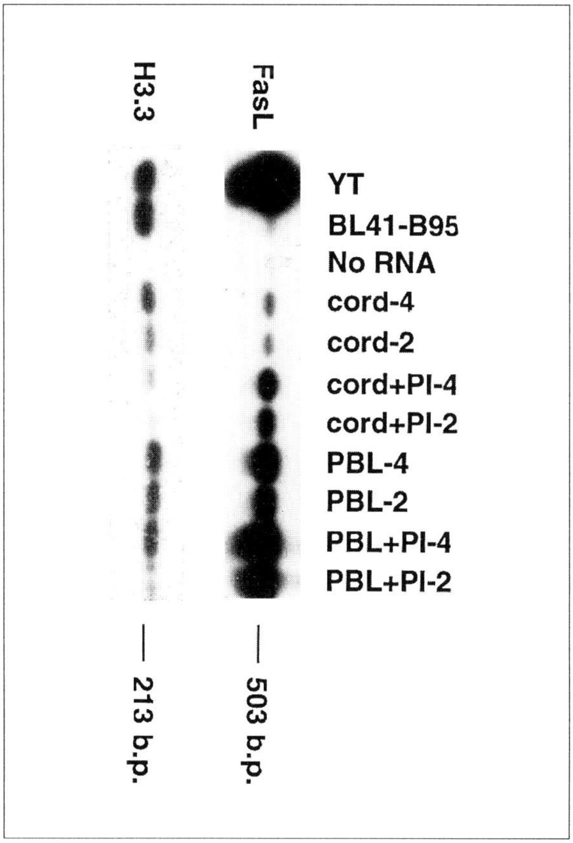

Figure 1. FasL message levels in umbilical cord blood cells are increased by PMA/ionophore (PI) stimulation. Total RNA was extracted from 2 cord blood samples (cord-2, cord-4), 2 normal PBLs, as Fas ligand positive control cell line (YT) and a Fas ligand negative control B cell line (BL41-B95) that were incubated either in CM alone or in CM containing PMA (20 and 40 ng/ml, PI-2 and PI-4, respectively) and ionophore (1 µg/ml) for 1 hr at 37°C. Total RNA was reverse transcribed using an oligo-p(dt)$_{15}$ primer. A 503 bp fragment of FasL cDNA or a 213 bp fragment of histone H3.3 cDNA was amplified, electrophoresed on an agarose gel, transferred to a nylon membrane, probed with ^{32}P-labeled FasL or H3.3 PCR products, an exposed to film.

In conclusion, we have shown that: (1) fresh UCBC do have the message for the Fas Ligand; (2) the message is increased by PIO treatment; (3) sensitive Fas+ TC can be lysed in 18 hour ^{51}Cr-release assays but not in 4 hour assays. These results indicate that Fas lysis may require the presence of another "facilitating" molecule besides the FasL for full activity.

References

1. Webb B, Bochan M, Montel A, Padilla LM, Brahmi Z. The lack of cytotoxicity associated with fresh HUCB may be due to the presence of soluble HLA in the serum. *Cell Immunol* 1994; 159:246-61.
2. Rouvier E, Luciani MF, Goldstein P. Fas involvement in Ca^{2+}-independent T cell-mediated cytotoxicity. *J Exp Med* 1993; 177: 195-200.
3. Arase H, Arase N. Fas-mediated cytotoxicity by freshly isolated natural killer cells. *J Exp Med* 1995; 181 :1235-8.
4. Montel AH, Bochan MR, Hobbs JA, Lynch D, Brahmi Z. Fas involvement in cytotoxicity mediated by human NK cells. *Cell Immunol* 1995; 166:236-46.
5. Eichen CM, Schilling JD, Lynch D, Krammer PH, Leibson PJ. Fc receptor-induced expression of Fas ligand on activated NK cells facilitates cell-mediated cytotoxicity and subsequent autocrine NK cell apoptosis. *J Immunol* 1996; 156: 2693-9.
6. Brahmi Z, Bray RA, Abrams SI. Evidence for an early calcium-independent event in the activation of the human natural killer cell cytolytic mechanism. *J Immunol* 1985; 135:4108-13.
7. Alderson MR, Tough TW, Braddy S, David-Smith T, Roux E, Schooley K, Miller S, Lynch DH. Regulation of apoptosis and T cell cytolytic mechanism. *Int Immunol* 1994; 6:1799-806.

Symposium communications

HLA Diversity

HLA typing and sequencing

Function of HLA

Transplantation biology and medicine

HLA and Diseases

Transplantation biology and medicine

Allorecognition. Tolerance and immunosupression in transplantation

Contents

The influence of HLA antigens on the T cell receptor repertoire

B. Gulwani-Akolkar[1], W. Bias[2], N. Kashiwagi[4], M. Kotb[3], M. El Demellawy[3], A. Kotby[5], M.S. Leffell[2], F. Obata[4], J. Silver[1]

1 North Shore University Hospital, Cornell U Med Coll, 300 Community Drive, Manhasset, New York 11030, USA
2 Johns Hopkins University, Baltimore, MD, USA
3 University Tennessee, Memphis,TN, USA
4 Kitasato University School of Medicine, Sagamihara, Japan
5 Ain Shams University Cairo, Egypt

The fine specificity of T cells is determined by a receptor for antigen displayed on the cell surface which is a heterodimer composed of an α chain and a β chain. The variable regions of these chains are responsible for antigen recognition and are encoded by juxataposed variable (V), diversity (D) (for β chains), and joining (J) gene segments. The enormous repertoire of T cell receptor (TCR) specificities is partially created by the random rearrangement of germline V, D and J region genes. Additional diversity is generated by the random insertion and deletion of nucleotides at the Vα-Jα and Vβ-D-Jβ junctional regions. The Vα-Jα and Vβ-D-Jβ junctional residues of the T cell receptor form the CDR3 region which is believed to be involved primarily with the recognition of peptides while the remainder of the V gene segment is thought to play a predominant role in MHC recognition [1].

Studies in mice have shown that the murine MHC, also known as H-2, plays a prominent role in shaping the TCR repertoire [2]. Once rearrangement occurs, most T cells undergo a selection process in the thymus in which autoreactive cells are deleted and cells with the potential to recognize foreign peptides presented by self-MHC molecules are allowed to further develop and emigrate to the various lymphoid organs and peripheral blood. Thus, during the thymic education process there is selection for, or against, particular V segments depending upon the HLA type of the individual. In addition, several other factors play important roles in determining the final TCR repertoire. These include mutations in the germline TCR genes which can dramatically alter the levels of particular V gene segments and, exposure to environmental antigens, which can also significantly skew the TCR repertoire [3, 4].

Previous studies have demonstrated that HLA can profoundly influence the TCRBV repertoire with little or no effect on the TCRAV segment usage [5-7]. To further document these observations the relative frequencies of T cells expressing various V segments was determined in individuals of selected families by three color staining using BV- and AV-specific mAb.

Materials and methods

Cell isolation and staining

Mononuclear cells were isolated from peripheral blood by Ficoll/Hypaque density gradient centrifugation and suspended in phosphate buffered saline containing 1 % BSA and 0.02 % NaN3 at 5 x 106 cells/ml. One hundred µl were incubated simultaneously with TCR-FITC, CD45 RO-PE, and CD4-PE Cy5 or CD8-PE Cy5 mAbs, for 30 min at 4°C, washed three times with PBS containing 1% BSA and 0.02 % NaN3 and fixed in PBS containing 2% formaldehyde. Fifteen mAb specific for BV2, BV3, BV5S1, BV5S2/S3, BV6S7, BV8, BV12, BV13, BV14, BV16, BV17, BV20, BV22, AV2 and AV12 were generously provided by T Cell Sciences and Immunotech and used in this study. The cells were analysed by gating on lymphocytes using forward and side scatter parameters and 50,000 cells were analysed using a live gate.

HLA typing

HLA typing for class I and class II Ag was performed by conventional microcytotoxicity or by sequence analysis.

Results and discussion

Previous studies analyzed the TCR repertoires of related and unrelated individuals by staining with BV-specific mAb in order to assess the influence of genetic (*e.g.* HLA) factors on the TCR repertoire [5-7]. These studies

Table I. Relative levels of expression of TCR V-segments in CD4+ and CD8+T cells

	CD4					CD8			
V-segments	AK	AM	JP	KB	V-segments	AK	AM	JP	KB
TCRBV5S1	2.6±1.1	3.7±1.1	2.7±1.0	3.2±1.8	TCRBV5S1	3.8±3.6	4.4±3.1	3.7±2.8	3.9±1.8
TCRBV6	5.7±2.8	9.8±3.1	1.9±1.3	4.7±3.2	TCRBV6	3.9±1.6	7.5±4.8	1.1±0.8	4.2±2.3
TCRBV8	5.1±3.5	14.2±7.1	5.2±2.3	9.5±4.9	TCRBV8	5.7±3.5	12.8±6.3	3.5±1.4	10.4±7.9
TCRBV12	2.4±0.7	2.9±1.3	2.6±2.1	2.9±1.6	TCRBV12	2.8±2.7	4.7±3.0	1.5±0.7	4.6±3.7
TCRBV13	5.9±2.7	8.4±2.3	6.0±4.2	7.9±3.7	TCRBV13	5.0±2.5	9.1±4.4	4.5±1.9	6.8±3.1
TCRBV20	4.8±3.9	6.1±4.0	2.4±1.3	5.7±3.7	TCRBV20	5.4±4.1	7.4±4.6	1.4±1.3	5.8±3.6
TCRAV2	3.3±1.3	5.7±2.3	3.2±1.4	5.3±3.5	TCRAV2	3.9±2.3	5.8±2.9	4.0±2.4	7.3±4.2

revealed a strong influence of HLA genes on the BV repertoire. For the purpose of this study four different ethnic groups were studied involving a total of ten families and eight pairs of HLA-identical siblings. They were the Japanese (JP), Amish (AM), Egyptian (KB) and the Long Island (AK) population. The average percentage of CD4+ and CD8+ T cells reacting with seven individual mAb, some of which showed an unusual population distribution, is shown in *Table I.* It was observed that the Japanese population had significantly fewer CD4+ and CD8+ cells reacting with mAb specific for TCRBV6S7 and TCRBV20 (Mann Whitney test). In contrast, the Amish and Egyptian population demonstrated a significantly higher number of T cells reactive with mAb for BV8 and BV12. The lower number of cells reacting with the mAb for BV6S7 in the Japanese population is very likely due to the fact that the OT145 mAb reacts with only one of the two alleles (allele a) of the BV6S7 gene product whereas the Japanese population is known to have a high frequency of the non-reactive BV6S7b gene product [8]. Similarly, the lower number of cells reactive with the BV20 mAb is very likely due to the high frequency of a BV20 "null" allele in the Japanese population [9]. The higher number of cells reacting with the mAb for BV8 and BV12 in the Egyptian and Amish populations cannot be similarly explained and may reflect "positive" selection by specific HLA alleles.

To determine whether HLA genes nevertheless could be shown to influence the TCR repertoire, similarities in repertoires between individuals were assessed by comparing the frequencies of T cells reacting with each of the fifteen V region-specific mAb in both the CD4+ and CD8+ populations. Thus, 30 parameters were used to compute a "Δ" score which represents the sum of the absolute differences between any two individuals for all 30 parameters. It was observed that the Δ scores, *ie.*, repertoire differences, were significantly lower ($p<0.001$ as determined by a two way analysis of variance) for HLA-identical siblings than forhaplo-identical siblings (*Figure 1*). These studies confirm the role of HLA genes on the TCR repertoire and also emphasize an important role for non-HLA genes on the repertoire [9, 10].

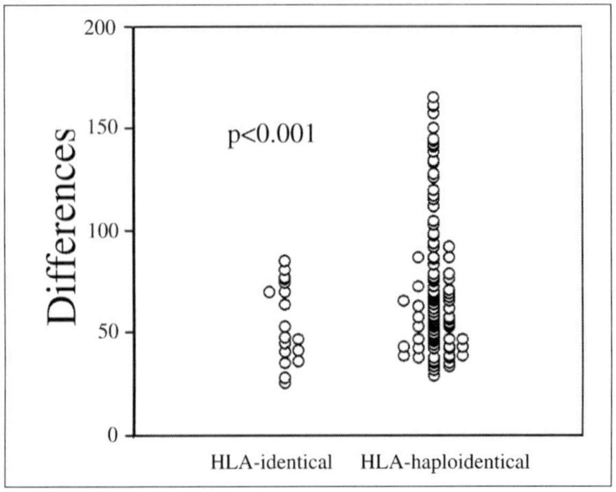

Figure 1. Distribution of "Δ" scores in pairwise comparisons of HLA-identical and HLA-haplo-identical individuals.

References

1. Marrack P, Kappler J. The T cell receptor. *Science* 1987;238:1073-8.
2. Bill J, Palmer E. Positive selection of CD4+ T cells mediated by MHC class II-bearing stromal cell in the thymic cortex. *Nature* 1989;341:649-51.
3. MacDonald HR, Lees RK, Schneider R, Zinkernagel RM, Hengartner H. Positive selection of CD4+ thymocytes controlled by MHC class II gene products. *Nature* 1988;336:471-3.
4. Fowlkes BJ, Schwartz RH, Pardoll DM. Deletion of self-reactive thymocytes occurs at CD4+8+ precursor stage. *Nature* 1988; 334:620-3.
5. Gulwani-Akolkar B, Posnett DN, Janson CH, Grunewald J, Wigzell H, Akolkar PN, Gregersen PK, Silver J. T cell receptor V-segment frequencies in peripheral blood T cells correlate with human leukocyte antigen type. *J Exp Med* 1991;174:1139-46.
6. Akolkar PN, Gulwani-Akolkar B, Pergolizzi R, Bigler RD, Silver J. Influence of HLA genes on T cell receptor V segment frequencies and expression levels in peripheral blood lymphocytes. *J Immunol* 1993;150:2761-73.
7. Gulwani-Akolkar B, Shi B, Akolkar PN, Ito K, Bias WB, Silver J. Do HLA genes play a prominent role in determining T cell receptor Vα segment usage in humans? *J Immunol* 1995;154:3843-51.
8. Li Y, Szabo P, Robinson MA, Dong B, Posnett D. Allelic variations in the human T cell receptor Vb gene products. *J Exp Med* 1990;171:221-30.
9. Malhotra V, Speilman R, Concannon P. Variability in T cell receptor Vβ usage in human peripheral blood lymphocytes. Studies of identical twins, siblings, and insulin-dependent diabetes mellitus patients. *J Immunol* 1992;149:1802-8.
10. Akolkar PN, Gulwani-Akolkar B, Robinson MA, Silver J. The influence of non-HLA genes on the human T-cell receptor repertoire. *Scand J Immunol* 1995; 42:248-56.

Self-restricted T cell recognition of donor HLA-DR peptides during graft rejection

Z. Liu, A.I. Colovai, S. Tugulea, J. Kinne, E.F. Reed, E.A. Rose, R.E. Michler, D. Cohen, M.A. Hardy, J. Molajoni, R. Cortesini, N. Suciu-Foca

College of Physicians and Surgeons of Columbia University, Department of Pathology, 630 West 168th Street, 14-401, New York, 10032, USA

The rejection of organ allografts is mediated by T cells which recognize the mismatched alloantigens of the donor either directly, *i.e.* without processing by host APC [1] or indirectly *i.e.* after processing and presentation of donor-derived allopeptides by host APC [2].
Direct recognition accounts for the strong, polyclonal T cell response seen *in vitro* in MLC and *in vivo* during early acute rejection episodes [1]. This process, however, does not explain the development of anti-HLA antibodies following transplantation since T cells recognizing processed forms of the allogeneic MHC molecules are required for generating specific help for allo-antibody producing B cells [3]. It is more likely that the humoral arm of the immune response to allogeneic transplants is activated *via* the indirect pathway.
Because the major threat to allograft survival is the development of anti-HLA antibodies [4], we have investigated the activation of the indirect recognition pathway following transplantation in 30 heart and 15 kidney allograft recipients.

Material and methods

LDA analysis of allopeptide reactive T cells in the graft and in the periphery

The method used for determining the frequency of donor-allopeptide specific T cells in the graft and in the periphery was the same with few exceptions [5]. PBMCs were obtained from the patients at weekly intervals during the first month and at two week intervals during the second and third month following transplantation. PBMC were counted and plated directly in 96-round bottom well trays at concentrations of 4, 2, $1x10^4$/well in 24 replicate-reactions. The cells were then expanded for 7 days in medium with IL-2, and tested over the next 3 days for reactivity to donor peptides in split-well assays. Biopsies were obtained at the same time intervals for histologic diagnosis of heart allograft rejection. Kidney allograft biopsies were not included in this study. The heart biopsy ($1mm^3$) was first cultured for 7-days in medium with IL-2 in order to generate a sufficient number of cells for testing. T cells were then harvested, counted, and plated in 96 well trays at various concentrations (8, 4 and $2x10^2$/well). After 7 days of expansion in medium with IL-2, the cells were tested in 3 day blastogenesis assay for reactivity to donor peptides. Blastogenesis was measured by ^{3}H[TdR] incorporation. The frequency of allopeptide reactive T cells was determined as previously described [6].

HLA typing

All recipients and donors were typed for HLA-DR antigens by conventional serology and by molecular methodology using PCR-SSOP (sequence specific-oligonucleotide probe).

Peptide synthesis

Synthetic peptides corresponding to residues 1-19, 21-39, 62-80 of DRβ1 chain from 32 HLA-DR alleles (DRβ1*0101, DRβ1*0102, DRβ1*0301, DRβ1*0302, DRβ1*0401, DRβ*0402, DRβ*0403, DRβ1*0404, DRβ*0405, DRβ1*0407, DRβ1*0408, DRβ1*0701, DRβ1*0801, DRβ1*0802, DDRβ1*0803, DRβ1*0804, DRβ1*0901, DRβ1*1001,DRβ1*1101, DRβ1*1102, DRβ1*1104, DRβ1*1201, DRβ1*1301, DRβ1*1302, DRβ1*1303, DRβ1*1401, DRβ1*1402, DRβ1*1501, DRβ1*1502, DRβ1*1503, DRβ1*1601, and DRβ1*1602) [7] were obtained from Chiron Mimotopes (San Diego, CA) and Peptide Innovation (Raleigh, NC). The purity of peptides was higher than 90%, as indicated by HPLC and mass spectrometry. Synthetic peptides were dissolved in RPMI 1640 medium at a concentration of 2mg/ml.

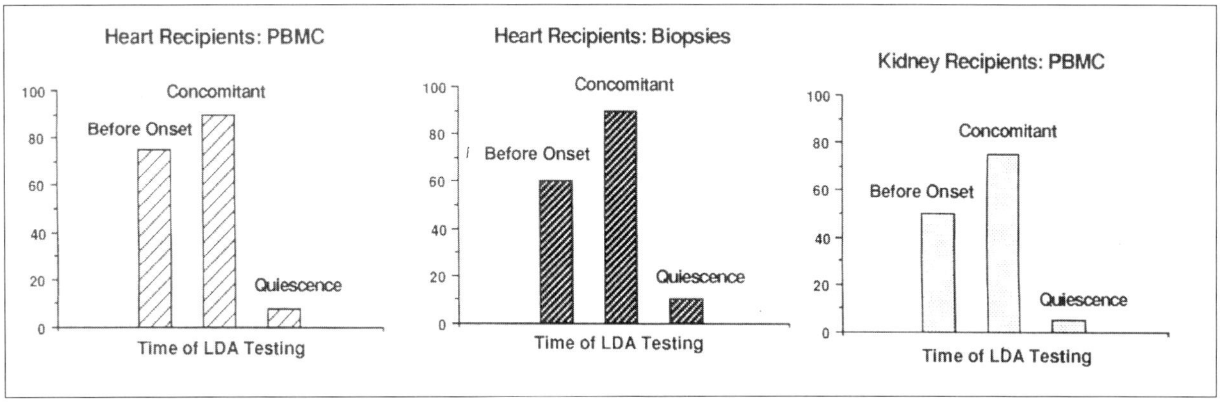

Figure 1. Relatonship between T cell reactivity to donor allopeptides and clinical status.

Results and discussion

To investigate the contribution of indirect recognition to allograft rejection we have monitored a population of 30 heart and 15 kidney allograft recipients for T cell reactivity to synthetic allopeptides corresponding to the hypervariable region of each HLA-DR antigen mismatched in the donor. In heart allograft recipients the presence of allopeptide reactive T cells in the periphery and in the graft showed a strong positive correlation with rejection episode. Analysis of Th precursor frequency showed that allopeptide reactive T cells were present in the circulation 7-14 days prior to the histologic diagnosis of rejection in 65% of the cases tested (N=26). Ninety percent of LDA performed at the time of rejection (N=30) revealed the presence of allopeptide reactive T cells in the periphery. In contrast, only 8% of the assays performed on PBMCs from patients in quiescence (N=50) showed allopeptide-reactivity (*Figure 1A*). The frequency of positive LDA obtained when T cells infiltrating the graft were tested for alloreactivity was 60% before histologic diagnosis of rejection, 90% at the time of diagnosis and 10% in patients in quiescence (*Figure 1B*).

Analysis of allopeptide reactive T cells in the circulation of renal allograft recipients yielded similar results. Allopeptide-reactive T cells were found in fifty percent of the LDA performed 7-14 days prior to the diagnosis of acute allograft rejection. During rejection, 75% of the LDA were positive while only 4% of the tests revealed the presence of allopeptide reactive T cells in patients who were in quiescence.

To identify the dominant epitope against which T cell alloreactivity was directed, T cell lines were generated from split LDA-cultures by stimulation with peptide mixture in the presence of autologous APCs. Testing of the lines for reactivity against each individual component of the peptide mixture in the presence of APCs sharing with the recipient a single HLA-DR antigen showed that the response was directed invariably against a sole peptide. This demonstrates that T cells immunized *in vivo* against allogeneic MHC molecule(s) recognize a single dominant allopeptide which is restricted by one of the host's HLA-DR antigens [2]. Furthermore, patients carrying a graft mismatched by two HLA-DR antigens recognized during primary acute rejection only peptides derived from one of the donor's HLA-DR proteins. Spreading of T cell alloreactivity to the second HLA-DR mismatch occurred only during recurrent rejections. This observation is consistant with studies on autoimmune diseases [8] as well as with the finding that the antibody response of transplant patients spreads from one alloantigen to another during multiple rejections [9].

This preferential recognition of a single dominant epitope from an allogeneic MHC-DR molecule is most likely due to differences in protein processing controlled by genes at the HLA-DM locus [10].

The finding that indirect allorecognition precedes and accompanies acute allograft rejection opens new avenues to the diagnosis and treatment of rejection. Thus, while the presence of allopeptide reactive T cells in the circulation can be used for predicting rejection, the administration of high concentrations of dominant allopeptide and/or of synthetic analogs is likely to permit the induction of specific immunologic tolerance to allogeneic organ allografts.

References

1. Sherman LA, Cattopadhyan S. The molecular basis of allorecognition. *Annu Rev Immunol* 1992; 11: 385-402.
2. Colovai AI, Renna Molàjoni E, Cortesini R, Suciu-Foca N. New approaches to specific immunomodulation in transplantation. *Int Rev Immunol* 1996; 13: 161-72.
3. Sawyer GJ, Dalchau R, Fabre JW. Indirect T cell allorecognition: a cyclosporin A resistant pathway for T cell help for antibody production to donor MHC antigens. *Transplant Immunol* 1993; 1: 77-81.
4. Suciu-Foca N, Reed E, Marboe C, Xi YP, Sun YK, Ho E, Rose E, Reemtsma K, King DW. Role of anti-HLA antibodies in heart transplantation. *Transplantation* 1991; 51: 716-24.
5. Liu Z, Harris P, Colovai AI, Reed EF, Maffei A, Suciu-Foca N. Indirect recognition of donor MHC-class II antigens in human transplantation. *Clin Immunol Immunopathol* 1996; 78: 228-35.
6. Sharrock, CEM, Kaminski K, Man S. Limiting dilution analysis of human T cells: a useful clinical tool. *Immunol Today* 1990; 11: 281-3.
7. Bodmer JG, Marsh SGE, Albert ED, Bodmer WF, Dupont B, Erlich HA, Mach B, Mayr WR, Parham P, Sasazuki T, Schreuder GM, Strominger JL, Svejgaard A, Terasaki PI. Nomenclature for factors of the HLA system. *Hum Immunol* 1994; 41: 1-20.
8. McRae BL, Vanderlugt CL, Cal Canto MC, Miller SD. Functional evidence for epitope spreading in the relapsing pathology of experimental autoimmune encephalomyelitis. *J Exp Med* 1995; 182: 75-85.
9. Suciu-Foca N, Reed E, D'Agati VD, Ho E, Cohen DJ, Benvenisty, AI, McCabe R, Brensilver JM, King DW, Hardy MA. Soluble HLA antigens, anti-HLA antibodies and anti-idiotypic antibodies in the circulation of renal transplant recipients. *Transplantation* 1991; 51: 593-601.
10. Morris P, Shaman J, Attaya M, Amaya M, Goodman S, Bergman C, Monaco J, Mellins E. An essential role for HLA-DM in antigen presentation by class II major histocompatibility molecules. *Nature* 1994; 368: 551-3.

Alloreactive helper T-lymphocyte precursor frequencies correlate with HLA-DRB1 antigen amino acid residue mismatches

N.T. Young, D.L. Roelen, M. Bunce, M.J. Dallman[1], P.J. Morris, K.I. Welsh

Nuffield Department of Surgery, University of Oxford, John Radcliffe Hospital, Oxford OX3 9DU,UK
1 Department of Biology, Imperial College of Science, Technology and Medicine, London, UK

The proliferation and maturation of primary alloreactive lymphocytes is directly influenced by regulatory lymphokines produced by helper T-lymphocytes (HTL) and antigen presenting cells (APC). Interleukin-2 (IL-2) is the principal lymphokine stimulating the growth of precursor lymphocytes and the acquisition of effector phenotype and characteristics by such cells. This lymphokine is produced by HTL of Th1 or Th0 subtype after antigen-specific stimulation of the T cell receptor (TCR) in conjunction with necessary non-antigen-specific costimulatory signals provided by APC [1]. The resulting generation of both cellular and antibody-mediated cytotoxicity is a major factor in allograft rejection and graft-versus-host disease. Recently, the estimation of alloreactive HTL precursor (HTLp) frequencies has been proposed as an *in vitro* correlate of *in vivo* alloresponsiveness in transplant donor:recipient pairs [2,3]. These quantitative cellular assays define HTLp as IL-2-producing cells and given the paradigmatic role of HLA molecules in the restriction of such responses, it might be expected that matching for these antigens should influence the level of alloreactive HTLp detected. In the present study we have examined the effect of HLA matching in limiting dilution assays for HTLp determination [4] derived from healthy blood donors. In addition to analysing the effect of matching for broad, serologically equivalent alleles of the HLA-A, -B, -Cw, -DR and -DQ loci, we have investigated the effect at the molecular level using HLA genotyping [5] and protein sequence comparisons to identify the number, location and influence of mismatched amino acid residues in the respective HLA molecules. The results were analysed for statistical significance using a two-tailed Mann Whitney U test and linear regression analysis.

Results

When analysed for HLA matching characteristics, it is immediately evident that frequencies of *in vitro* alloreactive HTLp are associated primarily with HLA-DR antigen mismatches in this set of responder:stimulator combinations. When assays are grouped according to HLA-DR mismatch, the mean frequency of HTLp detected in each group increases with the degree of HLA-DR antigenic disparity *(Figure 1A)*. Significant differences exist between the HLA-DR matched (n=6) and HLA-DR mismatched groups (n=24, p<0.02, Mann Whitney Test). This significant effect was evident when there were either one (n=10, p<0.02) or two (n=14, p<0.05) HLA-DR mismatches. Analysis of class I antigen matching in the thirty responder:stimulator combinations revealed that there were no significant differences between the mean number of HLA-A, -B and -Cw antigen mismatches in these groups. These values were 3.5 in HLA-DR matched combinations and 4.6 in HLA-DR mismatched. However, there appeared to be a subset of assay combinations in which the degree of class I antigen mismatch correlated almost exactly (n=6 of 30, r=0.99, p<0.0001) with HTLp frequency *(Figure 1B)*. All of these combinations were disparate at the HLA-DR locus with the highest HTLp frequencies detected in those assays which featured two HLA-DR antigen mismatches.

We analysed the HLA-DR matching effect in greater detail by examining HLA class II protein sequences in each responder and stimulator. Amino acid residue disparities in different combinations were identified by computerised sequence subtraction based on the results of molecular typing and known protein sequences. The

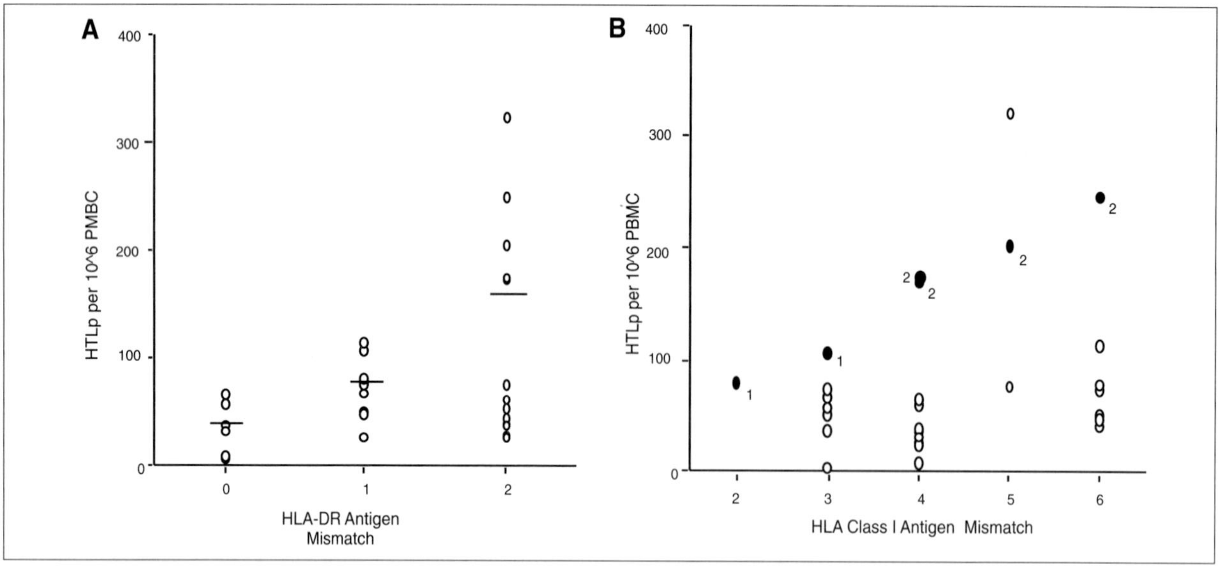

Figure 1. Alloreactive helper T-lymphocyte precursor frequency is significantly associated with the degree of HLA-DR antigen mismatching between responder and stimulator (Panel A). (o) represents individual frequency estimates, (—) indicates mean frequency value for each group. Significant differences are found between mean values in HLA-DR matched (n=6) and HLA-DR mismatched (n=24, p<0.02), HLA-DR matched (n=6) and HLA-DR one antigen mismatched (n=10, p<0.02), HLA-DR matched (n=6) and HLA-DR two antigen mismatched (n=14, p<0.05). Difference between HLA-DR one antigen and HLA-DR two antigen mismatched assays is non-significant. Relationship between class I (HLA-A, -B, -Cw) antigen mismatch and HTLp frequency reveals no significant association (Panel B) but identifies a subset of combinations (○) in which class I mismatch is highly correlated (r=0.99, p<0.0001). Numerals next to each data point refer to the number of HLA-DR antigen mismatches in each combination.

reason for the non-significant difference in HTLp frequency between one- and two-HLA-DR antigen mismatched assays is evident when the number of mismatched HLA-DRB1 amino acid residues in these groups are compared. Although these assay combinations differ in classically defined HLA-DR matching there is no significant difference between the two groups at the level of protein sequence differences, with a mean value of 14.2 mismatched residues (n=10, range 8-25) in the one DR antigen group and a mean value of 19.3 mismatched residues (n=14, range 10-29) in the two DR antigen group.

The data resulting from the sequence analysis was then analysed by linear regression analysis to assess the relationship between amino acid residue mismatches and HTLp frequency. The association between total class II (HLA-DRB1, -DRB3/4/5, -DQB1 and -DQA1) mismatches and frequency of alloreactive HTLp was positive but weak ($r = 0.28$, $p > 0.05$). However, the number of mismatched HLA-DRB1 residues correlated strongly ($r = 0.545$, $p < 0.002$) with this aspect of alloreactivity *(Figure 2)*. The greater significance of the correlation between HTLp frequency and mismatches in the beta sheet structural region of the HLA-DRB1 molecule (residues 9-48; $r=0.535$, $p<0.005$) than those located in the alpha helical region (residues 57-86; $r=0.467$, $p<0.01$) suggests that peptide located in the antigen-binding groove of HLA-DRB1 is a major factor in the stimulation of alloreactive HTLp.

Discussion

We have demonstrated that HLA-DRB1 antigen amino acid disparity is the immunodominant stimulus for production of the regulatory lymphokine IL-2 by primary alloreactive helper T-lymphocyte precursors. The results of our study suggest that antigenic peptide bound in the groove of HLA-DRB1 molecules is a major influence in this response. Our conclusions are supported by pre-

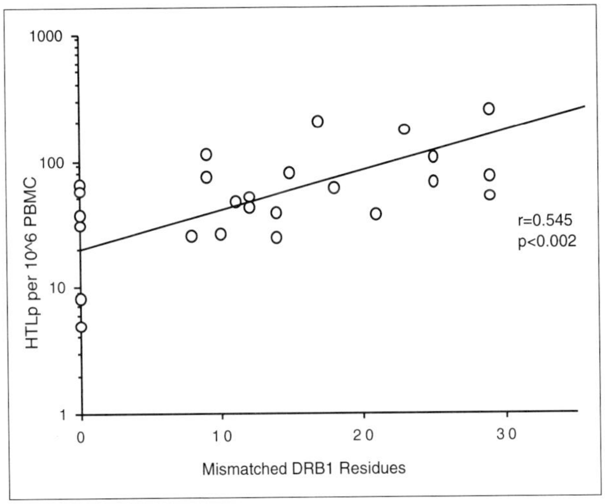

Figure 2. Correlation between HLA-DRB1 amino acid residue mismatch and HTLp frequency estimate (n=30; residues 1-237; r=0.545, p<0.002).

vious studies in mixed lymphocyte reaction of class I antigen matching [6], release of other cytokines such as IL-10 [7] and the reported restriction of T cell receptor Vβ CDR3 length in alloreactive lymphocytes [8].

The possible clinical relevance of our investigation is suggested by a recent study [9] which examined the relation between HLA-DRB1 amino acid mismatches and the occurrence of rejection episodes in the first year after cadaveric renal transplantation. The reported association of increased rejection with mismatched residues in the beta sheet and alpha helix sections of the HLA-DRB1 molecule parallels the results of our study. It is well known that matching of donor and recipient for the HLA-DR [10] locus greatly improves the subsequent survival of cadaver renal grafts. Mismatched antigens at the other class II loci may not play as important a role as HLA-DRB1 in this respect. Our description of a positive correlation between HLA-DRB1 molecular matching and HTLp frequency provides experimental support for the concept of functional matching in transplantation and, in conjunction with the results of a study relating such mismatches to the clinical outcome of renal transplantation, suggests that further investigation of alloreactive HTLp in recipients of solid organ transplants is warranted.

References

1. Janeway CA, Bottomly K. Signals and signs for lymphocyte responses. *Cell* 1994; 76: 275-85.
2. Schwarer AP, Jiang YZ, Brookes PA, Barrett AJ, Batchelor JR, Goldman JM, Lechler RL. Frequency of anti-recipient alloreactive helper T-cell precursors in donor blood and graft-versus-host disease after HLA-identical sibling bone marrow transplantation. *Lancet* 1993; 341: 203-5.
3. DeBruyne LA, Ensley RD, Olsen SL, Taylor DO, Carpenter BM, Holland C, Swanson S, Jones KW, Karwande SV, Renlund DG, Bishop DK. Increased frequency of alloantigen-reactive helper T lymphocytes is associated with human cardiac allograft rejection. *Transplantation* 1993; 56: 722-7.
4. Young NT, Roelen DL, Wood KJ, Dallman MJ, Morris PJ, Welsh KI. Enumeration of human alloreactive helper T-lymphocyte precursor frequencies by limiting dilution analysis of interleukin-2 production. *J Immunol Methods* 1996; 195: 50533-41.
5. Bunce M, O'Neill C, Barnardo MCNM, Krausa P, Browning M, Morris PJ, Welsh KI. Phototyping: comprehensive DNA typing for HLA-A, -B, -C,-DRB1, -DRB3, -DRB4, -DRB5 and DQB1 alleles by 144 PCR reactions utilising sequence specific primers (SSP). *Tissue Antigens* 1995; 46: 355-65.
6. Chouaib S, Bensussan A, Termijtelen AM, Andreeff M, Marchiol-Fournigault C, Fradelizi D, Dupont B. Allogeneic T cell activation triggering by MHC Class I antigens. *J Immunol* 1988; 141: 423-29.
7. Tongouz M, Denys CH, De Groote D, Andrien MC, Dupont EC. Optimal control of IFN-γ and TNF-α by IL-10 in response to one HLA-DR mismatch during the primary mixed lymphocyte reaction. *Transplantation* 1996; 61: 497-502.
8. DePalma R, Gorski J. Restricted and conserved T cell repertoires involved in allorecognition of class II major histocompatibility complex. *Proc Natl Acad Sci USA* 1995; 92: 8836-40.
9. Sada M, Hashimoto M, Kinoshita T. Ichikawa Y, Takahara S, Tada M, Fukunishi T, Tsuji T. Importance of HLA-DRB1 amino acid residue matching between recipient and donor in cadaveric renal transplantation. *Transplant Proc* 1995; 27: 698-700.
10. Opelz G, Mytilineos J, Scherer S, Dunckley H, Trejant J, Chapman J *et al.* Survival of DNA HLA-DR typed and matched cadaver kidney transplants. *Lancet* 1991; 338: 461-3.

Importance of a single amino acid substitution of the α-helices of class I MHC molecules for the induction of a primary allogeneic response

M. Reboul[1], G. Noun[1], V. Lacabanne[1], J.P. Abastado[2], P. Kourilsky[2], M. Pla[1]

1 Mouse Immunogenetics, INSERM U93 , Saint-Louis Hospital, 1, avenue Claude Vellefaux, 75010 Paris, France
2 INSERM U277 , Pasteur Institute, Paris, France

T cells recognize foreign antigens as peptides presented by major histocompatibility complex (MHC) molecules. The allogeneic response is one of the most thoroughly documented responses in immunology, yet it remains paradoxical and in particular it is still not well understood how the recognition of allogeneic MHC molecules relates to MHC-presented antigen recognition. It has been suggested [1] that alloreactivity may result from the recognition of other surface components (we would now say "peptides") in combination with MHC molecules. Involvement of peptides in T cell alloreactivity has indeed been reported in several cases (reviewed in [2-4]). Thus alloreactive TcR would recognize a peptide derived from cellular protein degradation in association with an MHC molecule. However, another model envisages that alloTcR might interact directly with the polymorphic residues on the surface of an MHC molecule, even in absence of peptide. Thus the polymorphic MHC residues may contribute to the determinants recognized by alloreactive CTL by dictating which peptides can bind in the peptide pocket, by dictating the conformation of a given peptide in the pocket, or by interacting directly with the TcR itself [5,6]. As a part of our continuing effort to study the antigenic structure of class I molecules, we have compared the capacity of various point mutants (α-helices or β-sheet of the α1 and α2 domains) of an H-2 class I molecule to induce a primary allogeneic response. We have used an in vivo model [7] based on the observation that injection of cells expressing allogeneic MHC molecules into the hind footpad leads to the development of sensitized prekiller T cells within the draining lymph nodes. We report here an application of this model allowing the analysis of the CTL induced in draining lymph nodes of mice carrying H-2K^d molecules by a local graft of cells expressing various mutant K^d molecules, thus ensuring that the incompatibility between donor and recipient is limited only to one amino acid.

Materials and methods

Animals

Mice were bred and maintained in our own colony. The F1 mice used in this work were obtained from the crosses of mice B10.BR (K^k D^k) with C3H.OL (K^d D^k).

Cells

Transfected cells are mouse L fibroblasts (H-2^k) expressing mutated H-2K^d molecules in addition to MALA-2 molecule (the murine equivalent of the human adhesion molecule ICAM-1). All mutations were single alanine substitutions, located either on the β sheet (at positions: 5, 9, 33, 34, 45, 95, 97, 99, 114, 116, 118, 123 or 124) or on the α helices (at positions : 58, 62, 65, 69, 72, 82, 145, 149, 154, 155, 163 or 166). For the mutant nomenclature, the number indicates the position of the mutated residue, the first and last letters are the single letter codes for wild-type and substituted residues, respectively. K^d-negative cells are L fibroblasts transfected only with the MALA-2 gene.

Generation of alloreactive CTL

Recipient F1 mice were injected with 10^7 irradiated (55 Gy) fibroblasts into the hind footpads. After three days the draining lymph nodes were dissected out, a cell suspension was prepared and the cells were cultured for 4 more days *in vitro* in the absence of any stimulating cells, in culture medium containing Con A-stimulated rat spleen cells supernatant as a lymphokine source (50 units IL-2/ml). The culture medium was MEM alpha-medium (Gibco) supplemented with 100 units/ml penicillin (Gibco), 100 µg/ml streptomycin (Gibco), 2 mM glutamine (Gibco), 5×10^{-5} M 2-mercaptoethanol (Sigma) and 10% heat-inactivated fetal calf serum (Gibco).

Cell-mediated lympholysis assay

Five thousand ^{51}Cr-labeled target cells were incubated with primary CTL at various effector : target ratios in round-bottomed wells for 4h. The percentage of specific lysis was calculated as: 100 x (cpm experimental release - cpm spontaneous release) / (cpm maximum release - cpm spontaneous release).

Results and discussion

Fibroblasts expressing the various mutant K^d molecules (K^{dm}) were tested for their ability to induce alloreactive T cells in mice expressing the native K^d molecule. The induction protocol we used reproduces a graft situation in that the first contact between stimulator and responder cells occurs *in vivo*: irradiated K^{dm}-expressing fibroblasts were injected into the hind footpads of (B10.BR x C3H.OL) F1 recipient mice. Lymphocytes isolated from the draining lymph nodes and further cultivated in the absence of any other cells were tested for an anti-K^{dm} cell-mediated lympholysis activity. Three to six independent experiments were performed for each of the K^d variants. As the standard deviation (SD) for the mean of lysis values obtained with K^d-negative cells was 7%, we considered that a given K^d mutant elicits an alloreactive response when the difference between the percentages of specific lysis of K^{dm}-expressing cells and K^d-negative cells exceeded 14% (*i.e.* twice the SD) at a 100:1 E:T ratio in three independently repeated experiments.

The results shown in *Figure 1* represent typical examples of CTL activities. Most of the mutated K^d molecules (18 out of the 25 molecules tested) failed to induce a primary CTL response (results concerning mutants at residues 97 and 114 are shown in *Figure 1*). 7 out of the 25 K^{dm} tested were able to induce a primary CTL response in K^d-positive mice. As shown in *Figure 1*, the fibroblasts with K^d molecules mutated at residues 62, 65, 69, 72, 155, 163 or 166 were consistently able to elicit significant cytotoxic response. Interestingly all these residues are located on the α-helices. The side chains of residues 62, 65, 69, 72, 163 and 166 are thought [8] to point up towards the TcR and not into the peptide binding groove and presumably do not affect the range of bound peptides. These mutants provoked alloreactive responses in T cells from mice expressing unmutated K^d molecules suggesting that the mutated residues might be directly involved in the TcR recognition. Another explanation might be that these CTL have broken tolerance to self peptides by seeing them in a new context of mutated K^d molecules. In a study made by Grandea *et al.* [9,10] K^b molecules mutated at residues 65 or 69 were able to provoke strong alloreactive responses in T cells from mice expressing the native K^b. It was shown that mutant-specific alloreactive CTL were specific for self peptides extracted from wild-type K^b and recognized in the context of the mutant K^b molecules. Thus, the T-cell repertoire is reactive to very subtle changes away from self.

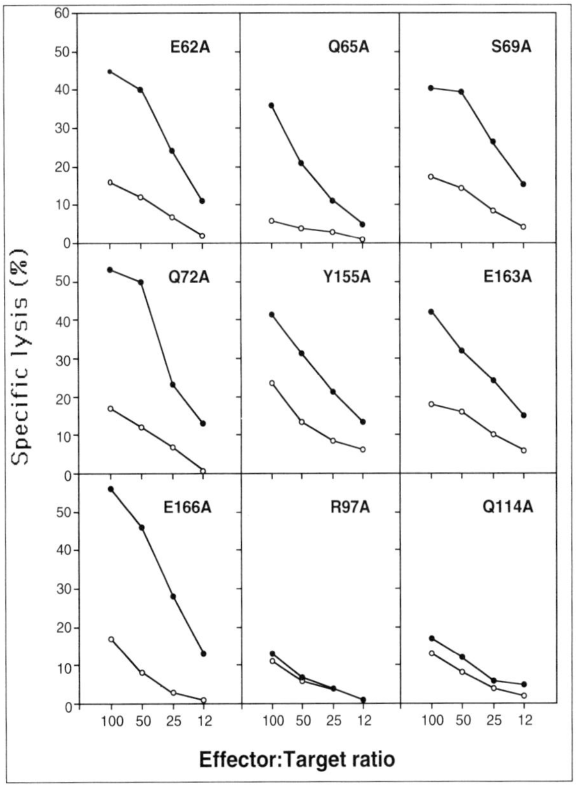

Figure 1. Induction of a primary cytotoxic T cell response by mutated K^d molecules.
(B10.BR x C3H.OL) F1 mice were injected into hind footpads with irradiated fibroblasts expressing mutated K^d molecules and draining lymph node cells were tested for cytotoxic activity on K^d-negative (○) and K^{dm}-expressing (●) fibroblasts. For the mutants nomenclature, the number indicates the position of the mutated residue, the first and last letters are the single-letter codes for wild-type and substituted residues, respectively.

The α-helices variants appear to be very immunogeneic, probably because all the self peptide-filled mutant molecules are potentially different from wild-type molecules bearing the self peptides. As for the β-sheet mutants, even if they do bind a new range of peptides as compared to wild-type molecules, these peptides would occupy only a fraction of the available molecules, and would thus be represented at a rather low density corresponding to that of conventional antigenic peptides. Therefore, the frequency of precursor T cells recognizing these peptides associated with the MHC molecule would be very low and undetectable in a primary response.

A unique advantage of the allorepertoire is that it can identify a variety of peptides associated with a specific MHC that could not, due to self-tolerance, be efficiently recognized syngeneically [4]. If an allospecific CTL sees a tumor or viral antigen associated with the MHC, then this CTL may, in theory, be useful in specific elimination of tumor or viral infected cells without harming normal cells in the individual.

References

1. Matzinger P, Bevan MJ. Hypothesis: why do so many lymphocytes respond to major histocompatibility antigens. *Cell Immunol* 1977; 29: 1-5.
2. Claverie JM, Kourilsky P. The peptidic self model: a reassessment of the role of the major histocompatibility complex molecules in the restriction of the T-cell response. *Ann Inst Pasteur/Immunol* 1986; 137D: 425-42.
3. Lechler RI, Lombardi G, Batchelor JR, Reinsmoen N, Bach FH. The molecular basis of alloreactivity. *Immunol Today* 1990; 11: 83-8.
4. Sherman LA, Chattopadhyay S. The molecular basis of allorecognition. *Annu Rev Immunol* 1993; 11: 385-402.
5. Hogan KT, Clayberger C, Bernhard EJ, Walk SF, Ridge JP, Parham P, Krensky AM, Engelhard GH. A panel of unique HLA-A2 mutant molecules define epitopes recognized by HLA-A2-specific antibodies and cytotoxic T lymphocytes. *J Immunol* 1989; 142: 2097-104.
6. Elliot TJ, Eisen HN. Cytotoxic T lymphocytes recognize a reconstituted class I histocompatibility antigen (HLA-A2) as an allogeneic target molecule. *Proc Natl Acad Sci USA* 1990; 87: 5213-7.
7. Rocca A, Degos L, Pla M. Analysis of primary HLA-specific cytotoxic T cell response in graft-draining lymph nodes. A transgenic mouse model for *in vivo* recognition of human MHC antigens. *Transplantation* 1991; 52: 1062-7.
8. Bjorkman PJ, Saper MA, Samraoui B, Bennet WS, Strominger JL, Wiley DC. The foreign antigen binding site and T cell recognition regions of class I histocompatibility antigens. *Nature* 1987; 329: 512-8.
9. Grandea III AG, Bevan MJ. Single-residue changes in class I major histocompatibility complex molecules stimulate responses to self peptides. *Proc Natl Acad Sci USA* 1992; 89: 2794-8.
10. Grandea III AG, Bevan MJ. A conservative mutation in a class I MHC molecule outside the peptide binding groove stimulates responses to self peptides. *J Immunol* 1993; 151: 3981-7.

Tolerizing effects of pretransplant exposure to donor HLA-DR antigen in random transfusion units for kidney recipients

A. Jackson, C. McSherry, K. Butters, M. Diko, S. Almond, A.J. Matas, N.L. Reinsmoen

Department of Surgery, University of Minnesota, Box 328 UMHC, 420 Delaware Street SE, Minneapolis, MN 55455, USA

During the 1970s and early 1980s, the introduction of deliberate transfusion protocols was responsible for a major improvement in renal transplantation. Early studies showed that transfusions increase the survival of first cadaver renal allografts by 15 - 20% over nontransfused patients [1]. However, in the mid 1980s, it was reported that the beneficial effect of blood transfusion had diminished following the introduction of cyclosporine [2-3]. Subsequent studies showed that improved graft survival in nontransfused patients is the main cause the transfusion effect has diminished, regardless of the immunosuppressive therapy used [4]. Recently, the results of the Transplant Registry of the University of California at Los Angeles demonstrated a considerable effect of blood transfusion [5]. This report showed that the transfusion effect can only be detected in HLA-DR-mismatched transplants and not in compatible transplants. It has also been shown that sharing of one HLA-DR antigen between the transfusion donor, and recipient may be crucial for improved graft survival [6]. In the following report we focused on HLA-DR sharing between the transfusion donor and the subsequent kidney donor. We analyzed whether pretransplant exposure to the same HLA-DR antigen *via* random blood transfusion and posttransplant *via* the transplanted organ influenced the development of donor antigen specific hyporesponsiveness.

We have used the *in vitro* assay of donor antigen-specific hyporeactivity as a useful marker for identifying solid organ transplant recipients (kidney, lung, or heart) at low risk of immunologic complications (*i.e.*, late acute rejection episodes and chronic rejection) [7,8]. We studied donor antigen-specific hyporeactivity at 1 year posttransplant by comparing pre- and posttransplant donor antigen-specific mixed lymphocyte responses to donor cells or homozygous typing cells (HTCs) expressing the donor antigens. We have identified donor antigen-specific hyporeactivity for 22% (47/215) of kidney, 35% (8/23) of lung, and 22% (6/27) of heart transplant recipients.

Anecdotal evidence from other institutions has suggested that the development of donor antigen specific hyporeactivity is observed more often in recipients who have received pretransplant blood transfusions. In this study we investigated whether pretransplant exposure to the donor HLA-DR antigen *via* the transfusion unit influenced the development of donor antigen-specific hyporeactivity and the occurrence of the transfusion effect. Our hypothesis is that the transfusion induces a state of specific T cell nonresponsiveness in recipients who are exposed to the same HLA-DR antigen pretransplant *via* the transfusion unit and posttransplant *via* the transplanted organ.

Material and methods

HLA-DR typing of transfusion units

HLA class II typing of the transfusion units were performed by a DNA-based sequence specific oligonucleotide probe (SSOP) technique to determine the HLA-DR alleles [DR1, 2, 3, 4, 5(11), 5(12), 6(13), 6(14), 7, 8, 9, 10]. Genomic DNA was be isolated using the Puregene DNA Isolation Kit (Mpls,MN). Utilizing the polymerase chain reaction (PCR) and generic primers which flank the second exon of the DRB1 gene, all alleles were amplified simultaneously [9]. The amplified DNA is denatured, anchored on to nylon membranes, and hybridized with 16 allele specific, digoxigenin 11-ddUTP (Boehringer Mannheim, Indianapolis,IN) labeled oligonucleotide probes [10]. The membranes are washed under stringent conditions to remove unbound probe, treated with an anti-

Digoxigenin alkaline phosphatase antibody, and immersed in Lumiphos 530 (Boehringer Mannheim). The resulting enzymatic reaction forms an unstable chemiluminescent intermediate detected by autoradiography. The hybridization pattern for each probe are then analyzed and DRB1 alleles assigned.

Identification of donor antigen-specific hyporeactivity

We define donor antigen-specific hyporeactivity as a significantly decreased post- *vs.* pretransplant MLC response to donor HLA-DR antigen using either donor cells or homozygous typing cells which express donor HLA-DR antigen. Our previous studies [7] have shown that a 60% double normalized value response or less indicates hyporeactivity to HTCs of donor specificity and a 60% decrease in the MLC reactivity to donor cells falls below the normal distribution of MLC responses observed in our laboratory. In this study we used both methods to define donor antigen-specific hyporeactivity.

Results and discussion

We analyzed whether receiving a random pretransplant blood transfusion sharing HLA-DR with either the transplanted organ or the transplant recipient had any effect on the development of donor antigen specific hyporesponsiveness. Included in the analysis were: examination of sensitization rates, time interval between transfusion and transplant, diabetes, and receipt of a cadaveric versus living donor organ. Sixty-five previously non-transfused patients awaiting primary kidney transplant were enrolled in this study. Each received two 150 ml pretransplant random blood transfusions. Azathioprine was administered at the time of transfusion and continued for two weeks. Recipients of living kidney donors received cyclosporine A one day prior, and prednisone and azathioprine day of transplant. Recipients of cadaveric kidneys were treated with anti-T cell antibody, prednisone and azathioprine at time of transplant, with delayed introduction of cyclosporine A. The sensitization rate (defined as PRA> or = 10%) was 4% or 3/ 65 patients in this study. One additional patient had a positive PRA prior to transfusion and was excluded from this percentage. Fifty-two of these 65 patients have gone on to transplant, including the 4 patients with positive PRA's. The HLA-DR of each random transfusion unit was determined retrospectively using PCR-SSOP. Twenty four patients who received a HLA-DR disparate kidney were assayed for donor antigen-specific hyporeactivity at one year posttransplant. Donor antigen-specific hyporeactivity developed in 7/24 (29%) patients analyzed, six of these hyporesponsive had pretransplant exposure to donor antigen *via* the random blood unit (*Table I,* p=0.04).

Table I. Transfusion unit containing a shared HLA-DR with the transplanted kidney

		Yes	No
Development of donor antigen-specific	Yes	6	1
Hyporeactivity	No	6	11
	p=0.04		

The single hyporesponsive recipient, who was not exposed pretransplant to the kidney HLA-DR, was exposed via transfusion to a HLA-DR known to share T-cell epitopes with the HLA-DR of the transplanted kidney (DR1 and DR10). HLA-DR sharing between the kidney recipient and the transfusion units did not enhance the development of donor antigen-specific hyporeactivity. None of the hyporesponsive patients shared a HLA-DR with the transfusates, whereas 10/17 responsive recipients did share a HLA-DR with at least one of their transfusion units. The time interval between transfusion and transplant ranged from 1-24 months; however the average time in both the hyporesponsive and responsive patients was similar (6 months).

These results show that pretransplant exposure to donor antigen increases the likelihood of developing donor antigen-specific hyporeactivity. However, other factors also play a role since not all recipients exposed to donor antigen pretransplant develop hyporeactivity. We are currently investigating whether the level of CD34+ stem cells in the transfusion units influences the development of donor antigen-specific hyporeactivity. Since recipients who develop donor antigen-specific hyporeactivity have a lower incidence of chronic rejection and improved graft survival, perhaps new strategies for induction of specific T cell unresponsiveness should be considered. We propose to HLA-DR type the transfusion unit donors and select units for each recipient such that each recipient is exposed to as many of the common DR types as possible.

References

1. Opelz G. Blood transfusion and renal transplantation. In: Morris PJ, ed. *Kidney Transplantation: Principles and Practice*. London: Grune and Stratton, 1984: 323.
2. Kahan BD, VanBuren CT, Flechner SM, Payne WD, Boileau M, Kerman RH. Cyclosporine immunosuppression mitigates immunologic risk factors in renal allotransplantation. *Transplant Proc* 1983; 15: 2469.
3. Lundgren G, Albrechtsen D, Flatmark A, Gabel H, Klintmalm G, Persson H, Groth CG, Brynger H, Frodin L, Husberg B, Maurer W, Thorsby E. HLA-matching and pretransplant blood transfusions in cadaveric renal transplantation - a changing picture with cyclosporine. *Lancet* 1986; 2: 66.
4. Opelz G. Improved kidney graft survival in non-transfused recipients. *Transplant Proc* 1987; 19: 149.
5. Iwaki Y, Cecka JM, Terasaki PI. The transfusion effect in cadaver kidney transplants: yes or no. *Transplantation* 1990; 49: 56.
6. Lagaaij EL, Henneman IPH, Ruigrok M, DeHaan MW, Persijn GG, Termijtelen A, Hendricks GFJ, Weimar W, Claas FHJ, VanRood JJ. Effect of one HLA-DR antigen-matched and completely HLA-DR mismatched blood transfusions on survival of heart and kidney allografts. *N Engl J Med* 1989; 321: 701.
7. Reinsmoen NL, Matas AJ. Evidence that improved late renal transplant outcome correlates with the development of *in vitro* donor antigen-specific hyporeactivity. *Transplantation* 1993; 55: 1017.
8. Reinsmoen NL, Bolman RM, Savik K, Butters K, Matas AJ, Hertz MI. Improved graft outcome in lung transplantation recipients who develop donor antigen-specific hyporeactivity. *J Heart Lung Transplant* 1994; 13: 30.
9. Saiki RK, *et al. Science* 1988; 239: 487.
10. ASHI Laboratory Manual, Afzal Nikaein, editor, Section IV.C.1.1.

Pregnancy can induce priming of cytotoxic T lymphocytes specific for paternal HLA-antigens, which is associated with antibody formation

G.J. Bouma[1], P. van Caubergh[1], F.P.M.J. van Bree[1], R.M.C. Castelli-Visser[1], M.D. Witvliet[1], P.M.W. van der Meer-Prins[1], J.J. van Rood[1,2], F.H.J. Claas[1]

1 Department of Immunohematology and Blood Bank
2 Europdonor Foundation, Leiden University Hospital, Building 1, E3-Q, PO Box 9600, 2300 RC Leiden, The Netherlands

Some transplant centers consider paternal HLA-antigens as unacceptable mismatches for mothers awaiting kidney transplantation. It is feared that a pregnancy may cause priming of the maternal immune response directed towards paternal HLA-antigens. Should a woman be transplanted with an organ from a donor who shared those paternal HLA-antigens, the risk of graft rejection might be increased.

If the rule is applied never to accept a mismatched HLA-antigen for transplantation that is shared by the husband, the number of donors suitable for transplantation may be reduced, especially if the husband has a common phenotype. Otherwise, husbands who volunteer to donate a kidney for their wives, may not even be taken into consideration. On the other hand, several reports show that kidney donation by a husband to his wife can result in a successful transplantation [1,2]. In general, graft survival of a kidney from a living donor is superior to that from a cadaveric donor [3]. This has also been reported for husband to wife transplantation, although graft survival was superior in women who had never been pregnant, compared to those which had been pregnant [2].

Method

Cellular immune responses can be quantified by performing limiting dilution analysis (LDA)-assays to determine precursor frequencies of T lymphocytes. T lymphocytes can also be distinguished qualitatively based on their state of activation, in naive and primed lymphocytes. Experimentally, *in vitro* primed cytotoxic T lymphocytes (CTL) are more resistant to inhibition by cyclosporin-A (CsA) [4] or anti-CD8 [5] than naive CTL.

More importantly, the distinction between naive and primed CTL by CsA or anti-CD8 could also be demonstrated after *in vivo* priming. Resistance of CTL to inhibition by CsA or anti-CD8 was correlated to rejection of kidney, heart and cornea allografts, while CTL responses that were sensitive to inhibition, coincided with a good graft function [6,7]. Also in highly immunized patients cellular responses against antigens that had induced antibody formation *in vivo*, were significantly more resistant to inhibition by CsA and anti-CD8 *in vitro* than CTL responses towards antigens that had not induced antibody formation [8].

It is known that some women, as a consequence of pregnancy, develop antibodies specific for paternal HLA-antigens [9]. To investigate whether a pregnancy can also prime the cellular immune response against paternal HLA-antigens and whether this occurs in all cases, the present study was set up. The results were related to implications for the selection of organ donors who carry HLA-antigens identical to paternal HLA-antigens. To that end, LDA-assays were carried out to determine the number of maternal CTL (CTL precursor frequency (CTLpf)) specific for paternal HLA-antigens. Differentiation between naive and *in vivo* primed cytotoxic T lymphocytes was made by performing these assays respectively in the absence and presence of anti-CD8. For comparison, also the CTL response against third party HLA-antigens was measured. To assess the nature of paternal-specific responses in more detail, paternal HLA-antigens were subdivided based on inheritance by children and their association with antibody formation *in vivo*. For statistical comparison of the data either the Mann-Whitney Test (MW) was used for unpaired CTLp frequencies or the Wilcoxon signed rank test (WSR) in case CTLp frequencies were paired.

Results

In general, the response of a mother against paternal HLA-antigens (PA), does not greatly differ from the response against third party HLA-antigens (3rd). However, CTLp frequencies and the inhibition thereof by anti-CD8 vary to a greater extent when paternal antigens are involved

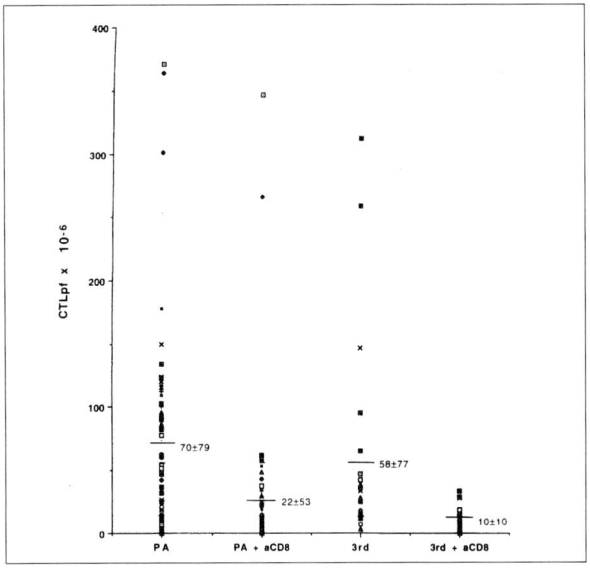

Figure 1. Maternal CTLp frequencies (CTLpf x 10^{-6}) were determined against paternal HLA-antigens (PA, n=68) and third party HLA-antigens (3rd, n=24), in the absence and presence (+aCD8) of anti-CD8. PA versus PA+aCD8: WSR p<0.0001, 3rd versus 3rd+aCD8: WSR p<0.0001, PA versus 3rd: MW p=0.42, PA+aCD8 versus 3rd+aCD8: MW p=0.72.

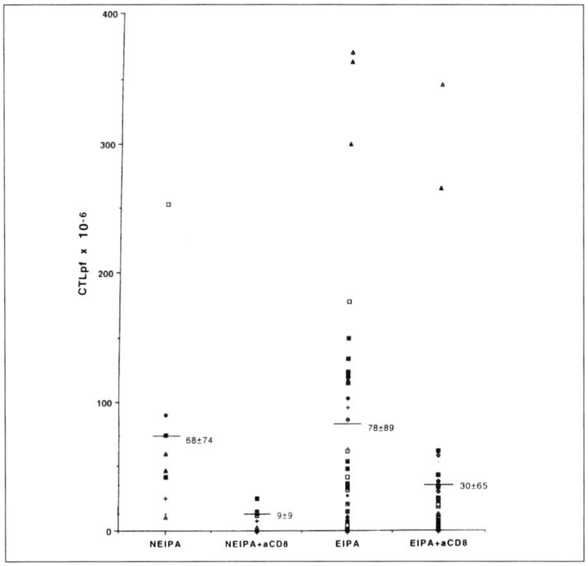

Figure 2. Maternal CTLp frequencies (CTLpf x 10^{-6}) were determined against paternal HLA-antigens which had never been inherited (NEIPA, n=9) and paternal HLA-antigens that had been inherited in one or more previous pregnancies (EIPA, n=43), in the absence and presence (+aCD8) of anti-CD8. NEIPA versus NEIPA+aCD8: WSR p=0.0039, EIPA versus EIPA+aCD8: WSR p<0.0001, NEIPA versus EIPA: MW p=0.96, NEIPA+aCD8 versus EIPA+aCD8: MW p=0.28.

(Figure 1). A division of paternal HLA-antigens based on inheritance was made into antigens that were never inherited (NEIPA) or were inherited in one or more previous pregnancies (EIPA). Responses against NEIPA were found to be quite homogeneous in contrast to those against EIPA *(Figure 2)*. Responses against NEIPA could be inhibited very well, while inhibition of CTLp frequencies raised against EIPA were found to range from complete to no inhibition at all.

HLA-specific antibodies induced by pregnancy in the women tested, were found to be directed towards EIPA and never towards NEIPA (results not shown). EIPA were further divided based on whether they had induced antibodies *in vivo*. CTLp frequencies raised against EIPA that had either or not led to antibody formation were compared *(Figure 3)*. The highest CTLp frequencies detected, were those against EIPA which had induced antibodies *in vivo*. On average, higher CTLp frequencies were found for EIPA that had led to antibody formation, than those that had not. This difference was statistically significant (MW p=0.034). The number of CTL remaining after anti-CD8 inhibition was similar for EIPA which had not led to antibody formation, for NEIPA *(see Figure 2)* and third party antigens *(see Figure 1)*. In contrast, the response against EIPA which had induced antibodies, could on average be blocked poorly by anti-CD8 indicating a primed cellular response. Significantly more CTL remained after anti-CD8 inhibition for EIPA which had led to antibody formation, compared with EIPA which had not led to antibody formation (MW p=0.045), with NEIPA (MW p=0.053), or with third party antigens (MW p=0.024).

Discussion

For highly immunized patients so called acceptable mismatches may be determined by performing a patient-specific screening assay [10]. An HLA-antigen may be defined acceptable if the patient has not formed antibodies against that antigen. It was found that cellular responses against these antigens were as sensitive to blocking by CsA or anti-CD8 *in vitro* as third party responses [8]. Since this is also the case for paternal HLA-antigens which have never been inherited, or those which have been inherited but have not induced antibodies, we propose to consider those paternal HLA-antigens as acceptable mismatches for the mother. In contrast, inherited paternal antigens which have led to

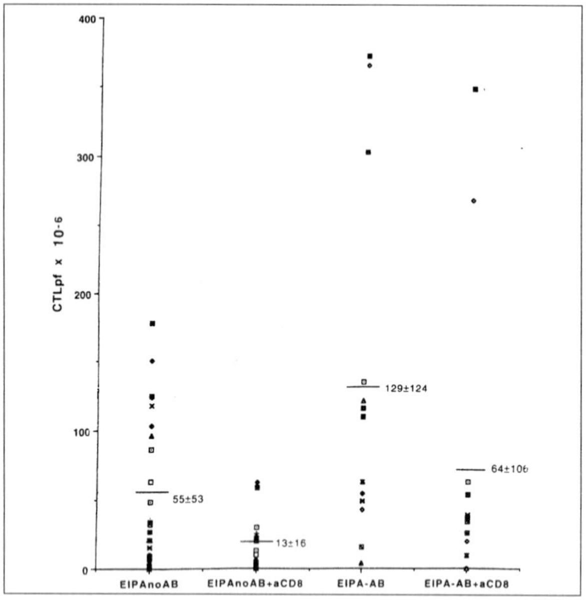

Figure 3. Maternal CTLp frequencies (CTLpf x 10^{-6}) were determined against paternal HLA-antigens which had been inherited in one or more previous pregnancies and which had not induced antibody *in vivo* (EIPAnoAB, n=27) and paternal HLA-antigens which had been inherited in one or more previous pregnancies and which had also induced antibody *in vivo* (EIPA-AB, n=14), in the absence and presence (+aCD8) of anti-CD8. EIPAnoAB versus EIPAnoAB+aCD8 : WSR $p<0.0001$, EIPA-AB versus EIPA-AB+aCD8: WSR $p=0.0006$, EIPAnoAB versus EIPA-AB: MW $p=0.034$, EIPAnoAB+aCD8 versus EIPA-AB+aCD8: MW $p=0.045$.

antibody formation in the mother, should not be taken into consideration as permissible mismatches in future transplants.

If the antibody-status of a woman has not been recorded since her pregnancies, the present *in vitro* assays might be applied to analyse the cellular immune response against specific paternal HLA-antigens, so as to indicate which paternal HLA-antigens may be acceptable or unacceptable for transplantation. Furthermore, the tissue-typing of the children can reveal those paternal HLA-antigens which have never been inherited. At least these antigens might be considered acceptable mismatches for transplantation.

To validate the clinical significance of the present findings we are performing a retrospective study, analyzing graft survival in mothers thereby differentiating HLA-mismatches identical to inherited paternal antigens from other mismatched antigens.

References

1. Albrechtsen D, Leivestad T, Fauchald P, Flatmark A, Sodal G, Thorsby E. Results of the National Kidney Transplantation Program in Norway. In: Terasaki PI, Cecka JM, eds. *Clinical Transplants 1992*. Los Angeles: UCLA Tissue Typing Laboratory, 1993: 207-13.
2. Terasaki PI, Cecka JM, Gjertson DW, Takemoto S. High survival rates of kidney transplants from spousal and living unrelated donors. *N Engl J Med* 1995; 333: 333-6.
3. Terasaki PI, Koyama H, Cecka JM, Gjertson DW. The hyperfiltration hypothesis in human renal transplantation. *Transplantation* 1994; 57: 1450-4.
4. Kabelitz D, Zanker B, Zanker C, Heeg K, Wagner H. Human cytotoxic T lymphocytes. II. Frequency analysis of cyclosporin A-sensitive alloreactive cytotoxic T-lymphocyte precursors. *Immunology* 1987; 61: 57-62.
5. MacDonald HR, Glasebrook AL, Bron C, Kelso A, Cerottini JC. Clonal heterogeneity in the functional requirement for Lyt-2/3 molecules on cytolytic T lymphocytes (CTL): possible implication for the affinity of CTL antigen receptors. *Immunol Rev* 1982; 68: 89-115.
6. Ouwehand AJ, Baan CC, Roelen DL *et al.* The detection of cytotoxic T cells with high-affinity receptors for donor antigens in the transplanted heart as a prognostic factor for graft rejection. *Transplantation* 1993; 56: 1223-9.
7. Roelen DL, Van Beelen E, Van Bree FPMJ, Van Rood JJ, Völker-Dieben HJ, Claas FHJ. The presence of activated donor HLA class I-reactive T lymphocytes is associated with rejection of corneal grafts. *Transplantation* 1995; 59: 1039-42.
8. Roelen D, Datema G, Van Bree S, Zhang L, Van Rood J, Claas F. Evidence that antibody formation against a certain HLA alloantigen is associated not with a quantitative but with a qualitative change in the cytotoxic T cells recognizing the same antigen. *Transplantation* 1992; 53: 899-903.
9. Regan L, Braude PR, Hill DP. A prospective study of the incidence, time of appearance and significance of anti-paternal lymphocytotoxic antibodies in human pregnancy. *Hum Reprod* 1991; 6: 294-8.
10. Claas FHJ, De Waal LP, Beelen J *et al.* Transplantation of highly sensitized patients on the basis of acceptable HLA-A and-B mismatches. In: Terasaki PI, Cecka JM, eds. *Clinical Transplants 1989*. Los Angeles: UCLA Tissue Typing Laboratory, 1990: 185-90.

The alloreactive CTL response to a single alloantigen involves CTL clones with diverse specificities

N. Cereb, H. Xiao, P. Muthaura, S.Y. Yang*

Memorial Sloan-Kettering Cancer Center, 1275 York Avenue, New York, NY 10021, USA
*Corresponding author

Alloreactive cytotoxic T lymphocytes (CTLs) recognizing HLA class I mismatches play significant roles in inducing graft-versus-host disease (GvHD) and graft rejection. The degree of matching required to avoid this complication is unknown. In certain cases a major mismatch for one locus can be tolerated [1], in others one amino acid mismatch can cause the rejection of the graft [2]. This variation may be a function of inter-individual differences in the TCR repertoire [3]. With the availability of DNA typing methods, it is now possible to type HLA class I molecules at the allelic level. The feasibility of finer matching for HLA class I should reduce the immunological complications of bone marrow transplantation. However, in the case of unrelated marrow grafts, mismatch transplants may be necessary because finding a matching donor can be very difficult due to the extensive HLA polymorphism in the population. In this study, we investigated the allostimulatory potential of micro- versus major-mismatches, using an *in vitro* system that allows us to examine the alloresponses to a single alloantigen at a time. An HLA null cell line K562 transfected with B*4403 was used as a stimulator [4] for the generation of alloreactive CTL lines from responders with different HLA backgrounds. The T cell clones isolated from the CTL lines were examined for their TCR repertoire.

Results and discussion

A CTL line was generated from one individual carrying B*4402 (GR: B*4402, B*4901), representing a micro-mismatch for B44 alleles that differs by one amino acid from B*4403. Two more were generated from two B44- individuals, AV (A*2402, A*6802, B*3503, B*4001) and JL (A*2601, A*2902, B*1401, B*3801), for a major antigen mismatch, by weekly stimulation with K562 expressing B*4403 molecules, as described previously [4] . A large number of T cell clones isolated from these three CTL lines did not kill the B*4403+ targets, the alloantigen which was used for stimulation *(Table I)*. The alloreactive CTL clones reactive with the B*4403+ targets were further analyzed for their allospecificity, using a panel of B-LCLs from the 10th International Histocompatibility Workshop core cell lines [5]. This panel included cell lines expressing, B*4402, the B44 crossreactive group (CREG) of antigens (B*4501, B*4901, B*5001) and other common B antigens (B*0702, B*0801, B*1302, B*1402, B*1501, B*1801, B*2705, B*3501, B*3503, B*3508, B*3701, B*3801, B*4001, B*4701, B*4201, B*5105, B*5301, B*5401, B*5701). Of the 55 B*4403-reactive AV clones analyzed, only one (clone AV6A1 in *Table II*) was found to be exclusively B*4403-specific. The rest were crossreactive towards at least one other antigen. The majority of the B*4403 reactive clones from JL were also crossreactive. By contrast, the monospecific clones obtained from the CTL line GR (elicited by the micro-mismatch), outnumbered the crossreactive ones. Almost all of the crossreactive clones recognized at least one of the B44 CREG antigens. These alloreactive T cell clones were further analyzed for T cell receptor usage of β and α chains by RT-PCR, using 5' BV or AV gene family-specific primers and a 3' Cβ or Cα region primer.

Table I. General characteristics of the CTL clones

CTL LINES	CLONES (%)			
	TOTAL	B*4403 REACTIVE		B*4403 NONREACTIVE
		Monospecific	Crossreactive	
AV(B*44⁻)	73	1 (1)	54 (74)	18 (25)
JL (B*44⁻)	54	4 (8)	11 (20)	39 (72)
GR(B*4402⁺)	33	9 (27)	5 (15)	19 (58)

Table II. TCR usage for B*4403

Clone	BSG	TCRBV	ASG	TCRAV	Specificity
AV6A1	4	BV13S6A1	1, 4	AV21S1, AV22S1	B*4403
GR6H11	1b	BV18S1	2	AV19S1	B*4403
GR7A11	1a	BV6S1A1		N.C	B*4403
JL1E2	4	BV13S1		N.C	B*4403
AV1A5	4	BV3S1	3	AV12	B*4403,B*4402,B*1501,B*3801
GR5A2	1a	BV8S1		N.C	B*4403,B*4901,B*5301
JL2G3	1c	BV5S4A2	3, 4	AV6, AV9	B*4403,B*5701,B*5301,B*4402

BSG and ASG: TCRBV and TCRAV subgroups, as defined by Chothia and co workers, respectively [6)] N.C: Not completed.

The DNA sequence of the amplified PCR products were determined using an ABI 373A DNA sequencer. The results from seven clones representing different specificities from AV, GR, and JL are summarized in *Table II*. A diverse TCR usage was observed among B*4403-monospecific T cell clones obtained from responders with different HLA background (*Table II*). However, the majority of the B*4403-specific clones isolated from donor GR, who had a micromismatch with the stimulating B*4403, used the TCRAV19S1BV18S1 combination (unpublished results). The TCR usage for the cross-reactive CTL clones were more diverse. However, all B*4403 reactive clones have BV gene segments that belong to subgroups 1 and 4 defined by Chothia *et al.* [6, 7]. This is consistent with the previous report on nonrandom usage of TCRs towards one class I alloantigen [8]. We are in the process of analyzing more B*4403 reactive clones for TCR gene segment usage to substantiate this finding. However, the degree of randomness of AV usage will be harder to determine because about 30% of T cells express two a chains.

Previous studies have suggested that the magnitude of alloresponses may depend on the stimulating alloantigen [9, 10]. The TCR repertoire is shaped by self MHC molecules during T cell development in the thymus where self-MHC reacting T cells are eliminated. A single MHC/peptide complex has the potential to interact with many different TCRs acquired *via* positive selection [11]. On the other hand, these potentially alloreactive T cells were shown to be eliminated by exposure to multitudes of self peptides during TCR selection [11]. Thus, the closer the HLA structures are between donor and recipient, the smaller the alloreactive T cell repertoire is likely to be. This is consistent with our findings where the CTL line and clones elicited by the micromismatch had narrower specificity with a more limited TCR usage than those generated by major mismatches that displayed wide crossreactivity and diverse TCR usage (*Table II*). Thus alloreactivity to a single alloantigen involves complex interactions, precluding the involvement of public TCRs. However, in most cases, an alloresponse to a micromismatch will be less complex than to a major mismatch. Analysis of all the clones generated from experiments described above is underway to determine the TCRs recognizing the alloantigens.

In this study, we have attempted to dissect the alloresponses to a single alloantigen with different combinations of mismatches. The knowledge of the allostimulatory potential of certain mismatch combinations will guide us to select better immunocompatible donors among candidates with various molecular disparities. Furthermore, pairwise examination of alloreactive TCR repertoire used for defined molecular disparities will also enable us to determine the feasibility of TCR-targeted prevention or treatment of graft rejection or GvHD.

References

1. Anasetti C, Beatty PG, Storb R, Martin PJ, Mori M, Sanders JE, Thomas ED, Hansen JA. Effect of HLA incompatibility on graft-versus-host disease, relapse, and survival after marrow transplantation for patients with leukemia or lymphoma. *Hum Immunol* 1990; 29 : 79-91.

2. Fleischhauer K, Kernan NA, O'Reilly RJ, Dupont B, Yang SY. Bone marrow allograft rejection by cytotoxic T lymphocytes recognizing a single amino acid at position 156 of HLA class I antigen. *N Engl J Med* 1990; 323: 1818-22.
3. Akolkar PN, Gulwani-Akolkar B, Pergolizzi R, Bigler RD, Silver J. Influence of HLA genes on T cell receptor V segment frequencies and expression levels in peripheral blood lymphocytes. *J Immunol* 1993; 150: 2761-73.
4. Cereb N, Yang SY. Induction of microvariant-specific CTL lines reactive to a single amino acid mismatch in bulk cultures using transfectant expressing a single class I HLA molecule. *J Immunol* 1996; 156: 18-26.
5. Yang SY, Milford E, Hammerling U, Dupont B. Description of the reference panel of B-lymphoblastoid cell lines for factors of the HLA system: the B-cell line panel designed for the Tenth International Histocompatibility Workshop. In Dupont B, ed. *Immunobiology of HLA: Histocompatibility Testing 1987*, vol. I. New York: Springer-Verlag, 1989: 11-9.
6. Chothia C, Boswell DR, Lesk AM. The outline structure of the T-cell alpha beta receptor. *EMBO J* 1988; 7: 3745-55.
7. Arden B, Clark SP, Kabelitz D, Mak TW. Human T-cell receptor variable gene segment families. *Immunogenetics* 1995; 42: 455-500.
8. Barber DF, Lopez D, Lopez de Castro JA. T cell receptor diversity in alloreactive responses against HLA-B27(B*2705) is limited by multiple-level restrictions in both α and β chains. *Eur J Immunol* 1995; 25: 2479-85.
9. Connolly JM. The peptide p2Ca is immunodominant in allorecognition of L^d by beta chain variable region $V\beta\ 8^+$ but not $V\beta\ 8^-$ strains. *Proc Natl Acad Sci USA* 1994; 91: 11482-6.
10. Sherman LA. Dissection of the B10.D2 anti-H-2Kb cytolytic T lymphocyte receptor repertoire. *J Exp Med* 1980; 151: 1386-97.
11. Ignatowicz L, Kappler J, Marrack P. The receptor of T cells shaped by a single MHC/peptide ligand. *Cell* 1996; 84: 521-9.

Relation between transfusion-associated graft-versus-host disease (TA-GVHD) and HLA

S. Uchida, Y. Yahagi, L. Wang, S. Mitsunaga, S. Moriyama, K. Tokunaga[1], K. Tadokoro, T. Juji

Department of Research, The Japanese Red Cross Central Blood Center, 4-1-31, Hiroo, Shibuya-ku, Tokyo 150, Japan
1 Department of Human Genetics, School of International Health, University of Tokyo, 7-3-1, Hongo, Bunkyo-ku, Tokyo 113, Japan

Transfusion-associated graft-versus-host disease (TA-GVHD) is a potentially fatal adverse reaction to blood transfusion with a mortality rate of 90 percent or higher [1]. It was estimated to have occurred in one out of 659 patients who underwent cardiac surgery in Japan [2]. The clinical manifestations of typical TA-GVHD are high fever, erythematous eruption, diarrhea, liver dysfunction and pancytopenia, and the patient dies from septicemia. TA-GVHD cases were initially termed as postoperative erythroderma with unknown aetiology, but later patients' symptoms were considered to be caused by GVH reaction in which lymphocytes contained in the transfused blood were accepted by the recipient and reacted with histoincompatible antigens of the host. TA-GVHD occurs not only in immunocompromised patients, but also in apparently immunocompetent patients. TA-GVHD in immunocompetent patients occurs mainly when lymphocytes from a human leukocyte antigen (HLA) homozygous donor are transfused into a HLA heterozygous patient who shares one haplotype with the donor [3]. We recently developed a definitive diagnostic test for TA-GVHD using polymerase chain reaction (PCR) amplification of highly polymorphic microsatellite repeat sequences [4]. Thirty-five cases of TA-GVHD among 98 patients who were referred to us through the Red Cross Medical Representative Network from October 1992 to December 1995 were diagnosed using this system. HLA alleles of the patient and the implicated donor were determined in 14 out of the 35 cases including 7 types for both class-I and class-II loci and 7 only for class-II.

Methods

TA-GVHD diagnosis

Diagnosis of TA-GVHD was confirmed by microsatellite DNA polymorphism analysis [4]. We extracted DNA from clippings of the patient's fingernails [5] and a sample of the patient's peripheral blood when TA-GVHD was suspected. Their PCR amplification products of five microsatellite loci were analyzed by polyacrylamide gel electrophoresis. Underlying diseases of TA-GVHD patients in this study are 6 cardiovascular siseases, 5 solid tumors, 1 prostatic hypertrophy, 1 head injury and 1 placenta previa.

HLA DNA typing

Genomic DNA prepared from clippings of the patient's fingernails and a sample of the patient's peripheral blood when TA-GVHD was suspected was subjected to HLA genotyping; the former was used for patient, and the latter for donor, HLA typing. HLA class-I (A,B) and class-II (DRB1,DQB1,DPB1) typing were performed using PCR-restriction fragment length polymorphism (RFLP) methods described previously [6].

Results and discussion

Figure 1 shows a typical result of microsatellite DNA analysis in a TA-GVHD patient. Peripheral blood DNA types determined after a patient developed symptoms of TA-GVHD have been found to differ from the fingernail DNA types. In other words, the patient's peripheral white blood cells had been replaced by exogenous lymphocytes during the development of TA-GVHD.

The results of HLA genotyping using DNAs from post-transfusion fingernail and peripheral blood samples are shown. *Table I* lists the HLA types of the patient and the donor for 14 cases of TA-GVHD in patients without evident immune deficiency. In each case, upper rows show HLA genotypes determined from DNA extracted from the clippings of the patient's fingernails and lower rows show HLA genotypes determined from DNA extracted from the sample of the patient's peripheral blood sample. At the DRB1 locus, the donors were homozygous for an allele for which the patients were heterozygous (one-way match) in all 14 cases. In cases 11-14, the donors' HLA haplotypes were homozygous of HLA-A24, B52, DR15. This donors'

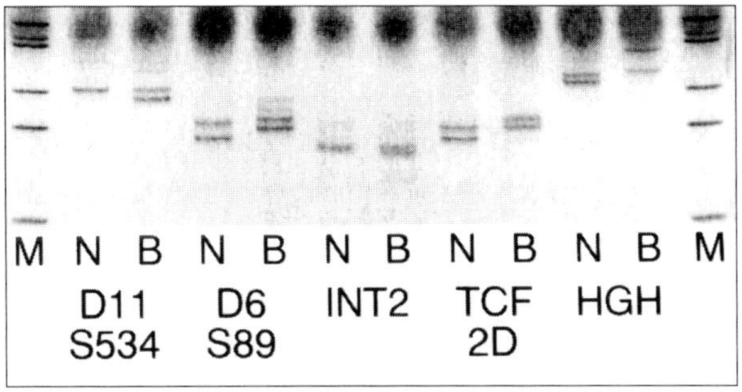

Figure 1. DNA polymorphism analysis in a TA-GVHD patient. Five sets of microsatellite primers (D11S534, D6S89, INT2, TCF2D and HGH) were used for PCR. Electrophoretic patterns of the PCR products derived from DNA extracted from fingernail (N) and peripheral blood cells (B) are shown. Lane M shows the DNA size marker ØX174 digested with HaeIII.

haplotype is a highest frequency (8.6%) in Japanese.

It is well established that a difference in both class-I and class-II antigens, but not in class-I or class-II antigens alone, triggers the donor T cells capable of inducing acute fatal GVHD in the mouse model [7]. However, we identified a patient with an atypical clinical course in which patient's class-I A and B loci were identical to those of the donor but the class-II DRB1 locus was one-way matched (*Table I*, case 8). These results suggest that fatal TA-GVHD might be induced by stimulation by class-II antigens only in humans. A one-way HLA match in class-II loci seems to be necessary for occurrence of TA-GVHD in immunocompetent patients.

Table I. Changes of HLA phenotypes in TA-GVHD patients

No	A	B	DRB1	DQB1	DPB1
1	n.t	n.t	02 04	n.t	n.t
	n.t	n.t	02	n.t	n.t
2	n.t	n.t	02 12	n.t	n.t
	n.t	n.t	02	n.t	n.t
3	n.t	n.t	1501 1502	n.t	0501 0901
	n.t	n.t	1502	n.t	0901
4	n.t	n.t	08 1502	n.t	0501 0901
	n.t	n.t	1502	n.t	0901
5	n.t	n.t	1501 1502	n.t	0201 0901
	n.t	n.t	1502	n.t	0901
6	n.t	n.t	0405 1502	0601	0402 0901
	n.t	n.t	1502	0601	0901
7	n.t	n.t	08032 1502	0601	0201 0901
	n.t	n.t	1502	0601	0901
8	0201	39 46	0802 1501	n.t	n.t
	0201	39 46	1501	n.t	n.t
9	2402	4002 52011	0901 1502	n.t	n.t
	24*	38* 61*	0901	n.t	n.t
10	2402 3301	40 44	1101 1302	n.t	n.t
	3301	44	1302	n.t	n.t
11	2402 2601	39 52	1201 1502	n.t	n.t
	2402	52	1502	n.t	n.t
12	0201 2402	4601 52011	1502 0901	n.t	n.t
	2402	52011	1502	n.t	n.t
13	02 2402	5201 59	0405 1502	0401 0601	n.t
	2402	5201	1502	0601	n.t
14	2402 3301	52011 44	1302 1502	0601	0401 0501
	2402	52011	1502	0601	0201 0901

* serological typing
recognizable antigens by donor cells are circled
n.t : not tested

References

1. Holland PV. Transfusion-associated graft-versus-host disease: Prevention using irradiated blood products. In: Garrarry G, eds. *Current concepts in transfusion therapy*. Arlington : American Association of Blood Banks 19858: 295-315.
2. Juji T, Takahashi K, Shibata Y, Ide H, Sakakibara T, Ino T, Mori S. Post-transfusion graft-versus-host disease in immunocompetent patients after cardiac surgery in Japan. *N Engl J Med* 1989; 321: 56.
3. Ito K, Yoshida H, Yanagibashi K, Shimada Y, Imamura M, Tobe T, Akiyama Y, Saji H, Maruya E, Hosoi T. Change of HLA phenotype in postoperative erythroderma. *Lancet* 1988; 20: 413-4.
4. Wang L, Juji T, Tokunaga K, Takahashi K, Kuwata S, Uchida S, Tadokoro K, Takai K. Polymorphic microsatellite markers for the diagnosis of graft-versus-host disease. *N Engl J Med* 1994; 330: 398-401.
5. Uchida S, Wang L, Yahagi Y, Tokunaga K, Tadokoro K, Juji T. Utility of fingernail DNA for evaluation of chimerism after bone marrow transplantation and for diagnostic testing for transfusion-associated graft-versus-host disease. *Blood* 1996; 87: 4015-6.
6. Mitsunaga S, Oguchi T, Moriyama S, Tokunaga K, Akaza T, Tadokoro K, Juji T. Multiplex arms-PCR-RFLP method for high-resolution typing of HLA-DRB1. *Eur J Immunogenet* 1995; 22: 371-92.
7. Rolink AG, Pals ST, Gleichmann E. Allosuppressor and allohelper T cells in acute and chronic graft-vs.-host disease. *J Exp Med* 1983; 157: 755-71.

Cyclosporin A (CyA) resistant alloimmunity measured *in vitro*

K.M.G. Haque[1], C. Truman[1], I. Dittmer[2], G. Laundy[1], T. Feest[2], B. Bradley[1]

1 University of Bristol, Department of Transplantation Sciences, Southmead Health Services, Westbury-on-Trym, Bristol BS10 5NB, UK
2 Richard Bright Renal Unit, Southmead Health Services, Bristol BS10 5NB,UK

Between 40-50% of renal transplant recipients develop a CyA resistant rejection crisis within the early post-transplant period. Some attempts have been made to develop *in vitro* correlates [1]. CyA appears to inhibit the transcription of genes encoding Interleukin-2 (IL-2), Interleukin-3 (IL-3) and Interferon-γ (IFNγ) [2]. It is also suggested that it inhibits transcription of the IL-2 receptor (IL-R) in naive CD8+ T cells. The inhibitory effects of CyA can be demonstrated in primary lymphocyte culture [3]. In theory, mature T cells expressing the high affinity IL-2 receptor (CD25) escape suppression by CyA if cultured in the presence of excess IL-2. In contrast, naive T cells are inhibited from responding to IL-2 because the CyA inhibits transcription of the genes for IL-2R [4]. We have therefore tested the inhibitory effect of CyA in the presence of excess IL-2.

Materials and methods

Patients with chronic renal failure on dialysis and/or awaiting transplantation (7 male, 4 female) and normal healthy adults (4 male, 1 female) were selected. 32 blood samples from other normal healthy adults were used as stimulator and third party targets. No attempts were made to HLA match. Peripheral blood mononuclear cells (PBMCs) were separated from heparinized blood by density gradient (Lymphoprep,1.077 g/ml, Nycomed) centrifugation and cryopreserved in liquid nitrogen.

CML-CyA assay

RPMI 1640 (Sigma-Aldrich Co Ltd, UK) was supplemented with 10% human AB serum (Sigma, heat inactivated at 56° C for 30 minutes) from normal healthy male donors and 3mM L-glutamine (Sigma). We did not use antibiotics. Powdered CyA was a generous gift from Sandoz Ltd, UK. A stock solution of 1mg/ml in absolute ethanol was stored at 4 °C. The CyA working solution was a 1:100 dilution dissolved in complete culture medium (CCM) with vigorous agitation. On day 0 an allogeneic one way mixed lymphocyte culture assay was set up. The cryopreserved cells were thawed and responder cells (4×10^4 per well) were co-cultured with irradiated (30 Gy) stimulator cells (5×10^4 per well) in 96 well U bottomed tissue culture plates (Falcon, 3077, Becton Dickinson). The responder cells were incubated at 37°C in a 5% CO_2 humidified atmosphere at varying concentrations of CyA (from 0 to 1500 ng/ml) in culture medium for one hour prior to the addition of irradiated stimulator cells. Specific radioimmunoassay for confirming CyA concentration in the culture medium was performed. To each culture well 25 Cetus units/ml of recombinant IL-2 (rIL-2, Eurocetus, Amsterdam) were added. 16- 24 replicates were set up and the culture was incubated for 7 days at 37°C in a 5% CO_2 humidified atmosphere. As a control, irradiated stimulator cells were cultured without the responder cells. On day 5 the cultures were refreshed by replacing the spent medium with fresh CCM containing rIL-2 (25 units/ml) and CyA (0 -1500 ng/ml). At the same time, as setting up the CML assay, PBMCs adjusted to 1×10^6 cells / ml were grown up as targets in CCM containing 20 units/ml rIL-2 and 2 µg/ml purified phytohaemagglutinin (PHA, Murex Diagnostics, UK) in a 24 well Costar plate (Cambridge, MA 02140). The PHA blasts were incubated for 7 days at 37°C in 5 % CO_2 humidified atmosphere. The blasts were examined microscopically , split and fed (usually on day 3 and 5) with freshly prepared CCM containing rIL-2 (20 units/ml). On day 7 of the assay, the PHA stimulated targets were labelled with Eu-diethylenetriaminopentaacetate (Eu-DTPA, Sigma) chelate and incubated for 15 minutes at 4°C [5,6]. After washing the highly fluorescent Eu-DTPA complex-labelled blasts were added to the 7 day cultured cells.

Label, released as a result of target cell lysis was measured by a Time Resolved Fluorimeter (1234, Arcus, Delfia, Finland). Each culture well was divided into two (split well analysis) and a cytotoxic assay was carried out for each replicate (responder /stimulator combination) using Eu labelled PHA targets from the *original stimulator cells*, *autologous cells* (original responder) and *third party* cells. Total release and spontaneous release Eu label was also measured for each target. Target cells were added to wells of split assay plates at a concentration of 5000 cells per well. Plates were gently centrifuged (1000 rpm for 1 minute at 18°-22°C) and incubated at 37°C in a 5% CO_2 humidified atmosphere for 3 hours. After incubation, plates were centrifuged (1800 rpm for 5 minutes at 18°-22°C). An aliquot of 20 µl supernatant from each well was transferred to low autofluorescent 96 well reader plates (Nunc) which were prefilled with 200 µl per well enhancement solution (Delfia, Finland) and the plates read by Time Resolved Fluorometry.

Data analysis

% lysis and % inhibition were calculated as follows:

$$\% \text{ lysis} = \frac{(\text{test value - spontaneous release}) \times 100}{\text{maximum release - spontaneous release}}$$

$$\% \text{ inhibition} = 100 - \left[\frac{(\text{test value - spontaneous release}) \times 100}{\text{value at nil CyA - spontaneous release}}\right]$$

Results

We observed that the CML against the original stimulator targets showed a wide variation of % lysis which quickly reduce with increased doses of CyA (*Figure 1*). The third party targets were also lysed but at a lower level indicating more than one clone of cross reactive alloimmune killer T cells (results not shown). Expressing the same CML values as % inhibition the results showed that, whereas in normal individuals and some patients CML was completely suppressed with therapeutic doses of CyA (50-250 ng/ml), other patients with no history of either blood transfusion or failed transplant showed partially resistant CML even to toxic doses of CyA (1000 ng /ml). Despite the wide variation of % lysis to original stimulator targets (at nil concentration CyA) we did not observe any significant correlation with % inhibition ($p > 0.05$).

Discussion

This CML-CyA sensitivity assay used random pairs of HLA mismatched cells. Consequently the % lysis in CML control (nil CyA) varied widely from 0% to 96% rendering the susceptibility to CyA difficult to interpret. By calculating % inhibition much of the variability between individuals was eliminated. When % inhibition was plotted (*Figure 2*) for all 16 individuals tested they appeared to fall into two patterns: a group (dotted Line) of 6 who were highly susceptible to low doses of CyA (50 - 250 ng/ml) and a group (solid Line) of 10 who were almost completely resistant to low doses and only partially inhibited by very high doses (1000-1500 ng/ml). Three hypothesis, which are not mutually exclusive, might explain these phenomena.

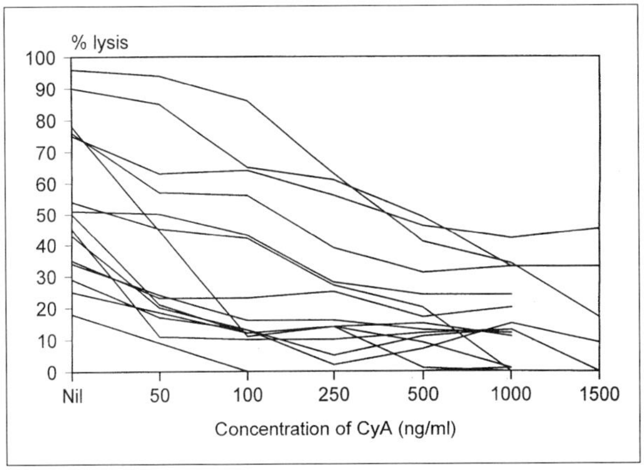

Figure 1. % lysis versus increasing concentration of CyA for 16 individuals.

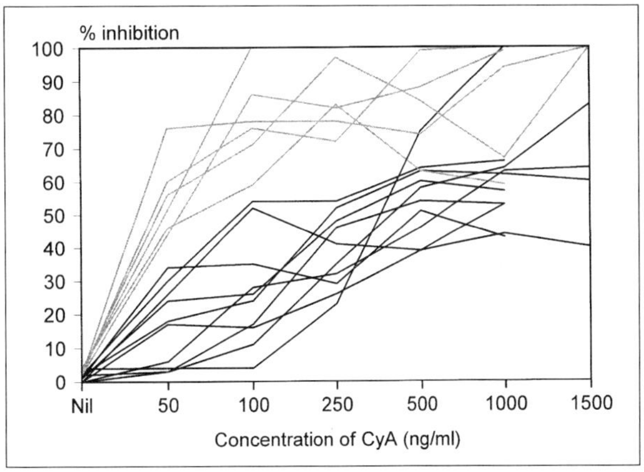

Figure 2. Same data as in *Figure 1* but recalculated as % inhibition versus increasing concentration of CyA.

Technical

IL-2R may be transcribed in the early stages of culture because insufficient time had been allowed for the CyA to penetrate and inhibit transcription.

Immunological

Through prior immunological experiences certain individuals may carry higher levels of mature T cell clones bearing IL-2R and would be resistant to CyA.

Genetic

Somewhere in the CyA inhibitory pathway (Calcineurin, NFAT, etc.) critical molecules may be transcribed at two different levels according to a biallelic system at the DNA level. It is possible these *in vitro* observations might be of prognostic value in renal transplantation.

Acknowledgements

KH is a recipient of a scholarship from the Association of the Commonwealth Universities in the UK. This work and CT are supported by a grant from the National Kidney Research Fund, UK (NKRF grant no.77/92). The authors thank all patients and blood donors who co-operated in this study. We gratefully acknowledged the support of the National Blood Service and the Clinical Chemistry Department, Southmead Health Services, Bristol.

References

1. Sander B, Brigati C, Moller E. Inhibition of *in vitro* alloreactivity by cyclosporin A: evidence for an inter-individual variation in sensitivity. *Scan J Immunol* 1986; 23: 435-40.
2. Schreiber SL, Crabtree GR. The mechanism of action of cyclosporin A and FK506. *Immunol Today* 1992; 13 (4): 136-41.
3. Haque K, Dittmer I, Truman C, Laundy G, Feest T, Bradley B. Dissection of cyclosporin- A sensitive and resistant T cell allo-immunity. Proceedings of the Spring Meetings of the British Transplantation Society. Oxford, March 1996 (abstract).
4. Roelen DL, van Bree SPMJ, van Beelen E, Schanz U, van Rood JJ, Claas FHJ. Differential inhibition of primed alloreactive CTLs *in vitro* by clinically used concentration of cyclosporine versus FK506. *Transplantation* 1993; 56: 190.
5. Bouma GJ, van der Meer-Prins PMW, van Bree FPMJ, van Rood JJ, Class FHJ. Determination of cytotoxic T lymphocyte precursor frequencies using Europium labelling as a non-radioactive alternative to labelling with chromium-51. *Hum Immunol* 1992; 35: 85-92.
6. Haque K, Truman C, Laundy G, Dittmer I, Denning-Kendall P, Bradley B. Optimisation of Europium (Eu) release T lymphocyte precursor frequency (CTLpf). Proceedings of the British Society for Immunology Spring Meeting. April 1996; 26 (abstract).

Vβ18-Dβ1-Jβ2.7 T-cell clonality in graft infiltrating cells in donor specific transfusion-induced allograft tolerance

P. Douillard[1], C. Pannetier[2], R. Josien[1], S. Menoret[1], P. Kourilsky[2], J.P. Soulillou[1], M.C. Cuturi[1]

1 ITERT, INSERM U437, 30, boulevard Jean Monnet, BP 1005, 44035 Nantes Cedex 01, France
2 Institut Pasteur, INSERM U277, 25, rue du Docteur Roux, 75724 Paris Cedex 15, France

Graft infiltrating T-cells (GITC) recognize allogeneic MHC antigens through their T cell receptor (TcR). Whereas it has been recently reported that T cells infiltrating a rejected allograft display a rather limited TcR repertoire diversity [1], little is known about T cells infiltrating a tolerated allograft. Heart allograft tolerance can be reproducibly induced in fully mismatched MHC congenic rats by donor-specific transfusion (DST) prior to transplantation [2]. The tolerated organ is highly infiltrated [3], suggesting an active process. In order to gain insight into the role of GITC in this tolerance induction, we have analysed their TcR β chain repertoire diversity.

Materials and methods

TcR β chain repertoire analysis was based on Immunoscope analysis [4] coupled, where necessary, to RNAse protection assay with multiset probes [5]. Briefly, total RNA from allografts and spleens was converted into cDNA, which was then amplified by PCR using a Cβ primer and one of the oligonucleotide primers specific for each of the twenty known rat Vβ subfamilies [6]. Each amplified product was used as a template for elongation reactions initiated with a Cβ oligonucleotide labeled with a fluorescent tag. The labeled run-off products, which have been elongated through CDR3 coding regions of various sizes, were loaded on polyacrylamide gels and subjected to electrophoresis in an automated DNA sequencer. Analysis with Immunoscope software yielded the VDJ size distribution and the intensity of the size peaks. Particular Vβ subfamilies were further characterized by using twelve Jβ-specific labeled primers to refine the analysis. To quantify Vβ family usage, RNase Protection Assay with multiset probes [5] was performed.

Results

LEW.1A ($RT1^a$) recipients rejected LEW.1W ($RT1^u$) heart allografts within 13.3±6 days. In this combination, two pretransplant DST induced specific tolerance. We assessed the TcR β chain diversity at the mRNA level in spleen and grafted heart by analysing the CDR3 length distribution for any Vβ-Cβ combination using the Immunoscope method [4]. Earlier studies in humans and mice have shown that, in each Vβ-Cβ combinations, there were six to ten size peaks spaced by three nucleotides corresponding to inframe transcripts [4, 7]. The area of each size peak is proportional to the quantity of TcR β transcripts displaying a CDR3 region of the corresponding size. Each peak corresponding to a given CDR3 length usually contains multiple distinct sequences. An increase in the height and area of a size peak commonly signals a monoclonal expansion over a polyclonal background. In rat spleens from naive animals, Vβ repertoire analysis revealed that, in all Vβ-Cβ combinations, the CDR3-size pattern was reproducibly distributed in a Gaussian-like fashion. In contrast, Vβ repertoire in GITC was characteristic for tolerant and rejecting animals, as much as some Vβ were almost absent while others expressed a preferential VDJ junction size. Interestingly, tolerated allografts reproducibly displayed a clonal expansion in Vβ18 subfamily; this expansion, corresponding to a 7 amino-acid CDR3 length, was present from day 1 to 30 post-graft. Direct sequencing of this PCR product revealed a conserved rearrangement at the nucleotide level among tolerant animals (n=8): the β chain of this clone used the Vβ18-Dβ1-Jβ2.7 combination. With RNase protection assay experiments, we were able to quantify the Vβ chain usage in allografts. Thus, in tolerated ones, Vβ18 was monoclonal and represented 5% of all Vβ. In contrast, in GITC from rejecting rats (n=9), Vβ18 was polyclonal in a non-Gaussian-like fashion, with expansions which were not reproducible between tested animals. Moreover, polyclonality was even seen when analysis was performed with the Jβ2.7 primer. Using a clonotypic labeled primer specific for this public Vβ18 rearrangement, we were able to detect the Vβ18-Dβ1-Jβ2.7 clone also in rejected allografts, though later in time, *i.e.* either from day 5 or from day 7 post-graft. Furthermore, since Vβ18 subfamily represented 3% of all Vβ in rejecting allografts, Vβ18 with a CDR3 size of 7 amino-acids (that comprises Vβ18-Dβ1-Jβ2.7) represented less than 1% of the whole repertoire in rejected allografts. With this clonotypic primer, we were able to detect the emergence of this clone in recipient PBL during transfusion time course, seven days after the first transfusion. Moreover, when transfusions were performed with LEW.1N ($RT1^n$) blood, we did not detect this clone, whereas when transfusions were performed with Wistar blood ($RT1^u$), we can detect it in recipient PBL. These results strongly suggest that this clone is specific of $RT1^u$ alloantigens. Finally, this rearrangement was detected in $CD8^+$ T cells.

Discussion

We have shown that graft infiltrating T lymphocytes displayed a limited Vβ repertoire in tolerated allografts. Moreover, the type of restriction seems to be mostly divergent between rejected and tolerated grafts, as profiles were different. Donors and recipients are congeneic; they shared the same genetic background but are mismatched for MHC antigens (class I and II). Our results strongly suggest that the same alloantigen (donor MHC) can induce different profiles of Vβ responses depending on the source, the way of administration and the timing of alloantigen presentation, *i.e.* either DST plus graft in tolerant animals, or graft only in rejecting ones. According to Shoskes and Wood [8], alloantigens from DST can be processed by recipient antigen presenting cells (APC) leading to indirect presentation pathway, whereas in rejecting situation, recipient infiltrating T lymphocytes directly recognize the alloantigens presented by donor APC presents in grafts, thus leading to rejection process; in parallel, recipient APC process alloantigens and stimulate alloreactive clones by the indirect pathway. Thus, we hypothesize that Vβ18-Dβ1-Jβ2.7 T cell clones could be preferentially restricted to indirect presentation, which would explain its strong and early presence in tolerated allografts, and also its later detection in rejecting ones. We have also performed Vβ repertoire analysis with primary mixed lymphocyte reactions which were known to represent direct allorecognition, and the specific Vβ18 clone was not detected, whereas Vβ-subfamilies specific for rejection situation were found (Douillard *et al.*, manuscript in preparation). Further experiments are in course in our lab to more precisely characterize the phenotype and functionalities of this clone in our model of allograft tolerance.

References

1. Shirwan H, Chi D, Makowka L, Cramer DV. Lymphocytes infiltrating rat cardiac allografts express a limited repertoire of T cell receptor Vβ gene. *J Immunol* 1993; 151: 5228-38.
2. Soulillou JP, Blandin F, Günther E, Lemoine V. Genetics of the blood transfusion effect on heart allografts in rats. *Transplantation* 1984; 38: 63-7.
3. Josien R, Pannetier C, Douillard P, Cantarovich D, Menoret S, Bugeon L, Soulillou JP, Cuturi MC. Graft infiltrating T-helper cells, CD45RC phenotype, and TH1/TH2-related cytokines in donor-specific transfusion-induced tolerance in adult rats. *Transplantation* 1995; 60: 1131-9.
4. Pannetier C, Even J, Kourilsky P. T-cell repertoire diversity and clonal expansions in normal and clinical samples. *Immunol Today* 1995; 16: 176-81.
5. Smith LR, Kono DH, Kammuller ME, Balderas RS, Theofilopoulos AN. Vβ repertoire in rats and implications for endogenous superantigens. *Eur J Immunol* 1992; 22: 641-5.
6. Smith AR, Kono DH, Theofilopoulos AN. Complexity and sequence identification of 24 rat Vβ genes. *J Immunol* 1991; 147: 375-9.
7. Pannetier C, Cochet M, Darche S, Casrouge A, Zöller M, Kourilsky P. The sizes of the CDR3 hypervariable regions of the murine T-cell receptor b chains vary as a function of the recombined germ-line segments. *Proc Natl Acad Sci USA* 1993; 90: 4319-23.
8. Shoskes DA, Wood KJ. Indirect presentation of MHC antigens in transplantation. *Immunol Today* 1994; 15: 32-8.

Modulation of HLA
Soluble HLA

Contents

IL-10 suppresses TAP function and makes cells NK sensitive

J. Charo[1], M. Petersson[1], F. Salazar-Onfray[1], G. Noffz[2], Z. Qin[2], T. Blankenstein[2], R. Kiessling[1,3]*

1 Microbiology and Tumor Biology Center (MTC), Karolinska Institute, Box 280, S-171 77 Stockholm, Sweden
2 Max-Delbruck Center for Molecular Medicine (MDC), 131 22 Berlin-Buch, Germany
3 Department of Experimental Oncology, Radiumhemmet, Karolinska Hospital, Stockholm, Sweden
* Corresponding author

Major histocompatibility complex (MHC) class I proteins present endogenous antigenic peptides to cytotoxic T lymphocytes (CTLs) [1], *via* transporter associated with antigen processing (TAP) [2], which are encoded by the TAP1 and TAP2 genes. Interestingly, tumor cells treated with recombinant IL-10 or transfected with the IL-10 gene showed phenotypical changes including: low but peptide inducible expression of MHC class I proteins; low sensitivity to specific CTLs mediated lysis and increased natural killer (NK) cell mediated lysis. Here in we found an IL-10 associated decrease in TAP function which might explain these effects. This is the first example to demonstrate that a cytokine could decrease the function of the TAP1/2 molecular complex. In more general terms it is the first example of a cytokine with a suppressive effect on the MHC class I antigen presentation pathway.

Results and discussion

Among several tested mouse tumor cell lines, the YAC-1 T-cell lymphoma constitutively express IL-10 message (by RT-PCR) and protein (by ELISA). This production was lost, however, following passage *in vivo* (YAC-1 asc) and was not regained in full until after at least three weeks of *in vitro* culture. YAC-1 cells IL-10 production levels varied inversely with surface H-2 expression and correlated directly with NK sensitivity [5] (*Table I*).

Since impaired TAP 1/2 expression was previously associated with decreased cell surface MHC class I levels [1],we employed the functional assay described by Neefjes *et al.* [6], to investigate possible association between IL-10 production and TAP activity. The mouse T lymphoma RMA, which normaly does not produce IL-10, was transfected with an IL-10 expression construct. This transfectant had lower levels of surface class I H-2 proteins and lower TAP activity relative to transfectants containing vector alone. As previously observed, these alterations coincided with an increase in sensitivity to NK cell-mediated cytotoxicity. Normaly NK resistent P-815 mastocytoma cells became NK sensitive following IL-10 transfection (*Table I*). In addition, YAC-1 cells maintained by passage *in vitro* were transfected with a retroviral vector encoding the mouse IL-10 gene in an anti-sense orientation. YAC-1 anti-sense transfectants were less sensitive to NK cell-mediated lysis and regained H-2 expression analogous to *in vivo* passaged cells (data not shown).

IL-10 gene expression has been detected in several tumor cell types [7], whereas TAP1/2 is often down regulated or lost in several tumor systems and in immunodeficient individuals [1,8,9]. These are correlates with tumor progression ([10] and references therein).We hope to have shed some light upon the mechanisms underlying these observations.

Acknowledgement
We are greatful for the critical reading of this report by Dr Ken Wasserman.

References

1. Heemels MT, Ploegh H. Generation, translocation, and presentation of MHC class I-restricted peptides. *Ann Rev Biochem* 1995; 64:463-91
2. Townsend A, Trowsdale J. The transporters associated with antigen presentation. *Semin Cell Biol* 1993; 4: 53-61.

Table I. Correlation between IL-10 production, TAP activity, H-2 expression and sensitivity to lysis by specific CD8+ T cells or NK cells

Cell line	IL-10 production*	TAP activity#	H-2 expression&	CTL sensitivity§	NK sensitivity§
YAC-1	45	38%	10%	-	47,37
YAC-1 2wk@	18	80%	52%	-	25,18
YAC-1 asc	0	100%	100%	-	14,9
RMA-neo	0	100%	100%	35,25	10,7
RMA-10	38	40%	40%	17,14	40,27
P815-neo	0	nd	100%	-	5,1
P815-10	27	nd	20%	-	19,16

@. two weeks *in vitro* cultured YAC-1 asc.

*. Unit /ml, determined by ELISA.

#, &. Expressed as relative values of maximum peptide translocation and H-2 expression (determined by FACS analysis) in the corresponding cell line where YAC-1 asc, RMA-neo and P815-neo are considered as reference lines for the corresponding derived cell lines (YAC-1, YAC-1 2wk, RMA-10 and P815-10 respectively) .

§. Percent of ^{51}Cr release at an effector: target ratio 50:1 and 25:1.

3. Matsuda M, Salazar F, Petersson M, Masucci G, Hansson J, Pisa P, Zhang QJ, Masucci MG, Kiessling R. Interleukin 10 pretreatment protects target cells from tumor- and allo-specific cytotoxic T cells and downregulates HLA class I expression. *J Exp Med* 1994; 180: 2371-6.
4. Salazar-Onfray F, Petersson M, Franksson L, Matsuda M, Blankenstein T, Karre K, Kiessling R. IL-10 converts mouse lymphoma cells to a CTL-resistant, NK-sensitive phenotype with low but peptide-inducible MHC class I expression. *J Immunol* 1995; 154: 6291-8.
5. Piontek GE, Taniguchi K, Ljunggren HG, Gronberg A, Kiessling R, Klein G, Karre K. YAC-1 MHC class I variants reveal an association between decreased NK sensitivity and increased H-2 expression after interferon treatment or *in vivo* passage. *J Immunol* 1985; 135: 4281-8.
6. Neefjes JJ, Momburg F, Hammerling GJ. Selective and ATP-dependent translocation of peptides by the MHC-encoded transporter. *Science* 1993; 261: 769-71.
7. Pisa P, Halapi E, Pisa EK, Gerdin E, Hising C, Bucht A, Gerdin B, Kiessling R. Selective expression of interleukin 10, interferon gamma, and granulocyte-macrophage colony-stimulating factor in ovarian cancer biopsies. *Proc Natl Acad Sci USA* 1992; 89: 7708-12.
8. De la Salle H,Hanau D, Fricker D, Urlacher A, Kelly A, Salamero J, Powis SH, Donato L, Bausinger H, Laforet M, Jeras M, Daniele S, Thomas B, Falkenrodt A, Cazenave JP, Trowsdale J, Tongio MM. Homozygous human TAP peptide transporter mutation in HLA class I deficiency. *Science* 1994; 265: 237-41.
9. Restifo NP, Esquivel F, Kawakami Y, Yewdell JW, Mule JJ, Rosenberg SA, Bennink JR. Identification of human cancers deficient in antigen processing. *J Exp Med* 1993;177: 265-72.
10. Seliger B, Hohne A, Knuth A, Bernhard H, Meyer T, Tampe R, Momburg F, Huber C. Analysis of the major histocompatibility complex class I antigen presentation machinery in normal and malignant renal cells: evidence for deficiencies associated with transformation and progression. *Cancer Res* 1995; 6: 1756-60.

Polymorphism in class II MHC dictates cytokine profile and clinical disease in mycobacterial infectious diseases

N.K. Mehra, D.K. Mitra, R. Rajalingam

Department of Histocompatibility and Immunogenetics, All India Institute of Medical Sciences, Ansari Nagar, New Delhi-110 029, India

The class II major histocompatibility complex (MHC) molecules are cell-surface glycoproteins that bind peptide fragments of foreign and self proteins and present these bound peptides to T lymphocytes. Polymorphism in these molecules determines the specificity of immune response and has been correlated with several diseases at the population level. We have earlier demonstrated an HLA-linked control of susceptibility to leprosy and pulmonary tuberculosis, the associated allele being HLA-DR2 (reviewed in [1]). Using the molecular techniques of PCR-SSOP hybridization, this association has now been confirmed in lepromatous leprosy (LL) and drug resistant pulmonary tuberculosis (PTB) [2,3]. The data is represented in *Figure 1*. On the other hand, HLA-DR2 did not show a significant deviation in patients with tuberculoid leprosy (TL) and drug responsive PTB. Molecular subtyping revealed that more than 97% of DR2+ves among patients and controls were either DRB1*1501 or *1502 suggesting that the presence of relevant epitope(s) on the DRB1*15 sequence may be important for lepromatous leprosy/drug failure PTB susceptibility. It implies that the single amino acid difference in DRB1*1501 and DRB1*1502 (Valine → Glycine) at codon 86 does not play a major role in influencing susceptibility to mycobacterial diseases. In a recent study done by our group in collaboration with the University of Pennsylvania (USA), a positive association of tuberculoid leprosy has been reported with HLA-DRB1 alleles (predominantly DRB1*1501 and *1502) that contain Arg [13] or Arg [70]-Arg [71] in the DRB1 first domain [4]. From the above, one can postulate that specific epitopes on the DRB1*15 molecule or cohesive epitopes on other non-DR15 molecules may be involved in preferential binding of pathogenic mycobacterial peptides (derived from either *M. tuberculosis* or *M. leprae*) leading to the stimulation of particular T cell clones that result in a detrimental immune response causing severe form of clinical disease.

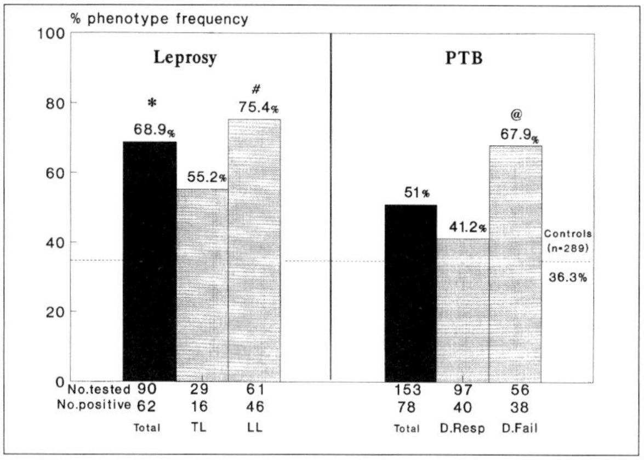

Figure 1. Association of HLA-DR2 with leprosy, pulmonary tuberculosis (PTB) and their clinical sub-groups like tuberculoid leprosy (TL), lepromatous leprosy (LL), drug responsive PTB (D.Resp) and drug failure PTB (D.Fail). Corrected probability (Pc) values: *<0.000002, Relative risk (RR)=3.9; #<0.0000006, RR=5.4; @<0.0003, RR=3.7). Control frequencies of HLA-DR2 are indicated by dotted lines.

Indeed, a corollary can be drawn between the drug resistant PTB and lepromatous leprosy. Both diseases appear to be immunologically similar with respect to the production of parasite-specific antibody, depressed cell mediated immunity, chronic presence of the parasite and ultimately chronic illness [5,6]. Observations on the increased occurrence of DR15 in both of them can be correlated with the type of immune response seen in them. Recently, different cytokine pattern (TH1 or TH2) was shown to be produced by CD4+ T cells responding to the same antigen in mice of different MHC genotypes [7].

Similar data has been obtained from our recent studies on the CD4+ T cell responses and HLA-DR restriction pattern in leprosy against *M. leprae* heat shock proteins,

HSP65, HSP18 and their trypsin digested fragments [8]. While all tryptic fragments of optimal digestion (TDB65-1,24kDa; TDB65-2, 18kDa; TDB65-3, 17kDa; TDB65-4, 14kDa and TDB18-1, 10kDa; TDB18-2, 5kDa; TDB18-3, 3kDa) and undigested HSPs (HSP65, HSP18) could stimulate CD4+ T cells from TL patients and healthy contacts, only two fragments, TDB65-2 (18kDa) and TDB18-3 (3kDa) triggered CD4+ T cells of anergic LL patients. Further, the cytokine release profile and MHC restriction have been studied in *M. leprae* HSPs primed CD4+ T cell cultures of polar leprosy patients to identify the relevant peptide responsible for the diversity in immune reaction elicited against the mycobacteria. HSP65 and HSP18 induced TH2 like activity when presented in the context of HLA-DR1 and DR7 respectively *(Table I)*. These proteins were restricted by multiple HLA class II determinants with HLA-DR15 providing the strongest restriction. However, when restricted by HLA-DR15 and other alleles like DR5 and DR8, TH1 like cytokine profile was obtained as determined by the release of IL-2 and IFN-γ. Further, 18kDa subunit of HSP65(TDB65-2) and 3kDa of HSP18(TDB18-3) induced only TH1 activity both TL as well as LL patients in the context of many DR alleles, DR15 being the main restriction element. Further details on this study have been published elsewhere [9]. The study provides direct evidence in the human system of the involvement of MHC class II phenotypes in governing the functional outcome of an immune response and ultimate disease phenotype in mycobacterial infectious diseases. Further, the induction of TH1 like activity in LL patients is indeed very important particularly in the light of the fact that such patients fail to recognize *M. leprae* antigens in general. The data is relevant for planning immune intervention therapy in leprosy.

Table I. Cytokine profile of CD4+T cells against *M. leprae* derived HSP65, HSP18 and their immunodominant tryptic fragments in patients with leprosy

M.leprae HSPs	Antigen Presenting HLA	Patients Category	Cytokine Response
HSP65*,	DR15,5,7	TL	TH1
TDB65-1,-3*,	DR1	TL	TH2
TDB65-2	DR15,5,7,4	TL,LL	TH1
HSP18*,	DR15,8	TL	TH1
TDB18-1*	DR7	TL	TH2
TDB18-3	DR15,1,5,8	TL,LL	TH1

* No CD4+ cell response observed in LL patients.
TH1 is ↑IL-2, ↑INF-γ, ↓IL-4 with INF-γ/IL-4 is >0.1.
TH2 is ↓IL-2, ↓INF-γ, ↑IL-4 with INF-γ/IL-4 is <0.1.

References

1 Mehra NK. Role of HLA linked factors in governing susceptibility to leprosy and tuberculosis. *Trop Med Parasitol* 1990; 41: 352-3.
2. Mehra NK, Rajalingam R, Mitra DK, Taneja V, Giphart MJ. Variants of HLA-DR2/DR51 group haplotypes and susceptibility to tuberculoid leprosy and pulmonary tuberculosis in Asian Indians. *Int J Lep* 1995; 63: 241-8.
3. Rajalingam R, Mehra NK, Jain RC, Myneedu VP, Pande JN. Polymerase chain reaction based sequence specific oligonucleotide hybridization analysis of HLA class II antigens in pulmonary tuberculosis: relevance to chemotherapy and disease activity. *J Infect Dis* 1996; 173: 669-73.
4. Zerva L, Cizman B, Mehra NK, Alahari SK, Murali R, Zmijewski CM, Kamoun M, Monos DS. Arginine at positions 13 or 70-71 in pocket 4 of HLA DRB1 alleles is associated with susceptibility to tuberculoid leprosy. *J Exp Med* 1996; 183: 829-36.
5. Ridley DS, Jopling WH. Classification of leprosy according to immunity: a five group system. *Int J Lepr* 1966; 34: 255-73.
6. Lenzini L, Rottoli P, Rottoli L. The spectrum of human tuberculosis. *Clin Exp Immunol* 1977; 27: 230-7.
7. Murray JS, Madri J, Tite J, Carding SR, Bottomly K. MHC control of CD4+ T cell subset activation. *J Exp Med* 1989; 170: 2135-40.
8. Mitra DK, Mehra NK, Maiti TK, Banerjee A, Taneja V, Rajalingam R, Ahuja RK, Bhattacharya BC. CD4+ T cell responses to recombinant HSP65, HSP18 of *M.leprae* and their trypsin digested fragments: diversity in HLA-DR restriction. *Int J Lep* 1995; 63: 518-28.
9. Mitra DK, Rajalingam R, Taneja V, Bhattacharya BC, Mehra NK. HLA-DR2 polymorphism modu lates the cytokine profile of *M. leprae* HSP reactive CD4+ T cells. *Clin Immunol Immunolpathol* 1997 (in press).

Effect of substance P and different cytokines on antigen presenting function of synoviocytes in RA

N.C. Lambert, B. Yassine Diab, P. Loubet-Lescoulié, B. Mazières, H. Coppin, A. Cantagrel

INSERM U395, Rheumatology Unit, CHU Purpan, BP 3028,31024 Toulouse Cedex, France

Inflammation of the synovial membrane in rheumatoid arthritis (RA) leads to a change in phenotype of fibroblastic synoviocytes. Thus, cytokine-rich microenvironment stimulates them to secrete proteolytic enzymes implicated in degradation of cartilage and to take an invasive or transformed phenotype [1]. Synoviocytes are themselves a major source of several inflammatory cytokines, which are believed to play a crucial role in migration and maturation of immune cells in the synovial tissue. Moreover, fibroblastic synoviocytes are sensitive to the neuropeptide substance P (SP), present at high level in the RA joint during the flare up of the disease. This sensory neuropeptide also increases their proteolytic enzyme secretion, enhances the action of IL1β on prostaglandin production and has an effect on synoviocyte proliferation [2]. This inflammatory microenvironment is also responsible for the expression of MHC class II molecules, and for the enhancement of adhesion molecules on the cell surface [3]. These observations led some authors to investigate whether this increase in expression had functional consequences for antigen presentation to T cells [4]. This work demonstrated the necessity of IFNγ induction to the MHC class II expression and suggested the important part of adhesion molecules in such functions.

To further investigate the role of synoviocytes on T cell activation, we first studied the effect of IFNγ, TNFα, IL1β and SP on the expression of several surface molecules : DR, ICAM-1, LFA-3, VCAM-1, B7.1 and B7.2. Secondly, we analysed the role of these cytokine-induced-molecules on antigen presenting function of synoviocytes in a peptide specific stimulation system.

Results and discussion

Effect of SP and cytokines on surface molecule expression

Flow cytometric analysis, performed by a two-step surface staining with the appropriate MoAbs and FITC-conjugated goat anti-mouse Ig (Immunotech S.A.), showed that rheumatoid synovial fibroblasts constitutively expressed ICAM-1 and LFA-3. Contrary to LFA-3, ICAM-1 was enhanced by IFNγ (100U/ml), TNFα (100ng/ml) and IL1β (10ng/ml) in this order of efficiency. Only IFNγ was able to induce MHC class II molecules. The costimulatory molecules B7.1 and B7.2 were never expressed on resting or cytokine -treated synoviocytes. Immunohistochemistry and a three stages immuno peroxydase technique indicated that resting synoviocytes expressed VCAM-1 and the three cytokines had an effect on this expression. By using the last method, we checked whether SP potentializes the effect of proinflammatory cytokines on the expression of ICAM-1 and VCAM-1 on RA fibroblastic synoviocytes. Synoviocytes were incubated 0, 6, 12 or 18 hours with TNFα or IL1β with or without SP. The expression of ICAM-1 and VCAM-1 was tested with monoclonal antibodies against these surface molecules or with a mouse monoclonal IgG1 as control and amplified with a biotinylated rabbit anti-mouse immunoglobulins and subsequently with streptavidin / biotinylated horseradish peroxidase complex.

Our results indicated that IL1β and TNFα had an effect on ICAM-1 and VCAM-1 molecule expression and this was observed as early as six hours of treatment. SP alone did not modify the expression of ICAM-1 molecules but at six hours induced expression of VCAM-1. Morever, SP significantly potentialized the action of TNFα and IL1β on the expression of VCAM-1 from the sixth to the eighteenth hour.

Recognition of MHC/Antigen complex alone is insufficient to fully activate most T cells. Induction of MHC class II by IFNγ on synoviocytes placed them in a potential antigen presenting role. Therefore, the presence of the adhesion molecules LFA-3, ICAM-1, VCAM-1, which facilitate physical interaction between APC and T cell, reinforced this role. Nevertheless, the lack of the costimulatory molecules B7.1 and B7.2 could hamper their function in activation of T cells, so, we tested the capacity of synoviocytes to induce T cell proliferation.

Assay of proliferative responses

Peripheral blood mononuclear cells (PBMC) derived from RA patients were stimulated with the peptide HA (306-318) derived from the influenza hemagglutinin (2 μg /ml). Seven days after antigenic stimulation, cells were fed with autologous irradiated PBMC and 20 U recombinant IL-2 /ml. They were then tested for their CD3 and CD4 expression prior to use in the T-cell proliferative assay. Proliferative T cell response was dependent of HA concentration and specific of the patient HLA typage.

Synoviocytes pretreated or not with cytokines were studied in an autologous system of co-culture with this peptide-specific T cell line. Our results showed that IFNγ treatment permitted synovial fibroblasts to serve as antigen presenting cells for the peptide specific T cell line. Without IFNγ treatment, TNFα, IL1β or SP did not correct the defect in antigen presenting cell function because of the incapacity of these three cytokines to induce MHC class II molecules (as described previously). So, the presence of MHC class II molecules on the synoviocyte surface was the *sine qua non* condition to a proliferative T cell response, but adhesion molecules such as ICAM-1 and VCAM-1 were not negligible. Their relative importance was demonstrated by the appropriate monoclonal antibodies during assays of proliferative responses. Addition of anti-DR inhibited T cell proliferation and that of anti-VCAM-1 or anti-ICAM-1 led to a partial reduction.

Finally, these results showed that synoviocytes can have an antigen presenting function and that this can be improved by cytokine-induced adhesion molecules.

Conclusion

This study allows us to understand the real implication of cytokines and the neuropeptide SP on surface molecule expression, and the consequences on the antigen presenting function of RA synoviocytes *in vitro*. This is also likely to occur *in vivo*, since substance P and the inflammatory cytokines are present at high levels in the synovial tissue. We already know how the milieu can have an effect on fibroblast function: Kundig *et al.* [5] have demonstrated that fibroblasts were efficient antigen presenting cells only in the cytokine-rich microenvironment of lymphoid organs. Thus, the synovial membrane could be seen as a privileged compartment where cytokines and the neuropeptide SP modify synoviocyte functions. Synoviocytes themselves are not common fibroblasts in that, contrary to dermal fibroblasts, they are able to express VCAM-1 molecules and to have costimulatory activity on resting T cells [6]. Our results showed that VCAM-1 played a crucial role by its SP-induced expression on synoviocytes and its costimulatory function in antigen presentation to T cells. This represents a pathway by which the nervous system might be directly involved in the inflammation of RA.

References

1. Lafiatis R, Thompson NL, Remmers EF, Flanders KC, Roche NS, Kim SJ, Case JP, Sporn MB, Roberts AB, Wilder RL. Transforming growth factor-beta production by synovial tissues from rheumatoid patients and streptococcal cell wall arthritic rats. Studies on secretion by synovial fibroblast-like cells and immunohistologic localization. *J Immunol* 1989; 143: 1142-8.
2. Lotz M, Carson DA, Vaughan JH. Substance P activation of rheumatoid synoviocytes: neural pathway in pathogenesis of arthritis. *Science* 1987; 235: 893-7.
3. Jia En Chin, Winterrowd GE, Krzesicki RF, Sanders ME. Role of cytokines in inflammatory synovitis. *Arthritis Rheum* 1990; 33:1776-86.
4. Boots AMH, Wimmers-Bertens AJMM, Rijnders AWM. Antigen presenting capacity of rheumatoid synovial fibroblats. *J Immunol* 1994; 82: 268-274.
5. Kündig TM, Bachmann MF, DiPaolo C, Simard JJL, Battegay M, Lother H, Gessner A, Kûhlcke K, Ohashi PS, Hengartner RM. Fibroblasts as efficient antigen-presenting cells in lymphoid organs. *Science* 1995; 268: 1343-7.
6. Looney RJ, Hooper M, Pudiak D. Costimulatory activity of human synovial fibroblasts. *J Rheumatol* 1995; 22:1820-4.

Inhibition of the alloimmune response by synthetic peptides derived from highly conserved regions of class II MHC alpha chain

B. Murphy, A.M. Waaga, C.B. Carpenter, M.H. Sayegh

Laboratory of Immunogenetics and Transplantation, Brigham and Women's Hospital, Harvard Medical School, 75 Francis Street, Boston, MA 02115, USA

The T cell receptor recognition of and interaction with the MHC + peptide complex is central to T cell activation. Variation in the nature of the peptide bound within the groove of the MHC molecule may result in an altered T cell response *in vitro* [1]. Since naturally processed peptides bound to MHC molecules have been shown to be derived from endogenous proteins, including the MHC molecules themselves, it has been suggested that they may play an immunoregulatory role [2]. Synthetic peptides representing non-polymorphic regions of class I MHC have been shown to inhibit cytotoxic T lymphocyte and NK function *in vitro*, and to prolong skin and cardiac allografts in several rodent models *in vivo*, either alone or in combination with low dose cyclosporine [3]. We have investigated the immunomodulating effects of synthetic class II MHC peptides on the alloimmune response. We initially synthesized two 25mer peptides derived from the non-polymorphic RT1.D (DR-like) alpha chain of the rat class II MHC molecule (peptide 1-residues 26-50, and peptide 2-residues 51-75). We found that peptide 2 inhibited the LEWxWF rat MLR and CTL generation in a dose response fashion [3]. Further experimentation indicated that the active peptide is a 15mer and corresponds to residues 61-75. In this study we compare the immunomodulatory capabilities of this 15mer peptide RT1.Dα (61-75) with those of 3 further peptides we synthesized, 2 derived from human class II MHC: HLA-DQα and HLA-DQβ, and 1 derived from rat: RT1.Bα (DQ-like). All 3 alpha chain peptides are derived from a region highly conserved across alleles and species. We found that these three peptides inhibited the rat LEWxWF MLR in a dose response fashion, while HLA-DQβ peptide did not. Both HLA-DQα peptide and RT1.Bα peptide resulted in 100% inhibition at a dose of 10 μg/ml; however, 250 μg/ml RT1.Dα peptide was required to produce a similar degree of inhibition. The inhibitory effect of the three peptides was independent of responder and stimulator haplotye. HLA-DQα peptide was a potent inhibitor of the human MLR with 100% inhibition at 100 μg/ml, while RT1.Bα peptide, which was an effective inhibitor of the rat MLR, only produced 42.6±10% inhibition of the human MLR at 100 μg/ml. The inhibitory effect of HLA-DQα peptide was not allele specific. Since HLA-DQα peptide inhibited both the rat and human MLRs we further studied the immunomodulatory function of this peptide, and compared it to the non-inhibitory peptide HLA-DQβ as control. We found that HLA-DQα peptide also inhibited the mouse MLR with 50% inhibition at 25 μg/ml and 100% inhibition at 100 μg/ml, further indicating that the inhibitory effect was not species specific. We examined the influence of both peptides on T cell mediated cytotoxicity. HLA-DQα, but not HLA-DQß, inhibited cytotoxic T cell generation (LEWxWF) in a dose response fashion. Neither peptide affected preformed effector cytotoxic T cells, indicating that the inhibitory effect of HLA-DQα is targeted at CD4+ T helper function. Mitogen induced T cell proliferation of human lymphocytes (PHA) was not inhibited by either HLA-DQα or HLA-DQβ peptide. When LEW lymphocytes were stimulated with mitogen (ConA) in the presence of HLA-DQα there was no significant inhibition of the proliferative response at 10 μg/ml, the dose which resulted in 100% inhibiton of the rat MLR. By increasing the dose of HLA-DQα ten fold only 62.3±1.7% suppression was achieved. Thus the inhibitory effect of HLA-DQα is neither toxic nor non-specific. We next examined the effect of HLA-DQα on cytokine production in the human. Supernatants were taken from human MLRs alone or following incubation with either HLA-DQα or

HLA-DQβ peptide. Time course and dose response studies were performed. We found that HLA-DQα at a dose of 100 μg/ml inhibited both IL2 and IFN-γ production throughout the 7 day study period, and this inhibitory effect was dose dependent. HLA-DQβ had no inhibitory effect on cytokine production. These data demonstrate that synthetic class II MHC peptides can alter T cell recognition of allo-MHC and inhibit the alloimmune response *in vitro*. The precise mechanism of action of these peptides, specifically the binding sites as well as the molecular mechanisms of their immunomodulatory action, are unknown at present, and is the subject of further investigation.

References

1. Eckels DD, Gorski J, Rothbard J, Lamb JR. Peptide mediated modulation of T cell allorecognition. *Proc Natl Acad Sci USA* 1988; 85: 8191-5.
2. Chicz RM, Urban RG, Gorga JC, Vignali AA, Lane WS, Strominger JL. Specificity and promiscuity among naturally processed peptides bound to HLA-DR alleles. *J Exp Med* 1993; 178: 27-47.
3. Murphy B, Sayegh MH. Immunomodulatory function of major histocompatibility derived peptides. *Curr Op Nephrol Hyper* 1996; 5: 262-8.

Antigen-specific T cell recognition of soluble divalent major histocompatibility analogs

S.M. O'Herrin, N.C. Barnes, J. Schneck

Johns Hopkins University School of Medicine, Department of Pathology, Ross Building, 664G, 720 Rutland Avenue, Baltimore, MD 21205, USA

Tracking and regulation of antigen-specific T cells are of critical importance in selective immunomodulation. Therefore, it would be useful to design reagents that are selective in a clonotypic fashion for T cells and that bind with sufficient affinity to: (1) allow the tracking of these T cells during an immune response and (2) effect their modulation. To this end, we made use of the natural specificity of peptide/major histocompatibility complexes (MHC) for their cognate ligands. To make these complexes soluble and increase their affinity for TCR, we constructed MHC/Ig chimeras. MHC/Ig chimeras were made soluble by virtue of secretion of Ig protein of the molecule and had increased affinity secondary to the divalent nature of the Ig chimeras. This was accomplished by ligating DNA encoding H-2K^b heavy chain to DNA coding for murine IgG1 heavy chain [1]. To study the interaction of soluble H-2K^b/Ig in antigen-specific, H-2K^b-restricted T cell responses, H-2K^b/Ig molecules were loaded with K^b-restricted peptide hen egg ovalbumin-derived peptide (ova; residues 257-264, SIINFEKL). These complexes, ^{ova}K^b/Ig, were immobilized on cells expressing cell surface anti-β_2m monoclonal antibody BBM.1 and incubated with the H-2K^b-restricted, anti-ova-specific T-cell clone, GA4. The results show that GA4 cells lyse BBM.1 cells incubated with ^{ova}K^b/Ig but not BBM.1 cells incubated with ^{vsv}K^b/Ig, K^b/Ig loaded with a control H-2 K^b-binding peptide derived from vesicular stomatatis nuclear protein (vsv; residues 52-59, RGYVYQGL). The ability of T cells to specifically interact with peptide loaded K^b/Ig indicates that these chimeric molecules may be useful for tracking and modulating antigen-specific immune responses.

This work was supported by grants from the National Institutes of Health (RO1 AI-29575) and the American Cancer Soceity (IM-736).

Results and discussion

Peptide loading of H-2K^b/Ig

To study the interaction of K^b/Ig with antigen-specific T cell clones, H-2K^b/Ig first had to be loaded with known H-2 K^b-binding peptides. Two parameters are important to assess the efficacy of peptide loading protocols: (1) the efficacy of stripping endogenous peptides resident in the K^b/Ig binding pocket; and (2) the proficiency of reloading peptides into "empty" K^b/Ig. These parameters can be assessed using mAb 20.8.4S [2], an H-2 K^b-specific mAb that recognizes a conformational, peptide-dependent determinant epitope on H-2K^b [3]. Using an ELISA assay based on recognition of K^b/Ig by both

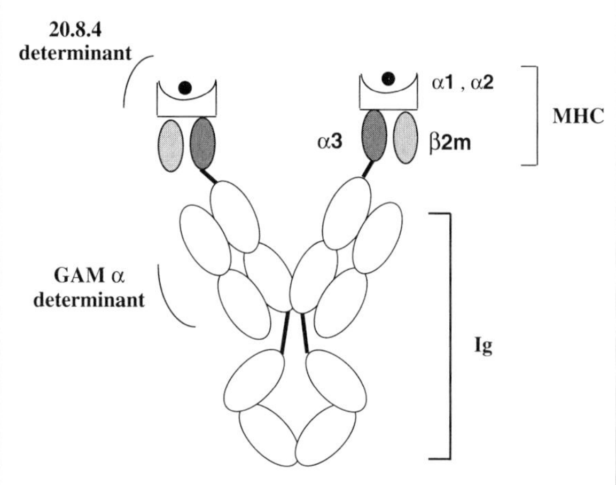

Figure 1. Hypothetical structure of H-2K^b/IgG molecule showing the determinants recognized by the antibodies used in ELISA's. The determinant recognized by mAb 20.8.4S is a conformationally-dependent one on the α-1 domain of H-2K^b [2,3]. The Ig λ determinant is recognized by the GAMλ-chain-specific polyclonal Ab. Construction and characterization of the H-2K^b/Ig chimera has been previously reported [1].

mAb 20.8.4S and goat-anti-mouse-λ (GAMλ), we could determine the amount of peptide loaded chimeric K^b/Ig molecules *(Figure 1)*.

A number of conditions were tested to assess the efficacy of stripping peptide from K^b/Ig and the receptivity of the "empty" K^b/Ig molecules for peptide loading. An acidic citrate phosphate buffer (pH 3.0) or a basic Tris buffer (pH 12.0) with 1M urea, while effectively stripping endogenous peptide, yielded recoveries of only 3-4% upon the addition of peptide (data not shown). The greatest recovery of K^b/Ig activity was obtained when K^b/Ig was incubated for 3-5 min at 25°C in a basic carbonate buffer (pH 11.5) followed by several washes with PBS (pH 7.4) in the presence of added peptide and an 18h or greater incubation at 4°C in the presence of peptide *(Figure 2)*. Using this protocol the stripping of endogenous peptide was about 90% effective as indicated by the amount of K^b/Ig recovered, approximately 10% when no peptide was added *(Figure 3)*. Yields of refolded peptide K^b/Ig were 75% of the initial amount of K^b/Ig when done in the presence of either the vsv or ova K^b-binding peptides *(Figure 3)*. The dependence of refolding on the addition of peptide was demonstrated when longer incubation of the stripped material in the absence of peptide did not increase yields (data not shown). These data demonstrate the usefulness of this protocol for obtaining preparations of K^b/Ig enriched for a population of molecules that contain a specific peptide in their antigenic-peptide binding pocket.

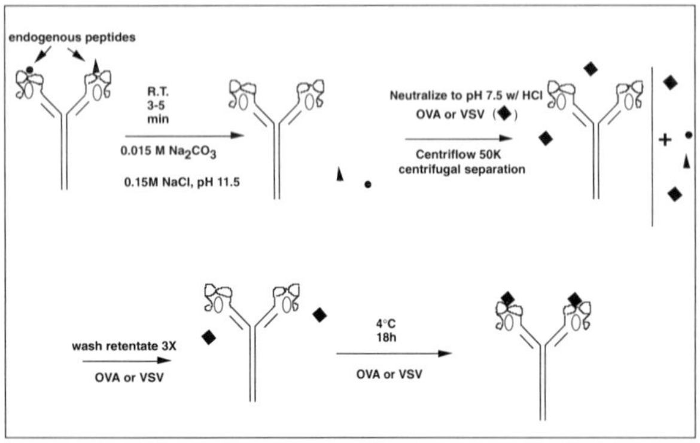

Figure 2. Denaturation and loading scheme for H-2Kb/Ig. K^b/Ig was diluted to 0.5 mg/ml before denaturation to reduce the potential for aggregate formation. Peptides were added (40 fold molar excess with respect to K^b molecules) immediately upon neutralization. Four centrifugal separation washes followed wherein 6 ml PBS was reduced to 1 ml during each wash. Peptide was added for each wash step. Final volumes were adjusted to give an estimated 0.5 mg/ml concentration.

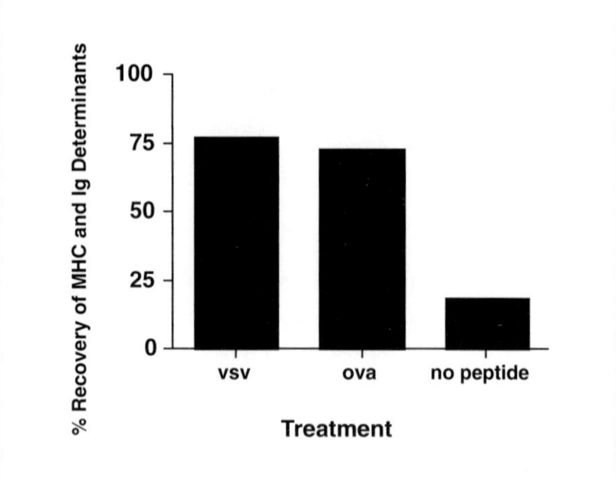

Figure 3. Stripping of endogenous peptide and loading with defined peptide are each efficient processes as indicated by high recoveries of specific determinants seen in ELISA's. The determinants which were assayed require both proper folding (20.8.4) and that H-$2K^b$ is covalently linked to Ig by the use of GAM λ. Plates were coated with 20.8.4 (10 μg/ml in carbonate buffer, pH 10.4). Blocking was performed in the same buffer with 1% fetal bovine serum for 1 hour. After the plates were washed three times [PBS/tween 20 (0.05%) fetal bovine serum (1%)], antigen was added and allowed to bind for 1h. After 3 washes, a GAMλ horseradish peroxidase conjugate (Sigma, St. Louis, Mo.) was added and the plates incubated for 30-40 minutes. Samples were developed using peroxide and TMB(3,3' 5,5'-tetramethlybenzidine dihydrocholride; Cappel, Durham, NC). All incubations were performed at 25°C. The results shown are the average of three independent experiments and are representative of several experiments.

Biological activity of peptide-loaded Kb/Ig

To assay the biological activity of peptide-loaded K^b/Ig, we analyzed the ability of antigen-specific T cells to recognize these complexes bound on the surface of target cells. The cell line BBM.1 expresses on its cell surface a mAb directed against human β_2m [4], the β_2m associated with K^b/Ig [1]. Thus, through the cell surface anti-β_2m mAb, the BBM.1 cells will bind K^b/Ig regardless of the peptide in the H-2 K^b antigenic-peptide binding groove. It is also likely that recognition of

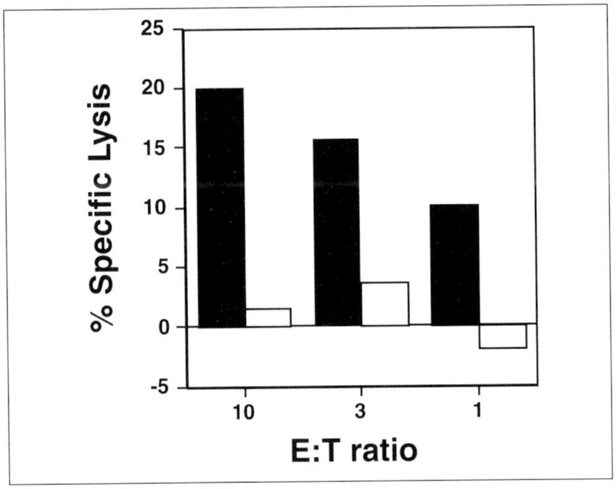

Figure 4. K^b/Ig binding an ova peptide directs antigen-specific killing of target cells by the ova- specific CTL, GA4. Targets (1 x 10^6 in 50 µl) were loaded with 100 µCi ^{51}Cr at 37°C for 1h. After three washes, cells were recounted and diluted to 5 X 10^4/ ml. Either $^{ova}K^b$/Ig or $^{vsv}K^b$/Ig (0.67 µmolar) were incubated with targets for 1h at 25°C. CTL assays were initiated by adding 100 µl of targets (5 x 10^3/well; see legend to *Figure 4*) to 100 µl of effectors at the ratios indicated. Plates were incubated at 37°C for 4h and harvested for counting on a gamma counter. Percent specific lysis was calculated according to [(experimental cpm - spontaneous cpm) /(maximum release cpm - spontaneous cpm)] x 100.

the determinant on β_2m will not interfere with the T-cell recognition of K^b/Ig due to its distance from the TCR interface.

A standard CTL assay was performed on BBM.1 target cells pulsed with peptide-loaded K^b/Ig. Cells pulsed with $^{ova}K^b$/Ig were recognized by the ova-specific, H-2 K^b-restricted CTL, GA4, while those pulsed with $^{vsv}K^b$/Ig were not *(Figure 4)*. Therefore preparations of K^b/Ig enriched for K^b binding a specific peptide are able to direct CTL-mediated lysis in a peptide-specific fashion. These results indicate that CTL recognize peptide-loaded soluble divalent MHC molecules in an antigen specific manner. Using this approach peptide-loaded soluble divalent MHC preparations can be tested in other biological assays for their ability to track or modulate immune responses of clonotypic effector cells.

References

1. Dal Porto J, Johansen TE, Catapovic B, Parfitt DJ, Tuveson D, Ulrik G, Kozlowski S, Fearon D, Schneck JP. A soluble divalent class I major histocompatibility complex molecule inhibits alloreactive T cells at nanomolar concentrations. *Proc Natl Acad Sci USA* 1993; 90: 6671.
2. Ozato K, Sachs DH. Monclonal antibodies to mouse MHC antigens. III. Hybridoma antibodies reacting to antigens of the H-2^b haplotype reveal genetic control of isotype expression. *J Immunol* 1981; 126: 317.
3. Catipovic BC, Dal Porto J, Mage M, Johansen TE, Schneck JP. Major histocompatibilty complex conformational epitopes are peptide specific. *J Exp Med* 1992; 176: 1611.
4. Brodsky FM, Bodmer WF, Parham P. Characterization of a monoclonal anti-ß2m antibody and its use in the genetic and biochemical analysis of major histocomapatibility antigens. *Eur J Immunol* 1979; 9: 536.

Mature neurons block induction of HLA class II by interferon-gamma and down regulate constitutive HLA class I in astrocytes

J. Boucraut, R. Steinschneider, H. Neumann, P. Delmas, M. Gola, H. Wekerle, D. Bernard

Laboratoire d'Immunopathologie, Faculté de Médecine La Timone, 26, boulevard Jean Moulin, 13385 Marseille Cedex 05, France

Astrocytes could play immunologic functions, by secreting cytokines [1] and by presenting peptides to CD8 and CD4 lymphocytes [2]. Indeed, *in vitro*, human astrocytes constitutively express HLA class I molecules and variable level of class II molecules [2]. In the presence of IFN-γ, astrocytes in culture express high levels of both class I and II molecules.

In vivo, immunohistochemistry of normal brain fails to detect any HLA class I or II expression in neural cells including astrocytes [3]. During CNS inflammatory diseases, HLA class I molecules are detected in astrocytes but HLA class II are not or seldom present in astrocytes [4]. These results suggested that, *in vivo*, astrocytes are under negative influence for expression of MHC molecules.

In order to understand the mechanisms that might be involved for the control of HLA expression in astrocytes in the brain, we established a coculture model with human astrocytes and rat embryonic neurons. We characterized this model by the following of the neuronal differentiation. We analyzed then the expression of HLA class II and class I molecules. We observed that mature neurons down regulates IFN-γ induced HLA class II expression and constitutive expression of MHC class I antigen.

Material and methods

Human astrocyte embryonic cultures

Human astrocyte embryonic cultures were performed as described by Aloisi [2] from 7-9 week-old human embryos, obtained from legal curettage abortions. Briefly, after removal of meninges, trypsinization and gentle mechanical disruption, we obtained a single cell suspension. Glial cell progenitors differentiated after 3 passages in type 1 astrocytes in MEM- D-valine (GIBCO) supplemented with 10% fetal calf serum. Neurons were obtained from 14-day-old (E-14) fetal Wistar rats cortex. Briefly, the cortices were dissociated after trypsinization at 37°C in presence of 0.1% DNAse. Neurons were almost pure and were cultured in serum-free media which limit glial cells proliferation. Under these conditions, cortical neurons rarely survived for more than 5 days and could not achieve synaptogenesis. After treatment with trypsin-EDTA, human astrocytes were harvested, washed twice in PBS, and in two-day-old neuron-cell cultures. Adding type 1 astrocytes (rat or human) to the culture permitted the seeding cortical neurons to survive over 3 weeks and promoted neuron maturation [5]. The maturation of the neurons was evaluated using the classical electrophysiological parameters : resting membrane potential, input resistance, excitability and synaptic activity [6]. In parallel, the cultures dishes were fixed in cold ethanol-acetic acid solution (95/5), and analysed, by immunocytofluoresence using a Cy3-labelled goat anti-mouse antiserum, for the expression of a neuronal differentiation marker MN2E4, which is a monoclonal antibody raised against a dephosphorylated heavy neurofilament (NF).

HLA class I and II expression

HLA class I and II expression was analyzed by FACS in astrocytes at different times of coculture with biotin-labelled anti-HLA class II or I monoclonal antibodies (IOT2a and IOT2, Immunotech, Marseilles, France) diluted at 10μg/ml in washing buffer (3 % FCS and 0.1% sodium azide in PBS). Human cells were specifically identified with a double staining procedure by adding a FITC-labeled mouse monoclonal antibody specific for a human membrane antigen (20C4, IgG2a, product in our laboratory) at 5μg/ml . It allowed us to discard the rat contaminant glial population which increased during coculture. The expression of HLA by astrocytes in coculture was compared with the expression by astrocytes alone cultured in the same medium.

Results

Characterization of the coculture model

After two days of rat neurons culture, human type 1 astrocytes were added in a 1/4 ratio (astrocytes/ neurons). They spreaded across the bottom of culture dishes under the neurons *(Figure 1, A)*. In these conditions, neurons survived for up to 3 weeks, as we observed with rat type 1 astrocytes [5].
MN2E4 labelling appears in the neuronal cell bodies at day 8 and in processes at day 9 *(Figure 1, B)*. In parallel electrophysiological whole cell recordings *(Figure 1,C)* were performed. All neurons were electrophysiologically silent up to day 4 of coculture and were therefore inexcitable. At day 6 of coculture, as the functional network formed, the number of neurons exhibiting spontaneous synaptic inputs increased. At day 8, almost all neurons (95%) were synaptically active. Later, the synaptic activity grew up in a more complex way. This mature pattern of activity did not change along the subsequent days. In conclusion, our coculture was divided in two periods : 0-6 "non active neurons" 6-later "active mature neurons".

Modulation of HLA expression in astrocytes cocultured with neurons

The human embryonic astrocyte population was cultured in serum-free medium and added to the neuron culture. Analysis for HLA expression was performed in parallel on the astrocytes alone or cocultured with rat neurons. IFN-γ (100 UI/ml) was added 48 days before each analysis. HLA class II expression was strongly positive in astrocytes at day 6 of coculture at a comparable level the astrocytes alone did *(Figure 2, a)*. IFN-γ enhanced strongly this expression *(Figure 2, b)*. Later, at day 10, when neurons are electrically active, HLA class II constitutive expression was only slightly reduced *(Figure 2, c)*. More significantly, IFN-γ inducibility was blocked at this period *(Figure 2, d)*. HLA class I analysis showed that IFN-γ inducibility was not affected at day 6 and day 10 *(Figure 3, a-d)*. Constitutive HLA class I expression was significantly reduced at day 10 compared to day 6 *(Figure 3, a, b)*. In conclusion, HLA class II IFN-γ but not HLA class I IFN-γ inducibility was negatively modulated in presence of active mature neurons. HLA class I spontaneous expression was reduced on astrocytes cocultured with electrically mature neurons.

Discussion

Our interspecies coculture is characterized by a well-timed neuronal maturation taking place in the first week, which is not possible with human embryonic neurons (not shown). Electrical activity and majority of neuromediators, potentially involved in our model, are common to human and rat neurons.The effect is specific for neurons. Indeed coculture with rat astrocytes did not

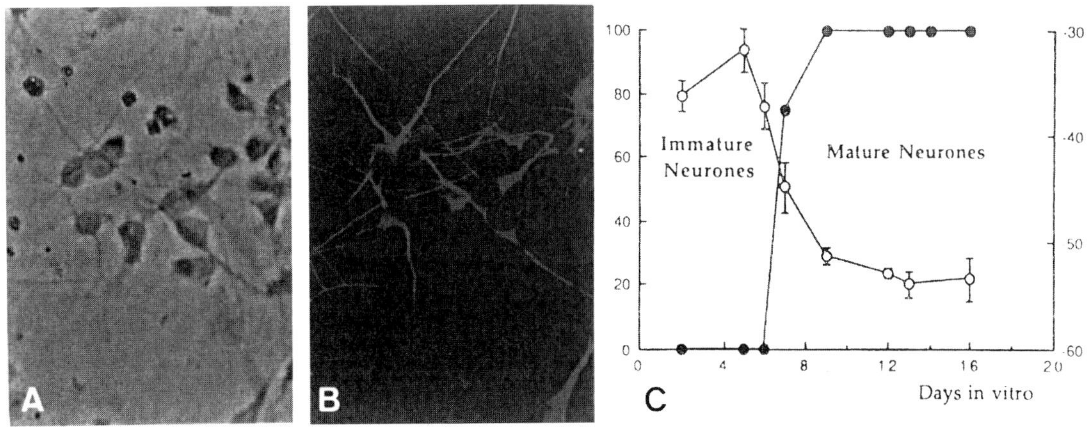

Figure 1. Phase contrast microphotograph of rat cortical neurons-human astrocytes coculture at day 9 (A). MN2E4 staining at day 9 of coculture (B). Time-related electrophysiological changes of cultured neurons (C) : open circles : resting potential (-30/-60 mV) black circles : number of excitable neurons (0-100 %).

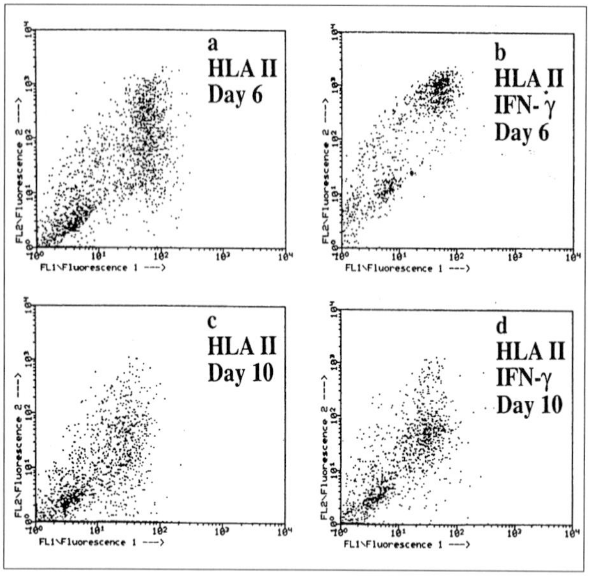

Figure 2. Double staining procedure: expression of the human membrane antigen (20C4) was measured on FL1 scale and HLA II expression on FL2 scale. Days of culture and presence of IFN-γ was noted in the dot representation.

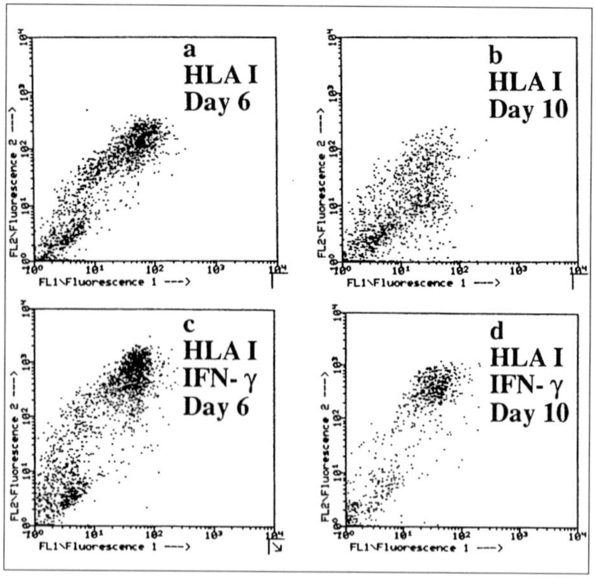

Figure 3. Double staining procedure: expression of the human membrane antigen (20C4) was measured on FL1 scale and HLA I expression on FL2 scale. Days of culture and presence of IFN-γ was noted in the dot representation.

reproduced the same effects and the down regulation effect on HLA class II IFN-γ inducibility disappeared when neurons degenerated (after 3 weeks).The mechanisms leading for this down regulation are still unknown. In our model, the down-regulation of the IFN-γ induction of HLA class II appears once the neurons were intensely electrically active and this effect was reversed in the presence of tetrodotoxin (not shown). It possibly involves the neuronal electrical activity by K+ release and subsequent depolarization of the glial cells as it is the case for GFAP expression [7]. Alternatively, active neurons may release substances. Astrocytes are closely associated with synapses and they express a wide repertoire of receptors to neuromediators [1]. Some neuromediators, glutamate [8], norepinephrin and VIP [9] are known to inhibit the induction of MHC class II expression on astrocytes by IFN-γ. As we found in our model, the induction by IFN-γ of MHC class I is not modified in presence of those neuromediators. The level of negative modulation on HLA class I constitutive expression varies from one experience to an other. It seems that those differences depend of the astrocyte differentiation state in culture. This modulation could be related to the neuron influence on glial maturation. Furthermore, Massa *et al.* have shown that gangliosides, which are highly expressed in neurons, reproduce similar effects on the constitutive HLA class I expression in astrocytes [10].

The coculture model described in this paper offers the possibility to compare astrocytes before and after the neuronal down regulation effect. It constitutes a useful tool for studying transduction and transcriptional regulation in target cells by separating human cells from rat cells using a specific human membrane marker.

References

1. Eddelston M, Mucke L. Molecular profile of reactive astrocytes: implications for their role in neurologic disease. *Neuroscience* 1993; 54: 15-36.
2. Aloisi F, Borsellino G, Samoggia P, Testa U, Chelucci C, Russo G, Peschle C, Levi G. Astrocyte cultures from human embryonic brain: characterization and modulation of surface molecules by inflammatory cytokines. *J Neurosci Res* 1992; 32: 494-506.

3. William KA, Hart DNJ, Fabre JW, Morris PJ. Distribution and quantitation of HLA ABC and DR(Ia) antigens on human kidney and others tissues. *Transplantation* 1980; 29: 274-9.
4. Bö L, Mörk S, Kong PA, Nyland H, Pardo CA, Trapp BD. Detection of MHC class II antigens on macrophages and microglia, but not on astrocytes and endothelia in active multiple sclerosis lesions. *J Neuroimmunol* 1994; 51: 135-46.
5. Steinshneider R, Delmas P, Nedelec J, Gola M, Bernard D, Boucraut J. Appearance of neurofilament subunit epitopes correlates with electrophysiological maturation in cortical embryonic neurons cocultured with mature astrocytes. *Dev Brain Res* 1997, in press.
6. Kowalski, C, Crest M, Vuillet J, Pin T, Gola M, Nieoullon A. Emergence of a synaptic neuronal network within primary striatal cultures seeded in serum-free medium. *Neuroscience* 1995; 6: 4979-93.
7. Canady KS Rubel EW. Rapid and reversible astrocytic reaction to afferent activity blockade in chick cochlear nucleus. *J Neurosci* 1992; 12: 1001-9.
8. Lee SC, Collins M, Vanguri P, Shin ML. Glutamate differentially inhibits the expression of class II MHC antigens on astrocytes and microglia. *J Immunol* 1992; 148: 3391-7.
9. Frohman EM, Frohman TC, Vayuvegula B, Gupta S, Van den Noort D. Vasoactive intestinal polypeptide inhibits the expression major of the MHC class II antigen on astrocytes. *J Neurol Sci* 1988; 88: 339-46.
10. Massa PT. Specific suppression of major histocompatibility complex class I and class II genes in astrocytes by brain-enriched gangliosides. *J Exp Med* 1993; 178: 1357-63

Amino acid residues in the α-helical portions of HLA-DR molecules can modulate T cell recognition of antigen

D.G. Doherty, D.M. Koelle, W.W. Kwok, S. Masewicz, M.E. Domeier, G.T. Nepom

Virginia Mason Research Center, 1000 Seneca Street, Seattle, WA 98101, USA, and University of Washington School of Medicine, Seattle, WA 98195, USA

The T cell antigen receptor (TCR) recognizes a complex composed of an antigenic peptide bound to a class I or class II major histocompatibility complex (MHC) molecule expressed on an antigen presenting cell (APC). Specific TCR engagement of a peptide-MHC complex can trigger the activation of various effector functions, including proliferation, cytolysis, and different patterns of cytokine release. These activation events are modulated by parameters such as density of the peptide-MHC complex, avidity of the TCR engagement, and the presence or absence of co-stimulation, often provided by accessory molecules on the APC. Several studies have demonstrated alterations in TCR recognition based on changes in the peptide component of the peptide-MHC complex, such that contact residue substitutions in the antigenic peptide engage the TCR, leading to different functional outcomes [1,2]. Since the interaction between TCR and peptide-MHC involves direct contact between the TCR and residues on both the MHC molecule and the bound peptide, we have explored the ability of alterations in residues on the MHC class II molecules, rather than on the peptide, to modulate TCR recognition.

Human CD4+ T cell clone ESL4.34 was derived from a donor heterozygous for DRB1*0402,*1301. This clone was generated by initial bulk stimulation of herpetic vesicle mononuclear cells (MNC) with phytohemagglutinin, a second bulk stimulation with crude herpes simplex type 2 (HSV-2) antigens and autologous peripheral blood MNC, and limiting dilution cloning in the presence of interleukin-2, as described previously [3,4]. The specificity of clone ESL4.34 for a peptide determinant corresponding to amino acids 393-405 of the HSV-2 virion protein VP16 was established using recombinant HSV-1 x HSV-2 viruses and overlapping peptides as described for other T cell clones [3,5]. Monoclonality of ESL4.34 was confirmed by polymerase chain reaction amplification of reverse transcribed mRNA using primers specific for TCR gene segments Vα 1-29 and Vβ 1-23, by nucleotide sequencing of the VDJ junctions of the Vα and Vβ PCR products, and by flow cytometry. Cytotoxic T cell (CTL) responses were measured using ^{51}Cr release assays with HLA-DR homozygous lymphoblastoid cell lines (LCL) pulsed with suboptimal concentrations of the VP16 393-405 peptide. Binding of biotinylated peptide to HLA-DR on whole cells was assayed by immuno-capture of peptide-DR complexes and detection using europium labeled streptavidin [6]. Generation and expression of site-specific mutants of DRB1*04 genes in LCLs has been previously described [7].

Cytolytic activity of T cell clone ESL4.34 was tested on DRB1*04 positive LCL pulsed with the VP16 393-405 peptide. As shown in *Table I*, DRB1*0402 presented the peptide efficiently, while DRB1*0401, *0404, and *0405 did not. These four closely related DRB1*04 alleles differ in the third hypervariable region of the DR second exon, encoding polymorphic amino acids at positions 67, 70, and 71. As shown in *Table I*, only the "IDE" motif in these positions supported cytotoxicity.

To explore the role of this "IDE" motif in supporting T cell recognition, we tested an extended panel of LCL's as APC. As listed in *Table I*, DRB1*13 and DRB1*11 groups of alleles contain natural variants which differ at positions 67, 70 or 71. DRB1*1301, which encodes the "IDE" motif, supported cytotoxicity, although at a lower level than DRB1*0402. In contrast, DRB1*1303, which differs from DRB1*1301 at residue 71, did not. Within the DRB1*11 cluster, only DRB1*1102, which carries the "IDE" motif, supported cytotoxicity. Even the single conservative change of isoleucine to phenylalanine at residue 67 abrogated CTL activity.

This restriction of cytotoxicity to MHC alleles expressing the "IDE" motif appears to be due to a direct interaction between TCR residues and the MHC polymorphic sites at 67, 70 and 71. This interpretation is based on the observation that some of the non-"IDE" alleles strongly bound the VP16 393-405 peptide, but did not present this peptide for cytotoxicity. For example, as shown in *Table I*, DRB1*1103 bound the VP16 peptide as well as, or better than, DRB1*1102 although, as noted above, it did not support cytotoxic recognition. Indeed, class II binding profiles for the VP16 393-405 peptide were fairly promiscuous, in that good peptide binding was seen with several alleles within the DRB1*04, *13, and *11 groups, except for those with charge substitutions at codon 71. In other words, class II molecules with substitutions at residues 67 and 70 continued to bind the peptide, but failed to support cytotoxicity. This was directly demonstrated by site-directed mutagenesis experiments, in which a mutated DRB1*0402 gene containing DRB1*0404 residue substitutions at codon 67, 70 or 71 was used for analysis. Only the wild-type DRB1*0402 allele supported cytotoxicity. Mutations at codon 67, 70 or 71 abrogated CTL recognition, and mutation at 71 also interfered with peptide binding. These results are also summarized in *Table I.*

These results confirm that the ability of ESL4.34 to lyse peptide pulsed targets is controlled in part by the presenting MHC molecule through specific interactions between residues on the TCR and the codon 67-71 region of the DR molecule. This is consistent with molecular modeling studies, in which this region of the DR molecule is predicted to contain side chains which are solvent accessible and available for TCR contact [8]. Indeed, it is of some interest that these same sites, codon 67, 70 and 71, have been implicated in susceptibility to autoimmunity, particularly in rheumatoid arthritis, where positive charged residues at these locations are highly associated with disease. We suggest that our observations with the ESL4.34 clone, although recognizing different residues at these positions, serves as a prototype to explain this disease susceptibility phenomenon, in that specific T cell recognition of antigen can be directly modulated by the specific amino acid residues in this shared epitope region of the HLA-DR molecule.

There is another aspect of this study which may have implications for immune recognition and autoimmunity. Studies of "altered peptide ligands" have documented examples whereby amino acid substitutions in the antigenic peptide can result in partial activation or altered T

Table I. DR specificities of antigen presenting cells, their position 67-71 amino acid sequences and VP16 393-405 peptide binding profiles, and cytotoxic responses of T cell clone ESL4.34

DRB1 allele	position 67-71 amino acids	cytotoxicity (specific lysis)	relative peptide binding
*0402	I L E D E	31	170
*0401	L - - Q K	0	12
*0404	L - - Q R	0	12
*0405	L - - Q R	0	11
*1301	- - - - -	13	30
*1303	- - - - K	0	40
*1101	F - - - R	0	12
*1102	- - - - -	32	70
*1103	F - - - -	0	95
*0402-Q70	- - - Q -	0	95
*0402-L67,Q70	L - - Q -	0	80
*0402-L67,R71	L - - - R	0	18
*0402-Q70,R71	- - - Q R	0	22

cell function, due to changes in the avidity of the specific trimolecular interaction [1]. We are intrigued by our observation that some DR alleles, such as DRB1*1103 and the mutant *0402 m70, for example, bind the same VP16 peptide as the closely related DRB1*1101 and DRB1*0402 alleles, but do not support cytotoxicity. We are currently investigating the possibility that presentation of the peptide on these altered self alleles may stimulate clone ELS4.34 along differential activation pathways. Preliminary data suggest the possibility that low level proliferation of the T cell clone ELS4.34 in the context of these "altered self ligands" may occur in the absence of cytolytic activity. We suggest that modulation of T cell recognition by altered self ligands, including naturally occurring polymorphic variants of class II molecules, may play an important functional role in determining the outcome of T cell activation.

References

1. Evavold BD, Sloan-Lancaster J, Allen PM. Tickling the TCR: selective T-cell functions stimulated by altered peptide ligands. *Immunol Today* 1993; 14: 602-9.
2. Evavold BD, Sloan-Lancaster J, Hsu BL, Allen PM. Separation of T helper 1 clone cytolysis from proliferation and lymphokine production using analog peptides. *J Immunol* 1993; 150: 3131-40.
3. Koelle DM, Corey L, Burke RL, Eisenberg RJ, Cohen GH, Pichyangkura R, Triezenberg SJ. Antigenic specificity of human CD4+ T cell clones recovered from recurrent genital HSV-2 lesions. *J Virol* 1994; 68: 2803-10.
4. Koelle DM, Abbo H, Peck A, Ziegweid K, Corey L. Direct recovery of HSV-specific T lymphocyte clones from recurrent HSV-2 lesions. *J Infect Dis* 1994; 169: 956-61.
5. Kwok WW, Domeier ME, Johnson ML, Nepom GT, Koelle DM. HLA-DQB1 codon 57 is critical for peptide binding and recognition. *J Exp Med* 1996; 183: 1253-8.
6. Kwok WW, Nepom GT, Raymond FC. HLA-DQ polymorphisms are highly selective for peptide binding interactions. *J Immunol* 1995; 155: 2468-76.
7. Hiraiwa A, Yamanaka K, Kwok WW, Mickelson EM, Masewicz S, Hansen JA, Radka SF, Nepom GT. Structural requirements for recognition of the HLA-Dw14 class II epitope: a key HLA determinant associated with rheumatoid arthritis. *Proc Natl Acad Sci USA* 1990; 87: 8051-5.
8. Penzotti JE, Doherty D, Lybrand TP, Nepom GT. A structural model for TCR recognition of the HLA class II shared epitope sequence implicated in susceptibility to rheumatoid arthritis. *J Autoimmun* 1996; 9: 287-93.

Transplantation biology and medicine

Immunologic monitoring of transplantation. HLA matching

Contents

HLA class II antibodies in highly sensitized patients awaiting renal transplantation

S.L. Saidman[1], D. Fitzpatrick[1], M. Mann[1], C. Comerford[1], L. Drew[1], M. Marrari[2], R. Duquesnoy[2]

1 Massachusetts General Hospital (MGH), Histocompatibility Laboratory, 32 Fruit Street, Room WHT 544, Boston, MA 02114-2690, USA
2 University of Pittsburgh Medical Center, Pittsburgh, PA, USA

A number of reports have demonstrated that B cell antibodies specific for donor HLA-DR antigens may lead to accelerated or hyperacute rejection [1-3]. We have screened highly sensitized renal transplant recipient sera submitted to the 12th International Histocompatibility Workshop against a B cell panel to determine the frequency and possible effects of such antibodies. We also present the results of B cell screens on patients awaiting transplant at the MGH.

Methods

B cell screens were performed using lymphocytotoxicity with immunobead isolated class II positive cells (Dynal). Sera and cells were incubated at 37°C for 30 minutes, followed by 60 minutes with complement at room temperature. T cell screens were performed by the AHG and/or Amos modified (4 wash) techniques using ficoll separated lymphocytes. Antisera were adsorbed with pooled platelets either prepared locally or purchased (Scantibodies Laboratory, Inc.). Packed platelets (0.4-0.6 ml) were mixed with 1 ml serum for 60 minutes at room temperature. Care was taken to prevent dilution of the sera by blotting all excess fluid from the platelets after a hard spin, prior to adding the sera. Adsorptions were repeated multiple times with each serum.

Results

Sera from 100 highly sensitized patients were submitted to the workshop for class I screening in 21 labs [4]. Nineteen sera were available in sufficient volume to allow B cell screening. The PRAs against a T cell panel (PRA-T) as reported by the submitting laboratories ranged from 50 - 99% (median 86%). All sera were initially adsorbed four times and 17/19 became negative with T cells. One of the remaining sera became T cell nonreactive after three additional adsorptions and one received no further treatment and therefore was not included in the analysis.

3/18 sera demonstrated significant B cell antibodies (PRA-B >5%). As seen in *Table I*, all three had DR specific antibodies. Serum HS048, obtained from the only patient who had received a prior transplant, was specific for the mismatched donor DR antigen.

B cell antibody screens were also performed with sera from patients awaiting renal transplantation at MGH

Table I. 12th Workshop sera from highly sensitized transplant patients with significant B cell reactivity

	HS025	HS048	HS058
Sensitization history*	0 tx, 4 p, >25 tr	1 tx, 0 p, 5 tr	0 tx, 0 p, ??tr
% PRA-T (Amos/AHG)	93/98	83/95	87/98
% PRA-B (platelet ads)	11	11	84
B cell antibody specificity	DR15	DR11	?DQ2, DQ3**
Prev. donor DR mismatch	-	DR11	-

*tx = previous transplants, p = pregnancies, tr = transfusions.
**antibody specificity not clearly defined due to high PRA, but serum reacted with all except DQI homozygous cells (serum donor was DQI).

Table II. Types of antibodies reactive with a B cell panel in the sera of patients awaiting renal transplantation

	1st transplant n (%)	Re-transplant n (%)
Total	158	35
Non-reactive	144 (91.1)	15 (42.9)
Sporadic/weak	7 (4.4)	2 (5.7)
Class I specific	4 ((2.5)	3 (8.6)
Undefined specificity	3 (1.9)	4 (11.4)
Class II specific	0	11 (31.4)
Previous donor class II unknown	0	5 (14.3)
Specific for previous donor class II	0	6 (17.1)

and 34/193 (18%) had significant B cell antibodies. 14/158 (9%) patients awaiting a first transplant had B cell reactivity (median PRA-B = 13%), whereas 20/35 (57%) awaiting re-transplant had such antibodies (median PRA-B = 57%). B cell reactivity in sera from patients awaiting a primary transplant was either sporadic and/or weak, class I specific (platelet adsorptions not done or incomplete), or strong but with undefined specificity (*Table II*). In comparison, the majority of the B cell reactivity found in sera from retransplant patients was class II specific and frequently specific for previous donor HLA-DR and/or -DQ alleles.

There was no correlation between %PRA-T and %PRA-B in re-transplant patients. In fact, five of the patients with significant B cell reactivity had no T cell reactivity, indicating that %PRA-T cannot be used to predict which patients will have B cell antibody.

There was some variation in the results of platelet adsorption between different patients and between different lots of pooled platelets. *Table III* shows data from both control and patient sera. Anywhere from two to seven adsorptions were required to remove class I antibodies from most sera, allowing HLA class II specific antibodies to be identified (*eg.* CR and MC). However, class I antibodies remained in some patients' sera even after seven adsorptions (*eg.* LD). A great deal of variability was found between lots of commercially prepared platelet pools. Class II antibodies were removed from a control serum (MGH 189) after seven adsorptions with one lot, whereas an equal number of adsorptions with locally prepared platelets had no effect on B cell reactivity.

Table III. Variation in results of pooled platelet adsorptions between different patients and between different lots of platelets

Serum	Platelet source*	# ads.	% PRA (T cell)	% PRA (B cell)	B cell antibody specificity
Patient CR	-	none	99	nd	
	M	4	0	27	DR11
Patient MC	-	none	100	nd	
	C.1	7	3	57	DQ3 (13/14)
Patient LD	-	none	82	nd	
	M	7	67	59	A2, 28
MGH 189	-	none	24	18	DR7 (6/6) + 1 extra
	C.2	4	0	16	DR7 (6/6)
	C.2	7	0	3	-
	M	4	0	27	DR7 (6/6)
	M	7	0	23	DR7 (5/5)

*Platelet source M=MGH, C=commercial (two different lots)

Discussion

This study demonstrates that patients who have lost a kidney allograft frequently have B cell reactivity, often specific for mismatched class II alleles from the previous donor. Even though HLA-DQ is thought to be less immunogenic, it is not uncommon for the antibodies to be DQ specific. Class II specific antibodies have been shown to be detrimental to renal allograft survival [3-5]. Routine B cell screening can be used to identify such antibodies and prevent unnecessary crossmatching with donors carrying the specific allele. Prior antibody identification and characterization is also useful in distinguishing HLA class II antibodies from non-specific B cell reactivity. The level of T cell reactivity cannot be correlated with B cell reactivity and therefore cannot be used to determine which patients should be screened. In addition, careful selection of platelet pools used for class I antibody adsorption is critical. Adsorption conditions must be optimized for each patient, and inclusion of controls is necessary to ensure that non-specific removal of class II antibodies does not occur.

References

1. Mohanakumar T, Rhodes C, Mendez-Picon G, Goldman M, Moncure C, Lee H. Renal allograft rejection associated with presensitization to HLA-DR antigens. *Transplantation* 1981; 31: 93-4.
2. Ahern AT, Artruc SB, Della Pelle P, Cosimi AB, Russell PS, Colvin RB, Fuller TC. Hyperacute rejection of HLA-AB identical renal allografts associated with B lymphocyte and endothelial reactive antibodies. *Transplantation* 1982; 33: 103-6.
3. Braun WE. Donor-specific antibodies: clinical relevance of antibodies detected in lymphocyte crossmatches. *Clin Lab Med* 1991; 11: 571-602.
4. Duquesnoy R, M. Marrari. In: Charron D, ed. *Genetic diversity of HLA. Functional and Medical Implication*, vol. I. Sèvres: EDK, 1997.

Monitoring of soluble HLA class I molecular weight variants and allotypes after liver transplantation*

V. Rebmann[1], M. Pässler[1], J. Erhard[2], F.W. Eigler[1], H. Grosse-Wilde[1]

1 Institute of Immunology, University Hospital of Essen, Wirchowstrasse 171, D45147 Essen, Germany
2 Department of General Surgery, University Hospital of Essen, Germany

Soluble HLA class I molecules (sHLA-I) are predominantly produced by the liver and have been identified in virtually all body fluids. sHLA class I molecules are thought to modulate alloimmune functions by blocking the T-cell receptor or by complexing HLA class I antibodies [1,2]. In view of these biological properties sHLA-I plasma levels have been monitored in patients after kidney, heart and liver transplantation [3-5]. These studies and our data demonstrated an increase in total sHLA-I plasma levels in correlation with clinical events such as cholangitis and graft rejection. We were interested whether monitoring of sHLA-I after liver transplantation (LTX) in terms of allotypes and weight variants is a useful tool to discriminate cholangitis from rejection.

Material and methods

Patients

A total of 22 patients were enrolled who received LTX at the local Transplant Centre from January 1993 - December 1995. Tissues typing of donors and recipients were performed either locally or by Eurotransplant affiliated laboratories. Graft function was monitored by laboratory serum parameters (alanine aminotransferase, total bilirubin, alkaline phosphatase and γ-glutamyltranspeptidase) and standard histopathology. In total, 24 biopsies were taken and indicated episodes of acute rejection and cholangitis in 16 and 8 cases, respectively.

Plasma samples

EDTA blood samples were obtained from each patient at daily intervals during the first two weeks after LTX and twice weekly thereafter (follow-up: minimum 14, maximum 58 days). After centrifugation (1.400 g, 10 min) the supernatant plasma was stored at -20° C until usage.

* supported in part by the DFG Grant Gr 608/7-1

Antibodies

For the ELISA format mab w6/32 (Serotec, Oxford, UK) specific for HLA class I plus β2-microglobulin (β2m) was used as capture antibody for whole sHLA-I molecules. Rabbit anti-human ß2m served as detection antibody. To visualise sHLA-I after one dimensional isoelectric focusing (1D-IEF) and SDS-PAGE, a rabbit antiserum towards denatured alpha chains (RaHC) and an alkaline phosphatase-conjugated goat anti-rabbit IgG (Dianova GmbH, Hamburg, Germany) were used.

Quantification of sHLA-I

Concentrations of sHLA-I molecules were analysed by ELISA as described previously [3] using recombinant HLA-B7 as standard reagent.

ID-IEF and SDS-PAGE analysis

The sHLA-I molecules of plasma samples were immunoprecipitated by mab w6/32 coupled to immunomagnetic beads (Dynabeads™ M280, Dynal, Hamburg, Germany). The 1D-IEF, SDS-PAGE, and Western blot were accomplished as described previously [6]. For the definition of sHLA allotypes two marker cell lines (M1 and M2 in *Figure 2*) with known HLA-A, B types were used. After SDS-PAGE and Western blot the intensities of the sHLA-I molecular weight variants were measured by densitometry.

Results and discussion

sHLA-I plasma levels after LTX

Based on bioptic results the plasma samples analysed were stratified into 3 groups: samples taken during episodes without clinical complications (group 1, n = 184); samples taken during episodes of cholangitis (group 2, n=68) and samples taken during episodes of acute rejection (group 3, n=88). Samples taken within 3 days before

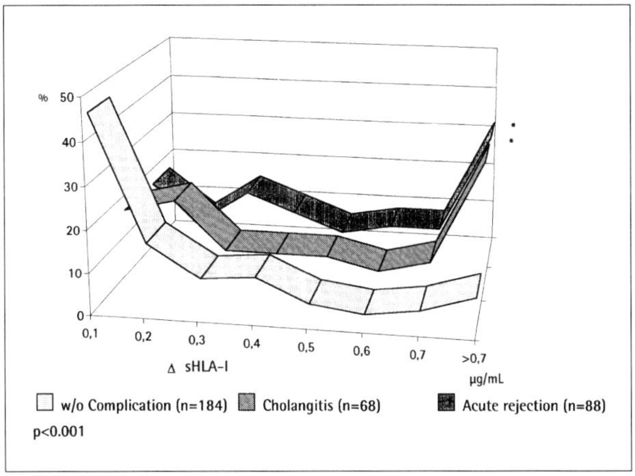

Figure 1. Increments of sHLA-I plasma levels in LTX patients (n=22).

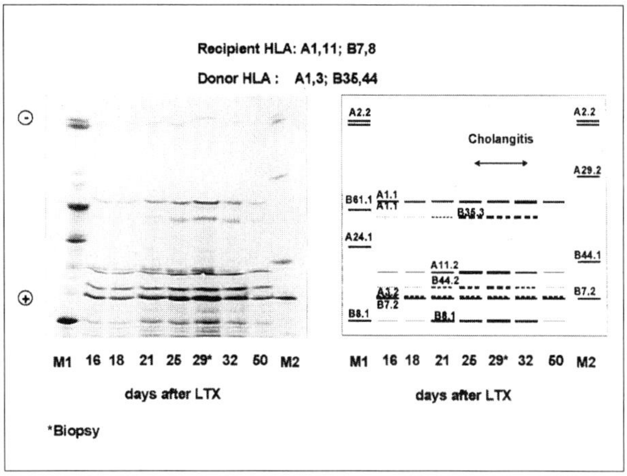

Figure 2. sHLA allovariants in plasma samples of a LTX patient.

and after biopsy were considered to belong to the episode under evaluation. For each patient the mean value of sHLA-I plasma concentration during episodes without clinical complications was determined. Based on these individual mean values the sHLA-I increments within each group were calculated and their distributions are given in *Figure 1*. For group 1 nearly 50 % of the samples revealed sHLA-I increments values of ≤ 0.1 µg/mL. This clearly demonstrates that only minor variations of sHLA-I plasma levels occur during episodes without complications. In groups 2 and 3, the distributions of increments shifted to the right with approximatively 30 % of samples contained sHLA-I > 0.7 µg/mL. Increases of sHLA-I concentrations above this level were significantly ($p<0.001$, χ^2-test) associated with both cholangitis and acute rejection. Thus, sHLA-I quantitation cannot discriminate between these two important clinical episodes.

Monitoring of donor and recipient sHLA allotypes

To follow recipient and donor derived sHLA class I allotypes after LTX, 1D-IEF and HLA class I specific Western blot were performed. Selected series of plasma samples from 12 patients were analysed covering 6 episodes of cholangitis and acute rejection, resp. After LTX in all samples recipient and donor derived sHLA allotypes were detectable. *Figure 2* demonstrates in the left part the 1D-IEF analysis of plasma samples from a LTX-patient sharing only HLA-A1 with the donor. The schematic drawing (*Figure 2*, right side) indicates the positions of sHLA allotypes (A1, 11.2; B7.2, 8) from the recipient and from the donor (A1, 3.2; B35.3, 44.2). During cholangitis (day 25-29 after LTX) recipient as well as donor derived sHLA-I allotypes clearly increased their intensities. Similar results were obtained during acute rejections (data not shown). The observed simultaneous occurrence of increased donor and recipient derived sHLA-I allotypes is most likely caused by shedding or release of these molecules from grafted liver cells and activated immune cells of the recipient. In contrast to other reports [4,5], we conclude from our 1D-IEF analysis that monitoring of donor and recipient derived sHLA-I allotypes is not an useful tool to discriminate between acute rejection and cholangitis.

Monitoring of sHLA-I molecular weight variants

sHLA-I molecules are heterogeneous with regard to their molecular masses. Three major sHLA-I variants are known with Mr of 43, 39, and 35 kD, respectively. To follow the distribution of sHLA-I molecular weight variants plasma samples of 22 patients were analysed by SDS-PAGE, HLA class I specific Western blot, and densitometry. *Figure 3* summarises the analysis of a LTX patient with acute rejection followed by cholangitis. During both episodes sHLA-I plasma levels were definitely increased. The corresponding SDS-PAGE revealed that the 35 kD variant of sHLA-I became the dominant molecular variant during acute rejection. During the following cholangitis episode none of the sHLA-I molecular variants appeared to be predominant.

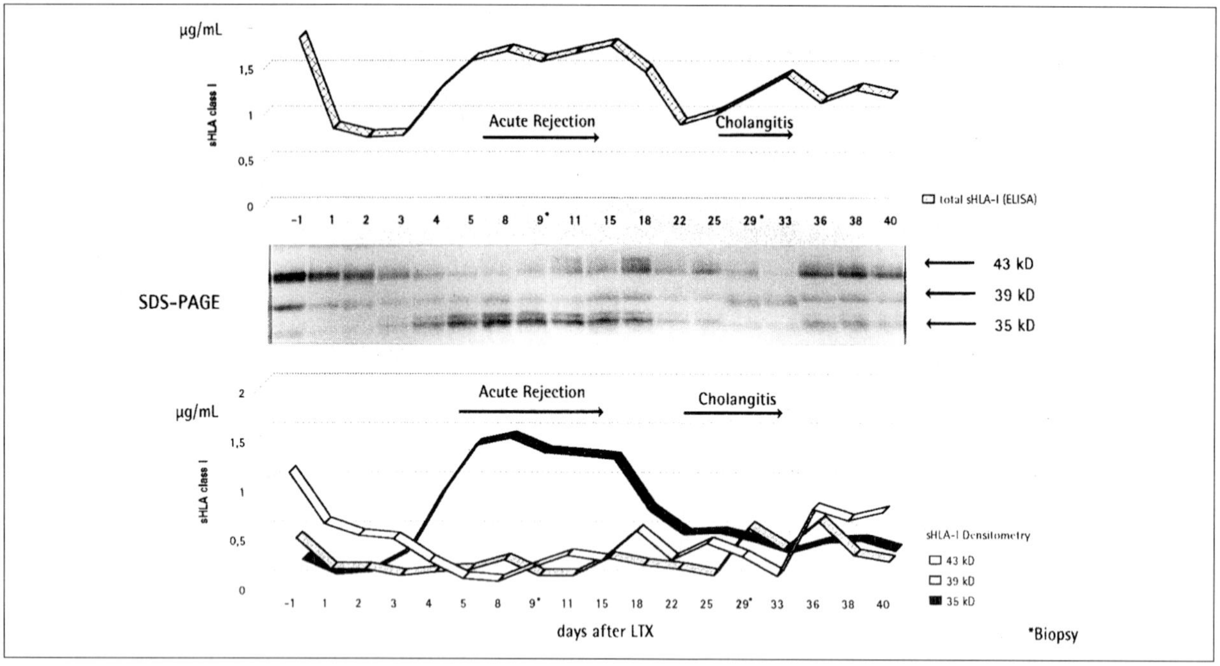

Figure 3. LTX patient with acute rejection followed by cholangitis.

To estimate the relative contribution of sHLA-I molecular variants the SDS-PAGE was subjected to densitometry and the optical densities were related to the sHLA-I plasma levels. From the lower panel of *Figure 3* it is obvious that during rejection the increased sHLA-I levels were mainly due to the 35 kD variant. To substantiate this observation all plasma samples subjected to SDS-PAGE (n = 236) were analysed by calculating the mean ratio ± SEM of 43 kD versus 35 kD. For groups 1 and 2 mean ratios (43kD : 35kD) of 13.4±2.3 and 8.4±2.9, resp. were obtained. In contrast to this, the ratio in group 3 was with 1.1±0.2 SEM statistically ($p<0.001$) reduced. Thus, only during acute rejection events sHLA-I molecules are predominantly shifted to the Mr 35 kD variant. The increase of this variant (Mr 35 kD) might be explained by an enhanced enzymatic degradation of membrane bound HLA class I molecules. In summary, monitoring of sHLA-I variants of 35 kD appears as a promising non-invasive parameter to identify episodes of acute rejection in LTX patients.

References

1. Buelow R, Burlingham WJ, Clayberger C. Immunomodulation by soluble HLA class I. *Transplantation* 1995; 59; 649-54.
2. Blasczyk R, Westhoff U, Grosse-Wilde H. Soluble CD4, CD8, and HLA molecules in commercial immunoglobulin preparations. *Lancet* 1993; 341; 789-90.
3. Tilg H, Westhoff U, Vogel W, Aulitzky WE, Herold M, Grosse-Wilde H. Soluble HLA class I serum concentration increase with transplant related complications after liver transplantation. *J Hepatol* 1992; 14; 417-20.
4. Pollard SG, Davies HS, Calne RY. Preoperative appearance of serum HLA class I antigen during liver transplantation. *Transplantation* 1990; 49; 659-63.
5. Zavazava N, Bottcher H, Mueller-Ruchholtz W. Soluble HLA class I antigens (sHLA) and anti-HLA antibodies in heart and kidney allograft recipient. *Tissue Antigens* 1993; 42; 20-4.
6. Kubens BS, Paeβler M, Grosse-Wilde H. Detection efficacy of soluble HLA-A, B antigens using 1D-IEF. *Eur J Immunogen* 1994; 21; 469-77.

Crossmatch testing of organ donors and recipients by Cross-Stat ELISA: clinical relevance of test results

F. Monteiro[1]*, H. Rodrigues[1], C. Viggiani[1], L.E. Ianhez[2], J. Kalil[1]

1 Laboratory of Transplantation Immunology, Heart Institute School of Medicine, University of São Paulo, R. Dr Eneas C. Aguiar 500, 3° andar, 05403-000, São Paulo SP, Brazil
2 Renal Transplant Unit, School of Medicine, University of Sao Paulo, Brazil
* Corresponding author

Pre-transplantation monitoring of potential allograft recipients includes the detection of anti-HLA antibodies. Especially important is the identification of anti-donor HLA class I IgG because such antibodies are harmful to the transplanted organ and, in the worst scenario, can cause hyperacute rejection. Traditionally, these antibodies are detected by complement mediated cytotoxicity (CDC). In general, CDC testing of donor and recipients has been very successful in minimizing the number of hyperacute rejections. However, Iwaki and Terasaki in 1987 [1] suggested that, for some patients, the lack of organ function may be due to anti-donor antibodies that could not be detected by conventional crossmatch techniques.

In search of improved specific crossmatch test procedures for clinically relevant antibodies, various modifications of the standard lymphocytoxicity and flow cytometry protocols have been evaluated. However, both, lymphocytotoxicity and flow cytometry are not standardized procedure and many different protocols are in use. In addition, several studies suggest that flow cytometry due to its high sensitivity can detect antibodies that are not harmful to the graft [2].

Recently, a standardized ELISA assay of anti-donor HLA class I antibodies was described [3]. A multicenter study demonstrated high reproducibility of test results and high correlation with lymphocytotoxicity and flow cytometry crossmatch assays. However, for some donor/recipient combinations ELISA results differed from those obtained by lymphocytotoxicity or flow cytometry. In the current study we evaluated the clinical relevance of these differences.

Material and methods

This study included 169 renal recipients (146 cadaveric donors and 23 living related donors) who underwent transplantation at our Institution between 1990 and 1994 and for whom pre-transplant serum specimens and donor cells were available. The patient's follow up was 12 months. Immunosupressive rejection prophylaxis consisted of classical triple therapy. Rejection episodes were diagnosed with a kidney biopsy when there was an unexplained rise in serum creatinine. The transplant failure was measured as return to dialysis, transplant nephrectomy or death of the recipient.

Lymphocytotoxicity testing

Lymphocytotoxic antibodies in serum specimens were detected by using NIH standard and AHG protocols. The recipient sera were tested against T and B donor cells before and after DTT treatment.

Detection of panel-reactive antibodies

Anti-HLA class I panel-reactive IgG antibodies were detected by ELISA using the PRA-STAT kit [4].

ELISA crossmatch

Anti-HLA class I IgG antibodies against donor were determined using the Cross-Stat kit [3]. A specific cut-off value determined with 1546 specimen pairs consisting of 32 kidney donors and 20-30 patient specimens was used to differentiate between positive and negative reactions. When donor-HLA was prepared from lymphocytes the used cut-off value was 1.0, when donor-HLA was obtained from a mixture of plasma, platelets and lymphocytes (PPL) prepared as recommended by the manufacturer, the used cut-off value was 1.2.

Results and discussion

Eighty seven of 169 recipients (51%) had 0-1 rejection episode, 67 recipients (40%) experienced more than one rejection episode and 15 patients (9%) lost their graft. In 10 of these 15 patients the transplanted kidney has never functioned. Acute vascular rejection (AVR) caused graft loss in

Table I. Characteristics of patients with graft loss

Patient ID	ELISA CM total IgG	CDC-CM	Clinical Event: Rejection episode #	Clinical Event: Loss Diagnosis
15	-	-	NF	AVR*
19	-	-	NF	ACR*
10	pos	B+	2	ACR*
22	-	-	NF	AVR*
14	pos	-	5	AVR*
6	pos	B+	NF	HR*
16	-	-	NF	Thrombosis*
18	-	-	NF	Thrombosis*
20	-	-	NF	Thrombosis*
7	pos	-	NF	Deceased**
23	-	-	-	Deceased**
24	-	-	-	Kidney Infection**
17	-	-	NF	Technical**
21	-	-	NF	Technical**
25	-	-	-	Technical**

NF : primary Non-Function Kidney
HR: Humoral Rejection
*Immune related graft loss
ACR: Acute Cellular Rejection
AVR: Acute Vascular Rejection
** Non-immune related graft loss

3 patients, acute cellular rejection (ACR) in 2, technical loss in 3, thrombosis in 3, kidney infection in 1, humoral rejection in 1 and 2 patients died. AVR, ACR, thrombosis and humoral rejection were considered immune related graft losses (9 patients) and technical loss, infection and patient death with functioning graft as non-immune related graft losses (6 patients - *Table I*).

All patients had been transplanted across a negative CDC T cell CM. Comparison between CDC and ELISA crossmatches revealed 12 of 155 donor/recipient pairs that had been tested negative by CDC were positive by ELISA. Two (n=2) additional CM pairs that tested positive by ELISA had been tested negative by CDC using T cells but positive using B cells. This corresponds to an overall agreement between CDC and ELISA of 93%, the specificity 93% and sensitivity 100%.

The presence of pre-transplant anti-donor class I antibodies detected by ELISA correlated significantly with an immune related graft loss within 2 months post- transplantation (p=0.031) (*Table II*). Analysis of pre-transplant ELISA crossmatch results showed 3 of 14 patients (21%) transplanted across a positive ELISA crossmatch lost their graft compared to 6 of 149 (4%) who were transplanted across a negative ELISA crossmatch.

Table II. Comparison of ELISA-CM and immune related graft loss

	ELISA-CM Pos	ELISA-CM Neg
Loss	3	6
No-Loss	11	143
	p = 0,031	

Out of those 14 patients who had been transplanted across a positive ELISA crossmatch (*Table III*), 3 patients (#6, #10 and #14) lost the graft probably due to antibody mediated rejection and can be characterized as follows: Patient #6 received a graft from a cadaveric donor and experienced antibody mediated hyperacute rejection. Anti-donor antibodies present in the patient's pre-transplant serum were detected in the ELISA crossmatch and the lymphocytotoxicity CM using B cell but not T cells. CDC-PRA was 11% before and 0% after DTT treatment and the ELISA-PRA was 67%. Patient # 10 lost his graft within 45 days due to acute cellular rejection. CDC-PRA was 0% before and after DTT treatment and ELISA-PRA was 83%. ELISA and CDC crossmatch results were similar to

Table III. Characteristics of patients with anti-donor HLA class I antibodies detected by ELISA

Patient ID	ELISA CM total IgG	PRA-STAT (%)	CDC-CM	Clinical Event Rejection episode N	Clinical Event Rejection episode Loss(day)
1	+	0	-	1	
2	+	87	-	1	
3	+	37	-	0	
4	+	9	-	0	
5	+	85	-	3	
6	+	67	B+	NF	HR(0)
7	+	83	-	NF	Deceased(7)
8	+	0	-	2	
9	+	35	-	2	
10	+	83	B+	2	ACR(45)
11	+	76	-	4	
12	+	0	-	1	
13	+	17	-	1	
14	+	7	-	5	AVR(56)

NF : primary Non-Function Kidney
ACR: Acute Cellular Rejection
AVR: Acute Vascular Rejection
HR: Humoral Rejection

that patient #6. Patient #14 received a graft from a living related donor. Graft loss due to an acute vascular rejection occurred 56 days after transplantation. All pre-transplant cytotoxicity tests were negative, however the ELISA-CM was positive. In addition, ELISA-PRA indicated the presence of anti-class I IgG antibodies albeit very few (PRA=7%).

Six of 149 (4%) who were transplanted across a negative ELISA crossmatch also, were negative using CDC protocols. Those patients lost their graft due to complications that were probably not antibody mediated (*Table I*).

In summary, the current study gave evidence of clinical relevance of anti-donor antibodies detected by ELISA-CM testing. Three patients that were transplanted across a positive ELISA-CM lost their graft earlier after transplantation. Nonetheless, one has to keep in mind that this study included patients who had been transplanted across a negative T cell crossmatch only. Therefore, it did not provide any information about patients with antibodies detectable by lymphocytotoxicity or flow cytometry but not by ELISA. A recent comparison of CDC, flow cytometry and ELISA crossmatch showed a very good agreement of the three assay procedures [3]. However, for a small number of specimen pairs discrepant results were obtained. These particular specimens may contain antibodies that can be detected under certain conditions only and additional studies will be necessary to analyze the clinical relevance of such antibodies.

References

1. Iwaki Y, Terasaki PI. Primary nonfunction in human cadaver kidney transplantation: evidence for hidden hyperacute rejection In: Najarian JS, Simons R eds. *Clin Transplant* 1987; 1: 125-9.
2. Thistlethwaite JR, Buckingham M, Stuart JK, Gaber AO, Mayer JT, Stuart FP. T-cell immunofluorescence flow cytometry crossmatch results in cadaver donor renal transplantation. *Transplant Proc* 1987; 19: 722.
3. Buelow R, Chiang TR, Monteiro F, Cornejo MC, Ellingson L, Claas F, Gaber O, Gelder F, Kotb M, Orosz C, Pouletty F. Soluble HLA antigens and ELISA: a new technology for crossmatch testing. *Transplantation* 1995; 60: 1594-9.
4. Buelow R, Mercier I, Glanville L, Regan J, Ellingson L, Janda G, Claas F, Colombe B, Gelder F, Grosse-Wilde H, Orosz C, Westhoff U, Voegler U, Monteiro F, Pouletty F. Detection of panel-reactive anti-HLA class I antibodies by ELISA or lymphocytotoxicity: results of a blinded, controlled multicenter study. *Hum Immunol* 1995; 44: 1-11.

Perforin and granzyme B expression, in peripheral blood lymphocytes associated to heart graft rejection

T. Langanay[1], B. Drénou[2], B. Lelong[1], B. Turlin[3], P. Menestret [1], L. Amiot[2], H. Corbineau [1], B. Sevray[1], A. Leguerrier[1], C. Rioux[1], M.P. Ramée[3], R. Fauchet [2], Y. Logeais[1]

1 Clinic of Cardiovascular and Thoracic Surgery
2 Hematology-Immunology Laboratory
3 Pathology Laboratory, University Hospital Pontchaillou, rue Henri le Guilloux, 35033 Rennes Cedex 9, France

Heart transplantation has become over the last ten years the elective therapie for end stage heart failure. But as it is virtually impossible to provide a donor heart perfectly matched to the host's immune system, acute rejection constitutes the main post-transplant complication and impairs significantly the first years survival. Routine rejection surveillance involves endomyocardial biopsies with histologic evaluation [1]. Though routinely done, it remains an invasive technique with potential complications (tamponade) and because the rejection may not affect homogeneously all the myocardium there might be false negatives.

Two functionnal markers of cytotoxic T lymphocytes and NK cells, granzyme B and perforin, have been used to identify activated lymphocytes in heart-infiltrates and also in the peripheral blood. These proteins are stored in and released by cytoplasmic granules of the lymphocytes. Perforin acts as a pore-forming protein [2] and granzyme B [3] belongs to a family of serine proteases which triggers synergistically with perforin an endogenous pathway of apoptosis, both leading to cell death.

In previous studies performed in kidney and heart transplantations, both in human and mouse, these proteins were shown to be markers for allograft rejection. Their expression on biopsies correlates with rejection [4-7], seems to have a predictive interest [8] and to be down-regulated by steroids and cyclosporin and increased by lymphokines [9].

Patients and methods

Patients

Between september 94 and june 95, 10 consecutive patients, 8 men and 2 women, aged 35 to 63 (mean 49) underwent an orthotopic heart transplantation at the University Hospital of Rennes (France) to treat an end stage heart failure. There was no inhospitality death and all patients received the current immunosuppressive therapy [10].

Data were prospectivelly collected from all patients until october 1995. Episodes of rejection were treated with increased doses of steroids and in refractory cases with lymphocyte antibody in hospital stay.

Biopsy and histologic grading

Routine rejection surveillance involves endomyocardial biopsies, done at weekly intervals for the first 4 weeks post transplantation, biweekly for the second month with a gradual reduction to once every 3 months. The histologic evaluation has been performed according to the International Society for Heart and Lung Transplantation grading system (grade 0 = no rejection; grade 4 = severe rejection) [1]. Four to 6 pieces of septal myocardium were sampled, two of them were snap-frozen in liquid nitrogen and stored at -80°C for monoclonal antibody analysis.

We also analysed the expression of perforin and granzyme in the graft infiltrating lymphocytes and in the peripheral blood lymphocytes (PBL).

Immunohistochemical studies

Analysis of myocardial biopsies was performed on frozen sections using: GB-42-PU (IgG1, anti-granzyme B) and PE-41-PU (IgM antiperforin) (Pharmacell), controls (IgG1 or IgGM Dako) with the Avidine - Streptavidine - phosphatase alcaline immunohistochemical technique (LSAB Kit - Dako).

Peripheral blood lymphocytes

Analysis is realised on whole blood using flow cytometry and the specific monoclonal antibodies, in a double layer technique (IgG antiF do'(2) (Silenus). Cell permeabilisation is performed before red blood cell lysis and the technical steps have been optimized to minimise the blood puncture.

Results

Analysis of heart biopsies (EMB)

118 EMB were studied using histological and immunohistochemical analysis. The results of histological grading of rejection were : grade 0 (no rejection): 19 biopsies - grade 1 (mild rejection) : 53 - grade 2: 40 - grade 3: 4 - grade 4 (severe acute rejection): 2. An increased coexpression of perforin and granzyme is found in the infiltrating T lymphocytes during the 2 episodes grade 4. In 3 of the 4 cases grade 3, there is a dissociation between perforin and granzyme and in one case, there is no increased expression at all (results are stated in percentage of lymphocytes expressing the proteins *(Table I)*.

Table I.

Patient	Grade	Day post-Transpl.	Lymphocytes Perforin +	Lymphocytes Granzyme B +
MAR...	4	18	9%	6%
	3	35	3,5%	<1%
	3	98	<1%	7%
PRO...	4	36	6%	13,5%
LEF...	3	96	6%	<1%
LEP...	3	70	<1%	<1%

Perforin and granzyme B expression in peripheral blood lymphocytes

Sixty consecutive EMB have been associated to the analysis of perforin and granzyme B in PBL. Ten «healthy» donors have been used as control and for 3 patients PBL pretransplant expression studied. The results are expressed in percentage of lymphocytes expressing the proteins *(Table II)*. In parallel to the increasing grades of rejection (ISHLT), there is also an increased expression of the proteins in the PBL. This has been shown to be statistically significant in different cases.

Perforin : grade 4 vs grades 0, 1, 2, 3 (p<0.001) and grade 4 vs controls (p<0.001).

Granzyme : grade 4 vs grades 0, 1 (p>0,02) and grades 2, 3 vs grade 0 (p<0,05).

In the 4 cases grade 3, the expression appears paradoxically very low and dissociated from the other results, without any clear explanation.

Table II.

Grade Rejection	Number of patients	% PBL Perforin +	% PBL Granzyme B +
0	9	0,6±1,1	22,2±13,3
1	35	2,9±4,9	31,8±26,7
2	10	3,8±4,3	50±32
3	4	1,05±0,7	46,3±22,8
4	2	26,1±1,85	81,3±11,3
Controls	10	1,2 %± 1,12	9,4% ± 6,92
Pretranspl.	3	1,8% ± 0,69	20,7% ± 15

In the 2 cases of severe acute rejection (grade 4) we have found a sharp increase of protein's expression at the time of biopsy *(Figure 1)* but also at the previous biopsies performed 8 and 15 days before, though at that time, it did not show any sign of rejection (grade 1A). After one week of treatment, the biopsies showed a disappearance of cellular infiltrates, coinciding with graft stabilization (grade 1A) and the protein's expression was also down regulated. More over, the proteins' expression never increased like that in any other case.

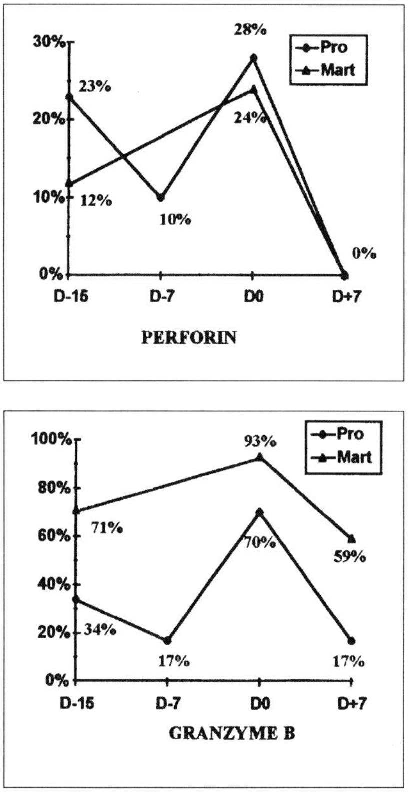

Figure 1.

Discussion

Despite the use of the potent immunosuppressive therapy, acute graft rejection remains the major post-transplantation complication. Graft stabilization coincided with a low expression of the functionnal markers in the peripheral blood lymphocytes, in contrast their expression increased in case of rejection and seemed to be down regulated by the immunosuppressive therapy. This observation suggests a relationship between heart rejection and the expression of perforin and granzyme in the PBL. Moreover, the analysis performed just before transplantation or in healthy donors showed a lower expression.

The dissociation between the PBL expression and the histological grading, observed 1 and 2 weeks before a severe rejection suggests that perforin and granzyme expression in PBL has a potential predictive interest.

The results, in grade 3, have to be reanalysed as they appear discordant from all the other cases. These data are only preliminary results which have to be confirmed on a larger scale. If so, monitoring of perforin and granzyme B expression in the PBL could reduce the need for myocardial biopsies and ultimately lead to earlier diagnosis of acute rejection, thus permissing to treat, earlier, episodes of rejection before the onset of severe histological damages.

Conclusion

A relationship between heart rejection and the expression of perforin and granzyme B in the infiltrating lymphocytes has been established by previous studies. These results suggest that this relationship could also be extended to the proteins'expression in the peripheral blood lymphocytes so that their monitoring in PBL could become an important element in the management of heart transplantation.

References

1. Billingham ME, Cary NRB, Hammond ME *et al.* A working formulation for the standardization of nomemclature in the diagnosis of heart and lung rejection: heart rejection study group. *J Heart Transplant* 1990; 6: 587 - 93.
2. Liu CC, Walsh CM, Young JDE. Perforin: structure and function. *Immunol Today* 1995; 16: 194-201.
3. Smyth MJ, Trapani JA. Granzymes: exogenous proteinases that induce target cell apoptosis. *Immunol Today* 1995; 16: 202-6.
4. Clément MV, Haddad P, Soulié A *et al.* Perforin and granzyme B as markers for acute rejection in heart transplantation. *Int Immunol* 1991; 3: 1175-81.
5. Griffiths GM, Namikawa R, Mueller C *et al.* Granzyme A and perforin as markers for rejection in cardiac transplantation. *Eur J Immunol* 1991; 21: 687-92.
6. Legros-Maïda S, Soulié A, Benvenuti C *et al.* Granzyme B and perforin can be used as predictive markers of acute rejection in heart transplantation. *Eur J Immunol* 1994; 24: 229-33.
7. Clément MV, Legros-Maïda S, Israël-Biet D *et al.* Perforin and granzyme B expression is associated with severe acute rejection. *Transplantation* 1994; 57: 322-6.
8. Alpert S, Lewis NP, Ross H, Fowler M, Valantine HA. The relationship of granzyme A and perforin expression to cardiac allograft rejection and dysfunction. *Transplantation* 1995; 60: 1478-85.
9. Mueller C, Shao Y, Altermatt HJ, Hess MW, Shelby J. The effect of cyclosporine treatment on the expression of genes encoding granzyme A and perforin in the infiltrate of mouse heart transplants. *Transplantation* 1993; 55: 139-45.
10. Logeais Y, Lelong B, Leguerrier A *et al.* Transplantation cardiaque. Étude clinique et résultats. À propos d'une série consécutive de 100 premières greffes. *Presse Med* 1994; 23: 23-7.

Limiting dilution analysis: increasing the sensitivity and specificity of the alloreactive T helper cell assay by abrogating unwanted IL-2 production

P. Hornick[1,2], P. Brookes[2], P. Mason[2], K.M. Taylor[1], M.Y. Yacoub[3], J.R. Batchelor[2], M. Rose[4], R.I. Lechler[2]

1 Department of Cardiothoracic Surgery
2 Department of Immunology, Royal Postgraduate Medical School, Hammersmith Hospital, Du Cane Road, London W12 OHS, UK
3 Department of Cardiothoracic Surgery
4 Department of Immunology, Harefield Hospital, Middlesex, UK

The most sensitive and quantitative technique for measuring T cell alloresponses is to determine their frequencies by limiting dilution analysis. Methods have been established for assaying the frequencies of alloreactive IL-2-secreting T helper cells (HTLf), sensitized by the direct pathway of allorecognition [1,2]. The key to maximising sensitivity and specificity of the assay is to eliminate extraneous sources of IL-2 production so that the only stimulus to IL-2 release is the direct anti-stimulator alloresponse of the responder cells. We have identified three sources of extraneous IL-2 production. Autologous mixed lymphocyte (AMLR) reactions may occur: (1) within the responder population, (2) within the irradiated stimulator population, and (3) "back presentation" by responder antigen presenting cells (APC's) to T helper cells resident within the donor population. Our solution has been to use monoclonal antibodies to deplete the responder population of antigen presenting cells, and the stimulator population of $CD4^+$ and $CD8^+$ T cells. These [1-3] cellular interactions do not now occur and unwanted IL-2 production is markedly reduced. These modifications have led to significant differences in T helper cell frequencies when compared to the results obtained using unseparated responder and stimulator cell populations. This strategy has produced a significantly improved, sensitive and specific assay, and is currently being used to investigate donor-specific alloreactivity following cardiac and renal transplantation

Materials and methods

Peripheral blood mononuclear cells (PBMC)

Preparation of responder PBMCs

Mononuclear cells were isolated by density gradient centrifugation from healthy volunteers. The responder cells were resuspended in a freezing mixture comprising serum from AB donors and 30% dimethyl sulphoxide (DMSO Analar BDK, Poole, England), to give a final concentration of 7.5% DMSO. Samples were stored in liquid nitrogen until required.

Preparation of stimulator cells

Portions of spleen were obtained during organ retrieval. Single cell suspensions were released by injecting cold sterile medium into the splenic substance with a syringe and were then frozen as above.

Antibody-mediated depletion

Stimulator cells

$CD4^+$ and $CD8^+$ T lymphocyte depletion of stimulators was carried out using anti-$CD4^+$- and anti-$CD8^+$- coated immunomagnetic beads (Dynabeads, Dynal AS, Oslo, Norway).

Responder cells

Purified, T cells were prepared using mouse anti-human monoclonal antibodies (MAb) against HLA DR, CD14, CD19, CD56, CD16 and CD33 (Becton Dickinson, San Jose, CA, USA). Following incubation on ice the cells were then washed with cold RPMI and incubated with goat-anti-mouse microbeads (Miltenyl Biotec GmbH, Germany). Depletion was achieved by running the cell suspension and microbeads through a MiniMacs separation column applied to a magnet (Miltenyl Biotec GmbH, Germany). Eluted cells were then used for subsequent experiments

Flow cytometry

In order to determine the efficiency of depletion, cells were stained with directly conjugated anti-CD3-FITC and anti-DR-PE (Simultest, Becton Dickinson, San Jose, CA, USA) then washed and fixed with 1% paraformaldehyde. Cells were subsequently analysed using a EXCEL flow cytometer (Coulter, Coulter Electronics, Bedfordshire, England). In all experiements T cell-depleted stimulator cells contained ≤ 4% CD3 and HLA class II- responders ≤ 1% DR^+ cells.

Maintenance of the interleukin-2 (IL-2)-dependent indicator cell line CTLL-2

The line was maintained in culture medium with the addition of human recombinant IL-2 (rIL-2, 10 U/ml, Boehringer, Mannheim, Germany) and 10% Foetal calf serum (FCS). The cells were subcultured every 3 days. Prior to use in a limiting dilution assay, the CTLL-2 cells were washed twice and cultured overnight in normal culture medium, but without rIL-2.

HTLf assay

Following the depletion processes the stimulator and responder cells were resuspended in RPMI with 5% AB serum. Graded numbers, 0.03125×10^4 to 5×10^4, of responder cells in 50 µl were added to 24 replicate wells of U-bottom 96-well microtiter plates (Flow laboratories, Irvine, Scotland). Stimulator cells were gamma-irradiated with 35 Gy using a ^{137}Cesium source (Gammacell 1000, Atomic Energy of Canada Ltd, Kanata, Canada), and 5×10^4 cells were added in 100 µl to each of the wells. Plates were incubated at 37°C in 5% CO_2 and 95% air for 72 hours. Following incubation the plates were irradiated with 25 Gy (8 MeV linear accelerator, Philips MEL, Crawley, England). The presence or absence of IL-2 production in each well was assessed by adding 1×10^3 CTLL-2 cells in 25 µl of medium. Eight hours later, 1 µCi of tritiated thymidine (^{3}H-TdR) (Amersham International plc, Amersham, England) in 25 µl of medium was added to each well. After a further 16-hr incubation, the cells were harvested onto glass fibre filter mats and the (^{3}H-TdR) incorporation by CTLL-2 was assessed by liquid scintillation spectrophotometry (1205 Betaplate, Pharmacia Wallac, Turku, Finland). Control wells for the calculation of background activity consisted of 24 wells containing irradiated stimulator cells alone. Wells were considered positive for IL-2 production when ^{3}H-TdR incorporation exceeded the mean of the background plus three standard deviations (SD). Other control wells contained responder cells in medium alone (negative control).

Statistical analysis

Frequencies of alloreactive Th cells were calculated using a maximum likelihood statistical programme using GLIM software (NAG Ltd., Oxford, UK), based on the method of Finney [3]. Frequencies were regarded as different if their 95% confidence limits (approximately two standard deviations) do not overlap. From the χ^2 values and degrees of freedom (the number of responder dilutions minus one), probability estimates ('p') may be calculated. P values ≥ 0.05 are statistically significant and show that the results follow 'single-hit' kinetics, *i.e.* that a single cell type, the alloreactive IL-2 producing Th cell, is limiting.

Results

Assessment of the contribution made to the HTLf assay by depleting the stimulator population of T cells

T depletion of the stimulator cells resulted in a lowering of the background such that there was an increase in the number of positive wells within the assay. In the example shown in *Table I*, this resulted in a change in frequency which is statistically significant.

Table I. Depletion of stimulator T cells affects the HTLpf assay

Responder Dilution (Cells/well)	Positive wells /24 Spleen cells	Positive wells /24 T depleted spleen cells
50000	23	24
40000	20	24
30000	17	23
20000	18	22
10000	11	18
5000	3	11
2500	3	7
1250	0	1
625	1	2
312.5	0	0
Frequency	1/19960	1/8257
	CI: 15984-24925	CI: 6494-10499
	p: 0.90-0.10	p: 0.95-0.90

Assessment of the contribution made to the HTLpf assay by depleting the responder population of HLA-class II+ cells

In this example, depletion of class II^+ cells within the responder population abolished the AMLR, and thus allowed a frequency to be estimated, as the assay now follows single-hit kinetics *(Table II)*.

Table II. Depletion of responder class II cells affects the HTLpf assay

Responder Dilution (Cells/well)	Positive wells /24 Responder PBMC	Positive wells /24 Class II+ depleted responder
40000	23	18
20000	23	15
10000	11	6
5000	11	4
1250	11	0
312.5	2	0
Frequency	1/8500	1/27513
	CI: 6408-11275	CI: 20172-37526
	p: <0.01	p: 0.90-0.110

Overall contribution to the HTLf assay by depletion of HLA class II+ cells from the responder population, and T cells from the stimulator population

The combined effect of T cell and HLA class II$^+$ cell depletion on responder and stimulator AMLR's and 'back-presentation' are illustrated in *Table III*. Prior to the depletion steps the assay does not follow single-hit kinetics, but a statistically valid frequency can be estimated once the extraneous sources of IL-2 production are eliminated.

Table III. Differences that responder depletion of HLA class II$^+$ cells and stimulator depletion of T cells can make to the overall frequency of the assay

Responder Dilution (Cells/well)	Positive wells /24 Responder PBMC and stimulator: spleen cells	Positive wells /24 responder Class II+ depleted cells and stimulator: spleen cells depleted spleen cells
40000	24	24
20000	24	22
10000	24	11
5000	23	5
1250	21	2
312.5	12	0
Frequency	1/715	1/12141
	CI: 482-1059	CI: 9182-16053
	p: <0.10	p: 0.90-0.10

Discussion

IL-2-producing T helper lymphocytes are central to the process of graft rejection and graft-versus-host disease [4-6]. The development of sensitive, specific and reproducible techniques that are able to quantify the direct anti-donor alloresponse allow assessment of sensitisation or tolerance induction following transplantation. We have used a functional definition of T helper cells in order to include CD8$^+$ HTL as reported by Joos [7]. IL-2 production due to cellular interactions other than direct responder anti-stimulator allorecognition affects the sensitivity and specificity of the alloreactive HTLf assay. IL-2 production by the T cells within the stimulator population has been addressed by Reisaeter *et al.* [8] using PBMC as stimulators. Their solution, in line with our own was to deplete the stimulator population of T cells. However, this fails to address the possibility of an AMLR reaction within the responder cell population. Furthermore, given the sensitivity of the assay [9], incomplete depletion of stimulator T cells leaves a residual risk of back-stimulation by HLA-class II$^+$ cells in the responder population, unless they are deliberately removed. We therefore use 35 Gy of irradiation to eliminate this possibility. We have shown that by depleting the responder population of HLA-class II$^+$ cells, and the stimulator population of T cells, the kinetics and the estimated frequency can significantly change. For some responder: stimulator pairs, such unwanted sources of IL-2 make little difference to the final estimation of frequency, however it is not possible to predict which stimulator: responder combinations will be in this group. We therefore advocate the depletion of responder APC's and stimulator T cells when performing an alloreactive HTLpf assay.

Acknowledgements

We would like to acknowledge the financial support given by the British Heart Foundation and the Royal College of Surgeons of England.

References

1. Deacock S, Schwarer A, Batchelor R, Goldman J, Lechler R. A rapid limiting dilution assay for measuring the frequencies of alloreactive, interleukin-2 producing T cells in humans. *J Immunol Meth* 1992; 147: 83.

2. Orosz C, Adams P, Ferguson R. Frequency of human alloantigen-reactive helper T cells lymphocytes. II. Method for limiting dilution analysis of alloantigen-reactive helper T cells in human peripheral blood. *Transplantation* 1987; 43: 718.
3. Finney D. Statistical method in biological assay. London: Charles Griffin, 1978.
4. Bishop DK, Shelby J, Eichwald EJ. Mobilisation of T lymphocytes following cardiac transplantation. *Transplantation* 1992; 53: 849.
5. Hall BM. Cells mediating allograft rejection. *Transplantation* 1991; 51: 1141.
6. Theobald M. Allorecognition and graft-versus-host disease. *Bone Marrow Transplant* 1995; 15: 489.
7. Joos J, Zanker B, Wagnar H, Kabelitz D. Quantitative assessment of interleukin-2-producing alloreactive human T cells by limiting dilution analysis. *J Immunol Meth* 1988; 112: 85.
8. Reisaeter A, Thorsby E, Brinchmann J. Analysis of alloreactive helper T lymphocyte precursor frequencies: influence of interleukin-2 produced by the stimulating cells. *J Immunol Meth* 1996; 189: 65-72.
9. Mason P, Robinson C, Lechler R. Detection of donor-specific hyporesponsiveness following late failure of human renal allografts. *Kidney Int* 1997 (in press).

Optimal control of IFN-γ and TNF-α by IL-10 produced in response to one HLA-DR mismatch during the primary mixed lymphocyte reaction

M. Toungouz, C. Denys, D. De Groote, M. Andrien, E. Dupont

Department of Immunology and Transfusion, Hôpital Erasme, Université Libre de Bruxelles, 808 route de Lennik, B-1070 Brussels, Belgium

IL-10 is an immunosuppressive cytokine (CK) produced by a variety of cell types including Th0 and Th2 subset of helper T cells, B cells, monocytes and macrophages. During the allogeneic reaction, exogenous IL-10 suppresses the production of many CKs including IFN-γ and TNF-α [1]. This activity is mostly due to an effect on antigen presenting cells (APCs). IL-10 downregulates MHC class I and II antigen expression [2] and IL-12 synthesis by APCs [3] resulting in suppression of the secretion of IFN-γ, a CK which is responsible for macrophage activation and subsequent TNF-α secretion during MLR [4]. We have shown that IFN-γ and TNF-α release is proportional to the level of DR incompatibility [5,6]. In the present study, we have analysed the HLA control of IL-10 production during MLR and its relationship with IFN-γ and TNF-α.

Results and discussion

Our work shows that the HLA-DR control of IL-10 differs from that of IFN-γ and TNF-α revealing unexpected aspects of the regulation of the allogeneic response. Comparison of pairs differing by one versus two DR antigens discloses a dissociation between patterns of IFN-γ and TNF-α secretion on one hand and pattern of IL-10 secretion on the other. Indeed, the two DR mismatched (MM) configuration failed to increase IL-10 production as it was observed for IFN-γ and TNF-α. In view of the regulatory capacities of IL-10, we hypothesised that the 1DRMM (or one DR matched) configuration constituted a situation in which the two pro-inflammatory mediators, *i.e.* IFN-γ and TNF-α, were optimally controlled by IL-10. In order to validate this concept, we performed blocking experiments using anti-IL-10 and anti-IFN-γ neutralising antibodies to compare the 1DRMM vs 2DRMM configurations *(Figure 1)*. The

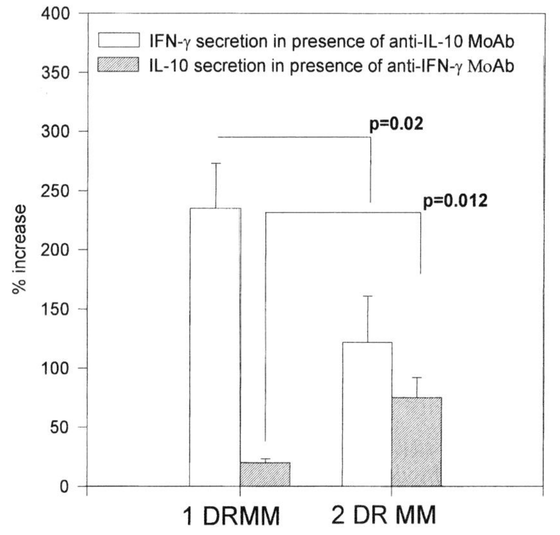

Figure 1. Influence of IL-10 (anti-IL-10) and IFN-γ (anti-IFN-γ) specific neutralising antibodies on IFN-γ and IL-10 production, respectively, in MLR involving subjects differing by one (1DRMM) or 2 (2DRMM) major HLA-DR disparities as defined by serology.

results of this analysis also favoured the hypothesis that IFN-γ constituted the triggering element of this immunoregulatory loop. Experiments using anti-IL-10 antibodies revealed that the 1DRMM setting was characterised by a much greater capacity of the antibody to increase IFN-γ and to a lesser extent TNF-α production than the 2DRMM setting. Conversely, neutralisation of IFN-γ restored the expected proportionality of IL-10 secretion according to the level of DR incompatibility. These data suggest that IFN-γ produced in a relative excess in the 2DRMM configuration is responsible for the unique pattern of IL-10 secretion. In order to evaluate whether other soluble suppressive factors such as IL-4 and TGF-β were involved in the control of MLR induced IFN-γ synthesis, we performed blocking experiments using anti-IL-4 and anti-TGF-β neutralising monoclonal antibodies. They were devoid of action ruling out an endogenous secretion of these CKs during MLR and suggesting that IL-10 constitutes the major suppressive factor controlling this process.

Based upon our experimental study, we propose the following scheme for the immunogenetic regulation of the allogeneic response and its relationship with HLA-DR molecules: the triggering of the TCR by the HLA-peptides complex induces IFN-γ secretion by T lymphocytes. This cytokine acting as a macrophage activating factor (MAF) induces the release of TNF-α which costimulates T cells. Macrophages also produce IL-10 which inhibits IFN-γ secretion and thereby constitutes a negative regulatory feed-back loop. IL-10 secretion is likely to be induced at least partially by TNF-α itself. The interaction between pro-inflammatory (IFN-γ and TNF-α) and anti-inflammatory (IL-10) CKs is differentially regulated by DR antigens. The fact that, in the 2DRMM configuration, neutralisation of IFN-γ produced in excess leads to maximal IL-10 secretion could represent the *in vitro* correlate of *in vivo* immunosuppression by ciclosporine and steroids which are agents inhibiting IFN-γ secretion. This could explain the apparent paradox of good functioning of some HLA-DR incompatible allografts. The optimal control of IFN-γ by IL-10 in the 1DRMM setting is reminiscent of the beneficial effect of one-DR-matched pre-transplant blood transfusion on allograft survival [7]. This *in vitro* finding could constitute the basis of functional assays aimed at the monitoring of planned blood transfusion prior to transplantation.

This work was supported by the Fonds National de la Recherche Scientifique (FNRS).

References

1. Bejarano MT, de Waal Malefyt R, Bigler M, Abrams JS, Bachetta R, de Vries JE, Roncarolo MG. Interleukin 10 inhibits allogeneic proliferative and cytotoxic T cell responses generated in primary mixed lymphocyte cultures. *Int Immunol* 1993; 12:1389-97.
2. De Waal Malefyt R, Haanen J, Spits H, Roncarolo MG, te Velde A, Figdor C, Johnson K, Kastelein R, Yssel H, de Vries JE. Interleukin 10 (IL-10) and viral IL-10 strongly reduce antigen-specific human T cell proliferation by diminishing the antigen-presenting capacity of monocytes *via* downregulation of class II major histocompatibility complex expression. *J Exp Med* 1991; 174:915-24.
3. D'Andrea A, Aste-Amezaga M, Valiante NM, Ma X, Kubin M, Trinchieri G. Interleukin-10 (IL-10) inhibits human lymphocyte interferon-γ production by suppressing natural killer cell stimulatory factor/IL-12 synthesis in accessory cells. *J Exp Med* 1993; 178:1041-8.
4. Toungouz M, Denys C, Andrien M, De Groote D, Dupont E. IL-12 unmasks HLA class I differences during MLR induced IFN-γ production. *Hum Immunol* 1995; 44:145-55.
5. Toungouz M, Denys C, Andrien M, De Groote D, Dupont E. Tumor necrosis factor-α and interleukin-6 production induced by variations of DR4 polymorphism during primary mixed lymphocyte reaction. *Transplantation* 1994; 58: 1393-8.
6. Toungouz M, Denys C, Andrien M, De Groote D, Dupont E. Optimal control of IFN-γ and TNF-α by IL-10 produced in response to one HLA-DR mismatch during the primary mixed lymphocyte reaction. *Transplantation* 1996; 61: 497-502.
7. Lagaaij EL, Hennemann PH, Ruigrok M, de Haan MW, Persijn GG, Termijtelen A, Hendriks GFJ, Weimar W, Claas FHJ, van Rood JJ. Effect of one - HLA-DR-antigen-matched blood transfusions on survival of heart and kidney allografts. *N Engl J Med* 1989; 321:702-5.

Is HLA-DP a kidney transplantation antigen ?

D.J. Cook, L. Roeske, D. Goldfarb, V.W. Dennis, A.P. Koo, A.C. Novick, E.E. Hodge

Transplantation Center, The Cleveland Clinic Foundation, 9500 Euclid Avenue, Cleveland, Ohio 44195, USA

HLA compatibility has been well established as a factor influencing the outcome of clinical kidney transplantation. Even with the powerful immunosuppressants now available, rejection and graft losses continue to occur, and it seems clear that it is the recognition of mismatched HLA antigens that initiates the immune responses that may result in the loss of the transplant. With the advent of molecular approaches for the determination of nucleotide sequences, it has become obvious that the HLA system is far more polymorphic than was thought, and this fact suggests that a reevaluation of the concept of "compatibility" in transplantation within the context of our current understanding of this histocompatibility complex is warranted.

Results and discussion

Of the testing performed for kidney transplantation, it is the crossmatch that has the greatest impact in terms of the selection of compatible donor-recipient pairs. With the rather wide range of sensitive techniques now available, it is not uncommon that positive anti-donor reactions are observed that are considered to be an acceptable risk when weighed against the potential benefit to the patient of proceeding with the transplant. We recently had such a case involving a sensitized candidate awaiting a third transplant and an HLA-A,B,DR zero antigen mismatch donor offered through the UNOS mandatory share program. The patient's first transplant was from his father, a second was from a cadaver donor, and his PRA at the time of the third transplant was 56% against a T cell panel and 88% against B cells. Donor and recipient were serologically matched for HLA-A (2,3), B (35,62) as well as for DR (8,13) and DQ (4,6), with a mismatch detected at HLA-C (patient 3,4, donor 3,7). Both T and B cell cytotoxic crossmatches were negative (one-wash technique), however flow cytometry revealed borderline T cell and a strong B cell reaction involving IgG. As it seemed unlikely that the patient would have a better opportunity for a compatible donor, the decision was made to perform the transplant. In addition to our standard quadruple immunosuppression (anti-thymocyte globulin, cyclosporine A, azathioprine and steroids), plasma exchange was initiated following the transplant, 3 times a week for 2 weeks.

The patient experienced delayed graft function in spite of the aggressive immunosuppression, with the serum creatinine reaching a nadir of 3.1 mg/dl on day 36, increasing soon after. Flow cytometry crossmatches utilizing serum samples obtained following the transplant revealed a decrease of approximately 60% of the binding to the donor B cells, and the levels continued to decrease during the period of plasma exchange. Detectable B cell reactions continued posttransplant, with no T cell reactions identified. As the original drop in B cell reactivity was most likely due to absorption of antibody by the transplanted kidney, these reactions may have been involved in the loss of the graft which occurred at 3 months without significant improvement in function.

After the transplant, both the donor and recipient were typed using a high resolution SSO approach for the DRB1, DQB1 and DPB1 loci. They were found to be identical for both DRB1 and DQB1, but mismatched at DPB1. In order to explore the possibility that the B cell reactivity that was noted against the donor cells may have been a result of presensitization due to mismatches common with one or both of the earlier transplants, cryopreserved lymphocytes from both the earlier cadaver donor (9 years before the current transplant) and the original transplant involving the patient's father five years prior to that, were used for SSO typing. The complete HLA types of the patient and all three donors are given in *Table I*. While both of the original transplants involved DPB1 mismatches, these mismatched antigens were not shared with the third donor.

Table I. HLA types of patient and donors

	A	B	C	DRB1	DQB1	DPB1
Patient	2	35	4	0801	0402	1901
	3	62	3	1301	0603	0401
Father	2	44	3	0401	0302	4701
	3	62	-	1301	0603	0401
CAD1	2	35	4	0101	0501	0401
	11	-	-	1104	0301	0301
CAD2	2	35	3	0801	0402	02012
(OMM)	3	62	7	1301	0603	0402

While HLA-DPB1 mismatches were identified in all three transplants, there were no HLA alleles that were previously mismatched that might explain the positive B cell crossmatch detected.

While we did not identify a DPB1 allele that might explain the observed positive crossmatch, we were able to examine antibody reactivity in sera obtained before and after the transplants using both of the original donors as targets. Only rather weak B cell reactions were identified by flow cytometry in serum obtained prior to the first transplant, however following the loss of this graft and prior to the second graft, strong T and B cell reactions were identified that persisted at the time of the third transplant. Of perhaps more interest were the reactions against the second transplant. The serum from the time of the first transplant was negative against this donor, but subsequent sera were all positive against B cells of this donor. It appears that this patient may have lost his second as well as third transplanted kidney at least in part due to alloantibodies with an apparent class II reactivity.

In an attempt to explain the apparent DPB1 reactivity, we observed that was not associated with previously mismatched DPB1 alleles, we examined the amino acid sequences of the pertinent alleles. As summarized in *Table II*, a number of amino acid differences were identified that were shared with one of the previous transplants and the OMM donor. Of the five possible shared amino acid sequences, it would seem that only the "DE" found at position 55 is a likely candidate for being involved in this case. This mismatch was present in the second donor (DPB1*0301) as well as in both of mismatched alleles of the OMM donor. The other sequences would not seem to be candidates, as the sequences identified were common with one of the patient's DPB1 alleles, although mismatched with the other. Given that there is little data available at this time regarding the immunogenicity of HLA differences at this level [1,2], it is at least conceivable that the mismatched sequences may have been responsible for the positive crossmatch that was detected

While this case certainly does not establish unequivocally whether or not HLA-DP mismatches are a significant factor in kidney transplantation, it does bring up some interesting issues. First, well matched kidney

Table II. DPB1 amino acid residues previously mismatched that were common to the OMM donor

DPB1	Allele	30 40	50 60	70 80 90
PAT	DPB1*0401	IYNREEF***AR***FDS	TELGRP***AA***EYWN	E***K***RAVPDRMCRHNYEL***GGPM***TLQ
	DPB1*1901	IYNREEFVRFDS	TELGRP***EA***EYWN	E***E***RAVPDRICRHNYELDEAVTLQ
LRD	DPB1*4701	IYNREEF***VR***FDS	TELGRP***EA***EYWN	E***E***RAVPDR***M***CRHNYEL***GGPM***TLQ
CAD1	DPB1*0301	IYNREEF***VR***FDS	TELGRP***DE***DYWN	E***K***RAVPDRVCRHNYEL***DEAV***TLQ
OMM	DPB1*02012	IYNREEF***VR***FDS	TELGRP***DE***EYWN	E***E***RAVPDR***M***CRHNYEL***GGPM***TLQ
	DPB1*0402	IYNREEF***VR***FDS	TELGRP***DE***EYWN	E***K***RAVPDR***M***CRHNYEL***GGPM***TLQ

Amino acids that were mismatched in the earlier transplants that were also found in phenotype of the third donor (shown in bold italic type). The mismatched "DE" at position 55-56 found in the DPB1 *0301 of the first cadaver donor and both DPB1 alleles of the OMM donor might explain the B cell crossmatch that was observed.

transplants such as those obtained under the UNOS mandatory share system, offer, in addition to excellent results [3], a cohort of transplants that may ultimately allow the study of both allele level mismatches, as well as examining the influence of loci not being considered by the algorithm such as HLA-C, DQ and DP. It would seem the best opportunity to examine the influence of mismatches at individual HLA loci will be in cases where there are no mismatches at the other loci. The clinical significance of mismatches only detectable at the DNA level is also a question that may be best studied in well matched grafts. This case also illustrates that even in a donor-recipient pair with no identifiable HLA mismatches, a positive crossmatch should not be considered to be without associated risk, particularly in cases involving regrafts. And finally, when considering the question of compatibility in organ transplantation, HLA-DP should not be forgotten. This highly polymorphic loci could be responsible for cases of rejection, but has not yet been implicated due to the fact that few laboratories are typing for HLA-DP.

References

1. Middleton D, Savage DA, Trainor F, Taylor A. Matching for various HLA class II loci in cadaveric renal transplantation using DNA techniques. *Transplantation* 1992;53:1138-41.
2. Middleton D, Mytillineos Y, Savage DA *et al.* Matching for HLA-DPB1 alleles in zero mismatched HLA-A,B and -DR renal transplants. *Transplant Proc* 1992;24:2439-501.
3. Takemoto S, Terasaki PI, Cecka JM *et al.* Survival of nationally shared, HLA-matched kidney transplants from cadaveric donors. *N Engl J Med* 1992; 327:834-9.

Impact of the "new" MHC-encoded genes (HLA-DMA,-DMB and LMP2) on kidney graft outcome

D. Chevrier[1], M. Giral[2], J.Y. Muller[1], J.P. Soulillou[2], J.D. Bignon[1]

1 Centre de Transfusion Sanguine, 34, boulevard Jean Monnet, BP349, 44011 Nantes Cedex, France
2 Institut de Transplantation et de Recherche en Transplantation, CHRU, Hôtel Dieu and INSERM U211, 44035 Nantes, France

In a previous study exploring the relationship between TAP1 and TAP2 gene polymorphism and compatibility on the fate of renal allograft, we showed that the currently described TAP1 and TAP2 gene polymorphisms did not influence the kidney transplant rejection outcome. Here we investigated for the first time whether the currently described polymorphism of HLA-DMA [1], -DMB [2], and LMP2 [3] genes are associated with differences in kidney graft outcome. In addition, we looked at the effect of these genes which could reflect the need for a more extended matching for this crucial genomic region in kidney allografting. For this purposes, 105 donors recipients couples were selected on the criteria of occurence of several rejection episodes and compared to 101 additional ones who never experienced rejection. Our data suggest that, in these clinical conditions tested, matching for all the new described HLA class II located genes does not influence the renal graft outcome. However, an increase of DMA*0102 allele was observed in the recipients of the rejection group when compared to those of the no-rejection group. This lattest observation could suggest a peculiar role of this specific allele in the exogenous pathway of class II presentation regarding the rejection of kidney transplant.

Patients, materials and methods

Patients and controls

We studied a selected population of 206 kidney recipients grafted in our institution between 1987 and 1993. They all received a sequential therapy with first, a bioreagent *(see below)*, steroïd and azathioprine followed by a maintenance treatment, based on cyclosporine A. This population was divided in two groups: (1) 105 patients with two or more acute cellular rejection episodes; and (2) 101 patients without any rejection episode.

One hundred healthy and geographically matched blood donors, previously HLA-DR,-DQ typed, were retrospectively typed for DMA, DMB, and LMP2 gene polymorphism and used as controls for frequency analysis.

DNA extraction

Genomic DNAs from recipients and controls were isolated from the peripheral blood lymphocytes by salting out extraction [4]. Genomic DNA from cadaveric donors was isolated from spleen cells by the same technic.

HLA-DMA, HLA-DMB and HLA class II typing

The HLA-DRB1 locus and the four HLA-DMA as well as the four HLA-DMB alleles were typed by PCR-SSO. We used oligonucleotide primers and oligoprobes previously described for HLA-DMA and DMB [5].

For LMP2 typing, PCR conditions were the same as for TAP gene [6,8], and following primers were specially designed :

LMP2-P1 : 5' TGATTTCTCGTATGGTAACTGCCTG 3'
LMP2-(ARG) : 5' CTGAACCAGAGAGTGCACAGTA-GAGGC 3'
LMP2-(HIS) : 5' GTCCCCGCTGCACGACCA 3'
LMP2-P4 : 5' TTGAACCAGGGAGGCGAAGT 3'

Statistical analysis

Statistical significances were determined by the chi-square test using the Yates correction when it was necessary.

Results

HLA-DR matching

The rates of HLA-DR mismatches (0 *versus* 2 mismatches) between recipients and donors were respectively of 18.1% and 29.5% for the rejection group *versus* 21.8% and 14.8% for the "no-rejection" group. These results indicate that HLA-DR matchings between recipients and donors were statistically different ($p<0.05$), between the "rejection" and "no-rejection" groups.

Typing of LMP2 and DMB alleles

In contrast to HLA-DR, we did not observed any effect of matching for these genes between the two groups. Moreover, the allelic distribution of LMP2 and DMB genes were not different neither between the two selected groups nor between recipients and donors of each group compared to controls (data not shown).

Typing of DMA alleles

As for the former genes studied (LMP and DMB), we did not observed any impact of DMA gene matching on the graft outcome. More interestingly, we observed *(Table I)* a significant increase of DMA*0102 allelic frequency in recipients of the rejection group when compared to that of the no-rejection group (14.8% *versus* 6.9%; pc<0.05).

Table I. HLA-DMA frequencies in recipients and controls

HLA-DMA alleles	Controls n=200	Rejection n=210	No-rejection n=202
DMA*0101	81%	78.1 %	87.1 %
DMA*0102	12 %	**14.8* %**	**6.9* %**
DMA*0103	2%	5.7 %	4.9 %
DMA*0104	5%	1.4 %	1.0 %

n=number of allele tested
*p=0.01 and pc<0.05.

Discussion

Since the discovery of new polymorphic genes TAP1, TAP2 and LMP2 involved in the classical pathway of presentation by MHC class I molecules, and HLA-DMA and -DMB involved in pathway of presentation by MHC class II molecules, we investigated the possible role of these polymorphisms in kidney allograft rejection. Typing DMA, DMB and LMP2 gene polymorphisms in two selected populations of kidney recipients (rejection and no-rejection), indicated, as we already described for TAP1 and TAP2, no impact of these donors and recipients gene matchings on the kidney transplant rejection outcome in contrast to the HLA-DRB1 locus matching.

Interestingly, we observed a significant increase of the DMA*0102 allele frequency in the recipients of the rejection group when compared to that observed in the no-rejection group. This difference did not seem to be explained by any linkage disequilibrium between HLA-DRB1 and DMA alleles. This observtion could define a peculiar role of this allele in the recipient immune response against the transplant, leating to an amplified host T-cell response. However, this data must be confirmed by other independant studies before to conclude to a pejorative effect of this DMA*0102 allele on kidney transplant outcome.

Work supported by grants from the European Communauty (BIO 2CT CT920300) and from Agence Française du Sang (FORTS).

References

1. Carrington M, Harding A. Sequence analysis of two novel HLA-DMA alleles. *Immunogenetics* 1994 : 40 : 165.
2. Carrington M, Yeager M, Mann D. Characterization of HLA-DMB polymorphism. *Immunogenetics* 1993 : 38 : 446-9.
3. Kelly A, Powis SH, Glynne R, Radley E, Beck S, Trowsdale J. Second proteasome-related gene in the human MHC class II region. *Nature* 1991: 353 : 667-8.
4. Kimura A, Sasazuki T. Reference protocol for the DNA-typing technique. *HLA, 11th International Histocompatibility Workshop,* vol.1. In Sasazuki T *et al.* eds. Oxford : Oxford University Press, 1992.
5. Teisserenc H, Charron D. Technical handbook of the twelfth international histocompatibility workshop. Addendum 12-1994. In Charron D, Fauchet R, eds. *HLA et Médecine,* 1994.
6. Newton CR, Graham A, Heptinstall LE, Powell SJ, Summers C, Kalsheker N, Smith JC, Markham AF. Analysis of any point mutation in DNA. The amplification refractory mutation system (ARMS). *Nucleic Acids Res* 1989 : 17 : 2503-16.
7. Powis SH, Tonks S, Mockridge I, Kelly AP, Trowsdale J. Alleles and haplotypes of the MHC encoded ABC transporters TAP1 and TAP2. *Immunogenetics* 1993 : 37 : 373-80.
8. Chevrier D, Giral M, Braud V, Bourbigot B, Muller JY, Bignon JD, Soulillou JP. Effects of MHC-encoded TAP1 and TAP2 gene polymorphism and matching on kidney graft rejection. *Transplantation* 1995 : 60 : 292-6.

HLA in Haematopoietic Cell Transplantation

Contents

Influence of donor-recipient HLA-Cw disparity on outcome of unrelated bone marrow transplants

Z. Tatari[1], H. Esperou[2], C. Chastang[3], C. Fortier[1], R. Tamouza[1], E. Gluckman[2], D. Charron[1], C. Raffoux[1]

1 Laboratoire d'Immunologie et d'Histocompatibilité, Hôpital Saint-Louis, 1, avenue Claude Vellefaux, 75010 Paris, France
2 Service de Greffe de Moelle, Hôpital Saint-Louis, Paris, France
3 Département de Biostatistique, Hôpital Saint-Louis, Paris, France

Allogeneic bone marrow transplantation (BMT) has been increasingly used to cure leukemia, aplastic anemia, immune and genetic disorders [1]. In clinical transplantation, donor and host are in general genotypically identical at the major histocompatibility antigens. The fate of marrow grafts depend on many factors, including conditioning regimens, immunosuppression after transplantation and the degree of histocompatibility between donor and recipient. However, allogeneic bone marrow transplantation is limited by the availability of suitable HLA-compatible donors, risk of donor-host immunologic reaction, especially graft rejection and GVHD, and risk of opportunistic infection. Clinically serious GVHD disease occurs in 20 to 50 percent of patients receiving marrow grafts from HLA identical siblings and some symptoms of the disease occur in 60 to 80 percent [2]. Successful engraftment of bone marrow is more likely if donor and recipient have identical HLA class I and II molecules [3]. Unfortunately the serological HLA-A,B,Cw, typing that has been practiced for the last twenty five years does not satisfy these requirements. Many of the serological antigens defined are not a unique allele but a group of alleles, which though closely related in structure have differences capable of stimulating alloreactive T cells [4]. Furthermore, some alleles cannot be defined by serology. These "blanks" alleles are particularly frequent at the HLA-Cw locus [5] and in non Caucasian populations. Indeed a recent analysis of donor recipient pairs in bone marrow transplantation showed that individuals typed serologically homozygous for HLA-C were heterozyous by DNA sequencing and that serologically matched individuals were mismatched on the basis of sequence [6]. As a consequence of the imprecision in HLA-C typing, the role of this locus as a transplantation determinant has not been defined. This report records the results of the 110 consecutive patients with malignant and nonmalignant disorders who have undergone an unrelated donor marrow transplantation. We compared Cw identical and Cw distinct pairs as observed by molecular biology typing of the HLA-Cw alleles by PCR-RFLP.

Patients and methods

Patients

110 patients who underwent allogeneic bone marrow transplantation in French hospitals between January 1988 to May 1994 with malignant (n=93) or non-malignant (n=17) hematologic diseases were studied for HLA-Cw genotyping. Diagnoses are summarized in *Table I.* The median age of patients was 27 years (range 6.0 m to 52.0 years). 61 patients were male and 49 were female. The median interval between inscription on the Bone Marrow Volunteer Donors Registries and transplantation was 11.8 months (range 2.0 to 44.0).

Table I. Disease distribution in 110 patients

Diagnosis	N=110
CML	52
ALL	28
ANLL (acute non lymphoblastic leukemia)	7
MDS (myelodysplasia)	6
Non malignant diseases	17

HLA typing

Serology was performed by complement-dependent cytotoxicity for HLA-A, -B loci. For patients and their selected unrelated donors, DRB1, DQA1 and DQB1 high resolution typing was performed by PCR-SSO using sequence specific probes from XIth Histocompatibility Workshop. For HLA-Cw typing PCR-restriction fragments length polymorphisms was used (5). HLA-A2 subtyping was performed by PCR-SSO [7] and HLA-B27 and -B44 were subtyped by DGGE (denaturing gel gradient electrophoresis) technique [8].

GVHD

Reports were based on observations from individual investigators. Criteria for diagnosis and treatment were based on institutional practice. The diagnosis of acute GVHD was made on the basis of appropriate clinical findings within 100 days of transplants and was confirmed by biopsy of skin and/or gastrointestinal tract and was graded according to the criteria of Sale *et al.* [9]

Engraftment and relapse

Criteria for diagnosis were haematological and were based on the absolute neutrophil count (ANC) $\leqslant 500/\mu l$ and platelet count $\geqslant 50\ 000/\mu l$ without transfusion. Time to relapse was defined as the time of reappearance of morphologic leukaemic blasts or reappearance of a specific chromosomal abnormality.

Data collection

Transplantation was performed at 4 French centres. Donors were provided through the European Donor Secretariat (EDS) and France Greffe de Moelle (FGM) located in Saint-Louis Hospital, Paris, France.

The major clinical criteria studied are acute and chronic GVHD and survival . Event times were measured from date of transplantation to date of neutrophil recovery, acute GVHD, relapse, death or last follow-up examination. Survival was defined as time elapsed until death. Event-free survival (for patients with malignant disease) was defined as time to relapse or death, whichever occurred first.

Results and discussion

HLA matching is an important factor to take into account in allogeneic bone marrow transplantation. The risk and severity of GVHD are correlated with recipient HLA incompatibility.

We have analyzed 110 donor recipient pairs transplanted between 1988 to 1994 with unrelated donors. The median fellow up is 4 years. All of the donor recipient pairs were HLA class I(A B) identical by serology and HLA-DRB1and DQB1 identical by molecular biology (PCR-SSO). The HLA-Cw genotyping was performed using the PCR-RFLP technique developed in our laboratory.

The study of the factors influencing GVHD shows that 3 factors significantly correlated with the incidence of the GVHD: age (p: 0.03) , hematological status of disease at the time of BMT (p:0.008) and especially HLA-Cw (p:0.002). The p value of HLA-Cw disparities is confirmed using a Cox model with age, risk and HLA-Cw disparity as covariates. The relative risk (RR: 1.943 CI: 1.216 - 3.106) of severe GVHD (grade > II) for the patient who have been transplanted with HLA-Cw mismatched donors is twice greater than patients grafted with HLA-Cw identical donor. However, a Cox model using risk and GVHD as covariates fails to suggest the role of HLA-Cw disparity on survival.

Furthermore, a subpopulation genotyped for HLA-A2 by PCR-SSO and for HLA-B44 and -B27 by DGGE (Denaturant Gradient Gel Electrophoresis) has been studied. The results show that among 28 patients grafted with HLA-Cw matched donors, only in one case, donor and recipient had an HLA-A subtype different. In contrast, among 27 patients transplanted with HLA-Cw mismatched donors, 10 cases of discrepancy for HLA-A or B have been observed.

In conclusion, HLA-Cw disparity influences the incidence of severe GVHD occuring after BMT with unrelated donors. However, we have not observed a significant correlation between the graft survival and GVHD incidence. Other factors as infection or toxicity directly influence the patients survival. Furthermore, this study shows clearly that HLA-Cw has a reliable value to predict the homogeneity or the disparity in the other class I loci, particularly concerning HLA-B disparities.

References

1. Gratwohl A, Hermans J. EBMT survey on bone marrow transplant activity in Europe: regional differences. *Bone Marrow Transplant* 1994; 13: 683-8.
2. O'Reilly RJ, Keever C, Kernan NA, Bordignon C, Flomenberg N. Graft host interactions following T-cell depleted marrow tranplants. In: Melchers F, *et al.*, eds. *Progress in immunology,* vol. 7. New York: Springer-Verlag, 1989: 1185-94.

3. Anasetti C, Amos D, Beatty PG, Appelbaum FR, Bensinger W, Buckner CD *et al.* Effect of HLA compatibility on engraftment of bone marrow transplants in patients with leukemia or lymphoma. *N Engl J Med* 1989; 320: 197-204.
4. Lòpez de Castro JA. HLA-B27 and HLA-A2 subtypes: structure, evolution and function. *Immunol Today* 1989; 10: 230-46.
5. Tatari Z, Fortier C, Babrynina V, Loiseau P, Charron D, Raffoux C. HLA-Cw allele analysis by PCR-restriction fragment length polymorphism: study of known and additional alleles. *Proc Natl Acad Sci USA* 1995; 92: 8803-7.
6. Santamaria P, Reinsmoen NL, Lindstrom AL, Boyce-Jacino MT, Barbosa JJ, Faras AJ *et al.* Frequent HLA class I and DP sequence mismatches in serologically (HLA-A, HLA-B, HLA-DR) and molecularly (HLA-DRB1, HLA-DQA1, HLA-DQB1) HLA-identical unrelated bone marrow transplant pairs. *Blood* 1994; 83: 280-7.
7. Tiercy JM, Djavad N, Rufer N, Speiser DE, Jeannet M, Roosnek E. Oligotyping of HLA-A2, -A3, and -B44 subtypes. Detection of subtype incompatibilities between patients and their serologically matched unrelated bone marrow donors. *Hum Immunol* 1994; 41: 207-15.
8. Tamouza R, Marzais F, Krishnamoorthy R, Besmond C, Raffoux C, Charron D. Rapid subtyping for HLA-B27 by denaturing gradient gel electrophoresis (DGGE). In: Charron D, ed. *Genetic diversity of HLA. Functional and medical implication*, vol. I. Sèvres, France: EDK, 1997.
9. Sale GE, Lertner KG, Baker EA, Shulman HM, Thomas ED. he skin biopsy in the diagnosis of acute graft versus host disease. *Am J Pathol* 1987; 389: 1197-203.

Sequence based detection of HLA class I mismatches for bone marrow transplantation

W. Hildebrand, L. Zhang, M. Ellexson, P. Chrétien, D. Confer

Department of Microbiology and Immunology, University of Oklahoma Health Sciences Center, PO Box 26901, Oklahoma City, OK 73190, USA

Understanding that serologic typing methods may fail to detect deleterious class I HLA polymorphisms in transplant patients [1], a host of molecular techniques are now being touted as "high resolution" alternatives to serologic class I HLA typing. In the research laboratory the most accurate class I type is obtained *via* HLA-A,B,C cloning, but the process of cloning and clone screening are too cumbersome and expensive for routine clinical HLA typing. However, two noteworthy developments have made it possible to obviate cloning for the development of a clinical DNA sequencing application. First, the fluorescent automated DNA sequencer has improved, simplified, and sped the collection of sequence data. Second, software advancements arriving with high throughput fluorescent DNA sequencing have simplified nucleotide sequence data collection and the comparison of collected sequences to a known database.

Building technological advances in DNA sequencing into a unique class I typing approach, cloning and the separation of clones into distinct populations have been eliminated from the class I DNA sequencing protocol (the methods applied are detailed in the sequence-based-typing component of the proceedings from the 12th IHWC). Briefly, RNA is extracted from the blood sample now collected for serologic class I typing, cDNA is synthesized, one PCR for each of the HLA-A,B,C loci is performed, and exons 2 and 3 from each locus are sequenced. The sequencing products are separated using a Pharmacia Biotech ALF DNA Sequencer, and heterozygote sequences are determined using the ALF manager base calling algorithm. Class I HLA subtypes are then automatically determined by the SBTyper software in a three step analysis process. First, the software automatically aligns the sample sequences at each locus with the concensus sequence derived from all alleles at that locus. Second, sample sequences are compared to all possible combinations of alleles contained in the database. Third, combinations of alleles that best match the sample sequences are listed in descending order. In total, 3 PCR reactions, 6 sequencing reactions, and 3 days are required to obtain a DNA sequence based HLA-A,B,C type with this approach.

Results and discussion

Applying this HLA-A,B,C sequence based typing technique for bone marrow transplant donor/recipient pairs, the bone marrow donor/recipient pair RD105U/RD105

Table I. Serologic and sequence based donor/recipient class I typing

	Donor RD105U		Recipient RD105	
Locus	Serologic	Sequence Based	Serologic	Sequence Based
A	A2,	A*0201,	A2	A*0201
	A24	A*2402	A24	A*2402
B	B7,	B*0702	B7	B*0702
	B39	***B*39011***	B39	***B*39062***
C	not typed	Cw*0702	not typed	Cw*0702

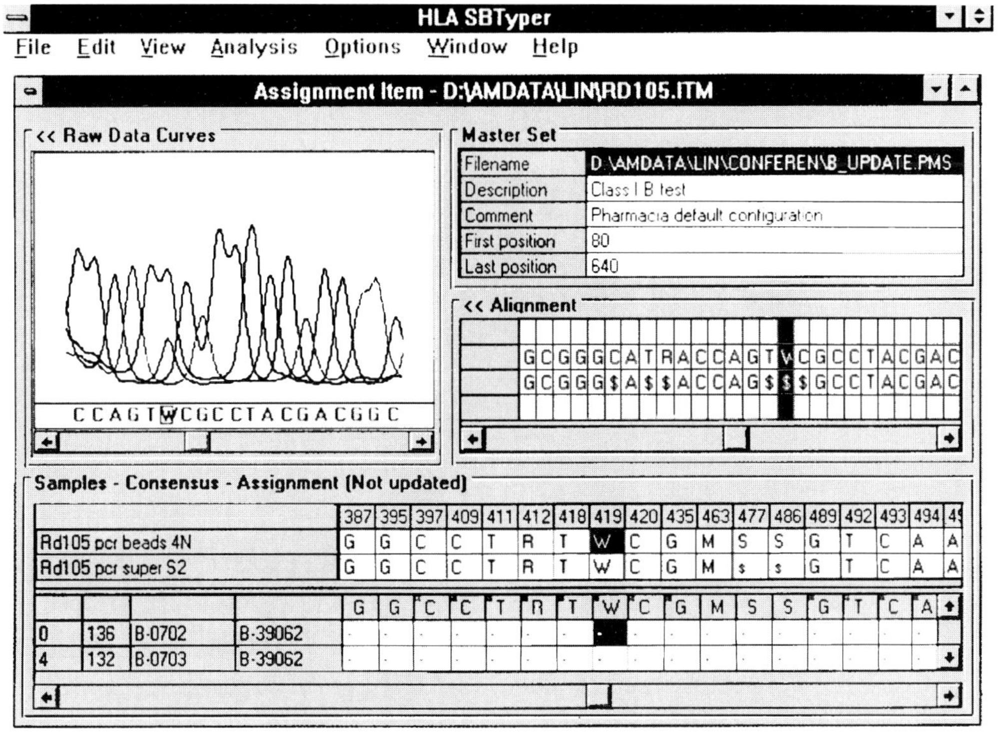

Figure 1. Screen capture of the Class I SBTyper software which assembles sequencing reads through exons 2 and 3 and compares the assembled sequence data to the class I HLA database. Note that in the bottom left hand rows of figure 1 the software determines which combination of class I alleles (in this case alleles B*0702/B*39062) best fits the data.

typed as A*0201/A*2402 and Cw*0702/Cw*0702 for both donor and recipient, while at the HLA-B locus B*0702/B*39011 was typed for the donor and B*0702/B*39062 for the recipient *(Table I).* Assigning HLA class I types to both donor and recipient was accomplished by loading raw DNA sequence data directly into the HLA SBTyper software package. An example of the typing result obtained with the HLA SBTyper is shown in *Figure 1:* the raw HLA-B sequence data for the transplant recipient RD105 was loaded into the SBTyper program, and in the bottom left portion of the screen-capture it can be seen that a class I type of B*0702/B*39062 was assigned with zero ambiguities. A view of the sequence chromatograms *(Figure 2)* confirms that the donor's B*39011 and the recipient's B*39062 alleles clearly differ (arrows, *Figure 2*). The data in *Figure 2* also demonstrates the ability of the ALF DNA Sequencer to accurately resolve positions of heterozygosity. The accuracy of the class I sequence based types were confirmed with traditional cloning and sequencing, and no discrepancies were observed between the results obtained.

Translating the alleles B*39011 and B*39062 reveals that the two class I heavy chains differ at amino acid positions 95 and 97 (Leu → Trp, Arg → Thr, respectively). Because patient RD105 suffers from chronic GVHD and was molecularly matched with the donor for DR/DQ, we questioned the role that the 95/97 mismatch might be playing in stimulating GVHD. Looking back to mouse studies, the donor-recipient B*39011-B*39062 mismatch becomes significant in terms of transplant success; mice differing only at amino acids 95 and 97 in the class I heavy chain reject reciprocal skin grafts [2]. Therefore, because mice differing solely at the positions where the RD105 BMT pair differ reject transplants, we hypothesize that the amino acid mismatches at positions 95 and 97 are contributing to the chronic GVHD in patient RD105, and the specificity of alloreactive cells gathered from the transplant recipient are being used to test this hypothesis.

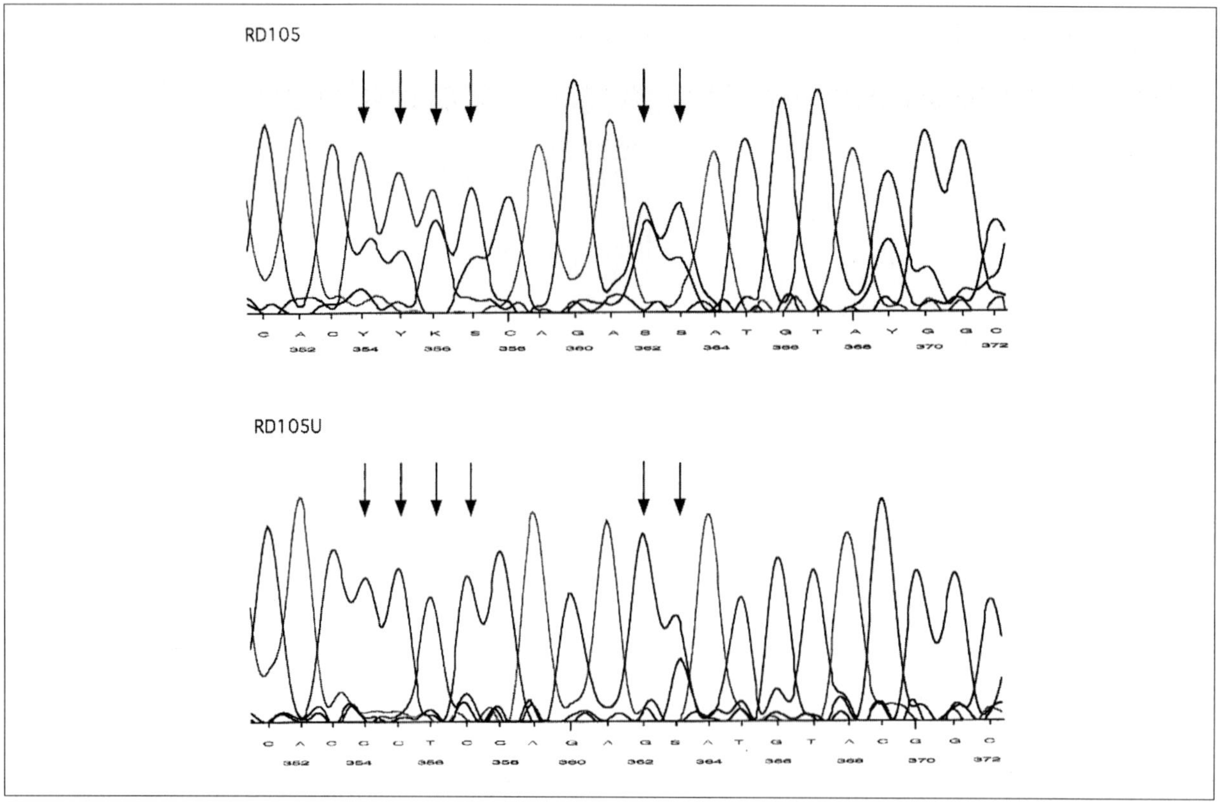

Figure 2. RD 105 and RD105U sequencing chromatograms. Heterozygous positions marked by arrows are apparent in the recipients B*0702/B*39062 combination (top panel) but absent in the donors B*0702/B*3901 combination (bottom panel).

In summary, we have developed a class I sequence-based method for the typing of bone marrow donor/recipient pairs. This method has the accuracy afforded by DNA sequencing and is coupled to a software package which facilitates the rapid assignment of a class I type. Thus, as demonstrated for the RD105U/RD105 donor/recipient pair typed herein, the HLA tissue typing community now has the option to provide an extremely accurate match for donor/recipient pairs with a straightforward DNA sequence-based approach.

References

1. Fleischhauer K, Kernan, NA, O'Reilly RJ, Dupont B, Yang SY. Bone marrow-allograft rejection by T lymphocytes recognizing a single amino acid difference in HLA-B44. *N Engl J Med* 1990; 323: 1818-22.
2. Horton RM, Hildebrand WH, Martinko JM, Pease LR. Structural analysis of H-2Kf and H-2Kfm1 using H-2K locus-specific sequences. *J Immunol* 1990; 145: 1782-7.

Evaluation of the limiting dilution cytotoxic T lymphocyte precursor frequency (fCTLp) assay in a multicenter study

J. Pei[1], C. Farrell[2], J.A. Hansen[1], T. Juji[3], C.A. Keever-Taylor[4], S. Knowles[5], B.D. Tait[6]

1 Fred Hutchinson Cancer Research Center, 1124 Columbia Street, Seattle, WA 98104-2092, USA
2 NSW Red Cross Blood Transfusion Service, Sydney, Australia
3 The Japanese Red Cross Blood Center, Tokyo, Japan
4 Medical College of Wisconsin, Milwaukee, USA
5 Red Cross Blood Bank, South Melbourne, Australia
6 Royal Melbourne Hospital, Parkville, Australia

The limiting dilution cytotoxic T lymphocyte precursor frequency (fCTLp) assay has been examined by a number of investigators as a histocompatibility test for donor selection based on the hypothesis that the frequency of donor CTLp responding to host alloantigens should predict graft-versus-host disease (GVHD) [1, 2]. However, published reports concerning the ability of fCTLp to predict GVHD have not been consistent [3, 4]. There may be differences in the way the assay is performed or intrinsic variation from assay to assay which may limit reproducibility. To assess inter-laboratory variation of fCTLp assay, two multicenter pilot projects were undertaken under the auspices of the 12th International Histocompatibility Workshop. Here we report the results of a collaborative pilot study undertaken by 6 Asian, Australian and North American laboratories.

Materials and methods

Peripheral blood mononuclear cells (PBMC) were isolated from 5 healthy individuals and cryopreserved in one laboratory, prior to distribution to each of the participating laboratories. Six CTLp assay combinations were selected to detect minor, class I or class II, and class I plus class II HLA disparities (*Table I*). Matching for HLA-A and B was based on phenotyping, and matching for DR and DQB1 was based on high resolution allele typing. These combinations were expected to generate a low, intermediate or high CTLp frequency.

Assays were set up by limiting dilution in U-bottom microculture plates containing responder PBMC in 50,000, 40,000, 30,000 and then in serial 2-fold dilutions from 20,000 to 1250 cells per well in 24 replicates, together with irradiated (3000 rad) stimulator PBMC at 50,000 cells per well. IL2, 15 U/ml in culture, was added on day 3 and 6. On day 10, effector cells were transfered to a new plate and assayed for cytolytic activity to 10,000 target cells (PHA blasts) in a 4 hour chrominum release assay.

The threshold for determing positive reactions was calculated by two methods:

1.Workshop method. 50,000 effector cells cultured with autologous target cells;

2. Kaminiski method. 10,000 target cells cultured alone.

The CTLp frequencies, 95% confidence intervals and

Table I. fCTLp assay combinations

fCTLp assay No.	Responder	Stimulator	Relationship*	Disparity from stimulator
1	01	02	R	Minor
2	01	03	UR	A23, B21, DRB1*0101
3	03	02	UR	Bw62
4	04	02	UR	DRB1*0401, DQw3
5	02	01	R	A32, B44
6	03	05	UR	B37, DRB1*0403

* R: responder and stimulator are related; UR: responder and stimulator are unrelated.

Table II. Results of fCTLp reported by participating laboratories*

Lab code	method	CTLp assay combination					
		No 1: 01x02	No 2: 01x03	No 3: 03x02	No 4: 04x02	No 5: 02x01	No 6: 03x05
A	Workshop	3 (1-5)	69 (55-83)	745 (525-966)	54 (39-68)@	117 (82-153)@	>2431
	Kaminski	15 (11-19)	209 (161-256)	209 (144-274)	155 (124-186)	161 (109-213)@	1253 (749-1758)
B	Workshop	14 (10-18)	257(138-376)	227 (180-275)	61 (45-76)	122 (87-157)	133 (103-163)
	Kaminski	8 (5-11)	221 (146-296)	234 (187-280)	98 (54-142)	91 (66-117)	186 (137-236)
C	Workshop	1 (0-3)	91 (70-112)	177 (117-238)@	27 (20-34)	55 (42-67)	68 (49-88)@
	Kaminski	1 (0-2)	57 (42-71)	139 (94-183)@	37 (27-47)	40 (30-50)	60 (43-76)@
D	Workshop	inv	inv	inv	62 (49-75)	inv	inv
	Kaminski	5 (3-7)@	21 (15-28)	45 (36-54)	31 (23-40)	4 (2-7)	21 (15-26)
E	Workshop	29 (23-37)	61 (48-77)	291 (218-387)	160 (108-211)@	35 (28-44)	101 (80-128)
	Kaminski	1 (0-2)	12 (9-16)	159 (109-20)	130 (90-170)@	21 (14-27)	27 (20-33)
F	Workshop	inv	inv	nd	nd	nd	nd
	Kaminski	1 (0-2)	6 (309)@	34 (27-42)	54 (41-68)	19 (14-24)	18 (13-23)

*results are CTLp per million of PBMC; ( ): 95% Confidence intervals of fCTLp; nd: not done; inv: invalid assay;
@: corrected fCTLp from invalid assay.

chi-square values were calculated by the minimum chi-square method of Taswell [5]. Each individual limiting dilution assay was considered to be valid if p value for the limiting dilution curve was greater than 0.05 by a linear regression analysis.

Results and discussion

Results of 32 assays analyzed by the Workshop method and 36 assays analyzed by the Kaminski method were reported by participating laboratories as shown above (*Table II*). Twelve of 32 (37.5%) Workshop assays and 7 of 36 (19.4%) Kaminski assays were invalid. From reviewing the data of the invalid assays it was apparent that some linear regression curves were skewed by a single abnormal data point. This was the case in 12 assays (5 involving Workshop method and 7 involving Kaminski method). After excluding the single aberrant data point the «corrected» limiting dilution curve gave an acceptable linear regression (corrected fCTLp marked «@»). There was substantial inter-laboratory variation in the estimated fCTLp per assay among the 6 laboratories regardless of which method was used to define background.

The *Table III* shows fCTLp median and rank for each assay analyzed by Kaminski method. The fCTLp were ranked from 1 (the lowest) to 6 (the highest) within individual laboratories. Rank is indicated by parentheses. Most laboratories correctly identified the assay generating the lowest fCTLp (assay No. 1) and the assay generating the highest fCTLp (assay No. 3). However, the fCTLp rank for the remaining assays was also variable from laboratory to laboratory. The rank order of fCTLp median was matched with overall rank for assay No.1 (the lowest) and No.3 (the highest), but not completely matched with these assays which fCTLp were in meddle. It also agrees that the lowest fCTLp and the highest fCTLp were easily to be identified in individual laboratory.

Table III. Comparison of fCTLp median and rank (Kaminski method)

	Lab code						fCTLp	
Assay No.	A	B	C	D	E	F	median	Overall rank*
1	15 (1)*	8 (1)	1 (1)	5 (2)	1 (1)	1 (1)	3	1
5	161 (3)	91 (2)	40 (3)	4 (1)	21 (3)	19 (4)	31	2
2	209 (4)	221 (5)	57 (4)	21 (4)	12 (2)	6 (2)	39	3
6	1253 (6)	186 (4)	60 (5)	21 (3)	27 (4)	18 (3)	44	5
4	155 (2)	98 (3)	37 (2)	31 (5)	130 (5)	54 (6)	76	4
3	209 (5)	234 (6)	139 (6)	45 (6)	159 (6)	34 (5)	149	6

( ): indicates the rank of fCTLp.
*: Overall rank is based on mean rank of each assay.

Conclusions

A standardized fCTLp assay was used to test aliquots of the same responder and stimulator pairs in 6 different laboratories. There was substantial inter-laboratory variation in the estimated fCTLp for same assay combinations, and also variation in the fCTLp rank order among six different responder-stimulator pairs tested from laboratory to laboratory. The assay generating the highest fCTLp and the assay generating the lowest fCTLp were able to be identified in most laboratories. These results indicate that further standardization should be achieved before the fCTLp assay can be reliably evaluated as a diagnostic tool for predicting GVHD in a multi-laboratory study.

References

1. Kaminski E, Hows J, Man S, Brookes P, Mackinnon S, Hughes T, Avakian O, Goldman JM, Batchelor JR. Prediction of graft versus host disease by frequency analysis of cytotoxic T cells after unrelated donor bone marrow transplantation. *Transplant* 1989; 48: 608-13.
2. Irschick EU, Hladik F, Niederwieser D, Nubbaumer W, Holler E, Kaminski E, Huber C. Studies on the mechanism of tolerance or graft-versus-host disease in allogeneic bone marrow recipients at the level of cytotoxic T cell precursor frequencies. *Blood* 1992; 79: 1622-8.
3. Fontaine P, Langlais J, Perreault C. Evaluation of in vitro cytotoxic T lymphocyte assays as a predictive test for the occurence of graft vs host disease. *Immunogenetics* 1991; 34: 222-6.
4. Van Els CACM, Bakker A, Zwinderman AH, Zwaan FE, Van Rood JJ, Goulmy E. Effector mechanisms in graft-versus-host disease in response to minor histocompatibility antigens. I. Absence of correlation with cytotoxic effector cells. *Transplant* 1990; 50: 62-6.
5. Taswell C. Limiting dilution assays for the determination of immunocompetent cell frequencies. I. Data analysis. *J Immunol* 1981; 126: 1614-9.

Molecular characterization of HLA-Cw incompatibilities recognised by alloreactive cytotoxic T lymphocytes

C. Grundschober, N. Rufer, M. Jeannet, E. Roosnek, J.M. Tiercy

Transplantation Immunology Unit, Division of Immunology and Allergology, Hôpitaux Universitaires de Genève, 1211 Geneva 4, Switzerland

The increased incidence of post-transplant complications after transplantation with bone marrow from unrelated donors reflects the high frequency of HLA incompatibilities that are not resolved by standard tissue typing. These serologically hidden mismatches are detected by cellular typing techniques, such as the mixed lymphocyte culture (MLC) for HLA class II and the cytotoxic T lymphocyte precursor frequency (CTLpf) analysis [1] for HLA class I. However full characterization of these mismatches can only be done by molecular typing methods. Clinical studies have shown an influence of HLA-AB [2-4] and DRB1 [5] matching on outcome in bone marrow transplantation (BMT) with unrelated donors, but poor serological definition of HLA-C antigens has precluded a thorough evaluation of their importance in BMT.

During the past few years we have been involved in the development of molecular and cellular typing techniques aimed at the precise characterization of HLA-A and -B incompatibilities that remain undisclosed by serology. We have previously shown that the degree of class I [6,7] and class II [8] incompatibilities in donor/recipient (D/R) pairs who were ABDR1-14-matched by serology was surprisingly high [1].

Since a number of CTLp-positive combinations could not be explained by HLA-A or B-subtype mismatches we have analysed HLA-C polymorphism by sequencing and by PCR/SSO-oligotyping. Our study demonstrates that HLA-C mismatches are recognised by CTLs and that the degree of HLA-C incompatibilities is high and varies as a function of ABDR haplotypes.

Patients, donors and methods

97 patients and their 272 unrelated donors selected from international registries were typed by serology for HLA-AB, and by SSO-oligotyping [9] and PCR-SSP for DRB1/B3/B5. Subtypes of HLA-A2, A3, B7, B35, B44, B51 were determined by oligotyping. For HLA-C oligotyping exons 2+3 were amplified [10] and hybridised with 27 DIG-labeled SSO probes identifying polymorphisms at codons H21, Q35, sP47 (s=silent substitution), A73, T73, S77, N77-K80, R91, I95, S99, C99, sY99, W97-F99, sP105, H113-L116, D114-S116, sT134, L147, A152, A152-Q156, T152, E155, W156, Q156, E163, L163, G170 [11]. Full length cDNA from a Cw*1601 bone marrow donor was transfected by electroporation in the class I-negative cell line 721.221 using the pBJI-Neo vector. After testing the expression of Cw*1601 by FACS analysis using the anti-class I antibody W6/32 the transfected cell line was used in a conventional cytotoxicity chromium release assay with the CTL clone. CTLpf analysis was done as described [1].

Results and discussion

High resolution typing of ABDR1-14 matched D/R pairs showed that <30% of the donors were compatible on the basis of AB-subtype, DRB1/B3/B5-oligo and of a negative CTLpf test. In particular 47% of the pairs displayed a positive pre-transplant CTLp test that was shown to correlate precisely with HLA-A or -B subtype incompatibilities. Oligotyping for allelic subtypes of antigens known to be frequently mismatched (A2, B7, B35, B44) have now been introduced in our unrelated donor selection procedure. Because of linkage disequilibrium, the rate of HLA-AB-subtype matching increases with the degree of matching for DRB1/DRB3/DRB5 [1,6,7].

We first performed exon 2 and 3 locus C sequencing on three positive CTLp combinations that were matched by oligotyping for AB-subtype and for DRB1/B3/B5. The results showed that the target molecules were HLA-C

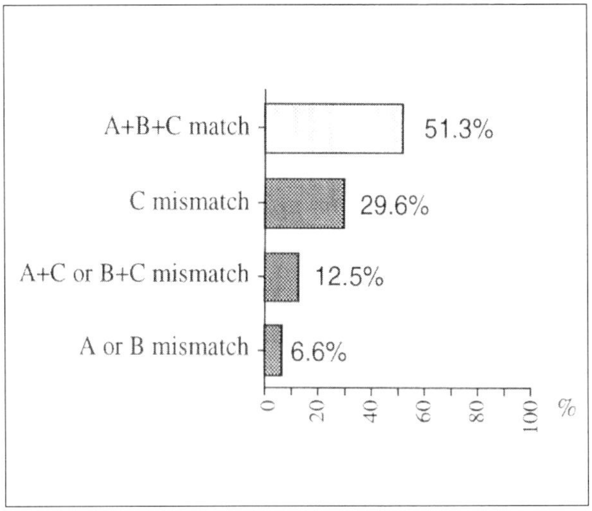

Figure 1. Degree of HLA matching in HLA-AB-sero and DRB1/B3/B5-oligo identical unrelated pairs.
73 patients and their 184 unrelated potential donors, selected on the basis of HLA-AB serology and DRB1/B3/B5 oligotyping identity, were subtyped for HLA-A2, A3, B7, B35, B41, B44, B51 and HLA-C by oligotyping. HLA matching was assessed in the resulting 287 pairwise combinations.

Table I. Linkage disequilibrium between HLA-B and -C

HLA-B		HLA-C *	% of B associated with C allele
B*0702	n=48	Cw*0702	100
B*13	n=17	Cw*0602	100
B*4001	n=17	Cw*0304	100
B*57	n=15	Cw*0602	100
B*14	n=19	Cw*0802	95
B*38	n=18	Cw*1203	94
B*08	n=45	Cw*0701	87
B*3501	n=52	Cw*0401	83
B*4402	n=62	Cw*0501	82
B62	n=34	Cw*0303	68
B*18	n=43	Cw*0701	60
B*4403	n=36	Cw*1601	50
B*5101	n=43	Cw*1502	42

* The HLA-C allele with the strongest association is shown.

antigens (Cw*1601, 1502 or 0702) that had escaped detection by serology. Direct recognition of the Cw antigen by CTL clones specific for the mismatched allele was demonstrated by lysis of the HLA class I-negative cell line 721.221 after transfection with the Cw*1601 cDNA. Specificity of the anti-Cw*1601 clones was high, since cells from a donor with the Cw*1602 allele that only differs at positions 77 and 80 were not lysed.
We then developed an oligotyping procedure allowing to discriminate 29 Cw alleles in order to type all patients and donors. Using this method we detected twenty-one Cw alleles in our panel of 369 individuals, The following alleles were not observed: 0402, 0801, 0803, 1301, 1403, 1504, and 1505. Serological blanks that turned out to be defined Cw alleles represent 50% of the CwX antigens.

Due to ABDR linkage disequilibrium the rate of HLA-C incompatibilities will be significantly affected by the stringency of matching for ABDRB1 antigens. To assess the degree of Cw matching we selected all pairwise combinations derived from 73 patients and their 184 potential donors matched for AB by serology and for DRB1/B3/B5 by oligotyping, the modern standard for compatibility in bone marrow transplantation. The results of 287 pairwise combinations are summarised in Figure 1. Whereas 51.3% of all pairs were HLA-C matched, 29.6% of the pairs were mismatched at locus C only, 12.5% at A+C or B+C loci, and 6.6% at locus A or B only. This rate of HLA-C incompatibility is comparable [12] or higher [13] to those observed previously. With 3 exceptions, currently under investigation, all HLA-C incompatibilities resulted in a positive CTLp test.
The rate of HLA-C incompatibility was significantly influenced by ABDR linkage disequilibrium (Table 1). As expected, the common haplotypes A1-B8-Cw*0701-DRB1*0301-DRB3*0101, A*0301-B*0702-Cw*0702-DRB1*1501-DRB5*0101, or Ax-B*4402-Cw*0501-DRB1*04 or 1501 can be considered as low risk haplotypes with respect to Cw incompatibility. However, Cw mismatches occurred frequently with B*4403, B*5101, B*18, and B62 haplotypes (*Table I*). For example only 50% of the B*4403-positive donors typed Cw*1601.
High resolution HLA class I and class II (DRB/DQB) typing is able to select the best matched donor, therefore decreasing mortality after unrelated BMT [14]. Because HLA-C incompatibilities are recognised by

alloreactive CTLs they might be as relevant as AB-subtype mismatches in transplantation. However further studies are required to asses the role of unique HLA-C incompatibilities in the outcome of unrelated bone marrow transplantation.

Acknowledgements

We are grateful to N. Adami, B. Kervaire, and P. Roux-Chabbey for contributing in oligotyping analyses, and to M. Bujan, V. Elamly, and C. Gonet for serological typing. We thank Dr. A. Madrigal for providing the modified pBJI-Neo vector and the 721.221 cell line. This work was supported by grants from the Swiss National Science Foundation (31-35247.92 and 31-45899.95).

References

1. Rufer N, Tiercy JM, Breur-Vriesendorp B, *et al.* Histoincompatibilities in ABDR-matched unrelated donor recipient combinations. *Bone Marrow Transpl* 1995; 16: 641-6.
2. Spencer A, Szydlo RM, Brookes PA, *et al.* Cytotoxic T lymphocyte precursor frequency analyses in bone marrow transplantation with volunteer unrelated donors. *Blood* 1995; 86: 3590-7.
3. Fleischhauer K, Kernan NA, O'Reilly RJ, Dupont B, Yang SY. Bone marrow allograft rejection by host-derived allocytotoxicT lymphocytes recognizing a single amino acid at position 156 of the HLA-B44 class I antigen. *N Engl J Med* 1990; 323: 1818-22.
4. Davies SM, Shu XO, Blazar BR, *et al.* Unrelated donor bone marrow transplantation. *Blood* 1995; 86: 1636-42.
5. Petersdorf EW, Longton GM, Anasetti C, *et al.* The significance of HLA-DRB1 matching on clinical outcome after HLA-A, B, DR identical unrelated donor marrow transplantation. *Blood* 1995; 86: 1606-13.
6. Tiercy JM, Djavad N, Rufer N, Speiser DE, Jeannet M, Roosnek E. Oligotyping of HLA-A2, A3, and B44 subtypes: detection of subtype-incompatibilities between patients and their serologically matched unrelated bone marrow donors.*Hum Immunol* 1994; 41: 207-15.
7. Gauchat-Feiss D, Rufer N, Speiser D, Jeannet M, Roosnek E, Tiercy JM. Heterogeneity of HLA-B35: oligotyping and direct sequencing for B35 subtypes reveals a high mismatching rate in B35 serologically compatible kidney and bone marrow donor/recipient pairs. *Transplantation* 1995; 60: 869-73.
8. Tiercy JM, Morel C, Freidel AC, *et al.* Selection of unrelated donors for bone marrow transplantation is improved by HLA class II genotyping with oligonucleotide hybridization. *Proc Natl Acad Sci USA* 1991; 88: 7121-225.
9. Cros P, Allibert P, Mandrand, Tiercy JM, Mach B. Oligonucleotide genotyping of HLA polymorphism on microtitre plates. *Lancet* 1992; 340: 870-4.
10. Cereb N, Maye P, Lee S, Kong Y, Yang SY. Locus-specific amplification of HLA class I genes from genomic DNA: locus-specific sequences in the first and third introns of HLA-A, -B, and -C alleles. *Tissue Antigens* 1995; 45: 1-11.
11. Kennedy LJ, Poulton KV, Dyer PA, Ollier WER, Thomson W. Definition of HLA-C alleles using sequence-specific oligonucleotide probes (PCR-SSOP). *Tissue Antigens* 1995; 46: 187-95.
12. Bishara A, Amar A, Brautbar C, Condiotti R, Lazarovitz V, Nagler A. The putative role of HLA-C recognition in graft versus host disease (GVHD) and graft rejection after unrelated bone marrow transplantation. *Exp Hematol* 1995; 23: 1667-75.
13. Petersdorf EW, Stanley JF, Martin PJ, Hansen JA. Molecular diversity of the HLA-C locus in unrelated marrow transplantation. *Tissue Antigens* 1994; 44: 93-9.
14. Speiser D, Tiercy JM, Rufer N, *et al.* High resolution matching associated with decreased mortality after unrelated bone marrow transplantation. *Blood* 1996; 87: 4455-62.

The probability of finding a haplotypically identical unrelated bone marrow donor

R.F. Schipper [1], J. D'Amaro [1], M. Oudshoorn [1,2]

1 Department of Immunohematology and Blood Bank,
2 Europdonor Foundation, Bldg. 1, E3-Q Leiden University Hospital, PO Box 9600, 2300 RC Leiden, The Netherlands

Prediction of the probability of finding a suitable donor for a patient in need of a transplant (Match prognosis, MP) is of interest to transplant organizations and physicians [1-3]. Several authors have explored methods to calculate so-called Match Prognostic Indices [1,2] for organ transplantation. Their MPs were based on bootstrap methods that matched patients against donors in a retrospective way. In this study we describe a method to estimate the number of haplotypically identical bone marrow donors for a particular patient, given a number of HLA-A, -B or -A, -B, -DR phenotypically identical (PhId) donors. We use the estimated haplotype frequencies (HF) of the Dutch bone marrow donor population to supply an example.
Large registries of bone marrow donors exist in many countries. HLA phenotype frequencies of most of these registries are compiled in the Bone Marrow Donors Worldwide (BMDW) registry. Related donors are usually searched for among the parents and siblings of the patient. Additionally, the extended family (blood-related uncles and aunts, cousins, etc.) of the patient can be searched [4]. Potentially suitable unrelated donors can be located by consulting the BMDW.
Matching donors and recipients for bone marrow transplantation (BMT) requires identity of HLA phenotypes. If no HLA-A, -B,-DR identical donors are listed in BMDW, one has to fall back on HLA-A, -B identical donors. HLA-DR typing for these donors has to be requested. The probability of an HLA-A, -B, -DR phenotypically identical (PhId) donor can be calculated from the frequencies of the patients HLA-DR antigens amongst all HLA-A, -B identical donors found in the donor pool. Such calculations can only be done on donor pools in which no selective HLA-DR typing of bone marrow donors has taken place [5].
Moreover, it has been suggested that marrow graft survival is higher when patient and donor share complete HLA haplotypes instead of just phenotypes [6]. Therefore it is of interest to know the probability that a PhId donor is also haplotypically identical (HId) to the patient.

Materials and methods

In order to test the validity of the estimation procedure, we selected 47 patients for which phenotypically identical HLA-A, -B typed donors were found in the Dutch donor pool. We determined their haplotypes by inspection of the HLA segregation patterns in their pedigrees. The estimated (expected) number of HLA-A, -B, -DR PhId donors for each of these patients was compared to the observed number, using the Pearson's Chi-square for goodness-of-fit test [7].
We estimated HFs using a file of 14,794 HLA-A, -B, -DR typed Dutch bone marrow donors that were included in the 22nd edition of the BMDW [8]. Maximum likelihood 2- and 3- locus HFs were estimated using the method of Yasuda and Tsuji [9].
The method for estimating HFs takes the hypothetical null antigen into account. The frequency of the null antigen represents the combined frequency of the undetected antigens in the sample. It can be used to calculate the probability of homozygosity for a particular antigen (i), using the formula:

$$P(hom.)_i = \frac{GF_i^2}{GF_i^2 + 2 \times GF_i \times GF_{null}}$$

This probability is necessary for calculation of expected number of HId donors because the occurrence of 'false homozygotes' in the sample can lead to very low probabilities of homozygosity for certain antigens. A large proportion of donors that appear homozygous for such an antigen will in fact be heterozygous.

The estimation procedure starts by determining if the patient is homozygous for any of the loci. If there is no homozygosity, the procedure simply takes into account the four possible haplotype combinations that can be formed of the patients 3-locus phenotype. The 2-locus phenotypes of the donors correspond with 2 possible haplotype combinations. *Table I* shows these combinations. Each set of two haplotypes leads to the same phenotype. The haplotype combination of the patient is marked with asterisks.

Table I. The four sets of two HLA-A, -B, -DR haplotypes that can form one phenotype and the probalities that these combinations occur. The haplotype combination of the patient is marked with asterisks. The patient is heterozygous at all three loci

Patient's phenotype: A_1 A_2 B_1 B_2 DR_1 DR_2 3-locus haplotypes	Probability of occurence
1: $A_1B_1DR_1$ 2: $A_2B_2DR_2$	2 x HF_1 x HF_2
3: $A_1B_1DR_2$ * 4: $A_2B_2DR_1$ *	2 x HF_3 x HF_4
5: $A_1B_2DR_1$ 6: $A_2B_1DR_2$	2 x HF_5 x HF_6
7: $A_1B_2DR_2$ 8: $A_2B_1DR_1$	2 x HF_7 x HF_8

If the patient is homozygous for one or more loci, the procedure takes into account extra haplotypes that have an undetected antigen on these loci. The probability that these haplotypes occur in a donor instead of the haplotypes that would lead to a real homozygous phenotype can be calculated from the probability of homozygosity. In order to calculate the probability that an HLA-A, -B, -DR PhId donor is HId, we can simply divide the probability of occurrence of the patient's haplotype combination (the one marked with an asterisk in *Table I)* by the sum of the probabilities of the four combinations that lead to the patient's phenotype. The number of expected HId donors is found by multiplying with the number of PhId donors:

$$Exp_{HId} = N_{PhId} \times \frac{P_{3,4}}{P_{1,2} + P_{3,4} + P_{5,6} + P_{7,8}}$$

Results

Comparison of the estimated number of HLA-A, -B, -DR phenotypically identical donors with the observed number for 47 Dutch patients with Pearson's Chi-square for goodness-of-fit resulted in a P-value of 0.1582 (χ^2 = 25.071, D.F. = 19), indicating that the observed and expected values do not differ significantly.
In *Table II* we give an example of the results of the calculations for a hypothetical patient with haplotypes A2 B35 DR1 and A3 B7 DR15. *Table III* gives an example of the calculations for a patient that is homozygous at the HLA-B and -DR loci.

Table II. Example of calculations. The haplotype combination of the patient is marked with asterisks

Patient's first haplotype	A2 B35 DR1		
Patient's second haplotype	A3 B7 DR2		
Haplotype combinations	**HF**	**HF**	**Exp. PF**
A2 B7 DR1 / A3 B35 DR2	2 x .0043 x	.0030 =	.000026
A2 B7 DR2 / A3 B35 DR1	2 x .0223 x	.0235 =	.001048
A2 B35 DR1 / A3 B7 DR2	2 x .0057 x	.0440 =	.000503 *
A2 B35 DR2 / A3 B7 DR1	2 x .0010 x	.0047 =	.000009
No. of ABDR id. donors: 17	Exp. no. ABDR HId:	5 (31.73 %)	

Discussion

The described procedure provides usefull additional information necessary for the location of suitable donors for BMT. In the ideal situation, the 3-locus HFs of all donor registries are available and the standard results of a search for donors in BMDW can be used to identify the registry that has the highest expected number of HId donors. Because of the substantial differences in HFs between donor populations, a small group of PhId donors from a particular registry may offer a higher expected number of HId donors than a much larger group from another registry. But even when the expected number of HId donors is higher in one registry, it will be much easier to find one in another, smaller registry that has a higher percentage of HId donors.
It may be expected that the results of MLC and CTLp tests will be more often negative with HId donors (van Rood, personal communication) and that they are also identical for HLA alleles as determined by DNA typing. In order to establish a beneficial effect on patient survival, long term follow-up analyses of these patients is required.

Table III. Example of calculations for a patient that is homozygous at the HLA-B and -DR loci. The haplotype combination of the patient is marked with asterisks

Patient's first haplotype A2 B7 DR2
Patient's second haplotype A3 B7 DR2

Haplotype combinations			HF	HF	Prob.	Exp. PF
A2 B7 DR2	/ A3 B7 DR2	2 x	.02229 x	.04402 x	0.96299 =	.001890 *
A2 B7 DR2	/ A3 B7 Null	2 x	.02229 x	.00021 x	0.03462 =	.000000
A2 B7 Null	/ A3 B7 DR2	2 x	.00012 x	.04402 x	0.03462 =	.000000
A2 B7 DR2	/ A3 Null DR2	2 x	.02229 x	.00001 x	0.00231 =	.000000
A2 Null DR2	/ A3 B7 DR2	2 x	.00000 x	.04402 x	0.00231 =	.000000
A2 B7 DR2	/ A3 Null Null	2 x	.02229 x	.00000 x	0.00008 =	.000000
A2 B7 Null	/ A3 Null DR2	2 x	.00012 x	.00001 x	0.00008 =	.000000
A2 Null DR2	/ A3 B7 Null	2 x	.00000 x	.00021 x	0.00008 =	.000000
A2 Null Null	/ A3 B7 DR2	2 x	.00000 x	.04402 x	0.00008 =	.000000

No. of ABDR id. donors: 18 Exp. no. ABDR HId: 18 (99.96 %)

The procedure will become efficient only when reliable HFs are available from many registries. Many bone marrow donor registries are actively improving the quality of the HLA phenotypes by non-selective HLA-DR typing and participating in typing laboratory accreditation programs.

In conclusion, one can optimize the chance of good bone marrow graft survival by selecting donors from the registry with the best chance of providing haplotypically identical donors.

Acknowledgments

The authors wish to thank Drs van Rood and Schreuder for criticaly reviewing the manuscript. The Europdonor foundation kindly suplied Dutch BMT donor phenotypes and results of matching Dutch BMT patients against unrelated donors. This work was supported in part by the J.A. Cohen Institute for Radio pathology and Radiation Protection (IRS) and the National Reference Center for Histocompatibility Testing.

Abbreviations

BMDW : Bone Marrow Donors Worldwide; BMT : Bone marrow transplantation; CTLp: Cytotoxic T lymphocyte precursor; HF: Haplotype frequency; HId : Haplotypically identical; HLA: Human Leukocyte antigens; MLC: Mixed lymphocyte culture; MP: Match prognosis; PhId: Phenotypically identical.

References

1. Thorogood J, Houwelingen JCv, Persijn GG, Rood JJv. Match prognostic index for predicting waiting time to renal transplantation. *Transplant Proc* 1993; 25: 1039-40.
2. Wujciak T, Opelz G. Computer analysis of cadaver kidney allocation procedures. *Transplantation* 1993; 55: 516-21.
3. McKinney S, Mickelson EM, Hansen JA. Assembly of an HLA-A,B,DR/DRB1 database and it's utility in unrelated donor searches. *Hum Immunol* 1995; 44 (suppl 1) : 107.
4. Schipper RF, D'Amaro J, Oudshoorn M. The probability of finding a suitable related donor for bone marrow transplant in extended families. *Blood* 1996; 87: 800-4.
5. Schipper RF, Oudshoorn M, D'Amaro J, Zanden HGMv, Lange Pd, Bakker JT, Bakker J, Rood JJv. Validation of large data sets, an essential prerequisite for data analysis: an analytical survey of the Bone Marrow Donors Worldwide. *Tissue Antigens* 1996; 47: 169-78.
6. Awdeh ZL, Eynon E, Stein R, Alper CA, Alosco SM, Yunis EJ. Unrelated individuals matched for MHC extended haplotypes and HLA-identical siblings show comparable responses in mixed lymphocyte culture. *Lancet* 1985; i: 853-5.
7. Pearson K. On the criterion that a given system of deviations from the probable in the case of a correlated system of variables is such that it can be reasonably supposed to have arisen from random sampling. *Phil Mag* 1900; L: 157.
8. Bone Marrow Donors Worldwide. Leiden: Europdonor Foundation, 1995.
9. Yasuda N, Tsuji K. A counting method of maximum likelihood for estimating haplotype frequency in the HL-A system. *Jpn J Hum Genet* 1975; 20: 1-15.

An optimal microsatellite analysis for donor and recipient cells after bone marrow transplantation

W.T.M. Van Blokland, M.G. Ignatiadis, E.C. Bosboom, L.F. Verdonck, D.F. Van Wichen, M.G.J. Tilanus, R.A. De Weger

Departments of Pathology and Hematology, University Hospital, PO Box 85.500, 3508 GA Utrecht, The Netherlands

After bone marrow transplantation (BMT) the presence of donor or recipient cells in the PBL is essential to study either the take of the graft, or study the recurrence of malignancy. As the donor and recipient are HLA matched before BMT, the cells can not be discriminated by HLA typing. Besides, the donor and recipient are often related as this maximizes a good result of the transplantation. Therefore, the best way to discriminate between donor and recipient cells is to analyse highly variable gene segments that are located on different chromosomes. For this purpose many microsatellite regions have been described [1-5]. We analysed by PCR in 50 healthy individuals and in 35 BMT cases, the use of microsatellites, *e.g.* variable number of tandem repeats (VNTR) repeats of >10 bp and short tandem repeats (STR) with 2 - 6 bp repeats. The PCR products were analysed by agarose electrophoresis and by gene-scanning using fluorescent-PCR primers. The best discrimination between donor and recipient cells was obtained by a combination of four 4 bp STR using gene-scanning.

Materials and methods

Patient material and DNA preparation

DNA from PBL or PBL fractions of 50 healthy individuals (all caucasians) and 35 patient and donor combinations before and after BMT were analysed. Heparinized blood was obtained and mononuclear cells (MNC) and polymorphonyclear cells were isolated by Ficoll-Hypaque density centrifugation. T- and non-T fractions were obtained after E-rozetting of the MNC. Cells were counted by Burker-Turk method and DNA was isolated by salting out.

Polymerase chain reaction

General information on the relevant microsatelites is summarized in *Table I.* Oligonucleotides for PCR were synthesized on an Applied Biosystems Synthesizer model 380B (Foster City CA). Data base searches and sequence analyses were performed using software made by PCGENE (Intelli-genetics). Primers used in PCR experiments are summarized in *Table I.* In case of gene-scanning the 5' primers were labelled with the fluorescent markers.

PCR was performed in 50 µl reaction mixture: milli-Q water, 10 x PCR buffer (500 mM KCl, 100 mM TrisHCl pH 8.4 en 5 mM $MgCl_2$), 4 µl 10 mM dNTP's, 0.2 unit Taq (Perkin Elmer Cetus, Norwalk, CT), 2 x 250 ng/ml of each primer and 0.5-1.0 µg DNA. PCR were performed in PE-Cetus thermal cycler. The different primer sets were used in different PCR procedures; each PCR was started with a denaturation at 95 °C for 5 min. Steps for the variable number of tandem repeats (VNTR) were: Apo B: 58 °C for 6 min and 95 °C for 1 min in 26 cycles. Steps for pMCT118 were: 65 °C for 1 min, 70 °C for 8 min, 95 °C for 1 min in 25 cycles. For pYNZ22 and SRY were: 55 °C for 1 min, 72 °C for 8 min and 95 °C for 1 min in 30 cycles. All STR PCR reactions were performed as follows: 25 µl PCR buffer (Perkin Elmer Cetus, Norwalk, CT, USA) containing dNTPs (0,1 mM final concentration), 2 mM $MgCl_2$ (Perkin Elmer Cetus), 2 x 1 pmol of each primer, 0,75 units Taq (Perkin Elmer Cetus) and 50 ng DNA. STR were amplified in 30 cycles; the amplification cycle profile was as follows, denaturation for 1 min at 95 °C; annealing for 1 min at 58 °C and extension for 1.5 min at 72°C. The amplification was preceeded by a hot start for 2 min at 95 °C and ended by a long extension for 10 min at 72 °C.

All PCR mixtures were covered by one droplet of mineral oil to prevent evaporation and then amplified on a DNA thermal cycler (Perkin Elmer Cetus) and were ended by an extra elongation step.

Table I. VNTR and STR primers

Name	Location	Primer	References
Variable number of tandem repeats			
APO-B	2p24-p23	CCTTCTCACTTGGCAAATAC ATGGAAACGGAGAAATTATG	Boerwinkle *et al.* [1]
pYNZ22	17p13.3	CGAAGAGTGAAGTGCACAGG CACAGTCTTTATTCTTCAGCG	Horn *et al.* [2]
pMCT118	1p36-p35	GTCTTGTTGGAGATGCACGTGCCCCTTGC GAAACTGGCCTCCAAACACTGCCCGCCG	Kasai *et al.* [3]
Tetrameric short tandem repeats			
D19S253	19p13.1	ATAGACAGACAGACGGACTG GGGAGTGGAGATTACCCCT	Urquhart *et al.* [5]
HUMTHO	11p15-15.5	GTGGGCTGAAAAGCTCCCGATTAT GTGATTCCCATTGGCGTGTTCCTC	Urquhart *et al.* [5]
HUMVWFA 31/A	12p13.3 -p13.2	CCCTAGTGGATGATAAGAATAATCAGTATG GGACAGATGATAAATACATAGGATGGATGG	Urquhart *et al.* [5]
388II	11p12 -p11.2	GGTAGCAGAGCAAGACTGTC CACCTTCATCCTAAGCGAGC	Phromchotikul *et al.* [4]

VNTR PCR products were analysed by gel electrophoresis in 2% agarose gels and visualized by ethidium bromide staining under UV-light. Both VNTR and STR products were analysed by gene scan analysis; 1 µl PCR product was combined with 0.5 µl of internal lane standard GS2500 (ABI) labelled with the dye ROX and 2.5 µl loading buffer. The samples were denautared before being loaded on a 6% polyacrylamide sequencing gel. Gels were electroforesed for 4 hrs at a constant power on an ABI373 automated DNA sequencer. Fragment sizes were determined automatically using ABI prism and genotyper software.

Results and discussion

Variable number of tandem repeats (VNTR)

The VNTR systems APO-B, pYNZ22, and pMCT118 analysed by agarose electrophoresis, showed a good heterogeneity and good discriminatory capacity between individuals (data not shown). When used in this combination of 3 VNTR systems, it was possible to analyse donor and recipient cells in the peripheral blood of the patient after family related BMT in 45 of 50 combinations. In some cases the SRY system was used in male female combinations to confirm the VNTR data.

Two base-pair short tandem repeats (STR)

The 2 bp repeat STR Mfd 38, Mfd 44, Mfd 154 and CFTR showed a good heterogeneity and good discriminatory capacity between individuals when analysed by gene-scanning. It was also possible to discriminate family related donors and recipients before BMT. However the 2bp STR always showed stutter bands, with a characteristic pattern, which do not hinder the discrimination of individuals. However, when tested after BMT the combination/ mixture of donor and recipient cells becomes complex due to these stutter bands, and makes the proper interpretation impossible.

Four base-pair short tandem repeats

The STR systems D19S253, HUMTHO, HUMVWFA31/A, and 388II (D11S554) showed a good hetero-

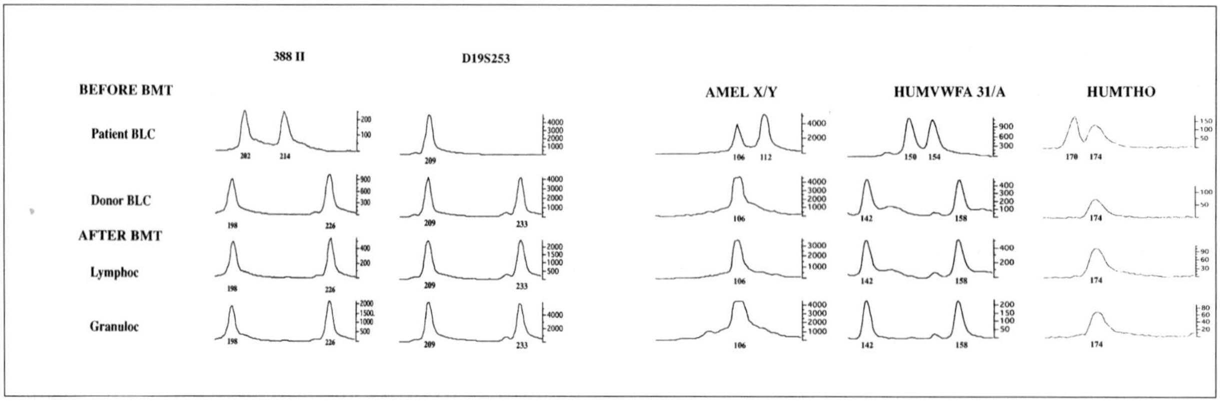

Figure 1. A representative example of the chimaerism analysis of PBL after BMT.
Blood cells (BLC) of the donor and recipient before transplantation and the blood lymphocytes and granulocytes after BMT, were analysed for the STR 388II, D19S253, HUMTHO, HUMVWFA 31/A and as this was a BMT with a male female combination, with Amel X/Y. In this particular situation only donor cells could be detected after BMT.

geneity and good discriminatory capacity between individuals when analysed by gene-scanning (data not shown). The 388II system was also analysed for the 50 individuals on agarose electrophoresis. Some alleles with small size differences could not be separated. However, by gene scanning these individuals often showed a clear heterogeneity in both their alleles. Similar findings were found for PMCT118.

When used in combination, these four STR were also able to discriminate between family related donors and recipients for BMT. Also after BMT (30 cases with a chimerism, have been analysed), these donor and recipient cells could be discriminated by one or more systems *(Figure 1)*. If only one 4bp STR was informative for donor and recipient analysis, an informative VNTR system or (in male female BMT combinations) the Amel X/Y system was used for confirmation.

In summary, our data show that four 4 bp STR, used in the combination of D19S253, 388II, HUMTHOI and HUMVWFA give a good capacity to discriminate patients and recipients, as often 2 or more sytems were informative. In few cases (1 to 2%) the combination of these 4 bp STR were not informative, and we had to add the VNTR systems (by gene-scanning). As these VNTR are larger, a longer running time is required then for STR.

References

1. Boerwinkle E, Xiong W, Fourest E, Chan L. Rapid typing of tandemly repeated hypervariable loci by the polymerase chain reaction: application to the apolipoprotein B 3' hypervariable region. *Proc Natl Acad Sci USA* 1989; 86: 212-6.
2. Horn G, Richards B, Klinger KW. Amplification of a highly polymorphic VNTR segment by the polymerase chain reaction. *Nucleic Acids Res* 1989; 17: 2140.
3. Kasai K, Nakamura Y, White R. Amplification of a variable number of tandem repeats (VNTR) locus (pMCT118) by polymerase chain reaction (PCR) and its application to forensic science. *J Forensic Sci* 1990; 35: 1196-200.
4. Phromchotikul T, Browne D, Litt M. Microsatellite polymorphisms at the D11S554 and D11S569 loci. *Hum Mol Genet* 1992; 1: 214.
5. Urquhart A, Oldroyd NJ, Kimpton CP, Gill P. Highly discriminating heptaplex short tandem repeat PCR system for forensic identification. *Biotechniques* 1995; 18: 116-21.

The genomic matching technique (GMT) A new tool for selecting unrelated marrow donors

H. Grosse-Wilde [1], N. Ketheesan[2], F.T. Christiansen [2], H.D. Ottinger [1], S. Ferencik [1], G.K. Tay [2], C.S. Witt [2], H. Teisserenc [3], M. Giphart [4], E.M. Freitas [2], D. Charron[3], R.L. Dawkins [2]

1 Institute for Immunology, University Hospital of Essen, Virchow Strass 171, D-45 147 Essen, Germany
2 Centre for Melocular Immunology and Instrumentation, The University of Western Australia, GPO Box F298, 6001 Perth, Australia
3 Laboratory for Immunology and Histocompatibility, Hopital Saint Louis, Paris, France
4 Department of Immuno-haematology, University Hospital of Leiden, The Netherlands

The recognition of ancestral haplotypes (AH) has led us to suggest that: (1) the human Major Histocompatibility Complex (MHC) consists of several polymorphic conserved blocks linked together to form haplotypes; (2) recombination preferentially occurs between the blocks [1,2] and (3) the haplotypes present for each individual are composed of DNA blocks each derived from a limited number or different remote ancestors. Each block consists of a hundred of more kilobases of sequence which encodes multiple polymorphic genes (HLA and non-HLA) [3,4]. The block around HLA-A has been designated "alpha block", whereas the "beta-block" includes HLA-B and HLA-C and the "delta block" HLA-DR and HLA-DQ.

Unrelated individuals with blocks derived from the same AH not only share the same HLA alleles, but probably the same DNA sequence for the entire block. In unrelated bone marrow transplantation (BMT) therefore, a donor might be either matched with the patient only for the particular HLA antigens tested or matched for the whole block including these HLA antigens.

The genomic matching technique (GMT) allows comparison of donor/recipient pairs on the block level. In brief, PCR amplification of the highly polymorphic but stable sequences of the alpha, beta- and delta blocks is performed using primers that correspond to flanking regions of relatively low variation. Since these regions are often replicated within the block, amplification results in a multitude of products. These products are resolved by gel electrophoresis and scanned using a gene scanner. The resulting polymorphic densitometric profiles serve as signatures for the block. By profile overlay the profiles of the donor and recipient can be compared and classified as the same (S), different (D) or uncertain (U) [5].

The present retrospective multicentre study was undertaken to evaluate whether: (1) GMT is reproducible between different laboratories; (2) block matching correlates with conventional HLA typing results and (3) unrelated donors matched with patient at the block level are preferable to donors only matched for the HLA antigens tested (differences in HLA-matched donor recipient pairs disclosed by GMT are an independent predictor of survival after unrelated BMT).

Materials and methods

The present retrospective multicenter study (Essen, Leiden, Paris, Perth) enrolled 147 patients who underwent unrelated BMT. Clinical data were available for all patients and included patient age, diagnosis, stage of leukemia, presence of acute GVHD and patient survival. Serological HLA class I and molecular genetic HLA class II typing of donors and recipients was undertaken by the submitting centres. In 33 pairs from Essen, biochemical (1D-IEF) HLA class I typing was also performed. All donors and recipients were evaluated in Perth using the GMT, but the evaluation of all pairs at all three blocks has not yet been completed. To evaluate the reproducibility of the GMT, DNA from a subset of these pairs were also tested in Paris (62 beta and 32 delta comparisons) and Leiden (45 beta comparisons) and the results were compared to those from Perth. All GMT tests were undertaken without knowledge of the clinical or HLA data or the test results in the other laboratories. Furthermore, GMT and HLA typing results were analyzed for correlation. For the analysis of the GMT against patient survival after BMT from HLA-matched donors, the GMT results from Perth were used.

Results and discussion

The GMT results obtained in Leiden or Paris compared to those obtained in Perth are summarized in *Table I.*

Table I. Beta and delta block matching is comparable between laboratories

Perth beta blocks	Leiden or Paris Beta blocks	
	Same	Different
Same	39	4
Different	0	44

Perth delta blocks	Paris delta blocks	
	Same	Different
Same	11	1
Different	0	13

Note: excluded are 20 cases (beta block) and 7 cases (delta block) classified uncertain in either laboratory - see text for details.

A total of 96 and 27 pairwise comparisons were made for the beta and delta blocks respectively. There was excellent concordance between the laboratories for those samples which could be classified as either S or D in both laboratories with a total of only five discordant results. In four of these cases a donor/recipient pair considered S in Perth was considered D in Paris. However, in 20 of 107 and 7 of 32 beta and delta block comparisons a laboratory was uncertain (U) in the classification mainly due to samples showing small differences in profile or inadequate amplification. Review of these cases suggests that the three centres have somewhat different thresholds in classifying profiles as D. Leiden classified more cases U and in all cases these were considered S or U in Perth. However, without exception all cases considered D in Leiden were also classified D in Perth. On the other hand Paris had fewer cases classified U but did classify 4 pairs D, which were all considered S in Perth and S (2 cases) or U (2 cases) in Leiden. Further work is required to standardize GMT in these difficult cases.

The matching obtained by GMT for the beta and delta blocks was compared to the results of conventional HLA typing (*Table II*). All cases mismatched by conventional typing were mismatched by GMT with only one exception for the beta block - a case where the donor and recipient were mismatched for HLA-B38 and B-39 by serology. Interestingly, however, some 39 % and 44 % of the cases matched by HLA typing were found to be mismatched by GMT at the beta and delta blocks respectively, indicating that currently many donor/recipient pairs are not matched at the genomic level. This, at least in part, may account for the poorer BMT outcome observed using unrelated donors [6,7].

Table II. Beta block matching subdivides HLA matched donor - recipient pairs

HLA DR + DQ typing*	Delta blocks	
	Same	Different
Matched	35	28
Mismatched	0	14

* by serology and DNA typing.

HLA-B#	Beta blocks	
	Same	Different
Matched	73	47
Mismatched	1	3

by serology and in some cases biochemistry.

The effect of beta and delta block matching by GMT on transplant outcome could be evaluated in 116 cases. Cases matched for both the beta and delta blocks had a significantly better survival than those mismatched at either or both blocks (*Table III*).

Table III. Beta plus delta block matching of donor and recipient result in improved survival following unrelated bone marrow transplantation

Survival-alive	Beta and delta blocks	
	Matched	Mismatched*
Yes	19	22
No	17	58

$p = 0.008$. * mismatched at either or both blocks.

This effect was evident even when analysis was confined to HLA-identical unrelated donor BMT and persisted after correction for patient disease stage as evidenced by mulivariate statistical analysis. Thus, GMT might appear as an independent risk factor beside disease stage and HLA match for overall survival after BMT from unrelated donors. Our present data on GMT results as an independent risk factor for BMT outcome, however, are preliminary, since serology is an unreliable method to prove HLA class I identify of the donor with the recipient. Hence, sequencing of all pairs classified as S by serology and D by GMT is underway. Anyway, GMT seems to be an appropriate tool for selecting unrelated donors matched at the genomic level for two MHC haplotypes with the recipient, since the projected two year survival in the block matched group of 58 % was similar to that found using HLA identical siblings [8].

Conclusions

This study shows that GMT can be applied in different laboratories with good concordance. However, further work is required to standardize those cases with poor amplification or minor differences and to determine the relevance of theses differences. It supports our previous finding that block matching identifies all patients mismatched by conventional techniques and that a large proportion of those donor-recipient pairs matched by conventional techniques are not matched at the genomic level [9]. In addition it supports our previous report that donor/recipient mismatches at the block level predict patient survival [10]. The improved outcome in patients transplanted with GMT matched donors might be due to better matching either for HLA class I and class II antigens or for non-HLA genes within the block. Further studies are necessary to distinguish between these alternatives. Either way GMT is inexpensive and rapid and can serve as a screening tool to identify suitable bone marrow donors.

References

1. Degli-Esposti MA, Leaver AL, Christiansen FT, *et al.* Ancestral haplotypes: conserved population MHC haplotypes. *Hum Immunol* 1992; 34: 242.
2. Dawkins RL, Degli-Esposti MA, Abraham LJ, *et al.* Conservation versus polymorphism of the MHC in relation to transplantation, immune reponses and autoimmune diseases. In Klein J ed. *Molecular Evolution of the Major Histocompatibility Complex.* Berlin: Springer Verlag, 1991; 391.
3. Leelayuwat C, Abraham LJ, Tabarias H, *et al.* Genomic organisation of a polymorphic duplicated region centromeric of HLA-B. *Immunogenetics* 1992; 36: 208.
4. Marshall B, Leelayuwat C, Degli-Esposti MA, *et al.* New MHC genes. *Hum Immunol* 1993; 38: 24.
5. Tay GK, Witt CS, Christiansen FT, *et al.* The identification of MHC identical siblings without HLA typing. *Exp Haematol* 1995; 23: 1655.
6. Horowitz MM, Bortin MM, *et al.* Results of bone marrow transplants from human leukocyte antigen - identical sibling donors for treatment of childhood leukemias: a report from the International Bone Marrow Transplant Registry. *Am J Paediatr Haematol Oncol* 1993; 15: 56.
7. Howard MR, Hows JM, Gore SM, *et al.* Unrelated donor marrow transplantation between 1977 and 1987 at four centres in the United Kingdom. *Tranplantation* 1990; 49: 547.
8. Ringden O, Sundberg B, Lundqvist B, *et al.* Allogenic bone marrow transplantation for leukemia: factors of importance for long term survival and relapse. *Bone Marrow Transplant* 1988; 3: 281.
9. Christiansen FT, Tay GK, Smith LK, *et al.* Histocompatibility matching for bone marrow transplantation donor/recipient pairs in the 4A011 cell panel. *Hum Immunol* 1993; 38: 42
10. Tay GK, Witts CS, Christiansen FT, *et al.* Matching for MHC haplotypes results in improved survival following unrelated bone marrow transplantation. *Bone Marrow Transplant* 1995; 15: 381.

Symposium communications

HLA Diversity

HLA typing and sequencing

Function of HLA

Transplantation biology and medicine

HLA and Diseases

HLA and Insulin Dependent Diabetes Mellitus

Contents

• HLA and Insulin Dependent Diabetes Mellitus

Presentation of an autoantigenic peptide in type I diabetes by an HLA class II protein protecting from disease

J.M. Bach[1] H. Otto[2], G.T. Nepom[3], G. Jung[2], H. Cohen[1], J. Timsit[1], C. Boitard[1], P.M. van Endert[1]

1 INSERM U25, Hôpital Necker, 161, rue de Sèvres, 75015 Paris, France
2 Institute of Organic Chemistry, Tübingen, Germany
3 Virginia Mason Research, Seattle, USA

Allelic polymorphism of HLA-class II DR and DQ molecules greatly modifies the risk to develop insulin-dependent-diabetes-mellitus (IDDM), and can be associated with highly elevated disease frequency (DR4/DQB1*0302 and DR3/DQB1*0201 haplotypes) or with moderately elevated risk (DR1 and DR8 haplotypes), but also with strongly decreased disease frequency, as in the case of the DR15/DQB1*0602 haplotype. One theory proposed to explain modification of risk for IDDM by HLA postulates that certain alleles are associated with high risk of IDDM because they present autoantigenic peptides with high efficiency [1]. Alternatively, the "determinant capture" theory proposes a competition between high and low risk alleles for binding of autoantigenic fragments of beta cell proteins. According to this hypothesis, protective alleles may bind crucial autoantigenic peptides preventing binding of these epitopes by high risk alleles [2,3].

To elucidate the mechanism underlying the effect of HLA class II polymorphism on IDDM risk, we have studied presentation by high and low risk alleles of an autoantigen which is likely to play an important role in the pathogenesis of the disease, the 65 kDa glutamate decarboxylase (GAD65) [4,5]. We have characterized GAD specific T cell lines (TCL) from two IDDM patients and determined two GAD-derived peptide epitopes presented by HLA-DR molecules to CD4+ T cells.

Patients

TCL were generated from two patients with recent-onset IDDM, patient A, 25 years old, and patient B, 49 years old. Both patients were diagnosed with IDDM in January 1994 and started on insulin treatment in January (patient A) or in May (patient B) 1994. PBMC showed vigorous proliferative responses to recombinant GAD65 at IDDM diagnosis.

TCL specific for GAD65

For each patient, GAD-specific TCL were generated from PBMC obtained at 4 different time points ranging from a few hours before to 6 months (patient A) or 8 months (patient B) after diagnosis. TCL were generated by successive stimulation cycles of PBMC ($2x10^6$ cells/well in 24-well plates) with recombinant human GAD65 (purified from insect cells infected with a recombinant baculovirus by binding to a chelating resin and used at 3 μg/ml), alternating with expansion cycles in IL-2 (5U/ml). TCL restimulations were performed with irradiated PBMC as antigen presenting cells (APC) and recombinant GAD65; $2\text{-}3X10^5$ TCL cells were added to 10^6 irradiated APC. The results obtained with the 4 independent TCL were equivalent for each patient. Lines maintained specific responsiveness to GAD65 for up to 8 rounds of stimulation. TCL from both patients were predominantly composed of single positive CD4 + T cells (>88%).

GAD65-derived epitopes recognized by the TCL

To characterize the GAD-peptides recognized by this lines, we used a set of 57 20-mer peptides and one 15-mer peptide spanning the entire human GAD65 protein with overlaps of ten amino acids. All peptides, used in this study, were more than 95% pure. We tested TCL in proliferation assays using fresh irradiated PBMC as APC that were preincubated with peptide or protein antigens (5-10x10^3 TCL cells + 5-10x10^4 APC/well in triplicates in round-bottom 96-well plates). Only peptide GAD 86-105 induced proliferation in TCL's from patient A above background level, while only peptide GAD 246-265 stimulated the lines from patient B.

To map the minimal epitopes and the critical residues in the two GAD-peptides for T cell stimulation, we used truncated variants and alanine- or glutamic acid-substituted analogs of both epitopes. The minimal epitope recognized by TCL is the 13-mer GAD 87-99 for patient A, and the 10-mer GAD 248-257 for patient B *(Figure 1)*. In both cases, we identified at least 8 residues as critical for TCL stimulation. These residues are likely either to bind to the HLA class II molecule or to contact the T cell receptor.

HLA restriction of the GAD65-derived epitopes

Proliferations in response to GAD65 or peptide of TCL from both patients were inhibited by a monoclonal antibody to HLA-DR (L243, used at 30 µg/ml), while the DQ-specific antibody SPV-L3 did not affect proliferations. Thus, both epitopes seem to be presented by HLA-DR. To determine which DR allele presented the epitopes, we used homozygous cell lines expressing only one of the two alleles of the patient. Epitope 87-99 is exclusively presented by cells expressing DRB1*0101, but not by other EBV-lines displaying any of the other three class II DR or DQ alleles carried by patient A. Thus, this epitope is presented by DRB1*0101.

Epitope 248-257 was not presented by lines expressing the DR13 haplotype. Therefore, it is presented by the DRB1*1501/DQB1*0602 haplotype. Because of the strict linkage disequilibrium between DRB1*1501 and DQB1*0602 among Caucasians, it was not possible to identify unequivocally the DR or DQ allele in this haplotype as the presenting molecule. However, the monoclonal antibody blocking experiments strongly suggested that this GAD-peptide is presented by an HLA-DR protein encoded in the DR15 haplotype.

The DR15 haplotype of patient B codes for two functional HLA-DRB proteins, DRB1*1501 and DRB5*0101. To decide which of these DR proteins presents epitope 248-257, we performed binding assays using HLA-DRB molecules purified from transfected L cell fibroblasts [6]. Various peptides comprising this epitope were used to compete against binding to HLA-DR of a biotinylated peptide derived from MBP, which binds with a similar affinity to both DR molecules encoded by the DR15 haplotype. As shown in *Figure 2*, two peptides containing the epitope competed very efficiently and with significantly higher avidity than unlabeled MBP reference peptide. Since binding competition for DRB5*0101 is 1000-fold more efficient than competition for binding to DRB1*1501, we concluded that DRB5*0101 presents this epitope.

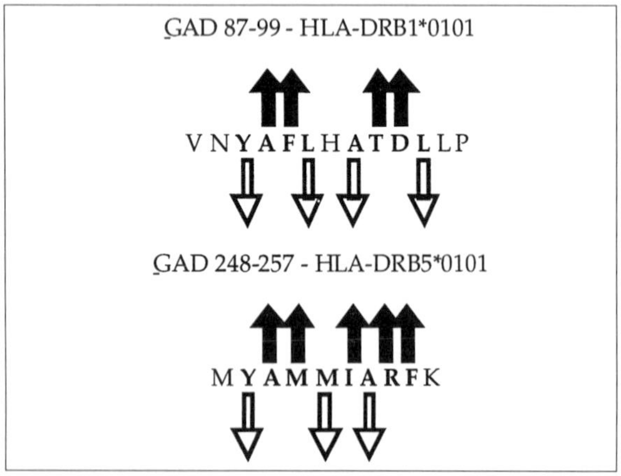

Figure 1. Minimal GAD-derived epitopes. White arrows show putative HLA anchors and black arrows correspond to putative T-cell contact residues.

Competitor peptide	IC50 for DRB1*1501 (nM)	IC50 for DRB5*0101 (nM)
MBP 84-102	100	100
SNMYAMMIARFK GAD 246-257	> 10 000	3
MYAMMIARFKMF GAD 248-259	10 000	5

Figure 2. Binding of GAD 248-257 to DR proteins encoded in the DR15 haplotype. Concentrations of unlabeled MBP 84-102 or GAD-derived competitor peptides required for 50% inhibition of binding of biotinylated peptide MBP 84-102 to DRB1*1501 and DRB5*0101.

For epitope 87-99, 4 of the residues crucial for TCL stimulation, match completely previously described residues found in the anchor positions P1, P4, P6 and P9, in the motif for binding to DRB1*0101 [7]. The other 4 critical residues are likely to interact with TCR of specific T cells. For epitope 248-257, an alignment with published data [7,8] suggests that tyrosine 249 represents the primary anchor for HLA-binding in the peptide *(Figure 1)*. In conclusion, we think to have shown for the first time that a peptide derived from an IDDM autoantigen can be presented with high efficiency by an HLA class II protein that is likely to protect from disease. Although, we do not know whether how representative this finding is for other epitopes and autoantigens, and which effect autoantigen presentation by protective HLA class II proteins has *in vivo*. We think that this observation argues in favor of an active role of autoantigen presentation by HLA class II in protection from diabetes.

References

1. Sinha AA, Lopez MT, McDevitt HO. Autoimmune diseases: the failure of self tolerance. *Science* 1990; 248:1380-8.
2. Nepom GT. A unified hypothesis for the complex genetics of HLA associations with IDDM. *Diabetes* 1990; 39: 1153-7.
3. Sheehy MJ. HLA and insulin-dependent diabetes. *Diabetes* 1992; 41: 123-9.
4. Tisch R, Yang XD, Singer SM, Liblau RS, Fugger L, McDevitt HO. Immune response to glutamic acid decarboxylase correlates with insulitis in non-obese diabetic mice. *Nature* 1993; 366: 72-5.
5. Atkinson MA, Kaufman DL, Campbell L, Gibbs KA, Shah SC, Bu DF, Erlander MG, Tobin AJ, McLaren NK. Response of peripheral-blood mononuclear cells to glutamate decarboxylase in insulin-dependent diabetes. *Lancet* 1992; 339: 458-9.
6. Kwok WW, Nepom GT, Raymond FC. HLA-DQ polymorphisms are highly selective for peptide binding interactions. *J Immunol* 1995; 155: 2468-76.
7. Rammensee HG, Friede T, Stevanovic S. MHC ligands and peptide motifs: first listing. *Immunogenetics* 1995; 41:178-228.
8. Vogt AB, Kropshofer H, Kalbacher H, Kalbus M, Rammensee HG, Coligan JE, Martin R. Ligand motifs of HLA-DRB5*0101 and DRB1*1501 molecules delineated from self-peptides. *J Immunol* 1994; 153: 1665-73.

Definition of antigenic determinant on glutamic acid decarboxylase molecule in HLA-DQ transgenic mice

N.F. De Souza Jr[1], E. Zanelli[2], S.B. Wilson [2], J.L. Strominger [2], S.R. Munn[1], C.S. David [2]

1 Departments of Immunology and Surgery, Mayo Clinic, 221 4th Avenue Sw, Rochester MN 55905, USA
2 Department of Molecular and Cellular Biology, Harvard University, Cambridge MA, USA

Insulin-dependent diabetes mellitus (IDDM) is a metabolic disorder resulting from the destruction of the insulin-producing B cells from the pancreatic islets of Langerhans by infiltrating autoreactive lymphocytes. There are more than a dozen self antigens on islet cells that are targets of the immune response in IDDM [1]. Each of these proteins, when processed by the antigen presenting cells, present multiple potentially immunogenic peptides which are capable of eliciting immune recognition and reach a level of inflammatory response able to destroy the pancreatic B cells. Glutamic acid decarboxylase (GAD 65) is the predominant serologically identified autoantigen in IDDM and is a target for specific cytotoxic T cells [2]. Antibodies against self-GAD antigens are found in the sera of most diabetic patients [3].
Genetic studies have permitted the identification of at least 13 loci that may play a role in IDDM predisposition [4]. Of these 13 loci, the MHC class II region carries the most important genetic factor in the susceptibility to IDDM [4]. Inside this region, the *HLA-DQB1* and *HLA-DQA1* loci are believed to be the genetic loci in this predisposition [5]. While HLA-DQ8 (DQB1*0302/DQA1*0301) is linked to IDDM, HLA-DQ6 (DQB1*0601/DQA1*0103) is negatively associated or protective. Through the use of HLA-transgenic mice expressing functional HLA-DQ8 and -DQ6 genes in the absence of endogenous mouse MHC genes [6], we have analyzed in the present study the HLA-DQ-restricted immunogenicity of GAD 65.

Results

The generation of DQ6.Ab° and DQ8.Ab° mice have been previously described [4]. DQ6.Ab° and DQ8.Ab° mice were immunized with 100 μg of human recombinant GAD 65 (rGAD 65), produced in a bacterial expression vector system, in complete Freund's adjuvant (CFA) using standard procedures. One week later, lymph node cells were prepared and challenged *in vitro* with rGAD 65 or 20-mer overlapping peptides derived from the mouse or human GAD 65 proteins. A strong T cell proliferation was observed against rGAD and human GAD peptides 467-487, 502-522, 507-527 in both DQ6. Ab° and DQ8.Ab° animals. However, only a weak, but significant, response was observed against mouse GAD peptides 507-527 (*Figure 1*). Sera collected at day 24 after immunization also showed a significant amount of rGAD 65-specific antibodies as detected by standard ELISA (data not shown).
When the same mice were immunized with the 20-mer self-GAD 65 peptides, themselves, T cell response was observed against peptides 507-527 and 537-557 (*Figure 2*).

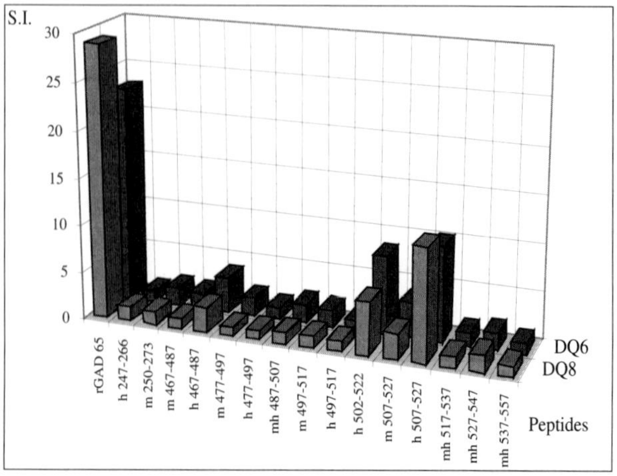

Figure 1. Immune response of lymph node cells from DQ6 and DQ8.Ab° mice immunized with rGAD.

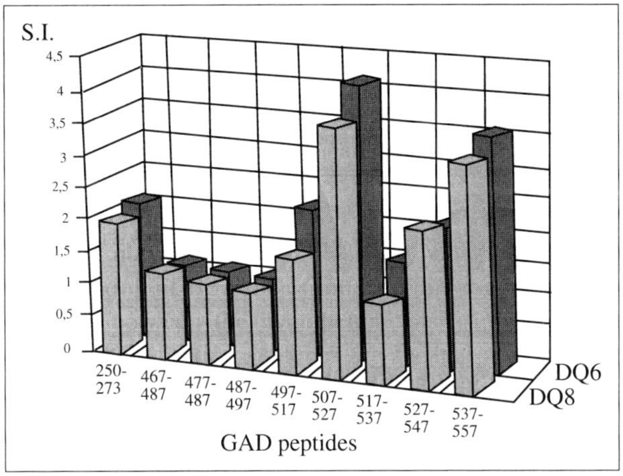

Figure 2. Immune response of DQ6 and DQ8.Ab^o to self-GAD 65 peptides.

Consistent with this weak reactivity against self-GAD determinants after rGAD immunization, blood glucose levels in both DQ6.Ab^o and DQ8. Ab^o mice remain normal, even six months after immunization, and no lymphocyte infiltration was observed in the pancreatic islets (data not shown).

Conclusions

Peripheral blood lymphocytes from IDDM patients and healthy individuals show reactivity against regions 161-243 and 473-555 of GAD 65. However, only reactivity against the latter region is significantly increased in patients compared to controls [7]. For this reason, we have concentrated our first study in HLA-DQ transgenic mice against this particular region. Our results show that, indeed, both DQ8 and DQ6 molecules are able to bind GAD peptides derived from this region. However, immunization with rGAD 65 fails to induce a strong T cell response against mouse determinants. Consistent with this result, HLA-DQ transgenic mice do not develop diabetes or insulitis after rGAD immunization.

Interestingly, GAD peptide 537-557 which is identical in mouse and human GAD 65 is immunogenic in these mice. Thus, this particular determinant is probably cryptic. Reactivity against self-peptides 507-527 and 537-557 show that self-reactive T cells exist in these mice, but mechanisms of peripheral tolerance are probably involved to prevent autoimmune manifestations.

Our results are consistent with findings in both mouse experimental models of diabetes, and studies in humans, and show that expression of an IDDM-associated HLA specificity in mice is not sufficient to induce destruction of the pancreatic islets [4, 8]. As already studied in the NOD model, other genes outside the MHC region are necessary for diabetes predisposition [8]. However, our study demonstrates the usefulness of transgenic mice expressing human MHC genes for mapping of antigenic determinants on autoantigens which are relevant to human diseases.

References

1. Eisenbarth GS. Type I diabetes mellitus: a chronic autoimmune disease. *N Engl J Med* 1986 ; 314 : 1360-8.
2. Tisch R, Yang XD, Singer SM, Liblau RS, Fugger L, McDevitt HO. Immune response to glutamic acid decarboxylase correlates with insulitis in non-obese diabetic mice. *Nature* 1993 ; 366 : 15-7.
3. Tuomilehto J, Zimmet P, Mackay IR, Koskela P, Vidgren G, Toivanen L, Tuomilehto-Wolf E, Kohtamaki K, Stengard J, Rowley MJ. Antibodies to glutamic acid decarboxylase as predictors of insulin-dependent diabetes mellitus before clinical onset of disease. *Lancet* 1994 ; 343 : 266-7.
4. Davies JL, Kawaguchi Y, Bennett ST, Copeman JB, Cordell HJ, Pritchard LE, Reed PW, Gough SC , Jenkins SC, Palmer SM. *Nature* 1994 ; 371 : 130-6.
5. Todd JA, Bell JI, McDevitt HO. HLA-DQ beta gene contributes to susceptibility and resistance to insulin-dependent diabetes mellitus. *Nature* 1987 ; 329 : 599-604.
6. Zanelli E, Krco CJ, Baisch JM Cheng S, David CS. Immune response of HLA-DQ8 transgenic mice to HLA-DQB1 HV3 peptides correlates with predisposition to rheumatoid arthritis. *Proc Natl Acad Sci USA* 1996 ; 93 : 1814-9.
7. Lohmann T, Leslie RDG, Hawa M, Geysen M, Rodda S, Londei M. Immunodominant epitopes of glutamic acid decarboxylase 65 and 67 in insulin-dependent diabetes mellitus. *Lancet* 1994 ; 343 : 1607-8.
8. Wicker LS, Todd JA, Peterson LB. Genetic control of autoimmune diabetes in the NOD mouse. *Annu Rev Immunol* 1995 ; 13 : 179-200.

Application of 10 novel microsatellites mapped in the MHC class III region to the study of susceptibility loci in type 1 diabetes

R.E. March, S.L. Hsieh[1], A. Khanna[2], S.J. Cross, R.D. Campbell

MRC Immunochemistry Unit, Department of Biochemistry, University of Oxford, South Parks Road, Oxford OX1 3QU, UK
1 Present address: Department of Microbiology and Immunology, NYMU School of Medicine, Shie-Pai 11221, Taipei, Taiwan, Republic of China
2 Present address: Sir William Dunn School of Pathology, University of Oxford, South Parks Road, Oxford, UK

The human MHC, which is located on chromosome 6p21.3, is conveniently divided into three regions. The class I and class II regions each include genes which encode highly polymorphic proteins involved in antigen presentation. The class III region, which is about 1.1 Mb long and lies between the class I and class II regions, also contains some genes that encode proteins involved in the immune response, such as the complement proteins C2, factor B and C4, three members of the heat shock protein 70 (HSP70) family and the cytokines tumour necrosis factor (TNF) and lymphotoxin (LT) A and B. In recent years over 55 additional novel genes have been mapped within the class III region, the functions of many of which are now being elucidated [1]. Many of these genes are potential candidates for involvement in type I diabetes, such as RAGE, the receptor for advanced glycosylation end products; G13, which encodes a potential member of the CREB family of transcription factors; G9a, which encodes a zinc-binding protein with 6 ankyrin repeats; and IkbL, a potential member of the I kappa B family, which interact with and regulate the NF kappa B family of transcription factors [2]. Because of the high density of genes in this region, it is particularly important to have highly informative markers that can be analysed by semi-automated technology in large numbers of individuals, in order to assess the effects of gene variants on disease, and we have therefore carried out a search for $(CA)_n$ repeats within the class III region.

Mapping of microsatellites in the class III region

Most of the class III region has been cloned into a minimum set of 23 overlapping cosmid clones. Southern blots derived from these cosmids were probed with a labelled $(CA)_{10}$ oligonucleotide, washed under stringent conditions, and positive fragments cloned into M13mp10 and sequenced. The most telomeric repeat, 62, is around 7 kb from the LTA gene, microsatellites 82-2 and 82-3 are in the B144 gene, microsatellite 82-1 is in the 5' region of the G1 gene, microsatellite T2 is in the 5' region of the G3 gene, microsatellites 9N-2 and -3 are in the G7 gene, microsatellite 9N-1 is in the G6 gene, microsatellite D3A is in the G14 gene region, and the LH1 microsatellite is within 100 kb telomeric of the DRA locus. It was subsequently discovered that the 62 microsatellite overlapped with the repeat sequence published by Nedospasov *et al.* [3], and designated TNFa and TNFb. The primers used in our laboratory amplify both TNFa, which is a $(CA)_n$ repeat, and TNFb, which is a $(TC)_n$ repeat, as well as the intervening 22 bp of non-perfect repeat sequence.

In an initial study, unlabelled PCR products amplified from DNA from 50 unrelated normal individuals were fractionated in non-denaturing gels and silver stained. These results were compared with sequenced products and used to estimate the size range, polymorphism information content (PIC) and heterozygosity index

Table I. Characteristics of 10 polymorphic $(CA)_n$ microsatellites in the class III region

Name	Range (bp)	Repeat sequence	N	HI	PIC
62	146-197	$(TC)_{10}$ - $CCT(C)_5$-$(TC)_3$-$(C)_3$-TGCAA-$(CA)_{15}$	14	82.4%	0.821
82-1	86-113	$(CA)_{13}$-CGCACG-$(CA)_{15}$	13	81.3%	0.740
82-2	113-135	$(CA)_{22}$	13	56.8%	0.504
82-3	140-174	$(CA)_{28}$	16	61.4%	0.571
T2	155-165	$(CA)_{21}$	14	65.1%	0.632
9N-1	87-103	$(CA)_{17}$	14	53.2%	0.479
9N-2	98-120	$(CA)_{23}$	7	72.3%	0.705
9N-3	80-126	$(CA)_{17}$	13	80.6%	0.797
D3A	113-144	$(CA)_{18}$-GAGA-$(CA)_4$-GA-$(CA)_3$	9	75.9%	0.739
LH1	79-103	$(CA)_{21}$	20	71%	0.699

HI = heterozygosity index; PIC = polymorphism information content; N=number of alleles.

(HI) of each $(CA)_n$ repeat *(Table I)*. We also checked that the $(CA)_n$ repeats were inherited in a Mendelian fashion in three-generation CEPH families (data not shown).

Application of the microsatellites to type 1 diabetes

Primers for five of the class III region microsatellites were fluorescently labelled and used to amplify DNA samples from 197 families (the BDA Warren DNA repository) with two or more sibs with type 1 diabetes. Primers for each set were labelled in a different colour, such that all PCR products for a single individual, together with a labelled size standard, could be run in one track and detected on an automatic ABI PRISM 377 DNA sequencer. Allele sizes were checked and exported to the GAS package version 2.0 [4], where they were numbered and tested for association with disease in a single-point transmission disequilibrium test [5]. These results were compared with the known HLA class II alleles for each individual *(Table II)*.

Alleles of all but one of the microsatellites tested were significantly associated with disease in this study, but the significance levels obtained were lower than those obtained for the class II alleles, except for microsatellite 62. The corrected significance level obtained with microsatellite 62 using the TDT analysis was higher than that obtained with DR3 and DR4, but not quite as high as those obtained with DQ2 and DQ8.

There are three possible explanations for this finding. First, the disease association found with the class III region microsatellites may be due to an independent biological effect of a class III region gene on disease susceptibility. Second, because the class III region is so closely linked to the class II region (1-2 cM) and because of the known linkage disequilibrium that extends across the MHC, alleles from the class III region microsatellites may be carried on an extended haplotype that is increased in frequency in the diabetic population, even if the biological effects of the class III region genes are neutral. Third, if variants of class III region genes carried on these haplotypes are not neutral, but have some biological effect on the disease process, they may augment the disease susceptibility of the haplotype carried by the class II genes. Further studies are in progress to distinguish between these different explanations.

In conclusion, we have mapped 10 novel polymorphic $(CA)_n$ microsatellites which we believe will greatly facilitate the identification of disease susceptibility genes within the class III region. Because of the small genetic distance

Table II. Results of transmission disequilibrium tests for association with type 1 diabetes

Marker	No. alleles tested	TDT probability	no.tests	corrected probability
DR3	458	1.6 x 10 -5	13	2.08 x 10-4
DR4	458	1.6 x 10 -5	13	2.08 x 10-4
DQ2	418	2.1 x 10-6	9	1.89 x 10-5
DQ8	418	1.6 x 10-6	9	1.44 x 10-5
D3A	416	6.9 x 10-4	6	4.14 x 10-3
82-1	516	4.5 x 10-4	12	5.4 x 10-3
82-2	392	1.4 x 10-4	8	1.12 x 10-3
82-3	468	ns	12	ns
62	638	4.2 x 10-6	11	4.6 x 10-5

ns = no allele was significantly associated with disease.

across the region and the relatively high level of linkage disequilibrium, we regard it as essential to have large numbers of affected families, informative markers such as we have described here, and semi-automated technology. These resources are enabling us to study the question of whether genes in the class III region represent an additional risk factor in the development of type 1 diabetes.

References

1. Aguado B, Milner CM, Campbell RD. Genes of the MHC class III region and the functions of the proteins they encode. In: Browning M, McMichael A eds. *HLA/MHC: genes, molecules and function.* Oxford: Bios Scientific Publishers, 1996: 39-76.
2. Albertella MR, Campbell RD. Characterization of a novel gene in the human major histocompatibility complex that encodes a potential new member of the I kappa B family of proteins. *Hum Mol Genet* 1994; 3: 793-9.
3. Nedospasov SA, Udalova IA, Kuprash DV, Turetskaya RL. DNA sequence polymorphism at the human tumor necrosis factor (TNF) locus. Numerous TNF/lymphotoxin alleles tagged by two closely linked microsatellites in the upstream region of the lymphotoxin (TNF-beta) gene. *J Immunol* 1991; 147: 1053-9.
4. GAS package version 2.0 (c) Alan Young, Oxford University, 1993: 5.
5. Spielman RS, Mcginnis RE, Ewens WJ. Transmission test for linkage disequilibrium: the insulin gene region and insulin-dependent diabetes mellitus (IDDM). *Am J Hum Genet* 1993; 52: 506-16.

DRB1, DQA1-QAP and DQB1-QBP haplotypes in 58 IDDM families

C. Carrier[1], F. Ginsberg [2], E. Russo [3], P. Rubinstein[1]

1 Immunogenetics Laboratory, New York Blood Center, 310 E67 TH Street, New York 10021, USA
2 Division of Pediatric Endocrinology, Mount Sinai School of Medicine, New York, USA
3 Division of Endocrinology, UNIFESP/Escola Paulista de Medicina, New York, USA

Structural variants of HLA-DQB1 dimers have major effects in determining susceptibility to IDDM and other autoimmune conditions but polymorphic promoter elements may also cause the association. Discrimination of their respective involvements is difficult because of the very high linkage disequilibrium.

We report here on the DQA1 and DQB1 structural and promoter "alleles" of haplotypes observed in IDDM-affected probands and normal siblings and parents, in 58 multiplex families from New York and São Paulo ("NY" and SP families, respectively).

HLA typing

HLA-A, B and C alleles were elucidated by serological methods. Class II and promoter typing used PCR amplification of the corresponding regions of the genes, followed by allele-specific hybridization with oligoprobes. High resolution typing implied group specific PCR using Workshop primers and probes. DQA1 and DQB1 promoter typing was done with Workshop reagents. Class II and promoter typing was done under locally-optimized conditions.

Results

In most NY and SP families, DR3 and/or DR4 were inherited by probands accounting for a large fraction of "affected" alleles (*i.e.*, inherited by the probands. "Unaffected" haplotypes are present in the parents but absent from all the patients in the pedigree). Six of 24 (25%) DR3 and 7/33 (27%) DR4 alleles were not affected. Each of the two DR3 haplotypes *(Table I)* had a different DQB1 allele with unique QBP variants, identical in NY and SP families. An exceptional affected haplotype, DRB1*0301, DQA1*0102|QAP 1.2, DQB1*0602|QBP (6.2/6.3) was inherited by a proband and a nonaffected sibling. There were nine different DR4-DRB1 subtypes, all with DQA1*0301|QAP 3.1 *(Table II)*. Affected DR4 haplotypes predominantly carried DQB1*0302, all of these with QBP 3.21. DR4 haplotypes with DQB1*0301 were mostly unaffected and had QBP 3.1. There were two exceptions, one each DRB1*0401 and *0402, with DQB1*0301|QBP 3.21, both affected. Thus, in DR4, DQB1 structural and promoter variants had similar population associations with IDDM. In the eclectic DQB haplotypes, both affected, the IDDM-associated promoter was coupled to the non-IDDM-associated structural allele, favoring the predominant importance of the promoter sequence. The scant supply of this combination and the absence of its reciprocal, prevents firmer conclusions at this time. DR2 haplotypes are not informative on the relative importance of promoter and structural sequences in IDDM susceptibility, because of strict linkage disequilibrium *(Table I)*.

Table I. IDD-Affected and -unaffected DRB1-DQA1-DQB1-QAP-DQB1-QBP haplotypes in New York and Sao Paulo multiplex families

	HAPLOTYPE					NY		SP	
	DRB1	DQA1	QAP	DQB1	QBP	N	AFF	N	AFF
DR1	*0101	*0101	1.1	*0501	5.(11/12)	9	5	3	2
	*0102	*0101	1.1	*0501	5.(11/12)	5	5	2	1
	*0103	*0101	1.1	*0501	5.(11/12)	-	-	2	-
DR2	1501	*0102	1.2	*0602	6.(2/3)	6	-	2	1
	1601	*0102	1.2	*0502	5.(11/12)	2	2	2	2
	1602	*0102	1.2	*0502	5.(11/12)	1	1	-	-
	1502	*0103	1.2	*0601	6.11	-	-	3	2
	1602	*0501	4.1	*0301	3.1	-	-	2	1
DR3	*0301	*0501	4.1	*0201	2.1	22	16	15	13
	*0301	*0102	1.2	*0602	6.12	1	1	-	-
	*0302	*0401	4.2	*0402	4.1	-	-	1	-
DR4	*0401	*0301	3.1	*0301	3.21	1	1	0	0
	*0401	*0301	3.1	*0301	3.1	7	1	1	1
	*0401	*0301	3.1	*0302	3.21	6	6	4	4
	*0402	*0301	3.1	*0301	3.21	1	1	0	0
	*0402	*0301	3.1	*0301	3.1	1	0	0	0
	*0402	*0301	3.1	*0302	3.21	5	4	1	1
	*0403	*0301	3.1	*0302	3.21	1	1	2	1
	*0403	*0301	3.1	*0301	3.1	0	0	1	1
	*0404	*0301	3.1	*0302	3.21	6	6	3	2
	*0405	*0301	3.1	*0302	3.21	2	1	8	7
	*0405	*0301	3.1	*0402	4.1	0	0	1	0
	*0407	*0301	3.1	*0302	3.21	1	0	0	0
	*0408	*0301	3.1	*0302	3.21	1	1	0	0
	*0410	*0301	3.1	*0302	3.21	0	0	1	1
	*0411	*0301	3.1	*0302	3.21	0	0	1	0
DR5	1101	*0501	4.1	*0301	3.1	4	2	3	1
	1104	*0501	4.1	*0301	3.1	3	-	1	-
	1201	*0501	4.1	*0301	3.1	1	1	-	-
DR6	1301	*0103	1.3	*0603	6.(2/3)	4	3	2	-
	1302	*0102	1.4	*0501	6.(2/3)	1	1	-	-
	1302	*0102	1.4	*0604	6.(2/3)	1	1	2	1
	1302	*0102	1.4	*0605/0606	6.(2/3)	-	-	2	1
	1305	*0501	4.1	*0301	3.1	-	-	2	-
	1406	*0501	4.1	*0301	3.1	-	-	2	2
DR7	7	*0201	2.1	*0201	2.1	6	4	4	3
	7	*0201	2.1	*0303.2	3.21	3	1	-	-
DR8	*0801/0805	*0401	4.2	*0402	4.1	4	3	1	1
	*0804	*0401	4.2	*0402	4.1	1	-	-	-
	*0803	*0501	4.1	*0501	3.1	-	-	1	1

Table II. IDDM susceptibility of DRB1-DQB1|QBP haplotypes

			NY		SP		Total	
DRB1	DQB1	QBP	Aff	Unaff	Aff	Unaff	Aff	Unaff
*0401	*0301	3.1	1	6	1	0	2	6
		3.21	1	0	0	0	1	0
	*0302	3.21	6	0	4	0	10	0
*0402	*0301	3.1	0	1	0	0	0	1
		3.21	1	0	0	0	1	0
	*0302	3.21	4	1	1	0	5	1
*0403	*0301	3.1	0	0	1	0	1	0
	*0302	3.21	1	0	1	1	2	1
*0404	*0302	3.21	6	0	2	1	8	1
*0405	*0302	3.21	1	1	7	1	8	2
	*0402	4.1	0	0	0	1	0	1
*0407	*0302	3.21	0	1	0	0	0	1
*0408	*0302	3.21	1	0	0	0	1	0
*0410	*0302	3.21	0	0	1	0	1	0
*0411	*0302	3.21	0	0	0	1	0	1

Molecular analysis of HLA DR-DQ-DP haplotypes in 180 Caucasian, multiplex IDDM families

J.A. Noble[1], A.M. Valdes[2], M. Cook[1], W. Klitz[2], G. Thomson[2], H.A. Erlich[1]

1 Department of Human Genetics, Roche Molecular Systems, 1145 Atlantic Avenue, Alameda, CA 94501, USA and Children's Hospital Oakland Research Institute, 747 Fifty-Second Street, Oakland, CA 94609, USA
2 Department of Integrative Biology, 3060 Valley Life Sciences Building, University of California, Berkeley, CA 94720-3140, USA

The association of HLA class II genes with insulin-dependent diabetes mellitus (IDDM) is well-established (for review, see [1]). While IDDM susceptibility is clearly multigenic [2], the HLA region genes have the greatest effect. The contribution of HLA to the total genetic risk for IDDM has been estimated at 44% [3]. To investigate the role of individual HLA alleles, genotypes, and haplotypes in IDDM susceptibility, we have used DNA-based HLA typing methods to identify class II alleles in 180 Caucasian, multiplex IDDM families. The Human Biological Data Interchange (HBDI, Philadelphia, PA) provided DNA from 166 families; DNA from the remaining 14 families was provided by Dr Donald Bowden (Bowman Gray School of Medicine, Winston-Salem, NC). DRB1, DQA1, DQB1, and DPB1 genotypes were determined for all families, and four-locus haplotypes were identifiable in 177 of the 180 families in the study. From analysis of these data, we were able not only to confirm previously-reported HLA effects but also to identify DPB1 associations with IDDM as well as a parental transmission effect.

DR-DQ effects

Consistent with other studies, the frequency of DR2 was greatly reduced in patients (.03) versus affected-family-based controls (.17) or CEPH family controls (.18) [4]. The dominant protection afforded by DR2 was limited, however, to the common haplotype DRB1*1501-DQA1*0102-DQB1*0602. The less common DR2 haplotype DRB1*1601-DQA1*0102-DQB1*0502 was found in nearly all DR2+ patients and was not decreased in patients compared to controls.

As found in previous studies, DR3/DR4 heterozygotes were greatly overrepresented in the patient population (~41% compared to ~ 2% in the general population). We examined individuals from affected sib pairs sharing zero parental HLA class II haplotypes, assuming that disease susceptibility in these individuals was least attributable to HLA genes and more likely to result from the effects of other, shared susceptibility loci. Even in this population DR3/DR4 individuals were present at >40%, illustrating the magnitude of the contribution of HLA to IDDM susceptibility.

The identity of the amino acid residue at position 57 in the DQβ1 chain has been implicated in IDDM risk [5,6], with particular emphasis on the role of the DQB1*0302 (Ala 57) allele found on DR4 haplotypes. In this study, the disease-predisposing effect of DQB1*0302 was dependent on genotypic context. In DR3/DR4 heterozygotes, as well as in DR4/DR4 and DR4/DR8 patients, nearly all DR4 haplotypes carried the high-risk DQB1*0302 allele, and the alternative DQB1*0301 (Asp 57) allele was rarely seen. In contrast, DR1/DR4 heterozygotes had a lower frequency of DQB1*0302 on their DR4 haplotypes (.72), similar to that found in CEPH controls (.71).

The reduced predisposing effect of the DQB1*0302 allele in DR1/DR4 heterozygotes was accompanied by an apparent increase in the contribution of the DRB1 locus. A hierarchy of risk is associated with individual DRB1*04 alleles; DRB1*0405 is most predisposing [7]. In these data, the distribution of DRB1 alleles on DR4 haplotypes in DR3/DR4 heterozygotes resembled that of control (CEPH) haplotypes [4]. The DR4 haplotypes of DR1/DR4 heterozygotes; however, had highly-predisposing alleles (DRB1*0405 and DRB1*0401) overrepresented. Overall, these data suggest that the relative effects of DRB1 and DQB1 alleles on disease predisposition are dependent on the genotypic context.

DP effects

Our PCR/SSOP typing system allowed determination of all DPB1 genotypes and, in most cases, assignment of DPB1 alleles to DR-DQ haplotypes. Genotype analysis indicated that several alleles show significant frequency differences in patients relative to controls. In some cases, these differences could be attributed simply to linkage disequilibrium, *i.e.*, a given DPB1 allele may be at increased frequency in patients because it is present on high-risk DR-DQ haplotypes. This is probably the case for DPB1*0202, which was found almost exclusively on DR3 haplotypes and, consequently, was increased in frequency in patient populations.

Of all the DPB1 alleles identified in these families, DPB1*0301 showed the most significant increase in patients relative to controls ($p < 0.001$, OR = 11.97). This allele was found on many different haplotypes in both patients and controls, suggesting that a simple linkage disequilibrium effect is an unlikely explanation for this increase. The idea that DPB1*0301 contributes to IDDM susceptibility is supported by a recent study of Mexican-American IDDM families in which a predisposing effect for DPB1*0301 was seen independent of linkage disequilibrium [8].

The allele with the most significant decrease in patient frequency for the DPB1 locus was DPB1*0402 ($p < 0.025$). Like DPB1*0301, DPB1*0402 was present on many different haplotypes in these data. Stratification analysis of DPB1 alleles on DRB1*0301, DRB1*0401, and DRB1*0404 haplotypes indicated a significantly-decreased transmission of DRB1*0301-DPB1*0402 haplotypes ($p < 0.005$). A similar decrease was not seen for DPB1*0402 on either DRB1*0401 or DRB1*0404 haplotypes. This suggests that, at least in some cases, the effect of a DPB1 allele on disease susceptibility may be dependent on its DR context. DPB1*0402 may mitigate the predisposing effect of DR3 haplotypes in some way but appears to have no effect on DR4 haplotypes.

DPB1*0101 was slightly increased in patients, but this increase did not achieve statistical significance. In addition, DPB1*0101 is in linkage disequilibrium with DR3, suggesting that this allele may be increased simply due to linkage disequilibrium. Transmission analysis, however, revealed that DR3-DPB1*0101 haplotypes were twice as likely to be of maternal origin than of paternal origin, whereas DR3 haplotypes carrying other DPB1 alleles showed no parent-of-origin effect.

Increased maternal transmission of DR3 in IDDM is a controversial issue [9]. Most analyses addressing this issue focus only on the DR and DQ loci. Extrapolating from the data in this study, one might conclude that the population frequency of the DPB1*0101 allele could determine whether increased maternal transmission of DR3 haplotypes would be observed in a given dataset. If the observation presented here holds true for populations other than Caucasian, then a population with a very high frequency of DPB1*0101 would be expected to show increased maternal transmission of DR3 haplotypes, while a population with a very low frequency of DPB1*0101 would not.

In conclusion, PCR/SSOP typing analysis of this very large dataset has allowed us to elucidate not only the very strong, striking effects of HLA on IDDM susceptibility, such as the increase in DR3/DR4 heterozygotes, but also more subtle effects, such as the dependence of DQB1*03 alleles (on DR4 genotypes) on genotypic context. In addition, effects of alleles too rare to evaluate in studies of fewer individuals can be seen in these data. The family-based samples allowed us to unambiguously assign alleles to haplotypes and analyze the transmission of those haplotypes uncovering previously-unreported parent-of-origin effects. Continuing analysis of these data, combined with data from additional families, will help clarify the contributions of HLA loci and may help determine the mechanism of HLA-based predisposition to and protection from IDDM.

References

1. Nepom GT, Erlich H. MHC class-II molecules and autoimmunity. *Annu Rev Immunol* 1991;9:493-525.
2. Owerbach D, Gabbay KH. The search for IDDM susceptibility genes. *Diabetes* 1996;45:544-51.
3. Risch N. Assessing the role of HLA-linked and unlinked determinants of disease. *Am J Hum Genet* 1987;40:1-14.
4. Begovich AB, McClure GR, Suraj VC *et al.* Polymorphism, recombination, and linkage disequilibrium within the HLA class II region. *J Immunol* 1992;148:249-58.
5. Todd JA, Bell JI, McDevitt HO. HLA-DQ beta gene contributes to susceptibility and resistance to insulin-dependent diabetes mellitus. *Nature* 1987;329:599-604.
6. Horn GT, Bugawan TL, Long CM, Erlich HA. Allelic sequence variation of the HLA-DQ loci: relationship to serology and to insulin-dependent diabetes susceptibility. *Proc Natl Acad Sci USA* 1988;85:6012-6.
7. Cucca F, Lampis R, Frau F *et al.* The distribution of DR4 haplotypes in Sardinia suggests a primary association of type I diabetes with DRB1 and DQB1 loci. *Hum Immunol* 1995;43:301-8.
8. Erlich HA, Rotter JI, Chang JD *et al.* Association of HLA-DPB1*0301 with insulin dependent diabetes mellitus in Mexican-Americans. *Diabetes* 1996;45:610-4.
9. Undlien DE, Akselsen HE, Joner G *et al.* No difference in the parental origin of susceptibility HLA class II haplotypes among Norwegian patients with insulin-dependent diabetes mellitus (letter). *Am J Hum Genet* 1995;57:1511-4.

Insulin-dependent diabetes mellitus in non-DR3/non-DR4 subjects

D. Dubois-Laforgue[1], J. Timsit[1], I. Djilali-Saiah[2], C. Boitard[1], S. Caillat-Zucman[2]

1. Diabetology Unit, Department of Clinical Immunology
2. Laboratory of Clinical Immunology, INSERM U25, Hôpital Necker, 161, rue de Sèvres, 75743 Paris Cedex 15, France

Insulin-dependent diabetes mellitus (IDDM) usually occurs as the consequence of an autoimmune disease leading to the specific destruction of β cells in the pancreatic islets of Langerhans [1]. In this context it is referred to as type 1 diabetes. IDDM is known to be associated with particular HLA alleles of the DR and/or DQ genes in the class II region of the MHC. In Caucasians it is strongly associated with DRB1* 03 and 04 and with DQB1* 0201 and 0302. Accordingly, it has been reported that over 95% of type 1 diabetic patients are DR3 and/or DR4 [2]. However, it must be underlined that the majority of the genetic studies of IDDM so far performed were conducted in pediatric patients, although IDDM occurs after the age of 20 in half of the patients [3]. In fact we have previously shown in a large group of IDDM patients that the percentage of non-DR3/non-DR4 increases with the age at onset, 26% of the patients in whom IDDM occurred after the age of 30 being non-DR3/non-DR4. Conversely, the proportion of DR3/DR4 heterozygotes decreases with age at onset [4]. This study raised the question of the aetiology of IDDM in non-DR3/nonDR4 patients the more so since the frequency of islet cell antibodies (ICA) was lower in this group than in patients below 15 yr at onset of diabetes. In the present study we have selected 77 non-DR3/non-DR4 patients with unambiguous IDDM to determine whether other associations could be found with other MHC class II alleles.

Subjects and methods

Subjects

Eighty-five subjects consecutively referred to our department for clinical IDDM and who were later found to be non-DR3/non-DR4 were studied. In these patients the diagnosis of IDDM was made on the basis of clinical presentation at onset (polyuria, spontaneous loss of body weight, ketosis or keto-acidosis, absence of family history suggesting maturity-onset of diabetes in the young, MODY). Diabetes secondary to hemochromatosis or chronic pancreatitis were ruled out. The presence of 3243 bp mtDNA point mutation, which is found in maternally transmitted diabetes [5], was ruled out in all subjects by mitochondrial DNA analysis performed on peripheral blood leucocytes. Non-caucasian patients were excluded from the study because of a particular syndrome ("flatbush diabetes") initially described in black patients comprising diabetes of acute presentation, increased frequency of DR3 and DR4 alleles, absence of anti-islet cell antibodies and late occurrence of remission of insulin-dependency [6]. Overall eight subjects were excluded from the study. The control population consisted of 272 non-DR3/non-DR4 healthy subjects.

HLA class II allele determination

HLA DRB1*, DQA1* and DQB1* typing was done by sequence specific oligonucleotide hybridization following DNA amplification by PCR according to the 12 th Workshop protocol.

Autoantibodies

Islet cell autoantibodies (ICA) were assayed by indirect immunofluorescence on cryostat section of human pancreas. Autoantibodies directed to glutamic acid decarboxylase (GADA) were determined by radioimmunoassay.

Statistical analysis

The odds ratio was calculated according to Woolf's formula and, by convention, expressed as a relative risk

Table I. DRB1 phenotypic frequencies (F) and relative risks (RR) in the control group (C), in non DR3/non DR4 diabetic patients (DB) and in the subgroup of patients positive for ICA and/or GADA (ICA+)

	C (n=272) %	DB (n=77) F	DB (n=77) RR	ICA+ (n=29) F	ICA+ (n=29) RR
DRB1*01	33.1	41.6		51.7	
DRB1*15	26.8	18.2		6.9	
DRB1*16	5.5	7.8		6.9	
DRB1*11	29.8	18.2		13.8	
DRB1*12	4	2.6		0	
DRB1*13	29.4	28.6		26.7	
DRB1*14	7.7	6.5		6.9	
DRB1*07	33.8	33.8		34.5	
DRB1*08	5.5	19.5	4.1*	27.6	6.8*
DRB1*09	2.6	3.9		3.5	
DRB1*10	3.7	1.3		0	

Only statistically significant RR are presented.
* Pc < 0.01

(RR). The statistical significance of the difference of RR from unity was tested by chi-square analysis with one degree of freedom. The level of significance was set to 0.05. P_c indicates a p value corrected by use of Bonferonni inequality method, by multiplying p by the number of alleles compared.

Results

The distribution of DRB1 alleles is shown on *Table I*. Only the frequency of DRB1*08 was significantly increased in diabetic patients compared to non-DR3/non-DR4 controls (19.5% vs 5.5%, $p_c < 0.005$, RR = 4.1). It must be underlined that DR1 that has been previously reported to be associated with IDDM was not increased in our population. Among DQB1 alleles only DQB1*0402 was increased in diabetic subjects (18.5%) compared to the controls (4%, $p_c < 0.005$, RR = 5.3). The frequency of DQA1*0401 was 14% in diabetic subjects and 4% in the controls ($p_c = 0.08$). No DRB1 allele appeared as "protective" in the present study. Particularly, the frequency of DRB1*15 was 18.2% in the diabetic subjects and and 26.8% in the control group (p = 0.14). The frequency of DQB1*0602 was similar in the two groups (21.5% and 22%).
We then stratified the patients acccording to the presence of serological markers of anti-islet cell autoimmunity, namely ICA and/or GADA. Because autoantibodies tend to disappear after onset of the disease in the majority of type 1 diabetic patients, we only considered the 44 patients who had had serum sampling within the first year of IDDM. Twenty-nine patients (66%) had ICA and/or GADA. In the patients with autoantibodies we found the same HLA class II associations as in the whole patient group. The RR were even higher in the former than in the latter (*Table I*). The frequency of DRB1*08 was 28.6% in the patients positive for ICA and/or GADA and 6% in the non-DR3/non-DR4 controls ($p_c < 0.005$, OR = 6.8). DQB1*0402 was increased in these patients (26.1%) compared to the controls (4%, $p_c < 0.01$, RR = 8.4). There was no difference in the distribution of DRB1*15 and of DQB1*0602 between the two groups. Lastly, the frequency of DQA1*0401 was increased in autoantibodies-positive diabetic subjects compared to the controls (26.3% and 4% $p_c < 0.02$, RR = 8.3). By contrast, patients negative for ICA and GADA were genetically identical to control subjects.
Analysis of genotype combinations did not reveal any preferential association of DRB1, DQB1 or DQA1 alleles, particularly in the DRB1*08 patients.

Since IDDM has been associated in Caucasians with DQB1* alleles encoding a non-aspartic acid at the position 57 of the DQβ chain [7] we assessed whether the same association was observed in the non-DR3/non-DR4 population. Despite the fact that the DRB1*08-DQA1*0401-DQB1*0402 haplotype encodes an Asp-positive Dqß57 chain we found a significant association with DQB1* non Asp57 alleles in the diabetic patients (80% vs 65% in the controls, $p < 0.04$, RR = 2.1). The association was even stronger when ICA and/or GADA positive patients were considered ($p < 0.01$, RR = 5.9, vs controls). This was due to the fact that all DRB1*08-DQB1*0402 patients had a non Asp57 allele on the second haplotype. By contrast with what previously reported in IDDM we found no predisposing effect of alleles encoding an arginine at the position 52 of the DQα chain.

Discussion

We analysed the immunogenetic characteristics of 77 non DR3/nonDR4 Caucasian patients presenting with typical IDDM. The prevalence of ICA (66%) in this diabetic population was the same as that we previously reported in DR3 and/or DR4 diabetic subjects [4]. Thus patients included in the present study shared common clinical and immunological features with an adult IDDM population.

Phenotypic analysis indicates that in non-DR3/non-DR4 subjects, only DRB1*08 confers significant susceptibility to IDDM. This association appears relatively weak since only 20% of the patients were DRB1*08 (compared to 6% of the controls). Weak associations of IDDM with DR1 and DR8 had previously been reported in non-DR3/non-DR4 Caucasien subjects [8]. In the present study DRB1*01 did not appeared as predisposing (41.5% in diabetics vs 33% in the controls). This discrepancy could be explained by the high frequency of this allele in our control population, or by differences in age or ethnic origin of the subjects studied.

Several studies have mapped IDDM susceptibility to DQ rather than to DR locus [2]. Whether susceptibility to IDDM is due to DRB1*08 or to DQB1*0402 cannot be solved by our study because of tight linkage disequilibrium between these two genes on the DRB1*08-DQA1*0401-DQB1*0402 haplotype. It might be argued that susceptibility was due to DRB1*08 because DQB1*0402 encodes a DQß57 Asp positive chain, while susceptibility to IDDM has been generally linked to nonAsp 57 encoding alleles in Caucasians. However, although no specific genotypic combination could be demonstrated in DRB1*08-DQB1*0402 patients, all were heterozygotes for the presence of a nonAsp 57 encoding allele. Predisposing DQ molecules may thus have resulted from transcomplementation, as suggested for DR3/DR4 heterozygotes in Caucasiens or in DR4/DR8 patients in other ethnic groups [9]. Nevertheless this observation suggests that the protective effect of the DQß57 aspartic acid is not dominant.

According to the presence of islet cell autoantibodies, we could distinguish two subgroups among non-DR3/non-DR4 patients. Patients positive for ICA and/or GADA had an increased frequency of the DRB1*08-DQA1*0401-DQB1*0402 haplotype, higher than that in the whole non-DR3/non-DR4 diabetic population. With regard to the role of MHC class II molecule in antigenic presentation, this finding suggests that different diabetogenic peptides, selected by different predisposing class II molecules, might be involved in the autoimmune process leading to ß cell destruction. Moreover, the nature of the peptide could modulate the phenotypic expresion of the disease, since non-DR3/non-DR4 diabetic population is mainly constituted by patients with adult-onset disease. Contrasting with what observed in ICA and/or GADA positive patients, we could not demonstrate any association with MHC class II gene in patients negative for both autoantibodies. It is thus tempting to consider these patients with no serological marker of autoimmunity and no genetic susceptibility mapping at the MHC class II region as distinct from autoimmune type 1 diabetic subjects, despite they present clinically as IDDM subjects. Evidence of non autoimmune diabetes that ressembles IDDM, as flatbush diabetes (in black subjects), mitochondrial diabetes and MODY 3, has recently emerged. These three kind of diabetes could be excluded in our patients because of our selection criteria. One may assume that other particular forms of diabetes that mimic type 1 diabetes will be recognized in the next years. This will probably give some light on the aetiology of diabetes in these non-DR3/non-DR4 autoantibody-negative patients.

In conclusion, we report in the present study that in non-DR3/non-DR4 subjects, the DRB1*08-DQA1*0401-DQB1*0402 haplotype is predisposing to IDDM, and that this association is evident only in patients positive for ICA and/or GADA. This finding first supports the immunogenetic heterogeneity of IDDM. It also indicates that the diagnosis of type 1 diabetes should be disputed in non-DR3/non-DR4 patients when serological markers of islet cell autoimmunity are absent, even though these subjects may appear clinically insulin-dependent.

References

1. Bach JF. Insulin-dependent diabetes mellitus as an autoimmune disease. *Endocrine Rev* 1994; 15: 516-42.
2. Jin-Xiong SHE. Susceptibility to type 1 diabetes: HLA-DQ and DR revisited. *Immunol Today* 1996; 17 : 323-9.
3. Melton LJ, Palombo RJ, Chu CP. Incidence of diabetes mellitus by clinical type. *Diabetes Care* 1983; 6 : 75-86.
4. Caillat-Zucman S, Garchon HJ, Timsit J, Assan R, Boitard C, Djilali-Saiah I, Bougnères P, Bach JF. Age-dependent HLA heterogeneity of type 1 insulin-dependent diabetes mellitus. *J Clin Invest* 1992; 90 : 2242-50.
5. Reardon W, Ross RJM, Sweeney MG , Luxon LM, Pembrey ME, Harding AE, Trembath RC. Diabetes mellitus associated with a pathogenic point mutation in mitochondrial DNA. *Lancet* 1992; 340: 1376-9.
6. Barneji MA, Chaiken RL, Huey H, Tuomi T, Norin AJ, Mackay IR, Rowley MJ, Zimmet PZ, Lebovitz HE. GAD antibody negative NIDDM in adult black subjects with diabetic ketoacidosis and increased frequency of human leukocyte antigen DR3 and DR4. Flatbush diabetes. *Diabetes* 1994; 43: 741-5.
7. Todd JA, Bell JI, Mac Devitt HO. HLA-DQb gene contributes to susceptibility and resistance to insulin-dependent diabetes mellitus. *Nature* 1987; 329 : 599-604.
8. Thomson G. HLA DR antigens and susceptibility to insulin-dependent diabetes mellitus. *Am J Hum Genet* 1984; 36: 1309-17.
9. Thorsby E, Ronningen KS. Particular HLA-DQ molecules play a dominant role in determining susceptibility or resistance to type I (insulin dependent) diabetes mellitus. *Diabetologia* 1993; 36: 371-7.

HLA associations in IDDM. HLA-DR4 subtypes may confer different degrees of protection

D.E. Undlien [1], T. Friede [2], H.G. Rammensee [2], K.S. Ronningen [1], E. Thorsby [1]

1 Institute of Transplantation Immunology, The National Hospital, Pilestredet 32, N-0027 Oslo, Norway
2 Deutsches Krebsforschungszentrum, Heidelberg, Germany

IDDM susceptibility associated with DQ8, either alone or in combination with DQ2, is greatly influenced by which DR4 subtype is also carried on the DQ8 haplotype. Our data together with those from others suggest that DRB1*0405, 0402 and 0401 are associated with susceptibility (in this decreasing order), while DRB1*0404, 0403 and 0406 are associated with an increasing degree of protection. The protection associated with DRB1*0403 and 0406 is dominant over the DQ8 associated susceptibility [1-5].

The β-chains of the susceptibility associated DR4 subtypes (0401, 0402, 0405) show several differences in terms of aacomposition. In particular the difference at position 71 (positively charged in DRβ1*0402 and negatively charged in DRβ1*0405 and 0401) has been shown to be very important for determining the charge of the aa which may be accommodated in pocket 4 (p4) of the DR4 molecule, and thus their peptide binding motifs [6-10]. This suggests that if DRB1*04 subtypes associated with susceptibility are assumed to exert an effect on IDDM susceptibility through binding of a potential diabetogenic peptide, one has to invoke several different peptides. In contrast the DRβ-chains of the more protective DR4 subtypes (0403, 0406 and 0404) appear much more similar; they are identical at the polymorphic positions 57, 67, 70, 71 and 86.

Information about peptide motifs of the involved DR4 subtypes is now available [6-10]. These data raise the possibility that a peptide which is a strong binder to the protective DR(α,β1*0403) and (α,β1*0406) subtypes may bind with lower affinity to DR(a,b1*0404) (mainly because of slightly different preferences at p4). Further, a strong binder to DR(α,β1*0403) and (α,β1*0406) should bind with an even lower affinity to the susceptibility associated DR(α,β1*0401) (different preferences at p4 and p1) and DR(α,β1*0402) subtypes (different preferences particularily at p7 and possibly also at p4), and maybe not at all to DR(α,β1*0405) (different preferences at p1 and in particular at p9, where DR(α,β1*0405) has a very strong preference for negatively charged aa's due to an Asp - Ser substitution at position 57 in DRβ1*0405). The binding of such a "protective" peptide could thus be envisaged to parallel the observed susceptibility pattern; binding with high affinity to the most protective DR4 molecules and with decreasing affinity to the more susceptible DR4 subtypes.

Taken together, we propose that the susceptibility associated with DR4-DQ8 haplotypes, alone or in com bination with DQ2, is mainly determined by the DQ(α1*03,β1*0302) or DQ(α1*03,β1*0201) heterodimers, while the associated DR4 subtypes confer different degrees of protection. This model is summarized in *Figure 1* (see also [5]).

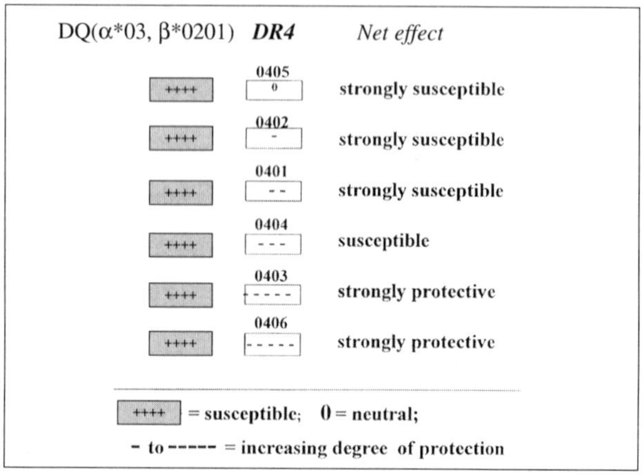

Figure 1. Susceptibility conferred by DR3-DQ2/DR4-DQ8 is the net effect of DQ encoded susceptibility and different degrees of DR4 encoded protection.

References

1. Caillat-Zucman S, Garchon HJ, Timsit J *et al.* Age-dependent HLA genetic heterogeneity of type 1 insulin-dependent diabetes mellitus. *J Clin Invest* 1992; 90: 2242-50.
2. Erlich HA, Zeidler A, Chang J *et al.* HLA class II alleles and susceptibility and resistance to insulin dependent diabetes mellitus in Mexican-American families. *Nature Genet* 1993; 3: 358-64.
3. Cucca F, Lampis R, Frau F *et al.* The distribution of DR4 haplotypes in Sardinia suggests a primary association of type 1 diabetes with DRB1 and DQB1 loci. *Hum Immunol* 1995; 43: 301-8.
4. Yasunaga S, Kimura A, Hamaguchi K, Ronningen K.S, Sasazuki T. Different contribution of HLA-DR and -DQ genes in susceptibility and resistance to insulin-dependent diabetes mellitus (IDDM). *Tissue Antigens* 1996; 47: 37-48.
5. Undlien DE, Friede T, Rammensee HG *et al.* HLA encoded genetic predisposition in insulin-dependent diabetes mellitus (IDDM). DR4 subtypes may be associated with different degrees of protection. *Diabetes* 1997, in press.
6. Wucherpfennig KW, Strominger JL. Selective binding of self peptides to disease-associated major histocompatibility complex (MHC) molecules: a mechanism for MHC-linked susceptibility to human autoimmune diseases. *J Exp Med* 1995; 181: 1597-601.
7. Hammer J, Gallazzi F, Bono E *et al.* Peptide binding specificity of HLA-DR4 molecules: correlation with rheumatoid arthritis association. *J Exp Med* 1995; 181: 1847-55.
8. Wucherpfennig KW, Yu B, Bhol K *et al.* Structural basis for major histocompatibility complex (MHC)-linked susceptibility to autoimmunity: charged residues of a single MHC binding pocket confer selective presentation of self-peptides in pemphigus vulgaris. *Proc Natl Acad Sci USA* 1996; 92: 11935-9.
9. Friede T, Gnau V, Jung G, Keilholz W, Stevanovic S, Rammensee HG. Natural ligand motifs of closely related HLA-DR4 molecules predict features of rheumatoid arthritis associated peptides. *Biochim Biophys Acta* 1997, in press.
10. Rammensee HG, Friede T, Stevanoviic S. MHC ligands and peptide motifs: first listing. *Immunogenetics* 1995; 41: 178-228.

HLA-DQB1 genotypes associated with IDDM risk in healthy schoolchildren positive for GAD65 and islet cell antibodies

J. Ilonen[1], M. Sjöroos[2], H. Reijonen[1], J. Rahko[3], P. Kulmala[3], P. Vähäsalo[3], M. Knip[3]

Turku Immunology Centre and
1 Department of Virology, University of Turku, Finland
2 Department of Biotechnology, University of Turku, Kiinamyllynkatu 13, FIN-20520 Turku, Finland
3 Department of Pediatrics, University of Oulu, Finland

Autoantibodies specific to pancreatic islet cells are associated with onset of insulin-dependent diabetes mellitus (IDDM) and can also be used in the prediction of the disease in relatives of diabetic patients (see [1]). These antibodies include the "classical" ICA detected by immunofluorescence as well as antibodies to defined autoantigens found in ß-cells like glutamic acid decarboxylase (GAD65), insulin and IA-2. The probability of clinical disease is increased when several types of antibodies are concurrently detected, when ICA are found at high titres and further when autoantibody positive subject have an HLA genotype associated with increased IDDM risk [2,3].

Population studies have generally shown that the frequency of ICA is much higher than the cumulative incidence of IDDM. This indicates a relatively low predictive value in the general population [4,5]. The aim of our present study was to look for the prevalence of both ICA and GAD65 antibodies (GAD65A) in healthy schoolchildren and analyse their association with the HLA alleles and genotypes defining an increased or decreased risk for IDDM.

Subjects and methods

Study subjects

Serum samples from 3662 healthy schoolchildren aged 7-16 years and living within two areas in Northern Finland were collected as well as EDTA treated blood samples used to prepare blood spots for HLA typing. The healthy reference population and children with IDDM used for comparisons were collected from various parts of Finland and data on them have been described elsewhere [6].

Autoantibody assays

ICA were determined by standard indirect immunofluorescence on sections of frozen human group O pancreas. Rabbit antihuman IgG (Behringwerke, Marburg, Germany) was used to detect ICA. End-point dilution titers were examined for the ICA-positive samples, and the results were expressed in Juvenile Diabetes Foundation units (JDF-U) relative to an international reference standard. The detection limit was 2.5 JDF-U.

GAD65A were analysed by the radioligand method described by Petersen *et al.* [7]. Human recombinant islet GAD65 cDNA was transcribed *in vitro* with the vector pB1882 and the transcribed RNA translated in a methionine free rabbit reticulocyte lysate in the presence of ^{35}S-methionine. Aliquots containing labelled GAD65 were incubated overnight with serum samples and immunocomplexes isolated by adding protein A-sepharose to each tube. GAD65A levels were expressed in relative units (RU) representing the specific binding of the labelled antigen by the test serum in relation to that by a positive standard serum. The cut-off limit for autoantibody positivity was 6.5RU (99. percentile in 372 nondiabetic children).

HLA typing

HLA-DQB1 alleles known to be significantly associated with IDDM risk or protection [6] were defined using a method described earlier in detail [8]. The polymorphic second exon of the HLA-DQB1 gene was amplified from blood spots using a biotinylated primer, and the amplification product was bound to streptavidin coated microtitre plate wells. After denaturation the products were allowed to hybridize with lanthanide (europium, samarium and terbium) labelled oligonucleotide probes and the specific hybridization detected by time-resolved fluorometry after washes and addition of enhancement solution. Chi-square test with continuity correction was used in comparisons of HLA allele or genotype frequencies between the groups.

Results

There were 104 (2.8%) children with ICA and 20 with GAD65A (0.5%) among 3662 screened schoolchildren. Fifteen (0.4%) of the children had both ICA and GAD65A, most GAD65A positive children were thus also positive for ICA. The frequencies of IDDM associated HLA-DQB1 alleles are shown in *Table I*. HLA-DQB1*0201 allele was significantly more common in ICA-positive children than in the reference population ($P<0.022$). The actual frequency of DQB1*0201 was higher in GAD65A positive and double antibody positive than in ICA positive children but statistical significance was not reached in these smaller groups. HLA-DQB1*0302 was even more increased among GAD65A-positive children and the frequency of 55% was significantly ($P<0.0015$) higher than among healthy controls. The protective DQB1*0602/0603 alleles were decreased among GAD65A-positive children enhancing their genetic similarity with IDDM children. *Table II* describes HLA-DQB1 genotypes in the same population of schoolchildren. These genotypes are grouped into four categories used to grade IDDM risk in the Finnish population (Ilonen *et al.*, 1996). The distribution of genotypes was highly significantly ($P<0.0001$) different in children with GAD65A and in those with both GAD65 and ICA compared to the reference population and resembled that of IDDM patients whereas children with ICA did not differ from controls. The main difference between GAD65A-positive subjects and IDDM children was that the protective genotypes were still more common among the GAD65A-positive controls ($p<0.013$).

Discussion

The number of ICA-positive healthy schoolchildren is somewhat lower than reported earlier from Finland but still relatively high and in concordance with the known high incidence of IDDM in Finland [9] . The frequency of 2.8% does still by far exceed the probability to develop IDDM which is around 0.6% before the age of 20 years confirming that most children positive for ICA do never progress to diabetes. This is in accordance with the HLA findings among these children. The distribution of HLA-DQB1 genotypes defined according to the associated IDDM risk did not differ from that found in the reference population although the HLA-DQB1*0201 allele associated with several autoimmune diseases was slightly increased among ICA positive children. Accordingly the process resulting in ICA production does not seem to be strongly influenced by the HLA genotype.

The number of GAD65A-positive children was much lower, actually even somewhat lower than the estimated probability of developing IDDM. The significance of these antibodies was strongly emphasized by the distribution of HLA-DQB1 genotypes which resembled that found among patients with IDDM. Only the frequency of protective genotypes was higher than in IDDM patients suggesting that the autoimmune process reflected by GAD65A may be more easily controlled in subjects with protective alleles. The presence of two antibodies, both ICA and GAD65A was also strongly associated with IDDM risk genotypes, but most of the GAD65A-positive children had also detectable ICA. It is thus difficult to estimate the significance of isolated GAD65A vs double antibody positivity, but the fact that GAD65A-positivity was usually associated with the presence of other autoantibodies migh further stress their predictive value at the population level.

In conclusion, the presence of GAD65A in unaffected schoolchildren may be associated with a considerable risk of IDDM as suggested by their low prevalence and close relation to HLA-DQB1 genotypes common among IDDM patients. Longitudinal follow-up studies are needed to confirm these assumptions and to make estimations of the actual risk.

Acknowledgements

We thank the skillful technical assistance of Terttu Laurén, Ritva Suominen, Päivi Ronkainen and Susanna Heikkilä. The study was supported by the Academy of Finland and the Foundation for Pediatric Research in Finland (Ulla Hjelt Fund).

Table I. HLA-DQB1 alleles [N (%)] associated with IDDM risk and protection in healthy school-children with ICA or GAD65A

Allele	ICA and GAD65A N=15	ICA N=104	GAD65A N=20	Controls N=756	IDDM N=649
*0201	7 (47)	36 (35)[1]	9 (45)	179 (24)	281 (43)
*0301	1 (7)	24 (23)	2 (10)	161 (21)	89 (14)
*0302	9 (60)[2]	25 (24)	11 (55)[3]	168 (22)	468 (72)
*0602/0603	3 (20)	52 (50)	3 (15)[4]	321 (42)	44 (7)

1P=0.022,2P=0.0017,3P=0.0015,4P=0.026 compared to healthy controls.

Table II. HLA-DQB1 genotypes [N (%)] associated with IDDM risk and protection in healthy schoolchildren with various combinations of autoantibodies. The distribution of genotypes in GAD65A positive schoolchildren as well as in those with both ICA and GAD65A was significantly different (P<0.0001) from that of healthy controls

Genotype	ICA and GAD65A N=15	ICA N=104	GAD65A N=20	Controls N=756	IDDM N=649
High risk	3 (20)	5 (5)	4 (20)	22 (3)	159 (24)
Moderate risk	5 (33)	12 (11)	5 (25)	86 (11)	243 (37)
Low risk	3 (20)	24 (23)	5 (25)	167 (22)	182 (28)
Decreased risk	4 (27)	63 (61)	6 (30)	481 (64)	65 (10)

High risk = DQB1*0201/0302; Moderate risk = DQB1*0302/x; Low risk =DQB1*0301/0302, 0201/0301, 0201/x and 0302/0602-3; Decreased risk = DQB1*0602-3/x,0301/0602-3,0201/0602-3,0301/x,x/x; x means an untyped allele or homozygosity for the marked allele.

References

1. Lernmark Å. Molecular biology of IDDM. *Diabetologia* 1994; 37: S73-81.
2. Lipton RB, Kocova M, LaPorte RE, Dorman JS, Orchard TJ, Riley WJ, Drash AL, Becker DJ, Trucco M. Autoimmunity and genetics contribute to the risk of insulin-dependent diabetes-mellitus in families - islet cell antibodies and HLA DQ heterodimers. *Am J Epidemiol* 1992; 136: 503-12.
3. Reijonen H, Vähasalo P, Karjalainen J, Ilonen J, Åkerblom HK, Knip M. The childhood diabetes in Finland (DiMe) study group. HLA-DQB1 genotypes and islet cell antibodies in the identification of siblings at risk for insulin-dependent diabetes (IDDM) in Finland. *J Autoimmun* 1994; 7: 675-86.
4. Landin-Olsson M, Karlsson A, Dahlquist G, Blom L, Lernmark Å, Sundkvist G *et al.* Islet cell and other organ-specific autoantibodies in all children developing type 1 (insulin-dependent) diabetes mellitus in Sweden during one year and in matched control children. *Diabetologia* 1989; 32: 387-95.
5. Karjalainen J. Islet cell antibodies as predictive markers for IDDM in children with high background incidence of disease. *Diabetes* 1990; 39: 1144-50.
6. Ilonen J, Reijonen H, Herva E, Sjöroos M, Iitiä A, Lövgren T, Veijola R, Knip M, Åkerblom HK. Childhood diabetes in Finland (DiMe) study group. Rapid HLA-DQB1 genotyping for four alleles in the assesment of IDDM risk in Finnish population. *Diabetes Care* 1996; 19:795-800.
7. Petersen JS, Hejnaes KR, Moody A, Karlsen AE, Marshall MO, Høier-Madsen M, Boel E, Michelsen BK, Dyrberg T. Detection of GAD65 antibodies in diabetes and other autoimmune diseases using a simple radioligand assay. *Diabetes* 1994; 43: 459-67.
8. Sjöroos M, Iitiä A, Ilonen J, Reijonen H, Lövgren T. Triple-label hybridization assay for type-1 diabetes-related HLA alleles. *BioTechniques* 1995; 18: 870-7.
9. Karvonen M, Tuomilehto J, Libman I, La Porte R. A review of the recent epidemiological data on the worldwide incidence of type-1 (insulin-dependent) diabetes-mellitus. *Diabetologia* 1993; 36: 883-92.

The HLA amino acids influencing IDDM predisposition

A.M. Valdes[1], S. McWeeney[1], H. Salamon[1], J. Tarhio[2], K. Ronningen[3], G. Thomson[1]

1 Department of Integrative Biology, University of California, 3060 Valley Life Sciences, Berkeley 94720 3140, USA
2 Department of Computer Science, University of Helsinki, Finland
3 Institute for Transplantation Immunology, The National Hospital, Oslo, Norway

The role of the human leukocyte antigen (HLA) region in insulin dependent diabetes mellitus (IDDM) has been known for more than twenty years (see [1]). Although the associations, linkage and genetic contribution to disease are all strong, the molecular basis of the role of HLA in IDDM has not been determined. The HLA component to IDDM displays a complex hierarchy of predisposing, neutral and protective effects at the allele, haplotype and genotype levels; a complete molecular model must explain all these features.

By 1980, the positive associations of DR3 and DR4 and negative association of DR2, as well as increased risk for DR3/DR4 heterozygotes, was well established [1]. A hierarchy of relative predispositional through protective effects was seen for the other DR alleles [2]. The ability of serologically typed DQ variation, and molecularly typed DQB1 sequence variation, to subdivide the DR4, DR2 and DRw6 haplotypes into susceptible and protective subtypes focused attention on the role of DQB1 in IDDM. There is a correlation of DQB1 alleles containing Asp at position 57 with protection, or low IDDM susceptibility, while alleles with a neutral position 57 residue (Ala, Val, Ser) correlate with increased susceptibility. Although the IDDM association of a haplotype can be predicted to some extent by the charge of the polymorphic residue at DQB1 position 57, not all DQB1 alleles with or without Asp 57 are "equally protective or predisposing"; in particular the 'neutral' DR7 haplotype (DRB1*0701 DQA1*0201 DQB1*0201) which has the same DQB1 allele as the predisposing DR3 haplotype (DRB1*0301 DQA1*0501 DQB1*0201) should be, but is not, predisposing (Ala) under the DQB position 57 hypothesis (reviewed in [3]).

Additional data, including Japanese and Chinese studies, implicated further HLA genetic variation, and led to the hypothesis that the joint presence of non-Asp at DQB1 position 57 and Arg at DQA1 position 52 was a strong IDDM predisposing factor (reviewed in [3]). However, by itself, this combination is insufficient to explain the HLA component of IDDM predisposition (see [3, 4]). Ethnic comparisons have been extremely useful in studying the HLA component to IDDM, especially given ethnic variation in disease prevalence and HLA associations (see [3]). Studies in Caucasian, Mexican American and Chinese populations have all implicated the role of DRB1 in IDDM, as well as DQB1 and DQA1. Various HLA DRB1, DQA1 and DQB1 amino acids, in addition to DQA1 #52 and DQB1 #57 have been hypothesized as involved in IDDM. However, no current molecular models of HLA fully explain the hierarchy of predispositional through protective IDDM allele, haplotype and genotype effects (reviewed in [5]).

Difficulty in the identification of specific disease predisposing and protective alleles at loci within the HLA region results from the fact that multiple genetic factors are involved, including genetic variants that are common in the general population. Also, amino acids, or a particular sequence of amino acids, involved in the disease process, are difficult to identify in the context of the high linkage disequilibrium common within the HLA region, in particular the very strong disequilibrium of the HLA class II DR and DQ genes.

Every HLA allele is defined by a unique DNA sequence in the exons. In the case of the HLA class II loci most of the variation is confined to hypervariable regions in the second exon, which affects the antigen binding pocket. The amino acids at variable sites in an allele typically occur in other alleles as well, which gives rise to the characteristic patchwork of variation seen when comparing the amino acid composition of HLA alleles.

Such patterns of amino acid site variability raise the possibility that HLA variation association with a disease may not be due to a given allele, but rather to one or more variable amino acid sites (shared epitopes) occurring on several alleles. Shared epitopes are suggested to be responsible for the HLA association with RA (reviewed in [1]). Here we investigate the role of HLA DR-DQ amino acids and IDDM.

Methods and results

The unique combinations method

The unique combinations method [6] involves an efficient computer program to detect all amino acid combinations (singles, pairs, triplets, etc.) which distinguish a particular sequence, or set of sequences, from another set of sequences. The unique combinations method utilizes an algorithm that isolates all patterns unique to a given sequence without investigating all possible $2^n - 1$ combinations of sites that characterize sequences of length n. This is necessary as even with the present day efficiency of computers, they cannot realistically calculate all possible combinations of sites when a locus is highly polymorphic, *e.g.*, as with HLA variation. In the case of disease; alleles, haplotypes or genotypes strongly predisposing to disease can be compared to those that are strongly protective. An example implementation of the unique combinations method yields greatly improved risk assessment over previously considered amino acids for IDDM in an analysis of HLA class II DQA1-DQB1 patient and control genotypes [6].

The haplotype method

The haplotype method for identifying disease predisposing amino acids [7] is a test of whether all relevant amino acids involved in disease have been identified. We consider separately the observed haplotypic amino acid combinations at putative predisposing sites. For each haplotype combination containing all the amino acid sites involved in the disease process, *e.g.*, amino acids a1 and b1 at sites A and B, the relative frequencies of amino acid variants at sites not involved in disease, *e.g.*, r_1 and r_2 at site R, are expected to be the same in patients and controls. That is, although the absolute frequencies of the haplotypes $a_1b_1r_1$ and $a_1b_1r_2$ will differ between patients and controls, the relative frequency of the ratio $a_1b_1r_1/a_1b_1r_2$ will be the same in patients and controls. Inequality of this ratio is expected if all sites involved in the disease process, and in linkage disequilibrium with the sites under study, have not been identified. The haplotype method has been shown to be robust for any number of amino acids involved in the disease process, provided they are all included in the haplotypes considered. Further, it is robust to mode of inheritance, penetrance of the disease and frequency of sporadic cases. The original application of the haplotype method was to allele frequency data [2]. Direct roles of HLA DR3 and DR4 in IDDM were excluded, since HLA B locus variation on these haplotypes was different in patients and controls.

Obviously, the haplotype method cannot distinguish between amino acid sites which are very highly correlated in a population, however ethnic comparisons can help identify the predisposing factors. Further, the method can unequivocally determine if all disease predisposing amino acid sites in a genetic region have not been identified. Of particular importance in defining disease predisposing factors when multiple sites are involved in a genetic region, is our result showing that the test statistic with use of the haplotype method gives a closer fit to the null expectation (all factors have been identified) when some, compared to none, of the true predisposing factors are included in the haplotype analysis [7]. Using a resampling technique, a statistical test has been developed which takes account of the non-independence of sites sampled.

We have applied the haplotype method to IDDM HLA DRB1-DQA1-DQB1 data from Norwegian, Sardinian, Mexican American, and Taiwanese populations. Our results prove that the combination DQA1 #52 - DQB1 #57, which has been proposed as an important IDDM agent, does not include all the IDDM predisposing elements [5, 7]. The combination of sites DRB1 #67, 86 DQA1 #47 DQB1 #9, 26, 57, 70 predicts the HLA class II DR-DQ component in these populations [5]. The frequencies and predisposing/protective effects of the haplotypes defined by these seven sites have been compared, and the effects on IDDM are consistent across the populations studied.

Discussion

The combination of sites DRB1 #67, 86 DQA1 #47 DQB1 #9, 26, 57, 70 predicts the predisposing component within the DR-DQ region in the Mexican, American, Norwegian, Sardinian and Taiwanese data considered. We do not claim to have identified all HLA DR-DQ amino acids, or highly correlated sites, involved in IDDM. However, the sites identified are strong predictors of IDDM in the populations studied.

The following sites, individually or in combination, have previously been suggested as IDDM components: DRB1 #57, 70, 71, 86 DQA1 #52, DQB1 #13, 45, 57 (DQB1 #13, 45 correlates 100% with #9, 26) (reviewed in [5]). We propose that DQA1 #47 is a better predictor of IDDM than the previously suggested DQA1 #52. DQA1 #47 and #52 divide the DQA1 alleles identically for *0101, 0102, 0103, 0104, versus *0201. However, while DQA1 #52 does not divide the remaining alleles, #47 distinguishes the DQA1 alleles *0301, 0302, from *0401, 0501, 0601. Specifically, it divides DR3 (DQA1*0501) haplotypes from the DR4 (DQA1*0301) haplotypes. Also, we add DRB1 #67 and DQB1 #70 to the HLA DR-DQ IDDM amino acids. There might well be other DRB1 sites involved in IDDM, and not identified in our study, such as DRB1 #57, 70, 71, but their effect is not as dramatic or evident in the populations we have studied. The application of the unique combinations and haplotype methods to other ethnic groups will prove very useful in discerning all DR-DQ sites involved and in keeping track of variation between ethnic groups in linkage disequilibrium within the HLA region.

It has been clearly demonstrated that other genes in the HLA region in addition to DR-DQ, and possibly spanning all of the HLA region contribute to IDDM (for review see [3, 4]). For example, using unaffected parents homozygous for DR3 haplotypes with two IDDM offspring, it is estimated that less than approximately 50% of HLA DR3 haplotypes (which are basically homogeneous for DRB1*0301 DQA1*0501 DQB1*0201) predispose to IDDM in Caucasians. This indicates that HLA region variation additional to DRB1, DQA1, and DQB1 is required to define IDDM predisposition and/or protection. This variation could be within, or outside of, the HLA class II DR-DQ region.

Although there are other HLA genes involved in IDDM, the results of our study reveal that a major factor is to be found within the DR-DQ region. The next step is to apply this method to a larger number of populations, and to move beyond the haplotype level to examine the interactions of amino acid sites at the genotype level (work in progress), including all aspects of the disease with respect to modes of inheritance, genetic heterogeneity, affected sib pair data, etc. (for review see [8]).

Acknowledgements
This work was supported by NIH grant HD12731.

References

1. Thomson G. HLA disease associations: models for the study of complex human genetic disorders. *Crit Rev Clin Lab Sci* 1995; 32: 183-219.
2. Thomson G, Robinson WP, Kuhner MK, Joe S, MacDonald MJ, Gottschall JL, Barbosa J, Rich SS, Bertrams J, Baur MP, Partanen J, Tait B, Schober E, Mayr WR, Ludvigsson J, Lindblom B, Farid NR, Thompson C, Deschamps I. Genetic heterogeneity, modes of inheritance and risk estimates for a joint study of Caucasians with insulin dependent diabetes mellitus. *Am J Hum Genet* 1988; 43: 799-816.
3. Harrison LC, Tait BD. Balliere's clinical endocrinology and metabolism, vol. 5. Genetics of diabetes, parts I and II. London: Bailliere Tindall, 1991.
4. Robinson WP, Thomson G, Barbosa J, Rich SS. The homozygous parents affected sib pair method of detecting disease predisposition effects: application to insulin dependent diabetes mellitus. *Genet Epidemiol* 1993; 10: 273-88.
5. Valdes AM, McWeeney S, Thomson G. HLA class II DR-DQ amino acids and IDDM. *Am J Hum Genet* 1997 (in press).
6. Salamon H, Tarhio J, Ronningen K, Thomson G. On distinguishing unique combinations in biological sequences. *J Comp Biol* 1997 (in press).
7. Valdes AM, Thomson G. The haplotype method for testing disease predisposing variants. *Am J Hum Genet* 1997 (in press).
8. Thomson G. Analysis of complex human genetic traits: an ordered notation method and new tests for mode of inheritance. *Am J Hum Genet* 1995; 57: 474-86.

T-cell receptor AV repertoire analysis of peripheral blood lymphocytes in antibody positive first degree relatives and type 1 diabetic patients

I. Durinovic-Bello, P. Ott, H. Naserke, A.G. Ziegler

Diabetes Research Institute and Academic Hospital München-Schwabing, Koelner Platz 1, 80804 Munich, Germany

Type 1 diabetes is a chronic cell-mediated autoimmune disease characterised by a silent prediabetic period of variable length during which the majority of insulin producing pancreatic ß-cells are destroyed. The clinical onset of type 1 diabetes is the end point of this destructive process. In pre-diabetes autoantibodies and T cells to several islet-cell-antigens, including glutamic acid decarboxylase (GAD), insulin and tyrosine phosphatase (ICA512/IA2) have been detected [1-3]. Moreover, we have recently demonstrated that peripheral blood mononuclear cells show reactivity to multiple islet-cell-antigens and membrane preparations of human pancreas in prediabetic subjects and to a lesser extend in newly diagnosed type 1 diabetic patients [2]. These observations point to the existence of oligoclonal antigen-specific T-cell populations represented by selected T-cell receptor (TCR) Vα (AV) and Vß (BV) families in the peripheral blood of prediabetic and early diabetic individuals. In previous years, two reports have been published on TCR BV repertoire analysis of peripheral blood lymphocytes. Both studies investigated patients with recent onset or long lasting diabetes and revealed no significant correlation with any of the BV families tested [4]. Moreover, the islet specific T-cell line which we previously generated from peripheral blood lymphocytes of type 1 diabetic patient - by restimulation with membrane preparation of rat insulinoma cells (BMA: beta membrane antigen) - did not show preferential usage of any of 24 BV families tested. Instead, two AV families (AV1 and AV12) were preferentially used [5]. Thus, for the first time, we concentrated on TCRAV repertoire analysis of peripheral blood lymphocytes in high risk non-diabetic first-degree relatives and type 1 diabetic patients at onset with the purpose to investigate the frequency and distribution of these families in early stages of the autoimmune process.

Subjects and methods

Blood samples were obtained with informed consent from 8 patients with newly diagnosed type 1 diabetes, 9 non-diabetic relatives at high risk of type 1 diabetes and 9 healthy individuals. Lymphocytes were isolated from heparinized blood by Ficol-paque (Pharmacia, Freiburg, Germany) density centrifugation for T-cell receptor repertoire analysis. Sera were tested for antibodies to islet-cells (ICA), insulin (IAA), glutamic acid decarboxylase (GADA) and tyrosine phosphatase (ICA512-Ab) as described previously [3]. DNA was obtained from EDTA blood for HLA-DR typing. All subjects are characterized in *Table I*. Patients with newly diagnosed diabetes were hospitalized at the 3rd Medical Department of the Academic Hospital München-Schwabing, Germany, and had a mean age at onset of 18±10 years (range 4 to 36 years). Type 1 diabetes was defined on the basis of a clinical diagnosis. Relatives of diabetic patients attending our hospital were routinely invited to participate in a screening programme for diabetes-associated antibodies. Nine relatives who were identified to be antibody positive (Ab+) in this screening programme were included into the study (3 relatives with 4 positive Abs, 3 relatives with 3 Abs, 2 relatives with 2 Abs, 1 relative with 1 Ab). In each case, antibody-positivity was confirmed by two or more consecutive serum samples. All 9 antibody-positive relatives (mean age: 29 ± 16 years, range 3 to 56 years) were followed for diabetes onset in 6 months intervals (1 to 6 years). To date, 1/9 relatives have developed overt type 1 diabetes confirmed by OGTT (2h blood glucose >200 mg%). Nine adult healthy individuals without family history of type 1 diabetes in first and second degree relatives, but with diabetes-associated HLA-DR alleles served as control subjects (mean age:

Table I. Characterization of type 1 diabetic patients, autoantibody-positive first degree relatives and healthy controls

				Autoantibodies				T-cell response (SI)			
Nr.	Age years	IDDM month	HLA-DR	ICA JDF U	IAA nU/ml	GADA U	ICA512 -Ab U	BMA	Insulin	GAD	ICA 512
Type 1 diabetic patients											
1	4	1	4,6	**>80**	**850**	**48**	**85**	**7**	**24**	**6**	1
2	7	12	3,3	**40**	**700**	**170**	8	nd	nd	nd	nd
3	11	3	1,3	**40**	**849**	**113**	**0**	nd	nd	nd	nd
4	11	0	3,4	**40**	14	**132**	**17**	**14**	**24**	nd	**5**
5	13	0	nd	**40**	nd	**91**	5	**8**	2	2	3
6	19	0	3,4	**>80**	**135**	nd	nd	nd	1	**5**	**7**
7	31	1	3,7	**40**	30	**317**	13	**7**	2	1	nd
8	36	12	nd	nd	nd	nd	nd	nd	nd	nd	nd
Antibody-positive first-degree relatives											
1	3		1,1	**40**	**1073**	6	0.2	1	2	2	1
2	5		2,11	**40**	**733**	**77**	7	nd	nd	nd	nd
3	5		3,11	**>80**	**1744**	**77**	**106**	**14**	1	1	**7**
4	6		4,4	**40**	**343**	8	**35**	**9**	**5**	**5**	**6**
5	12		3,13	<5	**360**	**65**	0	nd	nd	nd	nd
6	19		4,4	**40**	**72**	**55**	-4.9	nd	nd	nd	nd
7	19		7,1	<5	**66**	3	-10.3	nd	nd	nd	nd
8	22	12	4,4	**160**	**170**	**71**	**117**	nd	1	**3**	**8**
9	56		4,6	**10**	**136**	**86**	**24**	**5**	**11**	1	3
Controls											
1	19		3,13	<5	9	nd	nd	1	1	2	nd
2	20		4,8	<5	6	nd	nd	2	1	2	nd
3	21		3,15	<5	-12	nd	nd	2	2	1	nd
4	25		4,1	<5	10	nd	nd	1	2	1	nd
5	28		3,4	<5	17	0	3	1	1	1	3
6	29		4,1	<5	2	nd	nd	3	1	1	1
7	30		nd	<5	8	nd	nd	1	1	1	nd
8	32		3,8	<5	11	nd	nd	2	3	3	nd
9	47		3,3	<5	23	nd	nd	0	1	1	2

bold: positive antibody titers and T-cell responses; nd: not determined; BMA: membrane preparation of rat insulinoma cells; SI: stimulation index.

29 ± 8 years, range 19 to 47 years). They were negative for ICA and IAA respectively .

T-cell receptor repertoire analysis

Total RNA was prepared from $5x10^6$ peripheral blood lymphocytes (PBL) of each individual using RNAzol B (CINNA/BIOTECX, Houston, TX) and desolved in 7 µl of DEPC water (Sigma, Deisenhofen, Germany). Three micrograms of RNA was converted to cDNA by reverse transcriptase (Pharmacia, Freiburg, Germany) using external primers specific for the constant regions of the TCRA and TCRB locus (AC1 and BC1) in 50 µl final volume. Each of 18 TCRAV families were then individually amplified from 1µl of cDNA using one of the AV-gene 5'-oligonucleotides (15pM) paired with a 3'-oligonucleotide mat-

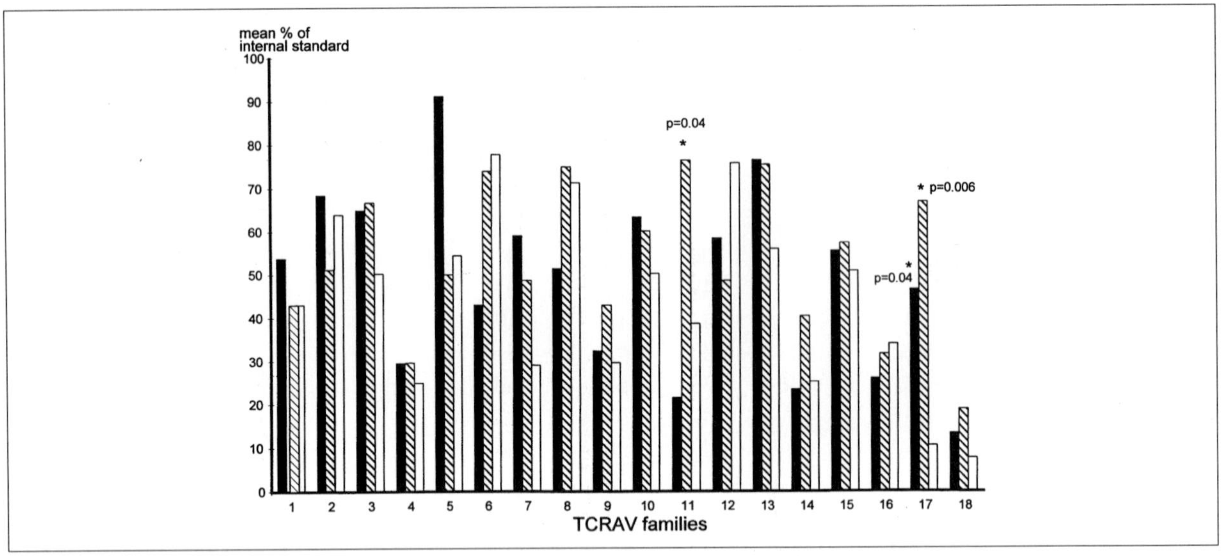

Figure 1. Mean TCR gene transcript level (mean % of internal standard) of each AV family in peripheral blood T-cells is illustrated for type 1 diabetic patients (black bars), antibody positive (Ab+) non-diabetic relatives (hatched bars) and control subjects (empty bars). Ab+ relatives and type 1 diabetic patients expressed significantly higher levels of AV17 gene families compared to healthy controls (p=0.006 and 0.04, respectively). The level of AV11 gene families was significantly increased in Ab+ relatives in comparison to controls (p=0.04).

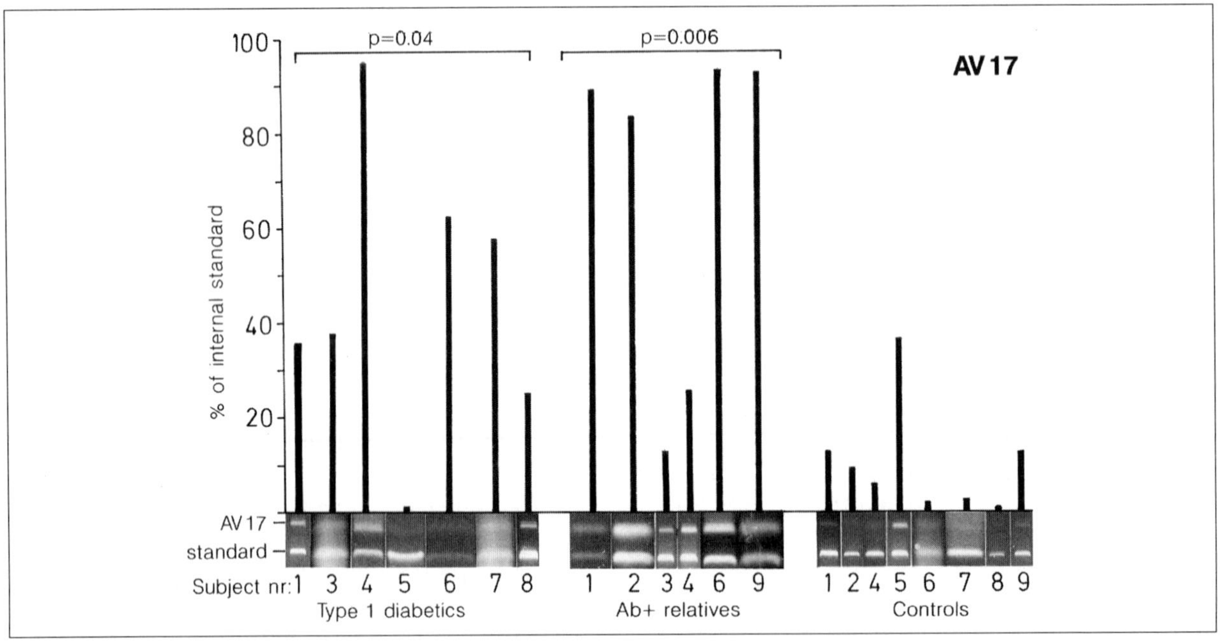

Figure 2. AV17 gene transcript levels (% of internal standard) of 8 type 1 diabetic patients, 6 Ab+ relatives and 8 control subjects are presented (patient numbers relate to numbers in table 1). For each individual gel imaging of amplification products of AV17 families and AC control fragments (internal standard) are shown. Ab+ relatives and type 1 diabetic patients express significantly higher median levels of AV17 gene transcripts compared to control subjects (p=0.006 and 0.04, respectively).

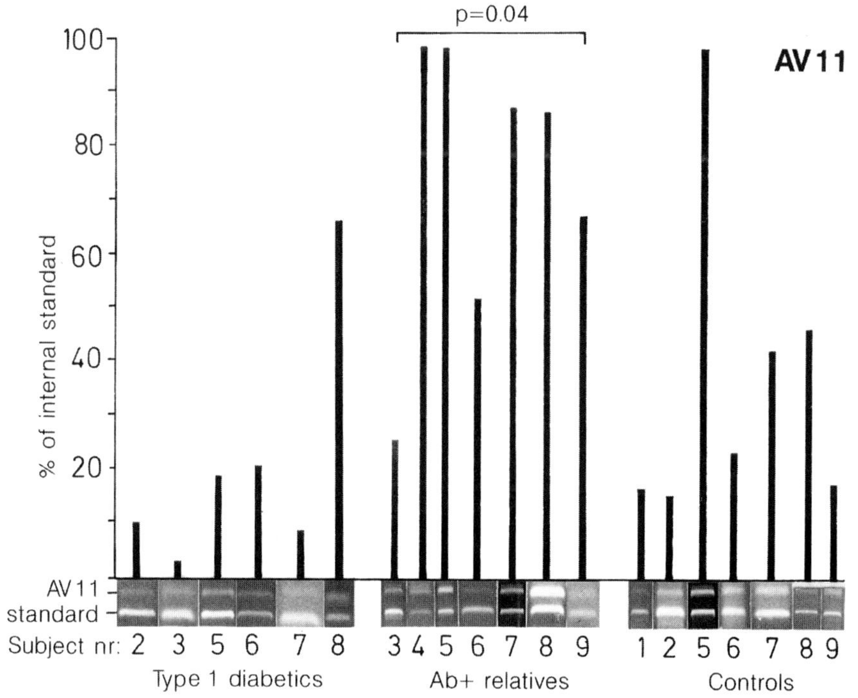

Figure 3. AV11 gene transcript levels (% of internal standard) of 6 type 1 diabetic patients, 7 Ab+ relatives and 7 control subjects are shown. Ab+ relatives show significantly higher median levels of AV11 gene transcripts compared to control subjects (p=0.04).

ched to the constant region of the AC gene (AC, 24 pM; [6]). Simultaneously in each tube two paired constant region oligonucleotides, 5'AC and 3'AC (9pM and 4.5pM, respectively [7]) were coamplified to be used as a internal standard. The linear range of amplification for every TCR VA family in combination with internal standard AC was tested individually in PCR reactions ranging from 25 to 35 cycles. Optimal amplification reaction was demonstrated for PCR reactions ranging from 30 to 35 cycles. The amplification mixture consisted of 10 mM Tris-HCl (pH 9), 50 mMKCl, 1.5 mM $MgCl_2$, 200 µM of each dNTP and 1 unit of Taq polymerase (Pharmacia, Freiburg, Germany) in a Perkin-Elmer-Cetus (Emeryville, CA, USA) thermocycler. Polymerase chain reaction (PCR) conditions were as follows: after an initial denaturation step at 95 °C for 5 min, 30 to 35 cycles were performed with three steps: denaturation at 94 °C for 60 seconds, annealing at 56 °C for 60 seconds and extension at 72 °C for 90 seconds. These reaction conditions allow for analysis of PCR products in the linear range of amplification as demonstrated by a dose-response relationship between initial amounts of cDNA and quantity of the final products.The specificity of the PCR amplification was assessed by the length of the PCR products and by Southern blotting and hybridisation with AC oligonucleotides (data not shown). PCR products were separated on 4% agarose gels, stained with ethidium bromide and photographed by Polaroid type 55 film (Sigma, Deisenhofen, Germany). The negative image of the gel was scanned using computer-based densitometer (Analysen-Technik Hirschmann, Neuried, Germany) and gel documentation software (Elscript-2D-Auswertesoftware V2.7). The amount of each TCRAV product was calculated as a percentage of the internal standard. The median intra-assay coefficient of variation calculated on the example of AV17 triplicate determinations was 6% (range 4% to 8,5%). The inter-assay coefficient of variation for the same AV17 family calculated for Ab+ relative Nr.4 of two blood samples taken 22 months apart was 12% (14% and 26%, respectively). Differences in the expression of single TCRAV families between the groups were analysed by Mann-Whitney U test.

Results and discussion

In this study we analysed the TCRAV repertoire of T-cells in the peripheral blood of type 1 diabetic patients, auto-antibody positive (Ab+) first degree relatives and healthy control subjects *(Figure 1)*. We demonstrated increased TCR AV17 and AV11 expression in Ab+ relatives (mean % of internal standard: 87% and 88%, respectively; p=0.006 and p=0.04) and increased AV17 expression in type 1 diabetic patients (mean 38%; p=0.04) compared to control individuals (mean 8% and 24%, respectively, *Figures* 2 and *3*). In order to correct our analysis for two diabetes associated HLA antigens DR3 and DR4, we reanalysed AV17 and AV11 data by comparing only DR3 and/or DR4 positive individuals. Despite smaller groups (AV17: 5 type 1 diabetics, 4 Ab+ relatives and 7 controls; AV11: 4 type 1 diabetics, 6 Ab+ relatives and 6 controls) the differences between patients and Ab+ relatives in comparison to the controls were still significant (AV17: diabetics p=0.007, Ab+ relatives p=0.04; AV11: Ab+ relatives p= 0.04). Furthermore, the levels of both AV families were higher in Ab+ first degree relatives than in type 1 diabetic patients at clinical onset, however, this did not reach statistical significance (*Figures* 2 and *3*). Since T-cells proliferate after interaction of their TÇR with the appropriate HLA-antigen complex, priming with specific antigen usually increases their frequency in circulation from ≈ 1/100 000 to ≈ 1/5 000 (20 times) [8]. Consequently, the increased expression of single TCRAV families in the peripheral blood of our Ab+ relatives and type 1 diabetic patients may be due to an antigen-driven stimulation of specific T cell populations since by them elevated T cell responses to different islet cell antigens have been found [1,2]. This could be explained as either the result of recirculation of in situ expanded T-cell specificities or of the expansion of T-cells upon contact with antigen in the periphery.

Restricted TCRAV and TCRBV gene usage of circulating T-cells or T-cells infiltrating affected organs was demonstrated in early stages of other autoimmune diseases like multiple sclerosis, rheumatoid arthritis and autoimmune thyroid disease [6,8,9]. By the use of the same technology, studies in type 1 diabetes did not reveal restriction of TCRBV usage in peripheral blood lymphocytes [4]. In contrast, analysis of TCRBV families through monoclonal antibodies showed increased proliferation of various BV-families tested [10]. Moreover, a study of islet-infiltrating lymphocytes in pancreas biopsies of type 1 diabetic patients described a dominant TCRAV usage of AV4 and AV6 families [11] and an other investigation of pancreas infiltrating T-cells in young patients who died at diagnosis revealed a prominent TCRBV7 expression [12]. All these results indicate that there is a considerable heterogeneity of T cell activation in different patients which may be in part influenced by the different time points of investigation during the long course of beta cell destruction.

This is the first report on TCRAV repertoire analysis in peripheral blood T cells of type 1 diabetic patients and high risk antibody positive relatives. In antibody positive relatives the early stage of the autoimmune islet-cell-destructive process is characterised by the simultaneous coexistence of specific T-cell populations reactive with multiple islet-cell antigens (including insulin, GAD and ICA512, [2]). The latter finding supports the idea that activated T cells in prediabetic individuals are heterogeneous and recognize a variety of epitopes on different dominant islet cell antigens. This, however, does not exclude the intriguing possibility that islet-cell-autoimmunity at an early stage is triggered by a single dominant antigen and later on due to 'determinant spreading' leads to diversification of the autoreactive T cell repertoire [13]. At this point we do not know whether AV17 and AV11 specific T-cell populations in prediabetic and type 1 diabetic subjects are islet cell specific. This important issue has to be further addressed by the isolation of AV17 and AV11 specific T-cells and the investigation of their antigen specificity. In the present study, we could not observe any association of increased AV17 or AV11 TCR levels with diabetes-associated HLA-DR3 and/or DR4 alleles *(Table I)*. Likewise, no correlation was found with age of the investigated subjects. In summary, our data indicate that TCRAV repertoire is restricted in the peripheral blood of patients with type 1 and pre-type 1 diabetes. Further investigations of TCR repertoire in very early stages of the autoimmune process - as near as possible to the time when β-cell autoimmunity is triggered - may help to understand immunological events which are responsible for the initiation of type 1 diabetes.

Acknowledgement
This work was supported by grants of the Deutsche Forschungsgemeinschaft (Zi310/5-2 and 310:6-7) and the German Diabetes Association. We gratefully acknowledge Prof. Dr. Dolores J. Schendel for providing oligonucleotides for the establishment of TCR repertoire analysis and for helpful comments. We also thank A. Steinle, P. Jantzer and C. Falk for advice in standardisation of TCR-PCR assays (all from Institiute of Immunology, Ludwig-Maximilians-University, Munich). The excellent technical assistance of S. Seggewieß is greatly appreciated. This study is part of the dissertation of P. Ott, Ludwig-Maximilians-University, Munich.

References

1. Tisch R, McDevitt H. Insulin-dependent diabetes mellitus. *Cell* 1996; 85: 291-7.
2. Durinovic-Bello I, Hummel M, Ziegler AG. Celular immune response to diverse islet cell antigens in type 1 diabetes. *Diabetes* 1996; 45: 795-9.
3. Roll U, Christie MR, Füchtenbusch M, Payton MA, Hawkes CJ, Ziegler A-G. Perinatal autoimmunity in offspring of diabetic parents: the German Multicenter 'BABY-DIAB' study. *Diabetes* 1997; 45 (in press).
4. Malhotra U, Spielman R, Concannon P. Variability in T cell receptor V beta gene usage in human peripheral blood lymphocytes. Studies of identical twins, siblings, and insulin-dependent diabetes mellitus patients. *J Immunol* 1992; 149: 1802-8.
5. Durinovic-Bello`I, Steinle A, Ziegler AG, Schendel DJ. HLA-DQ restricted, islet-specific T-cell clones of a type 1 diabetic patient; T-cell receptor sequence similarities to insulitis-inducing T-cells of nonobese diabetic mice. *Diabetes* 1994; 43: 1318-25.
6. Davies TF, Martin A, Concepcion ES, Graves P, Cohen L, Ben Nun A. Evidence of limited variability of antigen receptors on intrathyroidal T cells in autoimmune thyroid disease. *N Engl J Med* 1991; 325: 238-44.
7. Choi Y, Kotzin B, Herron L, Callahan J, Marrack P, Kappler J. Interaction of Staphylococcus aureus toxin "superantigens" with human T-cells. *Proc Natl Acad Sci USA* 1989; 86: 8941-5.
8. Goronzy JJ, Bartz Bazzanella P, Hu W, Jendro MC, Walser Kuntz DR, Weyand CM. Dominant clonotypes in the repertoire of peripheral CD4+ T cells in rheumatoid arthritis. *J Clin Invest* 1994; 94: 2068-76.
9. Oksenberg JR, Stuart S, Begovich AB, Bell RB, Erlich HA, Steinman L, Bernard CC. Limited heterogeneity of rearranged T-cell receptor V alpha transcripts in brains of multiple sclerosis patients. *Nature* 1990; 345: 344-6.
10. Kontiainen S, Toomath R, Lowder J, Feldmann M. Selective activation of T cells in newly diagnosed insulin-dependent diabetic patients: evidence for heterogeneity of T cell receptor usage. *Clin Exp Immunol* 1991; 83: 347-51.
11. Yamagata K, Hanafusa T, Nakajima H, Tomita K, Itoh N, Kono N, and Matsuzawa Y. Restricted heterogeneity of T cell receptor V alpha transcripts in the pancreas of newly diagnosed insulin-dependent diabetes mellitus. *Autoimmunity* 1993; 15: 52(abstr).
12. Conrad B, Weidmann E, Trucco G, Rudert WA, Behboo R, Ricordi C, Rodriquez Rilo H, Finegold D, Trucco M. Evidence for superantigen involvement in insulin-dependent diabetes mellitus aetiology. *Nature* 1994; 371: 351-5.
13. Lehmann PV, Forsthuber T, Miller AE, Sercarz E. Spreading of T-cell autoimmunity to cryptic determinants of an autoantigen. *Nature* 1992; 358: 155-7.

HLA and Rheumatism

Contents

• HLA and Rheumatism

The motif "DERAA" of HLA-DRB1*0402 is essential for DQ8-restricted T cell response in transgenic mice: implication for rheumatoid arthritis predisposition

E. Zanelli, C.J. Krco, C.S. David

Department of Immunology, Mayo Clinic, 221 4th Avenue SW, Rochester MN 55901, USA

Rheumatoid arthritis (RA)-associated DRB1*0101, DRB1*0102, DRB1*0401, DRB1*0404 and DRB1*0405 alleles share the motif Q(K/R)RAA in the region 70-74, while non-RA associated DRB1*0103 and DRB1*0402 alleles have the common DERAA motif. Based on this observation, it has been proposed that the third hypervariable (HV3) region of DRB1, the so-called "Shared Epitope", is the molecular basis for the HLA component of RA predisposition in humans. Albeit attractive, the mechanism by which the "Shared Epitope" affects RA manifestations remains unknown.

Like RA, predisposition to collagen-induced arthritis (CIA) in mice is controlled by genes inside the MHC class II region, namely *H2Aa* and *H2Ab*. Expression of a functional *H2Eb*^{d} gene in CIA susceptible *H2A*^{q} mice results in a dramatic reduction in both incidence and severity of arthritis [1]. Polymorphism of the first domain of the H2E molecule affects the protective effect on CIA, and a correlation exists between reduced severity and incidence of arthritis and H2A-restricted T cell response against HV3 peptides of the protective H2*Ebd* and H2*Ebs* molecules [2]. A correlation also exists between HLA-DQ8-restricted T cell response against DRB1 HV3 peptides and association with RA of the corresponding DRB1 alleles [3]. On the basis of these findings, we have proposed that the real RA predisposing molecule is HLA-DQ, and that the presentation of DRB1 HV3 peptides by RA-predisposing DQ molecules affects T cell response against joint components and prevents, or limits, the risk of developing RA [4].

Results

To better understand how a DRB1 HV3 peptide presented by HLA-DQ molecule could affect RA predisposition, we have analyzed in the present study the HLA-DQ8-restricted antigenicity of the peptide DRB1*0402 (65-79) of sequence KDILEDERAAVDTYC. This peptide is the strongest immunogen of all the DRB1 HV3 peptides [3]. Transgenic mice expressing functional DQB1*0302 and DQA1*0301 genes in the absence of endogenous MHC class II genes (DQ8.Ab°) have been previously described [4]. Mouse immunization and *in vitro* T cell assay were performed using standard methods [5].

When DQ8.Ab° mice were immunized with DRB1*0402 HV3 peptide, and lymph node cells were challenged 7 days later with DRB1*0402 peptides truncated of one or several amino acids at either ends, we found that the minimum determinant was the peptide DERAAVDTYC. Next, we performed similar experi-

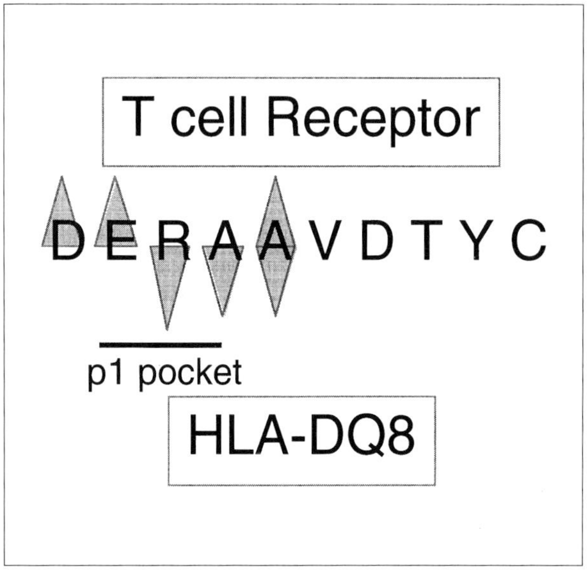

Figure 1. The motif DERAA guarantees DQ8-restricted immunogenicity.

Table I. Immunogenicity of DERAA-bearing peptides in DQ8.Abo mice

Species	Protein	Sequence	Δ cpm *
Homo sapiens	DRB1*0402	KDILE**DERAA**VDTYC	53,360
Streptomyces ribosidificus	Kan[c] resistance	EEWPE**DERAA**VVDAI	53,048
Chlamydia trachomatis	Omp	ETRLI**DERAA**HINAQ	33,618
Saccharomyces cerevisae	RNA pol III	LVNDN**DERAA**EVVKG	58,721
Homo sapiens	Vinculin	REEVF**DERAA**NFENH	34,438
Influenza A virus	Nucleoprotein	VFELS**DERAA**NPIVP	50,239

* mean cpm in experimental assays - mean cpm in control wells without peptide.

ments using peptides containing amino acid substitutions. The results can be summarized as shown on *Figure 1*. The motif DERAA contains enough information for both DQ8 binding and T cell recognition. On this motif, R is the main anchor residiue, while D and E are in strong interaction with the T cell receptor. The remaining motif VDTYC is mostly interacting with the T cell receptor, as many substitutions do not dramatically affect the T cell proliferation.

Speculating that the DERAA motif might be relevant to RA predisposition by affecting T cell response against different foreign and self peptides containing the same motif, we ran a search on the Swiss-Prot and EMBL databases. We found 14 matches including the human vinculin, constituent of a submembranal plaque interacting with the cytoskeleton, the outer membrane protein (Omp) of *Chlamydia trachomatis*, the kanamycin-resistance gene of *Streptomyces ribosidificus,* one of the RNA polymerase subunit of *Saccharomyces cerevisae,* and the nucleoprotein of the Influenza A virus *(Table I).* All these peptides were tested and found to be immunogenic in DQ8.Abo mice, confirming that the motif DERAA guarantees DQ8-restricted T cell response, independently of the adjacent amino acid residues *(Table I).* However no crossreactivity was observed among these peptides.

Discussion

The finding that the motif DERAA guarantees DQ8-restricted immunogenicity allows some interesting speculations on the role of HLA-DQ in RA predisposition. According to our model, DQ4, DQ7, DQ8 and DQ9 are RA-predisposing molecules. Interestingly, polymorphic residues among these four DQ molecules are outside the p1 pocket. It is therefore likely that peptides bearing the DERAA motif should bind all four DQ alleles. S4, D24, D26, E27 and E28 on the DQA1*0301 chain and E86 and T89 on the different DQB1 chains are probably essential in the use of R as main anchor residue of the peptide. Thus, it is conceivable that a common "arthritogenic" determinant could bind all four DQ molecules. This determinant could be the Omp peptide of *Chlamidia Trachomatis,* an agent already involved in the etiology of reactive arthritis [6]. Although no crossreactivity was observed among the DERAA-bearing peptides, it can also be speculated that presentation of DRB1*0402 peptide by DQ8 molecule in the thymus could lead to the negative selection of precursors of autoreactive T cells in the periphery. Our results offer several interesting opportunities to better clarify the role of the MHC class II region in RA, and define the nature of a potential causative infectious agent.

References

1. Gonzalez-Gay MA, Nabozny GH, Bull MJ, Zanelli E, Douhan III J, Griffiths MM, Glimcher LH, Luthra HS, David CS. Protective role of major histocompatibility class II Ebd transgene on collagen-induced arthritis. *J Exp Med* 1994; 180: 1559-64.
2. Gonzalez-Gay MA, Zanelli E, Krco CJ, Nabozny GH, Hanson J, Griffiths MM, Luthra HS, David CS. Polymorphism of the MHC class II Eb gene determines the protection against collagen-induced arthritis. *Immunogenetics* 1995; 42: 35-40.
3. Zanelli E, Krco CJ, Baisch JM, Cheng S, David CS. Immune response of HLA-DQ8 transgenic mice to peptides from the third hypervariable region of HLA-DRB1 correlates with predisposition to rheumatoid arthritis. *Proc Natl Acad Sci USA* 1996; 93: 1814-9.
4. Zanelli E, Gonzalez-Gay MA, David CS. Could HLA-DRB1 be the protective locus in rheumatoid arthritis? *Immunol Today* 1995; 16: 274-8.
5. Krco CJ, Beito TG, David CS. Determination of tolerance to self Ea peptides by clonal elimination of H-2E reactive T cells and antigen presentation by H-2A molecules. *Transplantation* 1992; 54: 920-3.
6. Kvien TK, Glennas AS, Melby K, Granfors K, Andrup O, Karstensen B, Thoen JE. Reactive arthritis: incidence, triggering agents and clinical presentation. *J Rheumatol* 1994; 21: 115-22.

Collagen induced arthritis in HLA-DR4/human CD4 transgenic mice

A.P. Cope, L.H. Fugger, W. Chu, G. Sønderstrup-McDevitt

Department of Microbiology and Immunology, Fairchild Bldg, Stanford University School of Medicine, California 94305, USA

Collagen induced arthritis (CIA) is an experimentally induced inflammatory polyarthritis in rodents, which shares many clinical and histopathological features with rheumatoid arthritis (RA) in humans. Collagen type II (CII) is a major component of cartilage matrix protein in synovial joints. Immunization with bovine CII in complete Freunds adjuvant (CFA) has been shown to induce an inflammatory arthritis in specific mouse and rat strains, while other strains are resistant to CIA; this susceptibility to CIA is linked to major histocompatibility (MHC) class II genes in both species [1,2]. Similarly, susceptibility to RA is associated with the MHC class II region [3], in particular, specific HLA-DR4 subtypes which share an amino acid motif from positions 67-74 of the HLA-DRB1 chain [4]. Other HLA-DR specificities confer susceptibility to RA since they too express this 'shared epitope' (reviewed in [5]). It should be emphasized that CIA is an experimentally induced disease, provoked by immunization with native xenogeneic CII molecules. CIA starts with an active inflammatory phase followed by spontaneous remission in the majority of mice, with residual destruction and ankylosis of synovial joints. CIA cannot be re-induced in animals once recovered from the disease. RA, on the other hand, is a spontaneous chronic inflammatory disease occurring in genetically susceptible individuals with unknown triggering events and, although remissions and relapses occur, progressive joint destruction is a characteristic feature.

We have generated triple transgenic (trg) mice expressing the HLA-DRA*0101, DRB1*0401 and human CD4 transgenes [6] for studying immune responses to cartilage autoantigens thought to be important in the pathogenesis of RA. Since 10% of RA patients have specific autoantibodies to type II collagen, we have pursued CII as a potential arthritis related autoantigen in RA using this transgenic mouse model. The value of this approach was recently investigated by immunization of HLA-DRB1(*0401) trg mice with bovine CII in CFA and the generation of collagen specific T cell hybridomas [7]. One of the immunodominant T cell epitopes generated from the trg animals mapped to the region p261-273, which is highly homologous to both murine and human CII sequences. Accordingly, we wished to characterize CIA in mice expressing RA susceptible MHC class II alleles as transgenes.

Methods and results

DBA/1J mice are susceptible to experimental CIA. Furthermore, the class II (H-2^{q}) loci of this strain only express an I-A element (HLA-DQ homologue) but no I-E elements (the HLA-DR homologue). This factor has allowed us to introduce human DRα and β chains into the H-2q haplotype without the generation of cross-species molecules of murine/human origin (DRα/I-Eβ). Since non-MHC genes contribute to arthritis in this model, the DR4 trg was back crossed to the DBA/1J strain at least 9 generations, and in preliminary experiments, non-transgenic littermates were found to develop arthritis indistinguishable from inbred DBA/1J mice, following immunization with CII. Two groups of animals, group I (11 non-trg), and group II (9 heterozygous HLA-DR4 trg) were immunized at the base of the tail with 200 μg bovine CII, purified in our laboratory as described in [8], emulsified in CFA (*Figure 1*). Clinical observation and scoring was performed biweekly by two independent observers with assessment of numbers of affected paws, single joints counts, and measurements of paw swelling using calipers as described in [8]. In this experiment all non-trg litter-

Parameter	Non-transgenic	Transgenic	p
incidence of arthritis	100% (11/11)	55% (5/9)	
onset of arthritis	20 days	33 days	
time for 50% to develop arhritis	33 days	50 days	
mean peak joint score*	6.7 ± 3.9	3.0 ± 4.4	< 0.035
mean peak joint index	6.5 ± 5.6	2.1 ± 2.4	< 0.015
mean peak ankle swelling (mm)	0.5 ± 0.5	0.14 ± 0.2	< 0.003

Table I. Characteristics of collagen-induced arthritis in HLA-DR4 (DRA*0101/DRB1*0401) transgenic DBA/1J mice and non-transgenic littermates.
* peak joint scores, indices and swelling were oberved 10-12 weeks after immunization.

Arthritis severity	Mouse genotype/phenotype		
	Non-transgenic	Transgenic (arthritic)	Transgenic (non-arthritic)
Total no. joints assessed	19	7	7
normal	0 (0)*	0 (0)	5 (71)
mild	5 (26)	5 (71)	2 (29)
moderate	10 (53)	2 (29)	0 (0)
severe	4 (21)	0 (0)	0 (0)

Table II.
Histopathological assessment of arthritic joints. Assessment: **mild** - minimal synovitis, cartilage loss, focal bone erosions;
moderate- synovitis and erosions present but normal joint architecture;
severe - synovitis, extensive erosions, and joint architecture disrupted.
* % data are shown in parenthesis.

Anti-collagen antibody isotypes

Isotypes	Non-transgenic (n=11)	Transgenic arthritic (n=5)	Transgenic non-arthritic (n=4)
IgG,A,M	1,626,139 ± 632,263	1,478,932 ± 533,431	619,287 ± 532,585
IgG1	584,141 ± 302,607	119,875 ± 83,785¶	78,008 ± 76,835¶
IgG2a	1,107,759 ± 535,358*	981,283 ± 436,054*	348,280 ± 296,845
IgE	10,400 ± 9,216	5,389 ± 1,181	5,747 ± 2,493

Table III.
Anti-collagen type II antibody isotypes in HLA-DR4 transgenic mice and non-transgenic littermates at 8 weeks following immunization
¶ $p < 0.0033$ versus non-transgenic mice.
* $p < 0.022$ versus non-arthritic mice.

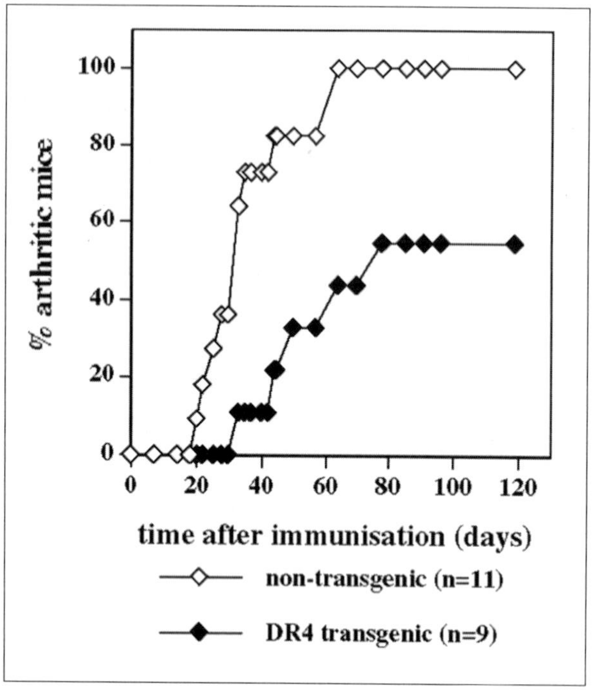

Figure 1. Collagen induced arthritis in HLA-DR4 transgenic mice and non-transgenic littermates.

mates developed arthritis (*Figure 1*); only 5 out of nine mice (55%) developed arthritis in the DR4 trg group, and the remaining four DR4 trg animals showed no clinical signs of arthritis.

Table I summarizes the arthritis data. It is clear that not only were there fewer DR4 trg animals developing arthritis (55% *versus* 100%), but the onset of disease in trg animals was delayed (33 *versus* 20 days). Additionally, disease severity was decreased with respect to joint score, joint index as well as mean peak swelling (*Table I*); differences were significant (non-paired t-test for > 95% confidence limits) for mean peak ankle swelling at 10 weeks (*Table I*).

Routine histopathological examination of hematoxylin and eosin stained sections were evaluated in 19 arthritic synovial joints from non-trg mice, 7 joints from arthritic DR4 trg animals, as well as 7 representative joints from non-arthritic DR4 trg group. Abnormalities were observed in all sampled joints from the non-trg group with histopathological scores ranging from mild (26%), moderate (53%), to severe (21%) (*Table II*). The arthritic HLA-DR4 trg animals had mild pathological changes in 71% and moderate severity in 29 % of sampled joints. While none of the joints in this group fell into the category of severe joint changes, neither were any of these joints normal (*Table II*). Only 2 (29%) of the sampled joints in the HLA-DR4 trg/non-arthritic group showed any histopathological changes, both of them falling within the category of mild joint disease (*Table III*). Only arthritic joints were collected from the non-trg and the HLA-DR4 trg/arthritic groups, while the seven joints from the non-arthritic HLA-DR4 trg group was chosen to match the seven joints collected in the HLA-DR4 trg arthritic group (a left wrist from the arthritic group matched with a left wrist from the non-arthritic group, etc.). The severity was assessed according to the degree of inflammatory infiltrate/pannus, and cartilage or bone erosion as described [8].

At 16 weeks both DR4 trg and the non-trg littermates showed similar CII specific T cell responses in proliferation assays (results not shown). In contrast, the collagen specific antibody responses were different between arthritic and non-arthritic mice. Collagen type II specific antibody levels were determined every 2 weeks from weeks 4 to 16 following immunization, with total CII specific antibody levels reaching maximal levels at 6 weeks and declining from 8-10 weeks (results not shown). The level of total (IgM, IgG and IgA) CII specific antibodies were similar in the non-trg and arthritic HLA-DR4 trg animals; but HLA-DR4 trg non-arthritic animals produced only about 30% the level of CII specific antibodies produced by the arthritic mice (*Table III*). Significantly higher levels of CII specific IgG2a antibodies were observed in arthritic mice at 8 weeks (*Table III*). The CII specific IgE antibodies were still increasing by week 10 in both arthritic and non-arthritic HLA-DR4 trg animals, whilst the IgE levels were found to decrease in the non-trg littermates (*Table III*). Collagen type II specific IgG1 antibodies were significantly lower in the HLA-DR4 trg animals as compared to the non-trg littermates, but no clear pattern emerged with respect to arthritis phenotype.

Discussion

Introduction of the HLA DR4 trg (I-E equivalent), which is associated with susceptibility to RA in humans seems to decrease both the frequency and the severity of arthritis. The antibody isotyping data indicate that the induction of a CII specific Th2 response, characterized by relative increases in IgE specific antibodies and lower levels of IgG2a specific antibodies in non-arthritic mice in the DR4 trg animals provide one possible explanation for disease protection. Similar mechanisms may operate in RA patients since not all HLA-DR4 subjects develop RA. The immunodominant epitope of CII presented by the HLA-DR4 and the I-Aq molecules are practically identical [7]; the anchor positions of the peptide in DRB1(*0401) are displaced three amino acids C-terminal as compared to I-A^q binding. This could potentially result in significant competition for peptide binding by the two MHC molecules, particularly if the binding affinity for HLA-DR4 was just slightly lower than for I-Aq. Additionally, the DR4 trg mice are known to express the HLA trg at a rather low level on a mouse class II positive background, which also can influence the direction of the T cell responses. In preliminary experiments with a transgenic rat model using exactly the same HLA-DR4 and human CD4 constructs, but choosing a trg rat line with a higher expression of the transgenes, the presence of the DR4 molecule seem to increase the severity of CIA in the DR4 trg animals compared to the non-trg littermates (Kremer *et al.*, unpublished).

It has also been suggested that the DRB1 locus is actually a protective allele, but HLA-DQ is the real susceptibility locus [9]. This notion has not been supported by any of the population genetic studies reported in the Workshops over the years; HLA-DQ8 associations have always been satisfactorily explained by linkage disequilibrium between HLA-DR and DQ. HLA-DQ7 has been found to be associated with more severe RA. Furthermore, HLA-DRB1(*0401) trg mice from our colony, when crossed onto a line of mice lacking murine class II genes [10], have developed severe CIA, which in some animals was severe enough to result in ankylosis of the joints.

References

1. Trentham DE, Townes AS, Kang AH. Autoimmunity to type II collagen: an experimental model of arthritis. *J Exp Med* 1977; 146: 857-68.
2. Griffiths MM, Eichwald EJ, Martin JH, Smith, CB, DeWitt CW. Immunogenetic control of experimental type II collagen induced arthritis. *Arthritis Rheum* 1981; 24: 781-9.
3. Stastny P. Mixed lymphocyte culture typing cells from patients with rheumatoid arthritis. *Tissue Antigens* 1974;4: 571-9.
4. Gregersen PK, Shen M, Song Q, Merryman P, Degar S, Seki T, Maccari J, Goldberg D, Murphy H, Schwenzer J, Wang C, Winchester RJ, Nepom GT, Silver J. Molecular diversity of HLA-DR4 haplotypes. *Proc Natl Acad Sci USA* 1986; 83: 2642-6.
5. Winchester R. The molecular basis of susceptibility to rheumatoid arthritis. *Adv Immunol* 1994; 56: 389-466.
6. Fugger L, Michie SA, Rulifson I, Lock CB, Sonderstrup-McDevitt G. Expression of HLA-DR4 and human CD4 transgenes in mice determines the variable region β-chain T-cell repertoire and mediates an HLA-DR-restricted immune response. *Proc Natl Acad Sci USA* 1994; 91: 6151-5.
7. Fugger L, Rothbard JB, Sønderstrup-McDevitt G. The specificity of the dominant HLA-DRB1*0401 restricted T cell response to type II collagen. *Eur J Immunol* 1996; 26: 928-33.
8. Williams RO, Feldman M, Maini RN. Anti-tumor necrosis factor ameliorates joint disease in murine collagen-induced arthritis. *Proc Natl Acad Sci USA* 1992; 89: 9784-8.
9. Zanelli E, Gonzalez-Gay MA, David CS. Could HLA-DRB1 be the protective locus in rheumatoid arthritis? *Immunol Today* 1995; 16: 274-8.
10. Cosgrove D, Gray D, Dierich A, Kaufman J, Lemeur M, Benoist C, Mathis D. Mice lacking MHC class II molecules. *Cell* 1991; 66: 1051-66.

Characterization of a MHC class I immune response gene controlling resistance to collagen induced arthritis

R.E. Bontrop, N. Otting, B. 't Hart

Department of Immunobiology, Biomedical Primate Research Centre,
PO Box 3306, 2280 GH Rijswijk, The Netherlands

Collagen induced arthritis (CIA) is an experimental animal model for studying immunoregulatory mechanisms that propagate an autoimmune disease. Upon intradermal immunization with type II collagen (CII), the major cartilage protein, Rhesus monkeys *(Macaca mulatta)* as well as several rodent strains develop CIA. This disease shares many pathological features with human rheumatoid arthritis (RA). Susceptibility to develop severe forms of human RA is associated with the HLA-DR1 and -DR4 specificities whereas in mice susceptibility to CIA has been mapped to particular alleles (I-A and I-E) encoded by the MHC class II region.

In this communication, we report on the genetic influence of MHC genes on the development of CIA in Rhesus monkeys. The animals used in this study were selected randomly from the BPRC colony which has an outbred character. Immunization of young-adult Rhesus monkeys (<10 years of age) with CII induced CIA in about 70% of the animals. In first instance, the animals were typed using specific alloantisera that were raised in Rhesus monkeys by active immunizations. These sera allow the identification of approximately ten alleles at each of the equivalents of the HLA-A, -B and -DR loci in Rhesus macaques [1]. Serological screening demonstrated that almost all resistant animals shared the serologically defined Mamu-A26 allele, which was found to be absent in all young Rhesus monkeys that developed CIA ($p<0.00002$). Thusfar, only two out of 30 resistant animals seem to lack the Mamu-A26 allele as it is defined by serological criteria.

It is generally accepted that during ageing the capacity of the immune system to maintain tolerance to autoantigens decreases. To study whether the association between Mamu-A26 and resistance to CIA is maintained in old animals, some aged animals (>22 years) were immunized with CII. The Mamu-A26 positive old animals developed a mild form of arthritis whereas, in contrast, the two Mamu-A26 negative animals developed a very severe arthritis [2]. These studies manifest that the protective effect of the Mamu-A26 marker seems to be less effective in old animals.

Biochemical methods were used to characterize the Rhesus monkey MHC class I gene products in more detail. The Mamu-A and -B locus encoded molecules were immunoprecipitated using monoclonal antibody W6/32. Precipitated molecules were separated on 1D-1EF gels. Such studies showed that Mamu-A and -B heavy chain isoelectric point differences correlate with serotypings. On top of that, it was found that Mamu-A26 is heterogeneous.

At this stage it is difficult to exclude between the possibilities that Mamu-A26 detects a gene product controling resistance or Mamu-A26 is just a marker detecting a closely linked gene. The latter alternative needs more scientific attention since serotyping demonstrate that the Mamu-A34 specificity is not only observed independent, but sometimes also in combination with Mamu-A11 or -A26. This implies that Mamu-A34 sera detect a class I gene product that is on the chromosome closely linked to the Mamu-A11 or -A26 genes. That this situation reflects reality is evidenced by gel electrophoretic analyses. This indicates also that some Rhesus monkey haplotypes encode multiple A locus products. As mentioned above Mamu-A34 is sometimes observed alone. Immunization studies demonstrate that such animals, but also Mamu-A11/A34 positive animals develop arthritis. Consequently, it seems unlikely that Mamu-A34 controls resistance to CIA.

At present, we are investigating the Rhesus monkey MHC class I region at the nucleotide level. By now we have characterized a large number of Mamu-A and -B genes. Comparitive analyses showed that our Mamu-A locus sera recognize the Rhesus macaque equivalents of the HLA-B locus (and *vice versa*). This implies that the Mamu-A26 sera are reactive with a B locus gene product. In humans, susceptibility to develop ankylosing spondylitis is strongly associated with HLA-B27. In Rhesus macaques, a particular B locus product seems to control resistance to an experimentally induced arthritic disease. The Mamu-A26 and HLA-B27 sequence do not share any significant degree of similarity. In conclusion, the MHC class I region plays an important role in maintaining/controlling tolerance to autoantigens. This non-human primate model will be instrumental in elucidating how this works mechanistically.

References

1. Bontrop RE, Otting N, Slierendregt BL, Lanchbury JS. Evolution of major Histocompatibility complex polymorphisms and T-cell receptor diversity in primates. *Immunol Rev* 195; 143: 33-62.
2. Bakker NPM, van Erck MGM, Otting N, Lardy NM, Noort· RC, 't Hart BA, Jonker M, Bontrop RE. Resistance to collagen-induced arthritis in a nonhuman primate species maps to the major histocompatibility complex class I region. *J Exp Med* 1992; 185: 933-7.

Polymorphism of the HLA-DM and DMB genes in rheumatoid arthritis

J.F. Eliaou[1], V. Pinet[1], O. Avinens[1], S. Caillat-Zucman[2], J. Sany[3], B. Combe[3], J. Clot[1]

1 Laboratoire d'Immunologie, INSERM U291, Hôpital Saint-Eloi, CHU de Montpellier, 34295 Montpellier Cedex 5, France
2 Laboratoire d'Immunologie, INSERM U25, Hôpital Necker, Paris, France
3 Fédération de Rhumatologie, Hôpital Lapeyronie, CHU Montpellier, Montpellier, France

Rheumatoid arthritis (RA) is an autoimmune disease characterized by a chronic inflammatory joint involvement. RA can also be identified as a complex multi-factorial disease with a strong genetic influence. Genes within the HLA genetic complex have been shown to determine susceptibility to RA. HLA-DR4 was first described to be associated with RA [1]. Advances in molecular biology permitted a more accurate definition of the various at-risk HLA-DRB1 alleles: DRB1*0401, *0404, *0405, *0408, *0101, and *0102. Although, the role of the HLA component in the susceptibility to RA is firmly established, the underlying molecular mechanisms are still unknow. In particular, the presence of particular amino acid motifs in position 70-74 of the HLA-DRβ1 molecule, determining the risk to develop the disease, cannot always account for the observed HLA-DRB1 gene distribution in patients. This is true especially when considering the disease phenotype and the genotypic configurations of the patients [2, 3].

The HLA-DMA and DMB genes are located within the HLA class II region between the DP and DQ gene regions. The α and β glycoproteins, respectively encoded by the DMA and DMB genes, are HLA class II- like molecules and form an heterodimer. The HLA-DM molecules have been localized in the endocytic compartment of the B lymphocytes where the peptides bind to HLA class II molecules [4]. Cellular mutants analysis have clearly demonstrated the direct involvement of the DM molecules in the HLA class II-dependent antigen presentation pathway (reviewed in [5]).

A limited nucleotide polymorphism has been described in the 3rd exon of the DMA and DMB genes [6] which does not involve the putative peptide-binding pocket but could influence the transport of the DM molecules in the cell. Linkage disequilibrium has been reported between certain alleles at the DM, DR and DQ loci [6]. However, these results were not found in an other study (S. Caillat-Zucman, personal communication).

In order to better understand the molecular basis of the association between the HLA class II component and RA, we compared the distributions of the DMA and DMB genes in RA patients and control individuals. We show that particular alleles at the DM loci are significantly associated with the susceptibility to RA.

Patients and methods

Patients and controls

All the patients and controls were from caucasian origin and from the same geographic area. The unrelated patient population consisted in 199 RA patients fulfilling the classical ACR criteria. Two unrelated control samples were used in this study. All were healthy volunteer bone marrow donnors. First, 147 individuals were randomly selected and typed for DR and DM. Second, to determine whether the association between RA and certain DM alleles resulted from direct influence of the DM genes or indirect influence through linkage disequilibrium with alleles at the DRB1 locus, a second group of control individuals was defined. This group of 218 individuals was closely matched for the HLA-DR genotype with the patients' group.

Methods

Genomic DNA was extracted from peripheral mononuclear cells following the classical salting-out procedure.

HLA-DR and -DQB typings were performed as previously described [7, 8]. DRB1*04 high-resolution typings were obtained by sequencing-based typings as described in the Volume I of the 12th IHWC proceedings.

The polymorphism of the DMA and DMB genes was determined following PCR amplification of genomic DNA using two pairs of primers *(Figure 1)*. Hybridization of the PCR products with the respective DMA and DMB pannel of sequence-specific oligonucleotide probes (SSOPs) was performed using a nonradioactive direct dot-blot procedure. The sequence of the SSOPs is given *Figure 1*. Four alleles have been defined for DMA and DMB. These alleles are named according the nomenclature for factors of the HLA system [9].

Statistical analysis

Odds ratios (OR) were calculated by the method of Woolf with Haldane's modification for small numbers. The significance of difference in allelic or genotype frequencies was determined by Fischer's exact tests. Corrected *p* values were calculated by the Bonferoni inequality method by multiplying *p* by the number of alleles compared. The level of significance was set to 0.05. Associations between HLA-DRB1 and DM alleles was assessed using the Δ value for nonrandom assortment of alleles [10].

Results

DMA *0103 and DMB *0104 alleles are associated with RA

When the distribution of the DMA and DMB alleles was compared between RA patients and randomly selected controls, no difference in the distribution of the DMA*0101 and DMB*0101 alleles was seen. However, although the frequency of these two alleles is quite high in both populations, alleles DMA*0103 and DMB*0104 are more frequent in RA patients (DMA*0103: 12.6% in patients vs 2.3% in controls, pc = 0.003, DMB*0104: 14.6% in patients vs 6.8% in controls pc = 0.03) *(Table I)*. The study of the distributions of the DMA and DMB genotypes gave similar results. The genotypes including respectively the DMA*0103 and DMB*0104 haplotypes were found to be more frequent in the patients' population (data not shown).

To entirely eliminate possible influences of a linkage disequilibrium between the DMA*0103, DMB*0104 and RA-associated DRB1 alleles, RA patients were compared to HLA-matched controls. No significant difference was observed between the patients' and controls' genotype distribution ($p = 0.16$, $\chi^2 = 7.9$ with 5 degrees of freedom). Again both DMA*0103 and DMB*0104 were found to be more frequent in patients than in HLA-matched controls (DMA*0103: 12.6% in patients vs 3.7% in controls, pc = 0.004, DMB*0104: 14.6% in patients vs 6% in controls pc = 0.02) *(Table I)*. Analysis of the genotype distributions gave similar results (data not shown).

Combined analysis of DM and DRB1 allele distributions in RA patients

It has been reported that the genetic risk associated with the various susceptibility DRB1 alleles was not equivalent [2, 3]. To determine whether difference in the distribution of the DMA and DMB alleles could be observed among the patients carrying the various DRB1 alleles, we categorized the patients and matched controls according to their DRB1 phenotypes and genotypes.

	HLA-DMA 3rd exon	HLA-DMB 3rd exon
Primer	5'-GGGTTTCCTATCGCTGAAGTG-3'	5'-CGGCCACCATCTGTGCAAGT-3'
	5'-CCAATAGGCAATTGCTGTGTA-3'	5'-CCAGTCCCGAAGGATGGGCTC-3'
SSOP	5'-CATCATTCCGTCCCTGTGG-3'	5'-GTGATGCTGGCCTGCTATG-3'
	5'-CATCATTCCATCCCTGTGG-3'	5'-GTGATGCTAGCCTGCTATG-3'
	5'-TGTCGATGGACTCAGCTTC-3'	5'-AGCAGCGCGCACAAGACGT-3'
	5'-TGTCGATGCACTCAGCTTC-3'	5'-AGCAGCGAGCACAAGACGT-3'
	5'-GAAATTGACCGCTACACAG-3'	5'-AGCAGCGTGCACAAGACGT-3'
	5'-GAAATTGACTGCTACACAG-3'	5'-GTAGAGCACATTGGGGCTC-3'
	5'-GAAATTGACCACTACACAG-3'	5'-GTAGAGCACACTGGGGCTC-3'

Figure 1. Sequence of the oligonucleotides.

Table I. Distribution of the DMA and DMB alleles in patients compared to the two control populations

	patients (N=199)	RC[1] (N=147)	MC[2] (N=218)	Comparisons patients vs RC		patients vs MC		RC vs MC	
	n (%)	n (%)	n (%)	*OR*	*Pc*	*OR*	*Pc*	*OR*	*Pc*
DMA*0101	194 (97)	146 (99)	217 (99)	-	ns	-	ns	-	ns
DMA*0102	29 (15)	33 (22)	43 (20)	-	ns	-	ns	-	ns
DMA*0103	25 (13)	4 (3)	8 (4)	*5.1*	*0.003*	*3.8*	*0.004*	-	ns
DMA*0104	2 (1)	4 (3)	1 (.5)	-	ns	-	ns	-	ns
DMB*0101	182 (91)	138 (94)	205 (94)	-	ns	-	ns	-	ns
DMB*0102	23 (12)	10 (7)	18 (8)	-	ns	-	ns	-	ns
DMB*0103	60 (30)	43 (29)	66 (30)	-	ns	-	ns	-	ns
DMB*0104	29 (15)	10 (7)	13 (6)	*2.3*	*0.03*	*2.7*	*0.02*	-	ns

[1]Randomly selected controls. [2]HLA-matched controls.

The DMA*0103 allele was found to be significantly more frequent in DRB1*01 patients than in controls *(Table II A)*. This difference is seen when both the DRB1*01 phenotype and the pooled genotypes DRB1*01/DRB1*01, DRB1*01/DRX (DRX standing for any DRB1 allele except the RA-associated DRB1*01 and DRB1*04 alleles) are considered (DRB1*01 phenotype: OR = 9, pc = 0.007, DRB1*01/DRB1*01 or DRB1*01/DRX genotypes: OR = 17, pc = 0.007), suggesting a combined effect of DMA*0103 and DRB*01. Indeed, in the DRB1*01/DRB1*01 or DRB1*01/DRX genotypes, the RA-associated DRB1*04 haplotypes are not taken in account. Strikingly, no difference in the DMB*0104 frequency was observed in this group of RA patients compared to matched controls.

The frequency of the DMB*0104 allele was higher in DRB1*04 patients than in matched controls. However no difference was found when DRB1*04/DRB1*04 or DRB1*04/DRX patients were considered *(Table II B)*.

Finally, in DRX/DRX patients the frequency of DMA*0103 allele is increased compared to matched controls, strongly suggesting that no linkage disequilibrium between DM and HLA-DRB1 could explain the effect of DMA*0103. This was confirmed by evaluating linkage disequilibrium, using Δ values for nonrandom assortment of alleles in control subjects. No significant linkage disequilibrium was found between DRB1*01 and DMA*0103 (Δ = 0.002, p =1).

Discussion

We show in this study that particular DMA and DMB alleles are associated with RA susceptibility. The influence of the DMA and DMB cannot be explained by a linkage disequilibrium with RA-associated HLA-DRB1 alleles. This was demonstrated both by the use of a HLA-matched control population and the determination of the Δ value for nonrandom assortment of alleles in controls.

The risk associated with the DMB*0104 allele can only be observed when the global population of patients is considered, suggesting a minor effect of this allele on the genetic susceptibility to the disease. On the contrary, DMA*0103 seems to play an important role on disease susceptibility since it is more frequent both in the overall RA population as well as in the DRB1*01 haplotype carrier patients. Moreover, the fact that DMA*0103 was not found to be increased in DRB1*04 haplotype carrier patients strongly suggests that this allele could be associated with the progression and the severity of RA in DRB1*01 and DRX patients. Indeed DRB1*04, and especially DRB1*04/DRB1*04 individuals have higher risk to develop severe disease than DRB1*01 or DRX patients [3]. The combined presence of DMA*0103 and DRB1*01 or DRX could represent a bad prognosis factor in patients expected to be at-low risk to develop a severe form of RA.

Although functional consequences of the polymorphism of the DM genes have not been demonstrated yet, it could be suggested that the class II-dependent antigen presentation pathway, involving the DM molecules could play a role in the pathophysiology of the disease, therefore representing an alternative molecular mechanism of the association between the HLA complex and RA.

Table II. Distribution of the DMA and DMB alleles in patients and HLA-matched controls according to the HLA-DR phenotypes and genotypes

A. HLA-DRB1*01[1] patients and controls

	DRB1*01 phenotype				DRB1*01/DRB1*01 and DRB1*01/DRX[2]			
	RA[3] (55) n (%)	MC[4] (59) n (%)	*OR*	*pc*	RA (39) n (%)	MC (44) n (%)	*OR*	*pc*
DMA*0101	52 (94)	59 (100)	-	ns	37 (95)	44 (100)	-	ns
DMA*0102	9 (16)	17 (29)	-	ns	6 (15)	13 (30)	-	ns
DMA*0103	13 (24)	2 (3)	*9.0*	*0.007*	11 (28)	1 (2)	*17.0*	*0.004*
DMA*0104	1 (2)	0	-	ns	1 (3)	0	-	ns
DMB*0101	52 (94)	57 (97)	-	ns	38 (97)	42 (95)	-	ns
DMB*0102	12 (22)	3 (5)	*5.2*	*0.04*	9 (23)	2 (4)	-	ns
DMB*0103	9 (16)	18 (30)	-	ns	5 (13)	14 (32)	-	ns
DMB*0104	7 (13)	4 (7)	-	ns	6 (15)	3 (7)	-	ns

B. HLA-DRB1*04[5] patients and controls

	DRB1*04 phenotype				DRB1*04/DRB1*04 and DRB1*04/DRX			
	RA (108) n (%)	MC (96) n (%)	*OR*	*pc*	RA (92) n (%)	MC (82) n (%)	*OR*	*pc*
DMA*0101	106 (98)	95 (99)	-	ns	91 (99)	81 (99)	-	ns
DMA*0102	17 (16)	14 (14)	-	ns	14 (15)	10 (12)	-	ns
DMA*0103	8 (7)	6 (6)	-	ns	6 (7)	5 (6)	-	ns
DMA*0104	0	1 (1)	-	ns	0	1 (1)	-	ns
DMB*0101	94 (87)	89 (89)	-	ns	76 (77)	75 (91)	-	ns
DMB*0102	11 (10)	9 (9)	-	ns	8 (9)	8 (10)	-	ns
DMB*0103	44 (41)	34 (34)	-	ns	40 (41)	29 (35)	-	ns
DMB*0104	18 (17)	5 (5)	*3.6*	*0.04*	17 (18)	5 (6)	-	ns

C. HLA-DRX patients and controls

	DRX/DRX			
	RA (52) n (%)	MC (78) n (%)	*OR*	*pc*
DMA*0101	51 (98)	78 (100)	-	ns
DMA*0102	6 (12)	16 (20)	-	ns
DMA*0103	6 (12)	1 (1)	*10*	*0.04*
DMA*0104	1 (2)	0	-	ns
DMB*0101	50 (96)	74 (95)	-	ns
DMB*0102	3 (6)	7 (9)	-	ns
DMB*0103	11 (21)	18 (23)	-	ns
DMB*0104	5 (10)	4 (5)	-	ns

[1]DRB1*01 includes all the RA-associated alleles: DRB1*0101, and *0102.
[2]DRX indicates any DRB1 allele except the RA-associated DRB1*01 and DRB1*04 alleles.
Number of RA patients[3], and HLA-matched controls[4].
[5]DRB1*04 includes all the RA-associated alleles: DRB1*0401, *0404, *0405, and *0408.

Acknowledgements
This work was partly supported by grants from the "Association de Recherche sur la Polyarthrite" and GREG (n° 88/94).

References

1. Stastny P. Association of the B-cell alloantigene DRw4 with rheumatoid arthritis. *N Engl J Med* 1978; 298: 869-71.
2. Dizier MH, Eliaou JF, Babron MC, Combe B, Sany J, Clot J, Clerget-Darpoux F. Investigation of the HLA component in rheumatoid arthritis by using the marker-association segregation chi-square (MASC) method: rejection of the unifying shared-epitope hypothesis. *Am J Hum Genet* 1993; 53: 715-21.
3. Weyand CM, McCarthy TG, Goronzy JJ. Correlation between disease phenotype and genetic heterogeneity in rheumatoid arthritis. *J Clin Invest* 1995; 95: 2120-6.
4. Denzin L, Robbins N, Carboy-Newcomb C, Cresswell P. Assembly and intracellular transport of HLA-DM and correction of the class II antigen-processing defect in T2 cells. *Immunity* 1994; 1: 595-606.
5. Roche P. HLA-DM: an *in vivo* facilitator of MHC class II peptide loading. *Immunity* 1995; 3: 259-62.
6. Carrington M, Stephens JC, Klitz W, Begovich AB, Erlich HA, Mann D. Major histocompatibility complex class II haplotypes and linkage disequilibrium values observed in the CEPH families. *Hum Immunol* 1994; 41: 234-40.
7. Eliaou JF, Palmade F, Avinens O, Edouard E, Ballaguer P, Nicolas JC, Clot J. Generic HLA-DRB1 gene oligotyping by a non-radioactive reverse dot-blot methodology. *Hum Immunol* 1992; 35: 215-22.
8. Eliaou JF, Humbert M, Balaguer P, Gebuhrer L, Amsellem S, Bétuel H, Nicolas JC, Clot J. A method of HLA class II typing using non-radioactive labelled oligonucleotides. *Tissue Antigens* 1989; 33: 475-85.
9. WHO Nomenclature Committee. Nomenclature for factors of the HLA system, 1995. *Hum Immunol* 1995; 43: 149-64.
10. Svejgaard A, Hauge M, Jersild C, Platz P, Ryder LP, Staub Nielsen LS, Thomsen M.The HLA system: an introductory survey. *Monogr Hum Genet* 1975; 7: 1-100.

Trans-regulatory Y box-binding nuclear proteins and susceptibility to rheumatoid arthritis

D.P. Singal, W.W. Buchanan, X. Qiu

Department of Pathology, McMaster University, 1200 Main Street West, Hamilton, Ontario, L8N 3Z5 Canada

Rheumatoid arthritis (RA) is a chronic inflammatory joint disease caused by tissue-destructive autoimmune response(s). We and others have shown that this aberrant immune response could be mediated by amino acid sequence motif QKRAA or QRRAA in HLA class II (HLA-DRB1) genes [1]. These associations between DRB1 genes and susceptibility to RA are however only partial in that about one-third of RA patients do not carry disease-susceptibility DRB1 epitope and not all disease epitope-positive individuals develop the disease. We therefore hypothesized that additional susceptibility gene(s) contribute to the development of RA. These include factors that regulate the level of expression of DR molecules on the cell surface, which may lead to an aberrant autoreactive class II-mediated immune response. In this regard, we have recently demonstrated that polymorphism at position -150 in the Y box of DRB promoters and the binding affinities of Y box-binding (NF-Y and NF-YB) nuclear proteins play a dominant role on the level of expression of DR genes [2,3]. In addition, we showed that the binding affinities of these Y box-binding proteins have inverse relationships to expression levels of DR genes. The objectives of the present investigation were to examine the role of Y box-binding nuclear proteins in susceptibility to RA.

Patients and methods

Twenty-five adult Caucasian patients with RA, who attended the rheumatology clinic at the McMaster University Medical Centre were studied. All patients had classical seropositive RA. Thirty-one unrelated Caucasian individuals, including eleven Epstein-Barr virus (EBV)-transformed homozygous typing cell (HTC) lines from the Tenth International Histocompatibility Workshop served as controls. Mononuclear cells from peripheral blood of RA patients and healthy subjects were separated by the Ficoll-Hypaque density gradient centrifugation. The enriched B lymphocyte population was obtained by the nylon wool adherent method and transformed with EBV by incubating B cells with EBV-containing supernatant derived from the marmoset cell line B95-8. Patients and normal healthy controls were typed for HLA-DR antigens by oligonucleotide typing of PCR-amplified genomic DNA.

Nuclear proteins were prepared from EBV-transformed B cell lines from RA patients, normal controls and HTCs, as described previously [4]. Two 20bp Y box oligonucleotides containing polymorphic nucleotide at position -150 were synthesized: YB1.1 = 5'-GCT-GATTGG TTCTCCAACAC-3' and YB1.2 = 5'-GCT-GATTCGTTCTCCAACAC-3'. Of these, YB1.1 carries an inverted CCAAT motif and YB1.2 has an imperfect inverted CCAAT sequence. Double-stranded oligonucleotides were end-labeled with DNA polymerase I, Klenow fragment. The gel mobility shift assays with double-stranded oligonucleotides and nuclear proteins were performed [3,4]. Competition experiments were performed with varying amounts of unlabeled double-stranded oligonucleotides. Samples were loaded on 5% polyacrylamide gels in 1 X TAE buffer. Gels were elctrophoresed at 4°C for 5h, dried and autoradiographed.

Results and discussion

The gel mobility shift experiments demonstrated that the *trans*-regulatory nuclear proteins bind specifically to two polymorphic Y box elements, one binding to YB1.1 motifs and the other to the YB1.2 sequence.

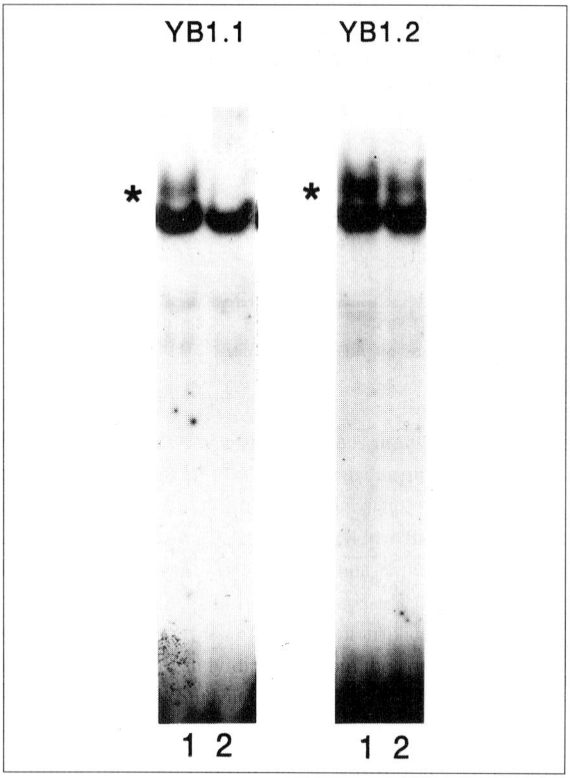

Figure 1. Gel mobility shift assay with two Y box double-stranded oligonucleotides (YB1.1 and YB1.2) and nuclear proteins from a normal individual (lane 1) and a patient with RA (lane 2). * = specific protein - DNA complex.

Competition experiments demonstrated that the *trans*-regulatory nuclear proteins have higher affinity for YB1.2 than for YB1.1 sequence.

The results from these experiments showed that when YB1.2 oligonucleotide was used as a probe, a specific protein-DNA complex was observed with nuclear proteins from all normal individuals, HTCs and RA patients *(Figure 1).* In contrast, when YB1.1 which contains an inverted CCAAT sequence was used as a probe, specific protein-DNA complex was observed in all healthy subjects and HTCs, but not in all patients. In fact, the *trans*-regulatory nuclear protein which binds to YB1.1 oligonucleotide was not detected in 11 of 25 patients with RA. The absence of YB1.1-specific nuclear protein in RA patients (44%) was significantly (Fisher's exact test, $p = 3x10^{-5}$; RR = 24.4) different from that in healthy individuals and HTCs (0%) *(Figure 2).*

We then analyzed our data on the prevalence of RA-susceptibility DRB1 epitope, carrying amino acid motif QKRAA or QRRAA at position 70 to 74 in DRB1 chain in patients and normal individuals *(Figure 2).* The prevalence of QKRAA or QRRAA motif in patients with RA (72%) was significantly (p=0.011; RR = 6.0) higher than that in normal healthy controls (30%). Further analysis of data demonstrated that all patients (100%) either carried the RA-susceptibility DRB1 amino acid sequence motif and/or lacked the *trans*-regulatory protein which binds to YB1.1 oligonucleotide, *i.e.* the Y box with an inverted CCAAT sequence. The relative risk associated with lack of nuclear protein that binds to the Y box with an inverted CCAAT sequence and/or the presence of RA-associated DRB1 amino acid motif for susceptibility to RA in unrelated subjects is 58.3 ($p = 2.3x10^{-7}$). In addition, the data demonstrated that all patients (n=7) negative for the RA-susceptibility amino acid sequence epitope lacked nuclear protein that binds to the YB1.1 oligonucleotide. Furthermore, the results show that five of these seven patients carry RA-resistance amino acid sequence motif, *e.g.* DERAA at position 70 to 74 in DRB1 chain.

We and others have identified two *trans*-regulatory nuclear proteins that bind to polymorphic Y box consensus motifs in DRB promoters and regulate the level of expression of DR molecules [3, 5]. Of these, *trans*-regulatory protein NF-Y has higher affinity for the Y box with an inverted CCAAT sequence (YB1.1) and NF-YB has higher affinity for Y box with an imperfect inverted CCAAT motif (YB1.2). In addition, we showed that the

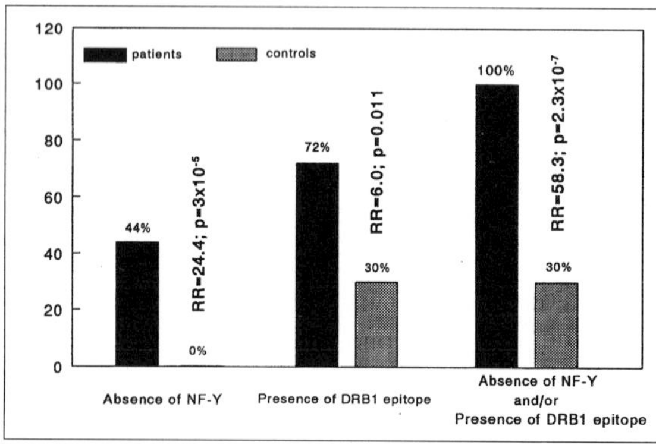

Figure 2. Frequency distribution of *trans*-regulatory nuclear protein NF-Y and HLA-DRB1 amino acid QKRAA or QRRAA motif in patients with RA and normal healthy individuals.

binding affinities of these Y box-binding proteins have inverse relationships with expression levels of DR molecules in the transfection experiments [3]. For example, lack of NF-Y protein will result in an enhanced expression of DR genes which carry an inverted CCAAT sequence in the Y box of their promoters, *i.e.* DRB1 (DR1,DR2), DRB3 (DR3,DR5,DR6) and DRB5 (DR2) genes. The results in the present study demonstrate that a number of patients with RA lack NF-Y protein. These data suggest that lack of NF-Y protein in patients will result in an enhanced expression of certain DR molecules or their expression on inappropriate cells, *e.g.* synovial tissue cells and T cells, thereby influencing presentation of both foreign and self antigens. These differences in antigen presentation by DR molecules will affect T cell responses and an aberrant tissue-destructive immune response skewed towards autoreactivity will cause susceptibility to RA.

A number of studies have reported associations between DRB1 genes and susceptibility to RA [1]. Since these associations are incomplete, it is likely that additional susceptibility gene(s) contribute to the development of RA. The results in the present study demonstrate that the *trans*-regulatory nuclear proteins that bind to the Y box which carry an inverted CCAAT sequence in DRB promoters are these factors that may cause susceptibility to RA. The present investigation has therefore demonstrated the clearest association between HLA class II genes and susceptibility to RA. These data show that the presence of DRB1 gene(s) with amino acid sequence QKRAA or QRRAA motif and the lack of *trans*-regulatory nuclear protein that binds to the Y box with an inverted CCAAT sequence cause susceptibility to RA.

Acknowledgement

This work was supported by a research grant from the Arthritis Society, Canada.

References

1. Singal DP, Buchanan WW. Human leucocyte antigens (HLA) and rheumatic diseases: HLA class II antigen-associated diseases. *Inflammopharmacology* 1993; 2: 47-62.
2. Singal DP, Qiu X. Polymorphism in the upstream regulatory region and level of expression of HLA-DRB genes. *Mol Immunol* 1994; 31: 1117-20.
3. Singal DP, Qiu X. Polymorphism in both X and Y box motifs controls level of expression of HLA-DRB1 genes. *Immunogenetics* 1996; 43: 50-6.
4. Singal DP, D'Souza M, Sood SK, Qiu X. Sequence-specific interactions of the nuclear proteins with polymorphic upstream regulatory regions of HLA-DRB genes. *Transplant Proc* 1993; 25: 180-2.
5. Emery P, Mach B, Reith W. The different level of expression of HLA-DRB1 and -DRB3 genes is controlled by conserved isotypic differences in promoter sequences. *Hum Immunol* 1993; 38: 137-47.

HLA-B27 alleles and susceptibility and resistance to ankylosing spondylitis (AS)

S. González-Roces[1], M.V. Alvarez[1], A. Dieye[2], C. López-Larrea[1]

1 Servicio de Immunología, Hospital Central de Asturias, Celestino Villamil s/n, 33006 Oviedo, Spain
2 Institut Pasteur de Dakar, Sénégal

HLA-B27 represents a family of nine closely related alleles (B*2701-B*2709) that differ in a restricted number of nucleotide substitutions that are mostly located in the C/F pocket *(Table I)* [1]. It appears to be the major genetic susceptibility factor for ankylosing spondylitis (AS). Although HLA-B27 is represented throughout nearly the whole world it shows a great difference in its distribution in different populations *(Figure 1).* It is strongly represented in Circumpolar and Subartic regions but it is barely present in Micronesian an Polynesian populations and practically absent in the native populations of Central and North America, Equatorial and Southern Africa and Australia [2]. Distribution of B27 subtypes has been studied by serological, isoelectrofocusing (IEF) and cytotoxic T lymphocyte typing methods. The HLA-B27 subtypes differ in their ethnic distribution which might be the result of different genetic and geographical origins. B*2705 was found in all ethnic groups studied. There is a North-South geographic decreasing gradient in the B*2705 distribution; it is over-represented in Circumpolar and Subartic regions of Eurasia and North America since it is the unique subtype present in Eskimo and North American natives; also B*2705 accounts for approximately 90% to 96% of HLA-B27-positive individuals in Euro-Caucasians. B*2702 has been described in Caucasians. B*2704, 06 and 07 have been found exclusively in Asians [3,4]. B*2703 was found to be over-represented in West African populations [5]. No data has been reported in relation to the distribution of B*2701, and 08 [2]. The results available indicate that only the alleles B*2701, 02, 04, 05 and 07 occur in patients [4,6]. We have recently described in Thai population that B*2706 is negatively associated with AS [4]. It has been suggested that B*2703 is negatively associated with the disease, but the evidence is still not conclusive [5]. B*2709, which has only been observed in Sardinians, was found to be absent in patients [7]. These negative associations with AS recently described, are ethnically and geographically restricted, and need to be confirmed in other populations [4,7].

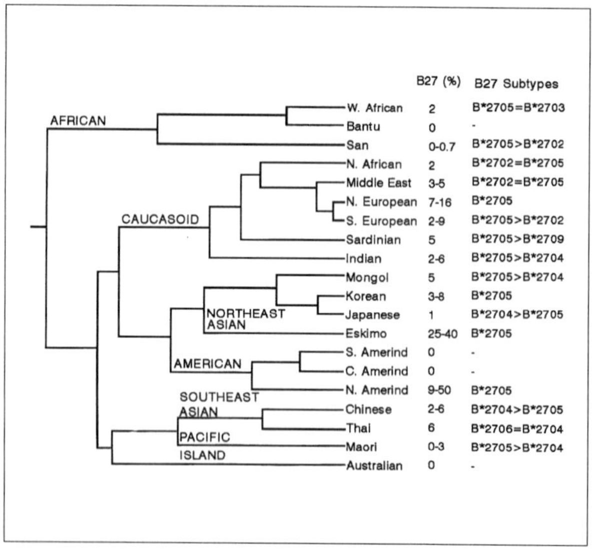

Figure 1. Genetic tree of 20 representative world populations with the prevalence of HLA-B27 and subtypes more represented in each population [12].

Material and methods

Populations

We have studied 800 B27 serologically typed samples from 17 populations with different ethnic origin, 476 of these were AS patients *(Figure 1).*

Table I. Polymorphic amino acid residues involved in formation of B27 pockets

Residues	59	74	77	80	81	82	83	97	113	114	116	131	152
Alleles													
B*2705	Y	D	D	T	L	L	R	N	Y	H	D	S	V
B*2701	-	Y	N	-	A	-	-	-	-	-	-	-	-
B*2702	-	-	N	I	A	-	-	-	-	-	-	-	-
B*2703	H	-	-	-	-	-	-	-	-	-	-	-	-
B*2704	-	-	S	-	-	-	-	-	-	-	-	-	E
B*2706	-	-	S	-	-	-	-	-	-	**D**	Y	-	E
B*2707	-	-	-	-	-	-	-	S	H	N	Y	R	-
B*2708	-	-	S	N	-	R	G	-	-	-	-	-	-
B*2709	-	-	-	-	-	-	-	-	-	-	**H**	-	-
Pockets	A	C/F	C/F	C/F	C/F			C/F	D	D/E	F		E

Residues from B27 alleles involved in each pocket are identified by their position number. A single letter amino acid code is used. The residues 114(D) and 116(H) corresponding to B*2706 (D/E pockets) and B*2709 (F pocket) appear in bold type. They could correlate with the disease susceptibility.

However, only three populations which are representative of B27-AS associations will be discussed here. So, these three populations with different genetic HLA structures were chosen to analyse the B27 subtypes involved in AS: Spaniards (Caucasians)(n=94), Thais (Orientals) (n=64) and Senegaleses (West Africans) (n=15) *(Table II)*.

The primers and SSOP (CL-1 to CL-12 and PAN-B27) used in this study have been previously reported [4,9]. The B*2709 subtype was defined by the CL-12 SSOP (codons 113-118, TACCACCAGCACGCCTAC). The definition of B*7301, which shares many structural features with B27, has also been included in this study (CL-11: codons 76-83, AGTGGGCCTGCGGAACCTGCGCGG).

Sequencing

DNA from HLA-B27 alleles, showing B*2703 and B*2706 patterns by molecular typing, were selected in order to confirm these subtypes by sequencing.

Results and discussion

The data compiled from the AS patients studied show that B*2705 and B*2702 were found to be associated with AS in Spanish (Caucasians), B*2705, B*2704 and B*2707 in Thai (Asians) and B*2705, B*2703 and B*2702 in Senegalese (Africans) populations *(Table II)*. The association of B*2703 with AS has not been previously reported, but is of remarkable interest since it has been suggested that B*2703 is negatively associated with the disease [5].

Non-significant differences were found between AS patients and controls in the population studied, excepting the Thai population, where B*2706 previously identified as a rare subtype present only in some Asian individuals, was found to be absent in the Thai AS patients but over-represented in the Thai control group (53% in C vs 0% in AS). The data available from this

Table II. Distribution of B27 alleles in the Spanish, Thai and Senegalese populations

	Populations					
	Spanish (n=94)		Thai (n=64)		Senegalese (n=15)	
Subtypes	Controls (n=30)	Patients (n=64)	Controls (n=19)	Patients (n=45)	Controls (n=3)	Patients (n=12)
B*2702	2 (7%)	6 (9%)	-	-	-	1 (8%)
B*2703	-	-	-	-	-	3 (25%)
B*2704	-	-	8 (42%)	41(91%)*	-	-
B*2705	28(93%)	58(91%)	1 (5%)	2 (4,5%)	3(100%)	8 (67%)
B*2706	-	-	10(53%)+	-	-	-
B*2707	-	-	-	2 (4,5%)	-	-

* pc=5.10-5; RR: 14; EF: 0,8
+ pc<10-6; PF: 1
The allelic frequencies are given in parenthesis.
pc: p corrected; RR: relative risk; EF: etiological fraction; PF: protective fraction.

Table III. B27 subtypes confering susceptibility and resistance to AS among different populations

	AS		
Subtypes	Susceptibility	Resistance	Populations
B*2701	+?	-	Caucasian
B*2702	+	-	Caucasian
B*2703	+	-	West African
B*2704	+	-	Oriental
B*2705	+	-	Caucasian
B*2706	-	+	Thai, Indonesian
B*2707	+	-	Oriental
B*2708	?	?	Caucasian
B*2709	-	+	Sardinian

The symbols +/- denote susceptibility or resistance to AS.
"?" indicates that insufficient data are available.

study indicate that B*2706 is not associated with AS in Thailanders, showing the maximum protective factor value (pc<10-6; PF=1). Moreover, in this same population B*2704 was estimated to be significantly increased in AS controls (91% in AS, 42% in C) [4], this is probably due to the absence of B*2706 in the AS group. In addition, the B*2709 subtype was found to be negatively associated with AS in Sardinian population [7].

The information now available on the B27 alleles conferring susceptibility and protection from AS among different populations is summarized in *Table III*. B*2701,02,03,04,05,07 occur in AS patients, whereas B*2706 has been described to be absent in Thai [4] and B*2709 in Sardinian patients [7]. This B*2706 negative association has recently been confirmed in a Indonesian population (T.E.W. Feltkamp, personal communication) It has been proposed that AS may be a product of a CTL-mediated response to a arthritogenic peptide or peptides found in joint tissue, which could be presented by the B27 molecule [8,10]. All the B27 subtypes bind peptides carrying Arg at P2 as the major anchor, however, variations among the B27 alleles may affect the binding of peptide side chains in other positions. Analysis of the anchor motifs shared from the B27 alleles indicate that the different subtypes can bind a common set of peptides, but allelic differences have also been observed [11]. The arthritogenic peptide(s) must be presented by all B27 subtypes know to be linked with the disease. Examination of B27 alleles indicate that the major differences between the hypothetical disease-linked and resistance-associated subtypes are located at pocket D (His114Asp for B*2706) and pocket F (Asp116Tyr for B*2706 and Asp116His for B*2709) *(Table I)*. The present study suggests that in addition to B pocket, the D and F pockets of B27 could play a prominent role in putative arthritogenic peptide(s) binding.

Acknowledgment
This work was supported by grants from the Spanish FIS 93/854 and CICYT SAF 96-0065.

References

1. López de Castro JA. Structural polymorphism and function of HLA-B27. *Curr Op Rheumatol* 1995; 7: 270-8.
2. Khan MA. HLA-B27 and its subtype in world populations. *Curr Op Rheumatol* 1995; 7: 263-9.
3. Breur-Vriesendorp BS, Dekker-Saeys AJ, Ivanyi P. Distribution of HLA-B27 subtypes in patients with ankylosing spondylitis: the disease is associated with a common determinant of the various B27 molecules. *Ann Rheum Dis* 1987; 46: 353-6.
4. López-Larrea C, Sujirachato K, Mehra NK, Chielwsilp P, Isarangkura D, Kanga U, Dominguez O, Coto E, Peña M, Setién F, González-Roces S. HLA-B27 subtypes in Asian patients with ankylosing spondylitis. *Tissue Antigens* 1995; 45: 169-76.
5. Hill AVS, Allsopp CEM, Kwiatkowski D, Anstey NM, Greenwood BM, McMichael AJ. HLA class I typing by PCR:HLA-B27 and an African subtype. *Lancet* 1991; 337: 640-2.
6. Choo SY. The HLA-B27 antigen family and disease susceptibility. In: molecular mimicry in HLA-B27 related arthritis. *Ann Intern Med* 1989; 111: 581-91.
7. D´Amato M, Fiorillo MT, Carcassi C, Mathieu A, Zuccarelli A, Bitti PP, Tosi R, Sorrentino R. Relevance of residue 116 of HLA-B27 in determining susceptibility to ankylosing spondylitis. *Eur J Immunol* 1995; 25: 3199-201.
8. Hermann E, Yu DT, Meyer zum Buschenfelde HM, Fleischer B. HLA-B27-restricted CD8 T cells derived from synovial fluids of patients with reactive arthritis and ankylosing spondylitis. *Lancet* 1993; 342: 646-50.
9. Dominguez O, Coto E, Martinez-Naves E, Choo SY, López-Larrea C. Molecular typing of HLA-B27 alleles. *Immunogenetics* 1992; 36: 277-82.
10. Benjamin R, Parham P. Guilt by association: HLA-B27 and ankylosing spondylitis. *Immunol Today* 1990; 11: 137-42.
11. Tanigaki N, Fruci D, Vigneti E, Starace G, Rovero P, Londei M, Butler RH, Tosi R. The peptide binding specificity of HLA-B27 subtypes. *Immunogenetics* 1994; 40: 192-8.
12. Cavalli-Sforza LL, Menozzi P, Piazza A. The history and geography of human genes. Princenton: Princenton University Press, 1994.

HLA-B27 in the Lebanese population: subtypes analysis and association with ankylosing spondylitis (AS)

R. Tamouza [1], H. Awada [2], F. Marzais [1], A. Toubert [1], C. Raffoux [1], D. Charron [1]

1 Laboratoire d'Imunologie et d'Histocompatibilité, Hôpital Saint-Louis, 1, avenue Claude Vellefaux, 75010 Paris, France and INSERM U396, Paris, France
2 Service de Rhumatologie, Hôtel Dieu, Beirut, Lebanon

Association between ankylosing spondylitis (AS), spondylarthropathies (SP), and HLA B27 was first described in 1973 and is extremely well documented [1]. This association which mecanism is not fully understood, is one of the few HLA-disease associations that is close to 100%. Evidence of HLA B27 subtypes has, however, raised the possibility of a more refined linkage analysis, especially because, up to now, the role of HLA B27 in disease has primarily been considered in the context of peptide presentation to cytolytic T lymphocytes. The B27 specificity represents at a molecular level, a group of nine presently known alleles (B*2701-09). The distribution of these alleles, has been studied in several populations [2]. B*2705, the most common allele, was found in all ethnic groups and seems to be the progenitor of other subtypes. B*2701 and 02 have been described in Caucasians, while B*2704, 06, and 07 have only been reported in Orientals. B*2703 is over-represented in West African populations. B*2708 and 2709 have been described recently in Caucasians. The linkage data between SA and the HLA B27 subtypes, has shown that the alleles B*2701, 02, 04, 05 and 07 are represented in patients who have a different percentage level of association among the studied populations.
In Lebanon, the prevalence of HLA B27 is low in the general population, varying between 1 to 2% [3], yet the prevalence of AS seems to be the same as in Europe [3-5]. Considering that a definitive conclusion of the B27 subtypes associated to AS would require specific typing of a large number of AS patients from different ethnic groups, the aim of this study was to assess the frequency of HLA B27 and the distribution of its alleles in the SP patients in Lebanon. The subtype distribution and the linkage with SP, have not been studied yet in any Arabic population of the Middle East.

Material and methods

Subjects

Three groups of subjects are studied in this work. A total of 69 SP patients (19 AS and 50 others Sp) have been defined according to the European Spondylarthropathy Study Group criteria (ESSG). The control group population included 139 subjects having non-inflammatory rheumatic diseases.
In addition, 16 B27 positive healthy blood donors were studied to ascertain the distribution of HLA B27 in the Lebanese population.

HLA typing

Serological typing of HLA A and B was performed by microlymphocytotoxicity using sera provided by the French National Reference Laboratory.

B27 subtyping

The B27 subtyping was carried out by PCR-SSOP, and was performed under the same conditions as described previously by Lopez-Larrea *et al.* [6].

Results and discussion

In the 69 SP patients, the prevalence of HLA B27 is 27.5%. Among these B27 positive patients, AS represents 37% of the total cases. This percentage is much lower than that observed in other populations studied.
The prevalence of HLA B27 in 1.4% of our control

population is comparable to that of 1 to 2%, previously reported in the general Lebanese population. Although this prevalence is low, the SP appears to be as frequent as in Europe. In other populations where the frequency of B27 is low, such as in Japan (1%) and in countries of the Middle East (3% in Israel and Irak), the prevalence of B27 remains high in AS (80% in Japan and 60% in Israel) [2,4].

On the other hand, in the 69 SP patients, no other HLA A or B is significantly associated with SP, including those previously described, to be additional susceptibility alleles [7,8].

HLA class II typing is in progress to better characterise our population.

In the 69 SP patients, the major disease associated subtype is B*2702 (52.5%), with a frequency more than double of the one found in the healthy control group (25%). B*2705, the most common Caucasian subtype, is much less represented in comparison with the healthy B27 positive group (15.8% *versus* 43.7%). B*2707, which is known to be rare, is as frequent as B*2705 (21.1% *versus* 15.8%).

One additional interesting point, is the presence of the B*2703 subtype among the SP patients even in one case.

The observed weak association between B27 and SP in the Lebanese anthropologically diverse heterogenous population, could suggest involvement of other linked or unlinked genes. In fact, the presentation of antigenic peptide by HLA class I molecules is a complex mechanism. It is dependent upon the function of other genes in the MHC region, such as LMP and TAP genes, encoding proteins needed respectively for the cleavage and the subsequent transport of antigenic peptides. Therefore, B27 alleles could be associated with particular TAP or LMP alleles which would selectively prevent delivery of the antigenic peptides to the HLA molecules in the endoplasmic reticulum. The study of TAP polymorphism will be achieved in this peculiar population to test this hypothesis.

The distribution of B27 alleles in the SP patients, might argue that other subtypes including B*2703 could be permissive to the developement of the disease.

Furthermore, we cannot exclude environmental factors which influence may be greater in Lebanon than in Nordic European populations.

Studies of other population groups in this region, as well as other potential candidates susceptibility loci will be of a particular interest.

References

1. Schlosstein L, Terasaki PJ, Bluestone R, Pearson CM. High association of HLA antigen W27 with ankylosing spondylitis. *N Engl J Med* 1973; 288: 704.
2. Khan MA. HLA-B27 and its subtypes in world population. *Curr Op Rheumatol* 1995; 7: 263-9.
3. Serre JL, Lefranc G, Loiselet J, Jacquard A. HLA markers in six Lebanese religious subpopulations. *Tissue Antigens* 1979; 14: 251-5.
4. Khan MA, Van Der Linden S. Ankylosing spondylitis and other spondylarthropathies. *Rheum Dis Clin North Am* 1990; 16: 551-79.
5. Mendelek V. La spondylarthrite ankylosante au Liban. *Rev Rhum* 1969; 36: 87-90.
6. Lopez-Larrea C, Sujirachato K, Mehra NK, Chiewslip P, Isarangkura D, Kanga U, Dominguez O, Coto E, Pena M, Setien F, Gonzalez-Roces S. HLA-B27 subtypes in Asian patients with ankylosing spondylitis. Evidence for new associations. *Tissue Antigens* 1995; 45: 169-76.
7. Robinson WP, Van Der Linden SM, Khan MA. HLA Bw60 increases susceptibility to ankylosing spondylitis in HLA-B27+ patients. *Arthritis Rheum* 1989; 32: 1135-41.
8. Yamaguchi A, Tsuchiya N, Mitsui H, Shiota M, Ogawa A, Tokunaga K, Yoshiniya S, Juji T, Ito K. Association of HLA-B39 with HLA-B27-negative ankylosing spondylitis and pauciarticular juvenile rheumatoid arthritis in japanese patients. *Arthritis Rheum* 1995; 38: 1672-7.

HLA-B27 subtypes in patients with rheumatic disease: molecular typing by PCR and subtyping by SSO

H. Kellner[1], B. Frankenberger[2], M. Ulbrecht[2], E. Albert[3], S. Scholz[3], E. Keller[3], M. Schattenkirchner[1], E.H. Weiss[2]

1 Medizinische Poliklinik, Klinikum Innenstadt, München, Germany
2 Institut für Anthropologie und Humangenetik, Richard Wagner strasse 101, 8033 München, Germany
3 Labor für Immungenetik, Ludwig-Maximilians-Universität, München, Germany

The striking association of HLA-B27 and seronegative spondyloarthropathies has been known for more than 20 years but the mechanism by which HLA-B27 determines susceptibility to rheumatic disease remains obscure. Over the past years, nine different HLA-B27 subtypes have been described and at least five of them, HLA-B*2701, 02, 04, 05, and 07 have been reported to be disease associated [1]. Several hypotheses have been proposed to explain this association but final clinical and scientific proof is still lacking [2]. New insights into the pathogenetic role of HLA-B27 was provided by the three-dimensional structure of this T cell restriction element and sequence determination of the HLA-B27 peptide ligands. Thus, it is very likely that the unique make-up of the HLA-B27 molecule determines its pathogenic role. The five disease-associated HLA-B27 subtypes differ by one to five amino acid substitutions. These substitutions are clustered mainly in the $\alpha 1$ (encoded by exon 2) and $\alpha 2$ (exon 3) domains which constitute the peptide binding groove, and thus influence the repertoire of the bound peptides. Consequently, not only HLA-B27 typing but additional HLA-B27 subtyping may be of diagnostic relevance. DNA typing techniques based on PCR have become available for class I and in particular HLA-B27 determination [3, 4] and amplification of an HLA-B27-specific motif in exon 2 allows group-specific DNA-typing of HLA-B27 [5]. We analysed a large panel of patients in order to compare HLA-B27 typing by MLCT detecting the HLA-B27 cell surface protein on lymphocytes, with gene typing on whole blood DNA. Subtyping was performed by hybridization of the exon 2 and exon 3 amplificates with sequence-specific oligonucleotide (SSO) probes. Additional 64 HLA-B27 positive patients were subtyped to search for a possible association between HLA-B27 variants and a certain type of HLA-B27 associated disease.

Patients

398 consecutive patients from the Rheumatology outpatient department were typed for HLA-B27 by the standard NIH microlymphocytotoxicity test (MLCT) and by PCR. Subtyping was performed in 142 HLA-B27 positive patients with seronegative spondyloarthropathies: 38 patients with ankylosing spondylitis (AS), 44 patients with reactive arthritis or Reiter´s syndrome, 45 patients with undifferentiated forms of spondyloarthropathies (uSpA), and in 15 patients with psoriatic spondylitis PsA). 125 HLA-B27 positive controls were obtained from a HLA-typing laboratory and consisted of healthy bone marrow donors.

Methods

Serological typing was performed using a standard two-stage MLCT with monoclonal antibodies on peripheral blood lymphocytes. PCR typing and subtyping was carried out as reported earlier [3].

Results

The serological and PCR typing results did not match in 17 patients. The MLCT result was equivocal in three patients and a possible cross-reaction due to HLA-B7 was possible in another 15 patients. DNA typing was positive in 2/3 equivocal cases and in 9/15 with possible cross-reactivity. Six patients in this cohort were negative by serology but tested positive by PCR, and the gene typing result was confirmed by direct sequencing of the amplificate. The calculated rate of false negative typing results in MLCT compared to the PCR was 2%, the false positive rate slightly lower (1.8%).
As expected, HLA-B*2705 was the most frequent subtype in the patient (85.9%) as well as in the control

group (90.4%). HLA-B*2702 was the only other subtype found in the studied population of southern Germany. Analysing the subtype frequencies with regard to the clinical diagnosis, the B*2702 subtype frequency in AS patients (23.7%) was significantly higher than in controls (9.6%). On the contrary, in uSpA patients the B*2702 frequency was reduced (6.7%), but the difference to the control group was not significant (chi-square method $p<0.04$)).

Discussion

HLA-B27 typing at the DNA level by PCR proved to be a reliable diagnostic tool in rheumatic disease. Compared to serological testing, false positive or negative typing due to ambiguous results or cross-reactivity with other HLA-B alleles can be avoided. In the patients of this study we did not find any individual with AS who is HLA-B27 negative. Moreover, we reanalysed, when available, all AS patients previously typed negative for HLA-B27, and they were positive by DNA typing. Thus, the association of HLA-B27 with AS could reach 100%.

The subtyping results confirmed the predominance of HLA-B*2705 in the German population. Interestingly, an increased frequency of subtype B*2702 was found in AS patients, whereas this allele seems to be underrepresented in uSpA. A similar study in an Asian population was published recently, in which an increased frequency of HLAB*2704 was found in AS patients and an increased B*2705 frequency in uSpA. Thus, a decrease of the common HLA-B27 subtype *2705 in AS patients and an increase of the other most frequent variant has been found in two populations. It is possible that the different HLA-B27 alleles may have an influence on the clinical course and probable outcome of the disease [6]. A reasonable explanation for the differences in disease development and phenotypical expression goes back to the diverse peptide repertoire of HLA-class I molecules. HLA-B*2702 and *2704 differ both from the *2705 subtype in amino acid position 77 [7]. The acidic aspartic acid (B*2705) is replaced by asparagine in B*2702 and by serine in B*2704. Amino acid 77 is part of the F pocket which buries the carboxy terminus of the bound peptide. Differences in this amino acid might influence the charge and configuration of the pocket and affect the peptide binding specificity or affinity. Differences in the C-terminal anchor of HLA-B*2705 and *2702 ligands have been observed [8]. It is not resolved whether this distinction is due to amino acid 77 since the two subtypes also differ in residues at positions 80 and 81.

Conclusion

Our results are in agreement with the arthritogenic-peptide hypothesis. For reactive arthritis HLA-B27 has been postulated to present a marker for disease severity rather than susceptibility [9]. Thus, it is conceivable that also individual HLA-B27 subtypes vary in the association with regard to disease severity.

References

1. Maclean IL, Iqball S, Woot P, Keat ACS, Hughes RA, Kingsley GH, Knight SC. HLA-B27 subtypes in the spondyloarthropathies. *Clin Exp Immunol* 1993; 91: 214-9.
2. Maclean IL. HLA-B27 subtypes: Implications for the spondyloarthropathies. *Ann Rheum Dis* 1992; 51: 929-31.
3. Dominguez O, Colo E, Martinez-Navez E, Choo S, Lopez-Larrea C. Molecular typing of HLA-B27 alleles. *Immunogenetics* 1992; 36: 277-82.
4. Steffens-Nakken HM, Zwart G, van den Bergh FA. Validation of allele-specific polymerase chain reaction for DNA typing of HLA-B27. *Clin Chem* 1995; 41: 687-92.
5. Olerup O. HLA-B27 typing by a group-specific PCR amplification. *Tissue Antigens* 1994; 43: 253-6.
6. Kanga U, Mehra NK, Larrea CL, Lardy NM, Kumar A, Feltkamp TEW. Seronegative spondyloarthropathies and HLA-B27 subtypes: a study in Asian Indians. *Clin Rheumatol* 1996; 15 (suppl 1): 13-8.
7. de Castro LJA. Structural polymorphism and function of HLA-B27. *Curr Op Rheumatol* 1995; 7: 270-8.
8. Rötzschke O, Falk K, Stephanovic S, Gnau V, Jung G, Rammensee HG. Dominant aromatic/aliphatic C-terminal anchor in HLA-B*2702 and B*2705 peptide motifs. *Immunogenetics* 1994; 39: 74-7.
9. Sieper J, Kingsley G. Recent advances in the pathogenesis of reactive arthritis. *Immunol Today* 1996; 17: 160-3.

Cytokine profiles and site-directed B27 mutation in the HLA-B27 transgenic rat

L. McLean[1], R.E. Hammer, J.D. Taurog

HC Simmons Arthritis Research Center, University of Texas Southwestern Medical Center, Dallas, Texas 75235-8884, USA
1 Present address: Department of Molecular Medicine, University of Auckland, Private Bag 92019, Auckland, New Zealand

Inbred rats transgenic (Tg) for HLA-B27 and human beta 2 microglobulin develop spontaneous multisystem inflammatory disease [1,2]. The spectrum is similar to the human spondarthropathies (SpA): arthritis, inflammatory bowel disease (IBD), and psoriaform skin lesions. Cell transfer experiments have shown that the disease needs T lymphocytes and a bone-marrow derived cell [3,4]. Development of IBD and arthritis require the presence of microorganisms [5].

HLA-B27 has an unusual unpaired cysteine at amino position 67 (Cys67). The B-pocket microenvironment is unique among the class I HLA alleles, and the sulphydryl (-SH) side chain may be chemically reactive on a proportion of B27 molecules [6,7].

To further explore the immunological basis of this model, we examined the cytokines produced within the inflammatory joint and gut lesions. The importance of Cys67 was investigated by producing rats Tg for HLA-B27 with the codon for Cys67 changed to that for serine (67CS mutation).

Methods

Cytokine production was assessed using semi-quantitative reverse transcriptase polymerase chain reaction (RT-PCR). Distal colon (DC) and synovium were harvested from the disease-prone 33-3 and 21-4H rat lines, and from 67CS mutant and control rats as below. Non-Tg littermates served as controls. RNA was obtained by acid phenol-chloroform extraction. Oligo-dT primed cDNA was amplified by PCR. Primers matched published cDNA or extronic DNA sequences for rat IL-1α, IL-2, IL-4, IL-6, IL-10, IFNγ, TNFα, TGFβ, MIP-2, and β-actin. IL-12 p40 primers were based on the murine sequence, and IL-8 on a combination of the human 5' and guinea pig 3' sequences. PCR products were vacuum dot-blotted to nylon membrane, probed, quantitated with an AMBIS system, and normalised against β-actin.

The codon for Cys67 on HLA-B27 was altered to that for serine [8]. A Tg rat line bearing the 67CS mutation was produced on a Lewis (Lew) strain background by the methods described previously [1], and was designated C133-1. Transgene content was established by quantitative dot-blot. Animals bearing the 67CS mutant transgene were examined clinically and histologically until over 40 weeks of age.

Cytokines were examined in DC of two 37 week-old homozygous C133-1 rats with established IBD. Controls comprised (1) two hemizygous C133-1 littermates; and age- and sex-matched rats with (2) a low copy number of the wild-type B27 transgene (21-3 line, 20 copies); (3) homozygous for the HLA-B7 gene (line 120-4, approx 46 copies); (4) a sick 21-4H rat; and (5) a non-Tg Lew rat. Cell surface expression of HLA transgenes on splenic lymphocytes was examined by flow cytometry. The systemic acute phase response was examined by Northern blot of hepatic mRNA with a probe for α1-acid glycoprotein (AGP), normalised against 18S ribosomal RNA.

Results

PCR products of appropriate length were obtained from lesional DC for all cytokines assayed. Consistent amplification of IL-4, IL-8, IL-12 and TNFα required high numbers of PCR cycles resulting in high backgrounds, poor triplicate replicates, and unreliable amplification linearity. These were not investigated further.

In lesional DC there were significant elevations of mRNA for IFNγ, IL-1α, IL-2 and the chemokine MIP-2 in comparison to littermate non-Tg DC. IL-6 was mildly elevated, whereas IL-10 and TGFβ1 were comparable to healthy non-Tg DC. In synovium from acutely arthritic joints, IL-6 levels were markedly higher those of either healthy or inflamed DC, whereas IL-1α, IL-2 and IFNγ were comparable to or lower than healthy, non-Tg DC. Synovial TGFβ1 was higher than healthy DC. Synovium obtained 2

weeks after the onset of arthritis showed the same profile (high IL-6, low IFNγ) as that obtained within 24 hours.
C133-1 rats hemizygous for B27 with the 67CS mutation carried an estimated 12 transgene copies, and remained healthy. Homozygotes developed typical IBD. The clinical and histological severity was comparable to the wild type B27 Tg lines (21-4H and 33-3, respectively 150 and 55 copies). Peripheral joint synovitis was observed in a low percentage of C133-1 animals.
Splenic lymphocyte surface expression of the 67CS mutant HLA-B27 molecule in C133-1 homozygotes was similar to that of wild type B27 on 21-4H lymphocytes and of B7 on homozygous 120-4 lymphocytes. Hepatic AGP mRNA levels in the homozygous C133-1 rats were similar to 21-4H. Distal colon IFNγ levels correlated with disease status.

Discussion

Interferon-γ, IL-1α, IL-2 and MIP-2 were elevated in the inflamed DC of HLA-B27 rats. IFNγ and IL-2 production is consistent with the involvement of lymphocytes of the T-helper 1 (Th1) type, whereas IL-1α and MIP-2 suggest activated macrophages. This is consistent with the mononuclear infiltrate seen histologically, and is similar to that in human IBD and in other animal models [9].
High interleukin-6 levels were found in inflamed synovium. Given the lack of IL-1α, synovial IL-6 may be produced by cells other than macrophages. The fibroblast-like synovial cell is a prominent candidate. The reciprocal cytokine patterns noted in the inflamed DC (IL-1α, IL-2, and IFNγ) and synovium (IL-6) suggest that different mechanisms act at the two sites of inflammation.
IBD of comparable severity developed in the wild-type HLA-B27 Tg and the homozygous C133-1 67CS mutant Tg rats. The latter also had a very low incidence of joint disease. These results suggest that Cys67 is not a critical residue for all aspects of the spondarthropathy of B27 rats.
Inflammatory bowel disease has also been produced in mice by targeted disruption of genes for IL-2, IL-10, T cell receptor, or MHC class II. IBD may be a "common pathway" outcome of immune dysregulation in a tissue undergoing constant exposure to a heavy microbial load, and in this model may represent a less specific effect of transgene expression. IBD seems necessary, but not sufficient, for the development of arthritis.
Fragments of bacteria have been identified within the joints of patients with reactive arthritis (ReA) triggered by mucosal infection. One model for human ReA invokes seeding of bacterial components to the synovium from mucosal breaches due to low grade chronic infection. HLA-B27 then has its main action in exacerbating inflammation within the joint. These results are consistent with this model.

References

1. Hammer RE, Maika SD, Richardson JA, Tang JP, Taurog JD. Spontaneous inflammatory disease in transgenic rats expressing HLA-B27 and human β2-m: an animal model of HLA-B27-associated human disorders. *Cell* 1990; 63: 1099-112.
2. Taurog JD, Maika SD, Simmons WA, Breban M, Hammer RE. Susceptibility to inflammatory disease in transgenic rat lines correlates with the level of B27 expression. *J Immunol* 1993; 150: 4168- 78.
3. Breban M, Hammer RE, Richardson JA, Taurog JD. Transfer of the inflammatory disease of HLA-B27 transgenic rats by bone marrow engraftment. *J Exp Med* 1993; 178: 1607-16.
4. Breban M, Fernandez-Sueiro JL, Richardson JA, Hadavand RR, Maika SD, Hammer RE, Taurog JD. T cells, but not thymic exposure to HLA-B27, are required for the inflammatory disease of HLA-B27 transgenic rats. *J Immunol* 1996; 156: 794- 803.
5. Taurog JD, Richardson JA, Croft JT, Simmons WA, Zhou M, Fernandez-Sueiro JL, Balish E, Hammer RE. The germfree state prevents development of gut and joint inflammatory disease in HLA-B27 transgenic rats. *J Exp Med* 1994; 180: 2359-64.
6. McLean L, Macey M, Lowdell M, Badakere S, Whelan M, Perrett D, Archer J. Sulphydryl reactivity of the HLA-B27 epitope: accessibility of the free cysteine studied by flow cytometry. *Ann Rheum Dis* 1992; 51: 456-60.
7. Whelan MA, Archer JR. Chemical reactivity of an HLA-B27 thiol group. *Eur J Immunol* 1993; 23: 3278-85.
8. El Zaatari, FA, Taurog JD. *In vitro* mutagenesis of HLA-B27: single and multiple amino acid substitutions at consensus B27 sites identify distinct monoclonal antibody-defined epitopes. *Hum Immunol* 1992; 33: 243-8.
9. Sartor, RB. Cytokines in intestinal inflammation: pathophysiological and clinical considerations. *Gastroenterology* 1994; 106: 533-9.

The human constitutive 73 kDa heat shock protein directly targets rheumatoid arthritis associated alleles HLA-DRB1*0401 and HLA-DRB1*1001 from endoplasmic reticulum to lysosomes

I. Auger[1], *J.M. Escola*[2], *J.P. Gorvel*[2], *J. Roudier*[1]

1 Laboratoire d'Immuno-Rhumatologie, Faculté de Médecine, 27, boulevard Jean Moulin, 13005 Marseille, France
2 CIML, Marseille, France

The QKRAA, QRRAA and RRRAA amino acid sequences in the third hypervariable region of HLA-DRB1*0401 and HLA-DRB1*1001 help the development of rheumatoid arthritis (RA) by an unknown mechanism. This mechanism may involve interaction of these sequences with a yet unidentified ligand. To identify such a ligand, we first screened bacterial proteins and we found that the QKRAA and RRRAA sequences specifically bind the bacterial 70 kDa heat shock protein, dnaK. We then observed that the human constitutive 73 kDa heat shock protein (hsp73) associates with HLA-DRB1*0401 and targets it from endoplasmic reticulum to lysosomes.
This suggests:
1. that HLA-DRB1*0401 and HLA-DRB1*1001 may have a particular intracellular route;
2. that HLA-DRB1*0401 and HLA-DRB1*1001 may present 70kDa HSPs (or fragments) to the immune system, possibly leading to anti HSP70 autoimmunization.

Shared HLA-DRB1 motif confers RA susceptibility

Rheumatoid arthritis (RA) is a chronic inflammatory disease of unknown etiology. RA was originally associated with HLA-DR4 [1]. However, susceptibility to RA is not carried by a single HLA-DR gene but by residues 70-74 of the third hypervariable region of different HLA-DRB1 chains [2]. Indeed, RA associated HLA-DRB1 alleles share a highly conserved motif in their third hypervariable region. This motif termed "shared epitope" is (according to the one letter code) QKRAA in HLA-DRB1*0401, QRRAA in HLA-DRB1*0404, 0405, 0408, 0101, 0102, 1402, and RRRAA in HLA-DRB1*1001. The QKRAA/ QRRAA/ RRRAA sequences are not associated equally with RA. The QKRAA sequence predisposes to a more severe disease than the QRRAA/ RRRAA sequences [3].
The mechanism by which the QKRAA sequence contributes to disease susceptibility and severity is not clear. It was proposed that the QKRAA sequence may be the site of a critical interaction with "arthritogen" antigens, T cell receptors or unknown ligands [4, 5].

The QKRAA sequence is a binding motif for dnaK, the bacterial 70 kDa heat shock protein

To identify a specific ligand of the QKRAA motif, we used total protein extracts from *Escherichia coli* and *Salmonella dublin.* These extracts were loaded on sepharose columns coated with peptides representing the third hypervariable region of various HLA-DRB1 alleles from residue 65 to residue 79. The bound ligands were eluted and analysed on SDS PAGE. We found that the DRB1*0401 peptide (but not DRB1*0402, 0403, 0404) bound a 70kDa protein from *Escherichia coli* and *Salmonella dublin* [6]. This protein was identified as dnaK, the bacterial 70 kDa heat shock protein, by amino acid sequencing and Western blotting.
Using synthetic peptides, we observed that the QKRAA motif was sufficient to interact with dnaK. The RRRAA sequence on HLA-DRB1*1001 shared similar properties.

Hsp73 coimmunoprecipitates with HLA-DRB1*0401 and HLA-DRB1*1001

We then investigated if HLA-DRB1*0401 and HLA-DRB1*1001 could bind human 70kDa heat shock proteins. HLA-DRB1 molecules from different HLA-DRB1 alleles were immunoprecipitated and analysed by Western blotting with monoclonal antibodies specific for the 70kDa heat shock proteins (including the constitutively expressed 73kDa heat shock protein, the inducible 72kDa heat shock protein, the ER-located chaperone, Bip). We observed that the constitutive 73kDa heat shock protein coimmunoprecipitated with HLA-DRB1*0401 and HLA-DRB1*1001 but not with 10 other HLA-DRB1 alleles.

Hsp73 targets HLA-DRB1*0401 from ER to lysosomes

To study the kinetic of the hsp73 association with HLA-DRB1*0401, we performed pulse chase experiments. We observed that Hsp73 associates early with AB Ii complexes. Hsp73 is known to be involved in the lysosomal transport and degradation of polypeptides that carry a KFERQ amino acid motif [7]. Our data suggested that the QKRAA motif acts in a similar manner in helping the transfer of polypeptides to lysosomes. To test this hypothesis, we performed the same experiments on lysosomal fractions. We detected hsp73 and HLA-DRB1*0401 in lysosomes after 5 minutes synthesis. This suggests that the interaction between Hsp73 and QKRAA on HLA-DRB1*0401 allows HLA-DRB1*0401 to reach the lysosomes immediatly after synthesis, bypassing the normal route through Golgi apparatus and endosomal compartments.

Potential role of hsp70s in RA

The binding of hsp73 to HLA-DRB1*0401 may have many consequences: for example it may cause degradation of HLA-DRB1*0401 into peptides, presentation of these peptides to the immune system and influence on the T cell repertoire [8].

Members of hsp70 family are important targets for the immune system. They may be cross reactive with type II collagen. It will be critical to determine whether T cell recognition of bacterial or human HSP70s is exaggerated in subjects who express HLA-DRB1*0401.

Acknowledgements

This work was supported by: Association pour la Recherche contre la Polyarthrite, Société Française de Rhumatologie, PHRC 1994, INSERM, CNRS.

References

1. Stasny P. Association of the B cell alloantigen DRw4 with Rheumatoid Arthritis. *N Engl J Med* 1978; 298: 869-71.
2. Gregersen PK, Silver J, Winchester RJ. The shared epitope hypothesis: an approach to understanding the molecular genetics of susceptibility to rheumatoid arthritis *Arthritis Rheum* 1987; 30: 1205-13.
3. Weyand CM, Mc Carthy TG, Goronzy J. Correlation between disease phenotype and genetic heterogeneity in rheumatoid arthritis. *J Clin Invest* 1995; 95: 2120-6.
4. Ollier W, Thomson W. Population genetics of rheumatoid arthritis. *Rheum Dis Clin North Am* 1992; 18: 741-59.
5. Roudier J, Rhodes G, Petersen J, Vaughan J, Carson DA. The Epstein barr virus glycoprotein gp110, a molecular link between HLA-DR4, HLA-DR1 and rheumatoid arthritis. *Scand J immunol* 1988; 27: 367-71.
6. Auger I, Escola JM, Gorvel JP, Roudier J. HLA-DR4 and HLA-DR10 motifs that carry susceptibility to rheumatoid arthritis bind 70-kDa heat shock proteins. *Nature Med* 1996; 3: 306-10.
7. Terlecky SR. Hsp70 and lysosomal transport. *Experientia* 1994; 50: 1021-5.
8. Salvat S, Auger I, Rochelle L, Begovich A, Geburher L, Sette A, Roudier J. Tolerance to a self-peptide from the third hypervariable region of HLA-DRB1*0401 in rheumatoid patients and normal subjects. *J Immunol* 1994; 153: 5321-9.

Association of HLA-DRB1 epitopes and alleles with rheumatoid arthritis in Koreans

M.H. Park[1], G.H. Hong[2], Y.W. Song[3], F. Takeuchi[4]

1 Department of Clinical Pathology, Seoul National University College of Medicine, 110744 Seoul, Korea
2 Department of Medicine and Physical Therapy, Faculty of Medicine, University of Tokyo, Tokyo, Japan
3 Department of Internal Medicine, Seoul National University College of Medicine, Seoul, Korea
4 Department of Medicine and Physical Therapy, Faculty of Medicine, University of Tokyo, Tokyo, Japan

Rheumatoid arthritis (RA) is a common autoimmune disease with unknown etiology. Both genetic and environmental factors are assumed to participate in its immune pathogenesis. Recently, several studies have shown that a conserved epitope in the third hypervariable region of the first domain of DRB1 may form the molecular basis of susceptibility to RA [1-4]. The sequences over this third allelic hypervariable region, which spans amino acid residues 70-74, have been shown to be QRRAA and QKRAA. These sequences in relation with RA have been found in susceptible DR4 subtypes (DRB1*0401, *0404 and *0405) as well as in other non-DR4 susceptibility alleles, such as DRB1*0101 and DRB1*1402 [1-10]. The association of HLA class II genes and RA has not been well studied in Koreans. In this report, we studied the association of HLA-DRB1 epitopes and alleles with RA in Koreans.

Materials and methods

Sixty-one adult Korean patients with RA (1987 revised criteria of the American Rheumatism Association) who attended the rheumatology clinic at the Seoul National University Hospital were studied. Eighty-two adult Korean healthy subjects served as controls.

HLA-DR serologic specificities (DR1-DR14) were identified using the microlymphocytotoxicity assay. For HLA-DRB1 epitope analysis, genomic DNA was amplified using primers for DRB generic amplification, and allelic sequences of amplified DNA were detected by oligonucleotide hybridization, using 6 digoxigenin-labeled sequence-specific probes (*Table I*) to the third hypervariable region of the DRB1 gene. Genotyping of HLA-DRB1 alleles (DR1, DR4 and DR8) was performed using the polymerase chain reaction-sequence specific conformational polymorphism (PCR-SSCP) method.

Results and discussion

PCR-amplified DNA segments from 61 patients and 82 controls were hybridized with 6 oligonucleotide probes to examine the association of certain polymorphic sequences with RA (*Table I*). The frequency of HLA-DR4 defined by probe 1 showed a significant increase in RA patients compared with controls (61% vs 29%, RR=3.7, p<0.0001). The relative risk obtained in this analysis is similar to those which have been reported for DR4 and RA in many other populations. Among the sequences encompassing the amino acid 70-74 of the DRβ1 chain, the frequency of QRRAA sequence defined by probe 2 was significantly increased in RA patients compared with controls (52% vs 21%, RR=4.2, p<0.0001), as well as that of QKRAA sequence defined by probe 5 (10% vs 1%, RR=8.8, p<0.05). These observations suggest that QRRAA was the major susceptible epitope and QKRAA also played a role in the pathogenesis of RA in Koreans. The frequency of the sequence defined by probe 3 (expressed by DRB1*0405 and DR8) was also increased in RA patients (54%) compared with the control subjects (30%), and this increase was mostly due to DRB1*0405 after genotyping of DR4 alleles. HLA-DR8 were mostly typed to DRB1*0803 in RA patients, and its frequency was decreased compared with controls (11% vs 22%), but it was not significant. DRB1*0802 was rare in both RA patients and controls. HLA-DR4 allele typing was done by the PCR-SSCP method and the results are shown in *Table II*.

Table I. Epitope analysis in patients with RA and controls in Koreans

Probe*	Corresponding aa[t] sequence of probe	RA (%) (n=61)	Control (%) (n=82)	Relative risk	p value
1	YFYHQEE(30-36)	37 (61)	24 (29)	3.7	<0.0001
2	QRRAAV(70-75)	32 (52)	17 (21)	4.2	<0.0001
3	RPSAEY(55-60)	33 (54)	25 (30)	2.7	<0.005
4	EDERAA(69-74)	4 (7)	19 (23)	0.2	<0.05
5	QKRAAV(70-75)	6 (10)	1 (1)	8.8	<0.05
6	QRRAEV(70-75)	7 (11)	14 (17)	0.6	NS

* Nucleotide sequence and DRB1* specificity:
Probe 1 (5'-TACTTCTATCACCAAGAGGA-3') for DR4;
Probe 2 (5'-GCAGAGGCGGGCCGCGGT-3') for *0101, *0404, *0405, *0408, *0410, *1402, *1406;
Probe 3 (5'-CGGCCTAGCGCCGAGTAC-3') for *0405, *0409, *0410, *0411, DR8;
Probe 4 (5'-GAAGACGAGCGGGCCGCG-3') for *0402, DR13;
Probe 5 (5'-CAGAAGCGGGCCGCGGTG-3') for *0401;
Probe 6 (5'-CAGAGGCGGGCCGAGGTG-3') for *0403, *0406, *0407.

[t] amino acid.
NS, not significant.

Table II. Association of DR4 alleles with RA in Koreans

DR4 alleles	RA[t] (%) (n=61)	Control (%) (n=82)	Relative risk	p value
DRB1*0401	6 (10)	1 (1)	8.8	< 0.05
*0402	0 (0)	0 (0)	0.0	NS
*0403	5 (8)	6 (7)	1.1	NS
*0404	1 (2)	2 (2)	0.7	NS
*0405	26 (43)	6 (7)	9.4	< 0.00005
*0406	2 (3)	8 (10)	0.3	< 0.05
*0410	1 (2)	1 (1)	1.4	NS

[t] Among RA patients, 4 were DR4 homozygote: 1 patient, DRB1*0404, *0405; 3 patients, DRB1*0401, *0405.
NS, not significant.

Significantly increased frequencies of the DRB1*0405 and *0401 alleles, which have the amino acid sequences QRRAA and QKRAA, respectively, at positions 70-74 of the DRβ1 chain were observed (43% vs 7%, $p<0.00005$; 10% vs 1%, $p<0.05$, respectively). Most of the QRRAA sequences in RA patients were defined as DRB1*0405, and DRB1*0404 and *0410 were very rare alleles in both patients and controls in Koreans. Genotyping analysis showed that all DR1 in RA patients was DRB1*0101 but its frequency was not significantly different from that of controls. The QKRAA sequence was exclusively defined as DRB1*0401. Among DR4+ control subjects, DRB1*0406 was the most common allele and its frequency was decreased in RA patients ($p<0.05$).

DRB1*0405 was shown to be a common type associated with RA in east Asian ethnic groups including the Japanese [3] and the Chinese [7], but was not a main type in Caucasians. In the present study, DRB1*0405 has been shown to be strongly associated with RA in

Koreans. DRB1*0404 was increased among Southern Chinese [7] RA patients, but not in Koreans and the Japanese. It is of interest that in the present study, DRB1*0401 which has been shown to be associated with RA mainly in Caucasians [5,6], is another allele denoting susceptibility to RA in Koreans.

Conclusion

Our results showed that HLA-DR4, especially DRB1*0405 and *0401 alleles, were associated with RA in Koreans. The QRRAA susceptibility epitope, which was mostly found in *0405, showed a significant increase in RA patients, together with an increase of QKRAA by *0401. Our observation confirmed the predominant importance of DRB1*0405 for the disease in east Asian ethnic groups. The findings in Koreans described here add further evidence to the "shared epitope hypothesis" for RA susceptibility.

References

1. Gregersen PK, Silver J, Winchester RJ. The shared epitope hypothesis: An approach to understanding the molecular genetics of susceptibility to rheumatoid arthritis. *Arthritis Rheum* 1987; 30: 1205-13.
2. Molkentin J, Gregersen PK, Lin X, Zhu N, Wang Y, Wang Y, Chen S, Chen S, Baxter-Lowe LA, Silver J. Molecular analysis of HLA-DR beta and DQ beta polymorphism in Chinese with rheumatoid arthritis. *Ann Rheum Dis* 1993; 52: 610-2.
3. Watanabe Y, Tokunaga K, Matsuki K, Takeuchi F, Matsuta K, Maeda H, Omoto K, Juji T. Putative amino acid sequence of HLA-DRB chain contributing to rheumatoid arthritis susceptibility. *J Exp Med* 1989; 169: 2263-8.
4. Nepom GT, Byers P, Seyfried C, Healey LA, Wilske KR, Stage D, Nepom BS. HLA genes associated with rheumatoid arthritis: identification of susceptibility alleles using specific oligonuceotide probes. *Arthritis Rheum* 1989; 32: 15-21.
5. Nepom GT, Seyfried CE, Holbeck SL, Wilske KR, Nepom BS: Identification of HLA-Dw14 genes in DR4+ rheumatoid arthritis. *Lancet* 1986; ii: 1002-5.
6. Wordsworth BP, Lanchbury JSS, Sakkas LI, Welsh KI, Panayi GS, Bell JI. HLA-DR4 subtype frequencies in rheumatoid arthritis indicate that DRB1 is the major susceptibility locus within the HLA-class II region. *Proc Natl Acad Sci USA* 1989; 86: 10049-53.
7. Seglias J, Li EK, Cohen MG, Wong RW, Potter PK, So AK. Linkage between rheumatoid arthritis susceptibility and the presence of HLA-DR4 and DR beta allelic third hypervariable region sequences in southern Chinese persons. *Arthritis Rheum* 1992; 35: 163-7.
8. Schiff B, Mizrachi Y, Orgad S Yaron M, Gazit E. Association of HLA-Aw31 and HLA-DR1 with adult rheumatoid arthritis. *Ann Rheum Dis* 1982; 41: 403-4.
9. Christiansen FT, Kelly H, Dawkins RL. Rheumatoid arthritis. In : Albert ED, Baur MP, Mayr WR, eds. *Histocompatibility Testing*. Berlin: Springer-Verlag; 1984: 378-83.
10. Willkens RF, Nepom GT, Marks CR, Nettles JW, Nepom BS. Association of HLA-Dw16 with rheumatoid arthritis in Yakima Indians: further evidence for the "shared epitope" hypothesis. *Arthritis Rheum* 1991; 34: 43-7.

Involvement of DPB1*0201 allele in the pathogenesis of juvenile chronic arthritis (JCA)

F. Mercuriali, M. Fare, C. Cereda, W. Ferraris[1], D. Gaboardi, F. Fantini[1]

Transfusion Center
1 Chair of Reumatology of the University of Milan, Centre for Rheumatic Children,
Istituto Ortopedico Gaetano Pini, Plaza C. Ferrari 1, 20122 Milan, Italy

Juvenile chronic arthritis (JCA) can be clinically subdivided into four subgroups according to EULAR [1]. (1) Early-onset (within 6 years) pauciarticular (EOPA) the most homogeneous subgroup is characterized by asymmetric arthritis in up to five joints without ocular manifestation. (2) Same clinical and articular characteristic and frequent complication of chronic iridocyclitis (EOPA+CIC). (3) Polyarticular form (PA) without articular manifestations with involvement of more than 5 joints. (4) Systemic onset (Syst) presents systemic symptoms (fever and rash). Several studies have revealed associations between many class I and class II alleles of the major histocompatibility complex (MHC) and JCA (EOPA, EOPA+CIC, PA) [2]. DPB1*0201 allele was found to have higher frequency [3, 4] in EOPA, EOPA+CIC and PA. There is not enough significant data about the relationship between the HLA system alleles and the systemic form [5, 6].
This study was aimed to verify whether the associations reported in the literature would hold true in a group of Italian children and to investigate whether the correlation with HLA determinants are the same in the four forms. Moreover the interaction between the HLA-DP, HLA-DR and HLA-DQ has been investigated to highlight the role of the DP2 antigen in JCA.

Materials and methods

Patients and controls

121 unrelated Italian JCA children have been studied: 31 EOPA, 31 EOPA+CIC, 31 PA and 28 Syst (*Table I*). Age of onset for EOPA, EOPA+CIC before the age of 6 and the Syst and PA before 12. Statistical significance was established against an Italian control population delivered from the XI International Histocompatibility Workshop (IHWS).

Isolation of DNA and typing

Genomic DNA was extracted from peripheral blood using the salting out method. Generic amplification of polymorphic second exon of the *DRB1, DQA1, DQB1,* and *DPB1* genes was obtained by polymerase chain reaction according to the protocol of the XII IHWS. DNA typing for DRB1, DQA1, and DQB1 was obtained by nonradioactive labelled sequence specific oligonucleotides (SSO) and chemiluminescent detection system. Reverse dot blot method using 24 biotinilated probes and colorimetric detection for *DPB1* gene.

Statistical analysis

For the associations the χ^2 test, based on a 2x2 table with Yates correction for discontinuity was used. The p-value, corresponding to the χ^2, was corrected by the number of alleles tested.

Table I. Characteristics of the series

Subgroup	N° patients	M/F	Factor R+	ANA+	Age of onset(y)
EOPA+CIC	31	3/28	0	27	<6
EOPA	31	9/22	0	29	<6
P.A.	31	7/24	4	15	<12
Syst	28	14/14	0	5	<12

Results

The comparision between DRB1, DQA1, DQB1 and DPB1 allele frequencies of the four forms and controls are shown in *Tables II, III, IV*: DRB1*1104 is significantly correlated in EOPA, EOPA+CIC and PA ($p<0.01$), the DRB1*0801 in EOPA and PA ($p<0.025$) and DRB1*0803 in EOPA+CIC ($p<0.05$). The DQA1*0501 allele is found in EOPA+CIC ($p<0.025$), while in the EOPA and PA subsets a significant association could only be found with DQA1 *0401 ($p<0.01$). The DQB1*0301 allele is strongly associated with EOPA+CIC ($p<0.01$) while DQB1*0402 was weakly associated with EOPA and PA ($p<0.025$). No statistically significant association between DR and DQ alleles was demonstrated in the systemic form. Moreover the statistical analysis shows an increase of the DPB1*0201 allele in all four forms, higher in the

Table II. Significance DRB1* allelic frequence (***=p<0.01, **=p<0.025, *=p<0.05)

		EOPA+ CIC	EOPA	PA	Syst
	Alleles	χ^2	χ^2	χ^2	χ^2
DRB1	*1104	30.14***	12.27***	9.52***	ns
	*0801	ns	9.46**	9.46**	ns
	*0803	5.17*	ns	ns	ns
	*0701	6.68**	3.27	ns	ns
	*0901	19.26***	ns	ns	ns

Table III. Significance DQA1* and DBQ1* allelic frequence (***=p<0.01, **=p<0.025, *=p<0.05)

		EOPA+ CIC	EOPA	PA	Syst
DQA1	*0401	3.93*	30.58***	11.66***	ns
	*0501	9.76**	ns	ns	ns
	*0601	8.13**	ns	ns	ns
	Alleles	χ^2	χ^2	χ^2	χ^2
DQB1	*0301	16.05***	5.81**	ns	ns
	*0402	ns	9.92**	9.92**	ns

EOPA+CIC and EOPA (p<0.01) lower in PA and Syst (p<0.025 and 0.05 respectively).

In *Figure 1* the two more frequent haplotypes of the forms are represented. Due to the very close linkage disequilibrium among DRB1, DQA1 and DQB1 it is possible to calculate the haplotypes without family data. The two haplotypes closely associated with JCA are: DRB1*11-DQA1*0501-DQB1*0301 and DRB1*08-DQA1*0401-DQB1*0402. The frequency of the DR11 haplotype is 43.33% in EOPA+CIC, 40.62% in EOPA and 32.26% in PA, the DR8 haplotype 6.67% EOPA+CIC, 10.00% EOPA, 11.29% PA. In the *Figure 1,* the systemic form is not represented due to the absence of any significant association with HLA DR-DQ.

The relationship between HLA DR/DP is reported in *Table V.* The frequency of the associations DR8/DP2 or DR11/DP2 in four different combinations is represented. In particular, the two (DR-DP) alleles are present together in 51.6% of the EOPA+CIC patients, in the 48.4% of the EOPA, in the 32.3% of the PA and in the 25% of the Syst, however it is unknown if the relationship is in *cis* or in *trans*. The DRB1 and DPB1 observed frequencies were compared with the expected and reported in *Table V*.

Discussion

The correlation between the HLA antigens and JCA reported in literature has been confirmed also in the Italian children. The EOPA, the EOPA+CIC and the PA are associated with the following alleles: HLA-DRB1*1104, *08, DQA1*0401, *0501 and DQB1*0301, *0402, in particular the molecular allele DRB1*1104, DQA1*0401 and DPB1*0201 are common in all three forms suggesting that these could represent the generic markers of the disease. The DRB1*0803 and DQA1*0601 allele is only present in EOPA+CIC and the DRB1*0801 and DQA1*0402 in the other two forms suggesting that DR8 identify the evolution to PA and DR11 to EOPA with or without ocular involvement. The only association demonstrated in the systemic form is with DPB1*0201 allele and the absence of association with DR and DQ alleles is confirmed. No protective allele was detected in any of the four forms [7]. Thus it can be assumed that EOPA+CIC, EOPA and PA can be considered as different subsets of the same disease while the systemic could be a different disease.

Our data also confirm the significant presence of DQA1*0501 and *0401 alleles. This is of particular rilevance as it has been demonstrated that *DQA1* gene codifies for an aminoacidic pattern (40-Gly, 47-Cis, 50-Val, 51-Leu, 52-Arg, 53-Gln) that is specific only for the DQA1 alleles associated with the disease. The discovery of this aminoacidic pattern provoked the study of the regulation of the *DQA1* gene. Kimura *et al.* [8] demonstrated that the promoter region (from -262 to +20 of the 5' end) of the *DQA* gene presents an extensive polymorphism that could, at times, cause a reduced expression of the α chain of the DQA molecules. Due to a strong linkage disequilibrium between the promoter alleles and the alleles of the gene codifing the α chain it is possible to correlate each DQA1 allele to its own promoter. P. Haas [9] showed that the DQA alleles significantly associated with JCA are those which carry a mutation in the Y-box

Table IV. Significance DPB1* allelic frequences (***=p<0.001, **=p<0.025, *=p<0.05)

		EOPA+ CIC	EOPA	PA	Syst
DPB1	**Alleles**	χ^2	χ^2	χ^2	χ^2
	*0201	24.41***	38.23***	5.48**	4.18*

Table V. Statistical significance of association DR8-DP2 and DR11-DP2

Disease form	DR11-DP2		DR8-DP2	
	χ^2	p<	χ^2	p<
EOPA+CIC	26.40	10^{-4}	NS	NS
EOPA	16.69	10^{-4}	4.02	0.05
PA	23.77	10^{-4}	5.59	0.025
Syst	18.96	10^{-4}	NS	NS

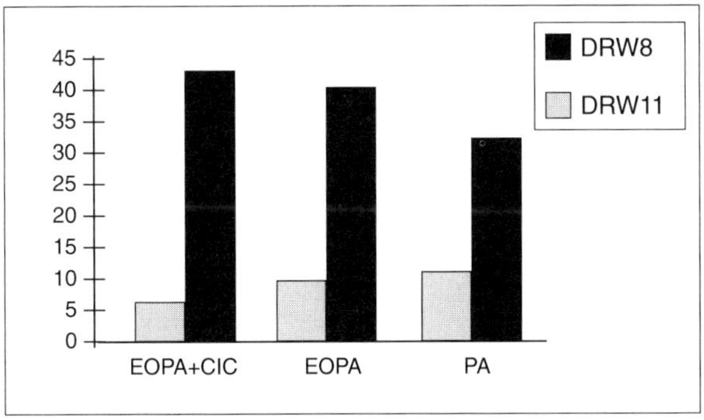

Figure 1. Patterns DRw8 and DRw11 in EOPA+CIC, EOPA and PA.

in the promoter region. This mutation causes a reduction in the expression of the α chain and therefore of the DQ4 and DQ7 heterodimers formed by the DQA1*0401-DQB1*0402 and DQA1*0501-DQB1*0301 alleles respectively. Our data confirms that all of the alleles significantly correlated are associated in two haplotypes: DRB1*11-DQA1*0501-DQB1*0301 and DRB1*08-DQA1*0401- DQB1*0402 which carry the QPA4.1 and QPA4.2 promoter alleles mutated in the Y-box respectively. As far as DPB1 is concerned a significant increase with DPB1*0201 allele in all forms with a significant dicrease in trend from EOPA to Syst has been documented. It was also been observed that when DPB1*0201 allele is present is always associated with DR11 and DR8 emphasizing that the disease is tied to particular haplotypes of class II and not to a single allele. These findings could fit with the hypothesis that JCA pathogenesis could be sustained by an arthritogenic peptide of autologous derivation presented by some DQ molecules [10]. In this case the arthritogenic peptide is represented by the DP2 molecule and as it is known that DPB1*0201 differs from DPB1*0402 allele by only one aminoacid in 69 position, this position could be responsable for binding of the peptide to the DQ molecules. In particular when the DPB1*0201 molecule is present with the DQ4 and DQ7 heterodimers the maximum expression of the disease is found in the subsets with articular involvement (EOPA, EOPA+CIC and PA) while if DPB1*0201 is present alone the disease manifests itself as the systemic form without arthropaty. It can be concluded that DPB1*0201 product being present in the four subsets of the disease could be interpreted as the molecule with a potential arthritogenic role while class II DQ heterodimers (DQ4, DQ7) act as a groove for arthritogenic peptide. To clarify the assumptions further investigations on the role of the DPB1 gene through cytofluorimetry study of DP molecule expression on lymphocytes and molecular study of DP promoter region are necessary. Moreover since it was been supposed that a reduced expression of the DQ molecules causes an insufficient degree of self-tolerance against the autoantigens a molecular study of the DQA promoter region will also be required.

References

1. Mathies H, Truckenbrodt H, Sänger L Diagnostische kriterien der juvenilen chronischen arthritiden. Basel : EULAR, 1988.
2. Fernandez-Vina MA, Fink CW, Stastny P. DQA1 and DQB1 alleles in patients with juvenile arthritis. *Hum Immunol* 1990; 11: 68-72
3. Odum N, Morling N, Friis J, Heilmann C, Hylding-Nielsen JJ, Jakobsen BK Pedersen FK, Platz P Ryder LP, Svejgaard A. Increased frequency of HLA-DPw2 in pauciarticular onset juvenile chronic arthritis. *Tissue Antigens* 1986; 28: 245-50.
4. Paul C, Schoenwald U, Truckenbrodt H, Bettinotti MP, Brunner G, Keller E, Nevinny-Stickel C, Yao Z, Albert ED. HLA-DP/DR interaction in early onset pauciarticular juvenile chronic arthritis. *Immunogenetics* 1993; 37: 442-8.
5. Glass DN, Litvin DA. Heterogeneity of HLA associations in systemic onset juvenile rheumatoid arthritis. *Arthritis Rheum* 1980; 23: 796-9.
6. Miller ML, Aarons S, Jackson J. HLA gene frequencies in children and adults with systemic onset juvenile rheumatoid arthritis. *Arthritis Rheum* 1985; 28: 146-50.
7. Haas JP, Nevinny-Stickel C, Schoenwald U, Truckenbrodt H, Suschke J, Albert ED. Susceptible and protective major histocompatibility complex class II alleles in early-onset pauciarticular juvenile chronic arthritis. *Hum Immunol* 1994; 41: 225-33.
8. Kimura A, Sasazuki T. Polymorphism in the 5'-flanking region of the DQA1 gene and its relation to DR-DQ haplotype. In: Tsuji K, Aizawa M, Sasazuki T, eds. *HLA 1991,* vol. II. Oxford: Blackwell 1992: 382-5.
9. Haas JP, Kimura A, Truckenbrodt H, Suschke J, Sasazuki T, Volgger A, Albert ED. Early-onset pauciarticular juvenile chronic arthritis is associated with a mutayion in the Y-box of the HLA-DQA1 promoter. *Tissue Antigens* 1995; 45: 317-21.
10. Altmann DM, Sansom D, Marsh SGE. What is the basis for HLA-DQ associations with autoimmune disease? *Immunol Today* 1991; 12: 267-70.

Rheumatoid arthritis association with a T-cell receptor genotype

F. Cornélis [1,2,3], L. Hardwick [4], R.M. Flipo [5], M. Martinez [1], S. Lasbleiz [3], J.F. Prud'homme [3], T.H. Tran [1,2,3], S. Walsh [4], A. Delaye [1,2,3], A. Nicod [4], M.N. Loste [6], V. Lepage [6], K. Gibson [4], K. Pile [4], S. Djoulah, P.M. Danzé [5], F. Lioté [2], D. Charron [6], J. Weissenbach [3], D. Kuntz [2], T. Bardin [2], B.P. Wordsworth [4]

1 INSERM U358, 75010 Paris, France
2 Laboratoire d'Histopathologie Synoviale, Centre Viggo-Petersen, 6, rue Patin, 75010 Paris, France (address for correspondence)
3 CNRS URA 192, Généthon, 9100 Évry, France
4 The Wellcome Trust Center for Human Genetics, Windmill road, Headington, Oxford, UK
5 Hôpital R. Salengro, 59037 Lille, France
6 Hôpital Saint-Louis, 75010 Paris, France

The T-cell receptor genes (TCRA and TCRB) are major candidates for contributing susceptibility to rheumatoid arthritis (RA). Their variable segments exhibit allelic variation affecting the amino-acid sequence [1-4]. Such variations were investigated systematically in this RA case/control study.

Material and methods

Genomic DNA of 1579 north-west European individuals, 766 patients with erosive and rheumatoid factor positive disease and 813 controls, was used. The systematic study of segments TCRAV6S1, TCRAV7S1, TCRAV8S1, TCRAV10S2 and TCRBV6S1, TCRBV6S7 relied on single-strand-conformation polymorphisms [2, 3]. The confirmation of the TCRAV8S1 association was performed with a RFLP (restriction-fragment length-polymorphism).

Results

In the systematic study (77 patients and 119 controls), only one significant association was found ($p<0.01$): an increase of TCRAV8S1 genotypes containing the allele *2 in patients [genotype 2(+)]. The significance of this finding was assessed in 2 further populations, one from France (212 patients and 254 controls) and one from Britain (477 patients and 440 controls). In both, the genotype 2(+) was increased in patients compared to controls, with a relative risk (RR) of 1.3 and 1.3, respectively. The similar RR allowed the data to be pooled with confirmation of the association (RR=1.3).

Discussion

These findings provide evidence for TCRA being a new RA susceptibility locus. The molecular explanation could provide a target for a therapeutic intervention in this disease. Together with similar findings in allergy [5, 6], it indicates new directions of research for other complex diseases of immune, infectious or malignant nature involving T-cells.

References

1. Posnett D, Wang C,Friedman S. Inherited polymorphism of the human T-cell antigen receptor detected by a monoclonal antibody. *Proc Natl Acad Sci USA* 1986; 83: 7888-92.
2. Cornélis F, Pile K, Loveridge J, Moss P, Harding R, Julier C,Bell J. Systematic study of human aßT-cell receptors V segments shows allelic variations resulting in a large number of distinct TCR haplotypes. *Eur J Immunol* 1993; 23: 1277-83.
3. Reyburn H, Cornélis F, Russel V, Harding R, Moss P, Bell J. Allelic polymorphism of human T cell receptor Valpha gene segments. *Immunogenetics* 1993; 38: 287-91.
4. Charmley P, Nickerson D, Hood L. Polymorphism detection and sequence analysis of human T-cell receptor V alpha -chain-encoding gene segments. *Immunogenetics* 1994; 39: 138-45.
5. Moffat M, Hill M, Cornélis F, Schou C, Faux J, Young R, James A, Ryan G, Le Souef P, Musk A, Hopkin J,Cookson W. Genetic linkage of the TCR alpha/delta region to specific immunoglobulin E responses. *Lancet* 1994; 343: 1597-600.
6. Moffat M, Young R, Faux J, Musk A, Cookson W. Involvement of TCR alpha/delta and HLA-DR in specific allergy. *Allergy* 1995; 50 (suppl): 164.

Genetics and specific immune response in Allergy and Asthma

Contents

HLA and immunity to allergens: therapeutic implications

H. Løwenstein[1], J. Lamb[2]

1 ALK, Bøge Alle 10-12, PO Box 408, DK-2970 Hørsholm, Denmark
2 Infection and Immunity Section, Department of Biology, Technology and Medicine, Imperial College of Science, London SW7 2BB, UK

It is now more than two decades since David Marsh and his colleagues first published the association between skin prick test reactions to the small molecule Amb a V from short ragweed and the HLA gene complex [1], and subsequently established specific IgE responsiveness was linked to the class II haplotype HLA-DR2 (DRB1*15; [2]). These findings prompted scientists to search for clear cut correlations between HLA phenotypes and sensitivity of allergic patients to identified aeroallergen molecules. So far a number of such associations have also been found but on several occasions these less strong linkages could not be verified [3], and a possible explanation might be the presence of multiple IgE reacting B cell epitopes on the allergen investigated. However, very recently the 3-dimentional structure of the major allergen of birch pollen, Bet v 1, has been derived by both X-ray crystallography and NMR technique [4]. From this structure it is evident that only part of the molecular surface is conserved in all isoforms thus identifing conditions for major IgE reacting epitopes. We, therefore, foresee that this additional knowledge of structure/function relationship at the molecular level also might create an additional basis for future studies of genetics of allergy.

The observation that IgE production is T cell dependent generated considerable interest in analysing the HLA restriction specificity of T-cell responses to allergens and how many HLA class II molecules, including those encoded by HLA-DP and -DQ as well as -DR, capable of restricting T cell recognition for a range of different allergens, have been reported (*eg.* [5]).

Now that information is available on the primary amino acid sequences of many allergens and the structure of HLA class II molecules has been defined by crystallography [6], it is possible to analyse the physical nature of allergen/class II molecular interactions in detail. However, the increase in our knowledge both from studying structure/function relationships at the molecular level and analysing HLA disease associations has had minimal impact on the practical aspects of treating allergic diseases. One area to which this information may contribute is in the design of subunit or peptide based vaccines for immunotherapy. In order to develop this approach to therapy both the identification of the dominant T cell epitopes and the determination of their HLA class II restriction specificity at the population is required. At present for the majority of allergens this information is lacking. However, the limited data that is available from the analysis of polyclonal and monoclonal T cell responses to allergens demonstrate that a given individual may recognise multiple T cell epitopes within a protein, which may be restricted by the same or different MHC class II molecules. In addition, there is also evidence that a single allergen derived T cell epitopes may be restricted by either HLA-DR or -DQ (*eg.* [5] and *Table I*).

Table I. Heterogeneity of the HLA class II restriction specificity of T cell responses to Der p 2 in a given individual

Peptide sequence	Stimulation index	HLA class restriction
1-15	0.9	
11-25	2.1	
21-35	7.3	**DRB1*1101/DQB*0301**
31-47	0.8	
41-55	0.8	
51-65	1	
61-75	1.02	
71-86	1.05	
81-96	2.8	**DQB1*0301**
91-105	0.9	
101-105	5.3	**DPB1*0402**
111-129	2.8	**DRB1*1101/DQB*0301**

Furthermore, an important parameter to consider in the development of peptide based immunotherapy is the potential of the allergen specific T cell repertoire to change over time. There are few reports in which the plasticity of the allergen reactivity of the human T cell repertoire has been determined in the context of epitope specificity (*eg.* [5, 7]). However, from *in vivo* experimental models there is evidence that immunisation with a dominant T cell determinant under conditions that result in the induction of T cell unresponsiveness will also downregulate the response to the entire protein, including all the minor T cell epitopes [8]. If such mechanisms of "infectious" T cell tolerance exist in man, temporal changes in the specificity of T cell responses may be less of a problem in the application of subunit vaccines. As opposed to inducing peripheral tolerance or anergy, the aim of immunisation with allergen derived peptides may be to prime naive T cells to adopt the characteristics of the Th1 functional phenotype. Indeed, the results of clinical trials using intact allergen preparations suggest that successful desensitisation is accompanied by the induction of a Th1 phenotype, however, serum levels of IgE may often remain high or are initially unaltered [9]. Therefore, it is likely that additional changes in the immune response are required to mediate the effects of allergen desensitisation. Although immunotherapy trials using defined peptides derived from Fel d 1 are in progress, what changes they induce in the qualitative nature of allergic immune responses in atopic individuals is unclear at present. Preliminary results on the desensitisation of bee venom patients using peptides has demonstrated reduced IL-4 and enhanced IFN-γ production together with an overall decrease in specific IgE [10]. However, whether or not peptide based immunotherapy will prove to be a long term viable approach to desensitisation in terms of safety and efficacy remains to be evaluated.

MHC molecules play an important role in shaping the T cell repertoire during development as well as in the recognition of allergen derived peptides by T cells in the periphery. This finding has prompted analysis of T cell antigen receptors (TCR) usage in order to determine if there is a bias towards the selection of particular Vβ and Vα segments in the response to specific allergens. For pollen and house dust mite (HDM) reactivity in atopic individuals there is some evidence to suggest the existance *in vivo* for the expansion of long lived T cell clones with a restricted range of specificities which have presumably been selected by chronic exposure to allergen [7]. In case of T cell recognition of HDM derived allergens, there was an indication of restricted usage of TCR-Vα8.1 [7]. Once again information on TCR usage at the population is too limited to evaluate at present. However, genetic linkage analysis indicates an association between TCR-Vα 8.1, DRB1*02 and Der p 2 specific IgE [11].

Asthma and rhinitis are immunological diseases involving Th2 derived cytokines and, therefore, proteins encoded by the HLA gene complex will contribute to the regulation of immune responses observed in individuals affected by these diseases. However, genetic susceptibility to allergic diseases is polygenic and other genes encoding TCR, cytokines, adhesion molecules and costimulatory receptors may be of equal or greater importance.

References

1. Marsh DG, Bias WB, Ishizaka K. Genetic control of basal serum immunologlobulin E level and its effect on specific reagenic sensitivity. *Proc Natl Acad Sci USA* 1974; 71: 3588.
2. Marsh DG, Hsu SH, Roebber M *et al.* HLA-Dw2: a genetic marker for human immmune response to short ragweed allergen Ra5 I. Response resulting primarily from natural antigenic exposure. *J Exp Med* 1982; 155: 1439.
3. Young RP, Dekker JC, Wordsworth BP, Schou C, Pile KD, Mathiessen F, Rosenberg WMC, Bell JI, Hopkin JM, Cookson WOCM. HLA-DR and HLA-DP genotypes and immunoglobulin E responses to common major allergens. *Clin Exp Allergy* 1994; 24: 431.
4. Gajhede M, Osmark P, Poulsen FM, Ipsen H, Larsen JN, Van Neerven RJJ, Schou C, Løwenstein H, Spangfort MD. X-ray and NMR structure of Bet v 1, the origin of birch pollen allergy. *Nature Struct Biol* 1997 (in press).
5. Verhoef A, Higgins JA, Thorpe C *et al.* Clonal analysis of the atopic immune response to the group 2 allergen of *Dermatophagoides* spp: identification of HLA-DR and -DQ restricted T cell epitopes. *Int Immunol* 1993; 5: 1589.

6. Stern LJ, Brown JH, Jardetzky TS, Wiley DC. Crystal structure of the human class II MHC protein HLA-DR1 complexed with an influenza virus peptide. *Nature* 1994; 368: 215.
7. Wedderburn LR, O'Hehir RE, Hewitt CRA, Lamb JR, Owen MJ. *In vivo* clonal dominance and limited T cell receptor usage in human CD4+ T cell recognition of house dust mite allergens. *Proc Natl Acad Sci USA* 1993; 90: 8214.
8. Hoyne GF, O'Hehir RE, Wraith DG, Thomas WR, Lamb JR. Inhibition of T cell and antibody responses to house dust mite allergen by inhalation of the dominant T cell epitope in naive and sensitised mice. *J Exp Med* 1993; 178: 1783.
9. Secrist H, Chelen, CJ, Wen Y, Marshall JD, Umetsu D. Allergen immunotherapy descreases interleukin 4 production in CD4+ T cells from patients from allergic individuals. *J Exp Med* 1993; 178: 2123.
10. Muller U, Fricker M, Caraballido J, Blaser K. Successful immunotherapy with T cell epitopes of bee venom phospholipase A2 in 2 patients with bee venom allergy. In: Ring J, Berendt H, eds. *New Trends in Allergy IV.* Hamburg, 1995.
11. Moffatt M, Schou C, Faux J *et al.* TCR-a restriction of immunoglobulin E responses to specific antigen. In: Charron D, ed. *Genetic diversity of HLA. Functional and Medical Implication,* vol. I. Sèvres: EDK, 1997.

TCR-α restriction of immunoglobulin E responses to specific antigen

M. Moffatt[1], C. Schou[2], J. Faux[1], W.O.C.M. Cookson[1]

1 Nuffield Department of Clinical Medicine, Oxford University, John Radcliffe Hospital, Headington, Oxford OX3 9DU, UK
2 ALK Research, Hørsholm, Denmark

People who are atopic differ in the antigens to which they react. The risk of development of clinical disease such as asthma is reliant on the particular antigen responses of an individual. Unlike grass pollen sensitisation, House Dust mite (HDM) sensitivity has been shown to carry an increased risk of asthma [1]. It is therefore of interest to establish what genetic and environmental factors are influencing the specificity of the IgE response. Understanding the genetic factors controlling specific allergy may result in the generation of a model system to investigate the restriction of the humoral response to exogenous antigens.

Two important candidates for the genetic control of the specific IgE response are the HLA class II genes and the T Cell Receptor (TCR) genes. Numerous studies have reported HLA allelic associations with particular allergen responses ([2] for review). However, many of these studies have involved a small number of subjects and have used, due to the high level of polymorphism in the HLA region, multiple tests of significance. The first association to be recognised was between the major allergen of ragweed, *Amb a* V, [3] and DR2 (HLA-DRB1*15). This association is the most secure having been consistently confirmed [4,5].

It is clear however, that the HLA genes alone cannot account for the differences in an individual's IgE reactions to allergens. The TCR repertoire is not random and is influenced by genomic polymorphisms. We have therefore investigated the role of the TCR genes. We have previously shown strong genetic linkage between a highly informative microsatellite repeat, associated with the TCR-α/δ locus, and IgE responses to a number of purified allergens [6]. The TCR-α/δ locus is very complex containing many elements that may potentially influence specific antigen recognition. We decided to carry on from our linkage study by looking for allelic associations with polymorphisms in the Vα gene segments. A previous study has suggested a dominant expression of Vα8 and Vβ3 genes in T cell clones reactive to allergens of the HDM [7]. A bi-allelic polymorphism in Vα8.1 has previously been described [8] and in the following study this has been investigated for its association with IgE responses to HDM antigens. Due to the important role of the HLA class II genes in antigen presentation, recognition and shaping of the TCR repertoire, we have also performed HLA-DRB1 typing. This has enabled us to investigate whether HLA and TCR interactions exist, restricting the IgE response to particular antigens.

Materials and methods

Subjects

413 Australians (Set A) from 88 nuclear families with 2 or more atopic siblings were identified from a general population sample of the country town of Busselton, Western Australia. In order to test any associations found for replication, a second set of 435 Australian subjects (Set B), from the same general population sample, were used. 30% of Set B had a positive RAST to HDM.

Phenotype analysis

For all subjects elevation of IgE titres to the whole allergen source *Dermatophagoides pteronyssinus* (HDM) was determined by the ImmunoCAP FEIA system (Pharmacia). Elevation of IgE titres to the major purified allergens of *D. pteronyssinus*, *Der p* I and *Der p* II, was determined by chemiluminescence assay using monoclonal anti-IgE (ALK Laboratories, Hørsholm, Denmark).

Table I. Vα8.1 allelic associations

a. Set A subjects

IgE PHENOTYPE	Vα8.1 ALLELES	n	MEAN (SE)	t	p
RAST HDM	1	316	1.630 (0.106)	-2.53	0.011
	2	490	1.984 (0.091)		
Der p I	1	316	1.133 (0.092)	-1.91	0.057
	2	490	1.367 (0.081)		
Der p II	1	316	0.620 (0.056)	-2.78	0.006
	2	490	0.833 (0.052)		

b. Set B subjects

IgE PHENOTYPE	Vα8.1 ALLELES	n	MEAN (SE)	t	p
Der p II	1	337	0.374 (0.044)	-2.17	0.030
	2	493	0.507 (0.042)		

c. Combined subjects

IgE PHENOTYPE	Vα8.1 ALLELES	n	MEAN (SE)	t	p
Der p II	1	653	0.493 (0.036)	-3.57	0.000
	2	983	0.669 (0.034)		

Table II. HLA-DRB1* allelic associations

Combined subjects

IgE PHENOTYPE	HLA-DRB1*1501	n	MEAN (SE)	t	p
RAST HDM	-ve	1421	1.372 (0.049)	-1.52	0.131
	+ve	228	1.588 (0.134)		
Der p I	-ve	1418	0.934 (0.041)	-2.02	0.044
	+ve	227	1.18[illegible] (0.115)		
Der p II	-ve	1418	0.553 (0.026)	-2.91	0.004
	+ve	227	0.788 (0.077)		

Table III. Interactions between Vα8.1, HLA-DRB1 and IgE titres to *Der p* II. Multiple regression analysis

Combined subjects

VARIABLE	B (Standard Error)	t	p
HLA-DRB1*1501	0.286 (0.073)	3.90	0.0001
Vα8.1	0.201 (0.052)	3.90	0.0001
Constant	-0.052 (0.130)	-0.41	0.68
			$R^2 = 0.0159$

Not signifiant: HLA-DRB1*01, *03, *04, *07, *11.

Genotype analysis

HLA-DRB1 typing was carried out by PCR amplification, dot blotting and then sequential hybridization to sequence-specific oligonucleotide probes as previously described [9]. Probes were labelled using the DIG labelling system (Boehringer, Mannheim) and hybridized accordingly. Typing of the single stranded conformational polymorphism (SSCP) in Vα8.1 was carried out as described previously [8]. 10% polyacrylamide gels were run in 0.5X TBE at 4°C for 22 hours. SSCP patterns were visualised by silver staining (BioRad).

Statistical analysis

Associations with quantitative phenotypes for the Vα8.1 polymorphism and HLA-DRB1 types were sought for by T-tests (SPSS 4.1 for VAX/VMS). Only the six most common HLA-DRB1 types were considered, HLA-DRB1*01, *02, *03, *04, *07 and *11. Multiple stepwise regressions were performed to confirm associations and reduce multiple comparisons to a single test of significance. Multiple stepwise regressions were also used to investigate whether interactions between Vα8.1 alleles and HLA-DRB1 alleles existed. Both forward and backward regressions gave identical results.

Results and discussion

In the Set A subjects, for the Vα8.1 polymorphism, a significant association with IgE titres to whole HDM (p=0.011) and to the major allergen *Der p* II (p=0.006) was seen *(Table Ia)*. Vα8.1 allele 2 (Vα8.1*2) was found to correlate with higher levels of IgE for the whole allergen source and the major purified allergen. A weak association with *Der p* I was seen (p=0.057). However, multiple regression analysis with Vα8.1 as the dependent variable revealed the association to be with *Der p* II only and not to whole HDM or *Der p I*. The association between Vα8.1*2 and IgE responses to *Der p* II was confirmed in the Set B subjects although with a somewhat lower level of significance - p=0.030 *(Table Ib)*. Pooling the two data sets the association was highly significant with a p value of 0.0000 *(Table Ic)*. IgE titres to *Der p* II were approximately 25% higher in individuals possessing Vα8.1*2.

Again using T tests and examining the six most common HLA-DRB1 types, a single DRB1 association was found. HLA-DRB1*02 (1501) was found to be positively associated with IgE responses to *Der p* II for both subject sets independently and combined (*Table II*, results for combined). For the pooled data sets, a weak association (p=0.044) was seen for IgE responses to *Der p* I. However, multiple regression analysis again showed the HLA-DRB1*1501 association to be only with *Der p* II and not with *Der p* I or HDM.

To investigate whether the HLA-DRB1*1501 association was independent of that seen for Vα8.1 a further multiple regression analysis was carried out. In the analysis, *Der p* II was the dependent variable with Vα8.1 and the six most common HLA-DR types as the independent variables. A single interaction was found in both subject sets independently and combined (*Table III*, results for combined shown) showing that the Vα8.1*2 and HLA-DRB1*1501 associations are not independent of one another. In the combined data, the mean IgE titre when Vα8.1*2 and HLA-DRB1*1501 were together in the same subject was 1.14±0.14 RAST units, compared to 0.56±0.025 when neither allele was present.

Further detailed genetic and functional studies are necessary however in order to determine whether the Vα8.1 polymorphism itself or an element in linkage disequilibrium is responsible for the association with IgE responses to *Der p* II. However, from this study it would appear that genomic polymorphisms within the TCR-α/δ locus restrict IgE responses to particular antigens. This restriction would appear to occur in the context of particular HLA-DR types. Investigation of additional polymorphisms within the TCR-α/δ locus may result in the finding of associations with different purified major allergens such as *Fel d* I from the domestic cat *Felis domesticus.*

References

1. Sears MR, Herbison GP, Holdaway MD, Hewitt CJ, Flannery EM, Silva PM. The relative risks of sensitivity to grass pollen, house dust mite and cat dander in the development of childhood asthma. *Clin Allergy* 1989; 18: 419-24.
2. Moffatt MF, Cookson WOCM. The genetics of specific allergy. In: *Monographs in allergy*, vol. 33. Basel: Karger, 1997, in press.
3. Levine BB, Stember RH, Fontino M. Ragweed hayfever: genetic control and linkage to HL-A haplotypes. *Science* 1972; 178: 1201-3.
4. Blumental MN, Awdeh Z, Alper C, Yunis E. Ra5 immune responses, HLA antigens and complotypes (abstract). *J Allergy Clin Immunol* 1985; 75: 155.
5. Marsh DG, Blumenthal MN, Ishikawa T, Ruffilli A, Sparholt S, Freidhoff LR. HLA and specific immune responsiveness to allergens. In: Tsuji K, Aizawa M, Sasazuki T, eds. HLA 1991, vol. I. *Eleventh International Histocompatibility Workshop and Conference*. Oxford: Oxford University Press, 1992: 765-7.
6. Moffatt MF, Hill MR, Cornélis F, Schou C, Faux JA, Young RP, James AL, Ryan G, le Soeuf P, Musk AW, Hopkin JM, Cookson WOCM. Genetic linkage of T-cell receptor α/δ complex to specific IgE responses. *Lancet* 1994; 343: 1597-600.
7. Wedderburn LR, O'Hehir RE, Hewitt CRA, Lamb JR, Owen MJ. *In vivo* clonal dominance and limited T-cell receptor usage in human CD4+ T-cell recognition of house dust mite allergens. *Proc Natl Acad Sci USA* 1993; 90: 8214-8.
8. Cornélis F, Pile K, Loveridge J, Moss P, Harding R, Julier C, Bell J. Systematic study of human αβ T-cell receptor V segments shows allelic variations resulting in a large number of distinct TCR haplotypes. *Eur J Immunol* 1993; 23: 1277-83.
9. Wordsworth BP, Allsop CEM, Young RP, Bell JI. HLA-DR typing using DNA amplification by polymerase chain reaction and sequential hybridization to sequence specific oligonucleotide probes. *Immunogenetics* 1990; 32: 413-8.

Evidence for the role of HLA-D alleles in the susceptibility of type I allergy to hevein of *Hevea* latex

H.P. Rihs, Z. Chen, R. Cremer[1], H. Allmers, X. Baur

Institute for Occupational Medicine (BGFA) at the Ruhr-University Bochum, Molecular Genetics, Buerkle-de-la-Camp Platz 1, D44789 Bochum, Germany
1 Children's Hospital, Cologne, Germany

Natural rubber latex from the rubber tree *Hevea brasiliensis* is the most important raw material in the production of latex devices. Due to the increased use of latex gloves in hospitals, the IgE-mediated reactivity to natural rubber latex has become a serious problem, especially among health care workers (HCWs) [1]. Furthermore, patients who need repeated surgery and/or long-term hospitalization have also a high risk of developing latex allergies, *e.g.* spina bifida (SB) patients [2,3]. Recently, Chen and coworkers described the 4.7 kDa polypeptide hevein of *Hevea brasiliensis* as a major latex allergen and developed an enzyme-linked allergosorbent test (EAST) permitting the measurement of hevein-specific IgE [4].

As a part of our efforts to elucidate the possible pathogenetic way of sensitization to certain latex allergens we decided to investigate the relationship between HLA class II alleles and the IgE-specific immune response to hevein of *Hevea brasiliensis.*

Subjects and methods

216 latex-exposed subjects were examined. The first group comprised 111 HCWs, the second one 105 SB patients. Additionally, we examined a group of 90 German blood donors (controls) without any sign of hypersensitivity when tested with 20 standard allergens by skin prick test excluding latex allergens. 130 subjects (79 HCWs, 51 spina bifida patients) showed positive anti latex-IgE values by the Pharmacia-CAP system or by EAST (>0.35 kU/l).

Out of this pool, 30 randomly selected latex-IgE-positive subjects (20 HCWs and 10 SB patients) were tested for their hevein-specific IgE concentrations by EAST.

In all cases, the target DNA was isolated from frozen white blood cells using the QIAamp blood kit (Qiagen) or the Dynabeads DNA direct kit (Dynal). PCR-amplification for DQB1 was performed with the primer pair DQ1: AGGGATCCCCGCAGAGGATTTCGTGT(A,T)FCC / DQ2: GAGCTGCAGGTAGTTGTGTCTGCA(C,T)AC (STAG, N.V., Belgium). For the amplification of DRB1,3,4,5, we applied the inosin-containing primer pair DRB5'-I: ACCGGATCGTTCITGTCCCCICAGCA/ DRB3'-I:CTCGCCICTGCACIGTIAAGC [5]. After controling PCR products by gelelectrophoresis, chemically denaturated, single-stranded DNA aliquots were put on a nylon membrane (Biodyne B; Pall) by dot-blotting and fixed by heat (80 °C, 30 min). All sequence-specific oligonucleotide probes (SSOPs) were end-labelled with DIG-11-ddUTP (Boehringer Mannheim) using methods as described recently [6,7]. Hybridization was carried out with 28 SSOPs for DRB1,3,4,5 and 18 SSOPs for DQB1 from the 11th IHWC [8] supplemented in a few cases by local SSOPs. Stringent washing conditions (data not shown) were found with control DNAs from another disease study [9]. The used method allows the identification of the broad DRB and DQB alleles equivalent to the serological specificities and in some cases a further subdivision.

Statistical analysis

Fisher's exact test (2-tailed) was used in all cases and carried out with the StatXact programme (Cytel Software). P-values were corrected for the number of comparisons (pc). The correction factor for DRB1 was 26 which corresponds to the 13 broad DRB1 antigens studied and the division into two groups (hevein-positi-

Table I. Phenotypic frequencies of DR antigens in latex-allergic subjects with and without hevein hypersensitivity and in healthy controls

DR antigen(s)	n	%	n	%	n	%
DR1	4	22	3	25	15	17
DR2 (15/16)	4	22	4	33	25	28
DR3	3	17	2	17	18	20
DR4	12	67[a,b]	0	0	22	24
DR5 (11)	1	6	3	25	10	11
DR5 (12)	0	0	0	0	4	4
DR6 (13/14)	5	28	2	17	33	37
DR7	3	17	6	50[c]	15	17
DR8	0	0	2	17	5	6
DR9	0	0	1	8	3	3
DR10	0	0	0	0	0	0

a Hevein-positive vs hevein-negative subjects: p=0.0003, pc=0.008.
b Hevein-positive subjects vs controls: p=0.0014, pc=0.036.
c Hevein-negative subjects vs controls: p=0.016, pc=n.s.

ve subjects vs hevein-negative subjects or vs controls). In the case of DQB1, the correction factor was 30 (15x2) corresponding to the 15 DQB1 alleles studied and division into two groups.

Results and discussion

18 out of the 30 latex IgE-positive subjects showed also hevein-specific IgE values > 0.35 kU/l when tested by EAST. The other 12 tested latex-positive subjects had no hevein-specific IgE antibodies. The statistical analysis of the generic HLA-DRB1 allele distribution revealed a signficantly elevated DRB1*04 (DR4) frequency (67%) in hevein-positive subjects when compared with the DRB1*04 (DR4) frequency in hevein-negative subjects (0, p=0.0003, p_c=0.008) and with that in controls (24%, p=0.0014, p_c=0.036). Furthermore, we observed that the frequency of DRB1*04 (DR4) was also elevated in the group of 79 latex-positive HCWs (44%) examined so far when compared with controls (24%, p=0.0089, p_c=n.s.). It is interesting that we found a decreased DRB1*04 (DR4) frequency (19%) in our studied 51 latex-positive SB patients comparable with that in unsensitized controls (24%). Additionally, we found a slightly increased DRB1*0701 (DR7) frequency in hevein-negative subjects. The distribution of the HLA-DR specificities in latex-positve subjects tested for hevein hypersensitivity is summarized in *Table I.*
Regarding the distribution of DQB1 alleles in the 18 hevein-positive subjects, we observed an elevated DQB1*0302 (DQ8) frequency (50%) when compared with the DQ8 frequency in hevein-negative subjects (0, p=0.004, p_c=n.s.) as well as in controls (18%, p=0.011, p_c=n.s.). These p-values did not withstand correction, however. The explanation for the elevated DQ8 frequency can obviously attributed to the linkage disequilibrium between DRB1*04 (DR4) alleles and DQB1*0302 (DQ8).

We showed recently that allergy to latex in HCWs is often associated with IgE-antibodies to hevein [4]. In this study, the hypersensitivity to hevein was identified in 16 out of 20 latex-positive HCWs (80%) and only in 2 out of 10 latex-positive SB patients (20%). Certain significant associations between HLA class II antigens and inhalative allergens with a small molecular weight like the grass pollen allergen Lol p 3 or ragweed pollen allergens Amb a 5 and Amb t 5 are well described (reviewed in [10,11]). The 4.7 kDa polypeptide hevein of *Hevea* latex seems to be a further inhalative allergen showing a strong association with a class II antigen.

Conclusions

Our preliminary results revealed strong evidence for an association between hypersensitivity to hevein and HLA-DRB1*04 (DR4). Furthermore, the difference of sensitization ratio to hevein between latex-allergic HCWs (high) and SB patients (low) leads to the assumption that differences in mode and intensity of latex exposure or a certain genetic selection pattern in SB patients play a role.

References

1. Yassin MS, Lierl MB, Fisher TJ, O' Brien K, Cross J, Steinmetz C. Latex allergy in hospital employees. *Ann Allergy* 1994; 72: 245-9.
2. Tosi LL, Slater JE, Shaer C, Mostello LA. Latex allergy in spina bifida patients: prevalence and surgical implications. *J Pediatr Orthop* 1993; 13: 709-12.
3. Konz KR, Chia JK Kurup VP, Resnick A, Kelly KJ, Fink JN. Comparison of latex hypersensitivity among patients with neurological defects. *J Allergy Clin Immunol* 1995; 95: 950-4
4. Chen Z, Posch A, Raulf-Heimsoth, Baur X. Isolation and identification of hevein as a major IgE binding polypeptide in latex from *Hevea brasiliensis. J Allergy Clin Immunol* 1996; 97: 982 (abstract).
5. Marsh DG, Blumenthal MN, Ishikawa T, Ruffilli A, Sparholt S, Freidhoff LR. HLA and specific immune responsiveness to allergens. In Tsuji K, Aizawa M, Sasazuki T eds. *HLA 1991: Proceedings of the 11th International Histocompatibility Workshop and Conference.* Oxford: Oxford IRL Press, 1992: 765-71.
6. Nevinny-Stickel C, Hinzpeter M, Andreas A, Albert ED. Nonradioactive oligotyping for HLA-DR1-DRw10 using polymerase chain reaction, digoxigenin-labelled oligonucleotides and chemiluminiscence detection. *Eur J Immunogenet* 1991; 18: 323-32.
7. Rihs HP, Thiele A, Perichon B, Krishnamoorthy R, Baur X. DNA typing with digoxigenin-11-dideoxyuridinetriphosphate-labelled oligonucleotide probes enables the non-radioactive analysis with a dual detection system: Application for screening HLA-DQA1 polymorphisms. *Int Arch Allergy Immunol* 1993; 101: 7-12.
8. Kimura A, Sasazuki T. Organization and design of the DNA component. In Tsuji K, Aizawa M, Sasazuki T eds. *HLA 1991: Proceedings of the 11th International Histocompatibility Workshop and Conference.* Oxford: Oxford IRL Press 1992; 395-419.
9. Tautz C, Rihs HP, Thiele A, Zwollo P, Freidhoff L, Marsh DG, Baur X. Association of class II sequences encoding DR1 and DQ5 specificities with hypersensitivity to chironomid allergen *Chi t*I. *J Allergy Clin Immunol* 1994; 93: 918-25.
10. Marsh DG, Zwollo P, Huang SK, Gosh B, Ansari AA. Molecular studies of human response to allergens. *Cold Spring Harbor Symp Quant Biol* 1990; 54:459-69.
11. Rihs HP, Baur X. Asthma and genetics. *J Invest Allergy Clin Immunol* 1994; 4: 324-8

HLA-D genes and the IgE immune responsiveness to a recombinant mite allergen

B. Martínez, S. Jiménez, G.B. Ferrara[1], L. Caraballo

Institute for Immunological Research, University of Cartagena, Bocagrande Cra 5, 7-77 Cartagena, Colombia
1 Institute for Advanced Biotechnology, Genova, Italy

In tropical and subtropical regions, allergens from the mites *Blomia tropicalis* (Bt) and *Dermatophagoides pteronyssinus* (Dp) are the most important inducers of allergic asthma (AA). Mite-induced asthma is the commonest form of AA and the specific IgE against mite allergens have been found to be essential for the type I inflammatory process to begin. Being AA a multifactorial disease, it is necessary, for prevention and control purposes, to identify most risk factors of the disease. IgE immune response is T cell dependent and HLA-restricted, so, the relative role of any of the HLA alleles in the etiology of AA is of considerable interest. To define an association with HLA genes controlling the specificity of immune response is better to use purified allergens instead of crude mite extract. In the present work we used, as a phenotype, the specific IgE response of asthmatic patients to a recombinant allergen from Bt. This allergen (BtM) was obtained from a cDNA library of Bt and is a small molecule of approximately 8 kDa that shares B epitopes with three important native allergens of Bt [1]. In addition to DRB1 and DQB1 loci, in this work we evaluated the role of TAP genes polymorphism in the control of specific IgE response to this recombinant allergen.

Subjects and methods

Both patients and controls were mulattos [2]. Ninety five Bt-induced asthmatics and 89 non-allergic controls were included in the study. All patients had atopic symptoms related to house dust exposure and were allergic to Bt and Dp, demonstrated by skin test (ST) and RAST. Controls were ST and RAST-negative to these allergens. RAST for IgE antibodies to Bt was made using allergen coated microtiter plates and ^{125}I labeled anti-human IgE. The IgE binding of sera to the recombinant allergen BtM was detected by plaque immunoassay [1]. HLA was typed by PCR/non-radioactive/sequence specific oligonucleotide (SSO). The set of DRB1, DQB1 and TAP SSOs were able to define 45, 17 and 8 specificities respectively. Hybridization conditions included washes of the hybridized membrane at room temperature and at 42 °C in TMAC. Probes for HLA-DRB1 were ddUTP-digoxigenine labeled.

Results

Seventy per cent of patients were allergic only to mites. The other 30% showed allergy to only two additional allergens (*Aspergillus* and cockroach). In the group of patients, 40 (42%) had IgE antibodies to the recombinant allergen BtM. Only 62 sera of the control group could be tested for IgE-binding to BtM, so they were random selected. Among them, 4 were positive. When comparing the frequency of HLA-DRB1alleles between the two main groups, a weak positive association of AA with HLA-DRB1*03 was found (p=0.05), which dissapeared when the p value was corrected by the number of alleles. However, analysing the distribution of HLA-DRB1*03 (including both *0301 and *0302 alleles) in the forty patients with IgE antibodies to BtM and the subgroup of 58 BtM-IgE-negative controls, an stronger positive association was evident (*Table I*): 42% of patients were HLA-DRB1*03 while only 7% of controls had the allele (p = 0.01). Regarding to HLA-DQB1 we found a weak negative association between DQB1*0601 and AA when the two main groups were compared but the association became stronger when the proportion of this allele were compared between the two subgroups of patients (allergic to the recombinant BtM) and controls (p = 0.005) (*Table I*). The frequencies of TAP alleles in patients and controls were: TAP1*0101: 80.2% and 72%; TAP1*02011: 37.5% and 48.4%; TAP1*0301: 9.3% and 7.2%; TAP1*0401: 13.5% and 8.2%. TAP2-A/E: 50% and 63%; TAP2-B/G: 62% and 68%; TAP2-C/D:28% and 23%; TAP2-H: 8.4% and

Table I. HLA and IgE responsiveness to the rBtM allergen

HLA	Patients IgE/BtM+ (n = 40)	Controls IgE/BtM- (n = 58)	p	O.R.
DRB1*03	17(42%)	7(12%)	0.01	5.4
DQB1*0601	5(12.5%)	22(37.9%)	0.005	0.23

Table II. Distribution of TAP alleles among AA patients and controls

	AA Patients	Controls	Pc
TAP1 ALLELES	n = 96	n = 97	
*0101	80.2%	72.0%	ns
*02011	37.5%	48.4%	ns
*0301	9.3%	7.2%	ns
*0401	13.5%	8.2%	ns
TAP2 ALLELES	n = 71	n =57	
A/E	50.0%		ns
B/G	62.0%		ns
C/D	28.0%		ns
H	8.4%		ns

3.5%. This non-significant distribution was almost the same when the subpopulations of allergic and non-allergic to the recombinant BtM were compared (*Table II*).

Discussion

Our study, performed in a mulatto population, shows a positive association between HLA-DRB1*03 and the IgE immune responsiveness to a recombinant allergen from Bt and a negative association between HLA-DQB1*0601 and the same response, supporting previous works that suggest a relationship between HLA and AA. HLA-DR3 has been also positively associated with other conditions with IgE-hyper responsiveness to allergens like grass [3], birch pollen [4] and acid anhydrides [5]. Previous studies have signaled that some HLA-DQ alleles may play a role in down regulating the immune response [6, 7]. Furthermore, DQB1*0601 has been reported to be significantly less frequent in patients with alopecia areata and IDDM than in the respective controls [8, 9]. Our previous work in the same ethnic group [10] also showed an association between HLA-DPB1*0401 and the resistance to mite induced AA. Analysing the amino acid sequence of this two alleles there is no evidence of homology at the region related with peptide presentation. In addition, we have no data supporting the existence of linkage disequilibrium between these alleles in mulatto population. So, these work and our results suggest a possible role of this gene in immunologically-mediated diseases. This study shows neither association between the IgE-hyperresponsiveness to mite allergens and TAP genes, nor linkage disequilibrium between these alleles and those HLA genes previously found associated with AA (data not shown). This supports the notion that HLA class II genes confer the primary HLA association described to such response.

References

1. Caraballo L, Avgioglu A, Marrugo J, Puerta L, Marsh D. Cloning and expression of cDNA coding for an allergen with common antibody binding specificities with three allergens of the house dust mite Blomia tropicalis. *J Allergy Clin Immunol* 1997 (in press).
2. Caraballo L, Marrugo J, Erlich H, Pastorizo M: HLA antigens in the population of Cartagena (Colombia). *Tissue Antigens* 1992; 39: 128-33.
3. Freidhoff L, Ehrlich-Kaustky E, Meyers D. Association of HLA-DR3 with human immune response to Lol p I and Lol p II allergens in allergic subjects. *Tissue Antigens* 1988; 31: 211-9.
4. Fisher G, Pickl W, Fae I. Association between IgE response against Bet v I, the major allergen of Birch pollen, and HLA-DRB alleles. *Hum Immunol* 1992; 33: 259-65.
5. Young R, Barker R, Pile K, Cookson W, Newman Taylor J. The association of HLA-DR3 with specific IgE to inhaled acid anhydrides. *Am J Respir Crit Care Med* 1995; 151: 219-21.
6. Matsushita S, Sasasuki T. Genetic control of IgE immune response. *Clin Rev Allergy* 1989; 7: 125-9.
7. Altmann DM, Sansom D, Marsh S. What is the basis for HLA-DQ associations with autoimmune diseases? *Immunol Today* 1991; 12: 267-70.
8. Welsh E, Clark H, Epstein S, Reveille J, Duvic M. Human leucocyte antigen DQB1*03 alleles are associated with alopecia areata. *J Invest Dermatol* 1994; 103: 758-63.
9. Chuang L, Jou T, Hu C, Wu H, Tsai W, Lee J, Hsieh R, Chen K, Tai T, Lin B. HLA-DQB1 codon 57 and IDDM in Chinese living in Taiwan. *Diabetes Care* 1994; 17: 863-8.
10. Caraballo L, Marrugo J, Jiménez S, Angelini G, Ferrara GB. Frequency of DPB1*0401 is significantly decreased in patients with allergic asthma in mulatto population *Hum Immunol* 1991; 32: 157-61.

HLA-DRB1* alleles as genetic risk factors in allergy to Parietaria. A multicenter linkage study

M. D'Amato, A. Picardi, A. di Pietro, P. Matricardi, B. Testa, R. Ariano, E. Maggi, A. Plebani, G. Sacerdoti, S. Poto, V. Santonastaso, A. Ruffilli

Istituto Internazionale di Biologia Cellulare, CNR, Roma, Italy
Istituto di Genetica e Biofisica, CNR, Via G. Marconi 10, 80125 Napoli, Italy
DASRS, Pratica di mare, Italy Ospedale Gesù e Maria, Napoli, Italy
Policlinico di Careggi, Firenze, Italy
Clinica Pediatrica Ospedali Civili, Brescia, Italy
II Facoltà di Medicina, Napoli, Italy
Ospedale Giovanni da Procida, Salerno, Italy

Allergy includes a group of clinical syndromes, mainly represented by asthma, rhinitis and eczema, which show a clear familial aggregation. The genetic control of allergy is multigenic and there is evidence that both cognate and non cognate mechanisms are involved [1]. It is also possible that allergy is genetically heterogeneous, diverse etiological processes causing partially overlapping clinical phenotypes.

The targets of non cognate mechanisms are probably multiple and include factors and processes able of influencing the expression of Th1/Th2-related cytokines at the microenviromental or generalized level. Candidate genes have been postulated in chr 5q 31.1-33.3 (a region including the TH2 cytokine loci cluster and the β2 adrenergic receptor locus) [2] and in chr 11q12-13 (β chain of high affinity IgE receptor) [3].

Cognate mechanisms are postulated to be responsible for the observed HLA association of the antibody response to certain allergens [4]. The best documented of these association is that of the minor Ambrosia pollen allergen, Amb a 5, with DR2. More recently, less stringent associations have been described (in some cases only in monosensitized patients) in the response to the insect allergen Chi t 1 (with DR1) and to the pollen allergens Ole e I (with DQ2) and Bet v I (DRB1 and B3 alleles sharing a YFH at pos 30-32) [5,6]. Linkage studies have shown excess sharing of HLA DR and DP haplotypes in sibling pairs responding to Fel d I and Alt a I (associated with DR1 and DR4 respectively) [7].

Allergy to the pollen of Parietaria is highly prevalent in Europe. The major pollen allergens from *P. judaica* and *P. officinalis*, are proteins of 12.5 kDa. Previously, we have shown that in the Italians IgG and IgE ab response to *Par o* I are positively associated with HLA-DRB1*1101 and 1104. The association was confirmed in a different (Spanish) study group [8]. To extend these studies, in the framework of an international study sponsored by the European Science Foundation, we have investigated genetic linkage between allergy to Parietaria and HLA DRB1* alleles. We report here the preliminary results of this study.

Subjects and methods

One hundred thirty one subjects from 29 nuclear families have been recruited through one or more sibs allergic to Parietaria in 10 Italian towns. The pedigrees contained 5O sib pairs. Ten parents of uncomplete families were added to the study group in some analyses. All subjects were informed volunteers.

Allergy was ascertained according to clinical history (using a standard questionnaire). All subjects were skin prick tested with extracts of common allergens. A wheal of diameter 2 mm or more greater than that of the negative control was considered a positive response. For 5 families the clinical documentation was not available.

Blood (70-30 ml) was drawn from each subject and plasma and cells separated by centrifugation. Total serum IgE level was measured in the serum (recovered from plasma) using standard procedures (Phadezym PRIST, Pharmacia). Par o 1 specific IgE and IgG ab level was determined using the double antibody radioimmunoassay (DARIA) and purified iodinated *Par o* 1.

HLA DRB1* alleles were typed using the heteroduplex methodology [9].

Linkage was ascertained through chi square analysis

Table I. Prevalence of selected HLA DRB1* alleles in 68 parents subdivided according to phenotypes

	number of subjects with allele (%)				
	IgE ab to Par o 1			IgG ab to Par o 1	
	+	-		+	-
HLA-DRB1*	(N=32)	(N=36)		(N=43)	(N=25)
01 (N=11)	4 (13)	7 (19)		9 (21)	2 (8)
1101/04 (N=38)	20 (63)	18 (50)	χ^2 3.7	26 (61)	12 (48)
03 (N=13)	6 (19)	7 (19)		4 (9)	9 (36)
04 (N=11)	6 (19)	5 (14)		8 (19)	3 (12)
07 (N=18)	10 (31)	8 (22)		13 (30)	5 (20)
13 (N=10)	2 (6)	8 (22)		7 (16)	3 (12)

Table II. Affected sibling per pedigree in 29 DRB1* typed families

Phenotype	N of pairs	N. of affected sibs		
		2	1	0
Parietaria ST positive*	48	18	22	8
with IgE ab to Par o 1	57	22	19	16
with IgG ab to Par o 1	57	33	13	11

*In 24 families.

Table III. Affected sib pairs sharing maternal or paternal alleles

Phenotype	Paternal allele		Maternal allele		
	N of pairs		N of pairs		
	sharing/not	sharing	sharing/not	sharing	χ^2
ST positivity to Par	11	5	7	9	
IgE ab to Par o 1	13	5	12	6	5.4 p=0.02
IgG ab to Par o 1	14	15	15	14	

performed on the assumption that the expected proportion of sibling pairs sharing an allele from the specified parent was 0.5 (identity by descent). Sibling pairs were included in the analysis only if the two alleles from the specified parents could be individually recognized. All sibling pairs from multiple sibships were considered as independent.

Results and discussion

Analysis of association

Taken toghether, the parents of the recruited families represented a sample of unrelated subjects from different areas of Italy. *Table I* reports the prevalence of selected HLA-DRB1* alleles in 68 parents subdivided according to the presence of IgG and IgE ab to *Par o* 1. There was an excess of DRB1* 1101/04 in subjects with ab to Par o 1 which was statistically significant for IgE ab, in agreement with our previous report [8].

Linkage analysis

Linkage was assessed in affected sibling pairs. The number and distribution of affected sibling pairs are represented in *Table II*. Sharing of parental alleles in sibpairs subdivided according to phenotype is reported in *Table III*. The excess sharing in sib pairs with IgE ab to *Par o* 1 was statistically significant.

In conclusion, this study confirms the association of IgE ab response to *Par o* 1 with HLA-DRB1*1101/04. Linkage analysis strongly suggests that the HLA DRB1* locus control Parietaria specific allergy. The analysis of a larger number of families is required to better investigate the pattern of inheritance and to ask the question of the interplay between atopy genes, presumably controlling non cognate probably polyclonal processes in the immune response and HLA genes which are involved in immune recognition.

References

1. Huang S, Marsh DG. Genetics of allergy. *Ann Allergy* 1993; 70: 347.

2. Marsh DG, Blumenthal MN, Ishikawa T, Ruffilli A, Sparholt S, Freidhoff LR. HLA and specific immune responsiveness to allergens. In: Tsujj T, Aizawa M, Sasazuki T eds. *XIth International Histocompatibility Workshop and Conference Book*. Oxford: Oxford University Press, 1992: 765-71.
3. Shirakawa T, Li A, Dubowitz M, Dekker JW, Shaw AE, Faux JA, Ra C, Cookson WOMC, Hopkins JM. Association between atopy and variants of the high-affinity immunoglobulin E receptor. *Nature Genet* 1994; 7: 125-9.
4. Marsh DG, Meyers DA, Bias WB. The epidemology and genetics of atopic allergy. *N Eng J Med* 1981; 305: 1551-9.
5. Cardaba B,Vilches C, Martin E, de Andres B, del Pozo V, Hernandez D, Gallardo S, Fernandez GC, Villalba M, Rodriguez R, Basomba A, Kreisler M, Palomino P, Lahoz C. DR7 and DQ2 are positively associated with IgE response to the main allergen of olive pollen (*Ole e* I) in allergic patients. *Hum Immunol* 1993; 38: 293.
6. Fisher GF, Pickl WF *et al.* Association between IgE response agaisnt Bet v I, the major allergen of birch pollen and HLA-DR alleles. *Hum Immunol* 1992; 33: 259.
7. Young RP, Dekker JW, Wordsworth BP, Schou C, Pile KD, Matthiesen F, Rosenberg WMC, Bell JI, Hopkin JM, Cookson WOCM. HLA DR and HLA DP genotypes and immunoglobulin E responses to common major allergens *Clin Exp Allergy* 1994; 24: 431-9.
8. D'Amato M, Scotto d' Abusco A, Maggi E, Sacerdoti G, Maurizio SM, Iozzino S, De Santo C, Oreste U, Tosi, D'Amato G, Baltadjeva D, Bjorksten B, Freidhoff LF, Lahoz C, Marsh DG, Reshev A, Ruffilli A. Association of responsiveness to the major pollen allergen of *Parietaria officinalis* with HLA-DRB1* alleles. A multicenter study. *Hum Immunol* 1997, in press.
9. D'Amato M, Sorrentino R. A simple and economical DRB1 typing procedure combining group-specific amplification, DNA heteroduplex and enzyme restriction analysis. *Tissue Antigens* 1994; 43: 295.
10. Moffat MF, Hill MP, Cornelis F, Schou C, Young RP, James AL, Ryan G, Le Souef P, Musk AW, Hopkins JM, Cookson WOCM. Genetic linkage of T-cell receptor alpha/delta complex to specific IgE responses. *Lancet* 1994; 343: 1597-600.

Family study of olive allergy: HLA class II, TcR and T epitope mapping

B. Cárdaba, A. Jurado, V. del Pozo, S. Gallardo, B. de Andrés, M. Cortegano, J.P. Albar[1], A. Plaza[2], F. Florido[3], P. Palomino, C. Lahoz

Department of Immunology, Fundación Jiménez Díaz, Avenida Reyes Católicos 2, 28040 Madrid, Spain
1 Biotechnology National Center (CNB), Autónoma University, Madrid, Spain
2 Department of Immunology, Clínica Pta de Hierro, Madrid, Spain
3 Allergy Department, Hospital General de Especialidades Ciudad de Jaen, Jaen, Spain

Olive tree (*Olea europaea*) is an specie widely distributed in Mediterranean area and its pollen is regarded as a major cause of respiratory allergy in those countries [1]. Several studies were carried out by different investigators in order to identified the olive pollen allergens, but were Lauzurica *et al.* [2, 3] who reported the identification and isolation of the two major allergens of this mediterranean tree: *Ole e* I and *Ole e* II, proteins of 17-19kD and 8kD respectively. Studies carried out lastly by Wheeler *et al.* [4] confirmed the reported characteristics of *Ole e* I and described its heterogeneous nature. Finally, this major allergen has been cloned and the complete amino acid sequence described by Villalba *et al.* [5, 6].

On the other hand, we have studied different aspects of the reactivity to olive pollen, in order to a better understanding of this allergic sensitization: Martín-Orozco *et al.* [7] using 6 isotyped and purified mAbs directed against the *Ole e* I found that *Ole e* I has at least, four epitopic determinants on its molecule identified by competition assays. The capacity of these epitopes to be also recognized by human IgE antibodies was in order of 20% assesed by binding inhibition assay.

Finally, we reported the relationship between HLA class II haplotypes and alleles, and the IgE antibody response to highly purified *Ole e* I, in two population (Spanish and Arab people) and we found a strong association between DR7 (DRB1*0701/2) and DQ2 (DQB1*0201) and this response [8, 9].

Results and discussion

In this study we try to go deeply into the three key points implicated in the antigen recognition for a better understanding of the response : HLA class II antigens, TcR and T cell reactive peptides (*Ole e* 1 peptides).

HLA class II

We studied 22 families (selected according to 12th Workshop HLA-Allergy criteria) composed by 4 members (n=88 subjects): parents non sensitized to olive pollen or only one of them, and two sibbling sensitized to olive, by skin test and RAST against olive pollen extract. The families were selected from Jaen, city in the south of Spain, were the olive tree is extensively distributed.

The final criteria of reactivity against *Ole e* 1 was: clinical manifestations of allergy, skin test and RAST positives, and significative levels of IgG and IgE a-*Ole e* 1. Following these criteria, 48 patients were IgE responders to *Ole e* 1.

The HLA class II antigens typing was performed in the 88 individuals: DNA was extracted from peripheral blood by "salting out method". The polymorphism of DRB1 locus was study by reverse dot-blot (Roche) and the polymorphism of DQB1 locus by PCR-SSO. The final results were that 17 families (77.2 %) showed the antigens DR7 and/or DQ2 (previously associated with *Ole e* 1 response by population studies) and 5 showed different antigens (22.7 %). When we analyzed the "informative families" (those whose parents showed allele differents for one or both loci, DRB1-DQB1) and compared the statistical signification in the presence of the relevant antigens (DR7, DQ2 and DR3), we only found a significative statistically increase in the DQ2 antigen ($p<0.05$ by Fisher's exact test): 14 families were informative for this antigen, and we found 21 sibbling compared with 14 that could be expect by probability. These results confirm the primary implication of DQ2 in the IgE antibody response against *Ole e* 1, as we have previuosly suggest by population studies [8, 9].

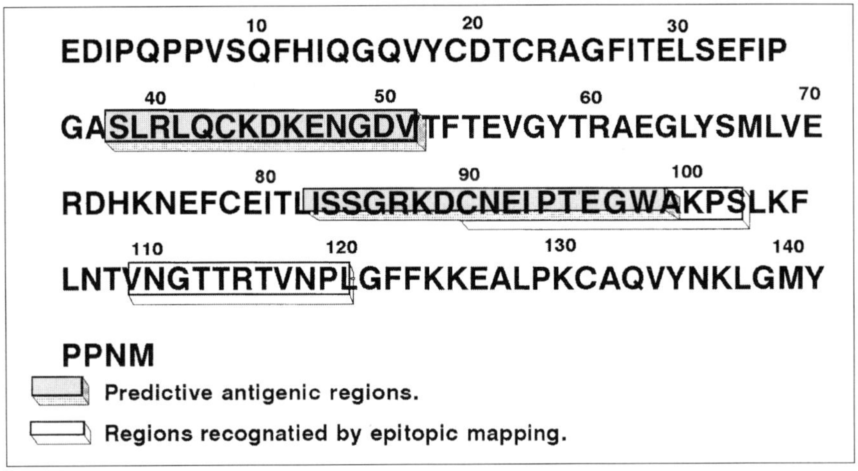

Figure 1. *Ole e* 1 sequence (Villalba *et al.* [6]).

Table I. Proliferation of PBLs to *Ole e* 1 peptides

	Peptides	1	2	3	4	5	6	7	9	10	11	12	13	14	15
Non allergics	P-55 (DR6)		+	+	+	+	+								
	P-56 (DR3-DR1)									+	+				
	P-11 (DR7-DR10)														
	P-12 (DR4)														
	P-19 (DR5-DR3)														
	P-91						+	+			+	+			
	P-20 (DR7-DR2)		+	+				+							
	P-92 (DR4-DR5)														
	P-93 (DR5-DR2)	N=9 (4 respond vs 5 non)													
Allergics	P-42 (DR7-DR5)									+					
	P-43 (DR3-DR5)											+			
	P-9 (DR4-DR10)							+		+					
	P-54 (DR6-DR3)									+		+	+		
	P-53 (DR6-DR3)										+	+	+		
	P-18 (DR7-DR5)	N=7(71.4% peptide 10,								+		+			
	P-RO (DR7-DR5)	57% peptide 12).								+	+		+		

TcR study

We selected two families (of the previous study) composed by 5 members (parents, two sibbling sensitized to olive pollen and one sibbling not allergic) and we studied the varibility in the Vßchain of TcR, in order to see if *a priori* there was some difference between "responders" and "non responders". The Vß polymorphism was analyzed in the PBLs of this subjects by flow cytometry, using 14 monoclonal antibodies (labeled with fluoresceine) that recognize: CD3, CD4, CD8, TcRaß, Vß2/CD3, 13.3, 17, 3, 5(a), 5(b), 5(c), 6(a), 8(a) and 12(a). The results showed that there are not any difference in the repertory of Vß between "reponders" and "non-responders" to *Ole e* 1.

T cell epitopes of Ole e 1

Finally, we search for the immunodominat epitopes in the *Ole e* 1 molecule, studyng the proliferative response of PBLs (from allergic and non-allergic subjects) to

15 *Ole e* 1 synthetic peptides (overlapping dodecapeptides, sintetized according the sequence described in 6). The proliferative response to this 15 peptides was study in 9 non-allergics and 7 *Ole e* 1 responders patients, previously typed. *Table I* shows the results of proliferation assays after 6 days in culture. The (+) means a positive proliferative response compared with a control (without any antigen). The assays were performed in triplicated and only considered the assays whose the SD was > 10%. The antigens were tested a different dosis (0.1, 1, and 5 micrograms/ml).

The results (*Table I*) showed that 4 from the 9 non allergic subjects respond to some *Ole e* 1 peptides (P-55, 56, 91, 20), but without any clear pattern of response. In contrast, all the allergics patients tested ("*Ole e* 1 responders") showed significant response to some *Ole e* 1 peptide, and 5 of the 7 (71.4 %) significativelly proliferated to peptide 10 (90-102 aa) and 4 of the 7 (57 %) respond to peptide 12 (109-121 aa). These preliminary results are very interesting for us, because previously, Villalba *et al.* [5, 6] described by predictiv analysis the possibility that two regions around (38-51 aa) and (83-99 aa) could be implicated in the antigenicity of this allergen (*Figure 1*). Our results could confirm these predition, and suggest that, the region around 90-99 aa of *Ole e* 1 could be a good candidate to localizate immunodominant epitopes on this antigen.

This work has been supported by European Science Foundation (ESF).

References

1. Bousquet J, Guerin B, Hewitt B, Lim S, Michel FB. Allergy in the Mediterranean area III:cross reactivity among *Oleaceae* pollens. *Clin Allergy* 1985; 15:439-48.
2. Lauzurica P, Gurbindo C, Maruri N, Galocha B, Díaz R, González J, García R, Lahoz C. Olive (*Olea europea*) pollen allergens-I. Immunochemical charactirization by immunoblotting, CRIE and immunodetection by a monoclonal antibody. *Mol Immunol* 1988; 25: 329-35.
3. Lauzurica P, Maruri N, Galocha B, González J, Díaz R, Palomino P, Hernández D, García R, Lahoz C. Olive (*Olea europea*) pollen allergens-II. Isolation and characterization of two major antigens. *Mol Immunol* 1988; 25: 337-44.
4. Wheeler AW, Hickman BE, Fox B. Heterogeneity of a major allergen from olive (*Olea europea*) pollen. *Mol Immunol* 1990; 27: 631-6.
5. Villalba M, Batanero E, López-Otín C, Sánchez LM, Monsalve RI, González de la Peña M, Lahoz C, Rodríguez R. Cloning and expression of *Ole e* I, the major allergen from olive tree pollen. *J Biol Chem* 1994; 269: 15217-22.
6. Villalba M, Batanero E, López-Otín C, Sánchez LM, Monsalve RI, González de la Peña M, Lahoz C, Rodríguez R. The amino acid sequence of *Ole e* 1, the major allergen from olive tree (*Olea europaea*) pollen. *Eur J Biochem* 1993; 216: 863-9.
7. Martín-Orozco E, Cárdaba B, del Pozo V, de Andrés B, Villalba M, Gallardo S, Rodríguez-García MI, Fernández MC, Alché JD, Rodríguez R, Palomino P, Lahoz C. Epitope mapping, cross-reactivity with other Oleaceae pollens and ultrastructural localization. *Int Arch Allergy Appl* 1994; 104: 160-70.
8. Cárdaba B, Vilches C, Martín E *et al.* DR7 and DQ2 are positively associated with the immunoglobuline-E response to the main antigen of olive pollen (*Ole e* I) in allergic patients. *Hum Immunol* 1993; 38: 293-99.
9. Cárdaba B, de Pablo R, Vilches C, Martín E, Geller-Bernstein C, de Andrés B, Zaharán Y, del Pozo V, Gallardo S, de Arruda- Chaves E, Waisel Y, Palomino P, Kreisler M, Lahoz C. Allergy to olive pollen: T cell response from olive allergic patients is restricted by DR7-DQ2 antigens. *Clin Exp Allergy* 1996; 26: 316-22.

HLA in Infectious Diseases

Contents

Anti-malarial HLA-B53 in Africa and common DNA type HLA-B*1513 in Malaysian aborigines share a C-terminal pocket of peptide binding groove

K. Hirayama, L.H. Sulaiman, A. Kimura, O.K. Joo,
M. Kikuchi, M.Z.A. Samah, N.H. Abdullah, S. Kojima, M.J. Wah

Department of Medical Zoology, Saitama Medical School, Moroyama, Saitama 350-04, Japan. Division of Immunology and Biotechnology Center, Institute for Medical Research, Kuala Lumpur, Malaysia. Department of Tissue Physiology, Division of Adult Disease,Medical Research Institute, Tokyo Medical and Dental University, Tokyo, Japan. Department of Parasitology, Institute of Medical Science, University of Tokyo, Tokyo, Japan

Natural selection has been proposed as a major cause generating the MHC polymorphism. Hill *et al.* [1] reported that an HLA- class I antigen HLA-Bw53 and an HLA-class II haplotype DRB1*1302-DQB1*0501, which are common in the West African population of The Gambia, were associated with resistance to severe malaria, suggesting that malarial infection had influenced the evolution of MHC in that area for over millions of years. In the restricted area of Peninsular Malaysia, several tribes of aborigine called Orang Asli have been living in jungle and maintaining their own culture. *Plasmodium falciparum* malaria, a fatal disease especially for small children, is endemic in jungle of Malaysia. Mass blood surveys for malaria studies are carried out regularly on all inhabitants of endemic areas. In certain areas, up to 20-30% of the blood slides from the Orang Asli have been found to be positive for *P. falciparum* and/or *P. vivax*. In fact, the people living in these areas are immune against severe malaria and do not develop any significant clinical symptoms such as fever, headache, and aneamia even in the presence of parasitaemia. Therefore, it is probable that the African HLA-B53-like HLA specificity may have been selected by this strong environmental pressure in Malaysia.

In this study, we analyzed 56 unrelated healthy individuals of Malaysian aborigines for their polymorphism in the HLA-B gene to search for an HLA-B53-like gene in Malaysia.

Results

After hybridization with 20 sequence specific oligonucleotide probes (SSOs) covering the 44th to 49th, and 62nd to 88th amino acids of a1 domain of HLA-B, one specific pattern that was similar to ECB75.1 except for the 77th amino acid substitution [2,3] but having the Bw4 motif instead of Bw6 was found to be very common. Serologically, B75 with a Bw4 epitope was reported in Thai [4] and was named B77 [5]. The whole cDNA coding sequence of the HLA-B77 heavy chain has recently been published as HLA-B*1513 [2]. Therefore, we tentatively call this Malaysian B*1513-like DNA type as ECB1513 (epitope combination of HLA-B*1513).

Table I shows the frequency of each ECB type in the Melayu Asli and in the Senoi. The ECB-1513, 18, 27.2, 7, and 62 were prevalent in the Melayu Asli and the ECB-35, 1513, 58, and 40 in the Senoi. The frequency of ECB1513 was not so much different between the two groups (Melayu Asli: 44%, Senoi: 25%). Another finding is that HLA-B53/B51 was only seen in one out of 56 individuals (AF=1.6%). In addition, this person was typed to have HLA-B51 and not B53 by serology. Therefore, none of the 56 individuals analyzed carried HLA-B53, suggesting a low frequency of B53 in Malaysian aborigines.

To confirm that the present DNA typing results were comparative with serological typing, the ECB types obtained here were compared with serological types in the 25 Senoi individuals *(Table II)*. The most significant difference between the serological B type and the DNA-ECB type was related to ECB1513. All of the individuals bearing ECB1513 were typed as HLA-B62 or B63 with Bw4 motif. The data corresponded well with results in the international cell exchange previously reported [2]. Another problem is that two individuals, S008 and S022, who bear the serological B46 could not be determined to have ECB46 by the DNA typing, even though we could amplify enough amount of Bw6 fragment from both individuals *(Table II)*. It is possible that

Table I. Antigen frequency of the unrelated Orang Asli population[a]

	Melayu Asli		Senoi		Total	
ECB[b]	n=31	Af[c]	n=25	Af	n=56	Af
1513	13	41.9	6	24.0	19	33.9
18	13	41.9	3	12.0	16	28.6
7	8	25.8	2	8.0	10	17.9
35	2	6.5	7	28.0	9	16.1
62	7	22.6	2	8.0	9	16.1
58	0	0	5	20.0	5	8.9
40	0	0	4	16.0	4	7.1
27.2	4	12.9	0	0.0	4	7.1
13	1	3.2	2	8.0	3	5.4
57	1	3.2	2	8.0	3	5.4
52	2	6.5	0	0.0	2	3.6
75.1	2	6.5	0	0.0	2	3.6
3802	0	0	2	8.0	2	3.6
44	1	3.2	0	0.0	1	1.8
51/53	0	0	1	4.0	1	1.8
others[d]	1	3.2	8	32.0	9	16.1

[a] Subjects. Finger prick EDTA blood samples (0.2-0.5ml) were obtained from inhabitants in Gapoi village, Bentong District which is about 115km east of Kuala Lumpur. A total of 114 individuals including family members were screened and 31 unrelated individuals (17 males and 14 females) with a mean age of 31.7 years (range: 10 to 73) were selected at random. They were of the Temuan tribe that belongs to the Melayu Asli. Twenty ml of heparinized venous blood samples for both HLA-DNA typing and serological HLA typing also were collected from patients admitted to the Gombak hospital, 18 km east of Kuala Lumpur. Twenty five unrelated individuals with the mean age of 28.8 years (range: 10 to 66) were selected for the population study. They were of the Semai and Temiar tribes that belong to the same ethnic group, the Senoi, living in the central area of peninsular Malaysia.

[b] Epitope combination of HLA-B. DNA typing of HLA-B gene was done by the method described by Yoshida *et al.* [3]. Each ECB type was determined by the PCR amplification for Bw4/6 and by the combination of SSOs positively hybridized. ECB-44, 49, 47, 58, 52, 37, 51/53, 57, 13, 59, 38, 27.2, 27.1, 40 (60, 61, 41, 45, 50), 48.2, 18, 35, 62, 75.1, 46, 75.2, 48.1, 8,14 (14, 39, 65), 70, 7 (7, 42, 55, 56, 67), 54 can be discriminated by the use of this method.

[c] Af: antigen frequency.

[d] Undefined type that was typed by serology but was not determined by the DNA typing.

we have detected a new B46 variant by the DNA typing. We then cloned HLA-B genes from two ECB1513 positive individuals to determine the structure of the ECB1513. Sequencing analysis of the cloned ECB1513 genes revealed that they were identical to HLA-B*1513 in the sequenced exons, from exon 1 to exon 4. It was, therefore, confirmed that HLA-B*1513 was a common HLA-B allele in this population.

Within the amino acids facing to the binding groove of HLA-class I molecule, those forming the B (P2) pocket and F (P9) pocket have been postulated to be important for predicting the shape of the antigenic peptide or its motif [6,7]. HLA-B*1513 had exactly the same amino acid sequences as HLA-B*5301 between 74th to 116th amino acids forming the F pocket *(Table III)*.

Finally, we have estimated their serum levels of IgG against *falciparum* malaria. As shown in *Figure 1*, HLA-B*1513 positive individuals showed significantly lower titer of antibody against the schizont form of malaria ($p<0.005$).

Discussion

DNA typing of the HLA-B gene in the peninsular Malaysian aborigines by using the SSOP method [3] was compared with conventional serological typing. Discordance was observed in rare cases as shown in *Table II* except for the HLA-B*1513 antigen. Because the DNA typing of HLA-B is not routinely used, there is not enough information about the distribution of each ECB type in the other ethnic groups in the regions around Malaysia. Given the information of serology in Thais, Singaporean Chinese,

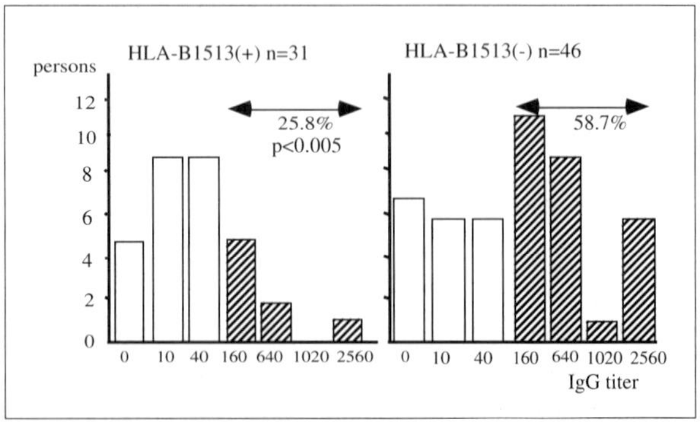

Figure 1. Negative association between the high IgG titer against p.falciparum schizont and HLA-B*1513.
The plasma levels of anti schizont IgG antibody were measured by the immunofluoscein staining. Cultured parasites were fixed on the glass slides and the serial dilutions (10x, 40x, 160x, 640x, 1280x, 2560x) of the plasma samples were added on the slides and incubated for 30 min. After washing with PBS containing 2% FCS, FITC labelled gout anti human IgG was added on the slides. After incubation at 37°C, the slides were washed and examined under UV microscopy.

Table II. Serology and DNA typing of the Malaysian aborigine population[a]

	Serology [b]			DNA typing		Serology		
No.	HLA-A	Bw	HLA-B	Bw	ECB	C	HLA-DR	DQ
S001	24, -	4,-	63, -	4,-	1513, -	BL	2,9	1,3
S002	24,34	-,6	-, 35	-,6	- ,35	4,6	2,-	1,-
S003	26,34	4,6	58,35	4,6	58,35	3,-	2,6	1,-
S004	24,34	-,6	62,61	-,6	40,62	6,7	4,-	3,-
S005	24,33	4,-	58, -	4,-	58, -	3,7	2,-	1,-
S006	2,11	4,6	62,38	4,-	1513, UND[c]	6,7	2,5	1,3
S007	24,11	4,6	38,60	4,6	3802,UND	3,7	2,-	1,-
S008	24,33	4,6	5, 46	4,6	58,UND	1,-	-	-
S009	2,-	4,6	62,18	4,6	57,18	7,-	2,9	1,3
S010	24,-	4,6	13,35	4,6	13,35	4,6	2,-	1,-
S011	24,-	4,6	62, -	4,6	1513,7	1,-	2,6	1,-
S012	2,24	4,-	13,63	4,-	1513,UND	3,4	2,-	1,-
S013	11,-	-,6	- ,60	-,6	-,40	6,7	2,-	1,-
S014	2,24	4,-	13,63	4,-	1513,UND	3,-	2,-	1,-
S015	1,24	4,-	13,38	4,-	13, 3802	3,7	2,-	1,-
S016	2,33	4,-	58,27	4,-	58,UND	3,-	2,8	1,3
S017	2,24	4,6	51,62	4,-	51,UND	BL	8,-	1,-
S018	24,34	-,6	22,60	-,6	40,7	1,3	2,-	1,-
S019	24,-	-,6	35,60	-,6	35,40	3,4	2,-	1,-
S020	2,24	4,6	35,63	4,6	1513,35	4,-	2,-	1,-
S021	24,34	-,6	62,-	-,6	62,-	7,-	2,-	1,-
S022	24,33	4,6	5,46	4,6	58,UND	1,3	-	-
S023	2,11	-,6	18,-	-,6	-,18	6,7	9,-	3,-
S024	24,-	4,6	63,35	4,6	57,35	4,-	5,-	3,-
S025	2,24	-,6	18,35	-,6	18,35	4,7	5,-	3,-

[a] The Senoi's unrelated population (n=25). Serology and HLA typing were performed independently.
[b] Serological typing. Mononuclear cells were separated by Ficoll-paque centrifugation. A part of them were stored at -80°C for DNA work and the residual cells were used for NIH microcytotoxicity test to type HLA-A,B,C and DR, except for HLA-B57 and B75 by using well established local and exchanged antisera, as described previously [2].
[c] Undefined types that was typed by serology but was not determined by the DNA typing.

Javanese, southern Hans, and Papua New Guinean populations reported in the XI th international HLA Workshop [8], HLA-B77 (B*1513) was indeed very rare around Malaysia. Because there are so many evolutionally related subtypes of HLA-B15 [2], it is interesting that HLA-B*1513 appears characteristic to the Malaysian aborigine population that is thought to be resistant against severe malaria. Hill *et al.* [9] reported that anti-malarial cytotoxic T cells from B53 positive donors recognized an antigenic peptide derived from Liver stage specific antigen 1 that contained a B53 binding motif but not a B35 motif. These findings combined with the strong association between B53 and resistance against malaria in Gambia suggest that HLA-B53 is effective in generating anti-malarial CTL due to its high affinity to some major antigenic peptide produced in the host hepatocyte while HLA-B35 is not so effective. Because the only difference between HLA-B*5301 and B*3501 is located in the F pocket due to the replacement of Bw4/6 epitopes [10], the shape of the C-terminal pocket should be critical for the development of immunity against malaria. Thus, the fact that B*1513 and B*1502 differ only in Bw4/6 within the a1 domain implies that the same kind of genetic events such as gene conversion may have happened during the course of evolution of the HLA-B gene in Malaysian aborigines. The specific shape of the F pocket shared by B*5301 and B*1513 might have some advantage to be maintained in the endemic areas for malaria, although it is practically impossible to compare the

allele distribution in the populations who have the same ancestral origin and reside in the non-endemic area.
In conclusion, HLA-B*1513 was independently found to be prevalent in the different groups of Malaysian aborigine and shared the C-terminal peptide binding pocket (pocket F) with an African resistant type against severe malaria, HLA-B*5301.

Table III. Peptide binding residues in the a1 and a2 domains of the HLA-B molecules

	P2 (B pocket[a])				P9 (F pocket[a])				
position	45	63	66	67	74	77	80	81	116
HLA-B*5301	T	N	I	F	Y	N	I	A	S
HLA-B*1513	M	-	-	S	-	-	-	-	-

Sequencing analysis of ECB1513. A DNA region of the HLA-B gene, from exon 1 to exon 4, was amplified by PCR from genomic DNAs of two ECB1513-positive individuals. Primers used in the PCR were ABC1F (5'-CAGAATCTCCTCAGACGCC-3') and B4R (5'-TGGAAGGTTCT(A/G)TCTCCT(G/C) CTGGT-3'). ABC1F was designed in the 5' untranslated region, from -23 to -5 upstream of the ATG codon, and B4R was designed in exon 4, positions from 797 to 724, to allow for a specific amplification of the HLA-B gene, because the 3' terminal nucleotide of B4R was matched to all known HLA-B alleles and not to HLA-A or -C alleles. PCR conditions were identical to those described above, except that 95 °C 1 min, 60 °C 1 min, and 72 °C 2 min steps were used. The PCR products of about 1 kb were cloned by using a TA cloning kit (Invitrogen, San Diego, CA) according to the manufacturer's instructions. At least 7 independent clones from each panel were sequenced for exon 1, 2, 3, and 4 by using a sequencing kit (Sequenase ver. 2, Amersham Japan, Tokyo) and sequencing primers; ABC2F (5'-CCCAGGCTCC-CACTCCATG-3'), ABC2SF (5'-CGACAGCGACGC-3'), ABC2SR (5'-TACTCCGGCCCCT-3'), ABC3SF (5'-CGG-CAAGGATTACA-3'), ABC3SR (5'-ACTTGCGCTGGG-3), and M13 universal -40 and M13 reverse primers (Amersham Japan, Tokyo).The sequences of HLA-B*5301 was obtained from the Gene bank nucleotide sequence database. Amino acids are represented by single letter code. Identities to HLA-B*5301 are indicated by dashes. [a]Silver, ML *et al.* 1992.

Acknowledgments

We thank the Director, Institute for Medical Research (IMR), Kuala Lumpur for permission to publish this paper. This study was supported in part by the IMR-Japan International Cooperation Agency (JICA) Project on Tropical Diseases technically managed by Dr. H. Tanaka, Chief Adviser and by Grant-in-Aid for Scientific Research on Priority Areas, from to the Ministry of Education, Science and Culture of Japan. We are grateful to Dr. Mohamad Ali M, Director, Gombak Hospital, and to Dr. Nik Shamsidah N.I. and Dr. Chan K.H. of Bentong Health Office for their cooperation and assistance.

References

1. Hill AVS, Allsopp CEM, Kwiatkowski D, *et al.* Common West African HLA antigens are associated with protection from severe malaria. *Nature* 1991; 352: 595-600.
2. Hildebrand WH, Domena JD, Shen SY, *et al.* HLA-B15: A widespread and diverse family of HLA-B alleles. *Tissue Antigens* 1994; 43: 209-18.
3. Yoshida M, Kimura A, Numano F, Sasazuki T. Polymerase-chain-reaction-based analysis of polymorphism in the HLA-B gene. *Hum Immunol* 1992; 34: 257-66.
4. Cambon-Tomsen D, Chandanayingyong M, Thomsen M, Hammond MG. Antigen report: HLA-Bw63 and other Bw4-associated variants of B15. In: Albert ED, ed. Histocompatibility Testing 1984. Berlin, Heidelberg: Springer-Verlag 1984; 171-2.
5. Nisperos BB, Chung KH, Hansen JA, *et al.* Antigen society reports No.108: HLA-B15, -B62, -B63, -B75, -B76, -B77, -B46. In: Tsuji K, Aizawa M, Sasazuki T, eds. *HLA 1991: Proceedings of the Eleventh International Histocompatibility Workshop and Conference*, vol. I. Oxford, New York, Tokyo: Oxford University Press, 1991; 310-5.
6. Silver ML, Guo H-C, Strominger JL, Wiley DC. Atomic structure of a human MHC molecule presenting an influenza virus peptide. *Nature* 1992; 360: 367-9.
7. Sidney J, Del Guercio MF, Southwood C, *et al.* Several HLA alleles share overlapping peptide specificities. *J Immunol* 1995; 154: 247-59.
8. Imanishi T, Akaza T, Kimura A, Tokunaga K, Gojobori T. Allele and haplotype frequencies for HLA and complement loci in various ethnic groups. In: Tsuji K, Aizawa M, Sasazuki T, eds. *HLA 1991: Proceedings of the Eleventh International Histocompatibility Workshop and Conference*, vol. I. Oxford, New York, Tokyo: Oxford University Press, 1991; 1065-119.
9. Hill AVS, Elvin J, Willis AC, *et al.* Molecular analysis of the association of HLA-B53 and resistance to severe malaria. *Nature* 1992; 360: 434-40.
10. Allsopp CEM, Hill AVS, Kwiatkowski D, *et al.* Sequence analysis of HLA-Bw53, a common West African allele, suggests an origin by gene conversion of HLA-B35. *Hum Immunol* 1991; 30: 105-9.

HLA and leprosy in Japanese

S. Joko[1,2], J. Numaga[1], K. Masuda[1], H. Maeda[2]

1 Department of Ophthalmology, University of Tokyo School of Medicine, 7-3-1 Hongo Bunkyo-ku, Tokyo 113, Japan
2 Blood Transfusion Service, Saitama Medical Center, Saitama Medical School, 1981 Tujido Kamoda Kawagoe, Saitama 350, Japan

Leprosy is a chronic infectious disease by Mycobacterium leprae and was reported to be positively associated with HLA-DR2 and DQ1 in several previous studies [1-6]. But there have been a few reports on the relationship between HLA class II genotypes and leprosy [5,7]. To the best of the author's knowledge, there have been no reports on the relationship between HLA class II genotypes except for HLA-DRB1*1501 and Japanese leprosy patients [5]. In the present study, we have analyzed HLA-DRB1, DRB5, DQA1 and DQB1 genotypes in the Japanese leprosy patients to investigate the immunogenetic background of the disease.

Materials and method

The subjects were 93 Japanese leprosy patients. All of them had been hospitalized in the National Leprosarium, Tama-Zensho-En, Tokyo, Japan. The diagnosis of leprosy was based on clinical manifestations, histological features, bacteriological examinations. 114 unrelated volunteers were randomly selected from the healthy unrelated Japanese blood donors at the Saitama Medical Center as controls. All subjects gave informed consent.

After serologic typing of HLA-DR and -DQ antigens, HLA-DRB1, DRB5, DQA1 and DQB1 genotypings were performed by using the polymerase chain reaction (PCR)-single strand conformation polymorphism and PCR-restriction fragment length polymorphism methods [8-10].

Fisher's exact test or chi-square analysis was employed to determine the statistical significance of the differences between patients and normal controls. Relative risk was estimated from the odds ratio.

Results

Table I shows the phenotype frequencies of HLA-DRB1, DRB5, DQA1 and DQB1 in the patients and controls. The frequencies of HLA-DRB1*1501, DRB5*0101, DQA1*0102 and DQB1*0602 were significantly increased in the patients. Relative risks for HLA-DRB1*1501, DRB5*0101, DQA1*0102 and DQB1*0602 were 4.6, 4.6, 3.0 and 4.6, respectively. The frequencies of HLA-DRB1*0405, *0803, *0901 and DQA1*03 and DQB1*0401 were significantly decreased in the patients. These alleles gave relative risks of 0.25 , 0.32, 0.47, 0.32 and 0.22, respectively.

Discussion

Previous studies demonstrated the associations of HLA-DR2 and DQ1 antigens with leprosy, but those studies

Table I. Phenotype frequencies of HLA-DRB1, DRB5, DQA1 and DQB1 alleles in patients and controls

HLA Genotypes	Patients n=93 n(%)	Controls n=114 n(%)	Relative Risk	P value
DRB1*1501	40(43.0)	16(14.0)	4.6	$< 5.0X10^{-6}$
*1502	30(32.2)	24(21.1)		
*0403	6(6.5)	9(7.9)		
*0405	9(9.7)	34(29.8)	0.25	$< 5.0X10^{-6}$
*0410	2(2.2)	5(4.4)		
*0802	3(2.2)	8(7.0)		
*0803	6(6.5)	20(17.5)	0.32	< 0.05
*0901	16(17.2)	35(30.7)	0.47	< 0.05
DRB5*0101	40(43.0)	16(14.0)	4.6	$< 5.0X10^{-6}$
*0102	30(32.2)	24(21.1)		
DQA1*0102	49(52.7)	31(27.2)	3.0	$< 5.0X10^{-4}$
*0103	37(39.8)	39(34.2)		
*03	40(43.0)	80(78.1)	0.32	$< 1.0X10^{-4}$
DQB1*0601	37(39.8)	38(33.3)		
*0602	38(40.9)	15(13.2)	4.6	$< 1.0X10^{-5}$
*0401	8(8.6)	34(29.8)	0.22	$< 5.0X10^{-4}$

were limited to serologic typing. In 1993, Rani and his colleagues reported that the frequencies of HLA-DRB1*1501, *1502 and DRB5*0101, *0102 and DQA1*0102, *0103 and DQB1*0601 were significantly increased in leprosy patients from North India as compared with normal controls [7]. These alleles gave relative risks of 7.6, 3.2, 7.6, 3.2, 2.9, 2.8 and 7.4, respectively. HLA-DRB1*0404, *0701, *1401 and DQB1*0503 were significantly decreased in the patients. These gave relative risks of 0.04, 0.3, 0.05 and 0.3, respectively.

Previously, we investigated only the DRB1 genes and described the positive association of DRB1*1501 in DR2-positive Japanese patients with leprosy [5]. In this study, we performed a DNA typing for HLA-DRB1, DRB5, DQA1 and DQB1 genotypes in the Japanese leprosy patients and compared our findings between the patients and controls. HLA-DRB1*1501, DRB5*0101, DQA1*0102 and DQB1*0602 were positively associated with the Japanese patients. The increased frequencies of HLA-DRB1*1501, DRB5*0101 and DQA1*0102 were found in both populations, whereas no consistent DQB1 allele was increased. From the viewpoint of relative risk, the most important genotypes were HLA-DRB1*1501 and DRB5*0101: relative risk for HLA-DRB1*1501 was 4.6 as well as DRB5*0101 in this study and 7.6 in Rani's, the greatest of all.

These findings indicate that HLA-DRB1*1501 and/or DRB5*0101 play more important role in the pathogenesis of leprosy than DQ alleles. However, it is difficult to determine which of two alleles is responsible for the leprosy susceptibility because of the strong linkage disequilibrium between HLA-DRB1*1501 and DRB5*0101.

On the other hand, HLA-DRB1*0405, *0803, *0901 and DQA1*03 and DQB1*0401 were negatively associated with the Japanese patients. These results were not consistent with Rani's report. Thus the other HLA, non-HLA gene and/or environmental factors may play critical role in resistance to leprosy.

References

1. Miyanaga K, Juji T, Maeda H, Nakajima S, Kobayashi S. Tuberuculoid leprosy and HLA in Japanese. *Tissue Antigens* 1981; 18: 331-4.
2. Kim SJ, Choi IH, Dahlberg S, Nisperos B, Kim JD, Hansen JA. HLA and leprosy in Koreans. *Tissue Antigens* 1987; 29: 146-53.
3. Todd JR, West BC, McDonald JC. Human leukocyte antigen and leprosy: study in northern Louisiana and review. *Rev Infect Dis* 1990; 12: 63-74.
4. Rani R, Zaheer SA, Mukherjee R. Do human leukocyte antigens have a role to play in differential manifestation of multibacillary leprosy: A study on multibacillary leprosy patients from North India. *Tissue Antigens* 1992; 40: 124-7.
5. Joko S, Numaga J, Fujino Y, Masuda K, Hirata R, Maeda H. HLA-DR2 alleles and uveitis in leprosy (in Japanese). *Jan J Lepr* 1995 ; 64: 112-8.
6. Joko S, Numaga J, Fujino Y, Masuda K, Hirata R, Maeda H. HLA and uveitis in leprosy (in Japanese). *J Jpn Ophthalmol Soc* 1995; 99: 1181-5.
7. Rani R, Fernandez-Vina MA, Zaheer SA, Beena KR , Stastny P. Study of HLA class ll alleles by PCR oligotyping in leprosy patients from North India. *Tissue Antigens* 1993; 42: 133-7.
8. Orita M, Iwahana H, Kanazawa H, Hayashi K, Sekiya T. Detection of polymorphisms of human DNA by gel electrophoresis as single-strand conformation polymorphisms. *Proc Natl Acad Sci USA* 1989; 86: 2766-70.
9. Ota M, Seki T, Fukushima H, Tsuji K, Inoko H. HLA-DRB1 genotyping by modified PCR-RFLP method combined with group-specific primers. *Tissue Antigens* 1992; 39: 187-202.
10. Saiki RK, Bugawan TL, Horn GT, Mullis KB, Erlich HA. Analysis of enzymatically amplified β-globin and HLA-DQα DNA with allele-specific oligonucleotide probes. *Nature* 1986; 324: 163-6.

HLA haplotypes associated with antibody non-responders to the present hepatitis B vaccine and with their response to a pre-S1 and pre-S2 containing hepatitis B vaccine

A.B. McDermott[1], J.N. Zuckerman[2], C.A. Sabin[2], A. Madrigal[1,2]

1 Anthony Nolan Research Institute
2 Royal Free Hospital School of Medicine, Pond street, Hampstead, London NW3 2QG, UK

Hepatitis B virus (HBV) infection is endemic in many regions of the world and represents a major public health problem. Current immunisation for protection against hepatitis B virus (HBV) infection is mediated by a vaccine containing a surface protein coded for by the 'S' region of the viral genome. Post vaccination an individual is considered, by WHO guidelines, to be 'protected' if the antibody titre (anti-HBs) is >100 IU/l, although in many countries production of 10 IU/l or more is considered a immune response. Approximately 5-10% of healthy vaccine recipients do not demonstrate a protective levels of antibody following repeated injections of 'S' containing vaccine. Aiming to increase immunogenicity a new vaccine, "Hep B-3", has been developed with the potential to enhance immunogenicity and efficacy. This vaccine contains the products of preS1 and preS2 regions of the viral genome which together with the S region code for the coat proteins of HBV. The addition of preS1 and preS2 antigenic components may mimic more closely the immune response associated with HBV infection. Studies in HBsAg non-responding mouse strains have demonstrated that immunisation with the additional components preS1 or preS2 elicits both cellular and humoral immune responses [1,2].

Several studies in humans have identified HLA haplotypes which are associated with antibody non-response to 'S' containing vaccine [3]. For example Craven *et al.* [4] studied 28 non-responding individuals and suggested that the common Caucasian extended MHC haplotypes B44; DR7; FC31 and B8; DR3; SC01 were frequently associated with non-response to HBsAg vaccines. They suggested that inheritance of the non-responder haplotype A1; B8; DR3 is a recessive trait in the Caucasian population [4,5]. In the Japanese population, non-responsiveness has been reported to be associated with the haplotype HLA-B54 DR4-DQ4 which is expressed at a high frequency in the population [6]. It has been reported that the cellular basis of non-response is associated with T-cells rather than a defect in antigen presentation [7]. In addition, individuals who fail to mount an adequate HBs-antibody response fail to proliferate *in vitro* to vaccine derived 'S' antigen [8].

For the purpose of a vaccine trial 86 true non-responders were recruited and revaccinated with Hep-B3 vaccine. From this we could study both HLA within (a) HBs-antibody non-response to vaccination and (b) the relationship of HBs-antibody response to revaccination with Hep-B3 vaccine. The control groups for this study consisted of 115 vaccine responders (HBs-antibody >100 IU/l) and 170 Caucasian individuals selected randomly from the Anthony Nolan donor register. All the trial subjects and controls were typed for HLA class I by serology and HLA class II by PCR-sequence specific oligonucleotides (SSO) typing method. The specific anti-HBs antibody titres were measured by two enzyme immunoassays (EIA), using commercial kits (Biokit, Spain and Ausab EIA, Abbott Laboratories, N. Chicago) according to the manufacturer's protocol. The frequencies of the antigens and alleles were compared using logistic regression methods. Also, we compare the odds ratio associated with being a trial subject to control subjects together with the associated p-value from the logistic regression *(Tables I - III).*

We identified 38 class I antigens and 30 class II alleles in our study population which are summarised in *Table I*. The number of HBs-antibody non-responder individuals expressing the allele DRB1*0701 was 52.3% which was significantly different from the expected 26.7% of the HLA control group and 24.8% of the HBs-antibody responder group. The allele DQB1*0201 is in linkage disequilibrium with DRB1*0701 and was also at a significantly higher frequency compared to controls. However, the antigen HLA-DQ1 was under-represented in the HBs-antibody non-responder population in comparison with both control groups. The HLA-DQ1 serotype is split into the molecular subtypes DQB1*0501-3 and DQB1*0601-5. From our data the frequency of HLA-DQB1*0602 was significantly

Table I. Relationship of HLA and Hbs-antibody non-response to vaccination

- HLA Antigen (HLA Allele)	HLA Control Group	Hep B-3 Trial Subjects			Vaccine Control Group		
	% with Antigen	% with Antigen	Odds Ratio	p-value*	% with Antigen	Odds Ratio	p-value*
B8	27.7	29.1	1.07	0.81	24.4	1.27	0.45
B44	33.5	40.7	1.36	0.26	24.4	2.13	0.01
DR1 (DRB1*0101/02/03)	21.4	11.6	0.48	0.07	28.7	0.33	0.005
DR3 (DRB1*0301)	28.2	32.6	1.23	0.50	21.8	1.73	0.10
DR7 (DRB1*0701)	**26.7**	**52.3**	**3.01**	**0.0002**	**24.8**	**3.34**	**0.0001**
DR8 (DRB1*0801)	3.1	2.3	0.76	0.75	5.0	0.46	0.36
DR15 (DRB1*1501)	31.3	27.0	0.36	0.005	31.8	0.80	0.59
DQ1 (DQB1*0501-3, DQB1*0601-5)	**62.8**	**40.0**	**0.4**	**0.001**	**62.1**	**0.41**	**0.003**
DQ2 (DQB1*0201)	**43.8**	**64.7**	**2.36**	**0.003**	**24.3**	**5.72**	**0.0001**

* p-value quoted from logistic regression analysis. This is not adjusted for multiple comparisons.

Table II. DQB1* subtypes

- HLA DQ1 (DQB1*)	HLA Control Group	Hep B-3 Trial Subjects			Vaccine Control Group		
	% with Antigen	% with Antigen	Odds Ratio	p-value*	% with Antigen	Odds Ratio	p-value*
0501	23.3	15.3	0.6	0.16	26.2	0.51	0.07
0502	0.8	2.4	3.08	0.36	1.0	2.46	0.47
05031	5.4	2.4	0.42	0.29	5.8	0.39	0.26
0601	0.8	0	0.02	0.68	1.0	0.01	0.66
0602	**28.7**	**9.4**	**0.26**	**0.001**	**23.3**	**0.34**	**0.01**
0603	6.2	5.9	0.95	0.92	8.7	0.65	0.46
0604	4.7	2.4	0.49	0.39	6.8	0.33	0.17
0605	2.3	5.9	2.63	0.19	2.9	2.08	0.32

* p-value quoted from logistic regression analysis. This is not adjusted for multiple comparisons.

lower in the HBsAg non-responder group than in the HLA control population *(Table II)*. We could not identify any significant relationship between class I antigens and HBs-antibody non-response. Within our HBs-antibody non-responder we identified a significant association with the haplotype B44;DR7 *(Table III)*. However, we could not see an association with the haplotype B8;DR3 as previously suggested [4,5].

Table III. Haplotype analysis

HLA Haplotype	HLA Control Group	Hep B-3 Trial Subjects			Vaccine Control Group		
	% with Antigen	% with Antigen	Odds Ratio	p-value*	% with Antigen	Odds Ratio	p-value*
B8; DR3	22.1	26.7	1.28	0.44	15.8	1.94	0.07
B44; DR7	**11.5**	**29.1**	**3.17**	**0.002**	**9.9**	**3.73**	**0.001**
B7; DR15	13.0	5.8	0.41	0.10	8.9	0.63	0.43
B44; DR4	13.7	16.3	1.22	0.61	9.9	1.77	0.2
B35; DR1	8.4	5.8	0.67	0.48	6.9	0.83	0.76

* p-value quoted from logistic regression analysis. This is not adjusted for multiple comparisons.

When the trial subjects were revaccinated with the additional immunogenic components in the Hep-B3 vaccine, 33.7% produced HBs-antibody of <10 IU/l. We analysed the correlation of HLA haplotypes and HBs-antibody non-response and 62% (18/29) expressed the haplotypes B8;DR3;DQ2 (34%) or B44;DR7 (28%). All individuals expressing the haplotype B7; DR15; DQ6 produced HBs-antibody of > 100 IU/l. A further analysis was carried out with the trial subjects grouped according to whether they exhibited a >50% decrease in HBs antibody titre between months 2 and 6 post vaccination *(Table IV)*. Of those individuals with a >50% decrease in HBs-antibody titre 50% (11/22) were either B8; DR3; DQ2 or B44; DR7; DQ2 haplotypes. In addition, no subjects with B7; DR15; DQ6 had a >50% decrease in HBs antibody titre. Preliminary *in vitro* assays revealed that HBs-antibody non-responders proliferate to Hep-B3 derived antigens. This cellular response is due to the products of preS1 and preS2 regions of the viral genome which are present in the vaccine.

Table IV. Transient antibody response

HLA Phenotype	>50% Decrease in titre	
	Number tested	% with phenotype
DR1; DQ5	22	9.1
DR15; DQ6	22	9.1
B7; DR15; DQ6	22	0.0
B44; DR7; DQ2	22	13.6
B8; DR3; DQ2	22	36.4

Therefore, despite the inclusion of additional immunogenic viral components, 2 common Caucasian haplotypes (B8; DR3; DQ2 and B44; DR7; DQ2) were associated with HBs-antibody non-response. These haplotypes were also associated with transient antibody responses. This has implications for the design of future HBV vaccine strategies.

References

1. Milich DR, Thornton GB, Neurath AR *et al.* Enhanced immunogenicity of the Pre-S region of hepatitis B surface antigen. *Science* 1985; 228: 1195-8.
2. Milich DR, Hughes JL, Mclachlan A *et al.* Importance of subtype in the immune to the response ro the pre-S2 region of the hepatitis B surface antigen. *J Immunol* 1990; 144 : 3535-43.
3. Walker M, Szmuness W, Stevens CE, Rubinstein P. Genetics if anti-HBs responsiveness: I HLA DR7 and non-responsiveness to hepatitis B vaccination. *Transfusion* 1981; 21: 601.
4. Craven DE, Awdeh ZL, Kunches LM *et al.* Nonresponsivenes to hepatitis B vaccine in health care workers. *Ann Intern Med* 1986; 105 : 356-60.
5. Alper CA, Kruskhall MS, Marcus-Bagley D *et al.* Genetic prediction of non-response to hepatitis B vaccine. *N Engl J Med* 1989; 321: 708-12.
6. Hatae K, Kimura A, Okubo R *et al.* Genetic control of nonresponsiveness to hepatitis B virus vaccine by an extended haplotype. *Eur J Immunol* 1992; 22: 1899-905.
7. Desombere I, Hauser P, Rosseau R *et al.* 1995; Nonresponders to hepatitis B vaccine can present envelope particles to T lymphocytes. *J Immunol* 1995; 154: 520-9.
8. Egea E, Iglesias A, Salazar M *et al.* The cellular basis for the lack of antibody response to Hepatitis B vaccine in humans. *J Exp Med* 1991; 173: 531-8.

HLA phenotypes in long term asymptomatics, HIV-infected adult individuals in France

I. Theodorou[1], B. Autran[1], A. Goubar[2], D. Costagliola[2], J.M. Bouley[1], F. Sanson[1], E. Gomard[3], Y. Rivière[3], C. Katlama[3], H. Agut[4], J.P. Clauvel[4], D. Sicard[4], C. Rouzioux[4], C. Raffoux[5], D. Charron[5], P. Debré[1]

1. Laboratoire Central d' Immunologie et URA CNRS 625 , Hôpital de la Pitié-Salpétrière, Bâtiment CERVI, 83, boulevard de l'Hôpital, 75013 Paris, France
2. Centre Cooperateur de Données Epidémiologiques sur l'Immunodéficience Humaine, INSERM SC4, Paris, France
3. The Immunoco study group
4. The ALT study group
5. Laboratoire d'Immunologie, Hôpital Saint-Louis, Paris, France

Many recent reports have focused attention on the relationship between the clinical variability of HIV-1 disease and HLA phenotype. Two different types of studies were conducted; one focusing on particular manifestations at advanced stages of HIV disease and another on disease free survival according to the patient's HLA phenotype [1-6]. Disease free survival studies have been performed in cohorts composed of less than 200 individuals and have drawn conclusions by comparing HLA haplotypes in rapid progressors compared to the general HIV population. Since most of the studies have been conducted in different ethnic groups, treated with different regimens, infected with different viral strains, presenting different risk factors, results are sometimes confusing. In order to clarify this issue, studies conducted in groups treated as homogeneously as possible should be performed. Concordance in the HLA haplotypes found in different ethnic populations infected with the same viral strains would strongly argue in favor of a protection by these particular HLA haplotypes or alleles probably due to more efficient presentation of viral peptides to T cell receptors. In this regard patients with a long and regular follow up with the same ethnic origin and not treated at all after the discovery of HIV infection constitute the best population to address this question.

In this study we analyzed HLA-A, HLA-B and HLA DRB1 gene frequencies in a population of long term asymptomatic (LTA) patients compared to a population of HIV infected individuals showing standard or rapid disease progression. LTA patients were selected among French Caucasians and fulfilled the following criteria: (a) Seropositive for more than 8 years (b) a peripheral blood CD4+ lymphocyte count of more than 600 per mm3 (c) a positive or null slope for the CD4+ count during the last two years (d) absence of clinical signs of disease progression (e) not treated with antiretroviral agents. 41 patients were included in this group. Patients with these characteristics represent less than 5% of the general HIV infected population in France. We used as a control population patients from the Immunoco cohort recruited at the Pitié-Salpetrière Hospital for the study of HIV specific CTL responses during HIV infection. Only patients presenting the same ethnic origins as the LTA patients, a known delay from the diagnosis of seropositivity and not fulfilling the LTA criteria were used as a control group. 111 patients were included in this latter group. In both cohorts the sex ratio, mean age and risk factors were comparable. HLA typing was performed with standard serological methods for HLA A and HLA B antigens for both LTA and Immunoco patients. For HLA DR molecules the Immunoco patients were also studied with standard serological methods while the LTA patients were typed with generic molecular typing. As shown in *Figure 1* A3, B27 and DR6 positive patients were statistically more frequent in the LTA group compared to the Immunoco group ($p<0,05$ according to Fisher's exact test). We also observed a striking increase of B5 positive individuals in LTA patients and a concomitant absence of B15 positive individuals. However these differences were not statistically significant. Both B27 and B5 increase in LTA is in accordance with previous studies suggesting a protective effect of these alleles in Caucasians. Increases in A3 and DR6 positive individuals among LTA individuals showing a normal CD8 count [7] is to our knowledge first reported in this study. This finding is probably due to different reasons. First, since LTA individuals represent less than 5% of the general HIV-infected population in France, the study of this cohort is equivalent to the study of at least 800 HIV-infected patients if one assumes that the Immunoco cohort is an adequate control for comparisons. In other terms we propose that in the LTA cohort the protective effect of particular HLA alleles is more informative than in cohorts containing very few patients with a prolonged survival [8]. This finding might also reflect ethnic differences between the different populations studied up to now and therefore addresses another question. Is it simply the antigen presenting function of HLA molecules that influences the outcome of HIV disease or alternatively an overexpression or underexpression of other polymorphic genes coding for complement proteins or cytokines in linkage disequilibrium with these alleles which are responsible for such finding [9,10]? We think that a more detailed functional analysis of antigen presentation of HIV proteins by these particular alleles should be a very promising alternative to address such question.

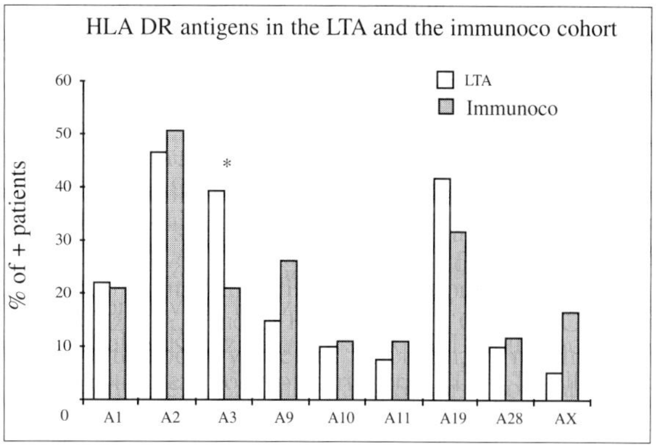

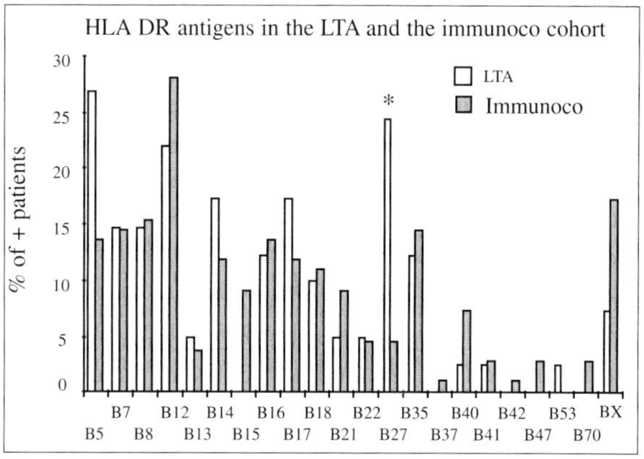

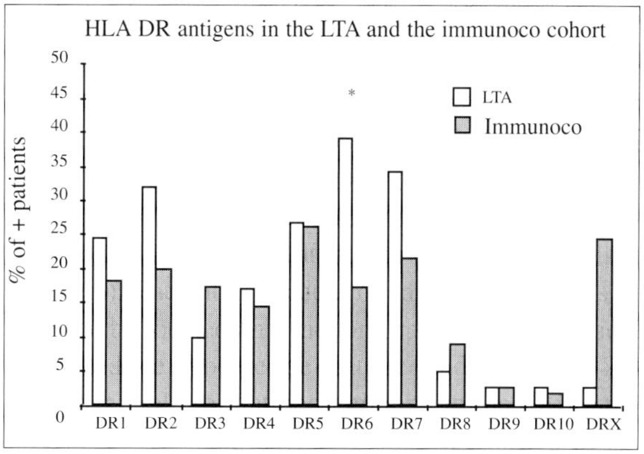

Figure 1. HLA A, B and DR distribution in LTA and Immunoco patients. Asterisks indicate alleles with statistically significant differences ($p<0{,}05$) between the two groups.

References

1. Scorza Smeraldi R, Fabio G, Lazzarin A, Eisera NB, Moroni M, Zanussi C. HLA-associated susceptibility to acquired immunodeficiency syndrome in Italian patients with human-immunodeficiency virus infection. *Lancet* 1986; 2(8517): 1187-9.
2. Kaslow RA, Duquesnoy R, Van Randen M, Kingsley L, Marrari M, Friedman H, Su S, Saah AJ, Detels R, Phair J *et al.* A1, Cw7, B8, DR3 HLA antigen combination associated with rapid decline of T helper lymphocytes in HIV-1 infection. A report from the Multicenter AIDS Cohort Study. *Lancet* 1990; 335: 927-30.
3. Mann DL, Murray C, O'Donnell M, Blattner WA, Goedert JJ. HLA antigen frequencies in HIV-1 related Kaposi's sarcoma. *J Acquir Immune Defic Syndr* 1990; 3 (suppl 1): S51-5.
4. Itescu S, Mathur-Wagh U, Skovron ML, Brancato LJ, Marmor M, Zelenich-Jacquotte A, Winchester R. HLA-B35 is associated with accelerated progression to AIDS. *J Acquir Immune Defic Syndr* 1992; 5: 37-45.

5. Klein MR, Keet IP, D'Amaro J, Bende RJ, Heckman A, Mesman B, Koot M, De Waal LP, Coutinho RA, Miedema F. Associations between HLA frequencies and pathogenic features of human immunodeficiency virus type 1 infection in seroconverters from the Amsterdam cohort of homosexual men. *J Infect Dis* 1994; 169: 1244-9.
6. Just JJ, Abrams E, Louie LG, Urbano R, Wara D, Nicholas SW, Stein Z, King MC. Influence of host genotype on progression to acquired immunodeficiency syndrome among children infected with human immunodeficiency virus type 1 *J Pediatr* 1995; 127: 544-9.
7. Itescu S, Rose S, Dwyer E, Winchester R. Certain HLA-DR5 and DR6 major histocompatibility complex class II alleles are associated with a CD8 lymphocytic host response to human immunodeficiency virus type 1 characterized by low lymphocyte viral strain heterogeneity and slow disease progression *Proc Natl Acad Sci USA* 1994; 91: 11472-6.
8. Kaslow RA, Carrington M, Apple R, Park L, Munoz A, Saah AJ, Goedert JJ, Winkler C, O' Brien SJ, Rinaldo C, Detels R, Blattener W, Phair JH, Erlich H, Mann DL. Influence of human major histocompatibility complex genes on the course of HIV-1 infection. *Nature Med* 1996; 2: 405-11.
9. Cameron PU, Mallal SA, French MA, Dawkins RL. Major histocompatibility complex genes influence the outcome of HIV infection. Ancestral haplotypes with C4 null alleles explain diverse HLA associations. *Hum Immunol* 1990; 29: 282-95.
10. Hentges F, Hoffmann A, Oliveira de Araujo F, Hemmer R. Prolonged asymptomatic evolution after HIV-1 infection is marked by the absence of C4 null alleles at the MHC. *Clin Exp Immunol* 1992; 88: 237-42.

MHC polymorphisms are associated with the rate of disease progression in HIV infection

N. Snowden[2], L. Pepper, S. Khoo[1], A. Hajeer, B.K. Mandal[1], E.G.L. Wilkins[1], W. Ollier

Molecular Immunogenetics Laboratory, ARC-ERU, University of Manchester, Manchester Medical School, Oxford Road, Manchester M13 9PT, UK
1 Infectious Diseases, North Manchester General Hospital, UK
2 Immunology Department, Hope Hospital, Salford M6 8HD, UK

The rate of immunological deterioration in HIV infection varies widely between individuals. Although the median time between acquisition and the development of AIDS is around 10 years, 5-10% of those infected lose CD4 T cells rapidly and develop AIDS within 3 years of infection whereas another 10-15% may show little or no loss of T cells at 10 years post-infection [1]. Some of this heterogeneity may be attributable to viral factors; subjects with rapid progression tend to have rapidly replicating, cytopathic, syncytium inducing strains of HIV with macrophage tropism. Coinfection with other pathogens (particularly CMV) can also stimulate viral replication and disease progression [1]. Variability in the host response to the virus seems likely to play a major role in determining the rate of immunological deterioration. The interaction between HIV and the host immune system is characterised by intense immunological activation, a vigourous CD8 T cell response to the virus, and massive turnover of CD4 cells and virus [2]. The CD8 response to HIV seems to be a major factor in slowing progression and loss of CD4 cells [3]. In contrast, the state of immunological activation associated with HIV infection seems to favour replication of HIV and possibly progression of disease. Even minor activation of the immune system (such as that associated with immunisation with a recall antigen) can increase the circulating viral load [4]. Immunological activation in HIV is associated with increased production of TNFα, TNFß, IL1, TNF receptors and markers of macrophage activation such as neopterin [5]. TNF α and β may play an important role in disease progression; both cytokines can stimulate viral replication and the production of TNF α and ß is in turn induced by HIV, suggesting a potential positive feedback loop between virus and cytokine [6].
We hypothesize that host genetic factors exert a major influence upon variability in the host T cell response to HIV and to the process of immunological activation in HIV infection. Several important candidate genes lie within the MHC. Class I, class II and TAP polymorphism have a potential profound influence upon the T cell response to the virus. Polymorphisms of the TNF loci within class III may be associated with variation in the interaction between TNF production, HIV replication and immunological activation. Previous studies have suggested that B35 and the A1 B8 DR3 haplotype predict rapid progression and that DRB1*1102 and 1301 are associated, in African American patients, with slow progression and a brisk CD8 response to the virus ([7,8] reviewed in [9,10]). TNF polymorphism has not been previously examined as a risk factor for progression, but it is of interest that the A1 B8 DR3 haplotype is associated with increased TNF production [11].

Study population and methods

We used a cross sectional approach to examine the importance of class II and class III polymorphism in 52 patients with HIV infection: 30 patients with slower progression (CD4>400/mm^3 at >7yrs post infection in the absence of specific antiviral therapy) and 22 with rapidly progressive disease (acquisition to CD4<100/mm^3 or AIDS in under 5 years). Groups were comparable in age and CMV seropositivity. All subjects were caucasoid and from the north west of England.
HLA DRB1, DQB1 and DQA alleles were defined using sequence specific oligotyping and TAP2 polymorphisms were identified using ARMS-PCR. Microsatellite typing of TNF a,b, c and d was performed using primers described by Udalova [12]. Primers were fluorescently labelled with HEX, 6-FAM or TET dyes and PCR products were sized on an ABI 377 automated genotyper [13]. TNF alleles were assigned using ABI genotyper software. Allele frequencies were compared with a geographically matched non-HIV infected control panel.

Table I.

	Slow N=23	Fast N=20	Controls N=102
TNFc1	87%	100%	94%
TNFc2	61%	15%	46%

TNFc Phenotype frequencies:

Fast vs slow OR 11.3 (95%CI 2.1-72)
Fast vs controls OR 4.9 (95%CI 1.25-99)

Results

Phenotypic frequencies for selected class II alleles and TNFc are summarised in *Tables I-IV*. The frequency of the TNF c2 allele was significantly decreased in the fast progressors compared to slower progressors and healthy controls. No significant association was demonstrated between progression and any TNF a,b or d allele or TAP2 allele. Minor differences were seen between the two HIV infected groups for DRB1*0101, DAB*1 0301, DQA1*0301 and DQA1*0501 but these did not achieve statistical significance. A significant decrease in both DQB1*0302 and DQB1*0303 was seen in fast progressors and DQB1*0303 was increased in slow progressors. DQB1*0603 was non-significantly increased in fast progressors. Certain class II alleles were over represented (DRB1*1301, DQA1*0102) or under represented (DRB1*0401, DQA1*03) in both HIV infected groups compared to controls.

Discussion

We have demonstrated a strong negative association between rapid progression of HIV infection and the TNF c2 allele. Negative associations were also demonstrated between rapid progression and two DQB1* alleles, 0302 and 0303. The size of our study population does not allow us to determine whether these associations are linked to a common haplotype or independent of each other, but preliminary analysis and previous data on the haplotypic association of TNF microsatellites and class II in UK populations [13], suggests that these effects may be independent; further data are required to examine this. It will also be of major importance to extend our study to an examination of class I polymorphism, since this is likely to exert a major influence on the CD8 T cell response to HIV. The association between rapid progression and the TNF locus is consistent with the hypothesis that an autoinductive positive feedback loop exists between HIV replication and TNFα and β production. TNF may also have the capacity to accelerate loss of CD4 cells in HIV by induction of apoptosis; recent studies suggest that TNFβ may play a central role in inducing apoptosis of uninfected lympho-

Table II.

DRB1* allele	Slow N=33	Fast N23	Control N=137
0101	15%	26%	15%
0301	18%	30%	29%
0401	3%	9%	25%
1301	15%	17%	4%

DRB1* Phenotype frequencies

1301
Fast vs controls OR 4.6 (95%CI 1.2-17.8)
Slow vs controls OR 3.9 (95%CI 1.1-13.7)

0401
Slow vs controls OR 0.095 (95% CI 0.013-0.72)

Table III.

DQA1* allele	Slow N=32	Fast N=23	Control N=69
0102	38%	44%	20%
03	31%	17%	55%
0501	28%	52%	36%

DQA1* Phenotype frequencies

0102
Fast vs controls OR 3.02 (95%CI 1.1-8.3)

Table IV.

DQB1* allele	Slow N=33	Fast N=23	Control N=137
0201	30%	57%	42%
0302	26%	0%	31%
0303	22%	0%	7%
0501	17%	38%	25%
0603	4%	24%	6%

DQB1* Phenotype frequencies

0302
Fast vs slow OR 8.3 p=0.007#

0303
Fast vs slow OR 6.3 p=0.03#
Slow vs controls OR 3.5 (95% CI 1.1-11)

0603
Fast vs controls OR 4.7 (95% CI 1.5-15.3)
#Fisher's exact test. 0302 &0303 Odds ratio is approximate as n=0 in the fast group

blasts following lymphocyte stimulation by HIV peptides [14]. This is of particular interest since the TNFc microsatellite is located in the first intron of the TNFβ gene and previous data have suggested that an NcoI polymorphism in this region predicts high or low TNFβ production [15]. Further examination of the relationship between TNF c alleles and TNFα and β production (particularly in response to HIV) is required.

The abnormal distribution of certain class II alleles in both fast and slow progressing groups (increased DRB1*1301, decreased DRB1*0401) is suggestive of a selective effect of HIV infection, possibly suggesting that these alleles may affect susceptibility to HIV. This requires further assessment in a broader sample of HIV infected subjects.

References

1. Levy JA. The transmission of HIV and factors influencing progression to AIDS. *Am J Med* 1993;95:86-100.
2. Wain-Hobson S. Virological mayhem. *Nature* 1995; 373: 102.
3. Cao Y, Qin L, Zhang L, Safrit J, Ho DD. Virologic and immunologic characterisation of long term survivors of HIV1 infection. *N Engl J Med* 1995; 332: 201-8.
4. Stanley SK, Ostrowski MA, Justement JS, *et al.* Effect of immunisation with a common recall antigen on viral expression in patients infected with HIV1. *N Engl J Med* 1996; 334: 1222-30.
5. Pantaleo G, Fauci AS. Tracking HIV during disease progression. *Curr Op Immunol* 1994; 6: 600-4.
6. Vyakernam A, McKeating J, Meager A, Beverly PC. TNFα and ß induced by HIV1 in peripheral blood mononuclear cells potentiate virus replication. *AIDS* 1990; 4: 21-8.
7. Kaslow RA, Carrington M, Apple R *et al.* Influence of combinations of human MHC genes on the course of HIV1 infection. *Nature Med* 1996; 2: 405-11.
8. McNeil AJ, Yaap PL, Gore SM *et al.* Association of HLA types A1-B8-DR3 and B27 with rapid and slow progression of HIV disease. *Q J Med* 1996; 89: 177-85.
9. Hill AVS. HIV and HLA: confusion or complexity? *Nature Med* 1996; 2: 395-6.
10. Mann DL, Carrington MN, Kroner BL. The human MHC and HIV-1 pathogenesis. *AIDS* 1994; 8 (suppl 1): S53-60.
11. Jacob CO, Fronek Z, Lewis GD, Koo M, Hansen JA, McDevitt HO. Heritable class II differences in production of TNFα: relevance to genetic predisposition to SLE. *Proc Natl Acad Sci USA* 1990; 87: 1233-7.
12. Udalova IA, Nedospasov SA, Webb GC, Chaplin DD, Turestskaya RL. Highly informative typing of the human TNF locus using 6 adjacent polymorphic markers. *Genomics* 1993; 16: 180-6.
13. Hajeer A, Worthington J, Silman AJ, Ollier WER. TNF microsatellite polymorphisms are associated with HLA-DRB1*04-bearing haplotypes in Rheumatoid Arthritis patients. *Arthritis Rheum* 1997, in press.
14. Clerici M, Sarin A, Berzovsky JA *et al.* Antigen stimulated apoptotic T cell death in HIV infection is selective for CD4+ T cells, modulated by cytokines and effected by lymphotoxin. *AIDS* 1996; 10: 603-11.
15. Messer G, Spengler U, Jung MC *et al.* Polymorphic structure of the TNF locus: An NcoI polymorphism in the first intron of the human TNFß gene correlates with a variant αα in position 26 and a reduced level of TNFß production. *J Exp Med* 1991; 173: 209-19.

Mapping of HLA-DR4 restricted T cell epitopes from the mycobacterial HSP60 with synthetic peptides

A.S. Mustafa[1], K.E.A. Lundin[2], F. Oftung[3]

1 Department of Microbiology, Faculty of Medicine, Kuwait University, PO Box 24923, 13110 Safat, Kuwait
2 Institute of Transplantation Immunology, The National Hospital, 0027 Oslo, Norway
3 Vaccine Department, National Institute of Public Health, 0462 Oslo, Norway

The mycobacterial 60 kDa heat shock protein (HSP60) is a major antigen recognized by mycobacteria reactive human CD4$^+$ T cells with lymphokine profiles and effector functions consistent with protective immunity [1-5]. In addition, the presence of a large number of T cell epitopes presented by several HLA class II molecules makes this antigen relevant to subunit vaccine design [6]. However, the results from animal models as well as human studies suggest that the mycobacterial HSP60 may induce T cell mediated autoimmune conditions [7]. In humans, the expression of HLA-DR4 represents a risk factor for rheumatoid arthritis and insulin autoimmune syndrome [7, 8]. These studies suggest that the HLA-DR4 restricted T cell epitopes of the mycobacterial HSP60 could be relevant to autoimmunity.

In this study, we established a large number of *M. leprae* and *M. tuberculosis* reactive CD4$^+$ T cell clones from HLA-DR4 positive healthy donors immunized with *M. bovis* BCG and killed *M. leprae*. By using these T cell clones, five HLA-DR4 restricted T cell epitopes of the mycobacterial HSP60 were identified. However, the amino acid sequences of these epitopes were highly divergent from the corresponding sequences in human HSP60 suggesting a lack of correlation between recognition of mycobacterial HSP60 in association with HLA-DR4 and autoimmunity.

Mycobacterial HSP60 reactive T cell clones

We have earlier shown that T cell lines established from three HLA-DR4 positive subjects recognized the mycobacterial HSP60 in association with HLA-DR4 [7]. In order to map the T cell epitopes and to determine their specificity for the mycobacterial HSP60, T cell clones were established from the T cell lines and tested for reactivity to the *M. leprae* and *M. tuberculosis* HSP60 and their peptides by using standard methods [1, 4]. From a total of 119 CD4$^+$ T cell clones established, thirteen T cell clones responded to the mycobacterial HSP60; eight of the thirteen T cell clones were specific for the *M. leprae* HSP60 and the remaining five clones responded to *M. leprae* and *M. tuberculosis* HSP60 [9].

Mapping of T cell epitopes with synthetic peptides

The epitopes recognized by the mycobacterial HSP60 reactive T cell clones were identified by testing the clones with 49 overlapping synthetic peptides (15 mers) covering the entire amino acid (aa) sequence of the *M. tuberculosis* HSP60 and 20 peptides (13 mers) covering most regions of the *M. leprae* HSP60 which are different from the *M. tuberculosis* sequence by one or more aa. The epitopes recognized by all of the five cross-reactive T cell clones were identified by using the *M. tuberculosis* peptides. One clone each responded to the peptides (331-345) and (441-455), respectively, and three T cell clones responded to a single peptide (501-515). The aa sequence of the peptides recognized by the cross-reactive T cell clones are completely identical in the *M. leprae* and *M. tuberculosis* HSP60 [9]. None of the *M. leprae* HSP60 specific T cell clones responded to the peptides of the *M. tuberculosis* HSP60 sequence. When tested with the peptide series of 13 mers from the *M. leprae* HSP60 specific sequence, the epitopes recognized by three *M. leprae* HSP60 specific T cell clones were identified. One T cell clone responded to the peptide (343-355) and two clones responded to the peptide (522-534). All of the peptides were recognized by the T cell clones in the presence of APC expressing HLA-Dw4 and Dw14 subtypes of HLA-DR4, except the peptide (343-355) which was presented to the T cells in the presence of HLA-Dw14 positive APC only [9].

Identification of a single aa position essential to HLA-DR4 binding

The peptide (522-534) differs between *M. leprae* and *M. tuberculosis* HSP60 by six aa residues, whereas the peptide (343-355) differs only by one aa residue [9]. Threonine at position 349 in the *M. leprae* HSP60 peptide (343-355) is replaced by glutamine in the corresponding *M. tuberculosis* HSP60 peptide [9]. This single amino acid substitution makes the relevant T cell clone a non-responder to the *M. tuberculosis* HSP60 and its peptide (341-355). The reason(s) for non-responsiveness of the T cell clone to the *M. tuberculosis* HSP60 peptide (341-355) could be that threonine at position 349 in the *M. leprae* HSP60 peptide (343-355) is critical either for binding of the peptide to the HLA-DR4, Dw14 molecule or for the recognition of the peptide by the T cell receptor. Experiments were done to differentiate between the two possibilities by using a peptide competition assay. Over a wide range of concentrations tested, the peptide (341-355) from *M. tuberculosis* HSP60 did not inhibit the proliferation induced by the peptide 343-355 from the *M. leprae* HSP60 *(Table I).*

Table I. Effect of the *M. tuberculosis* HSP60 peptide (341-355) on the proliferative response of the T cell clone responding to the *M. leprae* HSP60 peptide (343-355)

M. leprae peptide (343-355)	*M. tuberculosis* peptide (341-355)	Proliferation CPMx10^{-3}	% inhibition
10 ng/ml	Not added	30.5	-
10 ng/ml	10 ug/ml	24.5	19.7
10 ng/ml	1 ug/ml	24.4	20.0
10 ng/ml	100 ng/ml	32.3	-5.9
10 ng/ml	10 ng/ml	24.0	21.3
10 ng/ml	1 ng/ml	26.2	14.1
Not added	10 ng/ml	0.2	-

These results suggest that the *M. tuberculosis* peptide (341-355) was unable to bind to the HLA-DR4, Dw14 molecule and therefore it can be concluded that threonine at position 349 in the *M. leprae* peptide (343-355) was critical for binding of the peptide to the HLA-DR4, Dw14 molecule.
Sequence comparison of the mycobacterial HSP60 epitopes with the human HSP60.
To determine if any of the HLA-DR4 restricted T cell epitopes of the mycobacterial HSP60 may play a potential role in autoimmunity based on aa sequence homology, the identified peptide epitopes were compared with the aa sequences of the corresponding regions of the human HSP60 molecule. None of the epitopes recognized by the HLA-DR4 restricted T cell clones belong to the regions which show sequence homology between the mycobacterial and the human HSP60 [9, 10]. Thus these results do not suggest any direct correlation between T cell recognition of the mycobacterial HSP60 in the context of HLA-DR4 and autoimmunity based on crossreactivity to sequence homology regions of the self HSP60.

Acknowledgments
This study was supported by the Kuwait University Research Administration Grant MIO 73.

References

1. Mustafa AS, Oftung F, Gill HK, Natvig I. Characteristics of human T cell clones from BCG and killed *M. leprae* vaccinated subjects and tuberculosis patients. *Lepr Rev* 1986; 57 (suppl 2): 123-30.
2. Oftung F, Mustafa AS, Husson R, Young RA, Godal T. Human T cell clones recognize two abundant *Mycobacterium tuberculosis* protein antigens expressed in *Escherichia coli. J Immunol* 1987; 138: 927-31.
3. Mustafa AS. Identification of T-cell activating recombinant antigens shared among three candidate antileprosy vaccines, killed *M. leprae*, *M. bovis* BCG and *Mycobacterium w. Int J Lepr* 1988; 50: 265-73.
4. Oftung F, Mustafa AS, Shinnick TM, Houghton RA, Kvalheim G, Degre M, Lundin KEA, Godal T. Epitopes of the *Mycobacterium tuberculosis* 65-kilodalton protein antigen as recognized by human T cells. *J Immunol* 1988; 141: 2749-54.
5. Haanen JBAG, Malefijt RDW, Res PCM, Kraakman EM, Ottenhoff THM, deVries RRP, Spits H. 1991. Selection of a human T helper type-1 like subset by mycobacteria. *J Exp Med* 1991; 174: 583-92.
6. Mustafa AS, Lundin KEA, Oftung F. Human T cells recognize mycobacterial heat shock proteins in the context of multiple HLA-DR molecules: studies with healthy subjects vaccinated with *Mycobacterium bovis* BCG and *Mycobacterium leprae. Infect Immun* 1993; 61: 5294-301.
7. Van Eden W. Heat shock proteins and the immune system. *Immunol Rev* 1991; 121: 5-28.
8. Uchigata Y, Kuwata S, Tokunaga K, Eguchi Y, Takayama-Hasumi S, Miyamoto M, Omori Y, Juji T, Hirata Y. Strong association of insulin autoimmune syndrome with HLA-DR4. *Lancet* 1992; 339: 393-4.
9. Mustafa AS, Lundin KEA, Meloen RH, Shinnick TM, Coulson AFW, Oftung F. HLA-DR4- restricted T cell epitopes from the mycobacterial 60 000 MW heat shock protein (hsp 60) do not map to the sequence homology regions with the human hsp 60. *Immunology* 1996; 87: 421-7.
10. Jindal S, Dudani AK, Singh B, Harley CB, Gupta RS. Primary structure of a human mitochondrial protein homologous to the bacterial and plant chaperonins and to the 65-kiloDalton mycobacterial antigen. *Mol Cell Biol* 1989; 9: 2279-83.

HLA
and Diseases

HLA and Diseases

Contents

• HLA and Diseases

Molecular basis of HLA-DP-associated susceptibility to beryllium disease

G. Lombardi[1], J. Uren[1], W. Jones-Williams[2], C. Saltini[3], R. Lechler[1]

1 Departement of Immunology, RPMS, Hammersmith Hospital, Du Cane road, London W12 ONN, UK
2 Departement of Medicine, University of Wales, Cardiff, UK
3 Departement of Medical Science, Section Respiratory Disease, University of Modena, Italy

Chronic beryllium disease (CBD) is a granulomatous disorder leading to progressive lung fibrosis and severe respiratory dysfunction [1, 2]. It has been shown that Be-specific $CD4^+$ T cells accumulate in the lung of CBD patients [3, 4]. In addition, it has been demonstrated that mononuclear cells from CBD patients react against Be *in vitro* [5].

Recently, analysis of MHC class II genes in patients with CBD has shown a positive association with HLA-DPB1*0201 and a negative association with HLA-DPB1*0401 [6]. Furthermore, sequence comparison of DPβ chains suggested that susceptibility to CBD was conferred by expression of DPβ alleles with glutamic acid (Glu) at position 69.

In this study we have investigated the functional basis of HLA-DP susceptibility in Be diseases by generating T cell clones from patients with CBD. We have found that all the Be-specific T cell clones obtained were restricted by HLA-DP alleles with Glu at DPβ69, and that a single amino acid substitution at residue 69 in the β chain of the HLA-DP molecule completely abrogated their responses. These data elucidate the molecular basis of DP-associated susceptibility to CBD.

Methods

Beryllium, monoclonal antibodies, and cell lines

The beryllium sulphate tetrahydrate ($BeSO_4.4H_2O$) was purchased from the Aldrich Chemical Co Ltd (Sigma-Aldrich Co. Ltd., Dorset, UK).

The B7/21 (anti-HLA-DP), L2 (anti-HLA-DQ) and L243 (anti-HLA-DR), monoclonal antibodies (mAbs) were purified from hybridoma culture supernatants (ATCC).

Murine DAP.3 cell transfectants (DAP.3-Tx) expressing either HLA-DPB1*0201 (Workshop No: 8,301) or HLA-DPB1*0402 (Workshop No: 8,305), and Epstein Barr virus (EBV)-transformed lymphoblastoid B cell lines (B-LCLs) were obtained from the Xth International Histocompatibility Workshop (Xth IHW). DAP.3-Tx were maintained in DMEM with 10% FCS in the presence of appropriate drug selection, B-LCLs in RPMI 1640 with 10% FCS.

Generation and proliferation of Be-specific T cell clones

T cell clones were obtained by limiting dilution from blood of two patients with CBD, FC and NG, using PHA (2μg/ml), allogeneic irradiated PBMC and rIL-2. T cell clones were used for functional assays between 1 and 2 weeks after their last stimulation.

T cell clones (10^4 cells/well) were cultured with $3x10^4$ cells/well of either B-LCL or DAP.3-Tx pre-pulsed with $BeSO_4.4H_2O$ for 4 hours and then treated with 120Gy X-irradiation or with Mitomycin-C respectively. Wells were pulsed with 1μCi of ^{3}H-TdR (Amersham International, Amersham, UK), after 48 hours and the cultures harvested onto glass fiber filters 18 hrs. later.

Results

Be-specific T cell lines and clones generated from patients with CBD were preferentially restricted by HLA-DP with Glu at residue 69 of the DPβ chain. Of the T cell clones obtained 35% (13/37) from patient FC and 30% (3/10) from patient NG were specific for Be. A panel of B-LCLs expressing different DR, DQ and DP alleles was used to present Be to the T cell clones. The results strongly suggested that all the Be-specific clones were restricted by HLA-DP. The involvement of HLA-DP molecules in the responses of Be-specific T cell clones was further investigated using mAbs specific for

HLA-DR, DQ and DP *(Table I)*. All the T cell clones tested were completely inhibited by the presence of anti-HLA-DP mAb. In contrast, no inhibition was observed with the mAb against HLA-DQ molecules. In all the experiments performed the presence of the anti-HLA-DR mAb (L243) consistently led to 30 to 50% inhibition (Be41 and Be13). No inhibition in the presence of L243 was observed with a Tetanus Toxoid-specific T cell clone restricted by HLA-DPB1*0201 (D12).
In order to investigate the functional relevance of Glu at residue 69 in the β chain, we tested the response of Be-specific T cell clones to either B-LCL or DAP.3-Tx expressing HLA-DPB1*0201 and HLA-DPB1*0402 that shared the same DPα chain and differ only at position 69 in the β chain. All the Be-specific T cell clones obtained responded only to the APC with Glu at residue 69 *(Table II)*.
These data suggest that HLA-DP is the restriction element for Be-specific T cells and that the presence of Glu at residue 69 is essential for the reactivity of these clones to Be.

Discussion

The DP restriction of the Be-specific clones observed here suggests strongly that the DP association in CBD reflects the role of certain alleles of DP in presentation of Be to T cells. This is one of the first report of an HLA and disease association with a clear functional correlate. Despite the evidence of DP restriction for all of the Be-specific T cell clones examined, significant, although less impressive, inhibition was also seen with the anti-DRα mAb, L243. The reason for this inhibition is currently under investigation; it is possible that the DRα chain, contributes to the restriction element for some of the Be-specific T cell clones. As shown in Table I, the inhibition is not due to toxicity of the anti-DP mAb and is a peculiarity of the Be-specific T cell clones.
The immunogenetic analysis referred to above highlighted the importance of the Glu at position 69 in the DPβ chain. The functional importance of this residue was emphasised by the finding that none of the clones responded to Be presented by either B-LCL or DAP.3-Tx expressing DPB1*0402, an allele that only differs at position 69 in the DPβ chain.
In the light of these considerations it remains unclear as to how Be is recognised by T cells. Be can bind directly to the HLA-DP molecule leading to conformational alteration, or can interact with a self-peptide bound in the groove of the HLA-DP molecule leading to the display of «altered self». These two possibilities are under investigation.
To analyse the role of the Be-specific T cell clones *in vivo* the profile of cytokines produced by the clones was studied (data not shown). The results provide further evidence that these *in vitro* observed responses reflect *in vivo* events, in that the T cell clones appeared to be of the Th1 subset that would be predicted to be pathogenetic in a chronic inflammatory lung disease.

Table I. T cell clones specific for Be were restricted preferentially by HLA-DP

T Cell Clones	MAbs			
	-	anti-DP (B7/21)	anti-DR (L243)	anti-DQ (L2)
Be 41	19,149	0	8,977	22,102
Be 13	35,022	0	14,646	37,975
D12	5,776	0	9,458	8,456

T cell clones were cultured with B-LCL in the presence or absence of MAbs as described in M. and M. The data are expressed as Δcpm.

Table II. The presence of Glu at residue 69 in the DPβ chain is necessary for the T cell response to Be

T cell clones	Be (μM)	B-LCL		DAP.3-Tx	
		Glu 69	Lys 69	Glu 69	Lys 69
Be23	0	0	200	310	222
	30	10,687	534	10,512	70
	100	16,359	342	14,333	0
	300	21,916	180	17,237	0
	1000	33,401	343	20,410	0
	3000	31,097	71	18,565	0
Be41	0	206	314	381	251
	30	814	790	18,892	88
	100	2,083	217	38,698	77
	300	2,137	540	58,905	75
	1000	9,328	391	45,864	0
	3000	15,282	297	30,361	0

T cell clones were cultured with either B-LCL or DAP.3-Tx expressing Glu or Lys at residue 69 of the DPβ chain, as described in M. and M. The data are expressed as Δcpm.

All these results demonstrate that the preferential/exclusive use of HLA-DP as the restriction element in T cell recognition of Be accounts for DP-associated susceptibility to chronic beryllium disorders. Futhermore, from the pattern of cytokine production by the Be-specific clones suggests that these T cells are involved in the *in vivo* delayed type hypersensitivity reactions.

References

1. Freiman DG, Hardy HL. Beryllium disease. The relation of pulmonary pathology to clinical course and prognosis based on a study of 130 cases from the US beryllium case registry. *Hum Pathol* 1970; 1:25-44.
2. Hardly HL, Tabershaw JR. Delayed chemical pneumonitis occurring in workers exposed to beryllium copounds. *J Indust Hygiene Toxicol* 1946; 28: 197-211.
3. Saltini C, Winestock K, Kirby M, Pinkston P, Crystal RG. Maintenance of alveolitis in patients with chronic beryllium disease by beryllium-specific helper T cells. *N Engl J Med* 1988; 320:1103-09.
4. Saltini C, Kirby M, Trapnell BC, Tamura N, Crystal RG. Biased accumulation of T lymphocytes with "memory"-type CD45 leukocyte common antigen gene expression on the epithelial surface of human lung. *J Exp Med* 1990; 171: 1123-40.
5. Hanfin JM, Epstein WL, Cline MJ. *In vitro* studies of granulomatous hypersensitivity to beryllium. *J Invest Dermatol* 1970; 55: 284-8.
6. Richeldi L, Sorrentino R, Saltini C. HLA-DPB1 glutamate 69: a genetic marker of beryllium disease. *Science* 1993; 262: 242-4.

Association of type I psoriasis with the Cw*0802-DRB1*0102-DQB1*0501 haplotype in North-American multiplex families

S. Jenisch, R.P. Nair [2], T. Henseler [1], J.T. Elder [2], B. Marxen, M. Krönke, E. Westphal

1 Institute of Immunology, Department of Dermatology, University of Kiel, Michaelisstrasse 5, D-24105 Kiel, Germany
2 Department of Dermatology, University of Michigan, Ann Arbor, MI, USA

Psoriasis vulgaris (PsV) is a chronic hyperproliferative inflammatory disease affecting about 2% of Caucasians. Several associations between PsV and specific human lymphocyte antigens (HLA) have been described. The strongest association is found between psoriasis vulgaris and HLA-C antigens. The largest and most consistently reported relative risk has been related to HLA-Cw6, which also shows a strong association with age of onset and family history (PsV Type I) [1]. However, Cw6 by itself is not sufficient to explain the outbreak of PsV, since the prevalence of PsV in individuals positive for the implicated allele never exceeds 80%. Conversely, 90% of Cw6-positive individuals have no history of the disease. To further evaluate the nature of HLA association with PsV, the distribution and inheritance of HLA- antigens and -haplotypes was analyzed in 88 affected and 162 healthy family members of 16 families with high incidence of PsV.

Material and methods

Patients

88 affected and 162 healthy family members from a total of 16 north american families of caucasian origin were included into the study.

Methods

For serologic HLA-typing, EBV-transformed cell lines were used. HLA-A, -B and -C antigens were typed by the standard complement-dependent microlymphocytotoxicity technique (LCT). Additionally, HLA-C was typed by PCR-ARMS, using the primers proposed at the XII. Histocompatibility Workshop [2]. Subtyping of HLA-Cw8 was performed on a DNA sequencer (ABI 373A, Perkin Elmer, Norwalk, CT) after allele-specific amplification of the second, third and fourth exon of HLA-C [2,3]. HLA-DRB1 and -DQB1 alleles were defined by PCR with locus- and group-specific primers followed by hybridization with non-radioactive labelled sequence specific probes [4]. Whenever possible, HLA haplotypes were deduced manually by analysis of the inheritance of the HLA antigens.

Results

Frequency of HLA-Cw antigens

Using PCR-ARMS for typing of the HLA-C locus, 90.2% of the HLA-C alleles could be determined. *Table I* displays the detected antigen frequencies (af) of HLA-Cw-specificities. HLA-Cw8 was the only specificity showing a significant increase in affected probands ($p<0.05$), but only before correction of the p-value by the number of tested alleles. When compared to the af of Cw8 in the normal US population (4.7%)[5], Cw8 was highly overrepresented in diseased family members (p_{corr} <10-10).

Extended HLA class-I- and II- haplotypes

Analysis of the extended HLA class I and II haplotypes revealed, that Cw8 was linked with DRB1*0102-DQB1*0501 in 69.6% (16/23) of the affected and in 36,7% (8/22) of the unaffected HLA-Cw8 positive family members ($p<0.05$). Of all psoriatics under investigation, 18.2% carried this haplotype in contrast to 4.9% of the healthy probands ($p_{corr}<0.05$). The extended, HLA-Cw8-B65-DRB1*0102-DQB1*0501 haplotype is known as ancestral haplotype (AH) 65.1 [6].

Inheritance of HLA- antigens and -haplotypes

Table II illustrates the extended HLA-haplotypes cosegregating with disease. AH65.1 was found in 5 of the 16 families. In four families, AH65 was the haplotype sho-

Table I. Frequencies of HLA-Cw antigens

HLA-C antigen	affected (N=88)	not affected (N=162)	p-value
Cw*01	1 (1%)	3 (2%)	n.s.
Cw*02	6 (7%)	6 (10%)	n.s.
Cw*03	9 (10%)	28 (17%)	n.s.
Cw*04	22 (25%)	31 (19%)	n.s.
Cw*05	2 (2%)	18 (11%)	p<0.05
Cw*0602	33 (38%)	51 (31%)	n.s.
Cw*07	34 (39%)	67 (41%)	n.s.
Cw*08	23 (26%)	22 (14%)	p<0.05
Cw*1203	9 (10%)	19 (12%)	n.s.

n.s.: not significant; §: p-value not corrected.

wing the strongest cosegregation with PsV, in one family no segregation of AH65.1 was observed. In further five families, other Cw8-positive haplotypes were present. However, these haplotypes did not cosegregate with PsV *(Table III)*. A total of three families showed segregation of the Cw6-positive ancestral haplotype AH57.1, which was recently described to be highly associated with PsV Type I [7]. To further investigate whether the recognized association of HLA-Cw8 with PsV is related to genes within the haplotype AH65.1, the inheritance of Cw8 and AH 65.1 was analysed in greater detail. AH65.1 was transmitted to 16 of the 31 children with one parent heterozygous for AH65.1. Of those, 13 developed psoriasis, whereas only three stayed healthy. In contrast, haplotypes carrying Cw8 but not AH65.1 were inherited only to 4 affected, but to eight healthy family members (p<0.05). From the 15 children to whom AH65.1 was not transmitted, seven developed PsV and eight stayed healthy.

Age at onset

The age at onset of Cw6 positive (mean: 19.4; median: 17), Cw8 positive (mean: 22.4; median: 17), AH65.1 positive (mean: 15.9; median: 17) and of psoriatics negative for both Cw6 and Cw8 (mean 23.5; median 21) showed no significant difference.

Discussion

The association of Cw6 with PsV is well established but so far not sufficient to explain the outbreak of PsV. Recently, a population- and family-based study suggested, that juvenile onset Psoriasis is associated with the class I side of the Cw6-positive ancestral haplotype AH 57.1 [7]. In the current study, we describe an association of PsV Type I with another ancestral haplotype (AH65.1), which is positive for the Cw8-antigen. This haplotype has a very low frequency in caucasian populations of Northern Europe origin [8], where PsV is predominantly associated with AH57.1. Apparently, the association is not determined by HLA-Cw8, since only the inheritance of AH65.1

Table II. HLA-extended haplotypes cosegregating with PsV

HLA-Cw	HLA-B	HLA-DRB1	HLA-DQB1	ancestral haplotype	no. of families§
*0802	65	*0102	*0501	AH 65.1	4
*0602	57	*0701	*0303	AH 57.1	3
*0602	57	*0701	*0201/2		2
*07	8	*0301	*0201/2		2
*0602	70	*1401	*0501		1
*0602	13	*0701	*0201/2		1
*1203	38	*0402	*0302		1
*0602	37	*1302	*0604		1
*04	35	*1501	*0602		1
*03	62	*0801	*0402		1
*0602	13	*1301	*0603		1
*0602	37	*1001	*0501		1

§: number of families, in which the haplotype was cosegregating with disease.

but not of other Cw8-positive haplotypes is linked with the disease. The inherent problem of family-studies is a possible bias caused by the influence of ethnic groups. Because AH65.1 is most probably of mediterranean origin, the high prevalence of this haplotype in the analyzed families might be caused by stratification. However, analysis of the inheritance of HLA-extended haplotypes revealed a strong cosegregation of disease with AH65.1 in four, with AH57.1 only in three of the families.

In summary, our results demonstrate, that a novel association of the HLA-haplotype AH65.1 with PsV exists. The fact that this association is caused by the haplotype but not by the HLA-Cw8 antigen itself provides intriguing evidence that the outbreak of the disease is influenced by one or more genes centromeric to the HLA-C locus on chromosome six.

Table III. Cw8-positive, extended haplotypes found in more than one individual

Haplotype: (HLA-Cw*0802-B65-)	affected (N=88)	unaffected (N=162)	p-value	segregation
DRB1*0102-DQB1*0501	16 (18.2%)	8 (4.9%)	p<0.05	yes
DRB1*1303-DQB1*0301	1 (1.1%)	2 (1.2%)	n.s.	no
DRB1*0701-DQB1*0201/2	2 (2.3%)	4 (2.5%)	n.s.	no
DRB1*1501-DQB1*0602	3 (3.4%)	5 (3.1%)	n.s.	no

References

1 Henseler T, Christophers E. Psoriasis of early and late onset: characterization of two types of psoriasis vulgaris. *J Am Acad Dermatol* 1985; 13: 450-6.

2 Bunce M, Barnardo MC, Welsh KI. Improvements in HLA-C typing using sequence-specific primers (PCR-SSP) including definition of HLA-Cw9 and Cw10 and a new allele HLA-"Cw7/8v". *Tissue Antigens* 1994; 44: 200-3.

3 Santamaria P, Lindstrom AL, Boyce-Jacino MT, Myster SH, Barbosa JJ, Faras AJ, Rich SS. HLA class I sequence-based typing. *Hum Immunol* 1993; 37: 39-50.

4 Kimura A, Sasazuki T. Eleventh International Histocompatibility Workshop reference protocol for the HLA DNA-typing technique. In: Tsuji K, Aizawa M, Sasazuki T, eds. *HLA 1991. Proceedings of the Eleventh International Histocompatibility Workshop and Conference,* vol.1. Oxford-New York-Tokyo: Oxford University Press, 1993: 397-419.

5 Baur MP, Danilovs JA. Population Analysis of HLA-A,B,C,DR, and Other Genetic Markers. In:Terasaki PI, ed. *Histocompatibility Testing 1980.* Los Angeles: UCLA Tissue Typing Laboratory, 1980: 955-93.

6 Degli-Esposti MA, Leaver AL, Christiansen FT, Witt CS, Abraham LJ, Dawkins RL. Ancestral haplotypes: conserved population MHC haplotypes. *Hum Immunol* 1992; 34: 242-52.

7 Schmitt-Egenolf M, Eiermann TH, Boehncke WH, Ständer M, Sterry W. Familial Juvenile Onset psoriasis is associated with the human leukocyte antigen (HLA) class I side of the extended haplotype Cw6-B57-DRB1*0701-DQA1*0201-DQB1*0303: a population- and family-based study. *J Invest Dermatol* 1996; 106: 711-4.

8 Baur MP, Danilovs JA. Reference tables of two and three-locus haplotype frequencies for HLA-A,B,C,DR,BF, and GLO. In: Terasaki PI, ed. *Histocompatibility Testing 1980.* Los Angeles: UCLA Tissue Typing Laboratory, 1980: 994-1210.

A new microsatellite marker at the RFP locus on chromosome 6p22 locates the hemochromatosis gene at least one megabase telomeric to HLA-A

L. Malfroy[1], H. Coppin[1], L. Calandro[2], N. Borot[1], D. Baer[2], G. Sensabaugh[2], M.P. Roth[1]

1 CIGH, CNRS UPR 8291, CHU Purpan, 31300 Toulouse, France
2 Division of Public Health Biology and Epidemiology, University of California, Berkeley, USA

Genetic hemochromatosis is a common autosomal recessive disorder of iron metabolism characterized by excessive iron absorption through the duodenal mucosa and progressive iron overload in parenchymal organs. This results in the mid-life onset of severe clinical complications, including hepatic cirrhosis, arthropathy, diabetes, hypogonadotrophic hypogonadism, and myocardiopathy. With early diagnosis and phlebotomy treatment to reduce and maintain normal iron stores, all known complications due to hemochromatosis can be prevented. In contrast, a significant proportion of individuals who remain undiagnosed or tardily diagnosed will succumb to hepatocellular carcinoma or cardiac failure. The exact nature of the biochemical defect remains unknown. As yet, none of the main iron-related candidate proteins has proved to be the hemochromatosis gene product.

The gene for hemochromatosis has been placed on chromosome 6 based on studies showing association with the HLA-A3 antigen and linkage to HLA markers in affected pedigrees. Recent work demonstrating strong linkage disequilibrium between hemochromatosis and D6S105 [1, 3], a locus approximately 3 Mb telomeric to HLA-A [4], has pointed to a location for the hemochromatosis gene on the telomeric side of the HLA complex; the strength of the linkage disequilibrium has led some investigators to suggest that the hemochromatosis gene may in fact be telomeric to D6S105 [5, 6]. Recombinant data set the physical boundaries of the candidate region for the hemochromatosis gene at the HLA-F locus on the centromeric side [7] and the D6S109 locus on the telomeric side [1]; these loci are, respectively, 250 kb and an estimated 10-20 Mb telomeric to HLA-A. Therefore, with respect to physically localizing the gene, investigators must still contend with a candidate region spanning several megabases.

Efforts at mapping the hemochromatosis gene have been hindered by the lack of informative markers precisely localized in the region and a gap in the YAC contig covering the region between HLA-F and D6S105. However, several genes not functionally related to the immune system have recently been mapped to the distal part of the major histocompatibility complex (MHC). Among those are the gene encoding myelin oligodendrocyte glycoprotein (MOG), two genes encoding molecules bearing homology to olfactory receptors, OLF42 and OLF89, and the gene encoding the ret finger protein, RFP [8]. This latter gene is the most distal in the continuous physical map telomeric to the MHC and has been located 780 to 1130 kb telomeric to HLA-F [9]. Several microsatellite markers have recently been localized in the vicinity of the MOG gene [10], but no polymorphic marker was identified in the RFP region so far, leaving the region telomeric to MOG uncovered.

Results and discussion

The region surrounding the human RFP locus, isolated from cosmid ICRFc109O1720Q, was shown to contain a complex microsatellite, which we designated LM1. This microsatellite consisted of 11 repeats of the TC/AG dinucleotide and 20 repeats of the AC/TG dinucleotide in the cosmid DNA. Primers LM-1 and LM-2 were designed to amplify the repeated sequence. In the sample of 182 chromosomes from healthy unrelated individuals, ten alleles were identified, with frequencies of 0.203 (137 bp), 0.005 (147 bp), 0.159 (151 bp), 0.192 (153 bp), 0.071 (155 bp), 0.137 (157 bp), 0.148 (159 bp), 0.049 (161 bp), 0.022 (163 bp), and 0.011 (165 bp). The observed number of heterozygotes was 89%, and an exact test for fit to Hardy-Weinberg equilibrium did not show significant deviation (p=0.15). The RFP alleles segregated in a codominant manner in several three-generation CEPH families tested.

This RFP marker and the MOG locus microsatellite markers [10] have been used to map in greater detail the location of the recombinant event recently described by Calandro *et al.* [7]. Members of this recombinant family had been previously tested for serological types at the HLA-A and HLA-B loci, and for 13 microsatellite markers mapped to the region extending from DQA to F13A1. The MOGb locus was uninformative in this pedigree, yielding homozygous results in both parents.The typings at the MOGa, MOGc, and RFP loci showed alleles derived from one maternal chromosome whereas the D6S306 and more telomeric markers derived from the other. The cross-over point can thus be localized between RFP and D6S306, moving the centromeric boundary of the hemochromatosis gene region to RFP. This analysis also identifies a putative cross-over involving RFP in individual II-1. This individual showed the 157 bp allele on the maternally derived chromosome instead of the expected 151 bp allele. This could be accounted for by a tight double recombination event on both sides of the marker, or by gene conversion or mutation at the locus.

The interpretation placing the hemochromatosis gene telomeric to RFP would be brought into question if the proband's mother (I-2) were an unaffected hemochromatosis homozygote. However, as noted by Calandro *et al.*]7], her iron parameters are within normal ranges, and the proband's brother (II-4), who would have to exhibit similar incomplete penetrance, shows no irregularity in iron values at age 48. Assuming the genotypic status of I-2 is correct as characterized in the *Figure 1* below, the centromeric boundary for the candidate region can now be placed at least 1 Mb telomeric to HLA-A. Additional markers between RFP and D6S306 are needed to refine the site of cross-over and to further reduce the expanse of the candidate region.

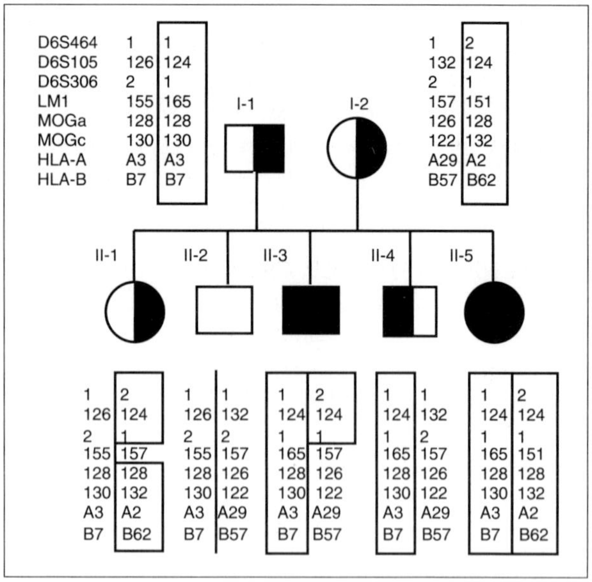

Figure 1. Chromosomal assignments of molecular and serological markers in the hemochromatosis pedigree (centromere to telomere). MOGa, MOGc, RFP and D6S105 allele designations are given in bp. Allele designations for microsatellite loci D6S306 and D6S464 are arbitrarily defined with 1 representing the smallest allele seen, 2 the next smallest, etc.

References

1. Jazwinska EC, Lee SC, Webb SI, Halliday JW, Powel LW. Localization of the hemochromatosis gene close to D6S105. *Am J Hum Genet* 1993 ; 53 : 347-52.
2. Camaschella C, Roetto A, Gasparini P, Piperno A, Fortina P, Surrey S, Rappaport E. Allelic association of microsatellites of 6p in Italian hemochromatosis patients. *Hum Genet* 1996 ; 94 : 476-81.
3. Gandon G, Jouanolle AM, Chauvel B, Mauvieux V, Le Treut A, Feingold J, Le Gall JY, David V, Yaouanq J. Linkage disequilibrium and extended haplotypes in the HLA-A to D6S105 region: implications for mapping the hemochromatosis gene (HFE). *Hum Genet* 1996 ; 97 : 103-13.
4. Stone C, Pointon JJ, Jazwinska EC, Halliday JW, Powell LW, Robson KJH, Monaco AP, Weatherall DJ. Isolation of CA dinucleotide repeats close to

D6S105; linkage disequilibrium with haemochromatosis. Hum Mol Genet 1994 ; 3 : 2043-6.

5. Raha-Chowdhury R, Bowen DJ, Stone C, Pointon JJ, Terwilliger JD, Shearman JD, Robson KJH, Bomford A, Worwood M. New polymorphic microsatellite markers place the haemochromatosis gene telomeric to D6S105. *Hum Mol Genet* 1995 : 1869-74.
6. Seese NK, Venditti CP, Chorney KA, Gerhard GS, Ma J, Hudson TJ, Phatak PD, Chorney MJ. Localization of the hemochromatosis disease gene: linkage disequilibrium analysis using an American patient collection. *Blood Cells Mol Dis* 1996 ; 22 : 36-46.
7. Calandro LM, Baer DM, Sensabaugh GF. Characterization of a recombinant that locates the hereditary hemochromatosis gene telomeric to HLA-F. *Hum Genet* 1995 ; 96: 339-42.
8. Isomura T, Tamiya-Koizumi K, Suzuki M, Yoshida S, Taniguchi M, Matsuyama M, Ishigaki T, Sakuma S, Takahashi M. RFP is a DNA binding protein associated with the nuclear matrix. *Nucleic Acids Res* 1992 ; 20 : 5305-10.
9. Amadou C, Ribouchon MT, Mattei MG, Jenkins NA, Gilbert DJ, Copeland NG, Avoustin P, Pontarotti P. Localization of new genes and markers to the distal part of the human major histocompatibility complex (MHC) region and comparison with the mouse: new insights into the evolution of mammalian genomes. *Genomics* 1995 ; 26: 9-20.
10. Roth MP, Dolbois L, Borot N, Amadou C, Clanet M, Pontarotti P, Coppin H. Three highly polymorphic microsatellites at the human myelin oligodendrocyte glycoprotein locus, 100 kb telomeric to HLA-F. Characterization and relation to HLA haplotypes. *Hum Immunol* 1995 ; 43 : 276-82.

Synergistic effect of two HLA heterodimers in celiac disease

F. Clerget-Darpoux[1], M.C. Babron[1], F. Bouguerra[2], F. Clot[1], I. Djilali-Saiah[3], F. Khaldi[2], A. Debbabi[2], S. Caillat-Zucman[3], S. Auricchio[4], J. Schmitz[3], L. Greco[4], J.F. Eliaou[5]

1 INSERM U155, château de Longchamp, Bois de Boulogne, 75016 Paris, France
2 Hôpital d'enfants, Tunis, Tunisia
3 Hôpital Necker, Paris, France
4 University Federico II, Naples, Italy
5 Hôpital Saint Eloi, Montpellier, France

The immunogenetic component of celiac disease (CD) is clearly demonstrated by the association of the disease with human leukocyte antigens (HLA). Patients usually carry the heterodimer DQ($\alpha_0\beta_0$) encoded by HLA-DQA1*0501 and DQB1*0201 [1] and the risk of developing celiac disease is significantly greater for individuals having a double dose of DQB1*0201 than for other dimer carriers [2]. Recently, we showed the role of the DRB4 gene in the genetic susceptibility of CD. Indeed, all patients not carrying the DQ($\alpha_0\beta_0$) heterodimer carry the DR($\alpha\beta$4) heterodimer formed with the β chain encoded by DRB4 and the invariant DRα chain [3, 4].
In the present study, we investigate the relative risk associated to these two heterodimers in the susceptibility to CD in three different populations : Italian, Tunisian and French.

Patient samples

Four groups of patients are studied: two samples of 50 and 35 Italian patients, (S1) and (S2) respectively, one of 94 Tunisian patients (S3) and one of 80 French patients (S4) The patients of S1, S3, S4 have been randomly selected ignoring familial history whereas all S2 patients have at least an affected sib. For all patients, the diagnosis of CD was established according to the criteria of the European Society for Pediatric Gastroenterology and Nutrition [5].

HLA typing

All patients were typed for DRB1 and DQB1. Only the French sample was typed for DQA1; in the other samples the DQA1 alleles were deduced thanks to the almost complete linkage disequilibrium between alleles at these 3 loci. Let α_0 represent DQA1*0501 and α all the other DQA1 alleles. Similarly let β_0 represent DQB1*0201 and β all the other DQB1 alleles. We denote by DQ($\alpha_0\beta_0$) the heterodimer encoded by α_0 and β_0 respectively. Genotypes of individuals who express the DRB4 gene in double dose are denoted by B4/B4, in single dose by B4/-. We denote by DR($\alpha\beta$4) the heterodimer encoded by the DRA gene and the DRB4 gene. Only individuals with a DRB1*04, DRB1*07 or DRB1*09 allele express the DRB4 gene.

HLA genotypes in patients

Six genotypes categories may be distinguished : the first five correspond to the DQ($\alpha_0\beta_0$) heterodimer carriers classified according to the number of α_0 and β_0 alleles and their cis-trans position. The sixth one represents all the non-DQ($\alpha_0\beta_0$) carriers. All patients of this last category express DRB4.

Method

The aim of the analysis is to estimate the differential risks associated to each of the 6 genotype categories.
For any value of these risks, the MASC program [6] provides the number of patients expected in the 6 categories. These expectations depend upon the allele frequencies in the population from which patients are sampled *(Table I)*. Minimizing the chi-square between observed and expected numbers gives an estimation of the relative risks. Several hypotheses are of interest and have been compared through the difference between their minimum chi-squares.

Results

Table II displays, for each sample, the number of individuals in each category and the risk estimates relatively to category V. The estimated relative risk is the highest for the second genotype category which corresponds to the presence of both heterodimers with β_0 in double dose. Comparing the different hypotheses gives evidence for :

(1) a different risk associated to the presence of the heterodimer DQ($\alpha_0\beta_0$) and that of DR($\alpha\beta4$); (2) a dose effect of β_0; (3) a synergistic effect of the two heterodimers.

Table I. DQA1-DQB1-DRB4 haplotype frequency in each population

	Italy [7]	Tunisia [8]	France [9]
$\alpha_0\beta_0$ –	0.10	0.21	0.14
$\alpha\beta_0$ – **B4**	0.14	0.10	0.14
$\alpha_0\beta$ –	0.27	0.17	0.14
$\alpha\beta$ – **B4**	0.07	0.12	0.11
$\alpha\beta$ –	0.42	0.40	0.47

Table II. Number of patients in each genotype category and risk estimates relatively to category V

Discussion

A major step in the understanding of the HLA observations in CD was achieved in 1989 by Sollid *et al.* [1] who showed that the heterodimer encoded by DQA1*0501 and DQB1*0201 was present in most CD patients (between 80-90%). Recently, we accomplished a further step by showing the additionnal role of the DR heterodimer encoded by DRA and DRB4. All our patients from 4 different samples carry at least one of these two heterodimers. In this study we quantify the respective contribution of each heterodimer. We confirm the double dose effect of β0. Moreover we give evidence for a synergistic effect of the two heterodimers.

Table II. Number of patients in each genotype category and risk estimates relatively to category V

Category	HLA-DQ	Number of patients				Relative risk			
		S1	S2	S3	S4	S1	S2	S3	S4
		(50)	(36)	(94)	(80)				
I	$\alpha_0\beta_0$-$\alpha_0\beta_0$	2	2	13	7	2.9	3.4	3.5	5.5
II	$\alpha_0\beta_0$-$\alpha\beta_0$	13	13	31	32	**6.7**	**7.8**	**9.0**	**10.0**
III	$\alpha_0\beta_0$-$\alpha_0\beta$	2	3	11	5	1.0	1.0	1.9	1.5
IV	$\alpha_0\beta$-$\alpha\beta_0$	20	11	6	10	3.8	2.5	2.5	2.5
V	$\alpha_0\beta_0$-$\alpha\beta$	8	6	18	16	1.0	1.0	1.0	1.0
VI	non DQ($\alpha_0\beta_0$) DRB4	5	1	15	10	0.3	0.1	0.6	0.3

The statistical arguments are reinforced by the existence of an homology between the sequence of the DQβ0 and the DRβ4 chain [3]. We can imagine, that beside the intra-isotypic heterodimers DQ(α0β0) and DR(αβ4), inter-isotypic formation of DRαDQβ0 and DQα0DRβ4 heterodimers is possible, and that these hybrid heterodimers confer a risk for CD.

Celiac disease is the first autoimmune disease for which the at risk HLA genotypes are so clearly delineated. It may provide a model for other autoimmune diseases.

Acknowledgments

Financial support was provided INSERM through réseau Nord-Sud #492NS1 and 5NS1 and by the Italian CNR : N9504648ST75.

References

1. Sollid LM, Markussen G, Ek J, Gjerde H, Vartdal F, Thorsby E. Evidence for a primary association of celiac disease to a particular HLA-DQ α/β heterodimer. *J Exp Med* 1989 ; 169 : 345-50.
2. Clerget-Darpoux F, Bouguerra F, Kastally R, Semana G, Babron MC, Debbabi A, Bennaceur B, Eliaou JF. High risk genotypes for celiac disease. *CR Acad Sci Paris Life Sci* 1994 ; 317 : 931-6.
3. Eliaou JF, Bouguerra F, Clot F, Babron MC, Auricchio S, Greco L. ClergetDarpoux F. A unifying explanation for the HLA susceptibility to celiac disease. *Proc Natl Acad Sci USA* 1997, submitted.
4. Bouguerra F, Babron MC, Eliaou JF, Debbabi A, Clot J, Khaldi F, Greco L, Clerget Darpoux F. Synergistic effect of two HLA heterodimers in the susceptibility to celiac disease in Tunisia. *Am J Hum Genet* 1997, submitted.
5. Meeuwisse GW Diagnostic criteria in cœliac disease. *Acta Paediatr Scand* 1970 ; 59 : 461-3
6. Clerget-Darpoux F, Babron MC, Prum B, Lathrop GM, Deschamps I, Hors J. A new method to test genetic models in HLA associated diseases: the MASC method. *Ann Hum Genet* 1988 ; 52 : 247-58.
7. Imanishi T, Akaza T, Kimura A, Tokunaga K, Gojobori T. Allele and haplotype frequencies for HLA and complement loci in various ethnic groups. In: Tsuji K, Aizawa M, Sasazuki T, eds. *Proceedings of the Eleventh International Histocompability Workshop and Conference : HLA 1991.* Oxford: Oxford Science Publications, 1991 : 1065-220.
8. Hmida S, Gauthier A, Dridi A, Quillivic F, Genetet B, Boukef K, Semana G. HLA class II gene polymorphism in Tunisians. *Tissue Antigens* 1995 ; 45 : 63-8.
9. Djilali-Saiah I, Caillat-Zucman S, Schmitz J, Chaves-Vieira ML, Bach JF. Polymorphism of antigen processing (TAP, LMP) and HLA classe II genes in celiac disease. *Hum Immunol* 1994 ; 40 : 8-16.

Narcolepsy susceptibility haplotype is defined by new markers: HLA-DQ promoter genes

E. Collina, E. Caldironi, G. Plazzi[1], F. Provini[1], M. Bragliani, E. Lugaresi[1], V. Mantovani

Tissue Typing Laboratory, Malpighi Hospital, via P. Palagi 9, 40138, Bologna, Italy
1. Neurology Institute, Bologna University, Bologna, Italy

Narcolepsy is a sleep disorder that is relatively common in several populations, characterized by excessive daytime sleepiness and cataplexy [1]. It is reported to cluster in families, although the genetic mode of transmission is not understood [2].

The major genetic component of the disease has been identified in HLA region [3,4].

There is agreement that narcolepsy is the disease most strongly HLA associated, but it is still controversial if this association is complete: in fact, this disease shows a total association with HLA DR2, DQ1 haplotype in Oriental narcoleptic patients, without exceptions. However, in Caucasian and Black patients some discrepant cases are reported [5].

As Narcolepsy does not seem an autoimmune disease, it is not likely that the DR2 itself is the candidate gene. One plausible explanation may be the *linkage disequilibrium* with HLA alleles and a putative narcolepsy-susceptibility gene.

The aim of our study was to try to better characterize the narcolepsy susceptibility haplotype, analyzing DQ promoter polymorphism beside classical HLA-class II polymorphism.

The upstream regulatory regions (URRs) of HLA DQA1 and DQB1 genes are QAP and QBP, extending upstream of the trancriptional start site [6, 7]. Although URRs are highly conserved, some hypervariable regions were found, and functional studies indicated that this allelic polymorphism could be associated with differences in transcriptional activity and affinity for DNA-binding proteins [8, 9].

Materials and methods

The study was carried out on 29 narcoleptic Italian patients and 56 controls, the latter selected from a local population of 607 healthy people for the presence of DRB1*1501 allele.

The polymorphism of DRB5, DRB1, DQA1, DQB1 genes was studied by PCR and radiolabeled sequence specific oligonucleotide method. Probes and primers were designed following the 12th International Histocompatibility Workshop recommended protocol.

For the typing of DQ promoter polymorphism, QAP and QBP genes were analyzed by using oligonucleotides provided through the 12th International Histocompatibility Workshop. The sequence-specific probes were labeled using digoxigenin-ddUTP [10] and for the hybridization detection a digoxigenin luminescent method was applied (Boehringer Mannheim GmbH, Germany).

This method allowed to be distinguished 10 alleles for QAP and 13 for QBP.

Results and discussion

Results of DQ promoter and DR-DQ polymorphism obtained in narcoleptic patients and controls are presented in *Table I*.

The haplotype DRB5*0101, DRB1*1501, DQA1*0102, DQB1*0602 was detected in all 29 narcoleptic patients. In addition, the presence of QAP 1.2 allele for DQA promoter and QBP 6.2 allele for DQB promoter was found in all patients.

In the 56 healthy controls, that were selected for the presence of DRB1*1501 allele, several combinations of different DQA-QAP and DQB-QBP alleles were observed. The analysis of DQA region showed two alleles for DQA1 gene (*0101, *0102), combined with the same QAP 1.2 allele. More variability was detected in DQB region, where four alleles were found for DQB1 gene (*0501, *0502, *0602, *0603), combined with four QBP alleles: 5.11, 5.12, 6.2, 6.3.

Table I. Haplotypes of DRB5, DRB1, DQA1, DQB1 genes and DQ promoters (QAP and QBP) detected in 29 narcoleptic patients and in 56 DRB1*1501 matched healthy controls. The relative haplotype frequences are shown in the last column

	DRB5	DRB1	DQA1	QAP	DQB1	QBP	Frequence %
Patients(n=29)	0101	1501	0102	1.2	0602	6.2	100
Controls(n=56)	0101	1501	0102	1.2	0602	6.2	62.5
	0101	1501	0102	1.2	0502	5.11	14.3
	0101	1501	0101	1.2	0602	6.2	12.5
	0101	1501	0102	1.2	0501	5.12	3.5
	0101	1501	0102	1.2	0603	6.3	1.8
	0101	1501	0101	1.2	0502	5.11	1.8
	0101	1501	0101	1.2	0603	6.3	1.8
	0101	1501	0101	1.2	0501	5.12	1.8

The DRB, DQA, DQB, DQ-promoter haplotype found in narcoleptic patients was the one more frequently found also in the DRB1 matched healthy controls (62,5 %).
Considering that the frequence of DRB1*1501 allele in our local population is 11,4%, the narcolepsy associated haplotype is solely owned by the 7% of the general population.
Our results indicate that narcolepsy in Italy is completely associated with HLA DR and DQ loci. This firm association extends as far as the promoter region of DQ genes, and QBP 6.2 results the most centromeric marker of the disease described to date.
The QAP 1.2 and QBP 6.2 alleles better define the narcolepsy susceptibility haplotype.
However, it rimains to be explained the nature of narcolepsy association with HLA. It is necessary to extend the studies to patients lacking one or more alleles of this haplotype to clarify whether a direct involvement of HLA or a narcolepsy gene in *linkage disequilibrium* with HLA are responsible of the disease.

References

1. Matsuki K, Honda Y, Juji T. Diagnostic criteria for narcolepsy and HLA-DR2 frequencies. *Tissue Antigens* 1987; 30: 155-60.
2. Guilleminault C, Mignot E, Grumet FC. Familial patterns of narcolepsy. *Lancet* 1989 ; ii : 1376-9.
3. Neely S, Rosemberg R, Spire JP, Antel J, Arnason BGW. HLA antigens in narcolepsy. *Neurology* 1987; 37: 1858-60.
4. Kuwata S, Juji T, Sasaki T, Honda Y, Wong H, Merwart HM, Haddad AP, Acton RD, Cross RA, Bing AJ, Mignot E, Grumet C. The first international collaborative study on narcolepsy. *Proceedings of the Eleventh International Histocompatibility Workshop and Conference 1991*, vol. II. Oxford: Oxford University Press, 1992: 730-7.
5. Andreas-Zietz A, Keller E, Scholz S, Albert ED, Roth B, Nevsimalova S, Sonka K, Docekal P, Ivaskova E, Schulz H, Geisler P. DR2-negative narcolepsy. *Lancet* 1986 ; ii: 684-5.
6. Morzycha- Wroblewska E, Harwood JI, Smith JR, Kagnoff MF. Structure and evolution of the promoter region of the DQA gene. *Immunogenetics* 1993; 37: 364-72.
7. Reichstetter S, Krellnar PH, Meenzen CM, Kalden JR, Wassmuth R. Comparative analysis of sequence variability in the upstream regulatory region of the HLA-DQB1 gene. *Immunogenetics* 1994; 39: 207-12.
8. Haas JP, Kimura A, Andreas A, Hochberger G, de La Paz Bettinotti M, Nevinny-Stickel C, Hildebrandt B, Sierp G, Sesasuki T, Albert E. Polymorphism in the upstream regulatory region of DQA1 genes and DRB1, QAP, DQA1, and DQB1 haplotypes in the german population. *Hum Immunol* 1994 ; 39 : 31-40.
9. Andersen LC, Beaty JS, Nettels JW, Seyfried CE, Nepom GT, Nepom B. Allelic polymorphism in trascriptional regulatory regions of HLA-DQB genes. *J Exp Med* 1991; 173: 181-92.
10. Nevinny-Stickel C, Bettinotti MdlP, Andreas A, Hinzpeter M, Muhlegger K, Schmitz G, Albert ED. Nonradioactive HLA class II typing using polymerase chain reaction and digoxigenin-11-2'-3'-dideoxy-uridinetriphosphate-labeled oligonucleotide probes. *Hum Immunol* 1991; 31: 7-13.

TAP1*0201 and HLA-DMA*0103 markers in severe forms of membranous nephropathy

D. Chevrier[1], M. Giral[2], D. Latinne[3], P. Coville[4], J.Y. Muller[1], J.D. Bignon1, J.P. Soulillou[2]*

1 Établissement de Transfusion Sanguine 44-85, Laboratoire HLA, 34, boulevard Jean Monnet, BP349 44011 Nantes Cedex, France
2 ITERT (Institut de Transplantation et de Recherche en Transplantation), CHRU, Immeuble Jean Monnet and INSERM U437 (Unité de recherche en Immunointervention dans les allo et xénotransplantations), 44035 Nantes, France
3 University of Louvain, Transplantation Immunology Laboratory, University of Louvain, avenue Hippocrate, 10, 1200 Brussels, Belgium
4 Centre Hospitalier Prosper Chubert, Service de Néphrologie-Hémodialyse, 56017 Vannes Cedex, France
*Corresponding author

Membranous nephropathy (MN) is the most frequent cause of the nephrotic syndrome in adults. MN has well defined histological features, essentially characterized by diffuse, subepithelial deposits consisting of immune complex aggregates. It has also clearly been established that MN is strongly associated with the HLA-B8, -DR3 haplotype of the major histocompatibility complex (MHC) [1].

Preliminary results suggested a possible association between TAP1*0201 allele and MN [2, 3]. Here, we present a more extensive study of this, and of the polymorphism of three other genes close to the TAP1 locus (HLA-DMA, HLA-DMB, LMP2 and LMP7) in this disease. In addition to the increased incidence of the HLA-DR3 phenotype in MN, the present study reveals a new association between MN and HLA-DMA*0103 allele. Furthermore, we show that TAP1*0201 allele could be associated with the most severe forms of this disease.

Patients, materials and methods

Patients and controls

Ninety-two adult patients with MN were included in this study. Patients were divided into two groups according to outcome. In group I (n=39), all patients had end-stage renal failure (ESRF). In group II (n=53), patients had no renal failure. One hundred randomly selected, healthy, geographically matched individuals were also typed for their HLA-DRB1, -DPB1, -DMA, -DMB, LMP2, LMP7, TAP1 and TAP2 gene polymorphisms and used as controls. Fifty other healthy HLA-DR3 positive individuals were also typed for these genes, and constituted the set of HLA-DR3 selected controls.

HLA and non-HLA gene typings

TAP1, TAP2 LMP2 and LMP7 alleles were typed by Amplification Refractory Mutation System PCR (ARMS-PCR) [4, 5]. HLA-DMA, -DMB, -DRB1, and -DPB1 were typed by PCR-SSO [6, 7].

Statistical analysis

Chi-squared tests, using the Yates correction when necessary, Fisher's exact test and relative risk (RR) were used in this study

Results

Association of HLA-DR3 with MN

We confirmed a significant increase in the frequency of HLA-DR3 phenotype in the whole series of patients with MN (65.2 %, versus 18% in the controls; p<10-10, with a relative risk of 8.5). There was, however, no difference in the proportion of patients with HLA-DR3 between group I (69.2%) and group II (62.2%).

Association of HLA-DMA*0103 with MN

An increased frequency of HLA-DMA*0103 phenotype in MN patients was observed (15.9% *versus* 4%: $p<0.006$, RR=4.5). This increased frequency was significant both in patients in group I (13.9 %; $p<0.05$) and in patients in group II (17.3 % ; $p<0.006$) as compared to the random control population (4%) *(Table I).*

Work supported by grants from the European Communauty (BIO 2CT CT920300).

Association of TAP1*0201 with severe MN disease (group I)

The frequency of TAP1*0201 phenotype *(Table II)* was no-significantly increased in the whole group of 92 MN patients (25%) as compared to controls (16 %). Surprisingly, this TAP1*0201 phenotype frequency was largely increased only in patients of group I (35.9%) comparatively to group II (17% : $p<0.04$; RR=2.7) or to controls (16% : $p<0.02$; RR=2.9).

Linkage disequilibria between HLA-DR3, HLA-DMA*0103, and/or TAP1*0201 alleles in control groups

No linkage disequilibrium were found neither between the HLA-DMA*0103 and HLA-DR3 alleles nor between TAP1*0201 and HLA-DR3 alleles.

Interdependence of MN risk factors

Since no linkage disequilibrium was observed between HLA-DR3 and DMA*0103 and between HLA-DR3 and TAP1*0201 alleles, in the control groups, a cumulative effect between these risk factors in MN patients was assessed. The calculated rate of patients expected to display both HLA-DR3 and HLA-DMA*0103 phenotypes was very similar to that observed (10.1 % vs 11.4 % respectively), further demonstrating independence between HLA-DR3 and HLA-DMA*0103 risk factors. In the same way, HLA-DR3 and TAP1*0201 were not found to act as cummulative factors in unfavourable evolution of MN disease.

Analysis of HLA-DP, -DMB , LMP2, LMP7 and TAP2 gene polymorphism in patients and controls

For these markers, no differences in the distribution of phenotypes were observed between patients of the two groups or between patients of the whole group compared to the controls (data not shown).

Table I. Frequency of HLA-DMA phenotypes in MN

Phenotype	controls	whole MN population	group I (ESRF)	group II
	n=100	n=88•	n=36•	n=52•
[DMA*0101]	97 %	98.9 %	97.2 %	100 %
[DMA*0102]	22 %	12.5%	11.1 %	13.5 %
[DMA*0103]	4 %[1] *+	15.9 %[1]	13.9 %*	17.3 %+
[DMA*0104]	9 %	5.7 %	0 %	9.6 %

• 4 patients (3 from group I and 1 from group II) were not tested.
[1] $P<0.006$ compared to controls, relative risk = 4.5.
* $P<0.05$ compared to controls.
+ $P<0.006$ compared to controls.

Table II. Frequencies of TAP1*0201 phenotypes in MN

	controls	whole MN population	group I (ESRF)	group II
Number of individuals	100	92	39	53
% [TAP1*0201]	16 %[1]*	25 %[1]	35.9 %*+	17 %+

[1] NS compared to controls (c2=2.4).
* $P<0.02$ compared to controls, relative risk = 2.9.
+ $P<0.04$ group I (ESRD) compared to group II, relative risk = 2.7.

Discussion

Association of MN disease with HLA-DR3 was hereby confirmed. This HLA-DR3 marker was equally distributed whatever the evolution of the disease. Interestingly, an increased frequency in TAP1*0201 phenotype was correlated with severe forms of the disease only. This association of TAP1*0201 with MN patients was checked not to be due to a linkage disequilibrium between TAP1*0201 and HLA-DR3. These two risk factors (HLA-DR3 and TAP1*0201 phenotypes) were not cumulative.

HLA-DMA*0103 phenotype, like HLA-DR3, was also significantly more frequent in MN patients both in groups I and II but again no linkage disequilibrium between these two alleles could be found to explain this association.These results suggest that DMA*0103 is also associated with MN (RR=4.5).

In summary, this study showed that TAP1*0201 was associated with severe forms of MN disease.

References

1. Papiha SS, Pareek SK, Rodeg RS, Morley AR, Wilkinson R, Roberts DF, Carre DN. HLA-A,B,DR and Bf allotypes in patients with idiopathic membranous nephropathy (IMN). *Kidney Int* 1987 : 31 : 130-4.
2. Chevrier D, Giral M, Braud V, Bourbigot B, Muller JY, Bignon JD, Soulillou JP. Effects of MHC-encoded TAP1 and TAP2 gene polymorphism and matching on kidney graft rejection. *Transplantation* 1995 : 60 : 292-6.
3. Chevrier D, Giral M, Braud V, Soulillou JP, Bignon JD. Membranous nephropathy and a TAP1 gene polymorphism. *N Engl J Med* 1994 : 331 : 133-4.
4. Powis SH, Tonks S, Mockridge I, Kelly AP, Trowsdale J. Alleles and haplotypes of the MHC encoded ABC transporters TAP1 and TAP2. *Immunogenetics* 1993 : 37 : 373-80.
5. Newton CR, Graham A, Heptinstall LE, Powell SJ, Summers C, Kalsheker N, Smith JC, Markham AF. Analysis of any point mutation in DNA. The amplification refractory mutation system (ARMS). *Nucleic Acids Res*1989 : 17 : 2503-16.
6. Kimura A, Sasazuki T. 11th International Histocompatibility Workshop reference protocol for the DNA-typing technique. In Sasazuki *et al.* eds. HLA, vol.1. Oxford: Oxford University Press, 1992.
7. Teisserenc H, Charron D. Technical handbook of the twelfth international histocompatibility workshop. Addendum 12-1994. In Charron D, Fauchet R eds. Publisher : HLA et Médecine, 15, rue de l'École de Médecine, 75006 Paris, France, 1994.

The contribution of two unlinked regions to genetic susceptibility in multiple sclerosis

L.F. Barcellos[1,2], P. Lin[1], J. Schafer[3,4], G. Sensabaugh[2], G. Thomson[1], W. Klitz[1]

1 Department of Integrative Biology
2 School of Public Health, University of California, 3060 Valley Life Sciences Building, Berkeley, CA 94720-3140, USA
3 Department of Neurology, University of California, Davis, USA
4 Medical Clinic of Sacramento, California, USA

Genes of the major histocompatibility complex (MHC) are implicated in inherited susceptibility to multiple sclerosis (MS). The strongest association is with the class II HLA region: molecular analyses among Northern European and North American Caucasians have identified the predisposing HLA-DR2 haplotype as HLA-DRB1*1501, DQA1*0102, DQB1*0602. A recent study of a large population-based sample of individuals with MS strongly suggests that variation in genetic, and not environmental factors are responsible for disease predisposition [1]. Because the HLA association accounts for only 10% of MS susceptibility [2], other genetic factors must also be responsible.

The apolipoprotein E/C1/C2 region on chromosome 19q13.2 has recently been identified as a possible candidate region for genetic susceptibility in Caucasian multiplex families [3]. The APOE locus within this region is polymorphic having three common alleles, E2, E3, and E4. Evidence suggests apo E dependent uptake of lipoproteins may play an important role in the development and maintenance of the nervous system, and in responses to both peripheral and central nervous system injury [4]. Here, we investigate APOE and nearby markers in a sample of Caucasian MS patients and controls, and find a significant association with a haplotype in this region. In addition, heterogeneity is detected when the patients and controls are subdivided by class II HLA DRB1*1501, suggesting a possible interaction effect between HLA and non-HLA loci in MS susceptibility. Unraveling the genetics of complex diseases, as this study initiates with MS, requires careful attention to interaction among contributing loci.

Subjects and methods

Patients

Caucasian MS patients (n=119) from California were recruited for this study. All were diagnosed as 'clinically definite' according to the criteria of Poser *et al.* [5]. The control population consisted of random Caucasian individuals (n=106) collected from the same area. DNA was extracted from whole blood samples using standard methods.

HLA class II typing

HLA-DRB1, DQA1 and DQB1 alleles were determined using PCR-SSOP methods as previously described [6].

APOE region loci

Four markers located in the 19q13.2 chromosomal region were typed as described in previous references (see methods *e.g.* [7]): APOE polymorphism, an anonymous (CA)n repeat marker D19S178, a (CA)n repeat polymorphism in the first intron of APOC2, and a HpaI RFLP in the 5' end of the APOC1 locus with a few modifications. Briefly, a 222 bp fragment encompassing the polymorphic HpaI restriction site was amplified and PCR product was denatured (0.5M NaOH/EDTA), dot-blotted in 96-well apparatus (Bio-Rad) and immobilized to nylon membrane by UV crosslinking. Oligonucleotide probes (5' biotinylated) were designed and used for hybridization and detection of the restriction site. Probe sequences are as follows: site (APOC1-S) 5'-CCTTCGTTAACTCA-3', no site (APOC1-N) 5'CCTTCCTTAACTCA-3'. Hybridization for both probes (2.5 pmole/ml hybe) was done in 2X SSPE/0.5%SDS at 37°C for 60 minutes followed by a washing step in 2X SSPE/0.1% SDS for 5 minutes at 37°C. The presence of hybridized probe was detected using horseradish peroxidase-streptavidin, HRP-SA, (Perkin-Elmer) and TMB as described elsewhere [6].

Statistical methods

The frequency of the HLA and Apo region alleles were compared using the chi-square test for heterogeneity in a contingency table of patient and control groups. All rows summing to less than three (rare alleles) were combined into a separate allelic class for the analysis. Haplotype frequencies were estimated in unrelated samples using a standard maximum likelihood method [8].

Results

The distribution of the 32 DRB1-DQB1 haplotypes identified in our study (data not shown) did not vary significantly between patients and controls using an overall test for heterogeneity. However, individual testing of the known predisposing MS haplotype, DRB1*1501-DQB1-*0602 was significant in the patient group (χ^2=7.94, p=0.005, OR=1.9). The distributions of 18 D19S178 alleles, 3 APOE alleles, 2 APOC1 alleles and 15 APOC2 alleles were also compared individually and not found to influence MS susceptibility; the frequency of the APOE E4 allele was slightly decreased in the patient group (14.7% vs. 18.4%). Genotype effects for each locus were not observed. APOC1 and APOC2 are located 10 and 40 kb telomeric, respectively, to the APOE locus, whereas D19S178 is centromeric to this region [7, 9].

Apo region haplotypes were determined and distributions were compared in patient and control populations. Of the 3 haplotype distributions examined between patients and controls (D19S178-APOE, APOE-C1, and APOE-C2), significant heterogeneity was observed with APOE-C2 (χ^2=27.19, df=16, p<0.05, shown in *Table I*). Analysis of the contribution of individual APOE-C2 haplotypes to this heterogeneity show that the frequencies of the E3-151 (15.0% of controls and 7.9% of patients, χ^2=5.19, p<0.02, OR=0.5) and E3-157 (no patients and 1.9% of controls, χ^2=4.49, p<0.05, OR=0.2) were reduced or absent in the patients suggesting a protective effect. The E3-147 haplotype (χ^2=4.36, p<0.05, OR=5.3) was found only in the patient population (2.1%).

Table I. Contingency table test for heterogeneity comparing the distribution of APOE-C2 haplotypes in MS patients to control population

APOE-C2	Patients*	Controls*	OR+
2-127	5.7	2.4	
3-127	29.1	18.0	
4-127	4.2	7.6	
3-135	25.9	23.8	
3-143	11.4	7.9	
3-145	0	3.0	
3-147	4.9	0	5.3
2-149	5.4	8.0	
3-149	42.5	37.2	
4-149	9.1	12.8	
3-151	18.9	32.2	0.5
4-151	6.6	3.7	
3-153	26.1	18.9	
4-153	8.5	8.1	
3-155	23.1	12.0	
3-157	0	4.0	0.2
$comb	16.6	12.4	
Total	238.0	212.0	

* Haplotype frequency estimates are not constrained to whole numbers.
$ All rows summing to less than 3.0 were combined into a separate allelic class for analysis
χ^2= 27.19, df=16, p<0.05
+ Odds ratio calculated when p<0.05.

Table II. APOE genotype by DRB1*1501 status in MS patients and controls

	Patients		Controls	
	*1501+	*1501-	*1501+	*1501-
APOE 2/3	10 (15.6%)	4 (7.3%)	1 (2.6%)	10 (14.7%)
3/3	37 (57.8%)	35 (63.6%)	17 (44.7%)	41 (60.3%)
3/4	14 (21.9%)	14 (25.5%)	16 (42.1%)	15 (22.1%)
other	3 (4.7%)	2 (3.6%)	4 (10.5%)	2 (2.9%)
Total	64	55	38	68

Summary : *1501+patients vs *1501+controls (χ^2=9.01, df=3, p<0.05)
*1501+controls vs *1501-controls (χ^2=10.33, df=3, p<0.05)

The interaction of HLA (DRB1*1501+/-) and APOE was also examined in this study. *Table II* compares APOE genotype by DRB1*1501 status in individual patient and control groups. No association was observed in the comparison of *1501- patients with *1501- controls. However, the distribution of APOE genotypes differed significantly when *1501+ patients were compared to *1501+ controls (X2=9.01, df=3, p<0.05). A difference was also detected between *1501+ and *1501- APOE genotype distributions (X2=10.33, df=3, p<0.05) in the controls, primarily due to a decrease in 2/3 and increase in 3/4 genotype frequencies. This was not observed when *1501+ and 1501- patient APOE genotype distributions were compared.

Discussion

In an effort to identify all of the genetic components associated with a complex disease, it is important to realize that (1) several independent (unlinked) genetic contributions are probably involved and that (2) understanding the particular relationships among these loci in producing disease will be critical to identifying some of these susceptibility loci. This is the first study investigating the role of both class II HLA loci and the c. 19 Apo region loci in determining MS susceptibility. The HLA component of MS is localized to the class II region. Our work replicated previous studies of Caucasian populations by demonstrating an association of MS with the DRB1*1501 DQA1*0102 DQB1*0602 haplotype, although at an odds ratio of only 1.9. Due to the strong linkage disequilibrium across this region, and the fact that in Caucasians these DR-DQ alleles are found almost exclusively on this haplotype, it is difficult to determine whether multiple genes or a single locus within this haplotype confer susceptibility.

A number of studies confirm association of the APOE E4 allele as a major risk factor for Alzheimer's disease [4]. Although no differences between our MS patient and control APOE allele frequencies were observed, the significant heterogeneity detected in frequency distribution of APOE-C2 patient and control haplotypes may be signaling an effect from another disease susceptibility locus nearby. Interestingly, a new gene (APOC4) has recently been identified in this region as a member of the apolipoprotein gene family, although its impact and importance for lipid metabolism has not yet been determined. These initial observations of Apo region association alone and when subdivided by HLA DRB1 *1501 status, deserve further exploration with an independent patient/control sample and additional chromosome 19 markers which are now available [10].

References

1. Ebers GC, Sadovnick AD, Risch NJ and The Canadian Collaborative Study Group. A genetic basis for familial aggregation in multiple sclerosis. *Nature* 1995; 377:150-1.
2. Hiller J. Human leukocyte antigen studies in multiple sclerosis. *Ann Neurol* 1994; 36 (suppl): 15-7.
3. Haines JL, Seboun E, Goodkin DE, Usuku K, Lincoln R, Rimmler J, Gusella JF, Roses AD, Pericak-Vance MA, Hauser SL. Genetic dissection of the multiple sclerosis genotype. *Am J Hum Genet* 1994; 53 : A266.
4. Kamboh MI. Apolipoprotein E polymorphism and susceptibility to Alzheimer's disease. *Hum Biol* 1995; 67:195-215.
5. Poser CM, Paty DW, Scheinber L, McDonald WI, Davis FA, Ebers GC, Johnson KP, Sibley WA, Silberberg DH, Tourellotte WW. New diagnostic criteria for multiple sclerosis: guidelineas for research protocols. *Ann Neurol* 1983; 13:227-31.
6. Erlich H, Bugawan T, Begovich A, Scharf S. Analysis of HLA class II polymorphism using polymerase chain reaction. *Arch Path Lab Med* 1993; 117:482-5.
7. Chartier-Harlin MC, Parfitt M, Legrain S, Perez-Tur J, Brousseau T, Evans A, Berr C, Vidal O, Roques P, Gourlet V, Fruchart JC, Delacourte A, Rossor M, Amouyei P. Apolipoprotein E, E4 allele as a major risk factor for sporadic early and late-onset forms of Alzheimer's disease: analysis of the 19q13.2 chromosomal region. *Hum Mol Genet* 1994; 3:569-74.
8. Baur MP, Danilovs J. Population genetic analysis of HLA-A, B, C, DR and other genetic markers. In: Terasaki PI, ed. *Histocompatibility Testing 1980*. Los Angeles: UCLA Tissue Typing Laboratory, 1980; 955-93.
9. Ashworth LK, Batzer MA, Brandriff B, Branscomb E, de Jong P, Garcia E, Garnes JA, Gordon LA, Lamerdin JE, Lennon G, Mohrenweiser H, Olsen AS, Slezak T, Carrano AV. An integrated metric physical map of human chromosome 19. *Nature Genet* 1995; 11:422-7.
10. Allan CM, Walker, D, Segrest JP, Taylor JM. Identification and characterization of a new human gene (APOC4) in the apolipoprotein E, C1, and C2 gene locus. *Genomics* 1995; 28:291-300.

Genetic susceptibility and anti-human platelet antigen 5b alloimmunization: role of HLA class II and TAP genes

C. Kaplan [1]*, T. Zazoun [1], M. Alizadeh [2], M.C. Morel-Kopp [1], B. Genetet, G. Semana [2]

1 Service d'Immunologie Leuco-Plaquettaire, INTS, 6, rue Alexandre Cabanel, 75739 Paris Cedex 15, France
2 Laboratoire Universitaire d'Immunologie, CRTS, rue Pierre-Jean Gineste, 35000 Rennes, France
*Corresponding author

Platelet alloimmunization results from exposure of normal individuals to allotypic determinants. Two well described clinical syndromes could be elicited by such an immunization: Post transfusion purpura (PTP) and fetal/neonatal alloimmune thrombocytopenia (NAIT) [1].
Since the time of the description of the first platelet specific antigen, five diallelic human platelet antigenic (HPA) systems have been defined [2] and a number of low frequency antigens. Progress in molecular biology has led to the identification of the polymorphisms responsible for several of the platelet allotypes (for example [3, 4]).
Neonatal alloimmune thrombocytopenia is a transient passive disease in an otherwise healthy newborn but there is a risk of intracerebral haemorrhage and therefore of neurological impairment or death during the thrombocytopenic period [5].
Among the platelet-specific alloantigens implicated in NAIT, HPA-1a is the most frequently involved in Caucasians. The incidence of NAIT linked to HPA-1a has been recently estimated to be 1 per 1000 live births [6].
HPA-5b is the second most frequent antigen implicated in Caucasians in NAIT [7] and PTP.
Understanding the mechanisms of platelet alloimmunization is a crucial step to define high risk groups and thus to allow developement of specific management for preventing adverse consequences. As it has been shown by retrospective and prospective studies that there is a strong correlation between the presence of HLA DRB3* 0101, and/or DQB1* 0201 and anti HPA-1a immunization [8, 9], it was of our interest to study the immune response against HPA-5b.

Patients and methods

Fifty women immunized against HPA-5b (n=47) or 5a (n=3) were included.

Antiplatelet immunization study
It was performed as previously described [7].

HLA class II DNA typing and TAP genotyping
HLA class II polymorphism was studied by reverse dot blot hybridization (Innolipa tests from Innogenetics) [10] and for TAP genotyping the methodology has been recently reported [11].

Results *(Table I)*

HLA class II gene typing
It was found that 74.5 % of immunized women carried a particular DRβ169-70 polymorphic sequence encoded by GAA-GAC versus 49 % of controls ($pc < 0.01$ RR = 2.95). Furthermore, 31.9 % of patients were homozygous for the DRβ1 GAA-GAC sequence versus 7.5 % of controls ($pc < 10^{-4}$, RR=5.7). Moreover, DRB5*0101 and *0102 alleles have also GAA-GAC sequence encoding Glu-Asp at position 69-70. Analysing simultaneously DRB1 and DRB5 genes showed that 85.1% of patients (40/47) versus 65% of controls (130/200) carried the GAA-GAC sequence ($pc<0.05$, RR=3.09) and that 40.4% of patients versus 11.5% of controls carried the GAA-GAC sequence in double dose ($pc<10^{-4}$, RR=5.25).
No predominance of a particular DRB3 or DQB1 or DPB1allele was found.

TAP1 and TAP2 genotyping
The signicative result we obtained concerned TAP 2 gene analysis. Homozygosity for Ile-Ile at position 379 was more frequent in patients (10.6 %) than in controls (3.8 %). When the 50 women immunized against the HPA-5 antigens were considered, homozygosity for this position in this group (16 %) was significantly different from the control population (3.8 %) ($pc < 0.02$ RR = 4.70). This TAP association was not due to a linkage desequilibrium with HLA-DRB1 locus.

Table I. HLA class II and TAP-2 results.

	Immunized women anti HPA-5b n=47		Controls n = 200		RR
	n	%	n	%	
DRB1*GAA-GAC 69-70	35	74.5 (pc < 0.01)	98	49.0	2.95
DRB1*GAA-GAC 69-70 homozygous	15	31.9 ($pc < 10^{-4}$)	15	7.5	5.70

TAP2 Position	Amino-acid	Immunized women against HPA-5b (n = 47)		Immunized women against HPA-5a or -5b (n=50)		Controls (n=183)	
		n	%	n	%	n	%
379	Ile-Ile	5	10.6	8	16 (pc < 0.02 - RR = 4.7)	7	3.8

Discussion

We have studied 50 women immunized against the HPA-5 antigens. Our results suggest a strong association of alloimmunization with a cluster of HLA DR molecules sharing a particular polymorphic amino acid sequence at position 69-70 (Glu-Asp encoded by GAA-GAC nucleotide sequence) of the DRβ1 chain (RR=2.95, RR=5.70 when patients were homozygous for this sequence), and a negative association with the DRB1*0301 allele (2.1% vs 28 %-RR=0.08). Furthermore an increased frequency of a TAP2 dimorphism at position 379 was observed in immunized women against the HPA-5 antigens (RR= 4.7).

The genetic background of alloimmunization against the HPA-5 antigens clearly differs from the anti HPA-1a alloimmunization where a major role has been attributed to DRB3 and DQB1 genes [8, 9].

In the clinical perspective, our findings, combined with those already published concerning other platelet antigens indicate that the nature of the polymorphism present in the platelet membrane glycoprotein could be of importance for the immune response. The implication of TAP genes is not clear. It could result from a linkage desequilibrium with another yet unknown but relevant gene located in this region, rather than a direct participation of TAP molecules. Definition of high risk group regarding antiplatelet alloimmunization should take into account not only the platelet antigens involved but also the particular immunogenetic background.

References

1. Shulman N, Marder V, Hiller M, *et al.* Platelet and leukocyte isoantigens and their antibodies. Serologic, physiologic and clinical studies. In : Moore C, Brown E, eds. *Progress in Hematology,* 4e ed. New York: Grune and Stratton, 1964; 222-304.
2. Von dem Borne AEGK, Decary F. Nomenclature of platelet specific antigens. *Br J Haematol* 1990 ; 74:2039-40.
3. Newman PJ, Derbes RS, Aster RH. The human platelet alloantigens, Pl^{A1} and Pl^{A2}, are associated with a leucine33/proline33 amino acid polymorphism in membrane glycoprotein IIIa, and are distinguishable by DNA typing. *J Clin Invest* 1989;83:1778-81.
4. Santoso S, Kalb R, Walka M, Kiefel V, Mueller-Eckhardt C, Newman PJ. The human platelet alloantigens Br^a and Br^b are associated with a single amino acid polymorphism on glycoprotein Ia (Integrin subunit α2). *J Clin Invest* 1993;92:2427-32.
5. Kaplan C, Morel-Kopp MC, Clemenceau S, Daffos F, Forestier F, Tchernia G. Fetal and neonatal alloimmune thrombocytopenia:current trends in diagnosis and therapy. *Transfus Med* 1992;2:265-71.
6. Durand-Zaleski I, Schlegel N, Blum-Boisgard C, Uzan S, Dreyfus M, Kaplan C. Screening primiparous women and newborns for fetal/neonatal alloimmune thrombocytopenia: a prospective comparison of effectiveness and costs. *Am J Perinatol* 1997 (in press).
7. Kaplan C, Morel-Kopp MC, Kroll H, Kiefel V, Schlegel N, Chesnel N, Mueller Eckhardt C. HPA-5b (Br^a) neonatal alloimmune thrombocytopenia - Clinical and immunological analysis of 39 cases. *Br J Haematol* 1991;78:425-9.
8. Valentin N, Vergracht A, Bignon JD, Cheneau ML, Blanchard D, Kaplan C, Reznikoff-Etievant MF, Muller JY. HLA DRw52a is involved in alloimmunisation against Pl^{A1} antigen. *Hum Immunol* 1990;27:73-9.
9. L'Abbé D, Tremblay L, Filion M, Busque L, Goldman M, Decary F, Chartrand P. Alloimmunization to platelet antigen HPA-1a (Pl^{A1}) is strongly associated with both HLA-DR3*0101 and HLA-DQB1*0201. *Hum Immunol* 1992;34:107-14.
10. Hmida S, Gauthier A, Dridi A, Quillivic F, Genetet B, Boukef K, Semana G. HLA class II gene polymorphism in Tunisians. *Tissue Antigens* 1995;45:63-8.
11. Moins-Teisserenc H, Semana G, Alizadeh M, Loiseau P, Bobrynina V, Deschamps I, Edan G, Birebent B, Genetet B, Sabouraud O, *et al.* TAP2 gene polymorphism contributes to genetic susceptibility to multiple sclerosis. *Hum Immunol* 1995;42:195-202.

Class I and II HLA antigens and Natural Selection Haplotypes (NSH) in Greek patients, males and females, with Graves' disease

F. Harsoulis[1], K. Adam[2], P. Lazidou[2], S. Lalaga[2], Z. Polymenidis[2]

1 Endocrine Unit, Second Propedeutic Department of Medicine, Aristotelian University of Thessaloniki,
2 Department of Immunology, National Regional Tissue Typing Laboratory, Hippokration General Hospital, 50 Papanastasioy Street, 54642 Thessaloniki, Greece

Graves' disease is the first autoimmune disease found to be associated initially with a higher frequency of HLA antigens [1]. The present study was undertaken for the following reasons (1) There are no published data available as yet on the HLA class II association of Graves' disease in Greek population, (2) the ethnology of Graves' disease in Greece has a historical and geographical consequence related to the HLA antigens frequency and (3) the Greek people has a particular identity among the European and Mediterranean nations [2, 4].

Subjects-methods

One hundred and five consecutive patients with Graves' disease (80 females, 25 males, from 18 to 67 years old), were included in this study. The patients consisted a fairly homogenous ethnic group coming from Northern Greece. One hundred and seventy (94 females, 76 males) normal, healthy, unrelated individuals matched for age and sex, coming from Northern Greece constituted controls for the study. All subjects were tested for HLA class I by serology and class II alleles with DNA-RFLP and the PCR-SSP "low resolution" methods [5, 6]. A 2x2 table analysis, chi-square test and relative risk were applied for the statistical evaluation. Haplotype frequency was determined by the antigen frequency in the same phenotype. Probability values were corrected (Pc) for the number of HLA alleles for each locus tested.

Results

Analysis of the HLA phenotypes of the 105 patients showed a non-significant increase of HLA-A1, B8, B15 and B39 among the patients. DNA analysis confirmed the serological assignment of the class II antigens, revealing a marked increase of the DRB1*16 and a significantly lower frequency of DRB1*14 among the patients compared with the controls *(Table I)*. The DRB1*0301 allele, well recognized in Caucasian populations, was not significantly different in patients and controls. A non-significant increase of DQA1*0102 and a significantly decrease of DQA1*0104 were found in the patients group. No differences in the distribution of DQB1 alleles were observed in Graves' patients. An increased frequency of the A1B8, B8DR3 and A1B8DR3 haplotypes was found in patients group when compared to the controls *(Table I)*. There is no difference in any HLA antigen or allele between the male group and the male controls, while HLA-DRB1*16 and DQA1*0102 alleles were increased in female patients

Table I. Frequency of HLA alleles and natural selection haplotypes among patients with Graves' disease and healthy controls.

HLA alleles-haplotypes	Patients Ī=105		Controls Ī=170*		x^2	Pc	RR
A1	31	(29.5%)	31	(18.2%)	4.11	(NS)	1.9
B8	21	(20.0%)	24	(14.1%)	1.23	(NS)	1.5
DRB1*16	31	(29.5%)	23	(13.5%)	9.53	0.026	2.7
DRB1*0301	28	(26.7%)	29	(17.1%)	3.08	NS	1.8
DRB1*14	4	(3.8%)	29	(17.1%)	9.57	0.026	0.2
DQA1*0102	43	(41.0%)	46	(27.1%)	5.10	NS	1.9
DQA1*0104	4	(3.8%)	36	(21.2%)	14.38	0.001	0.1
A1B8	16	(15.2%)	4	(3.3%)	8.49	0.003	5.3
B8DR3	18	(17.1%)	6	(4.9%)	7.55	0.006	4
A1B8DR3	14	(13.3%)	4	(3.3%)	6.40	0.01	4.5

*Family studies were available for 121 of the controls.

versus female controls (Pc=0.006, RR = 2.9 and Pc=0.02, RR=2.1 respectively). The DRB1*14 and DQA1*0104 alleles were significantly decreased in female patients compared with the female controls (Pc=0.002, RR=0.1 and Pc=0.0001, RR=0.08 respectively). When male patients are compared to female patients all but two (DRB1*14 and DQA1*0104) HLA antigens and haplotypes were found increased in females but this difference was not significant with the exception of DQA1*0102 allele (Pc=0.03). The DRB1*14 and DQA1*0104 alleles were decreased in female patients but the difference was still not significant.

Discussion

This study revealed a significant association of A1B8, B8DR3 and A1B8DR3 haplotypes in patients with Graves' disease. The class II haplotype DRB1*16 - DRB5*- DQA1*0102 is increased but not significantly and the class II haplotype HLA-DRB1*14 - DRB3*- DQA1*0104 is significantly decreased in patients group. The last one could be considered as protective Natural Selection Haplotype (NSH) [7], while the others as susceptible haplotype in Greek population. It seems that the ethnology of GD in Greek population depends on this NSH. The above mentioned differences are more distinct in female patients. Graves' disease is a multifactorial genetic disease in which there is a polygenic component consisting of several genes and possibly a dominant one, that interacts in a cumulative fashion [8]. The contribution of HLA region products in the pathogenesis of GD is different in various individuals, races, ethnic groups and sex as our study suggests.

References

1. Grumet FC, Payne RO, Konishi J, Kriss JP HL-A Antigens as markers for disease susceptibility and autoimmunity in Graves' disease. *J Clin Endocrinol Metab* 1974: 39: 1115-9.
2. Polymenidis Z. The identification of A and B locus in the HLA system in Greek population. Thesis, University Studio Press, Thessaloniki, 1978.
3. Piazza A, Fauchet R, Richiardi P, Carcassi C, Contu L. Anthropology report Belgian, French, Italian, Portuguese, Sardinian, and Spanish populations. *HLA 1991. Proceedings of the Eleventh International Histocompatibility Workshop and Conference*. Oxford : Oxford Science Publications, 1991: 1: 648 -51.
4. Cuccia M, Astoffi E, Gyodi E, Kastelan A, Papasteriades C, Salerno A, Suciu Foca. N. Veratti. A. HLA in five populations of southern Europe. *HLA 1991. Proceedings of the Eleventh International Histocompatibility Workshop and Conference*. Oxford : Oxford Science Publications, 1991 : 1 : 655-6.
5. Bidwell JL. DNA-RFLP analysis and genotyping of HLA-DR and DQ antigens. *Immunol Today* 1988: 9: 18-23.
6. Olerup O, Zetterquist H. HLA-DRB1 subtyping by allele-specific PCR amplification: a sensitive, specific and rapid technique. *Tissue Antigens* 1992: 37: 197-204.
7. Polymenidis Z, Adam K, Parapanisiou E, Sakellariou G, Papakyriazi E, Antoniadis A. Papadimitriou M. Importance of certain HLA-A,B haplotypes for the survival of grafts from living related donors. *Transplant Proc* 1992: 6: 2458-60.
8. Bias W, Reveille I, Beaty I, Meyers D, Arnett F. Evidence that autoimmunity in man is a mendelian dominant trait. *Am J Hum Genet* 1986: 39: 584 - 602.

HLA and Cancer

Contents

• HLA and Cancer

HLA class I alterations in laryngeal tumors

T. Cabrera, J. Salinero[1], M.A. Fernández, P. Jimenez, J. Cantón, F. Garrido

Departimento de Análisis Clínicos y
1 Departimento de Otorrinolaringología, Hospital Universitatio Virgen de las Nieves, Avenida Fuerzas Armades, 2, 18014 Granada, Spain

There is a great deal of information concerning the alteration of HLA class I expression in many different tumor systems [1-3]. HLA class I expression is frequently altered in tumors compared to the tissue from which they originate [4]. Given the central role of MHC products in the restriction of T-cell recognition and NK activity, regulation of tumor HLA expression might be a strategy for the evasion of immune surveillance by malignant cells.

Due to the difficulty of obtaining monoclonal antibodies against HLA alleles, these studies were carried out, until recently, only with monoclonal antibodies against HLA class I monomorphic and locus specific determinants. Previous studies have demonstrated that HLA class I antigens are down-regulated in around 30% of laryngeal tumors [5]. However, with the use of mAbs that define HLA alleles and work in cryostatic sections, we have been able to perform a more detailed analyses.

In this study, a total of 93 laryngeal tumors were evaluated in cryostatic sections using an immunoperoxidase technique. We found that 37% of the tumors had total or locus-specific loss *(Table I)*. Sixty-two tumors were only studied with mAbs defining HLA monomorphic and locus-specific determinants.

In 31 cases, we were able to type patient´s PBL and study these cases with allele-specific mAbs selected from the HLA and Cancer Component panel of the 12th International Histocompatibility Workshop. In this group, we found 3 tumors presenting total HLA-ABC loss, 6 with selective loss of HLA-A antigens, 5 tumors with absence of HLA-B antigens and 3 cases in which both HLA-A and B antigens were lost. The 14 tumors positive with monomorphic and locus-specific mAbs were then studied with allele-specific mAbs. Eight of the 14 tumors did not react with mAbs directed against HLA alleles *(Table II)*. Not all alleles could be studied because mAbs were not available against all specificities. We have included those tumors with a heterogeneous pattern (losses between 25-75%) in the group of negative tumors.

These results show that out of the 31 tumors studied with all the mAbs, 25 (80%) present some type of HLA class I alteration. Although, we detected HLA class I losses in 80% of the cases, we believe this figure is still an underestimate, given that in most of the 14 tumors studied for HLA allelic expression, we could not analyze all A and B, nor could we test any C alleles. For example, patient CL39 was considered HLA class I positive after we had analyzed the expression of A2 and Bw4 (*Table II*). However, the other alleles were not tested because no appropriate mAbs were available. Therefore the exact frequency of these HLA alterations in human tumors remains unknown.

We found a similar percentage of losses (88%) in 105 breast carcinomas using anti-HLA allelic class I mAbs [6]. In cervical carcinomas, losses of HLA allele expression in 73% of the patients have been reported [7].

Table I. HLA class I antigens in laryngeal carcinomas

n = 93*	
W6/32;b2m - negative	n = 17
HLA-A,B and AB - negative	n = 17
HLA allelic losses	n = 8 (out of 31**)
% of HLA class I losses = 80%**	

* We obtained a 37% of HLA class I losses using only anti HLA monomorphic and locus-specific mAbs.

** 31 of the 93 tumors were studied with mAbs against HLA alleles. The 80% of HLA class I losses was obtained from the group of 31 patients.

Table II. Detailed analysis of HLA expression of the 14 tumors previously found to be positive with anti-HLA class I monomorphic mAbs

TUMOR	LYMPHOCYTE TYPING		TUMOR TYPING					
CL10	A11,-,B14,-,Bw6		A11	-	B14	-	Bw6	
CL15	A2,-,B50,B35,Bw6	*	A2	-	B50	B35	Bw6	
CL22	A2,A29,B44,B18,Bw4,Bw6,Cw4,Cw5		A2	A29	B44	B18	Bw4	Bw6
CL33	A3,-,B7,B44,Bw4,Bw6	*	A3	-	B7	B44	Bw4	Bw6
CL38	A2,A30,B14,B18,Bw6,Cw5		A2	A30	B14	B18	Bw	
CL39	A2,A11,B39,B63,Bw4,Bw6,Cw7	*	A2	A11	B39	B63	Bw4	Bw6
CL41	A24,A25,B35,-,Bw4,Bw6,Cw4		A24	A25	B35	-	Bw4	Bw6
CL43	A2,A24,B63,B35,Bw4,Bw6,Cw7	*	A2	A24	B63	B35	Bw4	Bw6
CL47	A3,A31,B7,B27,Bw4,Bw6,Cw1,Cw7		A3	A31	B7	B27	Bw4	Bw6
CL49	A24,A26,B35,B41,Bw6,Cw4		A24	A26	B35	B41	Bw6	
CL53	A28,A29,B44,B14,Bw4,Bw6		A28	A29	B44	B14	Bw4	Bw6
CL54	A29,A33,B44,B14,Bw4,Bw6		A29	A33	B44	B14	Bw4	Bw6
CL55	A31,A34,B37,B41,Bw6,Cw1,Cw6	*	A31	A34	B37	B41	Bw6	
CL57	A11,A29,B35,B60,Bw6,Cw3,Cw4	*	A11	A29	B35	B60	Bw6	

The alleles in boxes are the ones we could study. White boxes indicate positive reaction and black boxes indicate negative reaction with the corresponding anti-HLA class I mAb.

References

1. Lopez-Nevot MA, Garcia E, Romero C, Oliva MR, Serrano S, Garrido F. Phenotypic and genetic analysis of HLA class I and HLA DR antigen expression on human melanomas. *Exp Clin Immunogenet* 1987 ; 5 : 203-12.
2. Garrido F, Cabrera T, Lopez-Nevot MA, Ruiz Cabello F. HLA class I antigens in human tumors. *Adv Cancer* Res 1995 ; 67 : 155-95.
3. Möller P, Mattfeldt T, Gross C, Schlosshauer P, Koch A, Koretz K, Moldenhauer G, Kaufmann M, Otto HF. Expression of HLA-A, -B, -C, -DR, -DP, -DQ, and of HLA-D-associated invariant chain (li) in non-neoplastic mammary epithelium, fibroadenoma, adenoma, and carcinoma of the breast. *Am J Pathol* 1989 ; 135 : 73-83.
4. Garrido F, Cabrera T, Concha A, Glew S, Ruiz-Cabello F, Stern P. Natural history of HLA antigens during tumor development. *Immunol Today* 1993 ; 14: 491-9.
5. Esteban F, Concha A, Delgado M, Pérez-Ayala M, Ruiz-Cabello F, Garrido F. Lack of MHC class I antigens and tumour aggressiveness of the squamous cell carcinoma of the larynx. *Br J Cancer* 1990 ; 62 : 1047-51.
6. Cabrera T, Fernandez MA, Sierra A, Garrido A, Herruzo A, Escobedo A, Fabra A, Garrido F. High frequency of altered HLA class I phenotypes in invasive breast carcinomas. *Hum Immunol* 1997 (in press).
7. Keating PJ, Cromm FV, Duggan-Keen M, Snijders PJF, Walboomers JMM, Hunter RD, Dyer PA, Stern PL. Frequency of down regulation of individual HLA-A and -B alleles in cervical carcinomas in relation to TAP-1 expression. *Br J Cancer* 1995 ; 72 : 405-11.

Comparison of the reactivity of frozen and formalin-fixed, paraffin-embedded sections of melanoma lesions with anti-HLA class I mAb

T. Kageshita, S. Hirai, T. Ono, S. Ferrone

Department of Dermatology, Kumamoto University School of Medicine, Kumamoto 860, Japan
Department of Microbiology and Immunology, New York Medical College, Valhalla, 10595 New York, USA

It has been known for some time that malignant transformation of cells may be associated with complete or selective loss of HLA class I allospecificities (for review, see [1]). These abnormalities may have a negative impact on the outcome of T cell based immunotherapy which is being used with increasing frequency in the treatment of malignant diseases. The realization of this possibility has rekindled interest in the analysis of HLA class I antigen expression in surgically removed malignant lesions. Immunohistochemical staining with anti-HLA class I mAb of surgically removed malignant lesions is becoming part of the battery of tests performed to select patients to be entered in some clinical trials of T cell based immunotherapy. This approach, which is likely to be applied with increasing frequency in the next years, has raised the question whether frozen or formalin-fixed tissue substrates should be used in immunohistochemical assays with anti-HLA class I mAb. We have addressed this question by comparing the reactivity of anti-HLA class I mAb with frozen and formalin-fixed, paraffin-embedded sections of primary and metastatic melanoma lesions.

Materials and methods

Tissue

Primary and metastatic melanoma lesions, obtained from patients who underwent surgery, were processed within 15 min following their surgical removal, as described [2].

mAb and conventional antisera

The mAb W6/32 to a monomorphic determinant expressed on β_2-μ associated HLA class I heavy chains, the mAb HC-10 to a determinant expressed on β_2-μ free HLA class I heavy chains and the anti-human β_2-μ mAb NAMB-1 were developed as described [3-5]. The Vectastain ABC kit and biotinylated anti-mouse Ig xenoantibodies were purchased from Vector Laboratories (Burlingame, CA). Target Unmasking Fluid (TUF) was purchased from Kreatech (Amsterdam, The Netherlands).

Indirect immunoperoxidase staining

Indirect immunoperoxidase staining of frozen and formalin-fixed, paraffin-embedded tissue sections with anti-HLA class I mAb was performed utilizing the Vectastain ABC kit according to the manufacturer's instructions with minor modifications, as described elsewhere [2]. Negative controls were performed by replacing primary antibody with supernatant from the murine myeloma cell line P3-X63-Ag8.653. Staining results were evaluated independently by two investigators. Variations in the percentage of stained cells enumerated by the two investigators were within a 10% range. Results were classified as -, ± and +, when the percentage of stained melanoma cells was less than 25%, between 25 and 75% and greater than 75%, respectively.

Results

The results of staining of frozen sections of 26 primary and 9 metastatic melanoma lesions with anti-β_2-μ associated HLA class I heavy chain mAb W6/32, anti-β_2-μ free HLA class I heavy chains mAb HC-10 and anti-β_2-μ mAb NAMB-1 and of formalin-fixed, paraffin-embedded sections of the same lesions with mAb HC-10 are summarized in *Table I*. Although the limited number of lesions tested invites one to exercise caution in interpreting the data, the following conclusions can be drawn.

Table I. Differential reactivity in the immunoperoxidase reaction of frozen and formalin-fixed, paraffin-embedded melanoma lesions with anti-HLA class I mAb

	Frozen sections						Paraffin sections	
Lesions	mAb W6/32		b-m mAb NAMB-1		mAb HC-10		mAb HC-10	
Primary	#	%	#	%	#	%	#	%
+[a]	24	92.3	23	88.5	22	84.6	14	53.8
±[b]	2	7.7	1	3.8	4	15.4	8	30.8
-[c]	0	0.0	2	7.7	0	0.0	4	15.4
Metastatic								
+	5	55.6	7	77.8	6	66.7	1	11.1
±	3	33.3	2	22.2	1	11.1	4	44.4
-	1	11.1	0	00.0	2	22.2	4	44.4

[a] Number and % of lesions in which the % of stained melanoma cells was greater than 75.
[b] Number and % of lesions in which the % of stained melanoma cells was between 25 and 75.
[c] Number and % of lesions in which the % of stained melanoma cells was less than 25.

1. The results of immunoperoxidase staining of frozen sections of primary and metastatic melanoma lesions with mAb recognizing distinct determinants expressed on the HLA class I complex and on its individual subunits are comparable, but not identical. The differences may reflect the differential expression of the antigenic determinants recognized by the mAb used and/or the characteristics of the mAb tested.

2. The reactivity of formalin-fixed, paraffin-embedded sections of both primary and metastatic melanoma lesions with mAb HC-10 is markedly lower than that of the corresponding frozen sections with mAb HC-10 as well as with mAb W6/32 and NAMB-1.

3. The difference in the reactivity with mAb HC-10 of frozen and of formalin-fixed, paraffin-embedded sections of melanoma lesions, as measured by the percentage of lesions classified as + and ±, is greater for metastatic than for primary lesions.

Discussion

The present study has shown a markedly lower reactivity with anti-HLA class I mAb of formalin-fixed, paraffin-embedded than of frozen melanoma lesions. This conclusion parallels similar results obtained by [6] who have compared the reactivity of mAb W6/32 and HC-10 with frozen and formalin-fixed cervical carcinoma lesions, respectively. Therefore, although the use of formalin-fixed, paraffin-embedded tissue sections of surgically removed lesions offers the advantage to preserve cellular details and to provide more representative information about the HLA class I antigenic phenotype of a lesion than frozen sections, it has the disadvantage to overestimate HLA class I antigen downregulation in surgically removed malignant lesions. An additional disadvantage of the use of formalin-fixed, paraffin-embedded tissue sections is represented by the fact that the few available anti-HLA class I mAb reacting with this type of tissue substrates recognize monomorphic determinants expressed on β2-μ free HLA class I heavy chains. Therefore, these reagents cannot detect loss of β2-μ as well as selective losses of HLA class I allospecificities which occur frequently in melanoma lesions [7-9].

The different reactivity patterns of formalin-fixed, paraffin-embedded primary and metastatic melanoma lesions deserve some comments. We believe that this difference reflects the worse preservation condition of metastases than of primary lesions because of their larger size. The larger size may also results in the detection of heterogeneity in the expression of HLA class I antigens in formalin-fixed sections, since they are more representative of the antigenic phenotype of a lesion.

Acknowledgements

The authors wish to acknowledge the excellent secretarial assistance of Mrs. Edwina L. Jones, Ms. Teresa L. Eley, Mrs. Harriett V. Harrison, Mrs. Donna D. James and Miss Naoko Ogata.

This investigation was supported by PHS grant CA67108 awarded by the National Cancer Institute, DHHS.

References

1. Garrido F, Cabrera T, Concha A, Glew S, Ruiz-Cabello F, Stern PL. Natural history of HLA expression during tumour development. *Immunol Today* 1993 ; 14 : 491-9.
2. Hicklin DJ, Kageshita T, Ferrone S. Development and characterization of rabbit antisera to human MHC-linked transporters associated with antigen processing. *Tissue Antigens* 1996, in press.
3. Barnstable CJ, Bodmer WF, Brown G, Galfre G, Milstein C, Williams AF, Ziegler A. Production of monoclonal antibodies to group A erythrocytes, HLA and other human cell surface antigens-new tools for genetic analysis. *Cell* 1978 ; 14 : 9-20.
4. Stam NJ, Spits H, Ploegh HL. Monoclonal antibodies raised against denatured HLA-B locus heavy chains permit biochemical characterization of certain HLA-C locus products. *J Immunol* 1986 ; 137 : 2299-306.
5. Pellegrino MA, Ng A-K, Russo C, Ferrone S. Heterogeneous distribution of the determinants defined by monoclonal antibodies on HLA-A and B antigens bearing molecules. *Transplantation* 1982 ; 34 : 18-23.
6. Cromme FV, Airey J, Heemels MT, Ploegh HL, Keating PJ, Stern PL, Meijer CJ, Walboomers JM. Loss of transporter protein, encoded by the TAP-1 gene, is highly correlated with loss of HLA expression in cervical carcinomas. *J Exp Med* 1994 ; 179 : 335-40.
7. Wang Z, Cao Y, Albino AP, Zeff RA, Houghton A, Ferrone S. Lack of HLA class I antigen expression by melanoma cells SK-MEL-33 caused by a reading frameshift in β_2-microglobulin messenger RNA. *J Clin Invest* 1993 ; 91 : 684-92.
8. Restifo NP, Marincola FM, Kawakami Y, Taubenberger J, Yannelli JR, Rosenberg SA. Loss of functional beta$_2$-microglobulin in metastatic melanomas from five patients receiving immunotherapy. *J Natl Cancer Inst* 1996 ; 88 : 100-8.
9. Kageshita T, Wang Z, Calorini L, Yoshii A, Kimura T, Ono T, Gattoni-Celli S, Ferrone S. Selective loss of human leukocyte class I allospecificities and staining of melanoma cells by monoclonal antibodies recognizing monomorphic determinants of class I human leukocyte antigens. *Cancer Res* 1993 ; 53 : 3349-54.

Down-regulated expression of HLA-B antigens in metastatic melanomas

A. Gasparollo, I. Cattarossi, A. Cattelan, M. Altomonte, M. Maio

Advanced Immunotherapy Unit, Centro di Riferimento Oncologico, INRCCS, Via Pedemontana Occidentale 12, 33081 Aviano, Italy

Immunotherapy of human melanoma has received new emphasis from the recent identification of melanoma-associated antigens (MAGE, BAGE, GAGE, p15), differentiation antigens of the melanocytic lineage (tyrosinase, gp100, gp75, Melan-A/MART-1) and unique melanoma antigens (CDK4, MUM-1) that are recognized by cytotoxic T lymphocytes (CTL) in the context of selected HLA class I allospecificities (for review, see 1). Different HLA-A alleles act as restricting elements for the presentation to T lymphocytes of the majority of the antigenic peptides deriving from the melanoma-associated antigens which have been so far identified [1]; in contrast, little is known on the role of HLA-B allospecificities in this phenomenon. The renewed interest in applying T cell-based immunotherapy to human melanoma has stimulated interest in the characterization of the expression of HLA class I antigens on malignant cells of the melanocytic lineage and on their structural and functional abnormalities [2] The majority of available studies investigated the expression of HLA class I antigens by immunohistochemical analysis of tissue specimens, demonstrating that about 10% and 70% of primary and metastatic melanomas show loss or down-regulation of HLA-A and/or HLA-B antigens expression [2]. The low sensitivity of immunohistochemical analyses may result in a high number of lesions classified as HLA class I-negative. In addition, the analysis of tissue sections does not provide reliable data on the quantitative expression of cell surface antigens. The latter information seems to be critical for applying T cell-based immunotherapy to melanoma patients. In fact, the heterogeneous lysis of HLA-A2 positive melanomas by a CTL clone recognizing the differentiation antigen Melan-A/MART-1 correlated with the amounts of HLA-A2 antigens expressed on the cell surface of neoplastic cells but not with that of Melan-A/MART-1 [3].

In view of the considerations above we performed a quantitative analysis of the expression of HLA-A and -B antigens on 14 primary cultures of metastatic melanomas by indirect immunofluorescence (IIF) followed by flow cytometry. Selected monoclonal antibodies (mAb) to HLA class I antigens, obtained through the HLA and Cancer section of the Twelfth Histocompatibility Workshop, were utilized for this study (*Table I*).

To minimize the potential influence of prolonged culture conditions, the analysis was performed between *in vitro* passages 5 to 10. The expression of HLA class I antigens on melanoma cells was compared to that of autologous HLA-typed Ficoll Hypaque-isolated peripheral blood mononuclear cells (PBMC). Data were analyzed by the Student's paired *t*-test.

Table I shows the mean values of mean fluorescence intensity obtained with the anti-HLA-A,-B,-C mAb W6/32, the anti-HLA-A mAb A 131 and the anti-HLA-B mAb YTH, for melanoma cells and autologous PBMC. All samples stained positive with used mAb. The expression of HLA class I, HLA-A and -B antigens was significantly ($p<0.05$) lower on melanoma cells compared to autologous PBMC. In addition, the mean ratio between the values of mean fluorescence intensity of HLA-B antigens expressed on PBMC and melanoma cells was significantly ($p<0.05$) higher than that of HLA-A antigens. The latter phenomenon being due to the consistently lower expression on melanoma cells of HLA-B antigens compared to HLA-A antigens.

Previous studies reported that the quantitative expression of the gene products of HLA-A and -B loci is genetically predetermined and varies among unrelated individuals [4]. However, the HLA-A/-B ratio was found to be constant on different non-malignant cell types of a given individual [5]. Therefore, we compared the HLA-A/-B ratio between melanoma cells and autologous PBMC. *Figure 1* shows that the HLA-A/-B ratio was low and homogeneous (range: 1.3 to 3.6) among the 14 PBMC analyzed. In contrast, it was high and heterogenous (range : 2.1 to 33) among the 14 autologous melanoma cells investigated.

Table I. IIF analysis of HLA class I antigens expressed on 14 melanoma cells and autologous PBMC[a]

mAb	Specificity	IIF (mean±SD)[b]		Ratio[c]
		PBMC	Melanoma	
34-1-2	Ctrl	4.3 ± 1.8	3.5 ± 1.0	1.3
64B4	Ctrl	4.1 ± 1	4 ± 1.1	1.1
W6/32	HLA-A,-B,-C	1467 ± 304	163 ± 103	13.0
A 131	HLA-A	1490 ± 471	279 ± 262	8.6
YTH	HLA-B	779 ± 410	35 ± 30	39.4

a Melanoma cells and Ficoll-Hypaque-purified PBMC were resuspended in PBS-0.1% bovine serum albumin-0.02% sodium azide and sequentially incubated with indicated mAb and with DTAF-conjugated $F(ab')_2$ fragments of goat anti-mouse or goat anti-rat IgG xeno-antibodies, cells were then analyzed in flow cytometry. A sample was considered positive when the mean value of fluorescence intensity with specific mAb was at least double than negative control mAb ;
b Data represent the mean values of mean fluorescence intensity (±SD) ;
c Data represent the mean ratio between values of mean fluorescence intensity of HLA-A and HLA-B antigens expressed on PBMC and autologous melanoma cells.

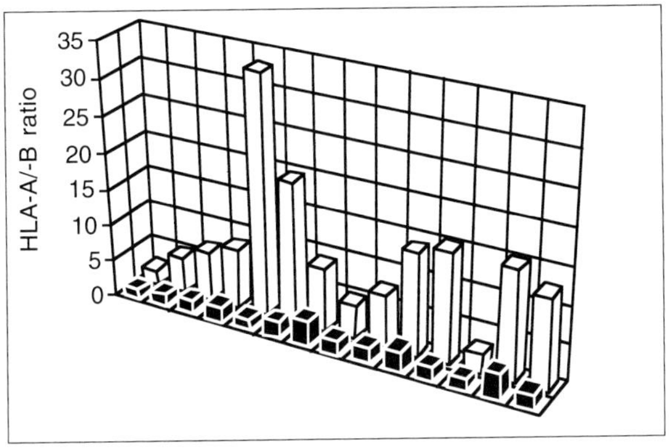

Figure 1. Ratio (y axis) between values of mean fluorescence intensity of HLA-A and HLA-B antigens expressed on melanoma cells (□) and autologous PBMC (■).

Altogether, our data demonstrate that low amounts of HLA-B antigens are expressed on metastatic melanoma cells. This phenomenon is likely due to an unbalanced regulation of HLA-B antigens expression as compared to HLA-A antigens in neoplastic cells. The functional significance of this observation in melanoma progression remains to be investigated. However, the demonstration of a quantitative correlation between HLA-A allospecificities and recognition of melanoma cells by antigen-specific CTL [3] and the identification of melanoma-associated antigens (MAGE-3, MUM-1) recognized by CTL in the context of HLA-B allospecificities (HLA-B44) [1] suggest that the down-regulated expression of HLA-B antigens may impair antigen recognition of melanoma cells by CTL and represent a limiting element for applying T cell-based immunotherapy to melanoma patients.

Acknowledgements
This work was supported by the Associazione Italiana per la Ricerca sul Cancro and by the Progetto Ricerca Finalizzata 1993 and 1995.

References

1. Parmiani G. Immunology of melanoma : an overview. In : Maio M, ed. *Immunology of Human Melanoma.* Amsterdam : IOS Press, 1996 : 1-10.
2. Ferrone S, Marincola FM. Loss of HLA class I antigens by melanoma cells : molecular mechanisms, functional significance and clinical relevance. *Immunol Today* 1995 ; 16 : 487-94.
3. Rivoltini L, Barracchini KC, Viggiano V, Kawakami Y, Smith A, Mixon A, Restifo NP, Topalian SL, Simonis TB, Rosenberg SA, Marincola FM. Quantitative correlation between HLA class I allele expression and recognition of melanoma cells by antigen-specific cytotoxic T lymphocytes. *Cancer Res* 1995 ; 55 : 3149-57.
4. Kao KJ, Riley WJ. Genetic predetermination of quantitative expression of HLA antigens in platelets and mononuclear leukocytes. *Hum Immunol* 1993 ; 38 : 243-50.
5. Kao KJ, Scornik JC, McQueen CF. Evaluation of individual specificities of class I HLA on platelets by a newly developed monoclonal antibody. *Hum Immunol* 1990 ; 27 : 285-97.

Transporter associated with antigen processing (TAP) downregulation in human melanoma cells

D.J. Hicklin, T. Kageshita, D. Dellaratta, S. Ferrone

Department of Microbiology and Immunology, New York Medical College, Valhalla, New York 10595, USA

The recent description of TAP1 loss in breast carcinoma, renal carcinoma, colorectal carcinoma, and cervical carcinoma [1-4] indicates that malignant transformation of cells may be associated with defects in the expression of molecules which play a role in HLA class I antigen processing. These findings have prompted us to investigate the expression of TAP1 and TAP2 in human melanoma cells and in surgically removed melanoma lesions. We have selected this malignancy for our studies since the potential role of immunological events in the pathogenesis of malignant melanoma [5] suggests that abnormalities in HLA class I antigen processing machinery in melanoma cells may have a negative impact on the clinical course of the disease. Furthermore, TAP1 and/or TAP2 downregulation may undermine the beneficial effects of T cell-based immunotherapy which is being used with increased frequency in malignant melanoma [6].

Loss of TAP expression by cultured melanoma cell lines

The expression of TAP1 and TAP2 in 27 human melanoma cell lines was tested by Western blotting analysis with anti-human TAP1 and anti-human TAP2 xenoantisera [7]. Representative results of Western blotting are shown in *Figure 1*. Five phenotypes of TAP expression were identified in the panel of melanoma cell lines tested: (1) constitutive expression of TAP1 and TAP2 was found in 17 cell lines; (2) lack of expression of TAP1 and TAP2 which could be induced by treatment with IFN-γ was found in 4 cell lines; (3) differential lack of TAP1 or TAP2 expression which could not be induced by treatment with IFN-γ was found in 2 cell lines; (4) differential lack of TAP1 or TAP2 expression which could be induced by treatment with IFN-γ was found in 2 cell lines and (5) lack of TAP1 and TAP2 expression which was not induced by treatment of cells with IFN-γ was found in 3 cell lines.

Distinct molecular mechanisms are likely to underlie TAP downregulation in the melanoma cell lines we have analyzed. Loss of TAP expression which could be induced by treatment with IFN-γ may reflect defects in the basal regulation of the TAP subunits. In contrast, structural abnormalities in the TAP genes and/or defects in their regulation may account for the lack of TAP expression which cannot be induced by IFN-γ.

TAP downregulation in surgically removed melanoma lesions

To determine whether defects in TAP expression identified in melanoma cell lines were also present *in situ*, we analyzed surgically removed melanoma lesions by immunohistochemical staining with affinity purified anti-TAP1 and anti-TAP2 xenoantibodies. Representative immunostaining patterns of melanoma lesions with anti-TAP1 and anti-TAP2 xenoantibodies are shown in *Figure 2*. Results are summarized in *Table I*. The expression pattern of TAP1 and TAP2 both in primary and metastatic lesions was similar but not identical. The discoordinate expression of TAP1 and TAP2 was more marked in metastases than in primary lesions. Furthermore, TAP1 and TAP2 downregulation was more marked in metastases than in primary lesions. This finding in conjunction with the association of the frequency of TAP subunit downregulation with clinical and histopathological parameters of the disease, *i.e.* disease stage and thickness of primary lesions, suggest that abnormalities in TAP expression may play a role in disease progression.

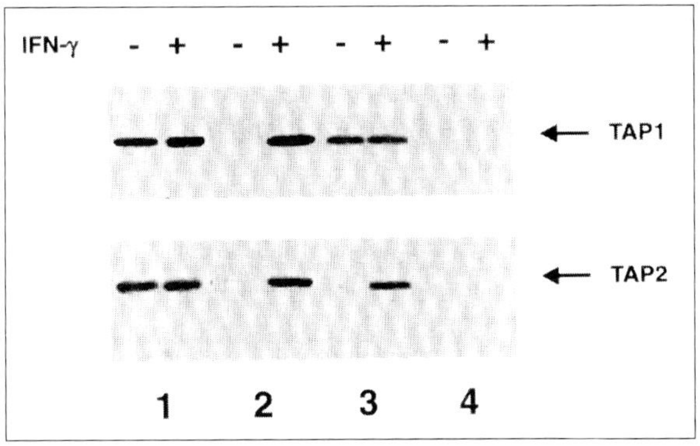

Figure 1. Differential phenotypic TAP1 and TAP2 expression by human melanoma cell lines. Cells were incubated in the presence (+) or absence (-) of IFN-γ (500U/ml) for 48hrs prior to detergent solubilization and Western blotting analysis with anti-TAP1 and anti-TAP2 xenoantisera. Distinct phenotypes of TAP1 and TAP2 expression identified in four melanoma cell lines are shown.

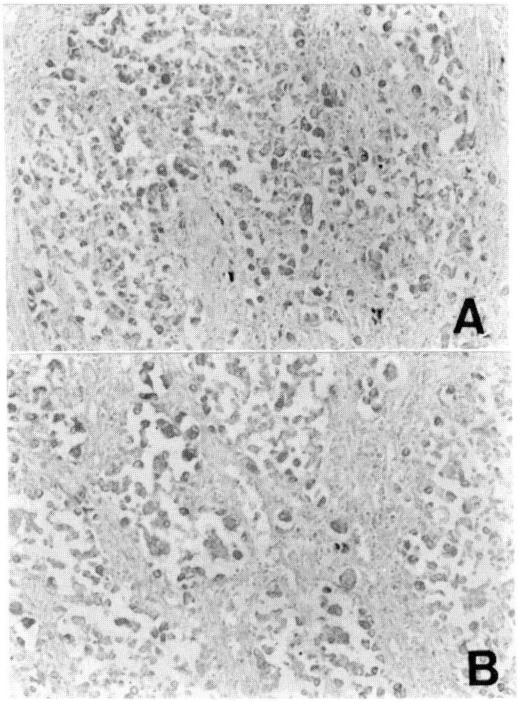

Figure 2. Heterogeneous expression of TAP1 and TAP2 in a surgically removed primary melanoma lesion. Formalin fixed, paraffin embedded sections of a primary melanoma lesion were stained in the immunoperoxidase reaction with affinity purified anti-TAP1 (A) and anti-TAP2 (B) xenoantibodies. Melanoma cells stained with a weak, heterogeneous pattern for both TAP1 and TAP2. x100.

Table I. Frequency of TAP1 and TAP2 downregulation in human melanoma cell lines and surgically removed melanoma lesions

TAP Subunit		Cell Lines[a]			Lesions[c] Primary			Lesions[c] Metastases		
		+	-	IFN-γ inducible[b]	+	+\-	-	+	+\-	-
TAP1	#	17	10	6	30	18	12	5	26	7
	(%)	(63)	(37)	(22)	(50)	(30)	(20)	(13)	(69)	(18)
TAP2	#	20	7	4	26	23	11	9	21	8
	(%)	(74)	(26)	(15)	(44)	(38)	(18)	(24)	(55)	(21)

[a] Expression of TAP1 and TAP2 was tested by Western blotting with xenoantisera elicited with TAP1- and TAP2-specific peptides.

[b] Melanoma cell lines were incubated with IFN-γ (500U/ml) for 48hrs at 37°C prior to analysis by Western blotting with anti-TAP1 and anti-TAP2 xenoantisera.

[c] Surgically removed lesions were tested in the immunoperoxidase reaction with affinity purified anti-TAP1 and anti-TAP2 xenoantibodies. Results were classified as +, +\- and - when the percentage of stained melanoma cells was greater than 75%, between 25 and 75% and less than 25%, respectively.

Conclusion

The present study has shown for the first time that malignant transformation of human melanocytes may be associated with TAP1 and/or TAP2 downregulation. Studies in progress indicate that abnormalities of the HLA class I antigen processing machinery in melanoma cells are not restricted to TAP1 and TAP2, since LMP2 and/or LMP7 downregulation has been found in melanoma cells in longterm culture and in surgically removed melanoma lesions (unpublished data). The molecular defects responsible for TAP and LMP downregulation in melanoma cells as well as the functional and clinical significance of these abnormalities are under investigation.

Acknowlegdements

The authors wish to acknowledge the excellent secretarial assistance of Mrs. Edwina L. Jones, Ms. Teresa L. Eley, Mrs. Harriet V. Harrison, and Mrs. Donna D. James. This investigation was supported by PHS grant CA67108 awarded by the National Cancer Institute, DHHS.

References

1. Kaklamanis L, Leek R, Koukourakis M, Gatter KC, Harris AL. Loss of transporter in antigen processing 1 transport protein and major histocompatibility complex class I molecules in metastatic versus primary breast cancer. *Cancer Res* 1995 ; 55 : 5191-4.
2. Seliger B, Hohne A, Knuth A, Bernhard H, Meyer T, Tampe R, Momburg F, Huber C. Analysis of the major histocompatibility complex class I antigen presentation machinery in normal and malignant renal cells : evidence for deficiencies associated with transformation and progression. *Cancer Res* 1996 ; 56 : 1756-60.
3. Kaklamanis L, Townsend A, Doussi-Anagnostopoulou IA, Mortensen N, Harris AL, Gatter KC. Loss of major histocompatibility complex-encoded transporter associated with antigen presentation (TAP) in colorectal cancer. *Am J Pathol* 1994 ; 145 : 505-9.
4. Cromme FV, Airey J, Heemels MT, Ploegh HL, Keating PJ, Stern PL, Meijer CJLM, Walboomers JMM. Loss of transporter protein, encoded by the TAP-1 gene, is highly correlated with loss of HLA expression in cervical carcinomas. *J Exp Med* 1994 ; 179 : 335-40.
5. Mastrangelo MJ, Baker AR, Katz HR. Cutaneous melanoma. In : DeVita VT Jr, Hellman S, Rosenberg SA, eds. *Cancer : Principles and Practice of Oncology*, vol. 2. Philadelphia : Lippincott, 1985 : 1371-422.
6. Bystryn JC, Ferrone S, Livingston P. Specific immunotherapy of cancer with vaccines. *Ann NY Acad Sci* 1993 ; 690 : 1-411.
7. Hicklin DJ, Kageshita T, Ferrone S. Development and characterization of rabbit antisera to human MHC-linked transporters associated with antigen processing. *Tissue Antigens* 1997 (in press).

A peptide from the known HLA class I restricted melanoma-specific tumor antigen GP100 is presented by HLA-DR in the melanoma cell line FM3

T. Halder [1], G. Pawelec [2], A.F. Kirkin [3], J. Zeuthen [3], H.E. Meyer [4], H. Kalbacher [1]

1 Medical and Natural Sciences Research Center, University of Tübingen, D-72070 Tübingen, Germany
2 Section of Transplantation Immunology, Medical Hospital, University of Tübingen, Germany
3 Department of Tumor Cell Biology, Division of Cancer Biology, Danish Cancer Society, Copenhagen, Denmark
4 Institute for Physiological Chemistry, University of Bochum, Germany

A number of HLA-class I restricted melanoma tumor antigens such as MAGE-1 and 3, MART-1/Melan-A, gp100 (Pmel17), gp 75 (tyrosinase-related protein) and tyrosinase have been characterized. Further, class I-restricted cytotoxic T cells specific for these tumor antigens and some of their corresponding peptide epitopes have been identified by several groups [for review see 1]. Thus far there is no direct proof if peptides derived from these antigens are also presented *in vivo* by HLA-class II molecules. To examine the class II-associated endogenous peptides we took the constitutively class II and CD80 expressing melanoma cell line FM3 (DR B1*0401, DR B1*02x, DQ B1*0301, DQ B1*0602). FM3 has been shown to possess effective antigen presenting cells in context with HLA-A2-restricted, $CD8^+$ cytotoxic T lymphocytes (CTL) but can also provoke a class II-restricted T cell response [2].

Isolation of DR-associated FM3 self peptides

The FM3 cells were cultured in RPMI supplemented with 5% FCS, 20 mM HEPES, 2 mM glutamine, and antibiotics in roller bottles up to 1 x 10^{10} cells. After harvesting, the cells were lysed with 2% NP-40 and the HLA-DR molecules were isolated by immunoaffinity chromatography using the mAb L243 coupled to CNBr-activated sepharose. The detergent was removed by washing the column with water. The elution was performed using TFA/water, pH 2.0. At this pH the bound peptides were released from the HLA molecules. To separate the eluted peptides from the HLA, an ultrafiltration step using a 20 kD membrane was added. The filtrate containing the DR-bound peptides was collected and lyophilized. The peptide pool was separated by HPLC with a C18/1 mm reversed phase column using a flat acetonitrile gradient (1%/min). The resulting chromatogram is shown in *Figure 1*. The peaks were collected and tested for purity by matrix assisted laser desorption mass spectrometry (MALDI-MS). Homogeneous peaks were directly sequenced by Edman degradation, inhomogeneous peaks were further purified by capillary chromatography with a C18/180 μm column and directly spotted on a PVDF sequencing membrane before submitting to the sequencer.

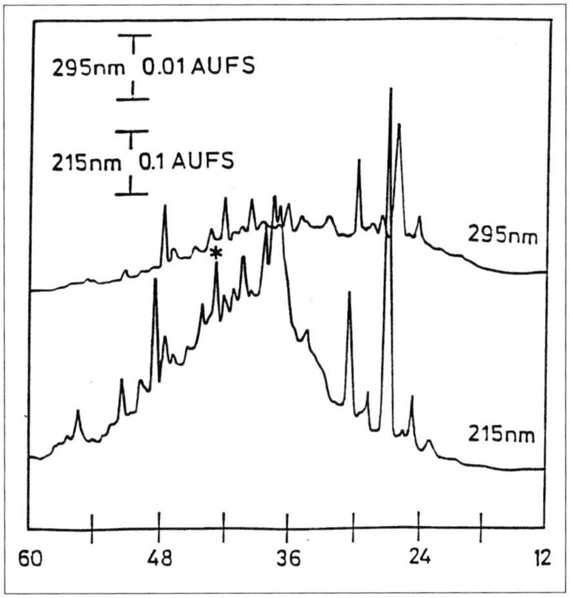

Figure 1. Reversed-phase HPLC separation profile of the HLA-DR-associated peptide pool from FM3. A C18/1mm column with a flow of 27 μl/min and a flat acetonitrile gradient (7-77% B, 1%/min) was used. Buffer A: 0.1% TFA, buffer B: 0.08% TFA/84% acetonitrile.

Characterization of the isolated peptides

The peak at 43 min seemed to be homogeneous. In MALDI-MS only one mass at [M+H]+ = 2121.1 was visible *(Figure 2)*. Sequencing of this fraction however proved the existence of at least three different peptides. The main sequence was identified by comparison with the Swissprot protein data base as a sequence from a grp78 (BiP)-homologous protein where the aminoterminal residue of the peptide was mutated from asparagine to alanine: AVMRIINEPTAAAIAYGLDK, position 194-213. The calculated mass was 2117.5. Further we subjected the same fraction to rechromatography and sequenced the separated minor peak. Now the sequence of a single peptide was clearly readable. We identified a 16mer peptide derived from the melanocyte specific protein gp100, position 44-59 with the sequence WNRQLYPEWTEAQRLD. The calculated peptide mass was 2105.3. The sequencing yield of the grp78-homologous peptide was 80 pmol, from the gp100 peptide 17 pmol were detected. So gp100 surely was not one of the most abundant peptides present in FM3.

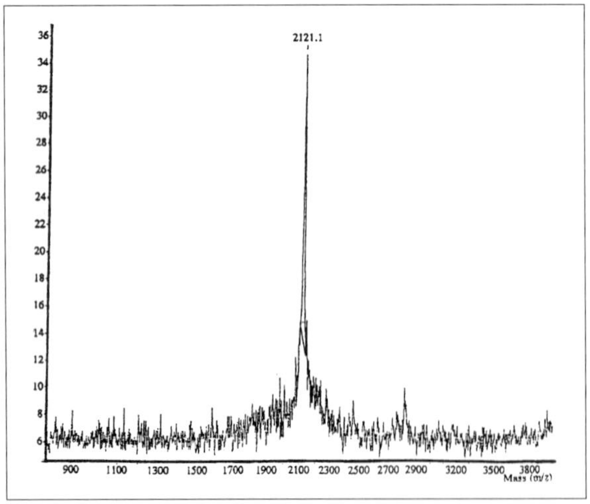

Figure 2. MALDI-MS of peak 43 (marked with an aterisk in *Figure 1*).

Specific binding of gp100, 44-59 to isolated DR molecules

To prove the specific binding of this peptide to different HLA-DR alleles we synthesized the peptide on a peptide synthesizer using the Fmoc/Bu^t-strategy and submitted it to our *in vitro* peptide binding/competition assay using gel filtration, isolated HLA-DR alleles and a 7-amino-4-methylcoumarin-3-acetic acid (AMCA) fluorescently labeled peptide [3]. *Figure 3* shows the result of this assay. The gp100 epitope showed highest affinity to one of the FM3 alleles, HLA-DR4 (DRB1*0401) with an IC50 of 7 µM compared to 90 µM to HLA-DR2 (DRB5*0101). Comparable binding was observed to HLA-DR1 (DRB1*0101), having an IC50 of 55 µM but not to HLA-DR3 (DRB1*0301) and HLA-DR11 (DRB1*1101) with an IC50 of 800 and 1000 µM respectively. Therefore it is very likely that gp100, 44-59 was isolated from DR4.

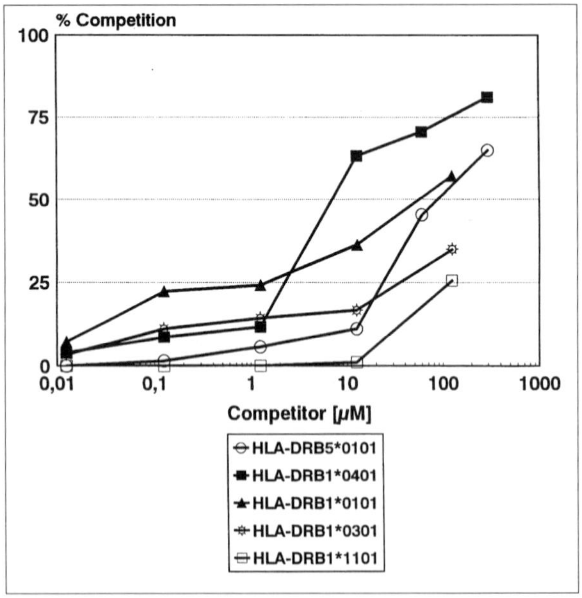

Figure 3. Competition by gp100, 44-59 for binding to different HLA-DR alleles:
The following fluorescently (AMCA)-labeled peptides were used at 1.5 µM: influenza hemagglutinin, 307-319, PKYVKQNTLKLAT for DRB5*0101, DRB1*0401, and DRB1*0101, hsp65, 3-13, KTIAYDEEARR for DRB1*0301and hsc70, 239-250, NHFIAEFKRKHK for DRB1*1101. Binders, competitors and HLA-DR isolates (0.2 µM) were incubated simultaneously with a cocktail of protease inhibitors for 40 hours at 37°C. Then the separation was performed using a high performance size exclusion (HPSEC) column.

Conclusions

This is the first reported HLA-DR-restricted epitope of a known tumor-associated antigen in melanoma. It is capable to bind to HLA-DR4 and should therefore be able to stimulate gp100-specific DR4-restricted $CD4^+$ T helper cells. For gp100 at least five different HLA-A2-restricted CTL epitopes are known so far, but none of them stems from the here identified region of the protein [4-6]. In this context it is interesting that an unknown epitope from the already known class I-restricted tyrosinase antigen is apparently also recognized by $CD4^+$ T cells [7].

These results document that the same gp100 molecule giving rise to a known class I-restricted tumor antigen recognized by CD8 cells provides a potential class II-restricted tumor antigen, derived from a different portion of the molecule which might be recognized by CD4 cells. Should these peptide/MHC complexes be recognizable by T cells, they may prove useful in future vaccination protocols for immunotherapy of melanoma.

References

1. Maeurer MJ, Storkus WJ, Kirkwood JM, Lotze MT. New treatment options for patients with melanoma: review of melanoma-derived T-cell epitope-based peptide vaccines. *Melanoma Res* 1996; 6 : 11-24.
2. Olsen AC, Fossum B, Kirkin AF, Zeuthen J, Gaudernack G. A human melanoma cell line, recognized by both class I and class II restricted T cells, is capable of initiating both primary and secondary immune responses. *Scand J Immunol* 1995; 41 :357-64.
3. Max H, Halder T, Kalbus M, Gnau V, Jung G, Kalbacher H. A 16mer peptide of the human autoantigen calreticulin is a most prominent HLA-DR4Dw4-associated self-peptide. *Hum Immunol* 1994; 41: 39-45.
4. Bakker ABH, Schreurs MWJ, de Boer AJ, Kawakami Y, Rosenberg SA, Adema GJ, Figdor CG. Melanocyte lineage-specific gp100 is recognized by melanoma derived tumor infiltrating lymphocytes. *J Exp Med* 1994 ; 179 : 1005-9.
5. Cox AL, Skipper J, Chen Y, Henderson RA, Darrow TL, Shabanowitz J, Engelhard VH, Hunt DF, Slingluff Jr DL. Identification of a peptide recognized by five melanoma-specific human cytotoxic T cell lines. *Science* 1994 ; 264 : 716-9.
6. Bakker AB, Schreurs MW, Tafazzul G, de Boer AJ, Kawakami Y, Adena GJ, Figdor CD. Identification of a novel peptide derived from the melanocyte-specific gp100 antigen as the dominant epitope recognized by an HLA-A2.1-restricted anti-melanoma CTL line. *Int J Cancer* 1995; 62 : 97-102.
7. Topalian S L, Rivoltini L, Mancini M, *et al.* Human $CD4^+$ T cells specifically recognize a shared melanoma-associated antigen encoded by the tyrosinase gene. *Proc Natl Acad Sci USA* 1994 ; 91: 9461-5.

HLA class II antigen presentation by melanoma

M.S. Brady[1], D.D. Eckels[3], S.Y. Ree[1], K.E. Schultheiss[1], J.L. Lee[2]

From the Department of Surgery[1] and Immunology Program[2], Memorial Sloan-Kettering Cancer Center, 1275 York Avenue, New York 10021, USA and the Immunogenetics Research Section[3], Blood Research Institute, Blood Center of South-eastern Wisconsin, Milwaukee, WI, USA

Normally, HLA class II molecules (HLA-DR, DP, and DQ) are only expressed on professional APCs of the immune system. Melanoma cell lines are unusual because, unlike most epithelial tumor cell lines, constitutive expression of HLA class II antigens is common [1,2]. Theoretically, HLA class II expression would allow the melanoma cell to present endogenous tumor antigens to CD4+ T cells. If naive CD4+ T cells recognize peptide presented by melanoma cells in the absence of co-stimulatory signalling, then T cell tolerance to melanoma antigens may be induced early in the disease [3]. Alternatively, antigen experienced CD4+ T cells may secrete anergy promoting cytokines in response to peptide presentation by HLA class II + melanoma.

Based on reports by others that HLA class II antigens on melanoma are non-stimulatory [4,5] and data to suggest that antigen presentation by HLA class II molecules on non-professional APCs results in T cell unresponsiveness [6], we predicted that CD4+ T cells would be unresponsive to peptide presented by HLA class II molecules on melanoma cells *in vitro*.

Results

We used HLA class II+ DR1/4-restricted melanoma cell lines (derived from metastases) and EBV-transformed autologous B cells as stimulators in co-cultivation experiments with HA1.7, a CD4+ T cell clone which proliferates in response to an influenza virus hemagglutinin (HA) peptide presented in the context of DR1/4 [7]. Stimulators (melanoma cells or B cells) were irradiated prior to co-cultivation. T cell responses to stimulators presenting HA were then measured using [^{3}H]-thymidine uptake. As shown in *Table I*, melanoma cell lines SKMEL-256, -113, -93 and -37 were able to present peptide efficiently to HA1.7, comparable to that seen with autologous B cells. We confirmed that the proliferative response of HA1.7 was HLA class II mediated by performing blocking studies using isotype matched monoclonal antibodies against HLA class II and I (L243 and W6/32, respectively).

We used whole HA protein to determine whether melanoma cells could process antigen for presentation. As

Table I. Proliferation of HA1.7 in response to peptide presentation by HLA class II positive melonoma cell lines and autologous B cells. Values shown are means of triplicate samples ± SEM

Cell line	No peptide	peptide	fold increase
SKMEL-256	5922±1334	64771±654	11
SKB-256	5119±25	36638±3685	7
SKMEL-113	6754±608	32327±1934	5
SKB-113	3513±262	6752±425	2
SKMEL-93	522±37	3549±249	7
SKB-93	1086±116	7602±633	7
SKMEL-37	5428±261	52671±806	10
SKB-37	2813±384	142190±4152	50

Table II. Cytokine production by HA1.7 responding to peptide presentation by melanoma or autologous B cells

Cell line	IL10 pg/ml	IFNy, pg/ml	proliferation
SKMEL-256,EXP#1	336	2160	34833
SKB-256,EXP#1	560	48000	37190
SKMEL-256,EXP#2	54	3000	44569
SKB-256,EXP#2	36	17520	36815
SKMEL-256,EXP#3	445	775	39153
SKB-256,EXP#3	415	2700	762
SKMEL-256,EXP#4	275	300	64460
SKB-256,EXP#4	180	1875	49926
SKMEL-113,EXP#1	225	775	47411
SKB-113,EXP#1	ND	ND	ND
SKMEL-113,EXP#2	180	450	34690
SKB-113,EXP#2	65	2770	10110

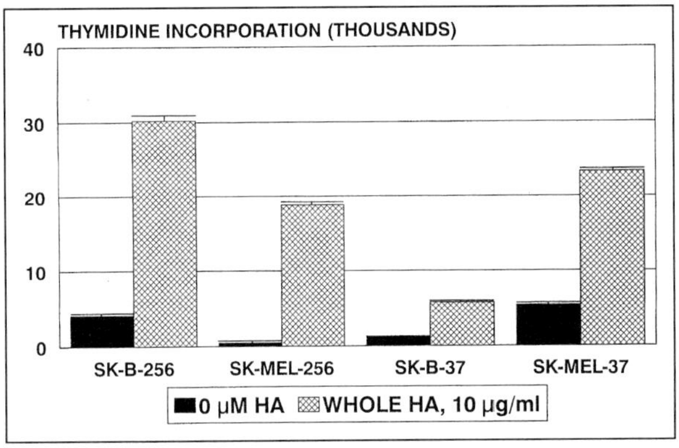

Figure 1. Melanoma cells (SKMEL-256 and SKMEL-37) were able to process whole HA into peptide for presentation, resulting in similar proliferative responses as seen with whole HA and autologous B cells (SKB-256 and SKB-37). Whole HA was used at a concentration of 10 μg/ml. Values represent the mean ± SEM of triplicate samples. All groups were significantly different from the control (0 μM HA) at the $p<.005$ level (Student's paired T test).

shown in *Figure 1*, all melanoma cell lines tested (SKMEL-256 and SKMEL-37) were able to process whole HA and present it to HA1.7 resulting in T cell proliferation significantly enhanced over no peptide controls. Autologous B cells were used as postitive controls for antigen processing.

We initially performed RT-PCR experients on supernatants obtained from the co-cultivation experiments to determine which cytokines were being produced by HA1.7 in response to either stimulator. These experiments demonstrated the presence of mRNA for IL10 and IFNγ but no significant amounts of IL2, IL4, IL12, or INFα. Subsequent ELISA analysis of supernatants from co-cultivation experiments confirmed significant production of IFNγ (up to 48 ng/ml) and IL10 (up to 500 pg/ml) but undetectable levels of IL2, IL4, or TNFα. HA1.7 cells produced IL10 and IFNγ whether responding to peptide presentation by melanomas or B cells although more IFNγ production occurred when responding to B cells, despite comparable levels of T cell proliferation (*Table II*).

We than analyzed cell surface expression of B7.1, B7.2 and ICAM-1 on our stimulator pairs by FACS analysis to determine the role of accessory or co-stimulatory molecules in the response of HA1.7. Melanoma cells did not express B7.1 or B7.2 by FACS analysis, while autologous B cells, as expected, expressed both. ICAM-1 was expressed by both B cells and melanomas. Interestingly, while the response of HA1.7 to melanoma and B cells was completely unaffected by blocking with CTLA-4Ig (a fusion protein which blocks CD28 ligation by B7.1 or B7.2), blocking antibody to ICAM-1 resulted in a decrease in T cell proliferation by >65% in response to peptide presentation by SK-MEL-256 but not autologous B cells, indicating that ICAM-1 plays a significant role in the response of CD4+ T cells to peptide presentation by melanoma (*Figures 2* and *3*).

Discussion

Previous investigators have suggested that HLA class II molecules on primary melanoma cells bind peptide and

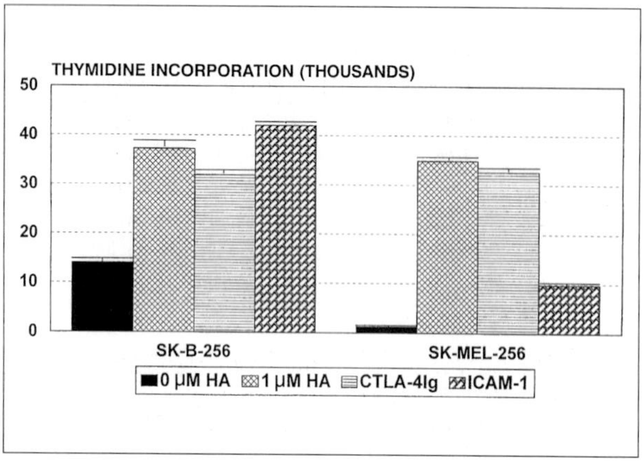

Figure 2. Proliferation of HA1.7 T cells in response to peptide presentation by B cells (SKB-256) and melanoma (SKMEL-256) was unaffected by blocking CD28 mediated signalling using CTLA-4Ig. Blocking antibody to ICAM-1 markedly diminished T cell proliferation in response to peptide presentation by melanoma (SKMEL-256) but not autologous B cells (SKB-256). Values represent the mean ± SEM of triplicate samples. All groups were significantly different from the control (0 uM HA) at the p<.005 level (Student's paired T test).

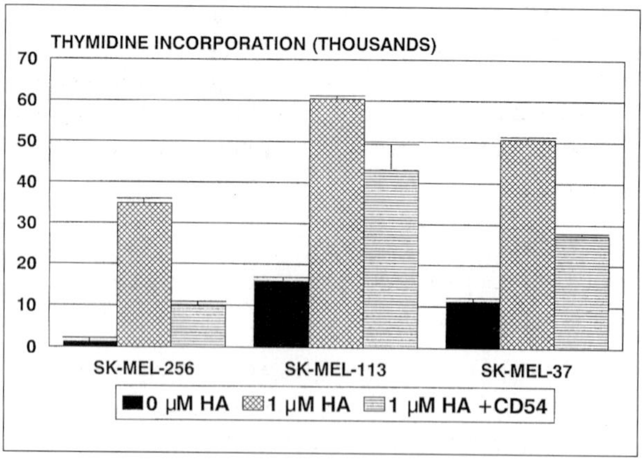

Figure 3. Blocking antibody to ICAM-1 markedly diminished T cell proliferation in response to peptide presentation by all three melanoma cell lines tested: SKMEL-256, SKMEL-113 and SKMEL-37. Values represent the mean ± SEM of triplicate samples. ICAM-1 blockade resulted in a statistically significant decrease in T cell proliferation compared to the peptide only group for all three cell lines at the p<.05 level (Student's paired T test).

stimulate a CD4+ T cell clone to proliferate, while those on metastatic clones lose their capacity to do so [5]. In contrast, our results indicate that melanoma cell lines, all derived from metastases, present peptide quite efficiently via HLA class II molecules to a peptide-specific CD4+ T cell clone. Indeed, the ability of melanoma cells to serve as APCs to these T cells is comparable to that seen with autologous B cells. Interestingly, Stohal *et al.* have demonstrated that the lymphocytic infiltration so common in early melanoma is composed largely of CD4+ cells [8]. This suggests that HLA class II molecules on the melanoma cells may interact in a negative fashion with these T cells and promote unresponsiveness to tumor. We propose that CD4+ T cells interact with endogenous peptides presented by HLA class II molecules on the melanoma cell but that a lack of effective co-stimulation results in a T cell response which promotes IL10 production and anergy to tumor. While our data do not address the question as to whether melanoma cells present endogenous «tumor» antigens *via* HLA class II molecules to T cells, recent work by Topalian *et al.* suggests that they do [9].

The low or absent expression of B7.1/B7.2 by our melanoma cell lines is consistent with the fact that expression of B7 is, in general, limited to professional APCs or activated T cells [reviewed in 10]. Interestingly, blocking ICAM-1 on the surface of the APC affected T cell proliferation in response to peptide presented by melanoma but not autologous B cells, demonstrating a qualitative difference in the T cell response to the two types of APC. The importance of ICAM-1 in the response of HA1.7 to the melanoma cells in our experiments suggests that it serves to facilitate the interaction of the T cell with the melanoma cell *in vivo*. Indeed, ICAM-1 expression is associated with malignant transformation, and is very rarely seen in benign melanocytic proliferation [11]. ICAM-1 expression increases, along with HLA-DR expression, as melanomas progress from early lesions to more invasive tumors [12]. ICAM-1 may actually facilitate an anergic T cell response by promoting the interaction of the naive T cell with a B7-deficient antigen presenting melanoma cell.

Most melanoma cell lines express HLA class II molecules constitutively, or can be made to do so upon exposure to IFNγ [2]. Our data demonstrate that human melanoma cells effectively process HA and present peptide to antigen experienced HA-specific T cells *in vitro via* HLA class II molecules. These findings, which refute the previously held belief that HLA class II molecules on metastatic melanoma cells are nonfunctional or nonstimulatory to T cells, may have important implications for the development of novel immunotherapeutic strategies based on HLA class II mediated antigen presentation.

References

1. Winchester RJ, Wang CY, Gibofsky A, Kunkel HG, Lloyd KO, Old LJ. Expression of Ia-like antigens on cultured human malignant melanoma cell lines. *Proc Natl Acad Sci USA* 1978; 75:6235-9.
2. Houghton AN, Thomson TM, Gross D, Oettgen HF, Old LJ. Surface antigens of melanoma and melanocytes. *J Exp Med* 1984; 160:255-69.
3. Jenkins MK, Ashwell JD, Schwartz RH. Allogeneic non-T spleen cells restore the responsiveness of normal T cell clones stimulated with antigen and chemically modified antigen-presenting cells. *Immunol* 1988; 140: 3324-30.
4. Alexander MA, Bennicelli J, Guerry D. Defective antigen presentation by human melanoma cell lines cultured from advanced, but not biologically early disease. *J Immunol* 1989; 142: 4070-8.
5. Becker JC, Brabletz T, Czerny C, Termeer C, Brocker EB. Tumor escape mechanisms from immunosurveillance: induction of unresponsiveness in a specific HLA-restricted CD4+ human T cell clone by the autologous HLA class II + melanoma. *Int Immunol* 1993; 5: 1501-8.
6. Bal V, McIndoe A, Denton G, Hudson D, Lombardi G, Lamb J, Lechler R. Antigen presentation by keratinocytes induces tolerance in human T cells. *Eur J Immunol* 1990; 20: 1893-97.
7. Lamb JR, Eckels DD, Lake P, Woody JN, Green N. Human T-cell clones recognize chemically synthesized peptides of influenza haemagglutinin. *Nature* 1982; 300: 66-9.
8. Strohal R, Marberger K, Pehamberger H, Stingl G. Immunohistological analysis of anti-melanoma host responses. *Arch Dermatol Res* 1994; 287:28-35.
9. Topalian SL, Rivoltini L, Mancini M, Markus NR, Robbins PF, Kawakami Y, Rosenberg SA. Human CD4+ T cells specifically recognize a shared melanoma-associated antigen encoded by the tyrosinase gene. *Proc Natl Acad Sci USA* 1994; 91: 9461-5.
10. June CH, Bluestone JA, Nadler LM, Thompson CB. The B7 and CD28 receptor families. *Immunol Today* 1994; 15:321-31.
11. Johnson JP, Stade BG, Holzmann B, Schwable W, Riethmuller G. *De novo* expression of intercellular-adhesion molecule 1 in melanoma correlates with increased risk of metastasis. *Proc Natl Acad Sci USA* 1989; 86:641-4.
12. Danen EH, van Muijen GN, Ruiter GJ. Role of integrins as signal transducing cell adhesion molecules in human cutaneous melanoma. *Cancer Surv* 1995; 24:43-65.

HLA and HPV polymorphism in cervical neoplasia

P.L. Stern, F. Clarke, J. Chenggang, M. Duggan-Keen, D.J. Burt, S. Glenville, J.S. Bartholomew

CRC Department of Immunology, Paterson Institute for Cancer Research, Christie Hospital NHS Trust, Manchester, M20 4BX, UK

Certain high risk types of human papillomaviruses (HPV) are involved in the aetiology of cervical cancer. The early region E6 and E7 gene products of these viruses are the major transforming proteins. They contribute to the development of cervical cancers by interacting with the cellular proteins p53 and Rb which play a pivotal role in the negative regulation of growth. During the neoplastic process, the viral genes are integrated in the host genome and their expression contributes to immortalization of epithelial cells in the transformation zone of the cervix. However, other changes in the cells are necessary for the development of an invasive carcinoma. There is evidence that cellular immune recognition of HPV is important in the elimination of virus infected cells. HPV (most commonly HPV 16) is associated with increased likelihood of malignant progression in cervical intraepithelial neoplasia (CIN) as well as with most carcinomas. Failure to control HPV infection may allow time for oncogenic transformation and tumour development to occur. The viral proteins are potential targets for immunological intervention throughout the pathological spectrum of the disease [1] and several vaccines aimed at inducing CTL responses are already being evaluated. However, for such approaches to be effective, viral peptides must be appropriately presented by MHC molecules expressed by the HPV infected/transformed cells to both activate and act as targets for specific T cells.

Any virus/disease-related alterations in MHC expression would critically influence immune surveillance of viral infection and have important consequences for the elimination of infected cells. We have used an extended set of allele and locus specific antibodies together with a knowledge of the patients' tissue type [2], to phenotype 154 cervical cancer biopsies at 76% of HLA-A and 87% of HLA-B alleles. This has shown that HLA-A and -B class I expression by cervical tumour cells is down-regulated at one or more alleles in at least 63% of carcinomas. There were 19 cases (12%) where there was no loss of any HLA-A or B allelic expression but in the remaining cases it is not known if there was any loss of expression. Until a set of antibodies recognising all the HLA class I allelic products is available only a minimum estimate of allele-specific loss can be made. Loss of expression for common alleles ranged from 9% to 55% (*Figure 1*) and such changes might be expected to influence specific immunogenic peptide presentation and consequent immune recognition.

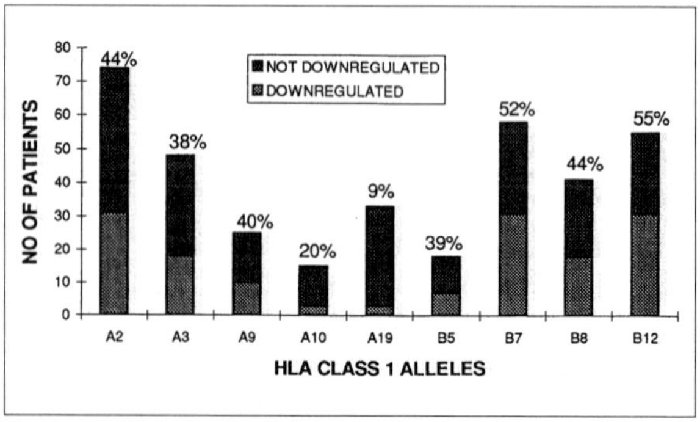

Figure 1. HLA class I allele expression in cervical carcinomas.

There is also evidence of an increased incidence of HLA class I down-regulation in cervical carcinoma lymph node metastases [3]. These observations are consistent with the selection of HLA class I negative cells during tumour progression. By contrast, in pre-invasive disease, complete loss of HLA class I expression in cervical premalignancy (CIN I-III) apparently occurs only rarely [4]. However, only a proportion of CIN III are likely to progress to carcinomas [5] and if these lesions alone show HLA class I loss then the proportion detected in a random sample of CIN would be very small. Analysis of allele specific expression in CIN in relation to progression or regression of the lesion would be the most appropriate study to ascertain whether HLA class I loss is important in the progress of events leading to malignancy.

The changes in HLA class I expression seen in cervical neoplasia could result from interference at any stage from the initiation of HLA class I gene transcription, through heavy chain assembly with β_2-microglobulin and peptide in the endoplasmic reticulum (ER) to the stability of cell surface expression [6]. Since some viral infections can directly interfere with HLA expression at various steps during class I assembly, it is of particular interest whether HPV gene expression directly or indirectly accounts for the observed down regulation of HLA in cervical cancer. Although no evidence has yet been obtained for direct effects of HPV gene expression on HLA class I modulation there are important consequences of the latter for immune surveillance of HPV in cervical malignancy. It is possible that the downregulation of HLA class I may be the result of immunoselective events, advantageous to the evolution of an invasive cancer. If this were true then it follows that those HLA allelic products capable of presenting target peptides of for example HPV 16 E6/E7 would be preferentially lost. If tumour growth is advantaged by failure to present particular immunogenic peptides then this could be effected by changes in the latter at key residues important in binding to the groove of HLA class I molecules. This has been shown to occur in the epitopes of several different viral proteins, including HPV16 E6, presented by particular HLA class 1 molecules [7]. The possibility that a specific mutation in a CTL epitope may influence the development of cervical cancer in the context of a particular HLA allele has important implications for our understanding of both the immunology and epidemiology of HPV-induced carcinogenesis. If particular HLA alleles offer protection against HPV infection and or tumour development, then this should be reflected by different antigen frequencies in patient versus control populations.There have been several reports documenting associations between particular HLA alleles and susceptibility or resistance to HPV 16 infection and/or cervical neoplasia. Thus far there is no overall consensus and very large studies are required to understand fully any relationship between HLA polymorphisms, HPV infection and cervical disease [1]. It is possible that more than one mechanism may be operating and more than one virus interacting, so clear-cut differences may be difficult to detect, even though they may exist.

The relevant CTL target antigens in cervical cancer may not be HPV derived but may be expressed as a result of virus infection. To examine this possibility, *in vitro* tumour cell lines have been established and the PBL or TIL from the patients used in attempts to isolate tumour specific cytotoxic cells [8]. *Figure 2* shows that such cervical carcinoma line cells can be used as stimulators in the generation of specific CTL clones, albeit at very low frequency. Importantly the HLA phenotype of such cell lines is frequently representative of the *in vivo* phenotype determined by immunohistochemistry, including any specific down-regulation of particular HLA class I expression. It might be necessary to reintroduce the lost HLA class I restricting elements to the tumour cells in order to isolate the relevant CTLs. If novel targets can be defined by such approaches (*e.g.* [9]) then immunological intervention in HPV associated cervical carcinoma might seek to expand target specific CTL *in vitro* with subsequent adoptive transfer [10].

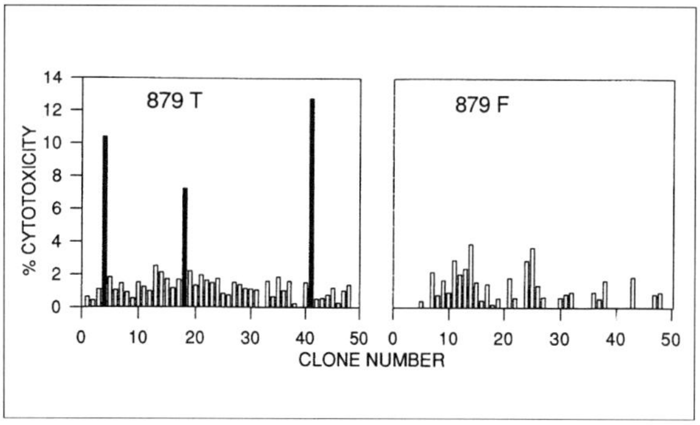

Figure 2. Autologous CTL clones kill tumour (T) not fibroblasts (F).

Supported by the Cancer Research Campaign, Joseph Starkey Fellowship and British Council.

References

1. Stern PL. Immunity to human papillomavirus associated cervical cancer.In: Klein G, Van de Woude GF, eds. *Advances in Cancer Research.* London: Academic Press, 1996; 67: 175-204.
2. Keating P, Cromme F, Duggan-Keen M, Snidjer PJF, Walboomers JMM, Hunter R, Dyer PA, Stern PL. Frequency of down regulation of individual HLA-A and -B alleles in cervical carcinomas in relation to TAP-1 expression. *Br J Cancer* 1995; 72 : 405-11.
3. Cromme FV, van Bommel P, Walboomers JMM, Gallee MPW, Stern PL, Kenemans P, Stukart MJ, Helmerhorst THJM, Meijer CJLM. Differences in MHC and TAP-1 expression in cervical cancer lymph node metastases as compared to the primary tumours. *Br J Cancer* 1994; 69: 1176-81.
4. Glew SS, Connor ME, Snijders, PJF, Stanbridge CM, Buckley CH, Walboomers JMM, Meijer CJLM, Stern PL. HLA expression in preinvasive cervical neoplasia in relationship to human papillomavirus infection. *Eur J Cancer* 1993; 29A: 1963-70.
5. McIndoe WA, MacLean MR, Jones RW. The invasive potential of carcinoma *in situ* of the cervix. *Obstet Gynaecol* 1984; 64: 451-8.
6. Garrido F, Cabrera T, Concha A, Glew S, Ruiz-Cabello F, Stern PL. Natural history of HLA expression during tumour development. *Immunol Today* 1993; 14: 491-9.
7. Ellis JRM, Keating PJ, Baird J, Hounsell E, Renouf DV, Rowe M, Hopkins D, Duggan-Keen MF, Bartholomew JS, Young LS, Stern PL. An HPV 16 variant is associated with cervical carcinoma in HLA-B7 positive women. *Nature Med* 1995; 1: 646-70.
8. Ghosh AK, Glenville S, Bartholomew JS, Stern PL. Analysis of tumour infiltrating lymphocyters in cervical cancer. In: Stanley M, ed. *Proceedings of the 2nd International Workshop of Immunology of Papillomaviruses.* New York: Plenum, 1994: 249-54.
9. Boon T, van der Bruggen P. Human tumour antigens recognized by T lymphocytes *J Exp Med* 1996; 183: 727-9.
10. Heslop HE, Ng CYC, Li C, Smith CA, Loftin SK, Krance RA, Brenner MK, Rooney CM. Long term restoration of immunity against Epstein-Barr virus infection by adoptive transfer of gene modified virus specific T lymphocytes. *Nature Med* 1996; 2: 551-5.

HLA DRB1*1301/02 is a possible protective allele against HPV associated carcinoma of the cervix in French women

M.N. Loste[1], X. Sastre-Garau[2], M. Favre[3], R. Ivanova[1], V. Lepage[1], D.Charron[1]

1 Laboratory of Immunology and INSERM U396, Hôpital Saint-Louis, 1, avenue Claude Vellefaux 75475 Paris Cedex 10, France
2 Departments of Pathology Institut Curie, Paris, France
3 Unité des Papillomavirus, Institut Pasteur, Paris, France

Specific types of human papillomaviruses (HPV 16 and 18) are associated with most cases of preinvasive and invasive neoplasia of the uterine cervix. HLA phenotype influences susceptibility and resistance to viral infections and may therefore influence the course of HPV-associated tumors. Some data suggest that specific HLA class II alleles may be associated with protection from or susceptibility to papillomavirus-associated lesions, but these results are still controversial. In order to favor a better understanding of the interactions between HPV and HLA types in the development of cervical neoplasia, we have analysed a series of 126 cases of infiltrative cervical cancers occurring in the French population. Using molecular probes, we have determined the *DQA1*, *DQB1* and *DRB1* HLA class II alleles in these cases. We have looked for significant associations of HLA class II genes, cervical cancer and HPV infection.

Material and methods

Patients

The population analysed corresponds to 126 unrelated Caucasian patients with invasive carcinoma of the cervix treated at the Institut Curie between 1986 and 1992. HPV typing was performed by PCR and Southern blot techniques using molecular probes. For Southern blot techniques, probes were mixtures of HPV DNA 6, 11, and 42, HPV DNA 16, 18 and 33, and HPV DNA 31, 35 and 39. For PCR, primers were specific for HPV6, 11, 16, 18 and 33.

HLA typing

An aliquot of DNA sample, extracted from tumoral tissue specimens for HPV typing was used for HLA typing. Locus DRB typing was performed by PCR SSO reverse dot blot (Innolipa*, Innogenetics, Haven, Belgium) [1]. Locus *DQA1* and *DQB1* were typed with SSO probes, respectively described by the XI International Histocompatibility Workshop (IHW) [2]. Controls were 165 healthy individuals, randomly selected, and previously typed.

Statistical analysis

The phenotype frequency of HLA *DRB1*, *DQA1*, *DQB1* was obtained by direct gene counting. HLA haplotype and phenotype were compared by chi-square analysis with Yates continuity correction.

Results

Viro-histological correlations

HPV sequences were detected in 104 of the 126 cases (83%), HPV16 in 66 cases (63%), HPV18 in 10 cases (9.6%) and 28 cases of others HPV types (27%).

HLA *DRB1*, *DQA1*, *DQB1* allele frequencies

The *DRB1*1301/02* frequency decreased significantly in patients (11%) as compared to controls (29%) (p= 0.0004, OR= 0.33, IC 95%= 0.17-0.65)

This decrease was linked to the HPV status of tumors: in HPV positive tumors, *DRB1*1301/02* frequency is 10%, significantly lower than that observed in controls (29%) (p=0.0003), whereas in HPV negative tumors, this frequency was 18% not significantly different from that observed in the controls (p=0,28).The same trends was observed with DQA1*0103 and DQB1*0603 alleles.

The *DQB1*03 (0301, 0302, 0303, 0304)* frequency observed was slightly higher in patients (70%) than in controls (58%) (p=0.03). This difference was most probably related to the *DQB1*0303* allele frequency which is 9% in HPV16 positive tumors and 2% in controls (Fisher = 0.03).

Allele frequencies, histology of tumors and course of diseases: In function of the histology of tumors, the above variations in allele frequencies were observed in the major group of SCC (squamous cell carcinoma). No

Table I. Allele frequencies in controls and patients. Analysis according to viral status and histology of tumors

					Virology								Histology			
	Controls n=165		All tumors n=126		HPV negative n=22		HPV positive n=104		HPV16 positive n=66		non HPV16 positive n=38		SCC n=110		others n=16	
DRB1*	n	%	n	%	n	%	n	%	n	%	n	%	n	%	n	%
01	34	20	17	13	2	9	15	14	8	12	7	18	15	14	2	13
1501	32	19	21	16	4	18	17	16	13	19	4	10	19	17	2	13
1502	3	2	2	1	0	0	2	2	1	1	1	3	2	2	0	0
1601/02	6	4	6	4	0	0	6	5	4	6	2	5	4	4	2	13
03	32	19	30	23	8	36	22	21	12	18	10	26	26	23	4	25
04	48	29	42	33	10	45	32	30	20	30	12	31	35	31	7	44
11	47	28	40	31	6	27	34	32	19	28	15	39	37	33	3	19
12	2	1	5	3	0	0	5	5	3	4	2	5	5	4	0	0
1301/02	48	**29**	15	**11***	4	18	11	**10****	9	**13**	2	**5**	13	11	2	13
1303/04	2	1	5	4	1	4	4	4	2	3	2	5	5	4	0	0
1401/07	15	9	12	9	3	13	9	8	6	9	3	7	10	9	2	13
07	31	18	29	23	4	18	25	24	19	28	6	15	26	23	3	19
08	10	6	6	4	0	0	6	5	5	7	1	2	4	3	2	13
09	2	1	2	1	0	0	2	2	2	3	0	0	2	2	0	0
10	0	0	3	2	1	4	2	2	2	3	0	0	2	2	1	6
DQA1*	n	%	n	%	n	%	n	%	n	%	n	%	n	%	n	%
0101	48	29	32	25	7	31	25	24	15	20	10	26	27	24	5	31
0102	49	29	37	29	8	36	29	27	20	30	9	23	31	28	6	38
0103	35	**21**	8	**6**	1	4	7	**6**	6	**9**	1	**2**	8	7	0	0
0201	30	18	29	23	4	18	25	24	19	28	6	15	26	23	3	19
0301	48	29	44	34	9	40	35	33	22	31	13	34	37	32	7	44
0401	9	5	7	5	1	4	6	5	5	7	1	2	4	3	3	19
0501	78	47	62	49	11	50	51	49	28	42	23	60	55	50	7	44
0601	2	1	3	2	0	0	3	3	2	3	1	3	3	3	0	0
DQB1*	n	%	n	%	n	%	n	%	n	%	n	%	n	%	n	%
0501	35	21	21	16	4	18	17	16	10	15	7	18	18	16	3	19
0502	5	3	8	6	1	4	7	6	4	6	3	7	7	4	1	6
0503	16	9	9	7	3	13	6	5	3	4	3	7	8	4	1	6
0601	3	2	3	2	0	0	3	3	2	3	1	2	3	2	0	0
0602	33	20	26	20	5	22	21	20	17	25	4	10	22	13	4	25
0603	29	**17**	6	**4**	1	4	5	**5**	5	**7**	0	**0**	6	5	0	0
0604	17	10	5	3	2	9	3	3	3	4	0	0	4	4	1	6
0605	1	1	2	2	0	0	2	2	0	0	2	5	1	1	1	6
0201	56	33	51	40	11	50	40	38	25	37	15	39	43	39	7	44
0301	65	39	57	45	10	45	47	45	26	39	21	55	51	46	6	38
0302	28	16	23	18	3	13	20	19	14	21	6	15	19	17	4	25
0303	4	**2**	8	6	0	0	8	7	6	**9*****	2	5	8	7	0	0
0304	0	0	1	1	0	0	1	1	1	2	0	0	1	1	0	0
0402	11	6	7	5	1	4	6	5	5	7	1	3	4	4	3	19

n = number SCC = squamous cell carcinoma [shaded] = statistically significant *: p = 0.0004 **: p = 0.0003 ***: Fisher = 0.03

significant variations in the frequency of alleles were observed when they were grouped according to initial clinical staging or to the course of the disease *(Table I)*.

Haplotype frequencies

The frequency of the *DRB1*1301/02-DQA1*0103-DQB1*0603* haplotype was lower in the group of patients (2%) than in controls (9%) (p=0.001) (OR= 0.25, IC= 0.08-0.7) . This decrease was linked to the viral status of tumors: it was significant between controls and HPV positive tumors (p=0.003).

Discussion

The observation that the *DQw03* allele was more frequent in patients with invasive cervical cancer (88%) than in the general population (50%)[3] has focused attention on the possibility of an HLA based predisposition to cervical cancer.

In a case control study of HLA *DRB1** and *DQB1** alleles and HPV infection in Hispanic women with invasive cervical carcinoma, an increase in the haplotype *DRB1*1501-DQB1*0602* in patients with HPV16 associated tumor was found [4].

Our analysis did not confirm the positive associations of cervical cancers with *DQB1*03* and *DRB1*15* alleles. Only a slight increase in the *DQB1*0303* allele was observed in the HPV16 associated group of patients. This discrepancy, also reported by others [5], may be related to the large number of cases analysed in our series

Our study shows a decrease in the frequency of the *DRB1*1301/1302-DQA1*0103-DQB1*0603* haplotype in patients compared to controls. This result confirms the negative association reported before on a different population of patients [3, 4] and indicates that the *DRB1*13* phenotype may provide a protective effect against HPV-associated tumors.

It is interesting to note that a protective effect of *DRB1*13* has also been reported in several infectious diseases such as severe malaria [6], thyphoïd and yellow fever [7]. Recently, an association between the *DRB1*1302* allele and clearance of the hepatitis B virus was observed [8].In a study about HIV infected infants [9] *DRB1* 13* alleles are preferentially associated with diminution in maternally transmitted HIV1 infection among black and hispanic children. A protective effect of this allele in insulin-dependent diabetes mellitus was also reported [10].Thus the *DRB1*13* might correspond to an effective phenotype in the presentation and processing of a variety of infectious antigens.

References

1. Buyse I, Decorte R, Baens M, Cuppens H, Semana G, Edmonds MP, Marynen P, Cassiman JJ. Rapid DNA typing of class II HLA antigens using the polymerase chain reaction and reverse dot blot hybridization. *Tissue Antigens* 1993 ; 41: 1-14.
2. Kimura A, Sasazuki T. Eleventh histocompatibility workshop reference protocol for the HLA DNA typing technique. In: Tsuji K, Aisawa M, Sasaki T, eds. *HLA 1991*. Oxford : Oxford University Press, 1992 : 397-419.
3. Wank R, Thomssen C. High risk of squamous cell carcinoma of the cervix for women with HLA-DQ3. *Nature* 1991 ; 352 : 723-5.
4. Apple RJ, Erlich HA, Klitz W, Manos M, Becker T Wheeler, C. HLA DR-DQ associations with cervical carcinoma show papillomavirus-type specificity. *Nature Genet* 1994 ; 6 : 157-62.
5. Glew S, Duggan-Keen M, Ghosh A, Ivinson A, Sinnott P, Davidson J, Dyer P, Stern P. Lack of association of HLA polymorphisms with human papillomavirus-related cervical cancer. *Hum Immunol* 1993 ; 37 : 157-64.
6. Hill AVS, Allsopp C, Kwiatkowski D, Anstey NM, Twumasi P, Rowe PA, Bennett S, Brewster D, McMichael AJ, Greenwood BM. Common West African HLA antigens are associated with protection from severe malaria. *Nature* 1991 ; 352 : 595-600.
7. De Vries RRP. HLA and disease: from epidemiology to immunotherapy. *Eur J Clin Invest* 1992 ; 22 : 1-8.
8. Thursz M, Kwiatkowski D, Allsopp C, Greenwood B, Thomas H, Hill A . Association between an MHC class II allele and clearance of hepatitis B virus in the Gambia . *N Engl J Med* 1995 ; 332 : 723-5.
9. Winchester R, Chen Y, Rose S, Selby J, Borkowsky W. Major histocompatibility complex class II DR Allele DRB1* 1501 and those encoding HLA DR 13 are preferencially associated with a diminution in maternally transmitted human immunodeficiency virus 1 infection in different ethnic groups: determination by an automated sequence - based typing method. *Proc Natl Acad Sci USA* 1995 ; 92 : 12374-8.
10. Caillat-Zucman S, Garchon HJ, Timsit J, Assan R, Boitard C, Djilali-Saiah I, Bougnères P, Bach JF. Age dependent HLA genetic heterogeneity of type 1 insulin-dependent diabetes mellitus. *J Clin Invest* 1992 ; 90 : 2242-50.

Both HLA-B7 and DRB1*1501 appear to be required to confer risk to HPV-16 associated invasive cancer, but function as independent risk factors for HPV16-associated severe dysplasia

R.J. Apple[2], P. Lin[1], T.M. Becker[1], H.A. Erlich[2], C.M. Wheeler[1]

1 University of New Mexico Cancer Center, Albuquerque New Mexico, USA
2 Roche Molecular Systems, Inc, 1145 Atlantic Avenue Alameda, CA 94501, USA

Human papilloma viruses (HPVs) are now considered to be the causative agents of most cervical carcinomas and cervical intraepithelial (CIN) lesions [1]. These lesions are graded according to morphologic features as CIN1, CIN2, and CIN3, and are the presummed precursors of cervical cancer. There are several types of HPV, which differ in their ability to transform the cervical epithelium. The high risk HPV types 16, 18, 26, 31, 33, 35, 39, 45, 51, 52, 55,56,58,59, and 68 are often observed in association with CIN2 (moderate dysplasia) and CIN3 (severe dysplasia/carcinoma *in situ*), as well as the majority of cervical cancers [1, 2]. In contrast, CIN1 lesions are more likely to be induced by HPV types other than the high-risk types, and often regress spontaneously [3]. However, cervical HPV infection does not always induce cellular abnormalities, and HPV infection is relatively common among cytologically normal women [4]. This observation suggests that additional environmental, immunological, or genetic cofactors are necessary in the development of cervical pathology and progression to invasive cancer.

HLA and cervical disease

We have been investigating the influence of the HLA class II antigens on the progression of HPV-mediated cervical disease. Specific alleles of the HLA region have been associated with a variety of diseases, including nasopharyngeal carcinoma [5] and Hodgkin's lymphoma [6]; each thought to be associated with the Epstein-Barr virus. We have conducted a study of HLA class II disease associations with cervical dysplasia [7] and cervical carcinoma [8] among Hispanic women of the southwestern United States using PCR-based DNA amplification and oligonucleotide probe strategies for HLA class II typing and HPV detection and identification. We have reported that certain class II haplotypes are negatively associated (or protective) with cervical carcinoma or for CIN3, while other class II haplotypes are positively associated with both CIN3 and cervical carcinoma. In particular we have noted that the haplotype DRB1*1501-DQB1*0602 is increased among women with HPV16-associated invasive carcinoma [8] and also HPV16-associated CIN3 [7]. This haplotype was not found to be increased among cancer cases or CIN3 cases that were associated with HPV types other than HPV16, relative to controls. This suggests that specific class II haplotypes influence the immune response to specific HPV-encoded epitopes and affect the risk of developing severe cervical disease and invasive cervical cancer.

HLA-B7 and cervical disease

However, the DRB1*1501-DQB1*0602 haplotype is known to be in linkage disequilibrium with the class I HLA-B7 serogroup [9]. The B7 serogroup has also been increased among Caucasian cancer cases in other studies [10]. To examine the role of this linked HLA-B serogroup to our reported associations with cervical disease, we have developed a DNA-based HLA-B7 screening assay using PCR and SSOPs. A nucleic acid polymorphism in the third exon of the HLA-B locus at position 65-82 is unique to HLA-B*0702, *0703, *0704, and *1510 alleles. This encodes the amino acid (a.a.) epitope GHDQY at position 112-116 of the HLA-Bα2 domain. Another polymorphism at nucleotide position 320-332 of exon 3 encodes the amino acid epitope DKLER at a.a. position 177-181 of the α2 domain. This

Table I. HLA-B7 and DRB1*1501 are both increased in HPV16-associated cervical disease

HLA	Control		HPV16-positive CIN3			HPV16-positive Cancer		
	n	(f)	n	(f)	p	n	(f)	p
B7+	19/220	(0.086)	11/41	(0.268)	0.002	12/53	(0.226)	0.004
1501+	14/220	(0.064)	10/41	(0.244)	0.001	13/53	(0.245)	0.00007

Table II. The relationship of HLA-B7 and DRB1*1501 differs among cervical disease groups

HLA	Control		HPV16-positive CIN3			HPV16-positive Cancer		
	n	(f)	n	(f)	p	n	(f)	p
B7+ 1501+	7/220	(0.032)	4/41	(0.098)	n.s.	10/53	(0.189)	0.00002
B7+ 1501-	12/220	(0.055)	7/41	(0.171)	0.016	2/53	(0.038)	n.s.
B7- 1501+	7/220	(0.032)	6/41	(0.146)	0.007	3/53	(0.057)	n.s.

DKLER epitope is present in the HLA-B*0702, *0703, *0704, *0705, *4001, *4007, *4801 and *8101 alleles. SSOPs for the GYEQH, and DKLER sequences, as well as a consensus exon 3 probe, were used as a HLA-B7 screen following amplification of a 200bp fragment of HLA-B exon 3. This small amplicon of the HLA-B locus allows the screening of DNA obtained from paraffin embedded tissues, and crude cellular lysates. Samples positive for all three probes were considered B7 positive. (The frequency of HLA-B*1510 among controls was 1/220 (0.005); therefore it is unlikely that a heterozygous genotype invoving *1510 and *4001,*4007, *4801, or *8101 affected our reported frequencies for HLA-B7.) This assay was used to detect HLA-B7 in our HPV-screened and class II typed Hispanic case/control study consisting of 98 invasive cancer cases, 128 dysplasia cases, and 220 control samples obtained from women with normal Pap smears, and no past history of cervical disease.

As seen in *Table I*, HLA-B7 was significantly increased among both HPV16-associated CIN3 cases and HPV16-associated cancers, relative to controls. However, as seen in *Table II*, the relationship of HLA-B7 to DRB1*1501 differed among the two HPV 16-associated disease groups. In comparing the B7+1501- and B7- 1501+ groups, it can be seen that both HLA-B7 and DRB1*1501 are independent risk factors for HPV16-associated CIN3. However, neither of these groups are increased in the HPV-16 cervical cancer cases. Instead, only the B7+ 1501+ group is significantly increased in the HPV16 cancer cases relative to controls. This suggests that HLA-B7 and DRB1*1501, although in linkage disequilibrium, interact to confer an increased risk for the development of invasive cervical cancer following infection with HPV16.

References

1. Schiffman MH, Bauer HM, Hoover RN, Glass AG, Cadell DM, Rush BB, Scott DR, Sherman ME, Kurman RJ, Wacholder S, Stanton CK, Manos MM. Epidemiologic evidence showing that human papillomavirus infection causes most cervical intraepithelial neoplasia. *J Natl Cancer Inst* 1993; 85:958-64.
2. Lorincz AT, Reid R, Jenson AB, Greenberg MD, Lancaster W, Kurman RJ. Human papillomavirus infection of the cervix: relative risk associations of 15 common anogenital types. *Obstet Gynecol* 1992; 79:328-37.
3. Lorincz AT, Schiffman MH, Jaffurs WJ, Marlow J, Quinn AP, Temple GF. Temporal associations of human papillomavirus infection with cervical cytologic abnormalities. *Am J Obstet Gynecol* 1990; 162:645-51.
4. Bauer HM, Ting Y, Greer CE, Chambers JC, Tashiro CJ, Chimera J, Reingold A, Manos MM. Genital human papillomavirus infection in female university students as determined by a PCR-based method. *JAMA* 1991; 265472-7.

5. Lu SJ, Day NE, Degos L, Lepage V, Wang PC, Chan SH, Simons M, McKnight B, Easton D, Zeng Y, de Thé G. Linkage of a nasopharyngeal carcinoma susceptibility locus to the HLA region. *Nature* 1990; 346: 470-1.
6. Klitz W, Aldrich CL, Fildes N, Horning SJ, Begovich, AB. Localization of predisposition to Hodgkin Disease in the HLA class II region. *Am J Hum Genet* 1994; 54: 497-505.
7. Apple RJ, Becker TM, Wheeler CM, Erlich HA. Comparison of human leukocyte antigen DR-DQ disease associations found with cervical dysplasia and invasive cervical carcinoma. *J Natl Cancer Inst* 1995; 87: 427-36.
8. Apple RJ, Erlich HA, Klitz W, Manos MM, Becker, TM, Wheeler, CM. HLA DR-DQ associations with cervical carcinoma show papillomavirus-type specificity. *Nature Genet* 1994; 6: 157-62.
9. Begovich AB, McClure GR, Suraj VC, Helmuth RC, Fildes N, Bugawan TL, Erlich HA, Klitz, W. Polymorphism, recombination, and linkage disequilibrium within the HLA class II region. *J Immunol* 1992; 148: 249-58.
10. Ellis JRM, Keating PJ, Baird J, Hounsell EF, Renouf DV, Rowe M, Hopkins D, Duggan-Keen, MF, Batholomew JS, Young LS, Stern PL. The association of an HPV16 oncogene variant with HLA-B7 has implications for vaccine design in cervical cancer. *J Natl Cancer Inst* 1997 (in press).

Major histocompatibility complex (MHC) class I antigen expression in non-Hodgkin lymphoma

B. Drénou, L. Amiot, B. Lanson, T. Lamy, I. Grulois, P.Y. Le Prisé, R. Fauchet

Laboratoire et service d'hématologie, CHRU Pontchaillou, Rue Henri Le Guilloux, 35000 Rennes Cedex France

Most of the genetic events that have been characterized during tumour development correspond to oncogenes activation contributing to the malignant phenotype. In some cases, the inactivation of tumour-suppressor genes is considered necessary for cell transformation. Major histocompatibility complex (MHC) class I molecules are major players in the immune recognition of malignant cells by their host. Structural and functional abnormalities of HLA antigen expression on tumoral cells have been characterized and may alter their recognition by cytotoxic T cells (CTL). Some informations are available concerning the alteration of HLA expression in many tumours such as melanoma, colon carcinoma, or cervical cancer [1, 3]. Total or selective HLA class I loss are clearly associated with tumour invasiveness and could appear in premalignant lesions as one mechanism to escape immune recognition and subsequent lysis. A few data are available in hematological malignancies [4]. In order to characterize HLA class I abnormalities, we analyzed class I molecules by flow cytometry in lymphoid malignancies .

Material and methods

To describe HLA class I abnormalities at the surface of lymphomatous cells, we have performed a biological prospective study by using flow cytometry (Cytoron, Ortho - Roissy France). A triple fluorescence staining is used with the following monoclonal antibodies (MoAbs) : W6/32 which recognize a monomorphic class I determinant is labeled with FITC. CD37 which is a pan-B monoclonal antibody (MoAb) is labeled with phycoerythrin and CD3 characterize T cells with P Cy5. W6/32 was purchased by Seralab (London UK) whereas CD37 and CD3 were purchased by Immunotech (Marseille, France). To compare HLA class I expression on B and T lymphocytes, we used the intensity of the W6/32 staining on CD37+ cells and CD3+ cells respectively. The intensity arbitrary value is detected by the use of the mean channel measured on a linearized scale. B or T tumoral cells from a pathological sample are compared respectively to T or B reactive lymphocytes. Ten normal blood samples and forty reactive lymph nodes were studied to obtain references. These cases were secondary to infectious diseases or non-hematological neoplasia. Eighty-two consecutive lymphoid malignancies cells were stained at diagnosis with the three MoAbs: 33 cases of B-chronic lymphocytic leukemias (B-CLL), 39 cases of low-grade non-Hodgkin lymphoma (NHL), 8 cases of high-grade NHL and 2 cases of hairy cell leukemias (HCL).

Results

No difference is found between normal B and T cells in the same sample. However a high difference is detected from one individual to another in normal blood as in reactive lymph nodes: the standard deviation is observed at 29 arbitrary units with a mean intensity at 72.

In lymphoid malignancies the absence of class I molecules at cell surface is a very rare event: it is detected in only one case out of 82. This case is associated with the diagnosis of secondary high-grade NHL after an indolent course of low-grade NHL. A significant decrease is observed in a quarter of the cases in comparaison to normal cells. By contrast, high class I intensity is detected in 10% of the cells especially in HCL.

Discussion

A difference was previously reported between B and T class I expression [5]. This study did not find such a discreapancy by using a simple and reproducible methodology. A significant decrease of class I molecules is observed in a quarter of NHL by using a MoAb (W6/32) which recognized a monomorphic determinant. These results are in accordance with reported data in several tumours [1-4]. The use of allele specific MoAbs would increase the percentage of abnormal cases. The mechanisms involved to explain such dysregulation in hematological malignancies are to be investigated in regard to β2 microglobulin or TAP genes expression. Immunohistological studies in different carcinomas show a relationship between HLA loss and tumour progression. Loss of class I molecules expression is similarly observed in high grade lymphomas. An increase of class I expression is observed in a few cases. The high staining with W6/32 observed in HCL could be explain by the peculiar villous aspect of the cell membrane: thus flow-cytometry measure an absolute intensity and not a cell surface density.

A quantitative approach using indirect immunofluorescence with standardized beads would allow to compare analysis from one laboratory to another.

Conclusion

The decrease of class I molecules in lymphoid malignancies would affect tumoral cell immune recognition and participate to their oncogenic potential. The association between these results and clinical data suggest that loss of class I MHC molecules may be a «second event» in the lymphomatous process. However, this preliminary results need to be precised by using different allele specific Mo-Ab.

References

1. Ferrone S, Marincola FM. Loss of class I antigens by melanoma cells: molecular mechanisms, functional significance and clinical relevance. *Immunol Today* 1995; 16 : 487-94.
2. Garrido F, Cabrera T, Concha A, Glew S, Ruiz-Cabello F, Stern PL. Natural history of HLA expression during tumour development. *Immunol Today* 1993; 14 : 491-9.
3. Cromme FV, Airey J, Heemels MT, Ploegh HL, Keating PJ, Stern PL, Meijer CJLM, Walboomers JMM. Loss of transporter protein, encoded by the TAP-1 gene, is highly correlated with loss of HLA expression in cervical carcinomas. *J Exp Med* 1994; 179: 335-40.
4. D'Alfonso S, Savoia P, Pitti G, Peruccio D, Pozzi C, Crepaldi T, Falda M, Ficara F, Resegotti L, Richiardi P. Quantitative expression of class I molecules in acute non-lymphoblastic leukaemia cells. *Eur J Immunogenet* 1993; 20: 165-73.
5. Trucco M, De Petris S, Garotta G, Ceppellini R. Quantitative analysis of cell surface HLA structures by means of monoclonal antibodies. *Hum Immunol* 1980; 3: 233-43.

Population and family study of histocompatibility antigens in acute leukemias and aplastic anemia

*A.M. Sell, E.A. Donadi, J.C. Voltarelli, V.C. Oliveira, A.C. Biral, E.M. Thomas, S.R. Brandalise, L.A. Magna, M.P. Teixeira, V.L. Aranega, M.H.S. Kraemer**

Department of Clinical Pathology, Immunogenetic Transplant Unit, UNICAMP, Campinas and Immunogenetic Unit, School of Medicine of Ribeirão Preto-USP, Ribeirão Preto, rua Aristides Lobo 255, Campinas Sao Paulo 13083-060, Brazil
*Corresponding author

It has been suggested that aplastic anemia (AA) may be a pre-leukemic disorder. Myelotoxic agents such as radiation and benzene can cause AA and leukemia. The later development of acute leukemia has been described in patients with chloramphenicol or phenylbutazone-induced marrow hypoplasia. Fanconi anemia and other causes of congenital AA may be followed by malignant manifestations which include acute myelogenous leukemia (AML) and acute lymphoblastic leukemia (ALL) [1]. On the other hand, HLA molecules and alleles have been associated with AA, AML and ALL. HLA-DR2 antigen has been reported to be significantly increased in AA patients [2]. HLA-Cw3 and HLA-Cw4 antigens have been positively associated with either AML and ALL [3, 4]. Children ALL patients have an increased frequency of HLA-DPB1*0201 allele [5]. In mice, homozygosity for the MHC haplotype H-2k has been associated with increased susceptibility to spontaneous or virus-induced leukemia [6]. In order to search whether AA and acute leukemias share or not immunogenetic markers we performed HLA-A, -B, -C, -DR and -DQ serological typing in 3 series of patients and respective unaffected siblings with AA, AML and ALL. A total of 786 individuals from 230 Brazilian families recruited from two Brazilian Clinical Centers (Campinas and Ribeirão Preto) with just one case of each: AA (97), AML (72) and ALL (61) were studied. The number of siblings for each of the above diseases were 223, 185 and 148, respectively. A total of 560 control individuals, 313 typed for HLA class I antigens and 247 typed for HLA class II antigens, from the same geographical area and of similar ethnic background were also studied. The p value obtained using the two-tailed Fisher exact test was corrected (pc) according to the number of antigens tested and comparisons made. Relative risk (RR), etiologic fraction (EF) and preventive fraction (PF) were also estimated.

Results and discussion

The frequency of HLA-A, -B, -Cw, -DR and -DQ antigens observed in patients, siblings and control individuals is shown in *Tables I* and *II*. Regarding the comparisons of HLA frequency between patients and controls, HLA-Cw1 antigen was underrepresented in the 3 groups of patients; however, statistical significance was reached only for AA patients ($pc = 0.002$, $RR = 0.04$). Likewise, HLA-DR52 and HLA-DR53 antigens were also underrepresented in all these series (AA: DR52 $pc < 0.001$, $RR = 0.1$, $PF = 67\%$, DR53 $pc < 0.001$, $RR = 0.04$, $PF = 39\%$; AML: DR52 $pc < 0.001$, $RR = 0.05$, $PF = 0.71$, DR53 $pc < 0.001$, $RR = 0.11$, $PF = 47\%$; ALL: DR52 $pc = 0.001$, $RR = 0.23$, $PF = 57\%$, DR53 $p = 0.009$, $RR = 0.36$, $PF = 33\%$). HLA - DR5 antigen was significantly increased only in AML patients ($pc < 0.001$, $RR = 11.5$, $EF = 30\%$). Regarding the comparisons of HLA frequency between patients and unaffected siblings, HLA-B17 and HLA-DQ7 antigens were significantly increased in AML patients ($pc < 0.001$, $RR = 59.2$, $EF = 13\%$ and $pc < 0 .001$, $RR =6.7$, $EF = 6\%$, respectively), and HLA-A33, HLA-B39 and HLA-B50 were significantly increased in ALL patients ($pc < 0.001$, $RR = 7.6$, $EF = 1\%$; $pc < 0.001$, $RR = 12.9$, $EF = 3\%$; and $pc < 0.001$, $RR = 7.6$, $EF = 1\%$, respectively). No HLA class I susceptibility marker was found in association with AA, AML and ALL on this study;however, HLA-Cw1 was found to be a protective marker. HLA-A19 antigen has been previously described as conferring protection against the development of ALL in Caucasoids [3]. As HLA-Cw3 and -Cw4 have been shown positively associated with several types of leu-

Table I. Frequency (%) of HLA-A, -B and -C antigens in patients with aplastic anemia (AA), acute myelogenous leukemia (AML), acute lymphoblastic leukemia (ALL) and controls (C)

HLA-A	AA	AML	ALL	C
A1	26 (15)	24 (25)	20 (13)	19
A2	46 (55)	46 (42)	41 (34)	49
A3	13 (14)	19 (21)	11 (19)	16
A9	10 (18)	15 (20)	16 (15)	5
A10	3 (3)	4 (2)	1 (7)	4
A11	12 (7)	15 (10)	6 (7)	8
A19	3 (4)	5 (9)	5 (8)	7
A23	6 (3)	5 (6)	10 (9)	6
A24	11 (9)	7 (7)	18 (15)	18
A25	2 (2)	1 (1)	3 (3)	5
A26	5 (2)	3 (3)	3 (2)	3
A28	12 (15)	12 (10)	11 (10)	16
A29	1 (5)	5 (7)	5 (7)	8
A30	4 (2)	7 (1)	6 (8)	4
A31	0 (1)	4 (2)	3 (2)	1
A32	3 (1)	1 (1)	1 (3)	2
A33	3 (1)	3 (3)	1 (0)	3
A34	1 (0)	1 (1)	0 (3)	1
A36	1 (1)	0 (0)	0 (1)	1
A66	1 (0)	0 (0)	0 (0)	0
A68	0 (0)	0 (0)	0 (0)	1
A69	2 (2)	0 (0)	0 (0)	1
A74	1 (1)	0 (0)	0 (0)	0

HLA-B	AA	AML	ALL	C
B7	10 (12)	21 (19)	16 (19)	14
B8	11 (5)	11 (11)	8 (6)	10
B13	9 (6)	8 (7)	3 (5)	5
B14	16 (11)	8 (14)	11 (8)	8
B15	2 (7)	0 (9)	5 (5)	4
B16	2 (4)	5 (9)	3 (7)	2
B17	9 (10)	12 (0)	15 (12)	7
B18	5 (4)	19 (14)	3 (3)	10
B21	8 (8)	7 (9)	3 (3)	2
B22	0 (0)	1 (1)	0 (0)	1
B27	0 (2)	3 (4)	0 (0)	4
B35	22 (26)	19 (20)	23 (20)	19
B37	0 (0)	1 (2)	2 (0)	3
B38	0 (0)	0 (0)	0 (0)	3
B39	6 (2)	3 (1)	5 (0)	5
B40	5 (5)	8 (7)	5 (5)	3
B41	4 (1)	1 (1)	0 (1)	2
B42	0 (1)	0 (0)	2 (5)	1
B44	25 (27)	12 (16)	24 (31)	23
B45	2 (1)	1 (2)	0 (1)	2
B47	0 (0)	0 (0)	2 (5)	1
B48	1 (0)	1 (1)	0 (0)	0
B49	5 (3)	1 (1)	2 (1)	6
B50	1 (0)	1 (2)	2 (0)	1

HLA-B	AA	AML	ALL	C
B51	14 (19)	10 (7)	20 (9)	24
B52	2 (0)	0 (0)	0 (0)	1
B53	2 (3)	1 (1)	0 (0)	2
B54	1 (0)	0 (0)	0 (0)	1
B55	1 (1)	4 (1)	0 (0)	1
B56	0 (0)	0 (0)	0 (0)	1
B57	1 (1)	0 (0)	0 (0)	4
B58	0 (0)	0 (0)	0 (0)	2
B60	1 (1)	3 (1)	0 (0)	6
B61	0 (1)	0 (0)	0 (0)	1
B62	1 (0)	3 (4)	0 (1)	5
B63	2 (1)	1 (1)	0 (0)	1
B73	0 (1)	0 (1)	0 (1)	0

HLA-C	AA	AML	ALL	C
Cw1	0 (0)	0 (0)	3 (0)	20
Cw2	9 (6)	4 (12)	9 (16)	8
Cw3	11 (14)	30 (38)	6 (9)	22
Cw4	30 (50)	33 (21)	22 (53)	23
Cw5	6 (8)	11 (9)	6 (3)	18
Cw6	9 (6)	15 (3)	3 (7)	20
Cw7	26 (19)	52 (35)	31 (37)	35
Cw8	15 (0)	0 (0)	0 (0)	7

Table II. Frequency (%) of HLA-DR and -DQ antigens in patients with aplastic anemia (AA), acute myelogenous leukemia (AML), acute lymphoblastic leukemia (ALL) and controls (C)

HLA-DR	AA	AML	ALL	C
DR1	22 (26)	28 (19)	20 (25)	25
DR2	40 (42)	36 (27)	30 (39)	23
DR3	30 (25)	20 (17)	25 (32)	22
DR4	19 (15)	18 (23)	17 (20)	33
DR5	8 (13)	33 (23)	12 (6)	3
DR6	8 (7)	8 (16)	5 (7)	2
DR7	20 (15)	16 (28)	32 (24)	16
DR8	7 (5)	11 (8)	2 (1)	4
DR9	4 (3)	5 (3)	2 (2)	4
DR10	0 (0)	0 (1)	0 (0)	2
DR11	9 (11)	5 (4)	20 (16)	22
DR12	0 (0)	0 (0)	0 (0)	1
DR13	0 (0)	0 (0)	0 (0)	7
DR14	0 (0)	0 (0)	0 (0)	4

HLA-DR	AA	AML	ALL	C
DR15	1 (0)	0 (0)	0 (0)	1
DR52	23 (31)	13 (12)	40 (34)	74
DR53	19 (18)	10 (10)	27 (25)	51

HLA-DQ	AA	AML	ALL	C
DQ1	77 (72)	36 (50)	57 (60)	59
DQ2	33 (36)	36 (33)	23 (35)	16
DQ3	28 (24)	50 (47)	29 (37)	42
DQ4	3 (4)	0 (3)	0 (0)	2
DQ5	8 (0)	0 (3)	5 (5)	4
DQ7	13 (11)	7 (0)	14 (7)	32
DQ8	13 (8)	0 (7)	5 (7)	1
DQ9	3 (4)	0 (0)	0 (0)	1

kemia, *i.e.*, AML, ALL and chronic myeloid leukemia (CML) [3,4], one can speculate that HLA-Cw molecules may participate in the pathogenesis of these diseases. At the family level, the most important association was with HLA-B17 antigen which conferred high RR and EF for patients with AML in relation to unaffected siblings. Although HLA-A33, -B39 and -B50 antigens were also overrepresented in ALL patients in relation to unaffected siblings, these associations were weaker since EFs for each antigen were low (1-3%). HLA-DR7 was the only HLA class II antigen which was more prevalent in AML patients than in unaffected siblings. A Russian study reported increased HLA-B17 and decreased HLA-DR7 antigen frequency in unrelated patients with ALL [7].

Certainly, the decreased frequency of HLA-DR52 and -DR53 antigens, shared by AA, AML and ALL patients, was the most remarkable finding of this investigation. Whether these molecules are decreased because of the lack of expression at the cell surface level, or respective HLA-DRB3 and HLA-DRB4 genes are down-regulated, or these molecules actually play a role in the protection against the development of these diseases are questions to be answered. The observation of decreased frequency of HLA-DR52 and -DR53 in patients and in unaffected siblings compared to controls suggest a familial segregation. Conversely, other studies have shown association of HLA-DR53 antigen with AML, with early-onset CML, and with high relapse rate in ALL patients [6,8]. In addition, it has been suggested that murine and human leukemia share susceptibility genes, *i.e.*, the location of putative leukemia genes in murine and human MHC regions are similar, and there is serological cross-reaction between H-2EK and HLA-DR53 antigens [6]. Although the results regarding the frequency of HLA-DR52 and -DR53 antigens are controversial, they clearly indicate the importance of these molecules in the pathogenesis of AA and acute leukemias. HLA-DR5 was the only class II antigen found in association with Brazilian AML patients. Although several antisera anti-HLA-DR5, -DR11 and DR12 were used, in most of our AML patients the broad specificity HLA-DR5 could not be split as -DR11 or -DR12. Molecular studies may discriminate these specificities.

Conclusion

AA may be caused by an intrinsic defect of the hematopoietic stem cell, and it has been suggested a link between AA and clonal disorders, in this report, we have further observed that in AA and in acute leukemias (AML and ALL) the HLA-Cw1, HLA-DR52 and -DR53 antigens were shared protective markers against the development of these diseases. HLA-DR5 was a susceptibility marker for AML. Molecular studies are being conducted to improve the understanding of such associations.

References

1. Marsh JCW, Geary CG. Is aplastic anaemia a pre-leukaemic disorder? *Br J Haematol* 1991; 77: 447-52.
2. Nimer SD, Ireland P, Meshkinpour A, Frane M. An increased HLA-DR2 frequency is seen in aplastic anemia patients. *Blood* 1994; 84: 923-27.
3. Bortin MM, D'Amaro J, Bach FH, Rimm AA, van-Rood JJ. HLA association with leukemia. *Blood* 1987; 70: 227-32.
4. Baldaf C, Kubel M. HLA und leukamie. *Folia Haematol Int Mag Klin Morphol Blutforsch* 1989; 116: 123-32.
5. Taylor GM, Robinson MD, Binchy A, Birch JM, Stevens RF, Jones PM,Carr T, Dearden S, Gokhale DA. Preliminary evidence of an association between HLA-DPB1* 0201 and childhood common acute lymphoblastic leukaemia supports an infectious aetiology. *Leukemia* 1995; 9: 440-3.
6. Dorak MT, Chalmers EA, Gaffney D, Wilson DW, Galbraith I, Henderson N, Worwood M, Mills KI, Burnett AK. Human major histocompatibility complex contains several leukemia susceptibility genes. *Leuk Lymphoma* 1994; 12: 211-22.
7. Timonova LA, Rumiantsev AG. HLA-antigeny I i II klassov pri ostrom limfoblastnom leikoze u detei. *Gematol Transfuziol* 1989; 34: 19-22.
8. Dorak MT, Owen G, Galbraith I, Hendenson N, Webb N, Webb D, Mills KI, Darke C, Burnett AK. Nature of HLA-associated predisposition to childhood acute lymphoblastic leukemia. *Leukemia* 1995; 9:875-8.

HLA class II, (CA)n microsatellites markers and susceptibility to Hodgkin's disease

J.D. Bignon[1], A. Cesbron[1], M.J. Rapp[2], F. Bonneville[1], P. Herry[1], N. Jugeaux[1], P. Moreau[2], J.L. Harousseau[2], J.Y. Muller[1]

1 HLA Laboratory. Blood Bank, ETS, 34,boulevard Jean Monnet, 44011 Nantes, France
2 Clinical Haematology Department, CHU Hôtel Dieu, 44035 Nantes, France

The relationship between HLA and an increased risk of Hodgkin's disease (HD) is still debated. Random patients studies tended to support a role for a HLA-class II-linked susceptibility. Report from the 11th HLA Workshop (Yokohama) showed a weak but significant increase of the DPB1*0301 allele [1] and further studies objectivated an increase of the DRB1*11 alleles [2-4]. The aim of this study was to confirm the relationship between HLA and Hodgkin's disease (HD) susceptibility and to test if microsatellites markers located near HLA genes could confirm this association more steadily.

Patients and methods

This study included 158 patients with a diagnosis of HD and 100 geographically matched unrelated Caucasian individuals. Among 60 histologically classified patients (Rye classification), 44 of them were noted as Nodular Sclerosis (NS). The tested markers and the technics used were as follows : HLA-DRB1 (PCR-SSO reverse), HLA-DQB1 (PCR-SSO), HLA-DPB1 (PCR-SSO), HLA-DRB1*11 subtyping (PCR-SSP). Sequences of microsatellite primers were obtained from Gene Data Bank. Genomic DNAs were amplified by PCR and hybridization were performed with a ECL 5' thiol HRP modified CA11 probe. Microsatellite polymorphism was detected using the ECL gene detection kit. The microsatellites studied were selected for their genomic location : DQ CAR located between DQA1 and DQB1 shows more than 10 alleles in linkage disequilibrium with specific HLA-DR and DQ haplotypes [5], D6S 291.1 (7 alleles) and D6S 439 (10 alleles) located closed to DPB locus.

Results

Results are summarized in *Table I*. When antigenic frequencies were compared between HD and controls, the data showed a significant increase of DRB1*11 ($p < 0.01$) but no particular DR11 subtype was implicated (data not shown). HLA-DPB*0301 allele was also confirmed to be significantly increased ($p < 0.01$). Moreover, the combination of these 2 markers showed an even higher chi-square, suggesting a cumulative susceptibility effect of this combination ($p = 0.001$).
Antigenic frequencies have also been studied in patients with nodular sclerosis (predominant group), but no difference was observed compared to the whole patients group.
Concerning the microsatellites markers, those selected according to their location (closed to DPB1 locus) were observed with the same antigenic frequency in patients and controls.
The DQ CAR microsatellite showed 10 alleles including 2 partially linked to DQB1*0301. These 2 alleles (DQ CAR 2 and DQ CAR 4) were present with a high rate in HD but also in controls.

Discussion

The results of this study confirm that susceptibility to HD was influenced by more than one locus within the HLA-class II region. Taking account the 2 main HLA markers (DRB1*11 and DPB1*301) we observed more patients displaying both alleles than expected by calculation suggesting a cumulative susceptibility effect of this combination.
According to the amino acid sequence, there are similarities between these 2 alleles since several monoclonal

Table I. Antigenic frequencies of HLA class II and microsatellites markers observed in Hodgkin's patients (HD) and control population

	HD patients	Local controls	p	HD nodular sclerosis	Caucasoid population
HLA Class II	(n = 158)	(n = 100)		(n = 44/60)	
DRB1*11+	36.7%	20%	< 0,01	36.4%	19%
DPB1*301+	30.4%	15%	< 0,01	37.2%	17.4%
DRB1*11+ and DPB1*301+	13.9%	1%	= 0,001	14%	3%
Microsatellites	(n = 108)	(n = 74)			
D6S 291.1	no susceptible allele			NT	NT
D6S 439	no susceptible allele			NT	NT
DQ CAR 2+	40%	32.4%	NS	NT	NT
DQ CAR 4+	19.4%	13.5%	NS	NT	NT

NT : Not tested NS : Not significant

antibodies from the AHS18 of the 12th Workshop recognized an identical amino acid sequence namely "DE" in position 55-56 for DPB1 and DE in position 57-58 for DRB1. One can postulate that this epitope could play a peculiar role in the susceptibility to Hodgkin's disease.

The study of 3 microsatellites located in the HLA class II region did not show stronger association than DR11 and DP3.

Moreover, clinical aspects should be considered on the total population of the unrelated HD included in this study and a related cases study should be of great importance to explain inheritance susceptibility.

References

1. Bodmer JG, Tonks S, Oza AM, Mikata A, Takenouchi T, Lister TA. Collaborating centers (1992) Hodgkin's disease study. In : Tsuji K, Aizawa M, Sasazuki T eds. *HLA 1991.* Oxford : Oxford University Press, 1992 : 701-4.
2. Begovich AB, Mc Clure GR, Suraj VC, Helmuth RC, Fildes N, Bugawan TL, Erlich HA *et al.* Polymorphism, recombination and linkage disequilibrium within the HLA class II region. *J Immunol* 1992 : 148 : 249-58.
3. Cesbron A, Moreau P, Rapp MJ, Cheneau ML, Herry P, Bonneville F, Muller JY, Harousseau JL, Bignon JD. HLA-DPB and susceptibility to Hodgkin's disease. *Hum Immunol* 1993 : 36 : 51a.
4. Klitz WK, Aldrich CL, Fildes N, Horning SJ, Begovich AB. Localization of predisposition to hodgkin disease in the HLA class II region. *Am J Hum Genet* 1994 : 54 : 497-505.
5. Macaubas C, Hallmayer J, Kalil J, Kimura A, Yasunaga S, Grumet FC, Mignot E. Extensive polymorphism of a (CA)n microsatellite located in the HLA-DQA1/DQB1 class II region. *Hum Immunol* 1995 : 42 : 209-20.

Author Index

Author Index

A

B

C

D

E

F

G

H

I

J

K

L

M

N

O

P

Q

R

S

T

U

V

W

X

Y

Z

Achevé d'imprimer par Corlet, Imprimeur, S.A.
14110 Condé-sur-Noireau (France)
N° d'Imprimeur : 24219 - Dépôt légal : juin 1997

Imprimé en C.E.E.